AF677838

OBSTETRIC ANESTHESIA: **THE COMPLICATED PATIENT**

SECOND EDITION

OBSTETRIC ANESTHESIA: THE COMPLICATED PATIENT

SECOND EDITION

Francis M. James, III, M.D.
Professor and Chairman
Department of Anesthesia
Wake Forest University Medical Center
Winston-Salem, North Carolina

A. Scott Wheeler, M.D.
Professor of Anesthesiology
Chief, Special Services Division
Anesthesia Coordinator
Main Operating Room
The University of Alabama at Birmingham
School of Medicine
Birmingham, Alabama

David M. Dewan, M.D.
Associate Professor
Head, Section on Obstetric and Gynecologic Anesthesia
Department of Anesthesia
Wake Forest University Medical Center
Winston-Salem, North Carolina

F. A. DAVIS COMPANY • **Philadelphia**

Copyright © 1988 by F. A. Davis Company

All rights reserved. This book is protected by copyright. No part of it may be reproduced, stored in a retrieval system, or transmitted in any form or by any means, electronic, mechanical, photocopying, recording, or otherwise, without written permission from the publisher.

Printed in the United States of America

NOTE: As new scientific information becomes available through basic and clinical research, recommended treatments and drug therapies undergo changes. The author(s) and publisher have done everything possible to make this book accurate, up-to-date, and in accord with accepted standards at the time of publication. However, the reader is advised always to check product information (package inserts) for changes and new information regarding dose and contraindications before administering any drug. Caution is especially urged when using new or infrequently ordered drugs.

LIBRARY OF CONGRESS
Library of Congress Cataloging-in-Publication Data

Obstetric anesthesia : the complicated patient / [edited by] Francis M. James III, Alan S. Wheeler, David M. Dewan. — 2nd ed.
p. cm.
Includes bibliographies and index.
ISBN 0-8036-4914-2
1. Anesthesia in obstetrics. 2. Pregnancy, Complications of. 3. Labor, Complicated. I. James, Francis M. II. Wheeler, A. Scott. III. Dewan, David M., 1943– .
[DNLM: 1. Anesthesia, Obstetrical. 2. Pregnancy Complications. WO 450 O1426]
RG732.O266 1988
617'.9682—dc19
DNLM/DLC
for Library of Congress 88-6882
CIP

Authorization to photocopy items for internal or personal use, or the internal or personal use of specific clients, is granted by F. A. Davis Company for users registered with the Copyright Clearance Center (CCC) Transactional Reporting Service, provided that the fee of $.10 per copy is paid directly to CCC, 27 Congress St., Salem, MA 01970. For those organizations that have been granted a photocopy license by CCC, a separate system of payment has been arranged. The fee code for users of the Transactional Reporting Service is: 8036-4914/88 0 + $.10.

DEDICATION

We dedicate this book to our wives, Dell James, Debbie Wheeler, and Pat Dewan, the mothers of our children, whose continuing understanding, sacrifice, and support have served to encourage and sustain us for so many years during our medical careers.

FOREWORD TO THE SECOND EDITION

Forty-five years ago, when first I became involved in the administration of obstetric anesthesia, parturients were supposed to be "young and healthy." Many women with medical problems either did not survive to the childbearing age, accepted their physician's advice to avoid pregnancy, or succumbed during the course of pregnancy. Gravidae with tuberculosis, mitral valvular disease, or the sequelae of poliomyelitis were rare exceptions. Women suffering from "toxemia" were oversedated with barbiturates and had a high incidence of mortality. Intrapartum events such as hemorrhage, embolization, or uterine rupture were usually irreversible. Yet, the classification of a "complicated" obstetric patient was unknown.

Pain relief during labor consisted of morphine-scopolamine; analgesia for spontaneous vaginal delivery consisted of four breaths of 100 percent nitrous oxide followed by inhalation of room air. Operative vaginal deliveries and cesarean sections were managed with spinal block or general anesthesia using cyclopropane, diethyl ether, or 80 percent nitrous oxide – 20 percent oxygen-ether.

Anesthetic techniques and agents have changed and so has our "clientele." Pregnant women no longer want to be called "patients." Yet, many are not young, and even more are not healthy. Modern prenatal care has enabled women with sickle cell disease, scleroderma, lupus erythematosus, and so forth to weather pregnancy and parturition and enjoy the birth of a viable infant. Similarly, women in their forties have been able to deliver healthy babies. Thus, the "complicated" obstetric patient is no longer a rarity in our labor-delivery suites today.

The first edition of *Obstetric Anesthesia: The Complicated Patient* has been a great help to the concerned anesthesiologist. It has served as a teaching manual for residents and as a reference text for the practitioner. Such readily available information concerning anesthetic and obstetric management of common and rare complications has undoubtedly aided in reducing maternal morbidity and mortality and in improving neonatal outcome. Yet, in the 6 years since its publication, new knowledge and improved technology have been abundant. This second edition is therefore most welcome. Twelve chapters have been added to the 16 that appeared in the first edition, and all of the previous chapters have been updated. I am looking forward to adding this second edition to my own as well as to our departmental library.

GERTIE F. MARX, M.D.
Professor
Department of Anesthesiology
Albert Einstein College of Medicine
Yeshiva University
Bronx, New York

FOREWORD TO THE FIRST EDITION

There has never been such widespread interest in obstetric anesthesia as now. In the past few years, a half dozen major textbooks on this subject have been published. Now, with *Obstetric Anesthesia: The Complicated Patient,* we have a unique, original, and significant contribution to our specialty. Distinguished obstetric anesthesiologists from all parts of the United States and Canada have written chapters focusing on the anesthetic management of the leading medical and surgical diseases complicating pregnancy. The reader can quickly find information between the covers of this book that before now had been scattered throughout many textbooks and medical journals.

Professors Francis M. James, III, and Scott Wheeler were inspired to compile this textbook by their experience at one of the major obstetric anesthesia centers in the United States. Forsyth Memorial Hospital, the maternity facility of Bowman Gray School of Medicine of Wake Forest University, is a level III referral center having a delivery rate of more than 4,000 births a year. Obstetric anesthesia and research is performed by five faculty anesthesiologists, fellows in obstetric anesthesia, three anesthesiology residents, seven CRNAs, and several student nurse anesthetists. Residents in obstetrics and gynecology from several medical centers also rotate through the service. With a referral base of approximately 5 million people, the editors and their associates are exposed to a vast array of complicated obstetrics. This, I believe, explains the genesis of the book and the desire to consolidate the available information on high-risk parturients.

The reader can be grateful to have a textbook that treats all aspects of the anesthetic management of the complicated obstetric patient so completely, succinctly, and authoritatively.

Sol M. Shnider, M.D.
Professor of Anesthesia, Obstetrics,
Gynecology and Reproductive Sciences
Vice Chairman, Department of Anesthesia
University of California, San Francisco

PREFACE

Six years have passed since the first edition of *Obstetric Anesthesia: The Complicated Patient* appeared in 1982. During that time, continuing advances in obstetrics have presented the obstetric anesthesiologist with even greater challenges. Anesthesia personnel must continue to be aware of the peculiar physiologic characteristics of normal pregnancy and the special needs of the patient experiencing a complicated pregnancy.

This book focuses on problem pregnancies rather than on the anesthetic care of women with normal pregnancy and uncomplicated labor and delivery. In order to provide the reader with a broader scope of information, the second edition has not only been updated but expanded significantly. It was divided into five sections, and 12 new chapters were added, including such topics as anesthesia for "In Vitro Fertilization," "Fetal Surgery," "Obesity," "Orthopedic Disease," "The Traumatized Patient," and "Extremes of Age: The Teenager and the Elderly Parturient."

We have enlisted experts in obstetric anesthesia throughout the United States and Canada to help us with this endeavor and thank them for the time and effort they have expended in writing their chapters. In each chapter, the authors expressed their own opinions and recommendations, which do not necessarily reflect those of the editors.

Susan Margitic, Medical Editor for the Department of Anesthesia of the Wake Forest University Medical Center, deserves a special note of thanks. Her editorial help, careful attention to details, and skills with organization proved invaluable to the editors' efforts to create this book.

F.M.J.
A.S.W.
D.M.D.

CONTRIBUTORS

Diane R. Biehl, M.D., F.R.C.P.C.
Professor
Department of Anesthesia
University of Manitoba
Winnipeg, Manitoba
Canada

William G. Brose, M.D.
Department of Anesthesia
Stanford University Hospital
Stanford, California

John W. Bryant, M.D.
Assistant Professor of Anesthesiology
Department of Anesthesiology
University of Alabama at Birmingham
Chief of Anesthesia
Carraway Methodist Medical Center
Birmingham, Alabama

Theodore G. Cheek, M.D.
Assistant Professor of Anesthesiology and Obstetrics and Gynecology
University of Pennsylvania Medical Center
Philadelphia, Pennsylvania

David H. Chestnut, M.D.
Department of Anesthesia and Obstetrics and Gynecology
University of Iowa College of Medicine
Iowa City, Iowa

Sheila E. Cohen, M.B., Ch.B., F.F.A.R.C.S.
Professor of Anesthesia (Clinical)
Department of Anesthesia
Stanford University School of Medicine
Stanford, California

Salha S. Daniel, Ph.D.
Research Scientist in Anesthesiology
College of Physicians and Surgeons
Columbia University
New York, New York

Sanjay Datta, M.B., F.F.A.R.C.S. (Eng)
Associate Professor of Anesthesia
Harvard Medical School
Associate Director of Obstetric Anesthesia
Brigham and Women's Hospital
Boston, Massachusetts

David M. Dewan, M.D.
Associate Professor
Head, Section on Obstetric and Gynecologic Anesthesia
Department of Anesthesia
Wake Forest University Medical Center
Winston-Salem, North Carolina

James C. Eisenach, M.S., M.D.
Assistant Professor
Section on Obstetric and Gynecologic Anesthesia
Department of Anesthesia
Wake Forest University Medical Center
Winston-Salem, North Carolina

Mieczyslaw Finster, M.D.
Professor of Anesthesiology
Obstetrics and Gynecology
Department of Anesthesiology
Columbia University
New York, New York

Brett B. Gutsche, M.D.
Professor of Anesthesiology and Obstetrics and Gynecology
University of Pennsylvania Medical Center
Philadelphia, Pennsylvania

David D. Hood, M.D.
Assistant Professor
Section on Obstetric and Gynecologic Anesthesia
Department of Anesthesia
Wake Forest University Medical Center
Winston-Salem, North Carolina

Francis M. James, III, M.D.
Professor and Chairman
Department of Anesthesia
Wake Forest University Medical Center
Winston-Salem, North Carolina

Monica M. Jones, M.D.
Assistant Professor
Department of Anesthesiology
Assistant Professor
Department of Obstetrics and Gynecology
Baylor College of Medicine
Houston, Texas

Nancy Kenepp, M.D.
Associate Professor
Department of Anesthesiology
Temple University Hospital
Philadelphia, Pennsylvania

Gordon L. Mandell, M.D.
Assistant Professor
Section on Obstetric and Gynecologic Anesthesia
Department of Anesthesia
Wake Forest University Medical Center
Winston-Salem, North Carolina

Graham H. McMorland, M.B., Ch.B., D.A., F.R.C.P.
Clinical Professor
Division of Obstetric Anesthesia
University of British Columbia
Head, Department of Anesthesia
Grace Hospital
Vancouver, Canada

Hisayo O. Morishima, M.D., Ph.D.
Professor of Anesthesiology
College of Physicians and Surgeons
Columbia University
New York, New York

Richard J. Palahniuk, M.D., F.R.C.P.C.
Professor and Chairman of Department of Anaesthesia
University of Manitoba
Winnipeg, Manitoba, Canada

Hilda Pedersen, M.B., Ch.B., F.F.A.R.C.S.
Associate Professor of Clinical Anesthesiology
Department of Anesthesiology
College of Physicians and Surgeons
Columbia University
New York, New York

Michael H. Plumer, M.D.
Associate Clinical Professor of Anesthesiology
University of California
Davis, California
Director, Perinatal Anesthesiology
Sutter Memorial Hospital
Sacramento, California

Sivam Ramanathan, M.D.
Professor of Anesthesiology
Director of Obstetric Anesthesiology
New York University Medical Center
New York, New York

Douglas S. Richards, M.D.
Assistant Professor of Obstetrics and Gynecology
University of Florida College of Medicine
Gainesville, Florida

John William Seeds, M.D.
Associate Professor, Obstetrics and Gynecology and Radiology
University of North Carolina at Chapel Hill
Chapel Hill, North Carolina

William Clyde Shelley, M.D.
Staff Anesthesiologist
Research Medical Center
Kansas City, Missouri

Fred J. Spielman, M.D.
Assistant Professor of Anesthesiology, Obstetrics and Gynecology
University of North Carolina School of Medicine
Chapel Hill, North Carolina

Frank R. Storniolo, M.D.
Section Head of Obstetric Anesthesia
Georgia Baptist Medical Center
Atlanta, Georgia

Herman Turndorf, M.D.
Professor and Chairman
Department of Anesthesiology
New York University Medical Center
New York, New York

A. Scott Wheeler, M.D.
Professor of Anesthesiology
Chief, Special Services Division
Anesthesia Coordinator
Main Operating Room
The University of Alabama at Birmingham
School of Medicine
Birmingham, Alabama

William D. Writer, M.B., Ch.B., F.F.A.R.C.S. (Eng), F.R.C.P.C.
Professor, Department of Anaesthesia
Dalhousie University
Halifax, Nova Scotia
Chief of Anaesthesia
Grace Maternity Hospital
Halifax, Nova Scotia

CONTENTS

PART 1

BACKGROUND

CHAPTER 1

MATERNAL PHYSIOLOGIC CHANGES DURING PREGNANCY

DIANE R. BIEHL, M.D., F.R.C.P.C.

For anesthesiologists providing analgesia or anesthesia to women during gestation the physiologic adaptations to pregnancy have important implications. Like the pediatric patient, the obstetric patient qualifies as "different"; though in most circumstances, the differences are not truly appreciated until a complication occurs. Because most obstetric patients are young and healthy, they often overcome the effects of suboptimal treatment. The pregnant patient with medical or obstetric complications may not be so fortunate. To obviate hazards that may confront the "complicated" obstetric patient the anesthesiologist must fully understand the normal physiologic changes of pregnancy. This chapter presents important maternal adaptations during pregnancy and emphasizes those that have implications for the anesthesiologist. The discussion centers primarily on changes in the cardiovascular, respiratory, and gastrointestinal systems because these alterations most often produce anesthesia-related problems. Each section relates physiologic changes to necessary adjustments in anesthesia management for parturients and for pregnant patients who require anesthesia prior to term.

Cardiovascular Changes

CIRCULATING BLOOD VOLUME

In the first trimester, probably as early as the 5th to 8th week of gestation,[1] the blood volume of the pregnant woman begins to increase. Although the precise underlying mechanism is unknown, changes in hormonal interaction probably contribute to this blood volume alteration.[2,3,4] Increasing circulating levels of progesterone plus alterations in the renin-angiotensin-aldosterone system may play a role.

The greatest increase occurs in the circulating plasma volume, which starts to increase early in pregnancy, reaches a maximum at 30 to 32 weeks' gestation, and remains at that level until term.[1] The overall increase approximates 40 to 50 percent, depending on the patient's size and weight and the weight gain during pregnancy.[5] Patients carrying multiple fetuses show a greater increase than those with a singleton pregnancy.[6] Figure 1–1 presents a comparison of plasma volume changes.

The composition of plasma also changes with

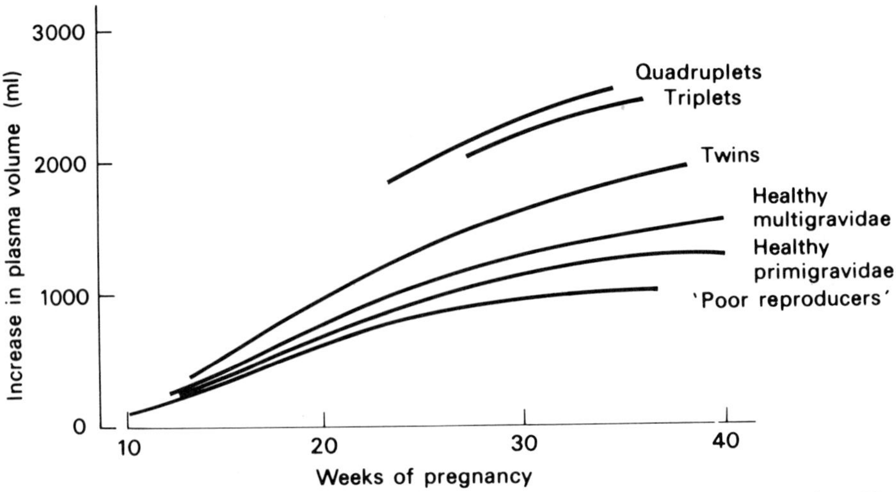

Figure 1–1. Increases in plasma volume during pregnancy in various patient groups. (Adapted from Hytten, F and Chamberlain, G (eds): Clinical Physiology in Obstetrics. Blackwell Scientific Publications, London, 1980, p 46.)

pregnancy. The increase in water exceeds that of colloid components,[6] which may have important implications for distribution and binding of drugs. The serum proteins, especially albumin, are present in lower concentrations than in the nonpregnant patient, possibly resulting in a decrease of plasma oncotic pressure.[7]

The red-cell mass of blood also increases in a parallel manner to that of the plasma volume, but not to the same extent (Fig. 1–2). By the middle of the second trimester, the patient develops the "physiologic anemia" of pregnancy,[8,9] as her actual hemoglobin concentration falls from 14 to 12 g per dl.

The maximum increase in the circulating blood volume occurs by the 30th week of gestation. When calculated on a volume-per-kilogram basis, circulating blood volume increases from 60 to 65 ml per kg before pregnancy to 80 to 85 ml per kg and remains at this level from 30 weeks until delivery. Blood volume reverts to normal levels by the sixth week postpartum.[9]

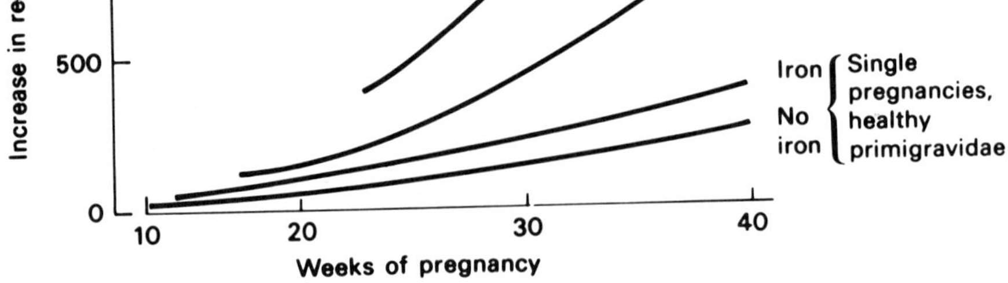

Figure 1–2. Increases in red cell mass during pregnancy in various patient groups. (Adapted from Hytten, F and Chamberlain, G (eds): Clinical Physiology in Obstetrics. Blackwell Scientific Publications, London, 1980, p 47.)

PERIPHERAL CIRCULATION

During pregnancy, the peripheral circulation undergoes significant changes, most likely as a result of the same influences that produce the increase in blood volume.[2,4] The literature on this subject is inconsistent, and many studies rely on measurements that have a considerable degree of inaccuracy.[10,11] Basically, however, investigators believe that a decrease in peripheral vascular resistance at the arteriolar level compensates for increased blood volume and cardiac output, so that arterial blood pressure does not increase in normal pregnancy. In fact, studies[12,13] on blood pressure in the second trimester demonstrate a significant decrease in diastolic pressure. Blood pressure values are more difficult to evaluate in the third trimester because a significant number of patients develop pregnancy-induced hypertension, which increases the average values of both systolic and diastolic pressures in any population.[14] Exclusion of hypertensive women poses a problem in prospectively designed studies. Currently the most common view holds that normal patients have no significant changes in systolic blood pressure throughout pregnancy. Diastolic pressure declines in the second trimester and gradually rises toward pregravid values by term. Clinicians consider patients who develop more than a 10- to 15-percent increase in either systolic or diastolic pressure after the 20th week of gestation to have gestational hypertension; the cause of such a blood pressure increase should be determined.[15]

Several studies also have investigated the venous side of the circulation, with equivocal or conflicting results. Generally, venous pressure as measured in the upper limbs remains constant in the first and second trimester.[16] In the lower limbs an increase in femoral venous pressure occurs by 20 weeks' gestation,[17] and by term this increase exceeds pregravid values by two or three times.[18,19] Venous pressure rapidly falls to normal soon after delivery. The factors responsible for increased venous pressure include: mechanical occlusion of the iliac veins and inferior vena cava by the gravid uterus, pressure of the fetal head on the iliac veins, and increased venous blood volume caused by outflow from the placental bed. The increased venous pressure in the lower limbs leads to some degree of edema in most women in the third trimester. Venous varicosities may be produced or exacerbated by pregnancy.[20]

Particularly in the late second and the third trimester, the obstruction to venous blood flow by the gravid uterus can compromise placental perfusion[21–23] and can produce adverse hemodynamic consequences, especially when the mother lies supine. In 10 to 15 percent of pregnant patients the impairment of venous return is sufficient to decrease right ventricular filling pressure, cardiac output, and arterial blood pressure[23] to the extent that the parturient becomes light-headed and nauseated when supine. Turning from the supine to the lateral position generally corrects the problem. Even if the mother does not develop symptoms of hypotension, the supine position produces obstruction of the inferior vena cava and iliac veins, which increases pressure in uterine veins and decreases placental perfusion pressure substantially.[24] During the second and third trimesters the supine position produces deleterious effects in both mother and fetus.

REGIONAL BLOOD FLOW

The most notable change in distribution of blood flow during pregnancy involves the increased flow to the uterus and adnexa.[25,26] Although measurements in human parturients are few,[27,28] these data, plus extrapolation from animal data,[29,30] indicate that uterine blood flow increases from approximately 85 ml per min in the nongravid uterus to 500 ml per min in the patient at 36 to 40 weeks' gestation. Figure 1–3 demonstrates a composite of human and animal data on uterine blood flow during gestation.

Uterine blood flow is distributed between the placenta (70 to 90 percent) and the myometrium (10 to 30 percent).[29] In the nonpregnant uterus control of myometrial blood flow resembles that in other smooth-muscle beds.[27] These vessels respond to adrenergic stimulation with vasoconstriction, while acetylcholine produces vasodilation. Reactive hyperemia in response to hypoxia or vasoconstriction also occurs in the myometrium of animal models.[30] The developing placenta, however, creates a large perfusion-passive vascular bed as fetal trophoblasts invade the spiral arteries. The smooth muscle in the arteriolar walls disappears, creating a low-

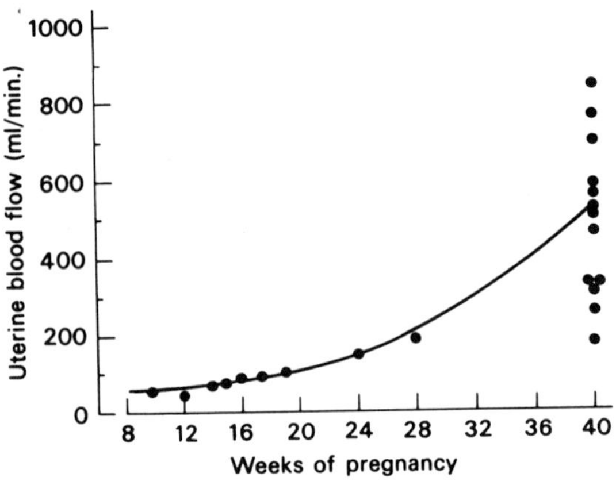

Figure 1–3. Changes in uterine blood flow during pregnancy. Data obtained from animal and human studies. (Adapted from Hytten, F and Chamberlain, G (eds): Clinical Physiology in Obstetrics. Blackwell Scientific Publications, London, 1980, p 21.)

resistance vascular bed.[27] With increasing placental size the pressure-passive nature of this vascular bed predominates, and by the second trimester uterine blood flow becomes primarily pressure passive, depending on maternal systemic blood pressure. Under normal circumstances placental blood flow is maximal and cannot be increased by pharmacologic manipulation. Placental blood flow decreases, however, when maternal hypotension occurs.[24] Aortocaval occlusion in the supine position represents the most common cause of decreased placental perfusion in the normal placenta.[23] Maternal hemorrhage will also decrease placental blood flow. Catecholamine release causes vasoconstriction of the larger arteries. Infusions of norepinephrine reduce uterine blood flow in both normotensive and hypotensive pregnant ewes.[31,32]

In pregnancies complicated by hypertension, a large low-resistance placental vasculature may not develop. A recent study,[33] using Doppler techniques to study resistance in the placental bed in parturients in the first and second trimester, suggests that patients with gestational hypertension do not show the same decrease in vascular resistance that occurs in normal pregnancies. This may explain their high incidence of intrauterine growth retardation and fetal distress.

Blood flow to the kidneys increases in early pregnancy to a level approximately 400 ml per min above the nongravid value.[34] In late pregnancy, assuming the supine position may substantially impair renal blood flow.[35]

Blood flow to the skin and subcutaneous tissues also increases markedly during pregnancy. In the upper part of the body, the increase is six to seven times nonpregnant values.[36] The effect of flow in the lower limbs is less predictable, however, as the position of the woman affects measurements to a large extent.

Pregnancy seems to influence blood flow to other organs much less than to the uterus, kidneys, and skin (Fig. 1–4). One study[37] demonstrates increased hepatic blood flow, but other investigations[38,39] fail to corroborate these findings during pregnancy.

PULMONARY CIRCULATION

The effect of pregnancy on the pulmonary circulation has not received detailed investigation in humans, but the studies that exist demon-

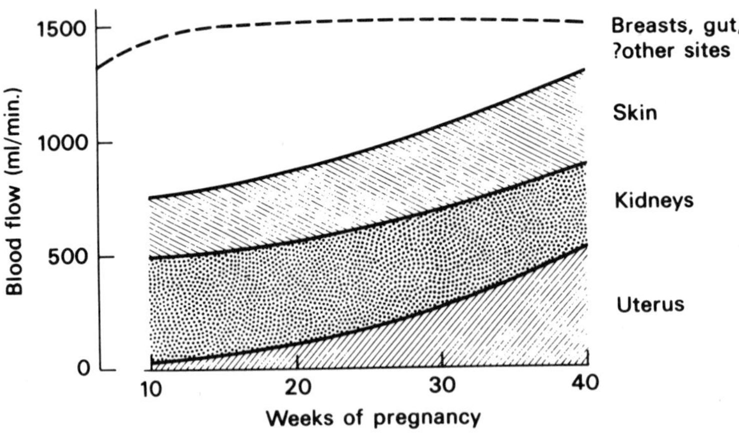

Figure 1–4. Blood flow to various organ systems during pregnancy. (Adapted from Hytten, F and Chamberlain, G (eds): Clinical Physiology in Obstetrics. Blackwell Scientific Publications, London, 1980, p 28.)

strate no change in pulmonary pressures during normal pregnancy.[40,41] This is not surprising, as the pulmonary circulation contains high-capacitance (or low-resistance) vessels. Capillary and arteriolar vasodilation occur to accommodate the increased blood volume flowing through the lungs. The characteristic roentgenographic appearance of increased vascularity and enlarged pulmonary vessels supports this process.[42] Although normal patients show no change in pulmonary vascular pressures, patients who have pulmonary hypertension prior to pregnancy usually fare poorly during pregnancy, especially after the first trimester.[41] The effects of a noncompliant pulmonary vasculature in these patients underscores the tremendous adaptive reserve of healthy pregnant patients.

THE HEART AND CARDIAC OUTPUT

All the changes in pregnancy outlined above must be accompanied by changes in cardiac output. Most authorities agree that cardiac output increases by 30 to 50 percent above normal during pregnancy. Ueland and coworkers[43] demonstrated that the increase begins in the first trimester and reaches a maximum at 28 to 32 weeks' gestation. From this time until term, measurement of cardiac output depends greatly on the mother's position.[44,45] Cardiac output is highest in the lateral position in the third trimester but declines somewhat by term (Fig. 1–5). In the supine position, cardiac output may be 12 to 20 percent lower than in the lateral position.[44] The two components of cardiac output, heart rate and stroke volume, both increase during gestation, although changes in stroke volume seem to predominate in the earlier stages of pregnancy. In Ueland's study,[43] mean pulse rate increased from 73.8 ± 9.5 beats per min at 20 to 24 weeks to 91.8 ± 17.2 beats per min at 28 to 32 weeks. The corresponding increases in stroke volume were 94.5 ± 15.6 ml at 20 to 24 weeks, followed by a decline to 72.4 ± 25.1 ml at 28 to 32 weeks.

The response of normal pregnant patients to graded exercise remains normal in the first two trimesters, but in the third trimester cardiac output increases less in response to exercise.[43] This implies that in late pregnancy cardiac reserve decreases even in normal patients.

Although cardiac output tends to fall, even when the woman is in the lateral position during the third trimester, marked increases occur with contractions, and catecholamine release in response to labor pain further augments cardiac output.[44–46] Cardiac output values peak during the second stage and in the immediate postpartum period at levels of 7 to 9 liters per min. The position of the patient in labor also influences the changes in cardiac output occurring with contractions. Regional anesthesia (caudal or lumbar epidural)[47] decreases the marked swings in cardiac output during labor, probably by removing the pain component but does not affect the overall increases that take place in stage 2. The course of labor affects both heart rate and stroke volume, but changes in stroke volume prove greater than pulse rate changes (in contrast to the findings during late pregnancy).[47]

In addition to the changes in cardiac performance accompanying pregnancy, other changes

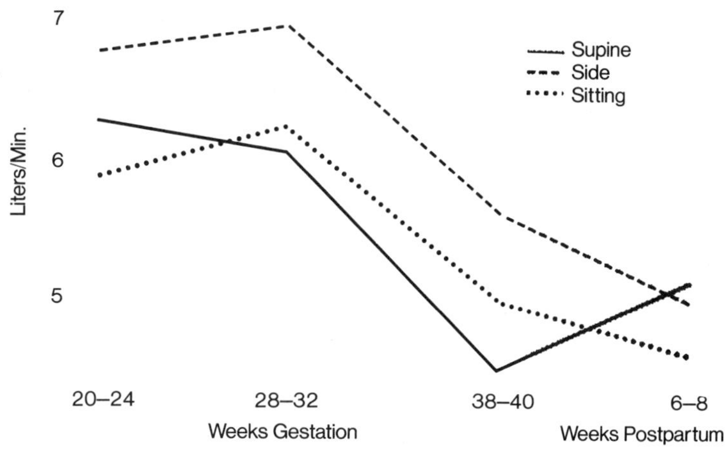

Figure 1–5. Changes in cardiac output related to various positions during pregnancy. (Adapted from Ueland, K, Novy, MG, Peterson, EN, and Metcalfe, J: Maternal cardiovascular dynamics. Am J Obstet Gynecol 104:856, 1969.)

sometimes confuse the clinician assessing a pregnant patient. Flow murmurs develop frequently, most notably over the pulmonary and aortic valves.[48] A fourth heart sound may develop normally in pregnancy, but a third sound constitutes a pathologic finding. As pregnancy advances, electrocardiography may detect rotation of the cardiac axis, often demonstrating left axis deviations of up to 15 to 20 degrees.[49] Nonspecific ST- and T-wave changes, which sometimes exist normally in pregnancy, should be investigated to rule out problems such as myocardial ischemia.[50] Pregnancy does not produce significant effects on the cardiac conduction system, but atrial and ventricular extrasystoles and increased susceptibility to supraventricular tachycardias have been reported.[51]

ANESTHETIC IMPLICATIONS

In summary, the adaptations of the cardiovascular system to pregnancy begin early in the first trimester, peak between 28 and 32 weeks' gestation, and generally remain elevated until term. During labor and delivery, marked swings in heart rate, blood pressure, and cardiac output sometimes accompany contractions, and the cardiac patient may have trouble tolerating the changes, which can persist into the puerperium. For the anesthesiologist attending such patients, the rapid cardiovascular changes may obscure other problems and may complicate cardiovascular assessment. Also, the anesthesiologist must remember the pronounced effect of maternal position on cardiovascular performance. Pregnant patients should assume the left lateral tilt position to prevent compression of the inferior vena cava and aorta,[52] especially during conduction of spinal, epidural, or deep planes of general anesthesia.

Respiratory Changes

Like those of the cardiovascular system, the respiratory changes of pregnancy usually begin in the first trimester and include alterations in anatomy and physiology.

ANATOMIC CHANGES

One of the most important changes involves the upper airway. Early in the first trimester, the effects of maternal hormones (estrogen, progesterone) become manifest in the nasal and oropharyngeal mucosa.[53] The mucosal linings become congested and swollen. As a result, many women complain of nasal stuffiness or "colds." Although this finding carries little significance for most physicians, it constitutes an important finding for anesthesiologists and nurse anesthetists because the increased swelling and vascularity may complicate tracheal intubation.[54] Edema of the epiglottis and glottis may be further accentuated in patients with pre-eclampsia.[55] Laryngeal edema, especially when accompanied by facial edema and breast enlargement, hampers efforts of the anesthesia team to correctly position the patient for easy intubation. Airway management of the pregnant patient often becomes considerably more challenging.[56] Avoiding the use of nasal airways prevents epistaxis.

Anatomic changes below the larynx also occur during pregnancy. The larger airways dilate as a result of the relaxant effects of progesterone and estrogen on airway smooth muscle,[57,58] and airway resistance decreases accordingly. As pregnancy progresses, the enlarged uterus displaces the diaphragm in a cephalad direction and the lower ribs flare outward.[59] Chest wall compliance, not significantly affected in slender patients, may decrease in obese mothers.[57] The recumbent or supine position produces a greater decrease in compliance than the sitting position.[60] Total compliance in all pregnant patients decreases by 30 percent at term.

PHYSIOLOGIC CHANGES

Pregnancy produces a state of continuous hyperventilation that becomes apparent as early as 6 to 8 weeks' gestation.[61] Tidal volume increases substantially so that minute ventilation increases by approximately 40 percent, a finding influenced significantly less by the rise in respiratory rate. In fact, some investigators suggest that respiratory rate during pregnancy is the same as the nongravid rate.[62] Alveolar ventilation increases because of the larger tidal volumes coupled with unchanged dead-space ventilation, and it exceeds nongravid levels by 50 to 70 percent.

The functional residual capacity (FRC) and the residual volume both decrease in pregnancy by approximately 20 to 30 percent. Therefore, the FRC decreases by 500 ml in the average-size woman. Figure 1–6 depicts the effect of pregnancy on all lung volumes. Pulmonary function tests performed during normal pregnancy show no significant change in maximum breathing capacity (MBC) or forced expiratory ventilation (FEV_1). Vital capacity increases, but total lung capacity (TLC) remains unchanged.[61,62] Studies on closing volumes in pregnancy yield varying results, but in some patients closing volumes may exceed FRC, especially in the supine position.[63,64] Such individuals are at risk for hypoxia during induction of general anesthesia.

Because of changes described above, alveolar mixing of gases and gas exchange prove more efficient in the pregnant than the nongravid patient, but oxygen reserves decrease because of the reduced FRC.

Gas Exchange During Pregnancy

As mentioned above, hyperventilation occurs throughout pregnancy. In the first trimester, arterial P_{CO_2} falls from 35 to 40 mmHg to approximately 30 mmHg. At the same time, arterial P_{O_2} usually increases from 90 to 95 mmHg to 95 to 105 mmHg.[65] Elimination of bicarbonate by the kidneys maintains plasma pH in the normal range (7.38 to 7.42). Since these changes occur in the first trimester, they are thought to result from respiratory stimulation centrally by progesterone rather than from an anatomic change.[66,67] A study by Templeton and Kelman[68] demonstrated no significant differences in pulmonary venous admixture, dead space–to–tidal volume ratio (V_D/V_T), or in alveolo-arterial oxygen gradients [$P(A\text{-}a)O_2$] in pregnant and nonpregnant subjects. Another study,[69] however, suggests that $P(A\text{-}a)O_2$ may increase when measured in pregnant women in the supine position. This finding likely results from the previously mentioned changes in FRC–closing volume differences.

A study by Artal and associates[70] examined pulmonary responses to exercise during pregnancy. Despite initially higher tidal volumes in pregnant patients, graded increases in exercise demonstrated less increase in minute ventilation than in nonpregnant controls. They concluded that pregnant patients had less pulmonary reserve than the nonpregnant controls.

Oxygen Consumption During Pregnancy

Several studies[71,72] demonstrated gradual increases in maternal oxygen consumption from 200 ml per min in early gestation to 250 ml per min at term. With labor, oxygen consumption

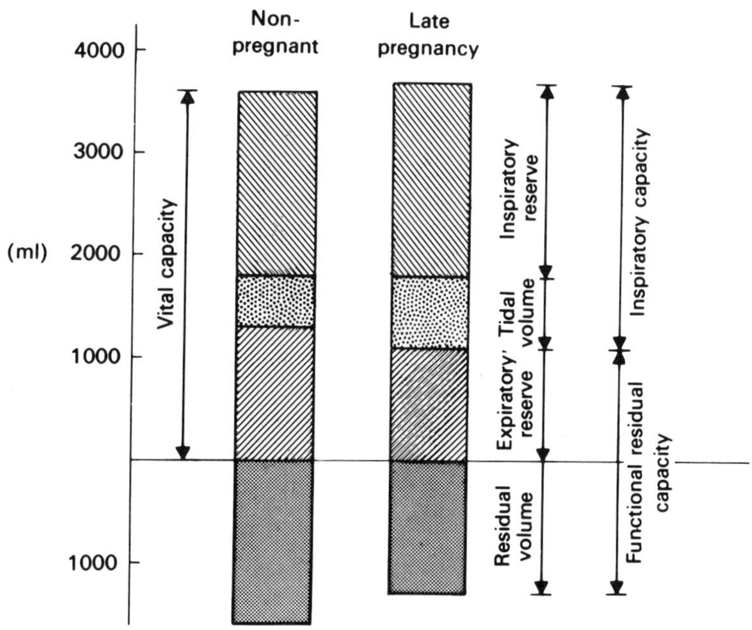

Figure 1–6. Changes in lung volumes from nonpregnancy to late pregnancy. (Adapted from Hytten, F and Chamberlain, G (eds): Clinical Physiology in Obstetrics. Blackwell Scientific Publications, London, 1980, p 47.)

may double to 500 ml per min, primarily as a result of increases in the work of breathing.[73] There is little documentation of carbon dioxide production in pregnant patients,[70] but it seems safe to assume that it must increase in parallel fashion to oxygen consumption. Rightward shift in the oxyhemoglobin saturation curve and increased cardiac output and perfusion of some tissues enhance oxygen delivery to and carbon dioxide transport from tissues (see Fig. 1–4).[71] For example, Kambam and coworkers[74] report an increase in the $Po_2 50$ from 26.7 mmHg in controls to 30.2 mmHg in maternal hemoglobin at term.

ANESTHETIC IMPLICATIONS

During pregnancy, a state of hyperventilation exists, with both alveolar ventilation and pulmonary gas exchange increasing, as reflected by the rise in arterial Po_2 and the fall in Pco_2. Balanced against this is a decrease in FRC and an increase in oxygen consumption, the latter becoming greatly accentuated by labor and delivery.

For the anesthesiologist respiratory changes during pregnancy may hinder airway management and tracheal intubation, thus promoting the development of hypoxia and hypercarbia. Also, oxyhemoglobin desaturates more rapidly during periods of apnea because of reduced FRC and pulmonary oxygen reserves and increased oxygen consumption. The supine position can expand the closing volume to exceed FRC and widen the $P(A\text{-}a)O_2$. Together, all these events may produce a rapid fall in arterial Po_2 during administration of general or regional anesthesia, particularly if they happen simultaneously with a decrease in venous return and cardiac output. The patient should be carefully positioned (avoiding the supine position) and supplemental oxygen should be administered during major conduction blocks for cesarean section. For the pregnant patient requiring general anesthesia, thorough preoxygenation must precede induction, and maintenance gases should contain at least 50 percent oxygen to assure adequate oxygenation of both mother and fetus. A pulse oximeter provides useful data regarding maternal oxygen saturation; capnography reliably assesses the degree of ventilation.

Gastrointestinal Changes

GASTRIC VOLUMES AND FUNCTION

Since the studies of Mendelson in 1946,[75] numerous investigations and editorial comments have addressed the dangers associated with gastrointestinal changes during pregnancy. Although the anesthesia team recognizes the implications of these alterations, no general agreement exists on their nature or on when during pregnancy they occur. Various teams[76–78] have studied gastroesophageal reflux, gastric secretion, and gastric emptying, but considerable differences in methodology among investigators make interpretation of results difficult. At present most authorities agree that many pregnant women experience reduced gastroesophageal sphincter tone and esophageal reflux.[77] Whether this results from relaxation of gastrointestinal smooth muscle during pregnancy or from decreased vagal tone remains unclear. Since symptoms of reflux often emerge early in pregnancy, the anesthesiologist must assume that gastroesophageal sphincter tone decreases throughout pregnancy and that reflux looms as a possibility during all stages of gestation and in the immediate puerperium.

The rate of gastric acid production apparently changes little during gestation. However, clear proof of this assumption is lacking. Some studies report gastric emptying to be normal while others find it delayed.[76,78] With advancing pregnancy, decreased gastrointestinal muscle motility and mechanical displacement of the stomach and duodenum by the gravid uterus may delay gastric emptying.

During labor, gastric motility irrefutably decreases, and pregnant patients may have gastric volumes in excess of 25 to 50 ml for many hours.[79,80] Roberts and Shirley[81,82] effectively demonstrated this during assessments of women undergoing labor and cesarean section. After several hours of fasting, gastric volumes actually increased because of delayed emptying combined with continued secretion of gastric acid. Patients were then at high risk, possessing high gastric volume of low pH.

Delayed emptying of the small and large bowel also may occur during pregnancy and with the onset of labor. Such effects presumably relate to both smooth muscle relaxation and decreased vagal tone. Feedback mechanisms, particularly from the duodenum, may further delay gastric emptying.[83]

ANESTHETIC IMPLICATIONS

Delayed gastric emptying and decreased gastroesophageal sphincter tone carry the threat of aspiration of gastric contents and aspiration pneumonitis. This problem has figured prominently in anesthetic morbidity and mortality for obstetric patients.[84] The administration of antacids to pregnant women prior to anesthesia has not eliminated the problem (see Chapters 4 and 7). Since there is no effective method to rapidly empty the stomach or to reduce acidity in emergency obstetric situations, all patients are treated as having a stomach full of acid contents. Meticulous attention must be paid to protecting the mother's airway by rapidly intubating the trachea with a cuffed tube during application of cricoid pressure. Pharmacologic methods such as the administration of clear antacids,[81] hydrogen blockers (cimetidine, ranitidine),[85,86] and metoclopramide[87] reduce maternal risk during more elective procedures but are not foolproof and do not obviate the threat of aspiration pneumonitis.

Hepatic and Renal Changes

HEPATIC CHANGES

During pregnancy, liver size and blood flow do not change. Mild elevations in serum glutamic oxaloacetic transaminase, lactic acid dehydrogenase, and alkaline phosphatase frequently occur, and serum cholesterol levels and bilirubin may also rise. Studies[88,89] show a decrease in both total circulating proteins and the albumin-to-globulin ratio.

The decline in serum cholinesterase activity during pregnancy and the postpartum period is of more concern to the anesthesiologist. Levels decrease by approximately 30 percent,[90] but prolonged muscle relaxation by succinylcholine rarely compromises the parturient.[91] However, Evans and Roe[92] studied 941 pregnant patients and found a significant number with enzyme levels low enough to produce delayed recovery from succinylcholine. Therefore, it seems prudent to monitor neuromuscular function with a peripheral nerve stimulator in a pregnant patient given succinylcholine during general anesthesia.

RENAL CHANGES

During pregnancy, renal blood flow (RBF) increases in parallel to increased cardiac output. By 32 weeks' gestation, RBF rises by approximately 40 percent.[93] Glomerular filtration rates climb similarly and account for a 20- to 40-percent decline in blood urea nitrogen (BUN) and serum creatinine. (The upper limits for BUN and serum creatinine are 9 mg per dl and 0.46 mg per dl, respectively.[94]) Creatinine clearance also increases, but values vary widely in women with normal renal function. Glucosuria (1 to 10 g per day) and proteinuria (300 mg per day) are common conditions found in parturients with normal kidneys.[93]

The renal calyces and ureters dilate early in pregnancy, possibly in response to increased circulating levels of progesterone.[95] In the third trimester, the enlarged uterus, compressing the ureters at the pelvic brim, may cause further dilation. These factors probably account for the increased incidence of cystitis and pyelonephritis in pregnancy.[96]

ANESTHETIC IMPLICATIONS

Most of the changes in hepatic and renal function, though not directly influencing the conduct of an anesthetic, may alter drug metabolism and excretion.[34] The increased volume of distribution of most drugs, in part, offsets these potential changes in drug pharmacokinetics, owing to the larger plasma and extracellular water volumes of pregnancy.[7] An increased volume of distribution decreases plasma concentration following a standard dose of drug, thus compensating for the increased clearance of drugs.

Hematologic Changes

The changes in red-cell mass during pregnancy have been previously discussed. An increased neutrophil count primarily accounts for the total white cell–count rise in early pregnancy,[97] which reaches 40.0×10^9 per liter during labor and delivery, but returns to normal by the 6th day postpartum.[98] The lymphocyte count is not markedly altered, and circulating levels of T and B cells remain unchanged.[99] However, pregnancy depresses lymphocyte activity and cell-mediated immunity.[100] Though this may benefit the fetus, it also decreases resistance to many viral infections.[101]

The platelet count diminishes during pregnancy for unexplained reasons.[99] A recent study[102] suggests that the diameter of platelets increases during pregnancy, indicating a greater rate of platelet turnover in pregnant than in nonpregnant individuals. However, platelet counts and function remain adequate in normal gestation. Additionally, circulating levels of clotting factors (VII, VIII, X), fibrinogen, and fibrin-fibrinogen complexes in maternal plasma increase, leading to a hypercoagulable state during pregnancy and during the first few days postpartum.[103,104] Generally, plasma fibrinogen levels exceed 300 to 350 mg per dl in normal pregnant women, and plasminogen-activator substances decrease.[103]

ANESTHETIC IMPLICATIONS

Most of the above changes do not directly affect anesthetic management of most parturients. The increased susceptibility to viral infections may have some significance, in that upper respiratory tract infections occur more commonly during pregnancy and may complicate airway management during general anesthesia. The increased susceptibility to infections with the herpes virus may heighten the risk of regional anesthesia, especially when there are lesions on the lower back and perineum.

The increased coagulability associated with pregnancy predisposes the mother to thromboembolic problems and may lead to high-risk situations like pulmonary embolism, which may occur during labor, delivery, or the immediate postpartum period. Chapter 14 discusses such problems.

Endocrine Changes

Most endocrine changes during pregnancy do not pose problems for the anesthesiologist, except for two areas: carbohydrate metabolism and thyroid function. Pregnancy induces complex changes in insulin kinetics and activity and is generally regarded as a diabetogenic state marked by the development of insulin resistance. During the third trimester, when fasting serum glucose concentrations normally fall below those occurring in the nonpregnant state, glucose utilization peaks with corresponding maximal decreases in serum levels.[105] However, the presence of insulin-resistant substances produced by the placenta exaggerates the response to the glucose tolerance test.[106] These alterations disappear quickly, usually within 24 hours after delivery. The anesthesiologist must remember that rapid infusions of intravenous fluids containing glucose prior to delivery often produce maternal hyperglycemia, which stimulates maternal and fetal insulin production[107] and promotes development of neonatal hypoglycemia several hours after delivery. Conversely, withholding solutions containing dextrose in the postpartum period may lead to dangerous degrees of maternal hypoglycemia as carbohydrate and insulin metabolism return to normal.

Thyroid function remains normal in pregnancy, although plasma levels of thyroxin-binding globulin increase.[108] Direct measurements of T_3 and T_4 demonstrate levels in the same range as for nonpregnant women. However, since pregnancy produces heat intolerance, increased metabolic rate, and a higher resting heart rate, it may mimic hyperthyroidism, making the diagnosis of the latter more difficult. Enlargement of the thyroid gland can occur during pregnancy, but in countries that supply iodized salt a toxic or true goiter seldom develops in a pregnant woman.[109]

Alterations in Drug Distribution and Metabolism

Changes in protein binding and increases in plasma volume (50 percent), extracellular water (2.5 liters), and adipose tissue mass (3 to 4 kg) affect drug distribution in the pregnant patient. Hepatic metabolism and clearance of drugs may decrease in response to competitive inhibitory effects of estrogen on the liver enzyme systems.[110] Increases in renal blood flow and glomerular filtration rate may enhance renal clearance of drug metabolites. Unfortunately, few studies have investigated the metabolism and elimination of anesthetic agents.[111,112] Morgan and coworkers[113] report that the volume of distribution of thiopental given for cesarean section increases, resulting in prolonged elimination of the drug.

Changes in Anesthetic Potency

The alteration of MAC values, which decrease by 25 to 40 percent for the inhalational anesthetics in pregnant animals, holds greater interest for the anesthesiologist[114] as this finding most likely applies to pregnant women as well. The explanation for decreased requirements of anesthetic gases remains unknown but may relate to increased levels of progesterone and/or β-endorphins in the central nervous system.[115,116]

Pregnancy also enhances the effects of local anesthetics, particularly during spinal and epidural anesthesia, so that local anesthetic requirements decrease by approximately 40 percent. This effect has been attributed to the decreased volume of the epidural and intrathecal spaces[117] and the influence of uterine contractions on the pressure in the subarachnoid space.[118] Recently, Datta and coworkers[119] presented evidence that nerve fibers exhibit more sensitivity to local anesthetics in pregnant than in nonpregnant mammals.

The anesthesiologist must remain aware of possible altered drug effects in the pregnant patient and make necessary adjustments, especially in regard to drug doses. While prevention of overdose represents the most important objective, drug effects may sometimes be less than anticipated in pregnant patients.

Summary

This chapter presents an overview of the physiologic adaptations that occur during pregnancy, especially those of concern to the anesthesia team. The most important changes involve the cardiovascular, respiratory, and gastrointestinal systems. If the anesthesiologist anticipates successful management of obstetric patients, he or she must remember:

1. The difficulties that can occur with the upper airway
2. The decreased oxygen reserve and rapidity of oxygen desaturation
3. The importance of tilting the patient so that the uterus does not impede venous return, cardiac output, blood pressure, or placental perfusion
4. That all pregnant patients have a full stomach and are at substantial risk for aspiration

References

1. Pirani, BBK, Campbell, DM and MacGillivray, I: Plasma volume in normal first pregnancy. J Obstet Gynaecol Br Commonw 80:884, 1973.
2. Verel, D, Bury, JD and Hope, A: Blood volume changes in pregnancy and the puerperium. Clin Sci 15:1, 1956.
3. Hytten, FE and Paintin, DB: Increase in plasma volume during normal pregnancy. J Obstet Gynaecol Br Commonw 70:442, 1963.
4. Ueland, K: Cardiorespiratory physiology of pregnancy. In Sciaria, JJ and Drigmuller, W (eds): Gynecology and Obstetrics, vol 3. Harper and Row, New York, 1979, p 31.
5. Campbell, DM and MacGillivray, I: Comparison of maternal response in first and second pregnancies in relation to baby weight. J Obstet Gynaecol Br Commonw 79:684, 1972.
6. Rovinsky, JJ and Jaffin, H: Cardiovascular hemodynamics in pregnancy I. Blood and plasma volumes in multiple pregnancy. Am J Obstet Gynecol 93:1, 1965.
7. Lewis, P: Drug metabolism in clinical physiology in obstetrics. In Hytten, F and Chamberlain, G (eds): Clinical Physiology in Obstetrics. Blackwell Scientific Publications, London, 1980.
8. Berlin, NI, et al: The blood volume in pregnancy as determined with ^{32}P-labelled red blood cells. Surg Gynecol Obstet 80:956, 1960.
9. Chesley, LC: Plasma and red cell volumes during pregnancy. Am J Obstet Gynecol 112:440, 1972.
10. Palmer, AJ and Walker, AMC: The maternal circulation in normal pregnancy. J Obstet Gynaecol Br Emp 56:337, 1954.
11. Bader, RA, et al: Haemodynamics at rest and during exercise in normal pregnancy as studied by cardiac catheterization. J Clin Invest 34:1524, 1955.
12. Ginsburg, J and Duncan, S: Direct and indirect blood pressure measurement in pregnancy. J Obstet Gynaecol Br Commonw 76:705, 1969.
13. MacGillivray, I, Rose, GA and Row, B: Blood pressure survey in pregnancy. Clin Sci 37:395, 1969.
14. MacGillivray, I: Hypertension in pregnancy and its consequences. J Obstet Gynaecol Br Commonw 68:557, 1961.
15. Perkins, RP: Management of the hypertensive pregnant patient. Clin Perinatol 7:313, 1980.
16. Theobold, GW and Lundborg, RA: Changes in limb volume and in venous infusion pressure caused by

pregnancy. J Obstet Gynaecol Br Commonw 70:408, 1963.
17. Hytten, FE and Taggart, N: Limb volumes in pregnancy. J Obstet Gynaecol Br Commonw 74:663, 1967.
18. Kerr, MG, Scott, DB and Samuel, E: Studies of the inferior vena cava in late pregnancy. Br Med J 1:532, 1964.
19. Kerr, MC: The mechanical effects of the gravid uterus in late pregnancy. J Obstet Gynaecol Br Commonw 72:513, 1965.
20. Robertson, EG: The natural history of oedema during pregnancy. J Obstet Gynaecol Br Commonw 78:720, 1971.
21. Howard, BK, Goodson, JH and Mengert, WF: Supine hypotension syndrome in late pregnancy. Obstet Gynecol 1:371, 1953.
22. Bieniarz, J, Crotlogini, JJ and Curacki, E: Aortacaval compression by the uterus in late human pregnancy. Am J Obstet Gynecol 100:203, 1968.
23. Marx, GF: Aortocaval compression: Incidence and prevention. Bull NY Acad Med 50:443, 1974.
24. Kauppila, A, et al: Decreased intervillous and unchanged myometrial blood flow in supine recumbency. Obstet Gynecol 55:203, 1980.
25. Assali, NS, Rauramo, L and Peltonen, T: Uterine and fetal blood flow and oxygen consumption in early pregnancy. Am J Obstet Gynecol 79:86, 1960.
26. Assali, NS, et al: Measurement of uterine blood flow and uterine metabolism. II: The techniques of catheterization and cannulation of the uterine veins and sampling of arterial and venous blood in pregnant women. Am J Obstet Gynecol 66:11, 1953.
27. Lewis, BV: Uterine blood flow. Obstet Gynecol Survey 24:1211, 1969.
28. Rekonen, A, et al: Measurement of intervillous and myometrial blood flow by an intravenous ^{133}Xe method. Br J Obstet Gynaecol 86:723, 1976.
29. Greiss, FC, Anderson, SG and Still, JG: Uterine pressure flow relationships during early gestation. Am J Obstet Gynecol 126:799, 1976.
30. Lander C, et al: Dynamics of uterine circulation in pregnant and nonpregnant sheep. Am J Physiol 218:257, 1970.
31. Greiss, FC: A clinical concept of uterine blood flow during pregnancy. Obstet Gynecol 30:595, 1967.
32. Anderson, SG, Still, JG and Greiss, FC: Differential reactivity of the gravid uterine vasculature: Effects of norepinephrine. Am J Obstet Gynecol 129:293, 1977.
33. Campbell, S, et al: Qualitative assessment of uteroplacental blood flow: Early screening test for high-risk pregnancies. Obstet Gynecol 68:649, 1986.
34. Dignam, WJ, Titus, P and Assali, NS: Renal function in human pregnancy. I: Changes in glomerular filtration rate and renal plasma flow. Proc Soc Exp Bio Med 97:512, 1958.
35. Chesley, LC and Sloan, DM: The effect of posture on renal function in late pregnancy. Am J Obstet Gynecol 89:754, 1964.
36. Ginsburg, J and Duncan, SLB: Peripheral blood flow in normal pregnancy. Cardiovasc Res 1:132, 1967.
37. Tindal, VR: The liver in pregnancy. Clinics Obstet Gynecol 2:441, 1975.
38. Munnel, EW and Taylor, HC: Liver blood flow in pregnancy—Hepatic vein catheterizations. J Clin Invest 26:952, 1947.
39. Lausko, L, et al: Hepatic blood flow in late pregnancy. Acta Obstet Gynecol Scand 50:175, 1971.
40. Bader, RA, et al: Haemodynamics at rest and during exercise in normal pregnancy as studied by cardiac catherization. J Clin Invest 34:1524, 1955.
41. Morgan, JA: Eisenmenger syndrome in pregnancy. Br Med J 1:1627, 1965.
42. DeSwiet, M: The cardiovascular system in clinical physiology in obstetrics. In Hytten, F and Chamberlain, G (eds): Gynecology and Obstetrics. Blackwell Scientific Publications, London, 1980.
43. Ueland, K, et al: Maternal cardiovascular dynamics IV. The influence of gestational age on the maternal cardiovascular response to posture and exercise. Am J Obstet Gynecol 104:856, 1969.
44. Vorys, N, Ullery, JC and Hanusek, GE: The cardiac output changes in various positions in pregnancy. Am J Obstet Gynecol 82:1312, 1961.
45. Lees, MM, Scott, DB and Kerr, MG: The circulatory effects of recumbent postural change in late pregnancy. Clin Sci 32:453, 1967.
46. Ueland, K and Hansen, JM: Maternal cardiovascular dynamics. II: Posture and uterine contractions. Am J Obstet Gynecol 103:1, 1969.
47. Hansen, JM and Ueland, K: The influence of caudal analgesia on cardiovascular dynamics during labour and delivery. Acta Anaesthesiol Scand [Suppl] 23:449, 1966.
48. Cutforth, R and MacDonald, CB: Heart sounds and murmurs in pregnancy. Am Heart J 71:741, 1966.
49. Landt, H and Benjamin, JG: Cardiodynamic and electrocardiographic changes in normal pregnancy. Am Heart J 12:592, 1936.
50. Oram, S and Hot, M: Innocent depression of the S-T segment and flattening of the T wave during pregnancy. J Obstet Gynaecol Br Commonw 68:765, 1961.
51. Burg, JR, et al: Alterations in systolic time intervals during pregnancy. Circulation 49:560, 1974.
52. Arbitol, MM, et al: Nonstress test and maternal position. Obstet Gynecol 68:310, 1986.
53. Marx, GR and Orkin, LR: Physiology of obstetrics anesthesia. Charles C Thomas, Springfield IL, 1967.
54. Mackenzie, AL: Laryngeal oedema complicating obstetric anesthesia. Anaesthesia 33:271, 1978.
55. Heller, PJ, Scheider, EP and Marx, GF: Pharyngolaryngeal edema as a presenting symptom in preeclampsia. Obstet Gynecol 62:523, 1983.
56. Tunstall, ME and Sheikh, A: Failed intubation protocol: oxygenation without aspiration. Clin Anaesth 4:171, 1986.
57. Sims, DC, Chamberlain, GVP and DeSwiet, M: Lung function tests in bronchial asthma during and after pregnancy. Br J Obstet Gynaecol 83:434, 1976.
58. Milne, JA, et al: Large airways function during normal pregnancy. Br J Obstet Gynaecol 84:448, 1977.

59. Cugell, DW, et al: Pulmonary function in pregnancy I. Serial observations in normal women. Am Rev Tuberc 67:568, 1953.
60. Eng, M, Butler, J, and Bonica, JJ: Respiratory function in pregnant obese women. Am J Obstet Gynecol 123:241, 1975.
61. Alaily, AB and Carrol, KB: Pulmonary ventilation in pregnancy. Br J Obstet Gynaecol 85:5128, 1978.
62. Weinberger, SE, et al: Pregnancy and the lung. Am Rev Resp Dis 121:559, 1980.
63. Bevan, DR, et al: Closing volumes and pregnancy. Br Med J 1:13, 1974.
64. Farebrother, MJB and McHardy, GIR: Closing volume and pregnancy. Br Med J 1:454, 1974.
65. Prowse, CM and Gaensler, EA: Respiratory and acid-base changes during pregnancy. Anesthesiology 26:381, 1965.
66. Lyons, HA and Antonio, R: The sensitivity of the respiratory centre in pregnancy and after administration of progesterone. Trans Assoc Am Physicians 72:173, 1959.
67. Kelman, GR and Templeton, A: Maternal blood gases during human pregnancy. J Physiol (London) 244:66P, 1975.
68. Templeton, A and Kelman, GR: Maternal blood gases ($PAO_2 - PaO_2$), physiological shunts and VD/VT in normal pregnancy. Br J Anaesth 48:1001, 1976.
69. Awe, RJ, et al: Arterial oxygenation and alveolar-arterial gradients in term pregnancy. Obstet Gynecol 53:182, 1979.
70. Artal, R, et al: Pulmonary response to exercise in pregnancy. Am J Obstet Gynecol 154:378, 1986.
71. Pernoll, ML, et al: Oxygen consumption at rest and during exercise in pregnancy. Respir Physiol 25:285, 1975.
72. Emerson, K, Saxena, BN and Poindexter, EL: Caloric cost of normal pregnancy. Obstet Gynecol 40:786, 1972.
73. Sangoul, F, Fox, GS and Houle, GL: Effect of regional anesthesia on maternal oxygen consumption during the first stage of labour. Am J Obstet Gynecol 121:1080, 1975.
74. Kambam, JR, et al: Effect of pregnancy on oxygen dissociation. Anesthesiology 59A:395, 1983.
75. Mendelson, DL: Aspiration of stomach contents into lungs during obstetric anesthesia. Am J Obstet Gynecol 52:191, 1946.
76. Wyner, J and Cohen, SE: Gastric volume in early pregnancy: Effect of metoclopramide. Anesthesiology 57:209, 1982.
77. Bainbridge, et al: Gastric-esophageal reflux in pregnancy: Altered function of the barrier to reflux symptomatic women during early pregnancy. Scand J Gastroenterol 19:85, 1984.
78. Davison, JS, Davison, MC and Hay, DM: Gastric emptying time in late pregnancy and labour. J Obstet Gynecol 77:37, 1970.
79. Grybhoski, WA and Sprior, MM: The effect of pregnancy on gastric secretion. N Engl J Med 255:1131, 1956.
80. Murray, FA, Erskine, JP and Fielding, J: Gastric secretion in pregnancy. J Obstet Gynaecol Br Empire 64:373, 1957.
81. Roberts, RB and Shirley, MB: Reducing the risk of acid aspiration during cesarean section. Anesth Analg 53:859, 1974.
82. Roberts, RB and Shirley, MB: The obstetrician's role in reducing the risk of aspiration pneumonitis with particular reference to the use of oral antacids. Am J Obstet Gynecol 124:611, 1976.
83. Parry, E, Shields, R and Turnbull, AC: Transit time in the small intestine in pregnancy. J Obstet Gynaecol Br Commonw 77:900, 1970.
84. Tomkinson, J, Turnbull, A and Robson, G: Report on Confidential Enquiries Into Maternal Deaths in England and Wales, 1976–79. Her Majesty's Stationery Office, London, 1982.
85. Hodgkinson, R, Glassenberg, R and Joyce, TH III: Comparison of cimetidine with antacid for safety and effectiveness in reducing gastric acidity before elective cesarean section. Anesthesiology 59:86, 1983.
86. Manchikanti, L, et al: Ranitidine and metoclopramide for prophylaxis of aspiration pneumonitis in elective surgery. Anesth Analg 63:903, 1984.
87. Brock-Utne, JG, et al: The effect of metoclopramide on the lower oesophageal sphincter in late pregnancy. Anaesth Intensive Care 6:26, 1978.
88. Seymour, CA and Chadwick, VS: Liver and gastrointestinal function in pregnancy. Postgrad Med J 55:343, 1979.
89. Tindall, VR: The liver in pregnancy. Clin Obstet Gynaecol 2:441, 1975.
90. Shnider, SM: Serum cholinesterase activity during pregnancy, labour and puerperium. Anesthesiology 26:335, 1965.
91. Blitt, CD, et al: Correlation of plasma cholinesterase activity and duration of action of succinyl choline during pregnancy. Anesth Analg 56:78, 1977.
92. Evans, RJ and Wroe, JM: Plasma cholinesterase changes during pregnancy. Anaesthesia 35:651, 1982.
93. Dunlop, W: Renal physiology in pregnancy. Postgrad Med J 56:642, 1979.
94. Davison, JM: Changes in renal function and other aspects of homeostasis in early pregnancy. J Obstet Gynaecol Br Commonw 81:1003, 1974.
95. Marcharte, DJ: Effects of pregnancy and progestational agents on the urinary tract. Am J Obstet Gynecol 112:487, 1972.
96. Mattingly, RF and Borkowf, HI: Clinical implications of ureteral reflux in pregnancy. Clin Obstet Gynecol 21:863, 1978.
97. Kewin, SF and Bhrecher, G: Differential neutrophil counts in pregnancy. New Engl J Med 266:877, 1962.
98. Gibson, A: On leukocyte changes during labour and the puerperium. J Obstet Gynecol 21:863, 1978.
99. Pitkin, RM and Witte, DL: Platelet and leukocyte counts in pregnancy. JAMA 242:2696, 1979.
100. Smith, JK, Caspray, EA and Field, EJ: Immune responses in pregnancy. JAMA 242:2696, 1979.
101. Sterrat, GM: The immunological system in clinical physiology in obstetrics. In Hytten, F and Chamber-

lain, G (eds): Gynecology and Obstetrics. Blackwell Scientific Publications, London, 1980, p 101.
102. Tygart, SG, et al: Longitudinal study of platelet indices during normal pregnancy. Am J Obstet Gynecol 154:883, 1986.
103. Howie, PW: Blood clotting and fibrinolysis in pregnancy. Postgrad Med J 55:362, 1979.
104. Hellgren, M and Blomback, M: Studies on blood coagulation and fibrinolysis in pregnancy, during delivery and in the puerperium. Gynecol Obstet Invest 12:141, 1981.
105. Spellacy, WN: Maternal and fetal metabolic inter-relationship in carbohydrate metabolism in pregnancy and the newborn. In Sutherland, HW and Flowers, JM (eds): Gynecology and Obstetrics. Churchill Livingstone, Edinburgh, 1975, p 42.
106. Forest, JC, et al: Reference values for the oral glucose tolerance test at each trimester of pregnancy. Am J Clin Pathol 80:828, 1983.
107. Datta, S and Kitzmiller, JL: Anesthetic and obstetric management of diabetic pregnant women. Clin Perinatol 9:153, 1982.
108. Osathanondh, R, Tulchinsky, D and Chopra, IJ: Total and free thyroxine and triiodothyronine in normal and complicated pregnancy. J Clin Endocrinol Metab 42:98, 1976.
109. Ramsay, ID: The thyroid gland in clinical physiology in obstetrics. In Hytten, F, and Chamberlain, G (eds): Gynecology and Obstetrics. Blackwell Scientific Publications, London, 1980, p 400.
110. Lewis, PJ: Drug metabolism in clinical physiology in obstetrics. In Hytten, F, and Chamberlain, G (eds): Gynecology and Obstetrics. Blackwell Scientific Publications, London, 1980, p 272.
111. McMorland, GH and Douglas, MJ: Systemic medication in labour and delivery. Clin Anaesth 4:81, 1986.
112. Fishburne, JI: Systemic analgesia during labour. Clin Perinatol 9:29, 1982.
113. Morgan, DJ, et al: Pharmacokinetics and plasma binding of thiopental: II. Studies at cesarean section. Anesthesiology 54:474, 1981.
114. Palahniuk, RJ, Shnider, SM and Eger, EI: Pregnancy decreases the requirements for inhaled anesthetic agents. Anesthesiology 41:82, 1974.
115. Merryman, W: Progesterone "anesthesia" in human subjects. J Clin Endocrinol Metab 14:1567, 1954.
116. Gintzler, AR: Endodorphin-mediated increases in pain threshold during pregnancy. Science 210:193, 1980.
117. Bromage, PL: Continuous lumbar epidural analgesia for obstetrics. Can Med Assoc J 85:1136, 1961.
118. Sivakumaran, C, et al: Uterine contractions and the spread of local anesthetics in the epidural space. Anesth Analg 61:217, 1982.
119. Datta, S, et al: Differential sensitivities of mammalian nerve fibres during pregnancy. Anesth Analg 62:1070, 1983.

CHAPTER 2

PERINATAL PHYSIOLOGY AND PHARMACOLOGY

HISAYO O. MORISHIMA, M.D., Ph.D.
SALHA S. DANIEL, Ph.D.

The Fetus

PHYSIOLOGY

Central Nervous System

Extensive investigations of the development of the central nervous system (CNS) in the human fetus (and in other species as well), with its billions of neurons and synaptic connections, have taken place during the last decade. In 1954, Flexner[1] first described a critical period of functional, histologic, and biochemical development in the mammalian CNS. Later studies[2,3] revealed that different components of the brain mature at different rates, which vary markedly among species. For example, rat neurons become functional near birth, whereas enzymes such as ATPase and succinic dehydrogenase do not mature until later. In guinea pig, sheep, rhesus monkey, and human fetuses, the development of cerebrocortical activity well before term appears to ensure a relatively mature brain at birth.[2,4,5] Cortical function in humans develops relatively early, but the appearance of spinal reflexes spans several months prenatally and postnatally.

Blood-Brain Barrier. Although some suggest that greater permeability of the blood-brain barrier exists during the perinatal period, in a wide variety of species including humans the barrier functionally resembles that of an adult.[4,5] For example, by 125 days' gestation (term 148 days) the fetal lamb's barrier functions in a manner resembling that of the adult sheep. The presence of kernicterus represents the only evidence for increased permeability between blood and brain in the human neonate,[6] although a recently reported[7] low protein level in the cerebrospinal fluid of the normal human newborn does suggest the early development of a barrier mechanism.

The relationship between administered anesthetics (or related drugs) in the blood and in the brain or cerebrospinal fluid remains poorly defined during the developmental stage. Noting that the introduction of ^{3}H-dihydromorphine into pregnant rats produces lower plasma concentrations of the drug in fetuses than in their

Acknowledgment: The authors thank Drs. M. Finster and H. Pedersen for their review of the manuscript and helpful criticism.

respective mothers, while the amounts of this drug in the fetal brain exceed maternal brain levels by a factor of three, investigators[8] concluded that the fetus lacks a blood-brain barrier. Others,[9] measuring meperidine brain levels in guinea pigs via electroencephalographic (EEG) response, offered the same explanation for their observations that maternal and fetal brains responded to the drug simultaneously, whereas fetal plasma levels remained substantially lower than those in the mother. In general, most anesthetics, having a high degree of lipid solubility, should readily cross the blood-brain barrier, in both the adult and the fetus.[10] Uptake in the brain depends on cerebral blood flow, plasma-protein binding, and the blood-brain partition coefficient, the latter depending on the chemical composition of the brain (which may change during development). Local anesthetics administered epidurally to the human adult appear in the cerebrospinal fluid within minutes, reaching a maximal level within 30 min, then declining at a rate similar to that in the plasma.[11-13] In general, lipid-soluble drugs easily enter CNS tissues, and return to the circulation nearly as rapidly, unless they are retained in the brain by processes such as "ion trapping."[14,15] Three excellent publications[10,14,16] review the current knowledge and concepts of the blood-brain barrier.

Cerebral Hypoxia. Many fetal and newborn mammals can withstand severe hypoxia better than adults.[17-19] The ability of the fetus and newborn to derive energy from an accelerated rate of glycolysis represents an early explanation for this phenomenon.[20,21] More recently, others[22] have emphasized the low energy requirement of the fetal and neonatal brain, which may account, in great part, for the capacity to withstand anoxia. This tolerance decreases with advancing maturity.[23] A striking adaptation to hypoxemia (and acidemia) involves a marked increase in the proportion of cardiac output distributed to the brain (and other vital organs) in both fetal monkeys and lambs.[24,25]

Cardiovascular System

Fetal Circulation. Nearly 350 years ago William Harvey described the difference between the circulation in the fetus and adult.[26] Well-oxygenated blood from the placenta flows into the fetus through the umbilical vein, to enter the inferior vena cava either via the ductus venosus or the hepatic microcirculation. The left atrium receives most of the inferior vena cava blood through the foramen ovale, and the left ventricle ejects this blood into the ascending aorta (Fig. 2–1). The relatively unsaturated blood in the superior vena cava, from the head, brain, and upper extremities, joins the remaining portion of inferior caval blood and enters the right atrium, then the right ventricle, to be pumped out into the pulmonary artery. A small volume of this venous blood traverses the pulmonary branches and returns to the left atrium via the pulmonary veins. Most of the right ventricular output is shunted through the ductus arteriosus into the thoracic aorta. Thus, the ductus arteriosus and the foramen ovale allow both sides of the fetal heart to work in parallel to pump blood from the great veins to the aorta.

Umbilical Blood Flow. Approximately 55 percent of the combined ventricular output flows to the placenta; 10 percent and 35 percent perfuse the lungs and other body tissues, respectively. Total umbilical blood flow increases with gestational age, but not in proportion to fetal weight. For example, in the fetal lamb, when calculated on the basis of perfusion rates per kilogram of body weight, umbilical blood flow decreases from 217 ml per min per kg at 87 to 95 days' gestation, to 170 ml per min per kg at 137 to 141 days.[27] During asphyxia, fetal arterial pressure and heart rate increase, and cardiac output decreases. The percentages of cardiac output distributed to the brain, heart, and adrenals increase significantly, while pulmonary, renal, and gastrointestinal blood flows decrease.[24,25] How long the fetus can tolerate the intrauterine asphyxia by making adjustments in its circulation has not been established. Our recent observations in the chronically instrumented sheep indicate that during a moderate degree of fetal asphyxia (PaO_2 15 mmHg), induced by partial umbilical cord occlusion, circulatory adaptation persists for as long as 4 to 5 hours.[28]

Autonomic Development. Various species resemble each other in the pattern of cardiac innervation; however, the development of sympathetic control of the fetal heart differs. For example, the term guinea pig fetus has a ma-

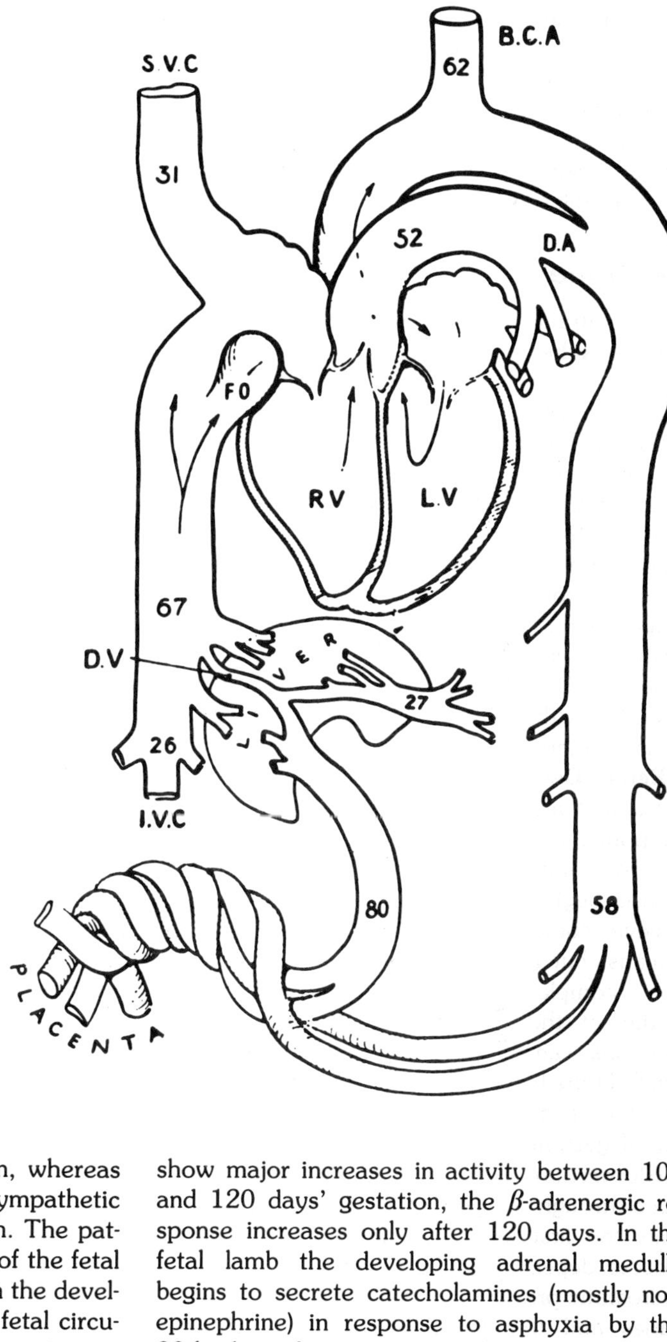

Figure 2 – 1. Diagram of the fetal circulation in the lamb. Numbers refer to percentage saturation of blood with oxygen. (From Born, GVR, et al: Cold Spring Harbor Symp Quant Biol 19:102, 1954, with permission.)

ture cardiac sympathetic innervation, whereas the rat and rabbit have no cardiac sympathetic nerves until about 1 week after birth. The pattern of parasympathetic innervation of the fetal heart is less well known. Research on the development of autonomic control of the fetal circulation has employed exogenous adrenergic agonists and specific autonomic adrenergic or cholinergic blocking agents. The presence of autonomic activity has been demonstrated in fetal lambs from 85 days' gestation.[29] Even at day 60, the fetal lamb exhibits a heart rate increase in response to isoproterenol. While parasympathetic and α-adrenergic systems show major increases in activity between 101 and 120 days' gestation, the β-adrenergic response increases only after 120 days. In the fetal lamb the developing adrenal medulla begins to secrete catecholamines (mostly norepinephrine) in response to asphyxia by the 80th day of gestation. In the same species, baroreceptors and aortic chemoreceptors begin to play a role in the control of fetal circulation at approximately 85 days' gestation.[30]

Pulmonary Vasculature. The fetal pulmonary blood flow is not constant, as the pulmonary vascular bed is sensitive to changes in arterial P_{O_2}, P_{CO_2}, and/or acidosis. Acute fetal asphyxia produces intense pulmonary vasoconstriction and a fall in blood flow. Injection of epinephrine or norepinephrine may also induce pulmonary vasoconstriction in experimental animal fetuses. In contrast, histamine, acetylcholine, and isoproterenol cause profound pulmonary vasodilation.

The Kidneys

During intrauterine life, the placenta, rather than the kidney, is the major regulatory organ of fetal internal environment. Nevertheless, the kidney serves to protect the fetus from acute disturbances in fetal or maternal fluid homeostasis and to maintain amniotic-fluid volume and composition.[31-33] The improved survival of immature infants has necessitated an understanding of the normal renal development in utero in order to provide a rational approach to their management. Most recent studies have been conducted in chronically instrumented fetal sheep, and the results compared, whenever possible, with those obtained from preterm human infants.

Renal Development. The metanephric or permanent mammalian kidney consists of two components, which develop in synchrony: the secretory and the collecting system.[34] Nephrogenesis begins early in the first trimester and achieves completion prior to term in sheep and humans, but continues postnatally in rats.[35,36] Once complete differentiation of the brush border of the proximal tubules occurs, the nephrons can begin filtration and reabsorption.[37] Urine formation in the human and in the sheep starts around the 9th week and the 55th day of gestation, respectively.

Glomerular Filtration Rate. Filtration of blood through the glomerular membranes represents the first stage in urine formation. This process depends on the balance between the hydrostatic pressure across the glomerular capillaries and the nonfilterable colloid osmotic pressure of capillary blood. Other factors influencing glomerular filtration rate (GFR) include the total capillary area, the permeability characteristics of the membrane, and the volume of blood circulating through the kidneys. A high intrinsic vascular resistance to flow primarily contributes to the low GFR in immature animals.[38] In addition, throughout most of gestation, systemic blood pressure in the fetus is only 40 to 50 percent of that in the adult. Sheep blood pressure increases slightly with gestation, and a positive correlation between GFR and arterial pressure does exist,[39-42] suggesting that the low arterial pressure partially accounts for the low GFR. The increase in GFR parallels change in fetal body or kidney weight up to 130 days in sheep and up to the 35th week of gestation in humans,[40,42,43] due to the appearance of new nephrons as well as the growth of existing ones. Several studies[44,45] provide evidence that demand influences the development of renal function.

Tubular Reabsorption. Reabsorption at various parts of the renal tubules of those glomerular filtrate components essential to the preservation of body fluids signifies the second stage of urine production. Despite a morphologic excess of glomerular to tubular elements in early life, reabsorption of at least 80 percent of the filtered load of water and electrolytes occurs as early as the second trimester. In general, the absolute amount reabsorbed proportionally follows the length and diameter of tubular structures. Reabsorption of the major components of glomerular filtrate, namely glucose, sodium (and chloride), and water, involves active transport. For each of these components, maturation of the transport mechanism depends on access of the transported substance to the carrier (protein), the number of active sites on the carrier, the energy available for transport, and concentration gradients.

Tubular Secretion. Maturation of various tubular secretory processes occurs at different rates. In general, active tubular secretion of organic acids or bases has not yet begun by the third trimester.[46] The small number of transport sites, due in great part to the underdevelopment of cortical nephrons, accounts for the low secretion rates of most substances.

Urine Composition During Gestation. As already stated, GFR and body size increase correspondingly in the fetal lamb. However, because of the different maturation rates of absorptive and secretory functions as gestation progresses, urine output per kilogram of body weight and osmolality remain essentially the same, while the concentrations of urea, potassium, phosphate, and ammonia increase and the concentrations of sodium, chloride, and bicarbonate decrease throughout gestation. Since absorption of bicarbonate and secretion of phosphate and ammonia contribute to urine acidification, urinary pH also changes with gestation, being greater than seven at the end of the second trimester and decreasing to 6.2 to 6.5 at 130 to 135 days' gestation.

Abrupt changes in fetal lamb urine composition occur a few days before delivery, including a fall in urine output to less than 0.1 per min per kg, a pH decrease to less than 6, and a rise in osmolality to over 300 mOsm per kg.[47] Changes in the hormonal level and/or sensitivity to hormones described during the last 3 to 4 days prior to the onset of labor may account for these transformations, since they occur regardless of gestational age at delivery.

Renal Homeostasis. Although the fetal kidney is not the primary organ of homeostasis and has limited function owing to the immaturity of several mechanisms, in sheep and in humans during the third trimester it processes 4 to 5 liters of glomerular filtrate and excretes 400 to 600 ml of urine per day. Recent studies with sheep demonstrated that the fetal pituitary, renin-angiotensin system, and kidney can respond to osmolar, volume, and pressure stimuli in a manner qualitatively similar to, though quantitatively smaller than, that in the adult.[32,33,48–53]

Release of vasopressin in response to osmolar or volume stimuli, as well as the kidney's response to vasopressin, increases as gestation proceeds.[33] The role of the renin-angiotensin-aldosterone system in regulating fetal sodium and fluid volume remains unclear.[32,42] Aldosterone crosses the placenta readily, but researchers[33,54] have reported no change in fetal aldosterone levels up to 120 days' gestation as a result of manipulation that increased production of maternal or fetal renin activity and angiotensin II.

The fetal lamb kidney also proves capable of responding to an acid load through increased excretion of phosphate, ammonia, and titratable acid; however, the fraction of acid excreted remains small, and the fall in urine pH measures only 0.4 pH units.[55,56]

Peripartum Renal Function. Little information exists concerning changes in fetal renal function during labor. Major changes occur in fetal sheep subjected to hypoxic or asphyxial episodes, including increased renal vascular resistance, decreased renal blood flow (and, to a lesser extent, GFR), a profound decrease in urine output, and a rise in urine osmolality and electrolyte concentrations.[57,58] These changes relate to the increased release of catecholamines, vasopressin, and the components of the renin-angiotensin system.

After delivery, the separation from the placenta results in a larger proportion of the neonatal cardiac output reaching the kidney. However, renal vascular resistance remains elevated, and renal blood flow and GFR remain relatively low. Tubular capacities, particularly reabsorption of electrolytes and water and acidification of urine, do not fully mature until several weeks after birth. Despite these limitations, the kidney in the healthy full-term neonate possesses homeostatic maintenance capabilities. In contrast the kidney of a premature or severely asphyxiated neonate has limited ability to control acid-base balance and plasma volume and composition.

Hepatic Function

During fetal life, large glycogen reserves accumulate in the liver, the concentration increasing as gestation advances to a maximum of 40 to 100 mg per g, or twice as much as in the adult. These serve as energy sources for the neonate until it adapts to the high-fat diet of milk. The fetus receives its glucose supply from the mother and carries out limited gluconeogenesis. Similarly, the placenta allows the fetus to eliminate many compounds, such as endogenously produced bilirubin and most maternally administered drugs without having to detoxify them through hepatic metabolic pathways. The hepatic microsomal enzymes, capable of metabolizing drugs and including cytochrome P-450, are absent in most animal fetuses but appear in the human fetal liver early during gestation. Workers[59–65] have documented oxidative metabolic reactions as early as 16 weeks, whereas other metabolic pathways such as reduction and conjugation remain poorly developed even in the human fetus. The greater threat of exposure to drugs and cigarette smoke for pregnant women (versus animals) raises concern for induction of hepatic enzyme systems in the fetus with resulting accumulation of toxic metabolites.[66]

Acid-Base Balance in Labor

Fetal Oxygenation. Early studies of fetal acid-base values obtained from human umbilical cord samples taken at delivery or from exteriorized fetuses led investigators[67] to conclude that the fetus exists in a hypoxic environment and derives at least part of its energy from anerobic metabolism. However, values from this study spanned a wide range, and some acid-base indices differed little between mothers and their respective fetuses. This suggested the presence of an unsteady acid-base state at birth, and led to the proposal that a number of factors, especially uterine contractions and compression of the umbilical cord, contributed to variable degrees of oxygen deprivation during the birth process.[68] Data obtained from chronically instrumented pregnant animals (mainly sheep) confirmed that the fetal acid-base environment was only slightly more acidotic than that of the mother. Although, in all species measured so far, fetal oxygenation falls below the adult standard, values of base deficit give no evidence of appreciable anerobic metabolism.

Fetal Scalp Samples. In the late 1960s Saling[69] introduced a new technique for sampling fetal capillary blood from the scalp during labor, which was later combined with recording of the fetal heart rate and uterine contractions to become a valuable tool for careful monitoring of the fetal condition. Sequential fetal pH determinations by scalp sampling showed that interruption of placental gas exchange during uterine contractions contributes to the gradual development of both respiratory and metabolic acidosis, as well as hypoxia during labor. Fetal pH and Po_2 decline most rapidly during the last stages of delivery.

Fetal pH and Neonatal Condition. The pH of capillary blood taken 30 min prior to delivery correlates significantly with an infant's clinical condition as evaluated by the 1-min Apgar score. In one study, 64 percent of all infants scoring seven or higher had fetal scalp pH values above 7.2 prior to delivery, while 18 percent scoring six or less had scalp pH values of less than 7.2.[70] However, 8 percent of the infants were not acidotic but depressed (false normals), while 10 percent of babies were acidotic but vigorous (false abnormals). Suggested reasons for the false normals included maternal medications, prematurity, or previous episodes of asphyxia from which the infant recovered with regard to acid-base state but not CNS responsiveness.[71,72] Maternal acidosis leading to harmless fetal acidosis accounted for most of the false abnormals.[72,73]

Maternal Ventilation and Acidosis. A negative oxygen gradient and positive hydrogen and carbon-dioxide gradients exist normally across the placenta from fetus to mother. Maternal hyperventilation almost immediately produces slight fetal hypocapnia, while excessive hyperventilation of the mother may lead to reduced uterine blood flow and fetal acidosis.[74,75] Maternal hypoventilation produces a rapid rise in fetal Pco_2 and a fall in Po_2. If the mother develops metabolic acidosis, the fetus eventually becomes acidotic, although this occurs more slowly than during maternal hypoventilation, since bicarbonate and fixed acids take longer to equilibrate across the placenta.

The acid-base state in the laboring mother usually does not change appreciably, the average change in pH from the first stage to the end of the second stage of labor being from 7.45 to 7.43.[70] However, the physical exertion of labor may produce some degree of metabolic acidosis, which can worsen if the mother becomes dehydrated or hypoglycemic.

Measurement of Fetal Po_2. Blood oxygenation, constituting the first of several acid-base indices that change during asphyxia, also represents one of the most important parameters influencing fetal heart rate (FHR). During the 1970s data obtained from a study[76] employing the continuous use of a transcutaneous Po_2 ($TcPo_2$) electrode generally showed good correlation between fetal scalp Po_2 and $TcPo_2$ values, the latter being approximately 2 mmHg lower than the former. Although uterine contractions have no consistent effect on $TcPo_2$ during early labor, they may cause a fall of 2 to 4 mmHg. Intermittent fetal scalp sampling,[76,77] has demonstrated that $TcPo_2$ falls gradually during normal labor and decreases most during the final stages, very low values occurring during the last 10 min before delivery. Basal FHR and fetal $TcPo_2$ did not correlate, except when FHR fell below 100 beats per min or exceeded 180 beats per min, when $TcPo_2$ was decreased.

$TcPo_2$ values may fall prior to the onset of fetal bradycardia, the start of the fall coinciding with an increase in FHR variability. Studies using the $TcPo_2$ electrodes have also confirmed a relationship between late FHR decelerations and fetal hypoxemia.

Administration of 100-percent oxygen to the mother during labor causes $TcPo_2$ in most cases to increase 10 to 82 percent, beginning after 1 to 6 min, and reaching a maximum by 10 min. The increase relates to the initial fetal $TcPo_2$, being least when fetal $TcPo_2$ is low. Nevertheless even in these cases, administration of high-oxygen mixtures to the mother can prevent severe fetal hypoxemia during strong contractions.[76,78] Between contractions, maternal hypoventilation often follows hyperventilation,[76] leading to a decline in fetal $TcPo_2$, indicating that intense hyperventilation during contractions may harm the fetus.

Measurement of Fetal Tissue pH. A modified subcutaneous pH electrode, developed in the late 1970s for use on the fetal scalp during labor,[79,80] showed good agreement between scalp and umbilical-artery pH measurements after introduction of improved methods of calibration and placement. Tissue pH (TpH) values generally average 0.04 pH units lower than capillary blood pH values and fall gradually as labor progresses, especially during the last 10 to 15 min prior to delivery.[81] TpH does not show the same variation with contractions as $TcPo_2$. When TpH does decrease during contractions, recovery proves much slower, indicating that a fall in TpH represents a more ominous sign.[82] Subcutaneous pH electrode use in the high-risk fetus yields TpH changes that correlate with FHR patterns in a manner consistent with current concepts of fetal distress.[83]

The difficulties of applying more than one skin electrode to the fetal scalp preclude simultaneous, continuous measurements of all components of acid-base balance in the fetus during labor. Results from a transcutaneous Pco_2 electrode, and combined transcutaneous Po_2/Pco_2 sensors, provide encouraging results in the area of fetal monitoring.[84–86] Further investigations will improve our assessment of fetal physiology and outcome in cases of intrauterine growth retardation, premature labor, and placental insufficiency.

PLACENTA

Function

Interposed between the maternal and fetal circulatory systems, the placenta performs many functions essential to fetal life, including respiration, excretion, and nutrition. Uterine blood supply originating from the uterine and ovarian arteries represents approximately 10 percent of the maternal cardiac output at term. The proportion of total uterine blood flow reaching the placenta exceeds 85 percent. Any reduction in placental perfusion may affect all the functions of this organ, particularly respiratory gas exchange.

Gas Transport. Oxygen and carbon dioxide exchange across the placental membranes occurs by simple diffusion, based on a concentration gradient without any expenditure of energy.

Fick's diffusion equation describes the factors governing placental gas transfer, for example oxygen.

$$Qo_2 = Ko_2 \cdot A \cdot \frac{Po_2(m) - Po_2(f)}{b}$$

where:

Qo_2 = quantity of O_2 transferred per unit time

Ko_2 = diffusion constant for O_2 in placental tissue

A = surface area of placenta

$Po_2(m)$ = mean O_2 tension of maternal blood in intervillous space

$Po_2(f)$ = mean O_2 tension of fetal blood in villous capillaries

b = mean distance separating maternal and fetal blood (i.e., thickness of placental tissue)

The factors influencing oxygen transport from mother to fetus include the blood flow on both sides of the placenta, Po_2 and oxygen affinity of maternal and fetal blood, hemoglobin concentration in both maternal and fetal blood, plasma diffusion capacity and vascular geometry, and oxygen consumption of the placental tissues. As the fetus grows the placental area enlarges to accommodate the increasing demand for oxygen and nutrients.

The hemoglobin concentration of human fetal

blood increases with gestational age, reaching 16.5 g per dl at term. The normal fetal arterial Po_2 ranges from 20 to 25 mmHg. The human fetus chronically deprived of oxygen responds by increasing its oxygen-carrying capacity, as exemplified by a hemoglobin concentration above 20 mg per ml for the growth-retarded fetus.[87] Increasing the hydrogen-ion concentration may influence oxygen exchange across the placenta by rightward shift of the fetal oxygen-dissociation curve (Bohr effect). The fetal oxygen-dissociation curve lies to the left of the maternal curve, resulting in a higher affinity of fetal red cells for oxygen at the prevailing low tensions. By shifting the oxyhemoglobin-dissociation curve fetal acidosis diminishes oxygen transfer to the fetus. Carbon dioxide has a higher lipid solubility and crosses the placenta more readily than oxygen, entering the maternal blood in one of three forms: dissolved carbon dioxide, bicarbonate ions, or carbaminohemoglobin. The transfer of oxygen from mother to fetus leads to dissociation of carbaminohemoglobin and facilitates carbon-dioxide elimination since reduced hemoglobin has a greater affinity for carbon dioxide than does oxyhemoglobin. Carbon-dioxide tension in fetal arterial blood approximates 40 mmHg, about 8 mmHg higher than that of maternal arterial blood.[88]

Transport of Other Substances. The passage of substances such as water involves a bulk flow mechanism dependent on hydrostatic or osmotic gradients. Specialized transport systems also exist, including active transport and facilitated diffusion. Active transport requires metabolic energy for the passage of substances (e.g., amino acids, water-soluble vitamins, and larger ions, such as calcium and iron) against their concentration gradients. During facilitated diffusion, the movement of molecules follows a concentration gradient, but the transfer rate exceeds that calculated according to physicochemical principles. The transfer of glucose and some other carbohydrates and certain endogenous substances occurs by this mechanism.

Although many investigators consider the placenta to resemble other lipid membranes in the body, it does not function simply as a semipermeable membrane.[89] Some endogenous substances are converted to more transportable compounds during their passage across the placenta. For example, glucose becomes phosphorylated and converted into fructose.[90] Riboflavin transfer involves the placental uptake of flavin adenine dinucleotide and conversion to free riboflavin before it enters the fetal circulation.[91] In the condition in vitro, a cigarette-smoking inducible enzyme system displays a capacity to deactivate benzpyrene. The placenta almost completely metabolizes catecholamines before their passage into the fetus. Research, however, has not yet documented the extent of placental metabolism in vivo of any analgesic or anesthetic agents commonly used in obstetrics.

Blood Flow

Adequacy of uteroplacental perfusion represents one of the most important determinants of fetal well-being. In the human at term, uterine blood flow approximates 700 ml per min. Maternal arterial blood flows into special arterioles in the basal plate, which enter into the intervillous space (Fig. 2−2). It then flows toward the chorionic plate, bathing the fetal villi in its passage and finally draining back by way of veins located in the basal plate. Maternal placental perfusion and umbilical blood flow both approximate 250 ml per min per kg.[92] The fetal umbilical arteries enter the placenta and ultimately divide into smaller vessels within the fetal villi, in which substances are exchanged between fetal and maternal blood.

Maternal placental blood flow is directly proportional to the net perfusion pressure across the intervillous space and inversely proportional to the intrinsic resistance of the spiral arterioles supplying the intervillous space and to the resistance imparted to the blood vessels by myometrial tension (Fig. 2−3). The net perfusion pressure amounts to the pressure within the spiral arterioles minus amniotic fluid pressure minus venous pressure. Thus, events such as maternal systemic hypotension, uterine hyperactivity, or vena caval occlusion reduce the net perfusion pressure. Increased intrinsic resistance may result from maternal anxiety and pain, as well as from injection of α-adrenergic agonists.

Under normal conditions, a sufficiently good circulatory reserve maintains fetal well-being during minor fluctuations in blood flow to the uterus and placenta. Indeed, such variations occur in nature according to a circadian rhythm,

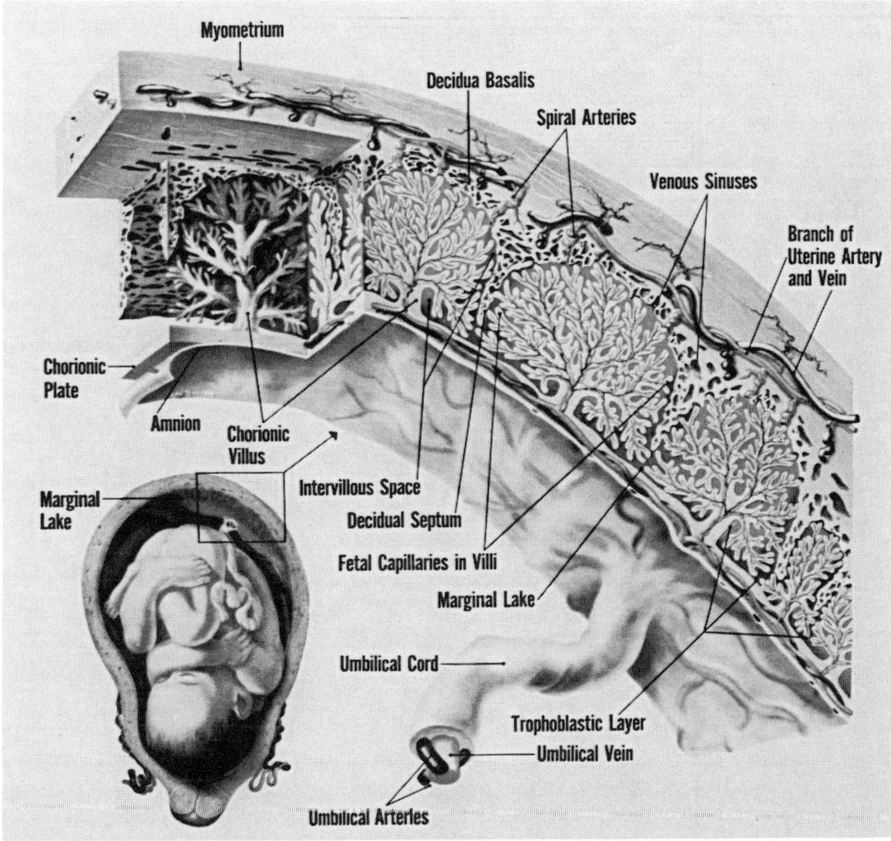

Figure 2–2. Placental circulation. (Reprinted with permission of Ross Laboratories, Columbus, OH 43216, from Clinical Education Aid, #2, 1960, © Ross Laboratories.)

and the normal fetus tolerates an estimated 50-percent reduction in uteroplacental blood flow. However, these reserves may be critically inadequate in disease states such as chronic hypertension, pre-eclampsia, diabetes mellitus, and renal disease.

Drug Transfer

As with oxygen and carbon dioxide, drugs administered to the mother cross the placenta by simple diffusion of unionized molecules. The transplacental gradient for these molecules depends on the following factors: the dose and kinetics of absorption, distribution, and metabolism in the mother; degree of maternal and fetal plasma-protein binding; degree of ionization of the drug; placental and umbilical blood flows, as well as the anatomic structure of the placenta; fetal metabolism and tissue uptake of the drug. The ability of a drug to cross the placental membranes correlates with its physicochemical properties, including its molecular weight and lipid solubility. Because most drugs used in obstetric anesthesia have high lipid solubility and low molecular weights (<500) the placenta presents no barrier to their diffusion. Muscle relaxants provide the only exception, since their relatively low lipid solubility and high degree of ionization allow transfer into the fetus only in low concentrations.

PHARMACOLOGY

Disposition of Drugs

Perforce, any drug carried across the placenta enters the fetal tissues, where its uptake depends on the tissue blood partition coefficient of

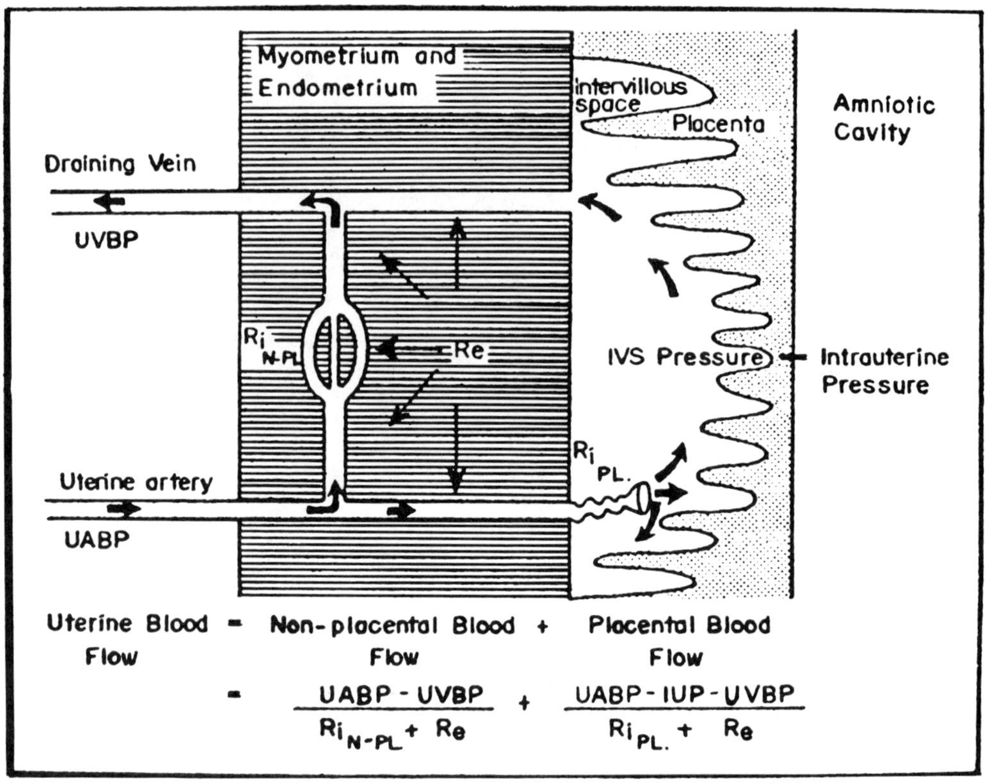

Figure 2–3. Factors determining placental and nonplacental uterine blood flow. (UABP = uterine arterial pressure; UVBP = uterine venous pressure; IUP = intrauterine (intra-amniotic) pressure; IVS = intervillous space; Ri_{PL} = intrinsic resistance of spiral arterioles; $Ri_{N\text{-}PL}$ = intrinsic resistance of nonplacental vasculature; Re = extrinsic vascular resistance imported by the myometrial tone.) (From Greiss, FC, Jr: MCV Q 8:60, 1972, with permission.)

the specific drug and the level of fetal tissue perfusion. For example, intravenous bolus injection of lidocaine into pregnant guinea pigs yields measurable concentrations of the drug in the fetal blood and tissues as early as 1 min after injection, reaching a maximum at 2 min.[93] Tissue assays revealed relatively high concentrations in fetal liver, myocardium, and brain, demonstrating the rapid distribution to highly perfused fetal organs. Only lidocaine levels in the fetal liver exceeded those in the mother. Investigations[94,95] have also shown substantial fetal hepatic accumulation of other anesthetic drugs, such as thiopental and halothane. The strategic location of the fetal liver relative to the umbilical circulation, combined with its high lipid content, explains the concentrations of anesthetic drugs found in this organ.

A reduction in drug concentration occurs during transit to the arterial side of the fetal circulation, as blood in the umbilical vein admixes with venous blood from the gastrointestinal tract, the lower extremities, the head, the upper extremities, and finally, from the lungs. This unique pattern of the fetal circulation produces a delay in drug equilibration between fetal tissues and blood, manifested by the persistent drug concentration gradient between the umbilical vein and the umbilical artery. This gradient emerges for a variety of anesthetics, including thiopental, lidocaine, and nitrous oxide.[96–98] The higher the tissue solubility of an anesthetic, the slower the equilibration within the fetus.

Lipid solubility greatly affects fetal tissue uptake of local anesthetics. In a study[99] comparing the characteristics of placental transfer of several local anesthetics in pregnant guinea pigs, the ratios of etidocaine and bupivacaine concentrations between the fetal and maternal blood fell substantially below those found for lidocaine, suggesting less placental transport of etidocaine and bupivacaine. However, the proportions of the injected doses recovered from fetuses over the first 60 min were remarkably similar for all three drugs studied. In contrast, the uptake of etidocaine or bupivacaine in the fetal myocardium, brain, and liver was substantially greater than the uptake of lidocaine. The relatively high tissue levels of these two long-acting agents in the fetus relate to the fact that bupivacaine is approximately 10 times, and etidocaine 50 times, more soluble in lipids than lidocaine. Greater protein binding of bupivacaine and etidocaine (which in guinea pigs is similar to that in humans) failed to limit their placental transfer. The greater tissue uptake of these drugs accounts for their relatively low fetal blood concentrations.

Experimental data gathered over the past few years indicate that the fetus may have the capability to metabolize and excrete certain drugs. For example, 2-chloroprocaine is rapidly hydrolyzed in plasma samples obtained from human umbilical vessels at birth, with a half-life of approximately 43 sec.[100] Although the human fetal liver at term contains microsomal enzymes capable of metabolizing amide-type local anesthetics, no direct evidence exists for human fetal metabolism of these drugs.

Effects of Drugs on the Fetus

Direct effects of drugs on the fetus frequently prove difficult to separate from the secondary effects of drug-induced placental or umbilical hypoperfusion. Postparacervical block bradycardia, originally attributed to depression of the fetal myocardium by local anesthetic transferred across the placenta,[101] was subsequently explained by the occurrence of fetal hypoxemia secondary to local anesthetic–induced uterine artery constriction.[102] Quantitative correlation between fetal drug effects and plasma concentrations became possible with the introduction of fetal scalp capillary blood sampling and microanalytic drug assays, as well as methods of continuous monitoring of the FHR and $TcPO_2$. Using this technology, investigators[103,104] found that following paracervical block (PCB), the maximal decrease in fetal $TcPO_2$ coincides with peak concentrations of local anesthetic in fetal plasma. An increase in FHR variability may occur after PCB or maternal administration of ephedrine,[103,105,106] while decreased variability may follow maternal medication with narcotics, tranquilizers (particularly diazepam), or local anesthetics.[107]

Intrauterine fetal breathing movements in animals and in humans occur in association with rapid-eye-movement (REM) sleep[108] and respond to alterations in fetal blood gases and glucose levels, and a variety of drugs. In fetal lambs, barbiturates and diazepam inhibit breathing activity, while administration of caffeine or doxapram has an opposite effect. Maternal cigarette smoking reduces the incidence of breathing activity in the human fetus.

The effect of maternal medication on animal and human fetal electrocortical activity reflects the rapidity with which anesthetic agents cross the placenta. Injection of thiopental into pregnant guinea pigs results in altered EEG patterns within 41 sec in the mother and 53 sec in the fetus.[109] These changes consist of an increase in voltage and wave frequencies, followed by slowing and voltage depression. Simultaneous maternal and fetal EEG recordings in pregnant guinea pigs also demonstrated the effects of meperidine.[110] Predictably, characteristic fetal EEG changes occurred more rapidly following maternal intravenous injection of meperidine, as compared with intramuscular and intraperitoneal injections. After infusion of lidocaine into the femoral vein of a fetal lamb near term EEG changes indicative of epileptiform activity appeared at a mean arterial drug concentration of 12 μg per ml.[111] Immature fetuses showed less susceptibility to this toxic effect of lidocaine.[112] In human fetuses monitored during labor, maternal PCB, induced with mepivacaine, produced a temporary reduction in the amplitude of the fetal EEG spectrum.[113]

Since fetal adaptation to asphyxia, as already stated, involves a relative increase in perfusion to the brain, heart, and placenta, much interest centers on whether anesthetic drugs have an adverse effect on this compensatory mechanism. Studies in sheep with chronically induced fetal asphyxia have produced conflicting data. The first report[114] suggested that maternal administration of 1-percent halothane results in marked reduction in fetal blood pressure and cerebral blood flow as well as aggravation of ongoing acidosis and oxygen desaturation. Subsequent studies[115,116] found that halothane does not affect fetal responses to asphyxia. In our own studies[28,117] lidocaine had no effect on the adaptation of the mature fetal lamb to asphyxia, but in the immature asphyxiated fetus, maternal infusion of the drug resulted in further deterioration in cardiac output and acid-base balance.

Neonate

PHYSIOLOGY

Adaptations at Birth

During this period and through the early hours and days of life, many morphologic and functional changes take place in the circulation, the lungs, the kidney, and the gastrointestinal tract. The cardiovascular and respiratory systems undergo the most dramatic alterations. In the normal newborn, two events occur almost simultaneously and within seconds of delivery: arrest of umbilical circulation through the placenta and expansion of the lungs. These events change the fetal circulation toward the adult type. Survival of the neonate depends primarily upon prompt expansion of the lungs and establishment of effective ventilation.

Cardiovascular Changes. The onset of respiration and expansion of the lungs opens up the pulmonary vascular bed, resulting in decreased resistance and a marked increase in pulmonary blood flow. A fetal pulmonary blood flow of 30 to 40 ml per min per kg of body weight increases to approximately 400 ml per min per kg shortly after birth, owing not only to the mechanical effects of lung expansion but also to the direct effects of oxygen and carbon dioxide on the blood vessels. Pulmonary vascular resistance decreases as oxygen tension rises and carbon-dioxide levels fall.

As soon as pulmonary perfusion increases, the foramen ovale, which constitutes a communication between the inferior vena cava (IVC) and the left atrium (LA), undergoes functional closure because of pressure changes across the valve of the foramen. Cessation of the umbilical circulation reduces pressure in the IVC and right atrium (RA), while the increase in pulmonary blood flow increases venous return and pressure in the LA. The ductus arteriosus (DA) does not constrict completely or abruptly after birth; functional closure may take hours, even days. Thus shunting still occurs in the neonatal period, its direction depending on relative resistances in the pulmonary and systemic vascular beds. The smooth muscle of the DA constricts in response to increased oxygen tension in the newborn's blood. Catecholamines, which exist in increased concentrations in the newborn, particularly during the first 3 hours of life also constrict the DA. In contrast, prostaglandins PGI_2 and PGE_2 produced by the wall of the DA relax the ductal smooth muscle. Administration of prostaglandin-synthesis inhibitors to fetal animals promotes constriction of the DA. Thus control of the DA involves a balance between constricting and relaxing substances.[118]

Cardiac output and its distribution also increase; left-ventricular output rises from approximately 150 to 400 ml per min per kg of body weight, whereas right ventricular output increases less significantly. Changes in cardiac output closely parallel the increase in oxygen consumption.[119,120] The redistribution of cardiac output also leads to increases in myocardial, renal, and gastrointestinal blood flow, while decreasing cerebral, adrenal, and carotid flows.

Pulmonary Changes. During fetal life, respiratory gas exchange takes place through the placenta. Delivery of the infant's trunk relieves thoracic compression, occurring within the birth canal, and the thorax and the lungs expand. The vast majority of infants initiate respiratory efforts a few seconds after birth. Following the first inspiration a cry usually results as the infant exhales against a partially closed glottis, thus increasing intrathoracic pressure significantly. Negative pressures in excess of 40 cm of water bring about the initial entry of air into fluid-filled alveoli. In the mature, normal neonate, the lungs expand almost completely after the first few breaths, and pressure volume changes achieved with each respiration resemble those of the adult. Following lung expansion, the functional residual capacity approximates 70 ml in the term newborn and changes little over the first 6 days of life. The tidal volume varies between 10 and 30 ml, the breathing frequency ranges from 30 to 60 times per min, and the minute ventilation exceeds 500 ml.

The factors responsible for the initial respiratory efforts to achieve expansion of the lungs and for the subsequent maintenance of rhythmic respiration, have been difficult to evaluate since many stimuli contribute simultaneously. The short time interval between birth and the onset of breathing suggests that impulses from peripheral receptors rather than the relatively slow changes in blood composition activate the respiratory centers. During delivery, the respiratory gas exchange across the placenta decreases drastically, resulting in varying degrees of acidemia and hypoxemia at birth. In the initial minutes of life, blood pH continues to fall while lactate concentration increases, but healthy infants re-establish normal acid-base balance at approximately 1 hour of life.

Thermal Regulation

During intrauterine life, heat exchange through the placenta regulates the fetal body temperature, which, under steady-state conditions, is approximately 0.5°C higher than that of the mother. Immediately after birth, the infant responds to cold stress by means of nonshivering thermogenesis, which entails increased metabolism of brown adipose tissue situated around the neck and between the scapulae. Although this mechanism plays an important role in body temperature regulation and heat production of neonates in several animal species, its importance in humans remains uncertain.[121,122] Despite the increased metabolism, the deep body temperature falls 2 to 3°C in the initial minutes after birth, primarily as a result of evaporation of amniotic fluid from the skin. In addition, the body mass of the neonate approaches 5 percent of the adult body mass, while the surface area approximates 15 percent that of the adult. This high ratio between body surface and mass, together with the greater curvature of body surfaces, facilitates thermal exchange by convection and radiation. Also, thin layers of skin and subcutaneous fat enhance thermal conductance. As a result, heat loss per unit of body weight in the newborn exceeds that in the adult approximately fourfold.[123]

Whether the fall in core temperature after birth favors or impedes adaptation to extrauterine life is unknown. Although thermal stimuli help initiate and establish breathing, prolonged cold stress causes progressive metabolic acidosis, while maintenance of body temperature immediately after birth exerts a beneficial effect on the rate of recovery from birth asphyxia.[124] Acute hypoxia and exposure to maternally administered drugs such as diazepam and meperidine impair the newborn's ability to maintain normal body temperature.

PHARMACOLOGY

Disposition of Drugs

With the cessation of umbilical circulation, neonates must dispose of drugs acquired transplacentally by their own mechanisms of distribution, metabolism, and excretion. The pharmacologic activity of a drug probably relates to the plasma concentrations of its free (unbound) form. Throughout gestation, fetal plasma concentrations of albumin and α_1-acid glycoprotein increase. At term, the fetal-maternal ratio for albumin is 1.2, while that for α_1-acid glycoprotein does not exceed 0.4.[125] These ratios affect the relative serum-protein binding of drugs between mother and baby. More extensive binding in the newborn serum occurs with diazepam, while most other drugs, including local anesthetics, d-tubocurarine, metocurine, propranolol, and meperidine, bind less extensively than in the mother.[126–129] Lower serum-protein binding, as well as the relatively high extracellular fluid volume, explains the large volume of distribution of local anesthetics and muscle relaxants in the neonate.[130,131] As already mentioned, many hepatic enzyme systems possess insufficient activity at birth. They develop rapidly during the neonatal period. For example, newborns achieve the adult capacity to oxidize phenytoin and pentobarbital within a few weeks.[132] Similarly, the ability to form sulfate and glucuronide metabolites of morphine increases dramatically within the first 2 months of life, as reflected by the clearance of morphine in 1- to 4-day-old infants, which approaches one half that in 17- to 65-day-old infants.[133] On the other hand, the hepatic clearance of fentanyl in infants exceeds that in children or adults, presumably because of the higher hepatic blood flow per kilogram of body weight in the neonatal period.[134,135]

In general, the neonate demonstrates poorly developed renal function, but urinary elimination of antibiotics approaches adult levels by 3 weeks. Neonates excrete a greater proportion of unmetabolized local anesthetic than adults. For example, the newborn kidney excretes approximately 20 percent of a dose of lidocaine unchanged, as compared with only 4 percent by the adult; for mepivacaine, the proportions are 43 percent and 3.5 percent, respectively.[136,137] Similarly, human neonates excrete more meperidine than normeperidine during the first 2 days of life.[138] By 3 days of age, the reverse occurs, indicating the neonate's capability for n-demethylation to normeperidine. The neonatal elimination of meperidine may continue for up to 6 days, and even longer for normeperidine.[139]

Data obtained from several human studies suggest a more prolonged elimination half-life ($t \frac{1}{2}\beta$) of commonly used amide-linked local anesthetics in the neonate than in the adult. For example, the $t \frac{1}{2}\beta$ for lidocaine is approximately 3 hours in the newborn, versus 1.75 hours in the adult; for etidocaine, approximately 6.5 hours in the newborn versus about 2.5 hours in the adult; and for mepivacaine, approximately 9 hours in the newborn and 2 to 3 hours in the adult. In our detailed pharmacokinetic study,[130] we injected lidocaine intravenously either into the newborn lamb or into nonpregnant adult sheep. The $t \frac{1}{2}\beta$ was approximately 60 percent longer in the newborn than in the adult (51 versus 31 min). Surprisingly, total body clearance and renal clearance were greater in the newborn than in the adult. Lower serum-protein binding of the drug and lower urinary pH accounted for the higher renal clearance of lidocaine in the newborn. Metabolic clearances, presumably hepatic, remained similar in the newborn and the adult (43 and 40 ml per min per kg) and nearly equal to hepatic blood flow. These data indicate that the newborn lamb metabolizes and excretes lidocaine as efficiently as the adult sheep. Thus, the longer elimination half-life of lidocaine in the newborn most likely results from a larger volume of distribution, so that, at any given time, the clearing organs have access to a smaller fraction of the drug. Other researchers,[136] administering lidocaine to premature human neonates by the subcutaneous route, have obtained similar results.

Effect of Drugs on the Neonate

Most drugs present in the maternal blood cross the placenta, possibly affecting the newborn. Maternal administration of hexamethonium produces paralytic ileus in the neonate; reserpine leads to neonatal nasal stuffiness, causing respiratory obstruction; and prilocaine, used for maternal regional anesthesia during labor, results in neonatal methemoglobinemia in a dose-related manner.[140–142]

Inhalation Agents. Maternal exposure to anesthetic concentrations of nitrous oxide or cyclopropane for more than 5 to 10 min leads to low 1-minute Apgar scores.[143,144] In contrast, the use of analgesic concentrations does not depress the newborn even after prolonged periods of maternal inhalation.

Barbiturates. Neonatal effects of transplacentally transmitted barbiturates depend on the dose and duration of exposure. Thus phenobarbital use throughout pregnancy in epileptic mothers produces sleepy and hypotonic newborns with poor sucking behavior.[145,146] Maternally administered induction doses of thiopental, not exceeding 4 to 5 mg per kg, have no discernible effect on the newborn's Apgar scores, regardless of the induction-to-delivery interval.[96] However, increasing the dose to 8 mg per kg produces neonatal depression, especially when the induction-to-delivery interval spans 3 to 7 min.[147]

Narcotics. Meperidine is the most commonly used narcotic in obstetrics. The possibility of neonatal depression depends on the dose, method of administration, and time interval between injection and delivery. For example, intramuscular injection of 50 mg causes newborn depression when delivery occurs 1 to 2 hours later.[148] Larger doses (75 to 100 mg) produce observable effects in neonates delivered even 3 hours later.

Tranquilizers. Chlorpromazine, if used during labor, may cause prolonged respiratory depression of the newborn.[149] Decreased neonatal muscle tone following premedication of the mother with promazine and promethazine prior to cesarean section may also occur.[150] Maternal administration of diazepam may produce neonatal hypothermia and hypotonia.[151,152] Midazolam, a new water-soluble benzodiazepine, appears to traverse the placenta less extensively than diazepam—probably due to rapid maternal elimination—and has less effect on the neonate.[153]

Muscle Relaxants. Although all muscle relaxants used in obstetric anesthesia reach the fetus, clinical doses given to the mother have no demonstrable effects on the newborn,[154] due to the already mentioned characteristics of relatively low lipid solubility and a high degree of ionization, which limit their transfer across the placenta. However, administration of succinylcholine to a mother with an abnormal variant of plasma pseudocholinesterase may yield significant fetal levels, with the development of prolonged apnea and muscle paralysis after birth.[155]

Local Anesthetics. Epidural administration of local anesthetics during labor may also produce neonatal depression, for example, when umbilical venous concentrations of mepivacaine or lidocaine exceed 2.5 to 3.0 μg per ml.[156,157] The suggestion that newborns appear to be more sensitive to the effects of local anesthetics than adults proves questionable, since infants inadvertently injected with mepivacaine during misguided placement of caudal needles stopped convulsing when the plasma drug concentration fell below 8 μg per ml, a level similar to the adult convulsive threshold.[158] In addition, our studies[159,160] of CNS and cardiac toxicity of local anesthetics infused into adult or newborn sheep show that significantly higher doses of local anesthetics are necessary to produce toxic symptoms in the lamb, while plasma drug concentrations associated with these symptoms are similar in both groups.

Hillman and coworkers[161] have demonstrated the ability of the newborn to recover from even a severe local anesthetic intoxication. They noted that, with proper treatment, infants inadvertently injected in utero with large doses of mepivacaine not only survive but apparently develop normally. Neurobehavioral[162,163] studies have identified subtle changes in newborn neurologic and adaptive functions following maternal anesthesia. In the case of most anesthetic agents, these changes prove minor and transient, lasting only 24 to 48 hours.

Summary

CLINICAL IMPLICATIONS

To meet the goal and the challenge of providing optimal pain relief for the mother with minimal effects in the newborn, clinicians must consider the physiology and pharmacologic characteristics of the fetus and newborn. To preserve uteroplacental blood flow, a factor of utmost importance, one should prevent or promptly treat maternal systemic hypotension and avoid the use of drugs that may stimulate uterine activity (large doses of ketamine, α-adrenergic agonists). Severe maternal apprehension or pain requires appropriate treatment.

Data from perinatal pharmacologic studies provide a wealth of information for the anesthesiologist. For example, when the mother receives a bolus of drug (e.g., thiopental) intravenously at the onset of uterine contraction, a reduced proportion will transfer to the fetus, as peak maternal plasma concentrations coincide with reduced placental perfusion.[164] Appropriate timing and reduction of the dose can minimize neonatal depression from maternally administered narcotics and sedatives. Nitrous oxide and volatile anesthetics should be administered in analgesic concentrations. However, uterine relaxation does call for higher concentrations of volatile anesthetics. Rapidly metabolized drugs such as chloroprocaine or long-acting agents such as bupivacaine, which require less frequent reinjection, can diminish fetal and neonatal accumulation of local anesthetic. In general, one should reduce the dose of narcotics and amide-linked local anesthetics in the face of fetal acidosis.

References

1. Flexner, LB: Enzymatic and functional patterns of developing mammalian brain. In Waelsch, H (ed): Biochemistry of the Developing Nervous System. Academic Press, New York, 1954, p 281.
2. Himwich, WA: Biochemical and neurophysical development of the brain in the neonatal period. In Pfeiffer, CC and Smythies, JR (eds): International Review of Neurobiology 4. Academic Press, New York, 1962, p 117.
3. Himwich, WA: Cerebral metabolism during growth of mammals. In Himwich, HE (ed): Brain Metabolism and Cerebral Disorders. Williams & Wilkins, Baltimore, 1976, p 65.
4. Reynolds, JM, Reynolds, ML and Saunders, NR: Development of blood-brain barrier mechanisms in the fetal sheep. In Comline, R, et al (eds): Fetal and Neonatal Physiology. Cambridge University Press, London, 1973, p 38.
5. Evans, CAN, et al: The development of a blood-brain barrier mechanism in foetal sheep. J Physiol 238:371, 1974.
6. Spatz, H: Die Bedeutung der vitalen Färbung für die

Lehre vom Stoffaustausch zwischen dem Zentralnervensystem und dem übrigen Körper. Arch Psychiatr Nervenkr 101:267, 1934.
7. Cole, VA, et al: Pathogenesis of intraventricular haemorrhage in newborn infants. Arch Dis Child 4: 722, 1974.
8. Sanner, JH and Woods, LA: Comparative distribution of tritium labelled dihydromorphine between maternal and fetal rats. J Pharmacol Exp Ther 148: 176, 1965.
9. Bleyer, WA and Rosen, MG: Meperidine-induced changes in the maternal and fetal electro-encephalograms of the guinea pig. Electroenceph Clin Neurophysiol 24:249, 1968.
10. Rapaport, SI: Blood-Brain Barrier in Physiology and Medicine. Raven Press, New York, 1976, p 153.
11. Lund, PC and Covino, BG: Distribution of local anesthetics in man following peridural anesthesia. J Clin Pharmacol 7:324, 1967.
12. Usubiaga, JE, LaTuppa, M and Moya, F: Passage of procaine hydrochloride and para-aminobenzoic acid across the human placenta. Am J Obstet Gynecol 100:918, 1968.
13. Wilkinson, GR and Lund, PD: Bupivacaine levels in plasma and cerebrospinal fluid following peridural administration. Anesthesiology 33:482, 1970.
14. Fenstermacher, JD, Blasberg, RG and Patlak, CS: Methods for quantifying the transport of drug across brain barrier systems. Pharmacol Ther 14:217, 1981.
15. Morishima, HO and Covino, BG: Toxicity and distribution of lidocaine in nonasphyxiated and asphyxiated baboon fetuses. Anesthesiology 54:182, 1981.
16. Brandbury, MWB, et al: Electrolytes and water in the brain and cerebrospinal fluid of foetal sheep and guinea pigs. J Physiol 227:591, 1972.
17. Kabat, H: The greater resistance of very young animals to arrest of the brain circulation. Am J Physiol 130:588, 1940.
18. Fazekas, JF, Alexander, FAD and Heinrich, HE: Tolerance of the newborn to anoxia. Am J Physiol 134:281, 1941.
19. Glass, HG, Snyder, FF and Webster, E: The rate of decline in resistance to anoxia of rabbits, dogs and guinea pigs from the onset of viability to adult life. Am J Physiol 140:609, 1944.
20. Himwich, HE, et al: Mechanism for the maintenance of life in the newborn during anoxia. Am J Physiol 124:287, 1942.
21. Himwich, HE: Brain Metabolism and Cerebral Disorders. Williams & Wilkins, Baltimore, 1951, p 127.
22. Mayman, C and Tijerina, MT: The effect of hypoglycemia on energy reserves in adult and newborn brain. In Briarley, JB and Meldrum, BS (eds): Brain Hypoxia. JB Lippincott, Philadelphia, 1971, p 242.
23. Myers, RE: Experimental models of perinatal brain damage: Relevance to human pathology. In Gluck, L (ed): Intrauterine Asphyxia and the Developing Fetal Brain. Year Book Medical Publishers, Chicago, 1977, p 27.
24. Behrman, RE, et al: Distribution of the circulation in the normal and asphyxiated fetal primate. Am J Obstet Gynecol 108:956, 1970.
25. Cohn, HE, et al: Cardiovascular responses to hypoxemia and acidemia in fetal lambs. Am J Obstet Gynecol 120:817, 1974.
26. Harvey, W: Exercitatio Anatomica de Motu Cordis et Sanguinis in Animalibus. Fitzeri, Francofurti, 1628.
27. Dawes, GS and Mott, JC: Changes in O_2 distribution and consumption of foetal lambs with variations in umbilical blood flow. J Physiol 170:524, 1964.
28. Morishima, HO, et al: Effects of lidocaine on the asphyxial responses in mature fetal lamb. Anesthesiology 66:502, 1987.
29. Vapaavouri, EK, et al: Developmental cardiovascular responses to autonomic blockade in intact neonatal and fetal lamb. Biol Neonate 22:177, 1973.
30. Dawes, GS, Mott, JC and Rennick, BR: Some effects of adrenaline, noradrenaline and acetylcholine on the foetal circulation in the lamb. J Physiol (Lond) 134:139, 1956.
31. Plentl, AA: The dynamics of the amniotic fluid. Ann NY Acad Sci 75:746, 1959.
32. Lumbers, ER and Stevens, AD: Changes in fetal renal function in response to infusions of a hyperosmotic solution of mannitol to the ewe. J Physiol 343:439, 1983.
33. Gomez, RA, et al: Developmental aspects of the renal response to hemorrhage during fetal life. Pediatr Res 18:40, 1984.
34. Grobstein, C: Inductive tissue interaction in development. Adv Cancer Res 4:187, 1956.
35. Vernier, RL and Birch-Andersen, A: Studies of the human fetal kidney. J Pediatr 60:754, 1962.
36. Arataki, M: On the postnatal growth of the kidney with special reference to the number and size of the glomeruli (albino rat). Am J Anat 36:399, 1926.
37. Gersh, I: The correlation of structure and function in the developing mesonephron and metanephron. Contrib J Embryology 26:53, 1937.
38. Gruskin, AB, Edelmann, CM and Yvan, S: Maturational changes in renal blood flow in piglets. Pediatr Res 4:7, 1970.
39. Robillard, JE, Weismann, DN and Herin, P: Ontogeny of single glomerular perfusion rate in fetal and newborn lambs. Pediatr Res 15:1248, 1981.
40. Robillard, JE, et al: Interrelationship between glomerular filtration rate and renal transport of sodium and chloride during fetal life. Am J Obstet Gynecol 128:727, 1977.
41. Yesberg, NE, et al: The effects of an angiotensin blocker (saralasin) on kidney function in dehydrated sheep. Q J Exp Physiol 67:97, 1982.
42. Stevens, AD and Lumbers, ER: The relationship between plasma renin activity and renal electrolyte excretion in the fetal sheep. J Dev Physiol 3:101, 1981.
43. Fawer, CL, Torrado, A and Guignard, JP: Maturation of renal function in full-term and premature neonates. Helv Paediatr Acta 34:11, 1979.
44. Edelmann, CM, Barnett, HL and Troupkou, V: Renal concentrating mechanisms in newborn infants. Effect of dietary protein and water content. Role of urea and responsiveness to antidiuretic hormone. J Clin Invest 39:1062, 1960.
45. Moore, ES, et al: Compensatory renal hypertrophy in

fetal lambs. Pediatr Res 13:1125, 1979.
46. Buddingh, F, et al: Long-term studies of the functional development of the fetal kidney in sheep. Am J Vet Res 32:1993, 1971.
47. Mellor, DJ and Slater, JS: Preparturient changes in the pH of urine from chronically catheterized foetal sheep. Res Vet Sci 13:89, 1972.
48. Weitzman, RE, et al: Arginine vasopressin response to an osmotic stimulus in fetal sheep. Pediatr Res 12:35, 1978.
49. Siegel, SR, et al: Effects of furosemide and acute salt loading on vasopressin and renin secretion in the fetal lamb. Pediatr Res 14:869, 1980.
50. Lingwood, B, et al: The effects of antidiuretic hormone on urine flow and composition in the chronically-cannulated ovine fetus. Q J Exp Physiol 63:315, 1978.
51. Daniel, SS, et al: Role of vasopressin in fetal homeostasis. Am J Physiol 242: F740, 1982.
52. Rurak, DW: Plasma vasopressin levels during hypoxaemia and the cardiovascular effects of exogenous vasopressin in foetal and adult sheep. J Physiol 277:341, 1978.
53. Iwamoto, HS and Rudolph, AM: Role of renin-angiotensin system in response to hemorrhage in fetal sheep. Am J Physiol 240:H848, 1981.
54. Siegel, SR, Oakes, G and Palmer, S: Transplacental transfer of aldosterone and its effects on renal function in the fetal lamb. Pediatr Res 15:163, 1981.
55. Daniel, SS, et al: Renal response to acid loading in the developing fetus, intact in utero. J Perinat Med 3:34, 1975.
56. Moore, ES, et al: Effect of Na_2SO_4 on urinary acidification in the fetal lamb. Am J Physiol 223:167, 1972.
57. Robillard, JE, et al: Developmental aspects of the renal response to hypoxemia in the lamb fetus. Cir Res 48:128, 1981.
58. Daniel, SS, et al: Renal response of the lamb fetus to partial occlusion of the umbilical cord. J Pediatr 87:788, 1975.
59. Yaffe, SJ, et al: The presence of a mono-oxygenase system in human fetal liver microsomes. Life Sci 9:1189, 1970.
60. Pelkonen, O, et al: Metabolism of chlorpromazine and p-nitrobenzoic acid in the liver, intestine and kidney of the human fetus. Acta Pharmacol Toxicol 29:284, 1971.
61. Pelkonen, O, et al: Drug metabolizing enzymes in human liver and placenta in early pregnancy. Scand J Clin Lab Invest [Suppl] 27:7, 1971.
62. Rane, A, et al: Drug metabolism in the human fetus. In Boreus, LO (ed): Fetal Pharmacology. Raven Press, New York, 1973, p 287.
63. Gurtoo, HL, et al: Population distribution of placental benzo(a)pyrene metabolism in smokers. Int J Cancer 31:29, 1983.
64. Pelkonen, O: Transplacental transfer of foreign compounds and their metabolism by the foetus. In Bridges JW and Chasseaud LF (eds): Progress in Drug Metabolism, vol 2. John Wiley & Sons, London, 1977, p 119.
65. Nau, H and Neuhert, D: Development of drug-metabolizing monooxygenase systems in various mammalian species including man: Its significance for transplacental toxicity. In Neubert, D, et al (eds): Role of Pharmacokinetics in Prenatal and Perinatal Toxicology. Georg Thieme, Stuttgart, 1978, p 1344.
66. Pelkonen, O: The differentiation of drug metabolism in relation to developmental toxicology. In Snell, K (ed): Developmental Toxicology. Croom Helm, London, 1982, p 167.
67. Eastman, NJ and McLane, CM: Foetal blood studies II. The lactic acid content of umbilical cord blood under various conditions. Bull Johns Hopkins Hosp 48:261, 1931.
68. James, LS: Acidosis at birth and its relation to asphyxia. Acta Paediatrica [Suppl 122] 49:17, 1960.
69. Saling, E: Die Blutgasverhältnisse und der Saure-Basen-Haushalt des Feten bei ungerstörtem Geburtsblauf. Z Geburtsh Gynaek 161:262, 1963.
70. Bowe, ET, et al: Reliability of fetal blood sampling. Am J Obstet Gynecol 107:279, 1970.
71. Adamsons, K, et al: The validity of capillary blood in the assessment of the acid-base state of the fetus. In Adamsons, K (ed): Diagnosis and Treatment of Fetal Disorders. Springer-Verlag, New York, 1968, p 175.
72. James, LS: Fetal blood sampling. Clin Perinatol 1: 141, 1974.
73. Daniel, SS, Adamsons, K, and James, LS: Lactate and pyruvate as an index of prenatal oxygen deprivation. Pediatrics 37:942, 1966.
74. Moya, F, et al: Influence of maternal hyperventilation on the newborn infant. Am J Obstet Gynecol 91:76, 1965.
75. Levinson, G, et al: Effects of maternal hyperventilation. Anesthesiology 40:340, 1974.
76. Huch, A, et al: Continuous transcutaneous monitoring of fetal oxygen tension during labor. Br J Obstet Gynaecol [Suppl] 84:4, 1977.
77. Lofgren, O: Continuous transcutaneous oxygen monitoring in fetal surveillance during labor. Am J Obstet Gynecol 141:729, 1981.
78. Willcourt, R and Queenan, JT: Fetal scalp blood sampling and transcutaneous Po_2. Clin Perinatol 8:87, 1981.
79. Stamm, O, et al: Development of a special electrode for continuous subcutaneous pH measurements in the infant scalp. Am J Obstet Gynecol 124:193, 1976.
80. Gilbert, S, et al: Continuous subcutaneous pH measurement in human fetuses: Correlations with scalp and umbilical blood pH. Am J Obstet Gynecol 128:901, 1977.
81. Lauersen, NH, Miller, FC and Paul, RH: Continuous intrapartum monitoring of fetal scalp pH. Am J Obstet Gynecol 133:44, 1979.
82. Young, BK, Katz, M and Klein, SA: Fetus, placenta, and newborn: The relationship of heart rate patterns and tissue pH in the human fetus. Am J Obstet Gynecol 134:685, 1979.
83. Young, BK, Katz, M and Wilson, SJ: Fetal blood and tissue pH with variable deceleration patterns. Obstet Gynecol 56:170, 1980.
84. Severinghaus, JW, Stafford, M and Bradley, AF: $TcPCO_2$ electrode design, calibration and tempera-

ture gradient problems. Acta Anesthesiol Scand 68:118, 1978.
85. Schmidt, S, et al: The influence of the progress of labor on the reliability of the transcutaneous PCO_2 of the fetus. J Perinat Med 13:195, 1985.
86. Schmidt, S, et al: Reliability of transcutaneous measurement of oxygen and carbon dioxide partial pressure with a combined PO_2-PCO_2 electrochemical sensor in the fetus during labor. J Perinat Med 13:127, 1985.
87. Battaglia, FC: Intra-uterine growth retardation. Am J Obstet Gynecol 106:1103, 1970.
88. Jacobson, L and Rooth, G: Interpretative aspects on the acid-base composition and its variation in fetal scalp blood and maternal blood during labour. J Obstet Gynaecol Br Commonw 78:971, 1971.
89. Waddell, WJ and Marlowe, GC: Biochemical regulation of the accessibility of teratogens to the developing embryo. In Juchau, MR (ed): The Biochemical Basis of Clinical Teratogenesis. Elsevier, New York, 1981, p 1.
90. Hagerman, DD and Villee, CA: Transport functions of the placenta. Physiol Rev 40:313, 1960.
91. Lust, JE, Hagerman, DD and Villee, CA: The transport of riboflavin by human placenta. J Clin Invest 33:38, 1954.
92. Stembera, ZK, Hodr, J and Janda, J: Umbilical blood flow in healthy newborn infants during the first minutes after birth. Am J Obstet Gynecol 91:568, 1965.
93. Finster, M, et al: Placental transfer of lidocaine (Xylocaine) and its uptake by fetal tissues. Anesthesiology 36:59, 1972.
94. Finster, M, et al: Tissue thiopental concentrations in the fetus and newborn. Anesthesiology 36:155, 1972.
95. Geddes, IC, et al: Distribution of halothane ^{82}Br in maternal and fetal guinea pig tissues. Brit J Anaesth 44:542, 1972.
96. Finster, M, et al: Placental thiopental concentrations in newborn following delivery under thiopental nitrous oxide anesthesia. Am J Obstet Gynecol 95:621, 1966.
97. Shnider, SM and Way, EL: The kinetics of transfer of lidocaine (Xylocaine) across the human placenta. Anesthesiology 29:944, 1968.
98. Marx, GF, Joshi, CW and Orkin, LR: Placental transmission of nitrous oxide. Anesthesiology 32:429, 1970.
99. Pedersen, H, Morishima, HO and Finster, M: Uptake and effects of local anesthetics in mother and fetus. In Stanton-Hicks, M d'A (ed): Regional Anesthesia: Advances and Selected Topics. Little, Brown & Co, Boston, 1978, p 73.
100. O'Brien, JE, et al: Metabolism and measurement of chloroprocaine, an ester-type local anesthetic. J Pharm Sci 68:75, 1979.
101. Gordon, HR: Fetal bradycardia after paracervical block: Correlation with fetal and maternal blood levels of local anesthetic (mepivacaine). N Engl J Med 279:910, 1968.
102. Freeman, RK and Schifrin, BS: Whither paracervical block? Advances in fetal monitoring and obstetric anesthesia. Int Anesthesiol Clin 11:2, 1973.
103. Petrie, RH, et al: Placental transfer of lidocaine following paracervical block. Am J Obstet Gynecol 120:791, 1974.
104. Miller, FC, et al: The effect of paracervical block on uterine activity and beat-to-beat variability of the fetal heart rate. Am J Obstet Gynecol 130:284, 1978.
105. Baxi, LV, Petrie, RH and James, LS: Human fetal oxygenation following paracervical block. Am J Obstet Gynecol 136:1109, 1979.
106. Wright, RG, et al: The effect of maternal administration of ephedrine on fetal heart rate and variability. Obstet Gynecol 57:734, 1981.
107. Finster, M and Petrie, RH: Monitoring of the fetus. Anesthesiology 45:198, 1976.
108. Wilds, PL: Observations of intrauterine fetal breathing movements: A review. Am J Obstet Gynecol 131:315, 1978.
109. Rosen, MG: Fetal electroencephalographic studies of the placental transfer of thiopental and ether. Obstet Gynecol 30:560, 1967.
110. Rosen, MG and Bleyer, WA: Bidirectional transfer of meperidine across the guinea pig placenta. Am J Obstet Gynecol 101:918, 1968.
111. Teramo, K, et al: Effects of lidocaine on heart rate, blood pressure, and electrocorticogram in fetal sheep. Am J Obstet Gynecol 118:935, 1974.
112. Teramo, K, et al: Gestational differences in lidocaine toxicity in the fetal lamb. Anesthesiology 44:125, 1976.
113. Peltzman, P, Goldstein, PJ and Battagin, R: Optical analysis of the fetal electroencephalogram. Am J Obstet Gynecol 116:957, 1973.
114. Palahniuk, RJ, et al: Maternal halothane anesthesia reduces cerebral blood flow in the acidotic sheep fetus. Anesth Analg 59:35, 1980.
115. Yarnell, R, et al: The effect of halothane anesthesia on the asphyxiated foetal lamb in utero. Can Anaesth Soc J 30:474, 1983.
116. Cheek, DBC, et al: The effect of halothane anesthesia on the asphyxiated fetal lamb. Anesthesiology 63:A356, 1985.
117. Morishima, HO, et al: Pharmacodynamics of lidocaine in the asphyxiated preterm fetal lamb. Anesthesiology 65:A372, 1986.
118. Heymann, MA, Iwamoto, HS and Rudolph, AM: Factors affecting changes in the neonatal systemic circulation. Ann Rev Physiol 43:371, 1981.
119. Klopfenstein, HS and Rudolph, AM: Postnatal changes in the circulation and responses to volume loading in sheep. Circ Res 42:839, 1978.
120. Lister, G, et al: Oxygen delivery in lambs: Cardiovascular and hematologic development. Am J Physiol 237:H668, 1979.
121. Hull, D and Segall, MM: The contribution of brown adipose tissue to heat production in the newborn rabbit. J Physiol 181:449, 1965.
122. Heim, T and Hull, D: The blood flow and oxygen consumption of brown adipose tissue in the newborn rabbit. J Physiol 186:42, 1966.
123. Adamsons, K, Gandy, GM and James, LS: The influence of thermal factors upon oxygen consumption of the newborn human infant. J Pediatr 66:495, 1965.
124. Gandy, GM, et al: Thermal environment and acid-base homeostasis in human infants during the first

few hours of life. J Clin Invest 43:751, 1964.
125. Krauer, B, et al (eds): Drugs and Pregnancy: Maternal Drug Handling—Fetal Drug Exposure. Academic Press, London, 1984, p 260.
126. Hamar, C and Levy, G: Serum protein binding of drugs and bilirubin in newborn infants and their mothers. Clin Pharmacol Ther 28:58, 1980.
127. Wood, M and Wood, AJJ: Changes in plasma drug binding and alpha$_1$-acid glycoprotein in mother and newborn infant. Clin Pharmacol Ther 29:522, 1981.
128. Thomas, J, et al: Plasma protein binding and placental transfer of bupivacaine. Clin Pharmacol Ther 191:426, 1976.
129. Nation, RL: Meperidine binding in maternal and fetal plasma. Clin Pharmacol Ther 29:472, 1981.
130. Morishima, HO, et al: Pharmacokinetics of lidocaine in fetal and neonatal lambs and adult sheep. Anesthesiology 50:431, 1979.
131. Fisher, DM, et al: Pharmacokinetics and pharmacodynamics of d-tubocurarine in infants, children and adults. Anesthesiology 57:203, 1982.
132. Neims, AH, et al: Developmental aspects of hepatic cytochrome P-450 monooxygenase system. Annual Review of Pharmacology and Toxicology 16:427, 1976.
133. Lynn, AM and Slattery, JT: Morphine pharmacokinetics in early infancy. Anesthesiology 66:136, 1987.
134. Singleton, MA, Rosen, JI and Fisher, DM: Pharmacokinetics of fentanyl for infants and adults. Anesthesiology 61:A440, 1984.
135. Johnson, KL, et al: Fentanyl pharmacokinetics in the pediatric population. Anesthesiology 61:A441, 1984.
136. Mihaly, GW, et al: The pharmacokinetics and metabolism of anilide local anesthetics in neonates. I: Lignocaine. Europ J Clin Pharmacol 13:143, 1978.
137. Moore, RG, et al: Pharmacokinetics and metabolism of the anilide local anesthetics in neonates. III: Mepivacaine. Europ J Clin Pharmacol 14:203, 1978.
138. Kuhnert, BR, et al: Meperidine disposition in mother, neonate, and non-pregnant females. Clin Pharmacol Ther 27:486, 1980.
139. Cooper, LV, Stephen, GW and Aggett, PJA: Elimination of pethidine and bupivacaine in the newborn. Arch Dis Child 52:638, 1977.
140. Hallum, JL and Hatchuel, WLF: Congenital paralytic ileus in a premature baby as a complication of hexamethonium bromide therapy for toxemia of pregnancy. Arch Dis Child 29:354, 1954.
141. Budnick, IS, Leikin, S and Haeck, LE: Effect in the newborn infant of reserpine administered antepartum. Am J Dis Child 90:286, 1955.
142. Lund, PC and Cwik, JC: Propitocaine (Citanest) and methemoglobinemia. Anesthesiology 26:569, 1965.
143. Moya, F: General anesthesia. In Shnider, SM (ed): Obstetrical Anesthesia: Current Concepts and Practice. Williams & Wilkins, Baltimore, 1969, p 88.
144. Finster, M and Poppers, PJ: Safety of thiopental used for induction of general anesthesia in elective cesarean section. Anesthesiology 29:190, 1968.
145. Rating, D, et al: Minor anomalies in the offspring of epileptic parents. In Janz, D, et al (eds): Epilepsy, Pregnancy and the Child. Raven Press, New York, 1981, p 283.
146. Rating, D, et al: Enzyme induction in neonates due to antiepileptic therapy during pregnancy. In Janz, D, et al (eds): Epilepsy, Pregnancy and the Child. Raven Press, New York, 1981, p 349.
147. Kosaka, Y, Takahashi, E and Mark, LC: Intravenous thiobarbiturate anesthesia for cesarean section. Anesthesiology 31:489, 1959.
148. Shnider, SM and Moya, F: Effects of meperidine on the newborn infant. Am J Obstet Gynecol 89:109, 1964.
149. Hodges, RJH and Bennett, JR: Some contributions to the use of chlorpromazine (with particular reference to obstetrical analgesia and anaesthesia). J Obstet Gynaecol Br Emp 66:91, 1959.
150. Crawford, JS: Anaesthesia for cesarean section: A proposal for evaluation with analysis of a technique. Br J Anaesth 34:179, 1962.
151. Scher, J, Hailey, DM and Beard, RW: The effects of diazepam on the fetus. J Obstet Gynaecol Br Commonw 79:635, 1972.
152. Kanto, JH: Use of benzodiazepines during pregnancy, labour, and lactation with particular reference to pharmacokinetic considerations. Drugs 23:354, 1982.
153. Kanto, JH, et al: Placental transfer and maternal midazolam kinetics. Clin Pharmacol Therap 33:786, 1983.
154. Abouleish, E: The placental transfer of drugs at term. Pa Med 78:56, 1975.
155. Baraka, A, et al: Response of the newborn to succinylcholine injection in homozyotic atypical mothers. Anesthesiology 43:115, 1975.
156. Morishima, HO, et al: Transmission of mepivacaine hydrochloride (Carbocaine) across the human placenta. Anesthesiology 27:147, 1966.
157. Shnider, SM and Way, EL: The kinetics of transfer of lidocaine (Xylocaine) across the human placenta. Anesthesiology 29:944, 1968.
158. Finster, M, et al: Accidental intoxication of the fetus with local anesthetic drug during caudal anesthesia. Am J Obstet Gynecol 92:922, 1965.
159. Morishima, HO, et al: Toxicity of lidocaine in adult, newborn and fetal sheep. Anesthesiology 55:57, 1981.
160. Morishima, HO, et al: Etidocaine toxicity in the adult, newborn and fetal sheep. Anesthesiology 58:342, 1983.
161. Hillman, LS, Hillman, RE and Dodson, WE: Diagnosis, treatment and follow-up of neonatal mepivacaine intoxication secondary to paracervical and pudendal blocks during labor. J Pediatr 95:472, 1979.
162. Hodgkinson, R, et al: Neonatal neurobehavioral tests following vaginal delivery under ketamine, thiopental and extradural anesthesia. Anesth Analg 56:548, 1977.
163. Kuhnert, BR, Linn, PL and Kuhnert, PM: Obstetric medication and neonatal behavior. Clin Perinatol 12:423, 1985.
164. Haram, K, et al: Transplacental passage of diazepam during labor: Influence of uterine contractions. Clin Pharmacol Ther 24:590, 1978.

CHAPTER 3

FETAL ASSESSMENT IN HIGH-RISK PREGNANCIES

DOUGLAS S. RICHARDS, M.D.
JOHN W. SEEDS, M.D.

Over the past half century maternal mortality in the United States has decreased dramatically from 600 maternal deaths per 100,000 live births in 1930 to 8.5 per 100,000 in 1981.[1] Given the relative rarity of maternal death, obstetricians have increasingly focused on identifying and treating disease in the other patient, the fetus. Numerous techniques for fetal assessment introduced since the late 1960s concentrated initially on identifying asphyxia during labor. Subsequently, the scope of prenatal diagnosis widened to include techniques for determining fetal compromise before labor, identifying fetal age and maturity, and detecting fetal structural and genetic abnormalities. Thanks in part to these fetal assessment techniques, the perinatal death rate (stillbirths and early neonatal deaths) has decreased notably, the current rate in the United States of 12.6 deaths per 1000 live births[2] representing approximately one fourth of the perinatal death rate observed in 1930.[1]

Fetal Heart Rate Monitoring

The first fetal monitoring techniques involved the detection and graphic display of the fetal heart rate (FHR). Marsac first heard fetal heart sounds in 1650, but the correlation between FHR abnormalities and fetal compromise did not become apparent until the current century.[3] The subsequent recognition of the importance of beat-by-beat variations in the FHR for indicating fetal condition prompted the development of electronic devices to detect and record instantaneous changes in the FHR.

BASELINE FHR

Beat-to-Beat Variability

The term "beat-to-beat variability" refers to the fluctuations of 3 to 8 beats per min that characterize a normal continuously recorded fetal heart rate. "Short-term variability" describes changes that take place from second to second, while "long-term variability" refers to fluctuations over longer periods of time (cycles of 10 to 20 sec duration). Classifications for beat-to-beat variability include normal, decreased, and absent (Fig. 3–1). Normal beat-to-beat variability

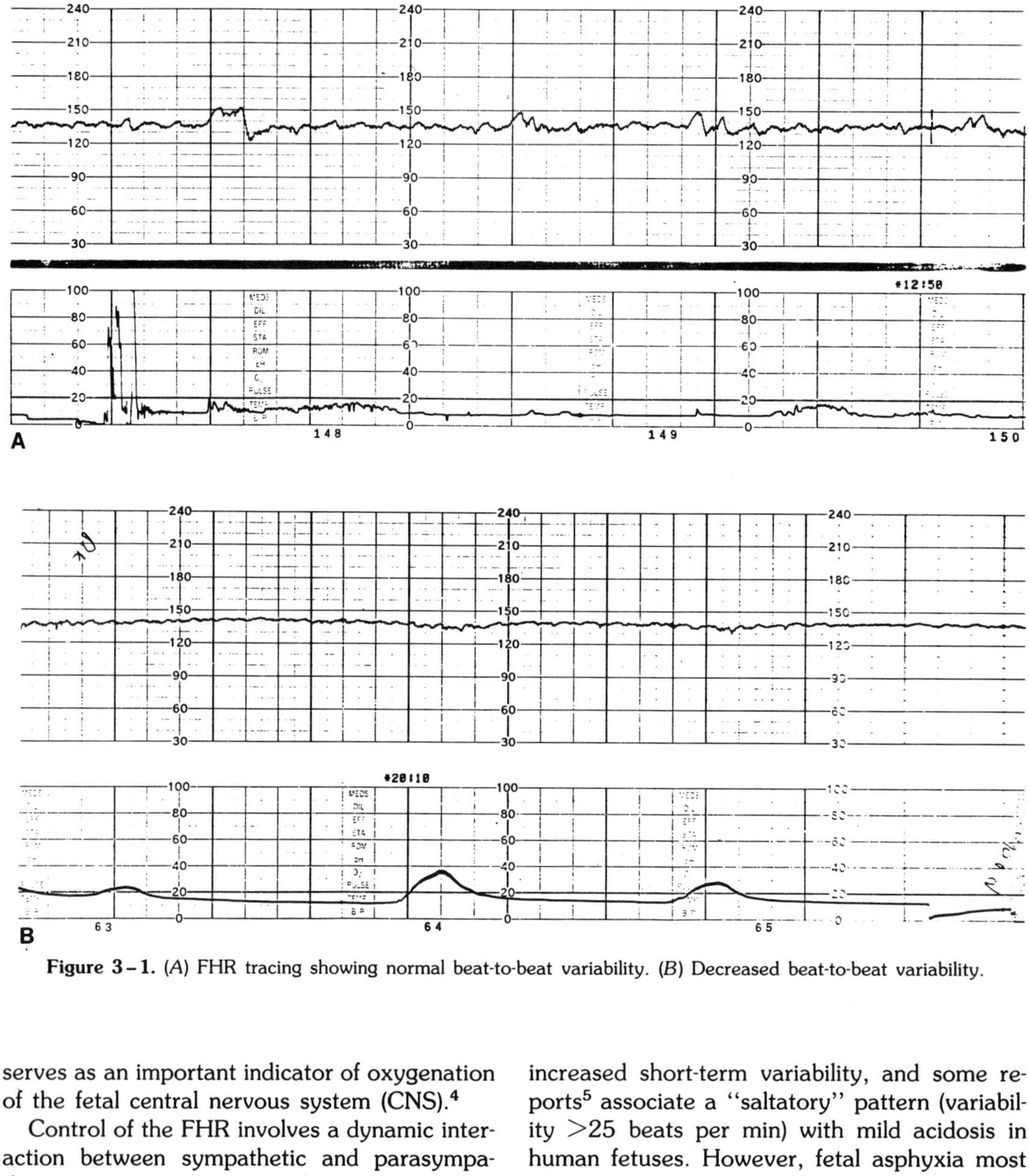

Figure 3–1. (*A*) FHR tracing showing normal beat-to-beat variability. (*B*) Decreased beat-to-beat variability.

serves as an important indicator of oxygenation of the fetal central nervous system (CNS).[4]

Control of the FHR involves a dynamic interaction between sympathetic and parasympathetic nervous system impulses originating in cardioaccelerator and cardiodepressor centers in the fetal brain stem. This dynamic interaction produces the beat-to-beat variability seen in a healthy fetus. Although the loss of beat-to-beat variability suggests fetal hypoxia, other factors, including fetal sleep states, CNS–depressant drugs, fetal tachycardia, and anomalies of the heart and CNS may also contribute to this condition.[5] Investigations[6] in sheep and monkeys show that acute fetal hypoxemia often produces increased short-term variability, and some reports[5] associate a "saltatory" pattern (variability >25 beats per min) with mild acidosis in human fetuses. However, fetal asphyxia most often produces decreased or absent beat-to-beat variability.

Sinus Tachycardia and Bradycardia

The baseline FHR normally ranges between 120 and 160 beats per min. Mild tachycardia occurs with a rate of 160 to 180, while rates in excess of 180 represent severe tachycardia. A baseline at 100 to 120 and rates below 100

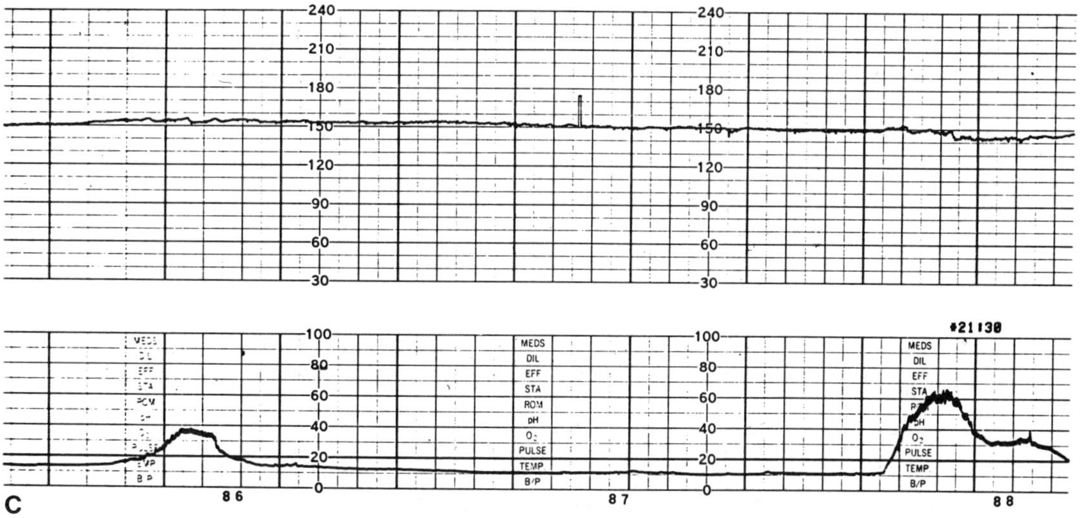

C

Figure 3–1. *Continued* (*C*) Variability is almost absent.

describe mild and strong bradycardia, respectively.[7] Deviations of the FHR from the normal range may correlate with significant pathology. For example, fetal tachycardia could signal early fetal hypoxia, especially when accompanied by decreased beat-to-beat variability. The ominous combination of fetal tachycardia, decreased beat-to-beat variability, and severe variable or late decelerations sometimes appears in preterminal fetuses.[8] Other causes of tachycardia include fetal infection, anemia, maternal fever, and maternal use of sympathomimetic drugs.[9] A sustained heart rate greater than 200 beats per min may result from a fetal supraventricular re-entry phenomenon.[9]

Vagal impulses from the cardiodepressor center in the fetal brain stem, resulting from hypoxia or cord compression, cause most episodes of fetal bradycardia. Hypoxic bradycardia usually develops by means of a reflex loop involving the carotid body, the cardiodepressor center, and the vagal nerves.[10] Bradycardia from direct myocardial depression results when hypoxia is severe. The mechanism of cord compression–induced fetal bradycardia is not completely understood, but probably involves fetal hypertension with stimulation of the carotid sinus, initiating a reflex bradycardia.[10] Several investigators[11] have demonstrated that head compression, usually in the setting of cephalic malposition, may elicit mild bradycardia (in the range of 110 to 120 beats per min). As long as normal beat-to-beat variability exists without ominous periodic decelerations, mild bradycardia is not associated with fetal morbidity.

Sinusoidal Pattern

The sinusoidal pattern, a special type of sustained FHR abnormality, occurs when three to five oscillations with a sine-wave configuration and an amplitude of 5 to 15 beats per min persists for more than 20 min (Fig. 3–2). The pattern, originally described in severely anemic fetuses, has also been observed in hypoxic fetuses and in fetuses whose mothers have received alphaprodine during labor.[12] Except in the final case, fetal jeopardy remains a possibility, indicating prompt evaluation.

Fetal Cardiac Arrhythmias

Complete fetal heart block may produce fixed bradycardia with a rate of 60 to 80 beats per min. Even then, cardiac output is usually sufficient for adequate tissue perfusion, and the persistent bradycardia does not imply hypoxemia. In most cases, complete heart block is associated with maternal circulating levels of anti–Ro (SS–A) antibody, an IgG antibody that crosses the placenta and may permanently dam-

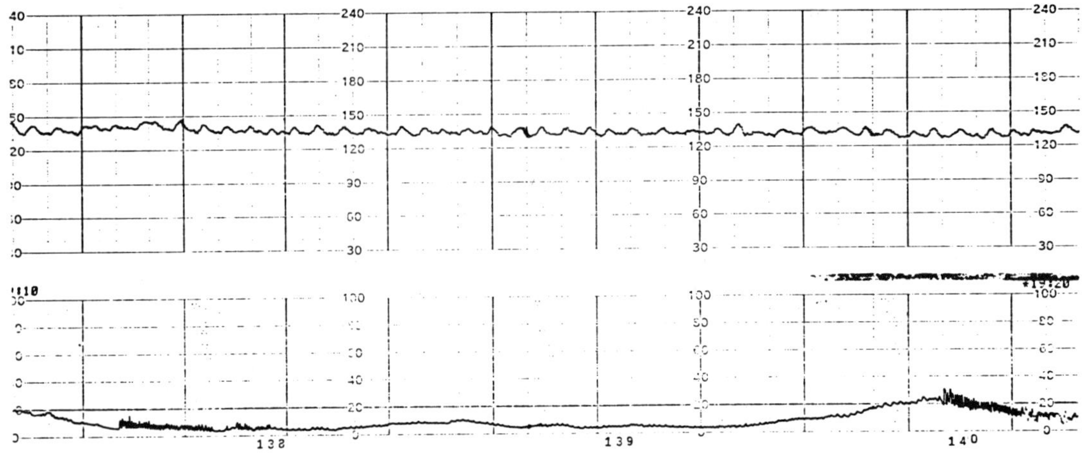

Figure 3–2. Sinusoidal fetal heart rate pattern. Note the sine wave–shaped undulations of the heart rate, with four cycles per minute. This tracing reflects the administration of alphaprodine to the mother.

age the fetal cardiac conduction system through deposition of antigen-antibody complexes.[13] Incomplete heart block can occur as well.

Supraventricular premature beats are common and usually resolve shortly after birth.[9] Although routine auscultation often uncovers these beats, they may come to attention when a characteristic spiking artifact appears on the electronic fetal monitor (Fig. 3–3). This happens when the microprocessor in the monitor measures an unexpectedly short R-R interval between successive beats. Although generally considered benign, premature beats occasionally evolve into potentially serious tachyarrhythmias, necessitating close fetal observation. Supraventricular tachycardias tend to revert to normal after birth[14] but can produce fetal heart failure if a rate greater than 200 beats per min persists over a prolonged period of time in utero.[15] Several reports[16,17] describe resolution of heart failure following successful pharmacologic cardioversion in utero of a tachyarrhythmia. Fetal tachyarrhythmias may complicate electronic fetal monitoring, since the monitor may interpret two or more heartbeats as various components of the same heart beat, thus recording values one half or one third of the true value. Such cases call for direct auscultation with a stethoscope to determine the true FHR.

Attempts at electrocardiographic (ECG) diagnosis of fetal arrhythmias by placement of elec-

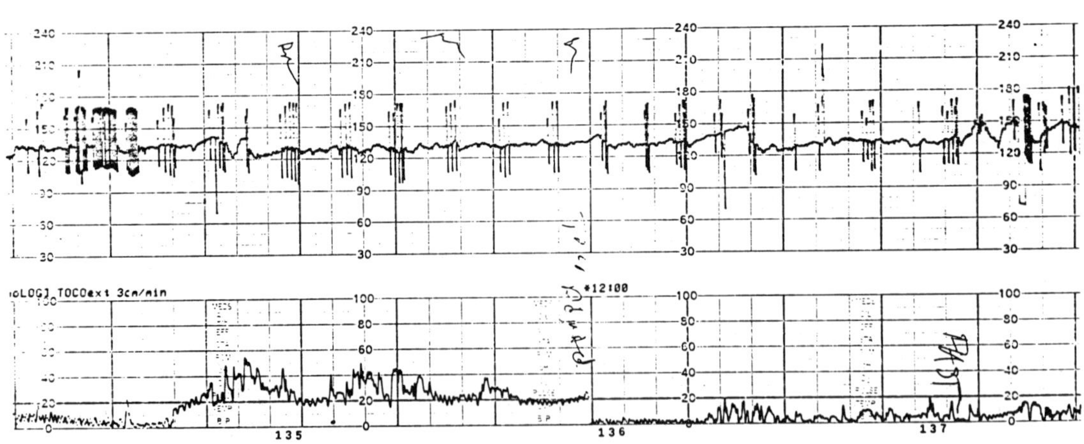

Figure 3–3. Monitor tracing showing the typical spiking artifact seen with a fetal arrhythmia.

trodes on the maternal abdominal wall have had limited success. Interference from maternal cardiac signals prevents precise isolation of fetal patterns. M-mode fetal ECG offers the opportunity to characterize arrythmias by visual discrimination of atrial and ventricular mechanical activity.[18] Additionally, it detects the presence of cardiac complications, such as heart failure, resulting from arrhythmias.

PERIODIC CHANGES IN THE FHR

Decelerations

Transient decelerations in the FHR fall into three categories depending on their shape and timing with respect to contractions. Some decelerations are benign, while others may indicate fetal compromise.

Early Decelerations. These mirror the shape of a contraction, starting with the onset of the contraction, reaching a nadir as the contraction peaks, and returning to baseline as the contraction ends (Fig. 3–4). Vagel stimulation from pressure on the fetal head accounts for early decelerations, which are not associated with fetal hypoxia.[19]

Late Decelerations. Late decelerations have the same configuration as early decelerations in that the heart rate gradually decreases and then increases, but the sequence is delayed with respect to the contraction (Fig. 3–5). The onset of the deceleration follows the onset of the contraction, the nadir occurs after the contraction peaks, and the tracing returns to baseline after the contraction has ended. In studies of mildly hypoxic sheep and monkey fetuses,[20,21] induced uterine contractions produced further decreases in the fetal Po_2, and triggered late decelerations of the FHR. In animals and in humans, late decelerations come about during the following chain of events:

1. Uterine contractions temporarily decrease intervillous space perfusion.
2. In the presence of marginal oxygenation between contractions, the temporary decrease in intervillous flow during contractions causes fetal Po_2 to fall below a critical level.
3. The carotid body senses the decreased Po_2 and activates the vagus system, with a resulting decrease in heart rate.
4. After the contraction ends and intervillous flow increases, fetal Po_2 gradually rises, and the heart rate gradually returns to baseline.

Causes of uteroplacental insufficiency with resulting late decelerations include static vascular abnormalities present in such diseases as hypertension or diabetes, or reversible conditions such as uterine hyperstimulation or maternal hypotension. In any event, late decelerations should always generate concern and require prompt evaluation and treatment.

Variable Decelerations. These are so named because of their variable timing relative to contractions, although they most commonly begin at the onset of contractions. Characteristically they begin with an abrupt drop off, and then return to the heart rate baseline equally abruptly. An associated "shoulder" often

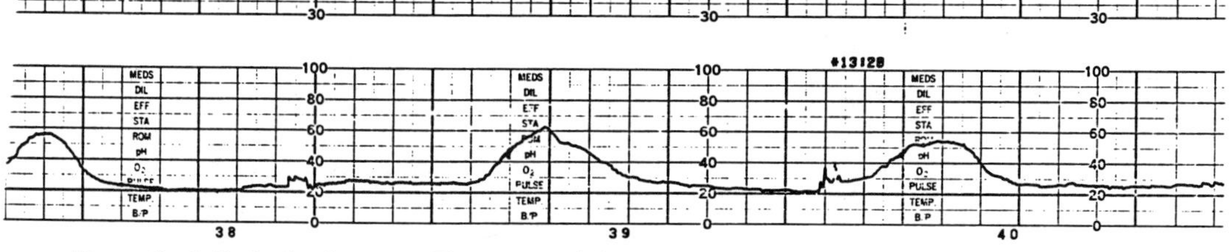

Figure 3–4. Early decelerations. The timing of the deceleration mirrors the timing of the contractions.

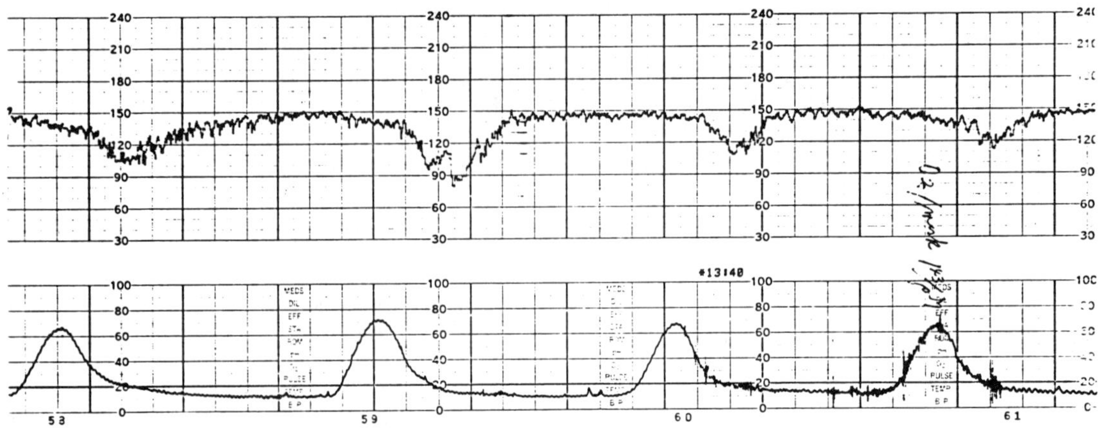

Figure 3–5. Late decelerations. Note the late onset and late return to baseline of the heart rate decelerations relative to the timing of the contractions. The preservation of beat-to-beat variability is a favorable sign.

occurs before and after the deceleration (Fig. 3–6). Variable decelerations result from cord compression by a mechanism not completely understood. Present theory[10] suggests that heart rate changes relate to alterations in fetal blood pressure, peripheral vascular resistance, and oxygenation of arterial blood, resulting in chemoreceptor and baroreceptor stimulation and reflex bradycardia. Classification of variable decelerations includes mild, moderate, and severe, depending on both degree and duration of heart rate decelerations (Table 3–1). Mild variable decelerations usually prove inconsequential; however, moderate variables may signal mild hypoxemia, while severe variables sometimes indicate frank fetal acidosis.[22]

Accelerations

The positive correlation between FHR accelerations and fetal health dates back to the early days of continuous electronic monitoring. Significant accelerations entail an increase in heart rate of at least 15 to 25 beats per min lasting 10 to 30 sec, commonly occurring during fetal movements. With the finding of a normal baseline heart rate, good beat-to-beat variability, and heart rate accelerations, the obstetrician can

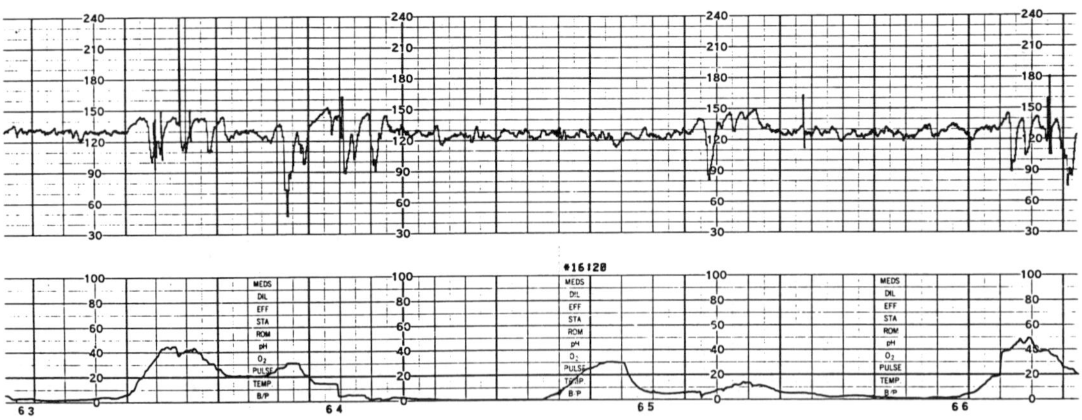

Figure 3–6. Variable decelerations. These FHR decelerations have a sharp drop-off and return to baseline. Note the brief accelerations or "shoulders" before and after the variable decelerations.

Table 3–1. DESCRIPTION OF VARIABLE DECELERATIONS

Mild	Duration <30 sec or deceleration of not less than 80 beats/min regardless of the duration
Moderate	<70 beats/min and lasting 30–60 sec OR 70–80 beats/min lasting >30 sec
Severe	<70 beats/min and lasting >60 sec

assume that the fetus is well oxygenated.[23] This association forms the basis for the antepartum nonstress test described later in this chapter.

Intrapartum Monitoring

INSTRUMENTATION

Electronic fetal monitors provide a record of the FHR and uterine contractions. Measurements are made with either external monitors strapped to the mother's abdomen or intrauterine systems (Fig. 3–7).

Heart Rate Monitors

External FHR Monitors. External FHR monitors employ either a phonocardiograph or Doppler ultrasound signal. Because of interference from other intra-abdominal sounds, the phonocardiograph is employed less frequently than Doppler devices, which detect the movement of the fetal cardiac chambers. With either device, a microprocessor measures the interval between heartbeats, and the heart rate is calculated and recorded from second to second. Older external FHR monitors accurately displayed the baseline heart rate and decelerations, but measurements of beat-to-beat variability proved inadequate. In contrast, current external monitors provide a more reliable representation of beat-to-beat variability; however, a direct fetal ECG signal remains superior in questionable cases. Change in maternal position often causes the fetus to change position with respect to the Doppler transducer; this is one of the major problems with external heart rate monitors. This requires frequent readjustment of the monitor and limits the mobility of the laboring patient. Obesity also makes it difficult to obtain a continuous representation of the FHR with an external monitor.

Internal Heart Rate Monitors. Internal heart rate monitoring utilizes a fetal scalp electrode (a fine spiral wire attached to the fetal scalp transvaginally) and a grounding plate attached to the mother's leg. This directly produces the fetal ECG. As with the external monitor, a microprocessor calculates the interval between successive R waves, giving an accurate representation of baseline FHR, accelerations and decelerations, and beat-to-beat variability. In comparison to the external monitor, the internal system produces a more accurate record of the FHR without gaps from fetal movement away from the transducer or confusing artifacts. In spite of these advantages external monitors remain quite useful because they provide fetal assessment when membranes are intact or the cervix has not dilated.

Contraction Monitor

The contraction monitor (tocodynamometer) also consists of either an external or internal system. The external device has a small plate that fastens to the mother's abdomen by a belt. Uterine contractions depress a central button fixed to the plate, generating a signal that is conveyed to the monitor. This device usually gives a satisfactory picture of the time, duration, and relative strength of contractions. As with the external fetal heart rate monitor, the external tocodynamometer requires frequent adjustments. In some patients, especially obese women, a satisfactory recording of the contraction pattern may be impossible.

When conditions call for an accurate measurement of the strength and frequency of contractions, an intrauterine pressure monitor proves superior to the external tocodynamometer. The internal system consists of a length of polyethylene tubing 2 mm in diameter, which is threaded through the cervix beside the fetal head into the uterine cavity. The catheter is filled with water and attached to a pressure transducer for direct measurements of baseline uterine tone as well as chronology and strength of contractions. This clear record of contractions proves particularly valuable during induced or augmented labor, and in labor with periodic decelerations wherein an external tocodynamometer would not accurately delineate

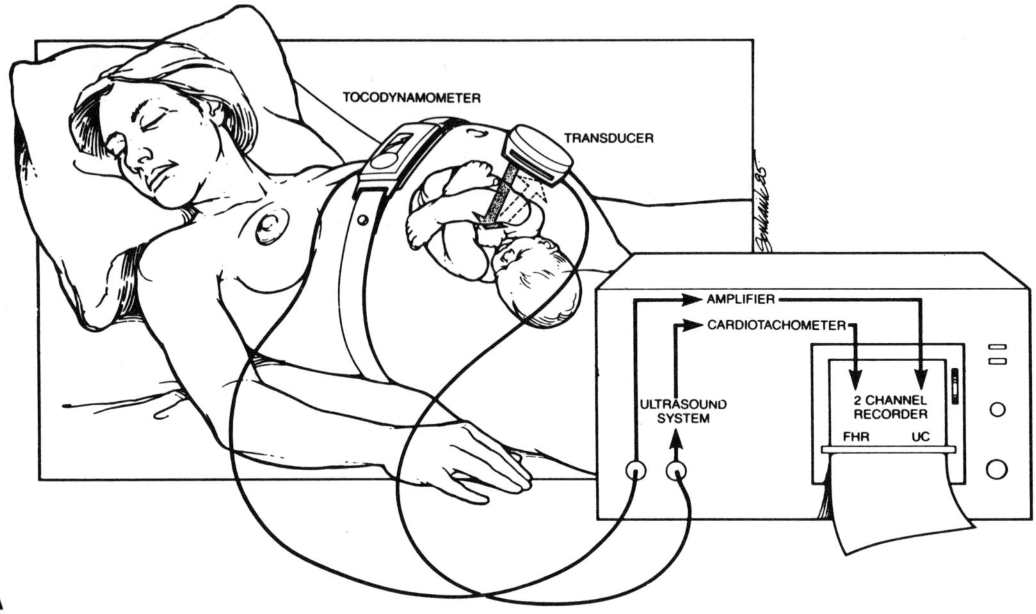

A

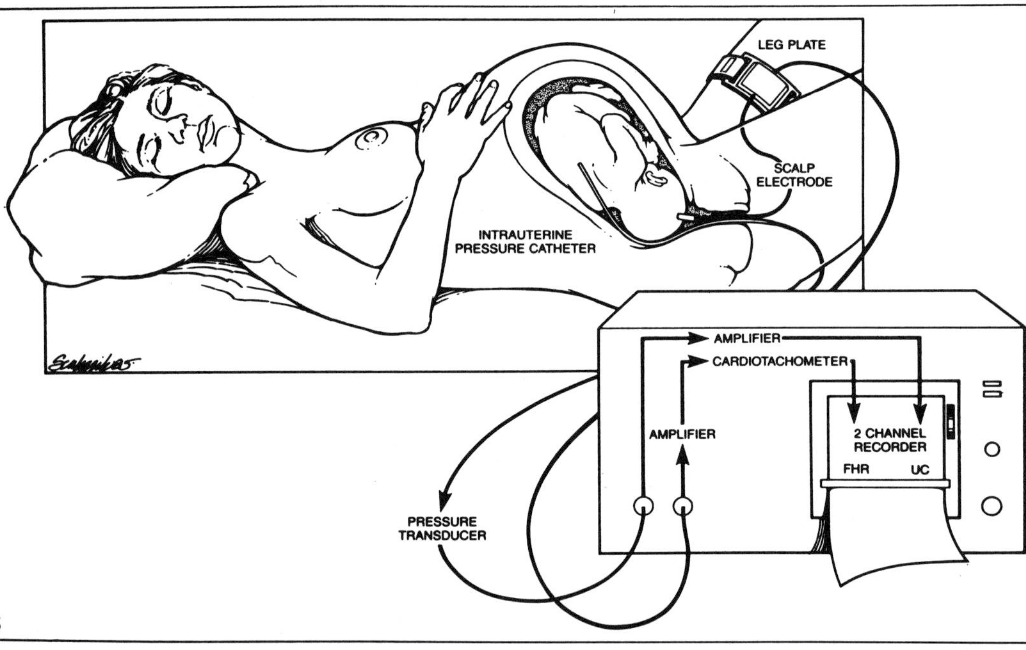

B

Figure 3–7. (*A*) External monitoring system. The tocodynamometer records uterine contractions (UC) and the Doppler transducer monitors the FHR. They are attached to the maternal abdomen with belts. (*B*) Internal monitors. The scalp electrode is attached directly to the fetus transvaginally. The pressure catheter is threaded through the cervix into the uterine cavity. (From Petrie RH: Intrapartum evaluation. In Gabbe, SG and Niebyl, J (eds): Obstetrics: Normal and Problem Pregnancies. Churchill Livingstone, New York, 1986 with permission.)

the relationship between decelerations and contractions.

Complications from Fetal Monitors

A low incidence of complications results from the use of internal fetal monitors. Localized scalp infections infrequently occur at the insertion site of the ECG electrode, possibly serving as the basis for neonatal sepsis in a few cases.[24] On occasion, the intrauterine pressure catheter perforates the uterus during insertion, possibly resulting in a broad-ligament hematoma. This complication likely occurs more often than is recognized.[24] Some authorities believe that, in long labors, the use of internal monitors increases the risk of chorioamnionitis. However, other studies[24,25] have shown no difference in risk when comparing outcome following long labors with or without the use of internal monitors. Because these complications rarely occur, they do not play a significant role in the obstetrician's decision to use internal devices.

Scalp pH Sampling

Although electronic assessment of FHR and contractions has reached a high level of sophistication, the method still does not always provide accurate diagnosis of intrapartum fetal distress. The incidence of poor fetal outcome stands considerably higher with an abnormal heart rate pattern than with a normal pattern; however, the predictive value of an abnormal tracing is only about 30 to 50 percent.[22] This implies that if clinical decisions depend solely on the use of heart rate monitoring, operative intervention for fetal distress will be inappropriate in a high percentage of cases.

The presence of significant fetal hypoxia initiates anerobic metabolism and systemic metabolic acidosis, which leads to decreased pH of capillary blood in the fetal scalp. Therefore, sampling fetal scalp blood for pH measurement assesses the degree of tissue ischemia, thus determining the clinical significance of abnormal FHR tracings during labor.[26]

Fetal blood sampling begins with visualization of the fetal scalp through a plastic tube inserted into the vagina. After mucus and amniotic fluid are cleared away and a small puncture with a 2-mm lancet is made, blood is collected in a capillary tube for pH measurement. Normal pH values exceed 7.25, indicating adequate tissue oxygenation; only persistent abnormal heart rate patterns call for repeated measurements. A pH value of 7.20 to 7.25 implies a preacidotic state, necessitating a second measurement in 15 min. An initial pH value below 7.20 signifies frank fetal acidosis (significant hypoxia), and a confirmatory result on a repeat sample usually mandates delivery.

Fetal scalp capillary pH correlates highly with cord blood pH when the fetus is delivered immediately.[22] The existence of a low scalp pH followed by delivery of a healthy fetus most likely relates to the presence of temporary respiratory acidosis occurring during sampling but clearing prior to delivery. Respiratory acidosis usually results from cord compression and often disappears within minutes. In comparison, metabolic acidosis resolves relatively slowly following restoration of fetal tissue oxygenation. Since most interests pertain to detection of a significant metabolic component, scalp sampling should not be performed during variable decelerations, and abnormal values warrant repeating the test.

Other potential causes of misleading results include contamination of blood with amniotic fluid and maternal acid-base disorders. Since the fetal pH increases and decreases in parallel with changes in maternal pH, a suspicion of a maternal acid-base disorder calls for obtaining a venous pH concurrently with the fetal sample for comparison.[27]

Fetal scalp sampling has several limitations. Intact membranes or cervical dilation less than 3 to 4 cm prevent the maneuver, while a high presenting part or contamination of the field by overabundant amounts of amniotic fluid complicate its completion. When a fetal scalp pH cannot be obtained in the presence of a worrisome FHR tracing, the "scalp stimulation test" has been proposed[28] and is based on the observation that if the FHR accelerates with fetal scalp stimulation (e.g., pinching the skin with an Allis clamp), the pH is almost always normal.

VALUE OF INTRAPARTUM MONITORING

Subsequent to initial use of continuous intrapartum electronic monitoring in the late 1960s, innumerable studies demonstrated an association between abnormal cardiographic tracings and abnormal fetal outcome. The obstetrician bases clinical application of electronic fetal monitoring on the assumption that, when abnormal heart rate patterns occur, he or she can intervene to prevent fetal asphyxia and death. Several large, uncontrolled studies strongly support the premise that electronic fetal monitoring in labor improves perinatal outcome.[29] At many institutions, perinatal death rates have decreased dramatically since the advent of intrapartum electronic fetal monitoring. For example, the perinatal death rate at the Los Angeles County–USC Medical Center fell from 54 per 1000 in the period from 1950 to 1969 (prior to electronic monitoring) to 21 per 1000 in 1974 (after introduction of continuous monitoring).[30] The apparent success of this technology in preventing intrapartum death has led to widespread use of continuous electronic monitoring in this country, including routine use in low-risk patients.

Unfortunately, electronic monitoring became the "standard of care" without adequate randomized controlled studies to define its usefulness. Prior to 1985, only five controlled studies of continuous intrapartum monitoring appeared in the literature; none demonstrated substantial benefit. However, these studies suffered from several deficiencies, the most important of which was an insufficient study size for demonstrating a clinically significant difference in outcomes, even if one had existed.[31] More recently,[32,33] two large controlled studies compared the value of continuous monitoring with intermittent auscultation in labor. A prospective study[32] of 35,000 deliveries reveals no difference in perinatal outcome with use of selective intermittent auscultation in low-risk pregnancies and that with universal continuous electronic monitoring in different months. MacDonald and coworkers,[33] who randomly assigned 13,000 women with previously healthy fetuses to one of two programs—continuous electronic fetal monitoring or intermittent auscultation of the FHR—found no difference in Apgar scores or frequency of perinatal death. A lower incidence of neonatal seizures appeared in the continuously monitored group. In both studies[32,33] an aggressive program of continuous monitoring and scalp sampling followed detection of FHR abnormalities.

Proponents and critics of electronic fetal monitoring generally agree that some form of fetal surveillance is necessary. Although the studies cited above demonstrate equivalent outcomes with the use of intermittent auscultation in low-risk pregnancies, it should be emphasized that this method must be used in a well-defined manner. Guidelines published by the American College of Obstetricians and Gynecologists[34] recommend as a minimum the auscultation of fetal heart tones during and after a contraction every 30 min during the first stage and every 10 to 15 min during the second stage of labor. If this auscultation uncovers abnormalities, continuous electronic monitoring should be initiated.

Ongoing debate centers on the question, "Is continuous electronic fetal monitoring a valuable tool which helps prevent harm, or does it represent a meddlesome, cumbersome imposition of technology that yields no benefit and causes unnecessary cesarean sections?" Although controlled studies fail to demonstrate a benefit of electronic monitoring over intermittent auscultation in low-risk pregnancies, the methods used to measure outcome in these studies may lack the sensitivity required for detection of more subtle forms of fetal damage. Electronic fetal monitoring does provide information about the fetus unobtainable in any other way. Convincing evidence demonstrates that this procedure identifies fetal distress and acidosis with a much higher frequency than intermittent auscultation. Unless one doubts the significance of fetal acidosis, the information obtained from electronic fetal monitoring has potential value. Admittedly, a clear need exists for methods that could better define when and how operative intervention should be used.

Even though intrapartum death and acute perinatal asphyxia have decreased since the advent of electronic fetal monitoring, a concomitant decrease in the incidence of cerebral palsy has not occurred.[35] Many authorities[36] now believe that most cases of cerebral palsy do not result from intrapartum asphyxia but rather from unknown causes, possibly genetic factors or episodic hypoxia remote from term. Much work remains to uncover the pathophysiology of fetal and neonatal neurologic problems.

Antepartum Monitoring

As perinatal deaths as a result of intrapartum complications have decreased, obstetricians have increasingly directed their attention toward preventing antepartum death and asphyxia. Certain risk factors of pregnancy are associated with uteroplacental insufficiency and increased fetal risk (Table 3–2). To determine health status of these fetuses antepartally, investigators have devised several tests that aim to detect minor degrees of intrauterine fetal compromise and to enable timely delivery before death or asphyxia occurs. Conversely, by using these tests, the clinician strives to safely delay delivery in high-risk pregnancies until sufficient fetal maturity develops and a favorable cervix exists for induction of labor.

CONTRACTION STRESS TEST

The first antepartum test to come into widespread use, the contraction stress text (CST), applies principles learned from intrapartum monitoring. The examiner looks for signs of uteroplacental insufficiency (late decelerations) by monitoring the FHR in the presence of artificially induced uterine contractions. As with spontaneous contractions during labor, these contractions produce a decrease in intervillous blood flow, and the Po_2 falls below a critical level in the marginally oxygenated fetus, which then manifests late decelerations.

The contraction stress test begins by obtaining a baseline fetal heart tracing, then administering incremental doses of oxytocin to produce uterine contractions. A positive CST, indicating an abnormal result, occurs when late decelerations develop with greater than 50 percent of contractions at a time when three contractions occur in a 10-min period. A negative CST denotes no late decelerations, whereas an equivocal result entails the finding of infrequent late decelerations (with <50 percent of contractions). Even the normal fetus develops late decelerations in response to uterine hyperstimulation, so the CST must be repeated in case of excessive oxytocic effects.

Table 3–2. CONDITIONS THAT INDICATE ANTEPARTUM MONITORING FOR FETAL WELL-BEING

Pre-eclampsia
Chronic hypertension and other cardiovascular diseases
Diabetes
Suspected intrauterine growth retardation
Postterm pregnancy
Previous unexplained fetal demise
Decreased fetal movement
Miscellaneous conditions with compromised uteroplacental blood flow or fetal tissue oxygenation

Several studies report a significant association between positive CSTs and adverse perinatal outcomes (i.e., fetal distress in labor, low Apgar scores, admissions to intensive care units, and perinatal deaths).[37] One assumes that prompt delivery in the face of a positive CST will prevent these adverse outcomes. Several investigators[8] demonstrated a decline in perinatal death rates after they started using the CST to monitor high-risk pregnancies. Unfortunately, no randomized studies using appropriate control groups have documented the true benefit of the CST. In a recent literature review of the CST Thacker[38] found that this method produced a false-positive rate of greater than 50 percent (incorrectly predicting adverse perinatal outcome) in more than half of the reports. Proponents[8] of the CST acknowledge this high false-positive rate but emphasize its low false-negative rate (i.e., the very high rate of normal outcomes after a negative CST). However, in spite of the low false-negative rate, the sensitivity for predicting adverse outcomes is less than 50 percent in most studies.[38] The physician must be aware that with any screening test for an uncommon event a low false-negative rate is to be expected, even if the screening test has low sensitivity.

An advantage of the CST is its theoretical ability to detect the marginally compromised fetus (i.e., the presence of poor placental reserve but only minimal fetal hypoxia). Inconvenience constitutes the major disadvantage of the CST which requires an intravenous (IV) line, fetal monitoring facilities, and 90 min for completion. To circumvent the need for an IV and to shorten the time required to perform the CST, recent studies[39] utilized nipple stimulation to produce uterine contractions and reported diagnostic accuracy equal to that with the oxytocin CST. The significant incidence of uterine hyperstimulation, occasionally producing fetal distress, necessitates performing this test near the labor and delivery unit.

NONSTRESS TEST

This simpler alternative to the CST has gained popularity over the past 15 years, becoming the most commonly used test for fetal health in the United States.[40] The nonstress test (NST) incorporates the observation that good beat-to-beat variability and FHR accelerations reflect fetal well-being. The procedure entails monitoring FHR and uterine activity while marking the tracing whenever the woman perceives fetal movements. Although no consensus prevails, the criteria for a reactive (normal) test commonly include the presence of two heart rate accelerations, each of 15 beats per min and lasting 15 sec, within a 20-min period (Fig. 3–8).[41] Accelerations are usually but not necessarily associated with fetal movements. Additionally, a normal baseline heart rate and normal beat-to-beat variability must exist. The absence of these criteria over 40 min constitutes a nonreactive test.

One of the main problems with the NST is that a normal fetus has active and quiet periods lasting 40 min or more, and a healthy but quiet fetus may have a nonreactive test.[42] For this reason, most authorities advocate that intervention not be based on a nonreactive NST alone and recommend further testing. Most frequently, the patient undergoes a CST, the results of which dictate subsequent management. Alternatively, a second NST performed later in the day and noted to be reactive indicates that the fetus was merely in a quiet period during the earlier test.[43] Another approach externally stimulates the fetus, either manually or with a vibroacoustic stimulus. Subsequent fetal movements and development of a reactive tracing predict a healthy baby as reliably as spontaneous reactivity.[44]

Like the CST, the NST has a disappointingly low sensitivity in predicting perinatal death or adverse outcome.[38] The false-negative rate is low, but again this may represent the low prevalence of poor outcomes rather than the sensitivity of the test. The high false-positive rate generates less concern, since the obstetrician performs further tests before contemplating intervention.

BIOPHYSICAL PROFILE

The NST, taken alone, strongly depends upon physiologic rest-activity cycles that may produce a nonreactive test in a healthy fetus. The biophysical profile serves to supplement the predictive value of the NST by observing other biophysical parameters, each of which correlates with fetal well-being. These include ultrasound assessment of gross body movements, fetal tone, fetal breathing movements, and amniotic fluid volume. Each of these four ultra-

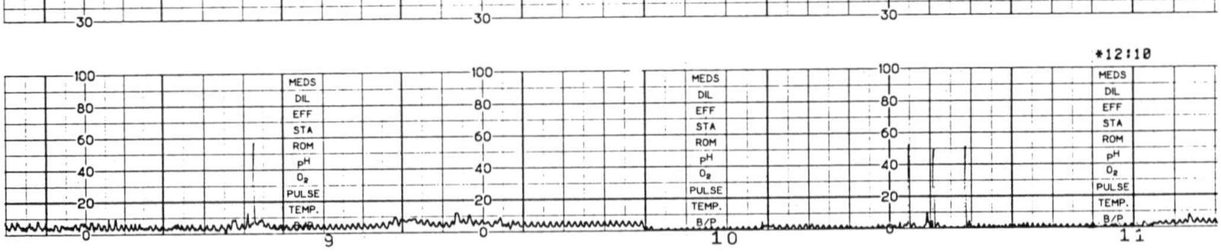

Figure 3–8. Reactive nonstress test. Note the accelerations of the fetal heart rate with fetal movements (FM). Also note the normal baseline rate and good beat-to-beat variability.

sound parameters as well as the NST receives a score of two if normal and zero if abnormal, for a composite score between zero and ten (Table 3–3). Manning and coworkers[45] report excellent correlation between the biophysical profile score and perinatal outcome, noting that a score of less than four is associated with a 50- to 100-fold increase in perinatal mortality. When the obstetric team notes the biophysical profile result and uses it for clinical management, the corrected perinatal mortality rate in a high-risk population decreases to 5 per 1000 (compared with 32 per 1000 in the blinded [unaware] group).[45] Although the five components of the biophysical profile receive equal weight in the scoring system, decreased amniotic fluid alone represents a critical risk factor, reflecting in one large retrospective study a 59-fold increase in perinatal mortality.[46]

FETAL MOVEMENT COUNTING

Daily fetal movement counting is a valuable but underutilized method of assessing fetal well-being. In a prospective controlled study of low-risk pregnancies, Nelham[47] found a significant reduction in perinatal mortality when women counted and recorded fetal movements during a designated period each day. In this and similar studies, various schemes have been suggested; all involve the counting of fetal movements within a designated period and instructions to call the hospital for further testing if the mother feels less than a specified number of movements. Because this technique involves no cost or invasive procedures, it is especially valuable for screening low-risk and high-risk patients. Some centers employ daily fetal movement counting in high-risk patients in addition to the more technically complex tests. Because the predictive value of this test remains largely undefined, most obstetricians use it for screening only and use results from more specific tests to formulate clinical management.

Table 3–3. COMPONENTS OF THE BIOPHYSICAL PROFILE

Test Parameter	Definition of Normal
Nonstress test	Two fetal heart accelerations in 20-min period
Gross body movements	At least three discrete movements in 30 min
Fetal tone	At least one episode of active extension and return to flexion
Breathing movements	Present for at least 30 sec in 30 min of observation
Amniotic fluid volume	>1-cm pocket measured in two planes

DOPPLER FLOW STUDIES

The presence of risk factors for uteroplacental insufficiency (e.g., diabetes, hypertension) usually indicates the use of the antenatal tests described above. In fact, a majority of women at risk for this disorder have normal uteroplacental circulation. Most tests of fetal status look for biophysical and cardiotocographic indicators of fetal hypoxia, factors that are imprecise and possibly abnormal even in a healthy fetus. A relatively new technique, using a Doppler device to obtain flow velocity wave forms in fetal and uterine blood vessels, shows promise of more accurate identification of uteroplacental insufficiency and fetal compromise. Several investigations[48] demonstrate the feasibility of making a direct diagnosis of uteroplacental insufficiency by measuring the flow in the arcuate branches of the uterine artery. As normal pregnancy advances, diastolic blood flow in these vessels progressively increases and constitutes a large portion of total blood flow. In some pathologic situations in pregnancy, flow in diastole diminishes sharply, leading to fetal compromise (Fig. 3–9). Doppler studies can identify abnormal uterine blood flow early in pregnancy and can predict subsequent complications such as intrauterine growth retardation and fetal distress in labor with a high degree of accuracy.

Flow velocity wave forms in fetal vessels, including the thoracic aorta and umbilical artery, can also serve as early indicators of fetal compromise.[49,50] When a fetus becomes hypoxic, blood shunting away from the lower extremities and umbilical circulation occurs to preserve blood flow to the heart and brain. In these instances tests such as the NST that indicate CNS hypoxia, may remain normal, while Doppler studies would show decreased flow in the fetal thoracic aorta and umbilical artery. For

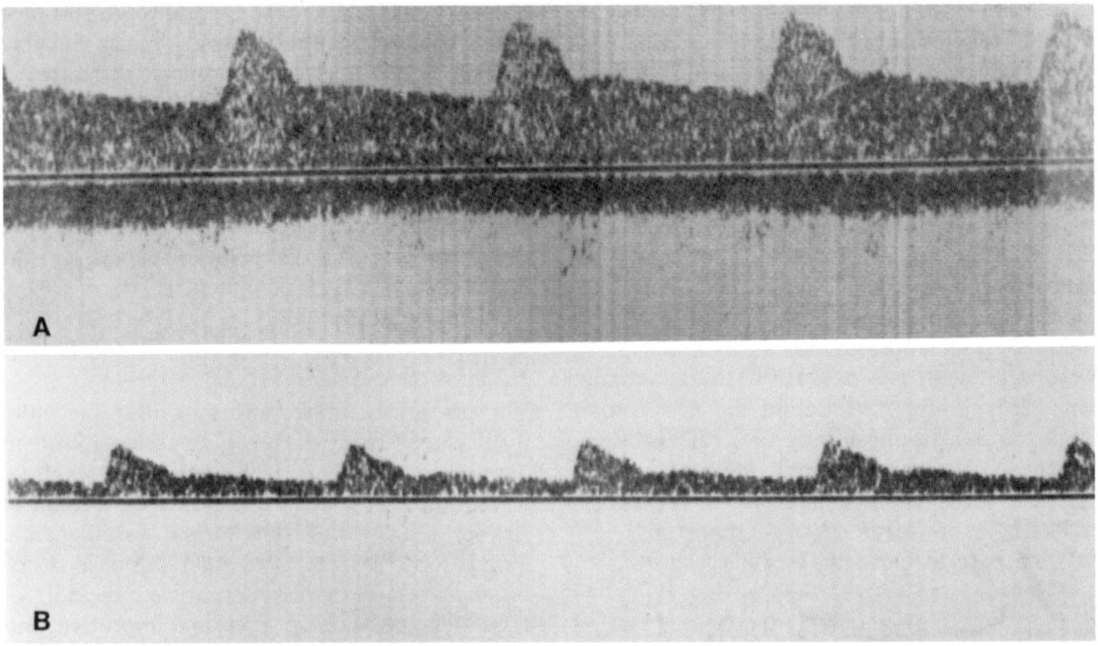

Figure 3–9. (*A*) A normal Doppler sonogram obtained from the arcuate branch of the uterine artery. Note the high end-diastolic velocities and low systolic-to-diastolic ratio. (*B*) Doppler sonogram of an abnormal arcuate artery. Compared with *A* there is a higher systolic-to-diastolic ratio, and decreased flow velocity in end diastole. (From Cohen-Overbeek, T, Pearce, JM and Campbell, S: The antenatal assessment of utero-placental and feto-placental blood flow using Doppler ultrasound. Ultrasound Med Biol 11:329, 1985 with permission.)

this reason, Doppler studies likely provide greater sensitivity than traditional tests of fetal status and, since they are independent of fetal sleep cycles, may be more specific as well. While Doppler flow studies show promise, the actual effectiveness for clinical purposes has not been fully evaluated, necessitating additional investigation.

Diagnostic Ultrasound

GESTATIONAL AGE ASSESSMENT

Depending on the population being studied, 25 to 40 percent of women have uncertain due dates based on menstrual data alone.[51] Possible reasons include inexact recollection of the time of the last menstrual period, recent oral contraceptive use, irregular periods, or bleeding in early pregnancy. In a recent study by Campbell,[52] only 65 percent of women with uncertain menstrual dates delivered within 2 weeks of their estimated date of confinement. In the modern practice of obstetrics, especially with high-risk pregnancies, proper management mandates accurate gestational age assessment. Even low-risk pregnancies require accurate dating since unpredictable complications such as premature labor and "postdatism" may develop.

In populations with "good dates" by menstrual history, 80 to 85 percent of women deliver within 2 weeks of their due date.[52] The fact that the remaining 15 to 20 percent deliver outside of this 4-week range results partly from the natural population variability in the onset of labor, which does not reflect "wrong dates." In the remainder, however, the data of conception is inaccurately estimated. Clinical parameters, such as serial fundal height measurements or the time of initial auscultation of fetal heart tones, help in either confirming secure menstrual dates or suggesting the need for ultrasound if a discrepancy occurs, but by themselves do not adequately determine gestational age. In a Swedish study,[51] 95 percent of women delivered within 2 weeks of a due date established with routine early ultrasound assessment. In another study[53] of routine ultrasonographic determination of gestational age, the incidence of postterm pregnancy was reduced to 1.9 percent compared with 8 percent in a control group. These studies underline the possible benefit of routine scanning of all pregnant women.

To establish gestational age with ultrasound, several different fetal body parts are measured and compared with available tables showing average measurements at different gestational ages. Because of the relative ease with which early equipment identified the biparietal diameter (BPD), this fetal measurement became the first widely studied parameter of fetal age. The BPD can be accurately measured starting at about 12 to 14 weeks' gestation (Fig. 3–10). Because the population variability of this and all other fetal measurements increases as pregnancy progresses, the earliest accurately measured BPD will best estimate gestational age.[54] By the third trimester, BPD measurements have a variability of plus or minus 3 weeks for estimations of gestational age.

With the recent advent of real-time imaging systems, the ultrasonographer can easily visualize and measure the fetal femur starting at about 12 to 14 weeks' gestation. The accuracy of femur length (FL) in assigning gestational age approximates that of the BPD through the 26th week. After this time, the FL appears to be superior for a number of reasons, including less biologic variability in the FL than in head size as gestation advances, the femur is not subject to distortion from molding, and it is almost always accessible, even when the head is engaged and the BPD cannot be visualized. As with the BPD, early femur measurements are superior to those later in gestation.

Before the 14th week of pregnancy, the crown-rump length (CRL) is used for ultrasound assignment of gestational age. Less biologic variability occurs with the CRL than with the

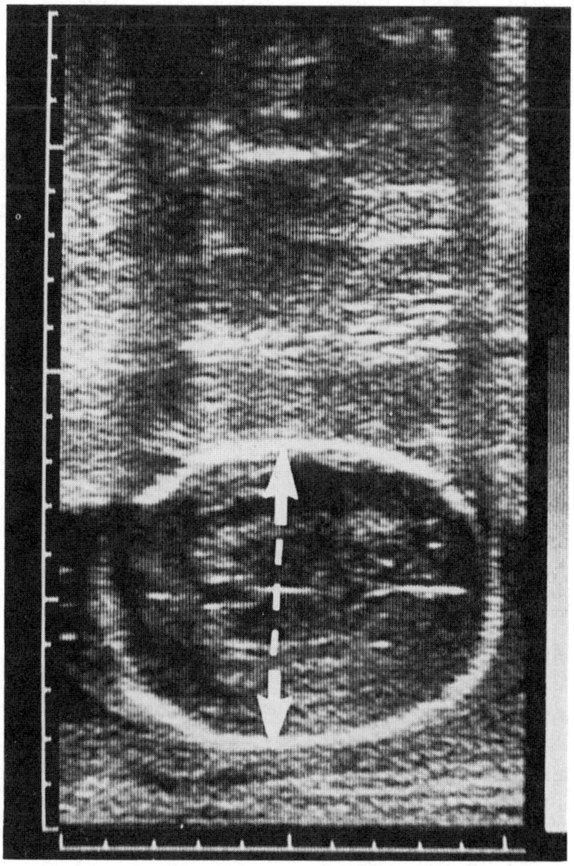

Figure 3–10. A transverse ultrasound view of the fetal head showing the biparietal diameter measurement.

BPD and FL, and, in research settings,[55] CRL has proved more accurate for estimating the EDC. However, in the clinical setting, the CRL is more subject to inaccuracies of measurement, and for this reason the BPD and femur measured in the second trimester predict the EDC at least as well as, if not better than, the CRL.[56]

Fetal weight estimates obtained from ultrasound measurements are important in the face of suspected macrosomia or intrauterine growth retardation. Reliable prediction of weight also improves management decisions in pregnancies where premature delivery is possible. Ultrasound is superior to clinical methods for weight estimates; however fetal weight estimates may differ by 10 percent or more from true fetal weight.[57]

OTHER USES OF ULTRASOUND IN ANTENATAL ASSESSMENT

Although gestational age assessment represents the principal use for ultrasound in current obstetric practice, other applications are gaining increasing importance. Improved ultrasound equipment has provided finer detail of fetal anatomy, enabling diagnosis of many structural abnormalities (Fig. 3–11*A*, *B*). Routine ultrasound for pregnancy dating reveals the majority of these, while others are noted when a family history of a defective fetus or inappropriate uterine size prompt the examination. The experienced sonographer detects a high percentage of fetal anomalies. Campbell and Pearce[58] assessed 2372 patients and correctly identified 405 of 425 congenital malformations. The advantages of diagnosing fetal anomalies before birth include the following:

1. The couple may have the option of pregnancy termination.
2. Continuing pregnancies can be followed at a referral center equipped to manage complications which accompany the fetal anomaly.
3. The presence of an anomaly may influence the timing and method of delivery.
4. Plans can be made for appropriate cytogenetic, pathologic, or biochemical studies on the newborn to establish the diagnosis and chance of recurrence.
5. The couple can prepare themselves psychologically for the birth of a baby with problems.
6. Cesarean delivery can be avoided if lethal abnormalities are present.
7. Therapy in utero may be possible with some disorders.

Despite the potential advantages of universal ultrasonographic screening to establish gestational age and to diagnose abnormalities of the fetus and placenta, it has not become a "standard of care." In 1984, a panel discussion at the National Institute of Child Health and Human Development[59] concluded that the data on safety are still inadequate to justify a recommendation for routine screening.

Fetal Pulmonary Maturity Tests

Good menstrual dates, confirmed by early ultrasound, allow elective delivery at term with minimal risk of unsuspected prematurity. As stated previously, the great biologic variability in fetal size in late pregnancy disallows reliable ultrasonographic assessment of fetal maturity with a single late study. When clinical or ultrasonographic documentation of gestational age is not available, the clinician may find it necessary to establish fetal pulmonary maturity by means of amniocentesis and analysis of amniotic fluid before proceeding with elective delivery. In complicated preterm pregnancies, amniotic fluid indicators of fetal pulmonary status strongly influence the decision to deliver or manage the fetus in utero to allow additional time for lung maturation.

COMMONLY USED TESTS

The most widely accepted amniotic fluid test for lung maturity is the lecithin-sphingomyelin ratio (L/S ratio). The concentration of sphingomyelin in amniotic fluid is relatively stable throughout gestation and provides an internal standard for levels of lecithin, a phospholipid quantitatively related to pulmonary surfactant. With an L/S ratio greater than 2.0, neonatal respiratory distress syndrome (RDS) rarely occurs.[60] However, an "immature" L/S ratio (<2.0) is often false-positive for RDS. For example, the chance of a baby developing RDS approximates only 50 percent when the L/S ratio is in the range of 1.5 to 1.9.[61] Performance of the L/S ratio con-

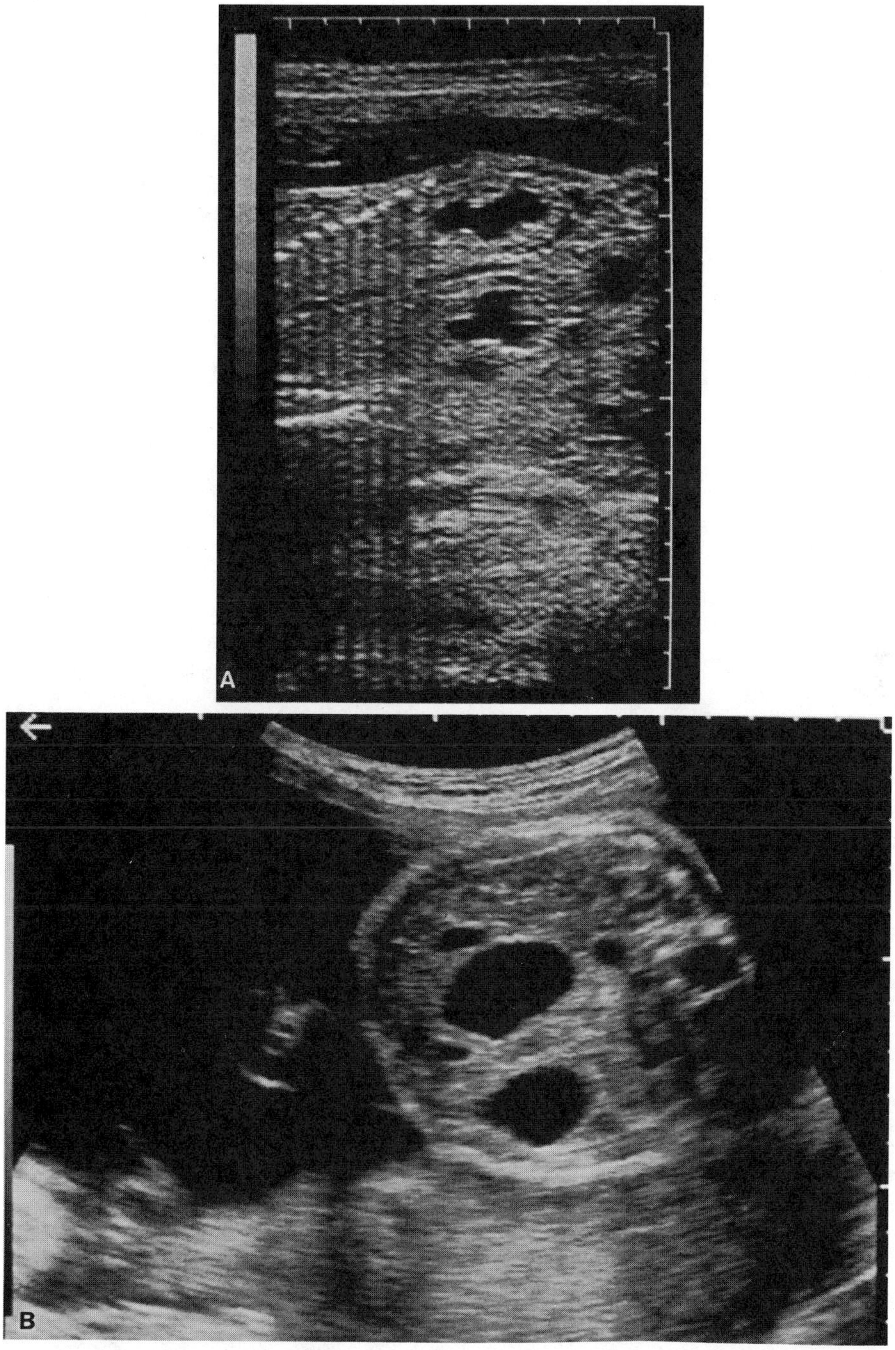

Figure 3–11. Examples of ultrasound diagnosis of fetal anomalies. (*A*) A coronal view of the fetal chest and abdomen showing bilateral dilation of the renal pelves secondary to bladder outlet obstruction. (*B*) A transverse view of the fetal abdomen with the "double bubble" sign characteristic of duodenal obstruction.

sumes substantial time and requires an experienced lab to achieve accurate results. A simpler method for measuring pulmonary phospholipid uses the radioimmunoassay of phosphatidyl glycerol (PG). The fetal lung produces PG at a more advanced stage of maturity than it does lecithin; hence, a positive test (PG present) better predicts pulmonary maturity than a mature L/S ratio.[62] Conversely, a negative PG less reliably predicts the development of RDS than an immature L/S ratio.

A third commonly used test is the foam stability index (FSI), a test of the functional ability of amniotic fluid to maintain bubbles in the presence of various concentrations of alcohol.[63] A "mature" result, when foam is stable at concentrations of alcohol above 47 percent, correlates with low rates of neonatal RDS. A commercially available kit allows rapid completion of the FSI by relatively unskilled laboratory technicians.

Because obstetricians have had extensive experience with the L/S ratio, it is the standard against which other tests of fetal pulmonary maturity are judged. Experience has shown that a positive result with any of the three tests described strongly predicts the absence of RDS. Because of the speed and convenience of the FSI and the PG radioimmunoassay many obstetricians now use these tests instead of the L/S ratio.

Summary

The intrauterine environment is no longer a black box wherein the fetal condition remains a mystery. In the majority of patients, spontaneous delivery of a normal healthy baby occurs at term without any attempt by the obstetrician to assess fetal well-being. However, as medical science advances, health-care professionals and the public alike expect virtually every baby to live and flourish, a goal that demands aggressive efforts to identify fetuses at risk. Although available techniques to establish fetal health remain imperfect and, in many cases, our ability to alter the eventual outcome is limited, much progress has been made. Considerable research continues in these areas, and our ability to assess fetal condition should continue to grow rapidly. Appropriate use of current methods, coupled with upcoming advances, should greatly facilitate ongoing efforts to produce the healthiest neonate possible.

References

1. Vital Statistics of the United States 1930–1983, vol 2. US Department of Health and Human Services, Washington, DC, 1984.
2. National Center for Health Statistics: Advanced Report of Final Natality Statistics. US Department of Health and Human Services, Washington, DC, 1983.
3. Fenton, AN and Steer, CM: Fetal distress. Am J Obstet Gynecol 83:354, 1962.
4. Paul, RH, et al: The evaluation and significance of intrapartum baseline FHR variability. Am J Obstet Gynecol 123:2, 1975.
5. Martin, CB, Jr: Physiology and clinical use of fetal heart rate variability. Clin Perinatol 9:2, 1982.
6. Parer, JT, et al: Increased fetal heart rate variability with acute hypoxia in chronically instrumented sheep. Eur J Obstet Gynecol Reprod Biol 10:393, 1980.
7. Miller, FC and Paul, RH: Intrapartum fetal heart rate monitoring. Clin Obstet Gynecol 21:561, 1978.
8. Freeman, RK and Garite, TJ: Fetal Heart Rate Monitoring. Williams & Wilkins, Baltimore, 1981, p 68.
9. Shenker, L: Fetal cardiac arrhythmias. Obstet Gynecol Surv 34:561, 1979.
10. Martin, CB, Jr: Regulation of the fetal heart rate and genesis of FHR patterns. Semin Perinatol 2:131, 1978.
11. Young, BK, et al: Fetal blood and tissue pH with moderate bradycardia. Am J Obstet Gynecol 135:45, 1979.
12. Modanlou, HD and Freeman, RK: Sinusoidal fetal heart rate pattern: Its definition and clinical significance. Am J Obstet Gynecol 142:1033, 1982.
13. Scott, JS, et al: Connective-tissue disease, antibodies to ribonucleoprotein, and congenital heart block. N Engl J Med 309:209, 1983.
14. Sugarman, RG, Rawlinson, KF and Schifrin, BS: Fetal arrhythmia. Obstet Gynecol 52:3, 1978.
15. Ramzin, MS and Napflin, S: Transient intrauterine supraventricular tachycardia associated with transient hydrops fetalis. Case report. Br J Obstet Gynaecol 89:965, 1982.
16. Kerenyi, TD, et al: Transplacental cardioversion of intrauterine supraventricular tachycardia with digitalis. Lancet 2:393, 1980.
17. Dumesic, DA, et al: Transplacental cardioversion of fetal supraventricular tachycardia with procainamide. N Engl J Med 307:18, 1982.
18. DeVore, GR: Fetal echocardiography: A new frontier. Clin Obstet Gynecol 27:2, 1984.
19. Hutson, JM and Mueller-Heubach, E: Diagnosis and management of intrapartum reflex fetal heart rate changes. Clin Perinatol 9:2, 1982.
20. Itskovitz, J, Goetzman, BW and Rudolph, AM: The mechanism of late deceleration of the heart rate and its relationship to oxygenation in normoxemic and chronically hypoxemic fetal lambs. Am J Obstet Gynecol 142:66, 1982.
21. Murata, Y, et al: Fetal heart rate accelerations and late

decelerations during the course of intrauterine death in chronically catheterized rhesus monkeys. Am J Obstet Gynecol 144:218, 1982.
22. Miller, FC: Prediction of acid-base values from intrapartum fetal heart rate data and their correlation with scalp and funic values. Clin Perinatol 9:2, 1982.
23. Lee, CV, DeLorenfo, PC and O'Lane, JM: A study of fetal heart rate acceleration patterns. Obstet Gynecol 45:142, 1975.
24. Ledger, WJ: Complications associated with invasive monitoring. Semin Perinatol 2:187, 1978.
25. Gibbs, DS, Listwa, HM and Read, JA: The effect of internal fetal monitoring on maternal infection following cesarean section. Obstet Gynecol 48:653, 1976.
26. Zalar, RW, Jr and Quilligan, EJ: The influence of scalp sampling on the cesarean section rate for fetal distress. Am J Obstet Gynecol 135:239, 1979.
27. Bowen, LW, et al: Maternal-fetal pH difference and fetal scalp pH as predictors of neonatal outcome. Obstet Gynecol 67:4, 1986.
28. Rice, PE and Benedetti, TJ: Fetal heart rate acceleration with fetal blood sampling. Obstet Gynecol 68:469, 1986.
29. Parer, JT: FHR monitoring: Answering the critics. Contemporary Ob Gyn 17:163, 1981.
30. Quilligan, EJ and Collea, JV: Fetal monitoring in pregnancy. Adv Pediatr 22:83, 1976.
31. Schifrin, BS: The fetal monitoring polemic. Clin Perinatol 9:399, 1982.
32. Leveno, KJ, et al: A prospective comparison of selective and universal electronic fetal monitoring in 34,995 pregnancies. N Engl J Med 315:615, 1986.
33. MacDonald, D, et al: The Dublin randomized controlled trial of intrapartum fetal heart rate monitoring. Am J Obstet Gynecol 152:524, 1985.
34. Standards for Obstetric Gynecologic Services, ed 6. American College of Obstetricians and Gynecologists, Washington, DC, 1985, p 34.
35. Jarvis, SN, Holloway, JS and Hey, EN: Increase in cerebral palsy in normal birthweight babies. Arch Dis Child 60:113, 1985.
36. Hensleigh, PA, Fainstat, T and Spencer, R: Perinatal events and cerebral palsy. Am J Obstet Gynecol 154:978, 1986.
37. Freeman, RK, Anderson, G and Dorchester, W: A prospective multi-institutional study of antepartum fetal heart rate monitoring. Am J Obstet Gynecol 143:771, 1982.
38. Thacker, SB and Berkelman, RL: Assessing the diagnostic accuracy and efficacy of selected antepartum fetal surveillance techniques. Obstet Gynecol Surv 41:121, 1986.
39. Huddleston, JF, Sutliff, G and Robinson, D: Contraction stress test by intermittent nipple stimulation. Obstet Gynecol 63:669, 1984.
40. Gabbe, SG: Antepartum fetal evaluation. In Gabbe, SG and Niebyl, J (eds): Obstetrics: Normal and Problem Pregnancies. Churchill Livingstone, New York, 1986, p 301.
41. Lavery, JP: Nonstress fetal heart rate testing. Clin Obstet Gynecol 25:689, 1982.
42. Patrick, J, et al: Accelerations of the human fetal heart rate at 38 to 40 weeks' gestational age. Am J Obstet Gynecol 148:35, 1984.
43. Phelan, JP, et al: Continuing role of the nonstress test in the management of postdate pregnancy. Obstet Gynecol 64:624, 1984.
44. Smith, CV, et al: Fetal acoustic stimulation testing II. A randomized clinical comparison with the nonstress test. Am J Obstet Gynecol 155:131, 1986.
45. Manning, FA, et al: Antepartum determination of fetal health: Composite biophysical profile scoring. Clin Perinatol 9:285, 1982.
46. Chamberlain, PM, et al: The relationship of marginal and decreased amniotic fluid volumes to perinatal outcome. Am J Obstet Gynecol 150:245, 1984.
47. Neldam, S: Fetal movement as an indicator of fetal well-being. Dan Med Bull 30:274, 1983.
48. Campbell, S, et al: New Doppler technique for assessing uteroplacental blood flow. Lancet 1:675, 1983.
49. Cohen-Overbeek, T, Pearce, JM and Campbell, S: The antenatal assessment of utero-placental and feto-placental blood flow using Doppler ultrasound. Ultrasound Med Biol 11:329, 1985.
50. Trudinger, BJ, Thompson, RS and Giles, WB: Doppler ultrasound and blood flow in obstetrics. In Sanders, RC and Hill, M (eds) Ultrasound Annual. Raven Press, New York, 1986, p 39.
51. Grennert, L, Persson, P-H and Gennser G: Benefits of ultrasonic screening of a pregnant population. Acta Obstet Gynecol Scand [Suppl] 78:5, 1978.
52. Campbell, S, et al: Routine ultrasound screening for the prediction of gestational age. Obstet Gynecol 65:613, 1985.
53. Eik-Nes, S, et al: Ultrasound screening in pregnancy: A randomized controlled trial. Lancet 1:1347, 1984.
54. Hadlock, FP, et al: Fetal biparietal diameter: A critical re-evaluation of the relation to menstrual age by means of real-time ultrasound. J Ultrasound Med 1:97, 1982.
55. Drumm, JE: The prediction of delivery date by ultrasonic measurement of fetal crown-rump length. Br J Obstet Gynaecol 84:1, 1977.
56. Kopta, MM, May, RR and Crane, JP: A comparison of the reliability of the estimated date of confinement predicted by crown-rump and biparietal diameter. Am J Obstet Gynecol 145:562, 1983.
57. Seeds, JW and Cefalo, RC: Practical Obstetrical Ultrasound. Aspen, Rockville, MD, 1986, p 85.
58. Campbell, S and Pearce, J: The prenatal diagnosis of fetal structural anomalies by ultrasound. Clin Obstet Gynaecol 10:475, 1983.
59. NICHD research highlights and topics of interest. ACOG Newsletter. May 1984.
60. Kulovich, M, Hallman, M and Gluck, L: The lung profile. Am J Obstet Gynecol 120:142, 1974.
61. Harvey, D, Parkinson, C and Campbell, S: Risk of respiratory distress syndrome. Lancet 1:42, 1975.
62. Garite, TJ, et al: A new rapid slide agglutination test for amniotic fluid PG: Laboratory and clinical correlation. Am J Obstet Gynecol 147:681, 1983.
63. Lipshitz, J, Whybrew, WD and Anderson, GD: Comparison of the Lumadex-foam stability index test, lecithin: sphingomyelin ratio, and simple shake test for fetal lung maturity. Obstet Gynecol 63:349, 1984.

CHAPTER 4

MATERNAL AND FETAL MORBIDITY AND MORTALITY

DAVID D. HOOD, M.D.

Maternal and neonatal morbidity and mortality increase in the complicated obstetric patient. Understanding maternal and neonatal complications should help modify obstetric and anesthetic care and improve outcome.

Maternal Mortality

ASSESSMENT

In the United States, maternal deaths are classified into three groups: direct obstetric deaths, indirect obstetric deaths, and nonobstetric deaths. Direct obstetric deaths result from complications of pregnancy or medical care during pregnancy. Maternal deaths caused by hemorrhage, infection, or pre-eclampsia represent direct obstetric deaths. Indirect obstetric deaths result from diseases that existed before or developed during pregnancy but were not produced by pregnancy. Pre-existing cardiac disease resulting in maternal death is an example of indirect obstetric death. Nonobstetric maternal deaths follow accidental or incidental causes unrelated to pregnancy or its treatment. Data on maternal mortality often combine direct and indirect maternal deaths. Traditionally only deaths that occur within 42 days of delivery are considered to be maternal deaths. However, over 50 percent of maternal deaths may occur 42 days or more following delivery, and current authorities recommend lengthening the reporting period to 90 days[1] or a year.[2]

Maternal death rates are underestimated in most United States reports. Rubin and coworkers[1] investigated maternal deaths in Georgia during 1975 and 1976. Using all available sources they identified 27 percent more maternal deaths than were reported by death certificates alone. Furthermore, extending the delivery-to-death interval to 90 days produced 50 percent more maternal deaths. Since 17 to 73 percent of maternal deaths may be mistakenly classified as nonmaternal, maternal mortality rates should use vital statistics and other sources.[1–4]

Preventable Maternal Deaths. Most authorities define the maternal mortality rate (MMR) as the number of maternal deaths divided by the number of live births. Until 1935 the United States MMR approximated 60 deaths per 10,000 births.[5] Since then, the MMR declined steadily to 1.5 per 10,000 in 1978.[2] An Ontario study,[6] reported an MMR of 0.85 per 10,000, yet 40 percent of all maternal deaths and 55 percent of direct maternal deaths were still "preventable." Similarly, a survey from England and Wales[7] reported preventable factors in 58 percent of maternal deaths, indicating that better results should be expected.

MAJOR CAUSES OF DEATH

Kaunitz and coworkers[2] recently conducted a national study of maternal mortality in the United States in which they obtained copies of maternal death certificates from the National Center for Health Statistics for the years 1974 to 1978, and pregnancy-related death certificates from state health departments (which were not included in the National Center for Health Statistics). Collaborative information included autopsy results, reports from state maternal mortality committees, and matched birth and fetal death certificates. All deaths occurring within 1 year of pregnancy were analyzed. The leading causes of maternal deaths were embolism (24 percent), hypertensive disease of pregnancy (20 percent), obstetric hemorrhage (16 percent), obstetric infection (10 percent), cerebrovascular accident (5 percent), and anesthetic complications (5 percent; Table 4–1).

From 1950 to 1971 the classic triad of hemorrhage, toxemia, and infection accounted for

Table 4–1. CAUSES OF MATERNAL MORTALITY IN THE UNITED STATES, 1974–1978

Classification	Number	Percent
Embolism	491	24
Thrombotic	271	
Amniotic fluid	189	
Air	25	
Other/unspecified	6	
Hypertension	421	20
Pre-eclampsia/eclampsia	396	
Other	25	
Obstetric hemorrhage	331	16
Postpartum	114	
Uterine rupture	71	
Abruptio placentae	55	
Nonuterine	39	
Retained placenta	33	
Placenta previa	19	
Obstetric infection	199	10
Upper genital tract	135	
Chorioamnionitis	18	
Postpartum intestinal rupture/ischemia	12	
External genitalia/perineum	4	
Other/unspecified	30	
Cerebrovascular accident	107	5
Postpartum	55	
Antepartum or intrapartum	19	
Other/unspecified	33	
Anesthesia/analgesia complication	98	5
Anoxia/hypoxia/hypoventilation	32	
Aspiration of gastric contents	28	
Cardiac arrest	25	
Other/unspecified	13	
Other and unspecified causes of maternal death	420	20
Total maternal deaths†	2067	100

†Pregnancies not associated with abortive outcomes.
(Reprinted with permission from the American College of Obstetricians and Gynecologists, Obstet Gynecol, vol 65, 1985, p. 65; supplemented with data from Cheek TG and Gutsche BB: Review: Causes of maternal mortality in the United States. Surv Anes 30:70, 1986.)

Table 4–2. PRIMARY CAUSES OF MATERNAL MORTALITY IN THE UNITED STATES, ENGLAND, AND WALES

Classification	United States 1974–1978 No.	%	Rate*	England & Wales 1979–1981 No.	%	Rate*
Embolism						
Thrombotic	271	10.9	1.7	23	13	0.9
Amniotic fluid	189	7.6	1.2	18	10	0.7
Hypertensive diseases	396	16.0	2.5	36	20	1.5
Obstetric hemorrhage	331	13.4	2.1	14	8	0.6
Obstetric infection	199	8.0	1.2	8	5	0.3
Anesthesia/analgesia complication	98	4.0	0.6	22	13	0.9
Cerebrovascular accident	107	4.3	0.7	(Included in Hypertensive Diseases)		

*Maternal deaths per 100,000 live births.
(From Kaunitz, et al,[2] and Turnbull, et al,[9] with permission.)

over 70 percent of maternal deaths.[8] However, between 1974 and 1978 infection accounted for only 8 percent of maternal deaths in the United States, and the triad currently accounts for only 36 percent.[2] Embolism (pulmonary or amniotic) now constitutes the leading cause of maternal death[2,9] (Table 4–2). In the United States, the increased percentage of deaths from embolism likely relates to improved obstetric management of the classic triad, resulting in fewer deaths from infection, hypertension, and hemorrhage and/or possible overreporting of embolism on death certificates.[2] For example, some deaths attributed to amniotic-fluid embolism in the United States were not supported by corroborative evidence obtained from maternal mortality records or autopsy reports.[2] Amniotic-fluid embolism is usually unpreventable, and medicolegal concerns may have influenced the diagnosis. In contrast, maternal deaths secondary to embolism in England and Wales[9] were confirmed histologically or at autopsy, and the MMR for amniotic-fluid embolism was one half that reported in the American study.[2]

Other factors associated with increased risk of death include delivery in small hospitals, race, and increasing maternal age.[2] When controlled for age, significantly higher maternal mortality rates are associated with the first pregnancy; increasing parity does not increase the risk of death.[8]

Method of Delivery

The risk of death associated with cesarean section decreased from 550 per 100,000 cesareans at the turn of the century[10] to approximately 300 per 100,000 in the late 1950s.[11] Recent studies[12–19] estimate 0 to 105 maternal deaths per 100,000 cesarean sections, while 0 to 62 of these deaths per 100,000 result directly from the operation (Table 4–3). These surveys also demonstrate wide variance regarding estimates of the relative risk of death for vaginal delivery (Table 4–4). The reported risk of death associated with cesarean section falls somewhere between 0 to 26 times greater than the risk associated with vaginal delivery.[9,12,13,15,17–19] The results of small studies or reports from different countries must be interpreted cautiously since differences in facilities and patient populations influence death rates. The reported risk of cesarean death probably is somewhere between two and four times the risk of vaginal delivery.[9,17]

Emergency abdominal delivery imposes major maternal risk. Emergency cesarean sections account for 12 of 13 maternal deaths[18] in Sweden and 67 of 87 in England or Wales.[9] The 1979 to 1981 England and Wales study reported a fivefold higher risk of direct maternal death following emergency cesarean section. Emergency cesarean sections account for a disproportionate number of obstetric and anesthetic deaths (Table 4–5).

Anesthesia Mortality

Unfortunately, improvements in obstetric anesthetic care have not kept pace with improvements in obstetrics. Despite reduced maternal mortality, the proportion of anesthesia-related

Table 4–3. MATERNAL MORTALITY RATE AFTER CESAREAN SECTION

Study	Years	Population	No.	Associated with C/S Deaths	Associated with C/S Rate*	Attributed to C/S Deaths	Attributed to C/S Rate*
Frigoletto et al.[15]	1968–1978	Boston Womens Hospital	10,231	0	0	0	0
Petitti et al.[19]	1975	California	41,237	8	19.4	—	—
Evrard and Gold[12]	1965–1975	Rhode Island	12,941	9	69.5	4	30.9
Rubin et al.[16]	1975–1976	Georgia	15,188	16	105.3	9	59.3
Amirikia et al.[14]	1965–1979	Hutzel Hospital	9,718	10	102.9	6	61.7
Turnbull et al.[9]	1979–1981	England & Wales	167,620	87	50.0	59	33.7
Moldin et al.[18]	1973–1979	Sweden	63,073	13	20.6	8	121.7

*Maternal deaths per 100,000 cesarean sections.

maternal deaths has increased. Airway problems during general anesthesia account for the majority of reported maternal deaths.

The triennial studies from England and Wales[7,9,20–24] provide detailed analysis of anesthesia-related maternal deaths. Difficult intubations account for a progressively larger percentage of maternal anesthetic deaths. For example, between 1973 and 1975, 23 percent of anesthetic deaths resulted from difficult intubation;[20] 53 percent of maternal deaths in the 1976 through 1978 triennium were the result of this complication.[7] During the latter period, persistent unsuccessful intubation attempts that produced fatal hypoxia or gastric aspiration, or esophageal intubation caused the majority of maternal deaths. Although the overall incidence of aspiration and difficult intubations declined in the 1979 to 1981 triennium, among 22 anesthetic deaths, eight were attributed to aspiration and eight to difficult intubation.[9] Gastric aspiration, alone or associated with difficult intubation, was the leading cause of anesthesia-related death.[9] All patients who developed fatal aspiration pneumonitis received antacid prophylaxis with the particulate antacid magnesium trisilicate[9] (see Chap. 7).

The incidence of regional anesthetic fatalities is unknown. Few regional anesthetic deaths were reported in the previously mentioned surveys, however, bupivacaine (for epidural analgesia) has been associated with 44 maternal cardiac arrests in the United States since its introduction in 1973.[25] Albright[25] estimates that the incidence of cardiac arrest approximates 1:50,000 to 1:100,000 bupivacaine anesthesias.

Similarly, no studies address the relative risks of regional and general anesthesia for parturition. Separating the inherent risks of the operative procedure from the risks of the anesthetic technique and the anesthetist's experience and skill are difficult.

Avoidable factors related to anesthesia

Table 4–4. MATERNAL DEATHS BY METHOD OF DELIVERY AND THE RELATIVE RISK OF DEATH

Study	Year	Vaginal*	Rate†	Cesarean*	Rate‡	Risk
Petitti et al.[17]	1970	204	20.4	69	113.8	5.6
Petitti et al.[17]	1974	174	15.2	72	62.9	4.1
Petitti et al.[17]	1978	100	9.8	72	40.9	4.2
Minkoff and Schwarz[13]	1977	—	17	—	108	6.4
Petitti et al.[19]	1973–1975	92	11	27	26	2.4
Evrard and Gold[12]	1965–1975	4	2.7	9	69.5	26
Frigoletto et al.[15]	1968–1978	6	7.2	0	0	0
Turnbull et al.[9]	1979–1981	229	13.4	87	50	3.7
Moldin et al.[18]	1973–1979	7	1.1	13	13	20.6

*Total maternal deaths *associated* with vaginal or cesarean delivery.
†Maternal deaths per 100,000 vaginal deliveries.
‡Maternal deaths per 100,000 cesarean sections.

Table 4–5. CESAREAN SECTION MATERNAL DEATHS ATTRIBUTED TO ANESTHETIC COMPLICATIONS

Procedure	Anesthetic Deaths	Total Cesarean Sections	Rate*
Elective cesarean	4	86,000	4.7
Emergency cesarean	15	81,000	18.5

*Maternal deaths per 100,000 cesarean sections.
(From Turnbull, et al,[9] with permission.)

deaths have increased from 50 percent of cases in 1961 to 1963, to over 90 percent in 1976 to 1978 (Table 4–6). This relative increase in preventable anesthesia mortality occurs at a time when the total maternal death rate has decreased; it results from: inexperience of the anesthetist; inadequate training and supervision of obstetric anesthesia personnel; and improper use or unavailability of necessary anesthetic equipment and monitors.[7,9]

Maternal Morbidity

LABOR PAIN

The woman's physiologic and psychologic response to severe, untreated labor pain may produce morbidity. Melzack and coworkers[26] reported excruciating pain in over 50 percent of primiparas and 40 percent of multiparas. In a Swedish study,[27] approximately 35 percent of primiparas reported severe to intolerable labor pain when interviewed after delivery, and almost 80 percent of this group were not judged by the medical personnel caring for them to have had painful labor. Prepared childbirth training primarily modifies the woman's overt response to pain but does not decrease the intensity of experienced pain.[26] Prepared childbirth training, which encourages women to believe that they will experience minimal pain, may result in significant psychologic disturbances during or after the labor period.[28,29] Thus, the failure to provide acceptable analgesia can produce undesirable changes in mother and fetus.

The physiologic responses to severe labor pain often include maternal hyperventilation,[30–33] hypoxemia between contractions,[33] excessive production of catecholamines,[34–36] increased cardiac output and blood pressure,[37,38] decreased uterine blood flow,[34,39,40] and dysfunctional labor.[34,35] Fetal effects resulting from these maternal changes include hypoxemia and heart rate abnormalities.[33]

ANESTHETIC MORBIDITY

Attempted relief of labor pain with systemic medications, regional analgesia, and prepared childbirth training may introduce additional maternal morbidity (see Chaps. 6 and 7).

Many clinicians, without substantiation, commonly attribute headache, backache, and micturition difficulties to epidural analgesia. However, the incidences of headache, backache, and urinary problems in normal vaginal deliveries performed with and without epidural analgesia are similar.[41] Crawford[42] reported a lower incidence of bladder dysfunction following epidural analgesia for vaginal delivery, while Moir and Davidson[43] reported no differences in the incidence of postpartum headache, backache,

Table 4–6. MATERNAL DEATHS DUE TO ANESTHETIC COMPLICATIONS IN ENGLAND AND WALES, 1961–1978

Year	Number of Anesthetic Deaths	Percent of True Maternal Deaths	Avoidable Factors Present (%)	Total Births	Total True Maternal Deaths
1961–1963[21]	28	4.4	50.0	2,550,252	692
1964–1966[22]	50	8.6	48.0	2,630,130	579
1967–1969[23]	50	10.9	68.0	2,457,444	455
1970–1972[24]	37	10.4	75.7	2,298,198	355
1973–1975[20]	31	13.2	90.3	1,940,689	235
1976–1978[7]	30	12.9	93.4	1,766,169	227
1979–1981[9]	29	12.6	—	1,942,859	176

or dysfunctional micturition following the use of forceps with epidural or pudendal anesthesia.

Epidural Analgesia and the First Stage of Labor

The effects of epidural analgesia on uterine contractility and the progress of labor are controversial. Many studies assess the problem but are complicated by supine positioning of the parturient and, possibly, by the addition of epinephrine to local anesthetic solutions. In early studies supine position commonly coexisted with and produced hypotension, decreased cardiac output, and uterine hypoperfusion, which impaired uterine activity.[44–47] Shellenberg[48] specifically avoided aortocaval compression and analyzed uterine activity following epidural top-up doses of bupivacaine. There were no significant changes in uterine performance. The beta effects of epinephrine decrease uterine contractility, and, in general, a 10- to 30-min reduction in uterine activity occurs following induction of epidural analgesia with local anesthetic solutions containing epinephrine,[49–53] even with the use of uterine displacement.[54]

The timing of epidural analgesia may also affect outcome. Early reports described caudal anesthesia during labor and suggested associated slowing of labor, especially if blocks were initiated early in the first stage.[55–59] However, these retrospective, uncontrolled studies allowed the supine position and the development of prolonged hypotension. Augmentation of labor with oxytocin was either not available or seldom used. Friedman and Sachtleben[59] retrospectively studied 681 women in labor and examined, among other factors, the effect of "early" administration of caudal anesthesia. They could not attribute slowing of labor to "early"-labor caudal analgesia.

Women who request epidural analgesia may have less efficient and more painful labor. When compared with women who did not request epidural analgesia, women who received epidural analgesia were found to have been admitted to the hospital with less cervical dilation and to have had longer courses of labor.[60–62] However, after initiation of the block the course of labor is similar to that of women who received no epidural analgesia.[61,62] Phillips[63] characterized labor curves in 598 women who received epidural analgesia as constant acceleration without slowing. Summarizing the previous studies; first stage epidural analgesia per se probably has little influence on labor progression.

Epidural Analgesia and the Second Stage of Labor

Epidural analgesia purportedly increases the duration of the second stage of labor and the forceps rate (see Perinatal Morbidity and Instrumental Delivery). However, early studies did not control for: different definitions of the second stage, oxytocin administration during the second stage, allowable durations of second stage prior to forceps delivery, the obstetrician's attitude concerning forceps delivery over a pain-free perineum, or the probable inclusion of more abnormal labor patterns in epidural studies. Other abnormal second-stage factors attributed to epidural analgesia include decreased uterine contractility; decreased urge and ability to push; and pelvic floor muscle relaxation, leading to abnormal fetal rotation and descent and necessitating forceps delivery.

Epidural analgesia can diminish the parturient's bearing down reflex and the reflex release of oxytocin during stretching of the cervix and vagina (Ferguson's reflex).[64–65] This decreased release of endogenous oxytocin may reduce uterine activity during stage 2. Supporting this hypothesis, Bates and associates[66] measured uterine activity during second stage labor and found activity significantly decreased in patients receiving epidural analgesia. Goodfellow and Studd[67] evaluated second-stage parameters in two groups of patients, both of whom received epidural analgesia. One group received increased oxytocin doses and delayed expulsive efforts for 1 hour or until the fetal head was visible; the other group encouraged to push immediately upon complete cervical dilation. Elective forceps deliveries followed 1 hour of pushing in both groups. Interestingly, the delayed pushing group required significantly fewer forceps deliveries. Other investigations also demonstrate that decreased uterine contractility or an impaired urge to push do not necessarily increase the forceps rate during epidural analgesia provided longer second stages of labor are allowed and/or oxytocin is administered.[60,68–75]

Many obstetricians believe that prolonged second-stage labors increase maternal and fetal morbidity and mortality. In 1952, Hellman and Prystowsky[68] reported increased postpartum hemorrhage and increased neonatal mortality when the second stage exceeded 150 min. As a result, many practitioners feel compelled to terminate stage 2 after 2 hours and condemn epidural analgesia for prolonging stage 2 labor. Cohen[69] analyzed second-stage labors in 4403 nulliparas whose fetuses were continuously monitored. Prolongation of second-stage labor in excess of 3 hours did not increase maternal or perinatal morbidity.

Even though prolonged second stages do not necessarily jeopardize the healthy mother and fetus, some authors[59,76] recommend discontinuing epidural analgesia to shorten the second stage. Hoult[76] reported a slightly lower incidence of instrument deliveries following discontinuation of epidural analgesia in the second stage, although he did not comment on the indications for his instrument deliveries and failed to randomly discontinue epidural analgesia. Thus, proper statistical analysis of effect could not be made. Two randomized, prospective studies[77,78] investigate the effect of allowing epidural analgesia to dissipate during stage 2. Phillips and Thomas[77] randomly continued or discontinued epidural analgesia in the second stage and found no prolongation of the second stage, less pain, fewer persistent fetal malrotations, and a marginally decreased forceps rate among women whose epidural analgesia was continued throughout labor and delivery. In the second study, Chestnut and coworkers[78] utilized a continuous epidural infusion of bupivacaine during labor and changed solutions to either saline or bupivacaine at 8 cm cervical dilation, in a randomized, double-blind controlled manner. The duration of second stage, the incidence of forceps deliveries, fetal acid-base values, and Apgar scores were similar in both groups.

The studies cited above demonstrate that epidural analgesia is not necessarily associated with increased maternal or fetal morbidity, especially in regards to effect on labor or method of vaginal delivery. A significant proportion of patients who request epidural analgesia have abnormal labor. Oxytocin administration when indicated, and allowing longer second stages if necessary, will result in similar outcomes for both stages of labor in women managed with and without epidural analgesia.

TRIAL OF LABOR AFTER PREVIOUS CESAREAN SECTION

In the United States, repeat cesarean sections account for much of the recent increase in the cesarean section rate.[79] The National Institutes of Health (NIH) conducted a Consensus Development Conference[79] in 1981 and recommended that vaginal birth be attempted after a previous cesarean section as a method of lowering the cesarean section rate. However, many practitioners fear the development of uterine rupture and unnecessarily elect to repeat cesarean section. Failure to distinguish between types of uterine "rupture" results in widely varied reported incidences (1:137 to 1:6107 deliveries).[80] Uterine rupture is of two general types: involvement of the entire thickness of the uterine wall, most frequently occurring in the unscarred uterus or the uterus scarred from a prior classic vertical cesarean incision and associated with pain, hemorrhage, and a high fetal and maternal mortality rate; and rupture of lower uterine segment scars, usually involving a partial separation of the uterine wall, often painless, with little or no hemorrhage, and associated with low fetal and maternal morbidity. Therefore, many obstetricians elect to allow a trial of labor following a previous cesarean section.

Flamm[81] reviewed the literature from 1980 to 1984 and reported that 86 percent of 10,000 trials of labor (TOL) resulted in vaginal births. No maternal deaths and only five fetal deaths were associated with uterine scar rupture in this survey. Shy and associates[82] studied the hypothetical risk of fetal death in 10,000 deliveries managed by either TOL or elective repeat cesarean section, and projected that elective repeat section would have produced 37 more fetal deaths than TOL.

Some clinicians, fearing that epidural analgesia will mask the pain of uterine rupture and lead to increased maternal and fetal morbidity, avoid epidural analgesia. However, only five uterine ruptures occurred in almost 800 TOL cases utilizing epidural analgesia.[81,83,84] Three of these patients experienced continuous pain despite epidural analgesia, and two patients were pain-free but fetal distress led to successful diagnosis and operative intervention. Whether pain would have been present without the epidural block is unknown. No maternal deaths occurred in this series.[81,83,84] Therefore, a trial of labor does not contraindicate epidural analgesia provided the patient care team employs continuous fetal heart rate (FHR) monitoring.

CESAREAN SECTION MORBIDITY

Maternal morbidity from cesarean section primarily relates to surgical complications. Nielsen and Hokegard[85] prospectively studied maternal outcome following cesarean section. Surgical morbidity occurred in 11.6 percent of cases. Of these sequelae, 82 percent were minor and 18 percent, major. Most complications, especially major morbidity, occurred in emergency cases (complication rate: 18.9 percent) rather than in elective procedures (4.2 percent). The factors most frequently associated with major complications in the emergency group included: station of the presenting part of the fetus, fetal prematurity (<32 weeks), previous rupture of membranes, previous cesarean section, labor prior to surgery, and an inexperienced surgeon (<2 years' training).

Infection

Infectious morbidity commonly follows cesarean section. In the first postpartum day, fever follows approximately 23 percent of abdominal deliveries and only 3.8 percent of vaginal deliveries.[86] Commonly cited risk factors for infection include protracted labor,[87–93] prolonged rupture of membranes,[90–94] internal fetal monitoring,[95,96] and general anesthesia.[97,98] However, most studies do not verify internal fetal electronic monitoring as a risk factor for postpartum infection.[90,91,93,94,98,99] Closer examination of the data[98] does not support anesthesia as a risk factor. For example, Anstey and coworkers'[98] general anesthetic group received antibiotics more often, and this factor accounted for their increased "infectious morbidity." Another study,[97] biased their conclusions by including more patients with prolonged rupture of membranes or who required emergency cesarean section in the general anesthetic group. Recent investigations[100,101] do not support an association between postoperative infection and the type of anesthesia.[100,101]

Hemorrhage

Average blood loss during vaginal and cesarean delivery is about 500 ml and 900 ml, respectively.[102] The normal physiologic expansion of maternal blood volume usually permits this degree of blood loss without requiring transfusion. Anesthesia may also influence intraoperative blood loss; regional anesthesia reportedly associated with less cesarean section blood loss[103,104] (see Chap. 6). Disregarding anesthetic method, approximately 3 percent of all cesarean section patients require transfusion[105–107] and risk factors include active bleeding, coagulopathy, oxytocin stimulation, overdistension of the uterus, and pre-eclampsia.[108]

CESAREAN SECTION/HYSTERECTOMY

Cesarean hysterectomies are classified as emergency or elective procedures. Blood loss and transfusions commonly produce morbidity in both cases. In various reports,[109–122] 12 to 92 percent of patients who undergo elective cesarean hysterectomy require transfusion and receive more blood than those who undergo cesarean section with tubal ligation.[114] Park and Duff[123] believe elective sterilization is not a valid indication for cesarean hysterectomy.

Prior to modern blood banking and antibiotics, early series reported high maternal mortality rates following cesarean hysterectomy. However, a large number of recent surveys report no maternal deaths.[112–114,116,118,121,122,124–127] Several investigators corrected maternal mortality rates for deaths related to emergency obstetric problems and compared results with those following cesarean section or abdominal hysterectomy alone. Comparable corrected mortality rates occurred in the three patient groups.[109,112,114,116,124–127]

Anesthetic Morbidity

Elective cesarean hysterectomy anesthetic complications commonly involve the increased duration of operation and hemorrhage. Cesarean hysterectomy requires almost twice the time of cesarean section. LaPlatney and O'Leary[128] reported that 22 percent of spinal anesthetics for cesarean hysterectomy require "augmentation with inhalation anesthesia because of prolonged surgery." Chestnut and Redick[129] reported similar results with epidural blockade, which initially produced satisfactory epidural anesthesia but frequently required conversion to general anesthesia intraoperatively. Although hemorrhage in the presence of sympathetic blockade induced by regional anesthesia may facilitate hypotension, none of Chestnut and Redick's[129] epidural anesthetics were converted to general anesthesia for this reason. No studies prospectively compare morbidity results with use of regional versus general anesthesia for elective cesarean hysterectomy.

ANESTHESIA AND CESAREAN SECTION

The major anesthetic complications that cause maternal morbidity are discussed in Chapter 7.

Regional or General Anesthesia?

In the United States, regional anesthesia has become the most popular method for cesarean section.[130,131] With the advent of epidural narcotics for postoperative analgesia, epidural anesthesia may become more popular. Many clinicians assume that regional anesthesia is associated with lower maternal morbidity and mortality. However, the complications of hypotension, total spinal, inadvertent intravenous administration of local anesthetics, and a higher incidence of anesthetic failure are associated with regional anesthesia, and merit consideration (see Chap. 7). Regional anesthesia may be associated with less postoperative maternal morbidity. Morgan and others[132] investigated postoperative morbidity following both regional and general anesthesia for elective cesarean section. Earlier mobilization and breast feeding, and less immediate postoperative pain and discomfort occurred in the epidural group. Fewer mothers receiving regional anesthesia were coughing, febrile, lethargic, or depressed by the 6th postoperative day.

Perinatal Mortality

In the United States, most studies underreport perinatal deaths.[133] However, between 1950 and 1981, the perinatal death rate declined from 32.5 to 12.6 per 1000 births. Between the years 1970 and 1980, 55 percent of the perinatal deaths in the United States involved neonates, of whom 84 percent expired within the first 6 days of life.[133-136]

The highest mortality in the United States exists among nonwhites. In 1981, the perinatal mortality for whites was 11.3 compared with 17.5 for other races.[137] Premature and low-birth-weight infants contribute significantly to the high perinatal mortality in the nonwhite population; low-birth-weight infants comprise 75 percent of all neonatal deaths.[137] Only 6 percent of white neonates weighed less than 2500 g, compared with 11 percent of babies of other races.[137]

Since 1983 neonatal mortality (birth to 28 days of age) has declined, while postneonatal mortality (28 days to 11 months) remains essentially unchanged.[138] Congenital anomalies are the leading cause of infant mortality, followed by sudden infant death (SIDS), respiratory distress, and prematurity. Peripartum hypoxia and birth trauma comprise only 3.3 percent of all infant deaths (Table 4–7).

Most of the recent decline in neonatal deaths result from decreased mortality rates in low- to very-low-birth-weight infants,[139-142] indicating greatly improved care of these babies. Antenatal referral of parturients to high-risk perinatal centers accounts for these encouraging results.[143,144] Paneth and others[145] remark that perinatal outcome parallels the obstetric and perinatal capabilities of the hospital. Iowa has an extensive regional health care system, with level 1, 2, 3 (tertiary) hospitals throughout the state. Hein and Brown[146] reviewed neonatal deaths in Iowa between the years of 1978 to 1979 and noted that approximately one half of all perinatal deaths occurred in level 1 facilities and were potentially preventable. Fatal perinatal asphyxia comprised 23 percent of deaths in level 1 institutions compared with only 3 percent of deaths in level 3 hospitals. A subsequent review[147] of outcome in 1982 to 1983 showed that referral of high-risk obstetric patients to

Table 4–7. INFANT MORTALITY*: SELECTED CAUSES OF DEATH

Age and Cause of Death	1984 (est.)	1983 (est.)	1982	1979
Total				
<1 year	1060	1091	1152	1307
<28 days	686	727	770	887
28 days–11 months	374	365	382	420
Congenital anomalies	228	232	245	255
Sudden infant death syndrome	132	130	143	151
Respiratory distress syndrome	104	101	110	156
Disorders of low birth weight (or prematurity)	93	93	98	100
Intrauterine hypoxia and birth asphyxia	26	32	41	40
Birth trauma	9	12	17	32

*Rates per 100,000 live births
(From National Center for Health Statistics,[138] with permission.)

level 2 and 3 centers markedly improved the neonatal mortality in level 1 hospitals. During this period 78 percent of all very-low-birth-weight infants were delivered in level 2 and 3 centers. However, asphyxia still accounted for 18.4 percent of neonatal deaths in level 1 hospitals compared to 9.9 percent in level 2 units.

Perinatal Morbidity

In 1980, there were over 63,000 perinatal deaths in the United States. Of the 3,412,000 children born alive, 18,000 to 23,000 suffered from severe mental retardation or physical handicaps resulting from cerebral palsy.[148] Assessments of fetal and neonatal morbidity are fallible. Electronic fetal monitoring (EFM), fetal scalp pH measurements, Apgar scores, and neurobehavior scores are frequently cited as objective measurements of perinatal outcome. However, the sensitivity and specificity of these evaluations must be understood when considering the effects of obstetric and anesthetic interventions.

ASPHYXIA

Perinatal asphyxia strongly correlates with increased mortality rates at all gestational ages and weights.[149–152] However, the incidence of neurologic impairment and death decreases with increasing gestational age.[153]

Estimates of significant long-term neurologic handicaps resulting from perinatal asphyxia vary from 6 to 22 percent.[154] Scott[155] retrospectively studied infants with Apgar scores of zero at 1 min or failure to establish spontaneous respirations within 20 min of birth. Fifty-two percent of the infants died. Initial neurologic problems occurred in 87 percent of the 23 surviving infants; however, 17 of the 23 survivors were neurologically normal on long-term follow-up. Obviously, perinatal hypoxia does not correlate well with long-term morbidity.[156–159]

Also controversial is the role perinatal asphyxia plays in the development of cerebral palsy. Nelson and Ellenberg[160] recently published an extensive, multivariate analysis of the antecedent risks for cerebral palsy in 54,000 pregnancies. Asphyxia correlated poorly with cerebral palsy. Prenatal risk factors accounted for 34 percent of cases of cerebral palsy, while intrapartum and neonatal events accounted for only 3 percent of the children with cerebral palsy. Prediction of infants at risk for cerebral palsy proved equally difficult. For example, only 2.8 percent of the infants at highest risk developed cerebral palsy; a 97-percent false-positive rate. Nelson and Ellenberg[160] concluded, "We probably do not know what causes most cases of cerebral palsy."

INSTRUMENT DELIVERY

As was previously discussed, some authors believe that epidural analgesia increases the forceps delivery rate. The perinatal consequences of forceps delivery have been greatly exaggerated in the press. Significant maternal or fetal morbidity does not result from the use of low or outlet forceps.[161–164] Similarly, when controlled for asphyxia, mid-forceps delivery does not influence short- or long-term perinatal morbidity and mortality.[164–167] The incidence of neonatal acidosis and low Apgar scores are comparable following matched cesarean section and mid-forceps deliveries performed electively or urgently (fetal distress).[164] Moreover, when compared with mid-forceps delivery, abdominal delivery does not reduce the incidence of birth trauma.[164,166,167] Contrary to a poorly controlled report by Freedman and associates,[162] most studies do not associate mid-forceps delivery with long-term impairment of childhood neurologic development or intelligence scores,[168–174] and well-selected forceps deliveries do not increase perinatal risk. Avoidance of epidural analgesia should not be based upon the fear of newborn effects of forceps delivery.

ELECTRONIC FETAL MONITORING

Perinatal mortality has improved since the advent of continuous electronic fetal monitoring (EFM). The incidence of unexpected stillbirths in labors monitored by auscultation every 30 min approximates 10 per 1000;[175] the incidence decreases to only 1 per 10,000 in continuously monitored labors.[176] EFM significantly reduces the incidence of intrapartum stillbirths and neonatal deaths.

Abnormal FHR tracings produce a high false-positive rate, resulting in the birth of normal infants 50 percent of the time,[177–180] and the majority of infants have no umbilical cord acidosis.[181–183] However, timely intervention based upon abnormal FHR tracings may avert the development of fetal acidosis. In contrast, 99 percent of infants with normal FHR tracings have normal 5-min Apgar scores.[177,184]

The value of EFM in high-risk parturients is generally accepted but debated in the "normal" laboring patient (see Chap. 3). Leveno and coworkers[185] prospectively evaluated the outcome of 35,000 labors using EFM for all patients or only the high-risk parturients (alternating months). The incidence of intrapartum stillbirths, low Apgar scores, the need for assisted ventilation of the newborn, admission to the intensive care nursery, and neonatal seizures were similar in both groups. This study found no further improvement in neonatal outcome with universal EFM. In fact, they reported a small, but statistically significant, increase in cesarean sections performed for fetal distress in the universal monitoring group.

EFM does decrease the incidence of intrapartum stillbirths and neonatal death in most studies. The high-risk parturient probably benefits from fetal monitoring, but the benefit of continuous monitoring in normal labors is less clear (see Chap. 3).

FETAL ACIDOSIS

Fetal pH values and metabolic acidosis reliably indicate the degree of perinatal asphyxia (see Chap. 3). Intrapartum fetal scalp pH values are recommended by many authorities to confirm the diagnosis of fetal distress based upon abnormal EFM tracings.[185–188] Seventy percent of infants with a scalp pH less than 7.20 have Apgar scores less than seven at 1 min.[178,189] Fetal acidosis exists in no more than 48 percent of cases in which EFM tracings suggest fetal distress.[178,190–192] This finding implies that the combined use of EFM and fetal scalp sampling increases the reliability of detecting significant fetal compromise. However, since no large prospective studies evaluate long-term outcome of transient neonatal acidosis, pH values are primarily utilized as an indicator of short-term fetal compromise.

APGAR SCORES

Many studies have evaluated Apgar scores and their relation to long-term outcome. Although originally designed to identify the depressed, mature neonate, Apgar scores are now inappropriately applied as a prognostic indicator. Table 4–8 shows the neonatal death rate associated with different Apgar scores and birth weights. As expected, low Apgar scores relate to an increased risk of death. However, low-birth-weight infants are significantly more likely to die than infants weighing more than 2500 g. An Apgar score of zero to three 20 min after delivery is associated with a 96 percent fatality rate in the low-birth-weight group compared with a rate of 59 percent in larger infants (>2500 g). These data show that other factors, besides the sole use of Apgar scores, influence risk of death, and that the predictive value of Apgar

Table 4–8. DISTRIBUTION OF APGAR SCORES AND DEATH RATES BY BIRTH WEIGHT

Time Period (*min*)	Birth Weight (*g*)	Apgar Score 0–3			Apgar Score 4–6			Apgar Score 7–10		
		No.	%	*Death 1st Yr** (%)	*No.*	%	*Death 1st Yr** (%)	*No.*	%	*Death 1st Yr** (%)
1	<2,500	762	15.5	48.2	969	19.7	14.2	3,186	64.8	3.8
	>2,500	2,002	4.5	5.6	5,783	13.1	1.6	36,298	82.3	0.9
5	<2,500	381	7.6	74.5	495	9.9	30.1	4,105	82.4	4.5
	>2,500	399	0.9	15.5	1,071	2.4	5.7	43,047	96.7	1.0
10	<2,500	235	17.5	85.5	299	22.3	43.8	806	60.2	10.5
	>2,500	122	2.5	34.4	345	7.1	12.5	4,370	90.4	1.8
15	<2,500	170	21.0	91.8	165	20.4	51.5	473	58.5	14.2
	>2,500	59	2.7	52.5	187	8.5	20.9	1,947	88.9	2.4
20	<2,500	139	22.5	95.7	121	19.6	57.0	357	57.9	14.8
	>2,500	39	2.2	59.0	112	6.4	23.2	1,593	91.3	2.4

*Comparison of death rates between birth weights—significant ($p < 0.001$) for all comparisons
(Data modified from Nelson and Ellenberg,[160] with permission.)

scores increases with time of assessment following delivery.

Apgar scores also poorly predict neonatal morbidity. Clinicians greatly overestimate handicaps for surviving infants with a 5-min Apgar score of three or less.[193] Severe acidosis, as measured by cord blood samples, correlates poorly with 1-min Apgar scores less than seven[181,194,195] and less than half the infants with 5-min Apgar scores less than seven have umbilical artery acidosis.[196]

In summary, Apgar scores do not reliably predict long-term neonatal morbidity or even acute acidosis. Rather they qualitatively measure basic reflexes and generalized neonatal depression or immaturity. Low Apgar scores, however, are predictive of neonatal mortality.

NEUROBEHAVIORAL SCORES

Neurobehavioral scoring systems assess the newborn's reflexes, motor tone, and behavior. Apgar scores and the presence of acidosis reflect only significant abnormalities and may not reveal more subtle neonatal changes. Although over 70 published studies use neurobehavioral testing, the results are often poorly controlled and contradictory. Additionally, no long-term studies assess the predictive value of neurobehavioral scoring systems. The importance of a presumed abnormal test result remains vague. Scanlon and coworkers[197] reported lower neurobehavioral scores in babies whose mothers received epidural block with lidocaine or mepivacaine. Women who received spinal anesthesia or local infiltration served as the control group, while nine cases in which lidocaine was used and 19 cases in which mepivacaine was used were combined into another group. Poor controls in this study permitted variable utilization of systemic maternal analgesics and sedatives and failed to compare infant neurobehavioral scores between the lidocaine, mepivacaine and spinal and local infiltration groups. Combining different local anesthetics into an "epidural" group and different delivery anesthetics into a "control" group biased this study. Following this poorly controlled study lidocaine and mepivacaine use decreased dramatically in obstetrics. Subsequent investigators[198–200] did not document different scores following lidocaine use compared with other local anesthetics. Lidocaine has enjoyed a resurgence of popularity for obstetric anesthesia. Major clinical decisions should not be based upon minor differences in neurobehavioral scores.

ANESTHESIA MORBIDITY

Several anesthetic factors influence perinatal morbidity: uterine displacement, maternal hypoxia and hyperoxia, induction-to-delivery (I–D) time, uterine incision-to-delivery (U–D) time, and hypotension. Uterine displacement prior to and during cesarean section improves neonatal oxygenation,[201,202] Apgar scores,[203] and acid-base status.[202–204] Left uterine tilt usually proves more effective than right uterine tilt.[103,205] Increased maternal arterial oxygenation improves fetal oxygen content,[206–209] which should theoretically increase fetal oxygen reserve during apnea and stress. However, evidence for improved morbidity is lacking, especially since many early studies purporting decreased 1-min Apgar scores in the absence of hyperoxygenation failed to control for other variables such as I–D time, U–D time, anesthetic agents, and uterine displacement. Although there is no conclusive information, most clinicians facilitate maternal and fetal hyperoxia, believing there is little potential for harm.

Many early reports concluded that longer anesthetic I–D times increased perinatal morbidity.[210–217] However, the use of the supine position, rather than anesthesia, could have produced these results. Depressed 1-min Apgar scores without corresponding fetal acidemia may also represent transient neonatal sedation following long I–D times during general anesthesia with nitrous oxide.[218] Crawford and associates,[219–221] employed table tilt and found no consistent deterioration in neonatal clinical status with I–D times of 10 to 30 min. In contrast, other investigators report that shorter I–D intervals (6 to 8 min) are associated with improved 1-min Apgar scores.[215–217] Prolonged U–D times may partially explain the confusion surrounding I–D times. Low 1-min Apgar scores and fetal acidemia are associated with U–D times exceeding 90 to 180 sec during general anesthesia and 180 sec during regional anesthesia.[217,218,221] Consequently, most authorities hold prolonged U–D intervals, rather than I–D times, as the most important factor in neonatal outcome.

Well-conducted anesthesia for cesarean section should not influence neonatal morbidity. Recent studies[103,222–225] comparing effects of regional and general anesthesia find no statistically significant differences in neonatal acid-base status or the incidence of low Apgar scores. Regional anesthesia has been traditionally regarded as relatively contraindicated for cases of fetal distress. Marx and coworkers[226] recently challenged this position, demonstrating comparable neonatal acid-base values and Apgar scores following the use of regional or general anesthesia for cesarean section indicated by fetal distress. The choice of anesthesia was based solely upon the mother's wishes, and the time from operative decision to incision was comparable in both anesthetic groups. Other confirmatory studies are required to confirm that well-conducted regional anesthesia for fetal distress produces comparable perinatal outcome.

Summary

Although maternal mortality and morbidity are declining, complications still occur. Improved obstetric and anesthetic care should further reduce maternal complications. Anesthetic care in particular, must be improved to minimize morbidity since it has lagged behind obstetric care. Unlike maternal morbidity and mortality, perinatal complications often occur without a single, identifiable precipitating event, and assessing potential morbidity is equally difficult. Recognizing the high-risk, complicated parturient and transporting her to an institution capable of providing advanced obstetric, anesthetic, and neonatal care will reduce maternal and fetal complications.

References

1. Rubin, G, et al: The risk of childbearing reevaluated. Am J Public Health 71:712, 1981.
2. Kaunitz, AM, et al: Causes of maternal mortality in the United States. Obstet Gynecol 65:605, 1985.
3. Friede, AM and Rochat, RW: Maternal mortality and perinatal mortality: An epidemiologic perspective. In Sachs, B (ed): Clinical Obstetrics: A Public Health Perspective. PSG Inc, Littleton, MA, 1986, p 1.
4. MMWR: Pilot surveillance in seven states. JAMA 255:184, 1986.
5. Jow-Ching Tu, E: Cohort maternal mortality: New York, 1917–1972. Am J Public Health 69:1052, 1979.
6. Steinberg, WM and Farine, D: Maternal mortality in Ontario from 1970 to 1980. Obstet Gynecol 66:510, 1985.
7. Tomkinson, J, et al: Report on Confidential Enquiries into Maternal Deaths in England and Wales 1976–1978. Her Majesty's Stationery Office, London, 1982, p 1.
8. Schaffner, W, et al: Maternal mortality in Michigan: An epidemiologic analysis, 1950–1971. Am J Public Health 67:821, 1977.
9. Turnbull, AC, et al: Report on Confidential Enquiries into Maternal Deaths in England and Wales 1979–1981. Her Majesty's Stationery Office, London, 1986, p 1.
10. Williams, JW: A critical analysis of twenty-one years' experience with cesarean section. Bull Johns Hopkins Hosp 32:173, 1921.
11. Johnell, HE: Cesarean section: A ten-year study. Acta Obstet Gynecol Scand 51:231, 1972.
12. Evrard, JR and Gold, EM: Cesarean section and maternal mortality in Rhode Island: Incidence and risk factors, 1965–1975. Obstet Gynecol 50:594, 1977.
13. Minkoff, HL and Schwarz, RH: The rising cesarean section rate: Can it safely be reversed? Obstet Gynecol 56:135, 1980.
14. Amirikia, H, Zarewych, B and Evans, TN: Cesarean section: A 15-year review of changing incidence, indications, and risks. Am J Obstet Gynecol 140:81, 1981.
15. Frigoletto, FS, Ryan, KJ and Rhillippe, M: Maternal mortality rate associated with cesarean section: An appraisal. Am J Obstet Gynecol 136:969, 1980.
16. Rubin, GL, et al: Maternal death after cesarean section in Georgia. Am J Obstet Gynecol 139:681, 1981.
17. Petitti, DB, et al: In-hospital maternal mortality in the United States: Time trends and relation to method of delivery. Obstet Gynecol 59:6, 1982.
18. Moldin, P, Hokegard, K and Nielsen TF: Cesarean section and maternal mortality in Sweden 1973–1979. Acta Obstet Gynecol Scand 63:7, 1984.
19. Petitti, D, Olson, RO and Williams, RL: Cesarean section in California: 1960 through 1975. Am J Obstet Gynecol 133:391, 1979.
20. Tomkinson, J, et al: Report on Confidential Enquiries into Maternal Deaths in England and Wales 1973–1975. Her Majesty's Stationery Office, London, 1979, p 1.
21. Walker, AL, et al: Report on Confidential Enquiries into Maternal Deaths in England and Wales 1961–1963. Her Majesty's Stationery Office, London, 1966, p 1.
22. Arthure, H, et al: Report on Confidential Enquiries into Maternal Deaths in England and Wales 1964–1966. Her Majesty's Stationery Office, London, 1969, p 1.
23. Arthure, H, et al: Report on Confidential Enquiries into Maternal Deaths in England and Wales 1967–1969. Her Majesty's Stationery Office, London, 1972, p 1.

24. Arthure, H, et al: Report on Confidential Enquiries into Maternal Deaths in England and Wales 1970–1972. Her Majesty's Stationery Office, London, 1975, p 1.
25. Albright, GA: Local anesthetics. In Albright, GA, Ferguson, JE II, Joyce, TH III, and Stevenson, DK (eds): Anesthesia in Obstetrics. Butterworth & Co., Boston, 1986, 115.
26. Melzack, R, Taenzer, P, Feldman, P and Kinch, RA: Labour is still painful after prepared childbirth training. Can Med Assoc J 125:367, 1981.
27. Nettlebladt, P, Fagerstrom, CF and Uddenberg, N: The significance of reported childbirth pain. Journal of Psychosomatic Research 20:215, 1976.
28. Stewart, DE: Psychiatric symptoms following attempted natural childbirth. Can Med Assoc J 127:713, 1982.
29. Lumley, J and Astbury, J: Birth Rites, Birth Rights. Sphere Books, Melbourne, 1980.
30. Gemzell, CA, Tillinger, K and Westman, A: Observations on circulatory changes and muscular work in normal labour. Acta Obstet Gynecol Scand 36:75, 1957.
31. Bonica, JJ: Maternal respiratory changes during pregnancy and parturition. In Marx, GF (ed): Parturition and Perinatology. FA Davis, Philadelphia, 1973, p 1.
32. Peabody, JL: Transcutaneous oxygen measurement to evaluate drug effect. Clin Perinatol 6:109, 1979.
33. Huch, A, et al: Continuous transcutaneous monitoring of foetal oxygen tension during labour. Br J Obstet Gynaecol 84S:1, 1977.
34. Lederman, RP, et al: Endogenous plasma epinephrine and norepinephrine in last-trimester pregnancy and labour. Am J Obstet Gynecol 129:5, 1977.
35. Lederman, RP, et al: The relationship of maternal anxiety, plasma catecholamines, and plasma cortisol to progress in labour. Am J Obstet Gynecol 132:495, 1978.
36. Shnider, SM, et al: Maternal catecholamines decrease during labor after lumbar epidural anesthesia. Am J Obstet Gynecol 147:13, 1983.
37. Ueland, K and Hansen, JM: Maternal cardiovascular dynamics: II. Posture and uterine contractions. Am J Obstet Gynecol 103:1, 1969.
38. Ueland, K and Hansen, JM: Maternal cardiovascular dynamics: III. Labor and delivery under local and caudal analgesia. Am J Obstet Gynecol 103:8, 1969.
39. Morishima, HO, Hey, M-N and James, LS: Reduced uterine blood flow and fetal hypoxemia with acute maternal stress: Experimental observation in the pregnant baboon. Am J Obstet Gynecol 134:270, 1979.
40. Shnider, SM, et al: Uterine blood flow and plasma norepinephrine changes during maternal stress in the pregnant ewe. Anesthesiology 50:524, 1979.
41. Jouppila, R, et al: Segmental epidural analgesia and postpartum sequelae. Ann Chir Gynaecol 67:85, 1978.
42. Crawford, JS: Lumbar epidural block in labour: A clinical analysis. Br J Anaesth 44:66, 1972.
43. Moir, DD and Davidson, S: Postpartum complications of forceps delivery performed under epidural and pudendal nerve block. Br J Anaesth 44:1197, 1972.
44. Vasicka, A, et al: Spinal and epidural anesthesia, fetal and uterine response to acute hypo- and hypertension. Am J Obstet Gynecol 90:800, 1964.
45. Milson, L, et al: Measurement of cardiac stroke volume by impedance cardiography in the last trimester of pregnancy. Acta Obstet Gynecol Scand 62:473, 1983.
46. Marx, GF, Gusain, FJ and Shiau, HF: Brachial and femoral blood pressures during prenatal period. Am J Obstet Gynecol 136:11, 1980.
47. Weaver, JB, Pearson, JF and Rosen, M: Posture and epidural block in pregnant women at term: Effects on arterial blood pressure and limb blood flow. Anaesthesia 30:752, 1975.
48. Shellenberg, JC: Uterine activity during lumbar epidural analgesia with bupivacaine. Am J Obstet Gynecol 127:26, 1977.
49. Lowenshon, RI, Paul, RH and Fales, S: Intrapartum epidural anesthesia: An evaluation of effects on uterine activity. Obstet Gynecol 44:388, 1974.
50. Craft, JB, Epstein, BS and Coakley, CS: Effect of lidocaine with epinephrine versus lidocaine (plain) on induced labor. Anesth Analg 51:243, 1972.
51. Raabe, N and Belfrage, P: Epidural analgesia in labour. IV. Influence on uterine activity and fetal heart rate. Acta Obstet Gynecol Scand 55:305, 1976.
52. Zador, G and Nilsson, BA: Low dose intermittent epidural anaesthesia with lidocaine for vaginal delivery. II: Influence on labour and foetal acid-base status. Acta Obstet Gynecol Scand [Suppl] 134:17, 1974.
53. Zador, G and Nilsson, BA: Continuous drip lumbar epidural anaesthesia with lidocaine for vaginal delivery. II: Influence on labour and foetal acid-base status. Acta Obstet Gynecol Scand [Suppl] 34:41, 1974.
54. Jouppila, P, et al: Fetal heart rate patterns and uterine activity after segmental epidural analgesia. Br J Obstet Gynaecol 84:481, 1977.
55. Nicodemus, RE, Ritmiller, LF and Ledden, LF: Continuous caudal analgesia in obstetrics on trial. Am J Obstet Gynecol 50:312, 1945.
56. Siever, JM and Mousel, LH: Continuous caudal anesthesia: Three hundred unselected obstetric cases. JAMA 122:424, 1943.
57. Ritmiller, LF and Rippmann, ET: Caudal analgesia in obstetrics: Report of thirteen years' experience. Obstet Gynecol 9:25, 1957.
58. Friedman, EA and Sachtleben, MR: Dysfunctional labor. II: Protracted active-phase dilatation in the nullipara. Obstet Gynecol 17:566, 1961.
59. Friedman, EA and Sachtleben, MR: Caudal anesthesia: The factors that influence its effect on labor. Obstet Gynecol 13:442, 1959.
60. Studd, JW, et al: The effect of lumbar epidural analgesia on the rate of cervical dilatation and the outcome of labour of spontaneous onset. Br J Obstet Gynaecol 87:1015, 1980.
61. Willdeck-Lund, G, Lindmark, G and Nilsson, BA: Effect of segmental epidural block on the course of

labour and the condition of the infant during the neonatal period. Acta Anaesthesiol Scand 23:301, 1979.
62. Jouppila, R, et al: Segmental epidural analgesia in labour: Related to the progress of labour, fetal malposition and instrumental delivery. Acta Obstet Gynecol Scand 58:135, 1979.
63. Phillips, JC, et al: Epidural analgesia and its effects on the "normal" progress of labor. Am J Obstet Gynecol 129:316, 1977.
64. Ferguson, JK: A study of the motility of the intact uterus at term. Surg Gynecol Obstet 73:359, 1941.
65. Goodfellow, CF, et al: Oxytocin deficiency at delivery with epidural analgesia. Br J Obstet Gynaecol 90:214, 1983.
66. Bates, RG, et al: Uterine activity in the second stage of labour and the effect of epidural analgesia. Br J Obstet Gynaecol 92:1246, 1985.
67. Goodfellow, CF and Studd, C: The reduction of forceps in primagravidae with epidural analgesia: A controlled trial. Br J Clin Pract 33:287, 1979.
68. Hellman, LM and Prystowsky, H: The duration of the second stage of labor. Am J Obstet Gynecol 63:1223, 1952.
69. Cohen, WR: Influence of the duration of second stage labor on perinatal outcome and puerperal morbidity. Obstet Gynecol 49:266, 1977.
70. Crawford, JS: Letter to the Editor. Br J Obstet Gynaecol 88:685, 1981.
71. Maresh, M, Choong, KH and Beard, RW: Delayed pushing with lumbar epidural analgesia in labour. Br J Obstet Gynaecol 90:623, 1983.
72. Hibbard, B, et al: Lumbar epidural analgesia in labour (correspondence). Br Med J i:286, 1987.
73. Friedman, EA: Letter to the Editor. Br J Obstet Gynaecol 88:464, 1981.
74. McQueen, J and Mylrea, L: Lumbar epidural analgesia in labour (correspondence). Br Med J i:640, 1977.
75. Bakhoum, S, Lewis, BV and Tipton, RH: Lumbar epidural analgesia in labour (correspondence). Br Med J i:641, 1977.
76. Hoult, IJ, MacLennan, AH and Carrie, LES: Lumbar epidural analgesia in labour: Relation to fetal malposition and instrumental delivery. Br Med J i:14, 1977.
77. Phillips, KC and Thomas, TA: Second stage of labour with or without extradural analgesia. Anaesthesia 38:972, 1983.
78. Chestnut, DH, et al: The influence of continuous epidural bupivacaine analgesia on progress of the second stage of labor: A randomized, double-blind, placebo-controlled study. Anesthesiology 65:A383, 1986.
79. The Cesarean Birth Task Force: National Institutes of Health consensus development statement on cesarean childbirth. Obstet Gynecol 57:537, 1981.
80. Beacham, W, Beacham, D, Webster, H and Fielding, S: Rupture of the uterus at New Orleans Charity Hospital. Am J Obstet Gynecol 106:1083, 1970.
81. Flamm, BL: Vaginal birth after cesarean section: Controversies old and new. Clin Obstet Gynecol 28:735, 1985.
82. Shy, KK, Logerfo, JP and Karp, LE: Evaluation of elective repeat cesarean section as a standard of care. Am J Obstet Gynecol 139:123, 1981.
83. Carlsson, C, Nybell-Lindahl, G and Ingemarsson, I: Extradural block in patients who have previously undergone caesarean section. Br J Anaesth 52:827, 1980.
84. Rudick, V, et al: Epidural analgesia for planned vaginal delivery following previous cesarean section. Obstet Gynecol 64:621, 1984.
85. Nielsen, TF and Hokegard, KH: Cesarean section and intraoperative surgical complications. Acta Obstet Gynecol Scand 63:103, 1984.
86. Filker, R and Monif, GR: The significance of temperature during the first 24 hours post-partum. Obstet Gynecol 53:358, 1979.
87. Gibbs, RS: Clinical risk factors for puerperal infection. Obstet Gynecol 55:178S, 1980.
88. D'Angelo, LJ and Sokol, RJ: Time-related peripartum determinants of postpartum morbidity. Obstet Gynecol 55:319, 1980.
89. Gibbs, RS, Listwa, HM and Read, JA: The effect of internal fetal monitoring on maternal infection following cesarean section. Obstet Gynecol 48:653, 1976.
90. Gibbs, RS, Jones, PM and Wilder, CJ: Internal fetal monitoring and maternal infection following cesarean section: A prospective study. Obstet Gynecol 52:193, 1976.
91. Rehu, M and Nilsson, CG: Risk factors for febrile morbidity associated with cesarean section. Obstet Gynecol 56:269, 1980.
92. Nielson, TF and Hokegard, KH: Postoperative cesarean section morbidity: A prospective study. Am J Obstet Gynecol 146:911, 1983.
93. Hawrylsyshyn, PA, Bernstein, P and Papsin, FR: Risk factors associated with infection following cesarean section. Am J Obstet Gynecol 139:294, 1981.
94. Ott, WJ: Primary cesarean section: Factors related to postpartum infection. Obstet Gynecol 57:171, 1981.
95. Perloe, M and Curet, LB: The effect of internal fetal monitoring on cesarean section morbidity. Obstet Gynecol 53:354, 1979.
96. Hagen, D: Maternal febrile morbidity associated with fetal monitoring and cesarean section. Obstet Gynecol 46:260, 1975.
97. Green, SL and Felix, SA: Risk factors associated with post cesarean section febrile morbidity. Obstet Gynecol 49:686, 1977.
98. Anstey, JT, Sheldon, GW and Blythe, JG: Infectious morbidity after primary cesarean sections in a private institution. Am J Obstet Gynecol 136:205, 1980.
99. Gassner, CB and Ledger, WJ: The relationship of hospital-acquired maternal infection to invasive intrapartum monitoring techniques. Am J Obstet Gynecol 126:33, 1976.
100. Chestnut, DH: Effect of anesthesia for repeat cesarean section of postoperative infectious morbidity. Obstet Gynecol 66:199, 1985.
101. Chestnut, DH and Noe, AL: Effect of anesthesia for primary cesarean section on postoperative febrile and infectious morbidity. Abstract presented to the Society for Obstetric Anesthesia and Perinatology (SOAP). Annual Meeting May 16, 1986.

102. Prichard, JA, et al: Blood volume changes in pregnancy and the puerperium. Am J Obstet Gynecol 84:1271, 1962.
103. James, FM III, et al: A comparison of general anaesthesia and lumbar epidural analgesia for elective cesarean section. Anesth Analg 56:228, 1977.
104. Moir, DD: Anaesthesia for caesarean section: An evaluation of a method using low concentrations of halothane and 50 per cent of oxygen. Br J Anaesth 42:136, 1970.
105. Patten, E and Alperin, JB: Type and screen: A safe and effective preoperative blood ordering policy with emphasis on its use in obstetrics and gynecology. Am J Obstet Gynecol 142:563, 1982.
106. Hill, ST and Lavin, JP: Blood ordering in obstetrics and gynecology: Recommendations for the type and screen. Obstet Gynecol 62:236, 1983.
107. Reisner, LS: Type and screen for cesarean section: A prudent alternative. Anesthesiology 58:476, 1983.
108. Danforth, DN: Cesarean section. JAMA 253:811, 1985.
109. Pletsch, TD and Sandberg, EC: Cesarean hysterectomy for sterilization. Am J Obstet Gynecol 85:254, 1963.
110. Alford, CD, Miller, AC and Simpson, JW: Cesarean section hysterectomy. A ten-year study. Am J Obstet Gynecol 82:644, 1961.
111. Prevedourakis, CN: Emergency cesarean hysterectomy. Int Surg 59:33, 1974.
112. Easterday, CL: Cesarean hysterectomy at the Boston Hospital for Women. Clin Obstet Gynecol 12:652, 1969.
113. Brenner, P, Sall, S and Sonnenblick, B: Evaluation of cesarean section hysterectomy as a sterilization procedure. Am J Obstet Gynecol 108:335, 1970.
114. Barclay, DL, et al: Elective cesarean hysterectomy: A five-year comparison with cesarean section. Am J Obstet Gynecol 124:900, 1976.
115. Morton, JH: Cesarean hysterectomy. Am J Obstet Gynecol 83:422, 1962.
116. Mickal, A, Begneaud, WP and Hawes, TP: Pitfalls and complications of cesarean section hysterectomy. Clin Obstet Gynecol 12:660, 1969.
117. Clark, SL, et al: Emergency hysterectomy for obstetric hemorrhage. Obstet Gynecol 64:376, 1984.
118. McNulty, JV: Elective cesarean hysterectomy: Revisited. Am J Obstet Gynecol 149:29, 1984.
119. Plauche, WC, et al: Cesarean hysterectomy at Louisiana State University, 1975 through 1981. South Med J 76:1261, 1983.
120. Sturdee, DW, Rushton, DI: Caesarean and post-partum hysterectomy 1968–1983. Br J Obstet Gynaecol 93:270, 1986.
121. Plauche, WC, Gruich, FG and Bourgeois, MO: Hysterectomy at the time of cesarean section: Analysis of 108 cases. Obstet Gynecol 58:459, 1981.
122. Chestnut, DH, et al: Peripartum hysterectomy: A review of cesarean and postpartum hysterectomy. Obstet Gynecol 65:365, 1985.
123. Park, RC and Duff, WP: Role of cesarean hysterectomy in modern obstetric practice. Clin Obstet Gynecol 23:601, 1980.
124. Aaro, LA and Saed, F: Low incidence cesarean section. Mayo Clin Proc 50:365, 1975.
125. Hofmeister, FJ: Tubal ligation versus cesarean hysterectomy. Clin Obstet Gynecol 12:676, 1969.
126. Langer, R, et al: Comparison of sterilization by tubal ligation and hysterectomy. Surg Gynecol Obstet 140:235, 1975.
127. Schneider, GT and Tyrone, CH: Cesarean hysterectomy. Surg Gynecol Obstet 130:501, 1970.
128. LaPlatney, DR and O'Leary, JA: Anesthetic considerations in cesarean hysterectomy. Anesth Analg 49:328, 1970.
129. Chestnut, DH and Redick, LF: Continuous epidural anesthesia for elective cesarean hysterectomy. South Med J 78:1168, 1985.
130. Gibbs, CP, et al: Obstetric anesthesia: A national survey. Anesthesiology 65:298, 1986.
131. Spielman, FJ and Corke, BC: Advantages and disadvantages of regional anesthesia for cesarean section. J Reprod Med 30:832, 1985.
132. Morgan, BM, et al: Anaesthetic morbidity following caesarean section under epidural or general anaesthesia. Lancet 1:328, 1984.
133. Kleinman, JC: Underreporting of infant deaths: Then and now (editorial). Am J Pub Health 76:365, 1986.
134. National Center for Health Statistics: Final mortality statistics, 1970. Monthly Vital Statistics Report 22(11):Suppl. Public Health Service Publication No. (HRA) 74-1120, Rockville, MD, 1974.
135. National Center for Health Statistics: Final mortality statistics, 1975. Monthly Vital Statistics Report 25(11):Suppl. Public Health Service Publication No. (HRA) 77-1120, Rockville, MD, 1977.
136. National Center for Health Statistics: Health, United States, 1983. Public Health Service Publication No. (HRA) 84-1232, Washington, DC, 1983.
137. Powell-Griner, E: Perinatal mortality in the United States: 1950–1981. Monthly Vital Statistics Report. Public Health Service Publication Number PHS 86-1120, Hyattsville, MD, 1986.
138. National Center for Health Statistics: Annual summary of births, marriages, divorces, and deaths: United States, 1984. Monthly Vital Statistics Report. Public Health Service Publication Number PHS 85-1120, Hyattsville, MD, 1985.
139. Lee, KS, et al: Very-low-birth-weight rate: Principal predictor of neonatal mortality in industrialized populations. J Pediatr 97:759, 1980.
140. Lee, KS, et al: Neonatal mortality: An analysis of the recent improvement in the United States. Am J Public Health 70:15, 1980.
141. McCormick, MC: The contribution of low birth weight to infant mortality and childhood morbidity. N Engl J Med 312:82, 1985.
142. Lee, KS, et al: Very-low-birth-weight rate: Principal predictor of neonatal mortality in industrialized populations. J Pediatr 97:759, 1980.
143. Cohen, RS, et al: Favorable results of neonatal intensive care for very-low-birth-weight infants. Pediatrics 69:621, 1982.
144. Modanlou, MD, et al: Perinatal transport to a regional perinatal center in a metropolitan area: Mater-

nal versus neonatal transport. Am J Obstet Gynecol 138:1157, 1980.
145. Paneth, N, et al: Newborn intensive care and neonatal mortality in low-birth-weight infants. N Engl J Med 307:149, 1982.
146. Hein, HA and Brown, CJ: Neonatal mortality review: A basis for improving care. Pediatrics 68:504, 1981.
147. Hein, HA and Lathrop, SS: The changing pattern of neonatal mortality in a regionalized system of perinatal care. Am J Dis Child 140:989, 1986.
148. Paneth, N and Stark, RI: Cerebral palsy and mental retardation in relation to indicators of perinatal asphyxia. Am J Obstet Gynecol 147:960, 1983.
149. MacDonald, HM, et al: Neonatal asphyxia. I: Relationship of obstetric and neonatal complications to neonatal mortality in 38,405 consecutive deliveries. J Pediatr 96:898, 1980.
150. Nelson, KB and Ellenberg, JH: Apgar scores as predictors of chronic neurologic disability. Pediatrics 68:36, 1981.
151. Jennett, RJ, et al: Apgar index: A statistical tool. Am J Obstet Gynecol 140:206, 1981.
152. Levine, DH, Michel, Y and Miller, JM: Another look at Apgars. Clin Res 30:885A, 1982.
153. Mulligan, JC, et al: Neonatal asphyxia. II: Neonatal mortality and long term sequelae. J Pediatr 96:903, 1980.
154. Brown, JK, et al: Neurological aspects of perinatal asphyxia. Dev Med Child Neurol 16:567, 1974.
155. Scott, H: Outcome of very severe birth asphyxia. Arch Dis Child 51:712, 1976.
156. Niswander, KR, Gordon, M and Drage, JS: The effect of intrauterine hypoxia on the child surviving to 4 years. Am J Obstet Gynecol 121:892, 1975.
157. Cushner, IM: Prolapse of the umbilical cord, including a late follow-up of fetal survivors. Am J Obstet Gynecol 81:666, 1961.
158. Drage, J, Berendes, H and Fisher, P: The Apgar scores and four-year psychological examination performance. Bull Pan Am Health Organ 185:222, 1969.
159. Steiner, H and Neligan, G: Perinatal cardiac arrest: Quality of the survivors. Arch Dis Child 50:696, 1975.
160. Nelson, KB and Ellenberg, JH: Antecedents of cerebral palsy: Multivariate analysis of risk. N Engl J Med 315:81, 1986.
161. Nyirjesy, L and Pierce, WE: Perinatal mortality and maternal morbidity in spontaneous and forceps vaginal deliveries. Am J Obstet Gynecol 89:568, 1964.
162. Friedman, EA, Sachtleben, MR and Bresky, PA: Dysfunctional labor. XII: Long term effect on infant. Am J Obstet Gynecol 127:779, 1977.
163. Niswander, KR and Gordon, M: Safety of the low-forceps operation. Am J Obstet Gynecol 117:619, 1973.
164. Gilstrap, LC III, Hauth, JC, Schiano, S and Connor, KD: Neonatal acidosis and method of delivery. Obstet Gynecol 63:681, 1984.
165. Richardson, DA, Evans, MI and Cibils, LA: Midforceps delivery: A critical review. Am J Obstet Gynecol 145:621, 1983.
166. James, DK and Chiswick, ML: Kielland's forceps: Role of antenatal factors in prediction of use. Br Med J 1:10, 1979.
167. Chiswick, ML and James, DK: Kielland's forceps: Association with neonatal morbidity and mortality. Br Med J 1:7, 1979.
168. Corston, JM: The end results in children delivered by mid or high forceps. Am J Obstet Gynecol 67:263, 1954.
169. Benaron, HB, et al: The remote effects of prolonged labor with forceps delivery, precipitate labor with spontaneous delivery, and natural labor with spontaneous delivery on the child. Am J Obstet Gynecol 66:551, 1953.
170. Fairweather, DV and Illsley, R: Obstetric and social origins of mentally handicapped children. Br J Prev Soc Med 14:149, 1960.
171. Barker, DJ: Low intelligence and obstetric complications. Br J Prev Soc Med 20:15, 1966.
172. Bishop, EH, Israel, SL and Briscoe, CL: Obstetrical influences on the premature infant's first year of development: A report from the collaborative study of cerebral palsy. Obstet Gynecol 26:628, 1965.
173. Browman, SH, Nichols, PL and Kennedy, WA: Preschool IQ: Prenatal and Early Development Correlates. L Eelbaum Associates, Hillsdale, NJ, 1975.
174. Greis, JB, Bienarz, J and Scommegna, A: Comparison of maternal and fetal effects of vacuum extraction with forceps or cesarean deliveries. Obstet Gynecol 57:571, 1981.
175. Beard, RW and Simons, EG: Diagnosis of foetal asphyxia in labour. Br J Anaesth 43:874, 1971.
176. Paul, RH and Hon, EH: Fetus, placenta, and newborn: Clinical fetal monitoring. V: Effect on perinatal outcome. Am J Obstet Gynecol 118:529, 1974.
177. Parer, JT: Fetal monitoring and neonatal outcome. In Gluck, L (ed): Obstetrical Decisions and Neonatal Outcome. Reports of the 78th Ross Conference on Pediatric Research. Ross Laboratories, Columbus, Ohio, 1981, p 71.
178. Schifrin, BS and Dame, L: Fetal heart rate patterns: Prediction of Apgar score. JAMA 219:1322, 1972.
179. Tejani, N, et al: Correlation of fetal heart rate: Uterine contraction patterns with fetal scalp blood pH. Obstet Gynecol 46:392, 1975.
180. Paul, RH, et al: Clinical fetal monitoring. VII: The evaluation and significance of intra-partum baseline FHR variability. Am J Obstet Gynecol 123:206, 1975.
181. Beard, RW, et al: The significance of the changes in the continuous fetal heart rate in the first stage of labor. J Obstet Gynecol Br Commonw 78:865, 1971.
182. Low, JA, et al: The relationship between antepartum fetal heart rate, intrapartum fetal heart rate, and fetal acid-base status. Am J Obstet Gynecol 154:769, 1986.
183. Gilstrap, LC III, Hauth, JC and Toussaint, S: Second-stage fetal heart rate abnormalities and neonatal acidosis. Obstet Gynecol 63:209, 1984.
184. Hon, EH: Detection of fetal distress. In Wood, C and Walters, WA (eds): Fifth World congress of gynaecology and obstetrics. Appleton-Century-Crofts, New York, 1967, p 58.
185. Leveno, KJ, et al: A prospective comparison of se-

lective and universal electronic fetal monitoring in 34,995 pregnancies. N Engl J Med 315:615, 1986.
186. Parer, JT: The current role of intrapartum fetal scalp monitoring. Clin Obstet Gynecol 23:565, 1980.
187. Antenatal diagnosis: Report of a consensus development conference. National Institute of Child Health and Human Development. Government Printing Office (NIH-79-1973), Washington, DC, 1979.
188. Saling, E: Fetal scalp blood analysis. J Perinat Med 9:165, 1981.
189. Wood, C: Fetal scalp sampling: Its place in management. Semin Perinatol 2:169, 1978.
190. Bowe, ET, et al: Reliability of fetal blood sampling: Maternal-fetal relationships. Am J Obstet Gynecol 107:279, 1970.
191. Young, DC, et al: Fetal scalp blood pH sampling: Its value in an active obstetric unit. Am J Obstet Gynecol 136:276, 1980.
192. Kubli, FW, et al: Observations on heart rate and pH in the human fetus during labor. Am J Obstet Gynecol 104:1190, 1969.
193. Paneth, N and Fox, HE: The relationship of Apgar score to neurologic handicap: A survey of clinicians. Obstet Gynecol 61:547, 1983.
194. Low, JA, et al: The prediction of intrapartum fetal metabolic acidosis by fetal heart rate monitoring. Am J Obstet Gynecol 139:299, 1981.
195. Sykes, GS, et al: Do Apgar scores indicate asphyxia? Lancet 1:494, 1982.
196. Silverman, F, et al: The Apgar score: Is it enough? Obstet Gynecol 66:331, 1985.
197. Scanlon, JW, et al: Neurobehavioral responses of newborn infants after maternal epidural anesthesia. Anesthesiology 40:121, 1974.
198. Kileff, M, et al: Neonatal neurobehavioral responses after epidural anesthesia for cesarean section using lidocaine and bupivacaine. Anesth Analg 63:413, 1984.
199. Abboud, TK, et al: Maternal, fetal, and neonatal responses after epidural anesthesia with bupivacaine, 2-chloroprocaine or lidocaine. Anesth Analg 61:638, 1982.
200. Abboud, TK, et al: Lack of adverse neonatal neurobehavioral effects of lidocaine. Anesth Analg 62:473, 1983.
201. Ansari, I, et al: Tilt caesarean section. Gynecol Br Commnw 77:713, 1970.
202. Downing, JW, et al: Lateral table tilt for caesarean section. Anaesthesia 29:696, 1974.
203. Crawford, JS, Burton, M and Davies, P: Time and lateral tilt at caesarean section. Br J Anaesth 44:477, 1972.
204. Crawford, JS, Burton, M and Davies, P: Anaesthesia for section: Further refinements of a technique. Br J Anaesth 45:726, 1973.
205. Buley, RJ, et al: Right versus left lateral tilt for caesarean section. Br J Anaesth 49:1009, 1977.
206. Ramanathan, S, et al: Oxygen transfer from mother to fetus during caesarean section under epidural anesthesia. Anesth Analg 61:576, 1982.
207. Baraka, A: Correlation between maternal and fetal Po_2 and Pco_2 during caesarean section. Br J Anaesth 42:434, 1970.
208. Marx, GF and Mateo, CV: Effects of different oxygen concentrations during general anaesthesia for elective caesarean section. Can Anaesth Soc J 18:587, 1971.
209. Newman, W, et al: Oxygen transfer from mother to fetus during labor. Am J Obstet Gynecol 99:61, 1967.
210. Teramo, K: Foetal acid-base values during caesarean section. Lancet 2:1146, 1968.
211. Fothergill, RJ, Robertson, A and Bond, RA: Neonatal acidaemia related to procrastination at caesarean section. Br J Obstet Gynecol 78:1010, 1971.
212. Magno, R, Selstam, U and Karlsson, K: Anesthesia for cesarean section. II: Effects of the induction-delivery interval on the respiratory adaptation of the newborn in elective cesarean section. Acta Anaesth Scand 19:250, 1975.
213. Stenger, VG, et al: Observations on pentothal, nitrous oxide, and succinylcholine anesthesia at cesarean section. Am J Obstet Gynecol 99:690, 1967.
214. Hodges, RJ, et al: General anaesthesia for operative obstetrics: With special reference to the use of thiopentone and suxamethonium. Br J Anaesth 31:152, 1959.
215. Kivalo, I, Timonen, S and Castren, O: The influence of anaesthesia and the induction-delivery interval on the newborn delivered by caesarean section. Ann Chir Gynecol 60:71, 1971.
216. Robertson, A, Fothergill, RJ and Bond, RA: Effects of propanidid and thiopentone on the acid-base status of babies delivered by elective caesarean section. S Afr Med J 48:1019, 1974.
217. Data, S, et al: Neonatal effect of prolonged anesthetic induction for cesarean section. Obstet Gynecol 58:331, 1981.
218. Shnider, SM and Levinson, G: Anesthesia for cesarean section. In Shnider, SM, Levinson, G (eds): Anesthesia for Obstetrics. Williams & Wilkins, Baltimore, 1979, p 254.
219. Crawford, JS, et al: A further study of general anaesthesia for caesarean section. Br J Anaesth 48:661, 1976.
220. Crawford, JS, Burton, M and Davies, P: Anaesthesia for section: Further refinements of a technique. Br J Anaesth 45:726, 1973.
221. Crawford, JS and Davies, P: Status of neonates delivered by elective caesarean section. Br J Anaesth 54:1015, 1982.
222. Downing, JW, Houlton, PC and Barclay, A: Extradural analgesia for cesarean section. Br J Anaesth 51:367, 1979.
223. Fox, GS, et al: Anesthesia for cesarean section: Further studies. Am J Obstet Gynecol 133:15, 1979.
224. Caritis, SN, et al: Fetal acid-base state following spinal or epidural anesthesia for cesarean section. Obstet Gynecol 56:610, 1980.
225. Hollmen, AI, et al: Neurologic activity of infants following anesthesia for cesarean section. Anesthesiology 48:350, 1978.
226. Marx, GF, Luykx, WM and Cohen, S: Fetal-neonatal status following caesarean section for fetal distress. Br J Anaesth 56:1009, 1984.

CHAPTER 5

PROBLEMS OF EARLY PREGNANCY

GORDON L. MANDELL, M.D.

Early pregnancy is defined as the period of gestation between fertilization and 24 gestational weeks. Anesthesia technique during these first two trimesters depends not only on specific disease processes — ectopic pregnancy, neoplastic trophoblastic disease, abortion, cervical incompetence — but also on the physiologic changes of early pregnancy. Anesthesia for cervical incompetence must also include fetal considerations.

Physiologic Changes During Early Pregnancy

These profound changes affect every organ system in the body, beginning soon after fertilization and increasing in magnitude as pregnancy continues. The three processes that alter maternal physiology during pregnancy are hormonal changes, increased metabolic demands of the growing fetus, and uterine enlargement. The first two are influential throughout pregnancy; the last is most important during the second and third trimesters. This section reviews only those physiologic changes taking place in the respiratory, cardiovascular, and gestrointestinal systems during early pregnancy, since Chapter 1 offers a thorough presentation of the physiology of pregnancy.

RESPIRATORY SYSTEM

Many changes occur in the maternal respiratory system during early pregnancy. The increased vascularity of the respiratory tract[1] produces generalized swelling of the pharynx, larynx, and trachea. Alveolar ventilation begins to increase in the first trimester,[2] increasing 25 percent by 16 weeks' gestation and 40 percent by 24 weeks' gestation in response to augmented tidal volume and respiratory rate. Progesterone probably accounts for this increased alveolar ventilation.[3] While the increasing metabolic demands of the growing fetus consume more maternal oxygen,[4] functional residual capacity decreases during pregnancy as the enlarging uterus elevates the diaphragm,[5] especially during the second and third trimesters, when the distended uterus expands beyond the pelvis. Pulmonary oxygen reserve decreases concomitantly.

These changes contribute to a greater risk for airway obstruction during early pregnancy, not only because of airway swelling from vascular congestion but also from generalized weight gain. Therefore, laryngoscopy and endotracheal intubation can be more difficult in the pregnant patient, necessitating a variety of endotracheal tubes and laryngoscopes. Nasal airways and nasotracheal intubation should be avoided because of the possibility of severe epistaxis.

Hypoxia develops quickly in the pregnant patient[6] owing to increased airway obstruction, increased oxygen consumption, and decreased oxygen reserve secondary to reduced functional residual capacity, especially in the second and third trimesters. Oxygenation prior to anesthetic induction, wise during the first trimester, is mandatory during the second and third trimesters.

The rate of induction of inhalational anesthesia increases in the pregnant patient for hyperventilation delivers more anesthetic to the alveoli and the reduced functional residual capacity produces less dilution of incoming gas. Thus inhalational anesthetics achieve a higher alveolar concentration more quickly. In addition, reduced minimal alveolar concentration (MAC) occurs during pregnancy,[7] possibly due to progesterone or to increased plasma endorphin levels.[8] These effects call for reducing doses of halothane, enflurane, or isoflurane to avoid overdose.

CARDIOVASCULAR SYSTEM

Maternal blood volume and cardiac output change to meet the increased metabolic demands of the growing fetus. Blood volume increases throughout pregnancy beginning between the 6th and 12th week of gestation.[9] Physiologic anemia results because plasma volume increases more than red-cell volume. The 15-percent increase in heart rate and 35-percent increase in stroke volume increase cardiac output during the first trimester by 40 percent.[10]

During the second trimester, when cardiac output continues to rise but at a slower rate, the effect of maternal position on cardiac output becomes important. Compression of the inferior vena cava by the enlarging uterus, occurring when the mother assumes the supine position,[11] decreases venous return and cardiac output and may lead to arterial hypotension. Approximately 10 percent of pregnant women become overtly hypotensive when supine. In the supine position, compression of the lower aorta may also occur, decreasing uterine blood flow.[12] The pregnant woman should avoid this position during the second and third trimesters to minimize these effects.

Several factors compensate for chronic aortocaval compression, including increased collateral venous return through the epidural venous plexus and azygos vein, hypervolemia, and increased peripheral vascular resistance. Hypervolemia occurs early during pregnancy, protecting the mother and fetus against impaired venous return and hemorrhage. Since increased peripheral vascular resistance also compensates for aortocaval compression, anything causing vasodilation (e.g., deep general anesthesia or regional anesthesia with extensive sympathetic blockade) will further reduce venous return.

As described previously, deep general anesthesia can occur quickly in the pregnant patient. Also, extensive sympathetic blockade can occur during regional anesthesia in this patient population because pregnancy affects the spread of local anesthetics. Epidural venous plexus engorgement secondary to aortocaval compression may increase local anesthetic spread by decreasing the size of the epidural and subarachnoid spaces.[13] Fragraeus and coworkers[14] demonstrated increased epidural spread after lidocaine administration to women in their first trimester of pregnancy, before aortocaval compression typically occurs. Perhaps progesterone increases the sensitivity of neural tissues to local anesthetics, augmenting spread even early in pregnancy.[15] Therefore, to avoid extensive blockade and hypotension, the anesthesiologist should reduce the dose of local anesthetics for spinal or epidural anesthesia. In addition, prior to induction of regional anesthesia, patients should receive adequate fluid pretreatment and, during the second and third trimesters, they should be positioned to produce uterine displacement.

GASTROINTESTINAL SYSTEM

The decreased tone and motility of the gastrointestinal tract during pregnancy prolong gastric emptying. Some investigators[16] report delayed gastric emptying early in pregnancy, while others[17] claim this does not occur until the third trimester. The presumed reason for delayed gastric emptying involves progesterone's inhibition of motilin, a peptide stimulant of stomach activity. As pregnancy progresses, increased gastric pressure, resulting from displacement of the stomach and intestines by the enlarging uterus, combines with decreased lower esophageal sphincter tone in some pregnant women to decrease barrier pressure. This can happen early during the second trimester.[18] In addition, elevated gastrin levels stimulate more acidic gastric contents.[19] Based on Roberts and Shirley's[20] criteria of risk for both gastric pH and volume, 37 percent of women with early pregnancies are at risk of aspiration pneumonitis.[21] However, one should consider all pregnant women during the second and third trimesters at risk, and take steps to avoid aspiration (see Chapters 1 and 7). When possible, use regional anesthesia to preserve airway reflexes. Should general anesthesia prove necessary, management must include pretreatment with a nonparticulate oral antacid, rapid-sequence induction with cricoid pressure, intubation with a cuffed endotracheal tube, and awake extubation.

Ectopic Pregnancy

Pregnancy begins with the fertilized ovum implanting in the uterine endometrium. Implantation anywhere else defines an ectopic pregnancy. In 1978, approximately 40,000 cases of ectopic pregnancy occurred in the United States, accounting for 5 percent of deaths associated with reproduction.[22] In most ectopic pregnancies, the fertilized ovum resides in some portion of the oviduct, giving rise to ampullar, isthmic, or interstitial tubal pregnancy. The ampulla is the most common site of ectopic implantation, followed by the isthmus. Interstitial pregnancies rarely occur. From these primary types, secondary forms of ectopic pregnancies (e.g., abdominal pregnancy) may develop.

DIAGNOSIS

Pritchard and coworkers[23] estimate that 10 to 50 percent of ectopic pregnancies terminate without complications by resorption or spontaneous abortion. However, many pregnancies end during the first trimester by tubal rupture. Before rupture or abortion, the clinical features of a tubal pregnancy vary greatly. With rupture of the oviduct, however, vaginal bleeding, accompanied by sudden severe lower abdominal pain, may occur. Examination of the abdomen reveals tenderness on palpation, and vaginal exam demonstrates pain on motion of the cervix. The obstetrician may palpate a boggy mass on one side of the uterus. If bleeding persists after tubal rupture, the patient may show signs of hemorrhage and hypovolemia.

The conditions most frequently confused with tubal pregnancy are acute or chronic salpingitis, threatened or incomplete abortion of an intrauterine pregnancy, rupture of a corpus luteum or follicular cyst with intraperitoneal bleeding, torsion of an ovarian cyst, appendicitis, gastroenteritis, and discomfort from an intrauterine device.

Because of the difficulty of diagnosing tubal pregnancy, many diagnostic aids are available, including pregnancy tests, sonography, culdocentesis, curettage, laparoscopy, culdoscopy, culdotomy or colpotomy, and laparotomy. With sonography, identification of a gestational sac in the uterus usually rules out a tubal pregnancy. Culdocentesis identifies a hemoperitoneum if tubal rupture has taken place. Curettage differentiates tubal pregnancy from a threatened or incomplete abortion. The obstetrician can perform culdocentesis and curettage with or without major regional or general anesthesia; however, culdoscopy, laparoscopy, culdotomy, and laparotomy require surgical anesthesia. Laparoscopy often proves necessary to diagnose disease of the pelvic viscera, including ectopic pregnancy. Culdoscopy is more difficult than laparoscopy. Culdotomy provides direct visualization of the oviducts and ovaries, allowing the performance of a salpingectomy. Laparotomy follows if any doubt remains.

RUPTURED OVIDUCT

Hypovolemia

When a patient presents with a suspected ectopic pregnancy, the clinician must assess intravascular fluid volume, since hypovolemia often accompanies oviduct rupture. Hypovolemia assessment can involve comparing blood pressure and heart rate in the sitting and supine position (a tilt test). A distinct decrease in blood pressure and rise in heart rate following a change from the supine to the sitting position may indicate hypovolemia. Decreased urinary output or low central venous pressure also suggests hypovolemia. Although a single hematocrit does not accurately diagnose acute hemorrhage, a decreasing hematocrit over several hours may more accurately reflect blood loss. Finally, the history and physical examination should look for diaphragmatic irritation, abdominal tenderness, and intestinal distention, since women with 500 ml or more of blood in the peritoneal cavity often demonstrate these findings.[24]

Preoperative Management

The patient with a suspected ruptured oviduct represents a surgical emergency. The surgical team should perform a brief history and physical examination, establish adequate intravenous access, send blood for hematocrit and type and crossmatch, and initiate fluid resuscitation with a balanced salt solution (see Chap. 15) while preparing the operating room for laparotomy. Because of the possibility of recent oral intake and the added risk of pregnancy, the patient should receive a nonparticulate oral antacid such as sodium citrate prior to induction of general anesthesia.

Surgical Anesthesia

In the operating room, oxygen is administered by face mask and a monitor is placed. The threat of sudden hypoxia in the pregnant patient necessitates preoxygenation, and monitoring oxygen saturation with a pulse oximeter is valuable. General anesthesia induction follows in a rapid-sequence fashion with cricoid pressure, then tracheal intubation with a cuffed endotracheal tube. Anesthesia may be induced with intravenous sodium thiopental, ketamine, or etomidate, and tracheal intubation is facilitated with intravenous succinylcholine. In the presence of hypovolemia etomidate or ketamine is the preferred induction agent. A light plane of halogenated agent combined with muscle relaxant, or a combination of nitrous oxide, narcotic, and muscle relaxant will maintain anesthesia. Note, however, that pregnancy decreases the minimal alveolar concentration and care should be taken to avoid overdose. At the conclusion of surgery, extubation of the trachea may take place once the patient has awakened, has stable vital signs, and has normal neuromuscular function. In the postanesthetic care unit, vital signs, hematocrit, and urinary output require close monitoring.

LAPAROSCOPY

Often, laparoscopy is performed to diagnose ectopic pregnancy. If the physician does not suspect tubal rupture, he may delay surgery briefly while a thorough preoperative evaluation is performed. However, the possibility of tubal rupture should preclude unnecessary delays. Most patients not needing laparotomy may return home the same day, so outpatient considerations influence the anesthetic technique. The section on anesthesia for abortion will discuss in more detail the special problems of the outpatient.

Anesthesia for Laparoscopy

Complications. In most centers, the gynecologist employs laparoscopy to confirm ectopic pregnancy. A pneumoperitoneum is required for laparoscopy. Carbon dioxide is the most soluble of the gases used for abdominal inflation and is widely used. Other gases used include nitrous oxide and air. Nitrous oxide is 68 percent as soluble as carbon dioxide, while air is the least soluble and most dangerous should gas embolism occur.[25] The use of carbon dioxide introduces the risk of hypercarbia during laparoscopy, caused by increased absorption of carbon dioxide across the peritoneal cavity.[26] Hypercarbia triggers the release of endogenous catecholamines which in turn can lead to hypertension and cardiac arrhythmias. Therefore, controlled ventilation (to avoid hypercapnia) and end-tidal carbon dioxide monitoring (when possible) should accompany laparoscopy.

Optimal visualization of pelvic structures often necessitates a steep Trendelenburg position. This position, in combination with a pneumoperitoneum, can affect arterial oxygenation.[27] Drummond and Martin[28] demonstrated a 19-percent decrease in functional residual capacity during laparoscopy in anesthetized, paralyzed women (nearly equal to the decrease in functional residual capacity a pregnant woman experiences at term). Reduced functional residual capacity can induce hypoxia as a result of a mismatching of ventilation and perfusion. Hypoxia can also occur if high intra-abdominal pressure decreases cardiac output. Controlled ventilation and oxygen saturation monitoring (when possible, with a pulse oximeter) help avoid hypoxia.

Laparoscopy can evoke profound circulatory effects. In humans, a pneumoperitoneum with intra-abdominal pressures of 15- to 20-cm water increases mean arterial blood pressure, central venous pressure, and heart rate without changing cardiac output.[29] Although mean arterial blood pressure, central venous pressure, and heart rate continue to increase as intra-abdominal pressure increases, cardiac output decreases. Ivankovich and colleagues[30] demonstrated this trend in dogs with intra-abdominal pressures of 40 mmHg, showing that as intra-abdominal pressure increases, venous return and cardiac output decrease. The elevated blood pressure occurs secondary to increased peripheral vascular resistance. During laparoscopy, intra-abdominal pressures exceeding 20 mmHg are potentially dangerous and should be avoided.

Other complications during laparoscopy include gas embolization, tension pneumothorax, pneumomediastinum, and perforation of organs and blood vessels with hemorrhage. The presence of hypotension in conjunction with a mill-wheel precordial murmur should raise suspicions of gas embolism. Acute reductions in end-tidal carbon dioxide levels and an increase in end-tidal nitrogen provide additional evidence.

Procedures. The anesthetic management of the patient undergoing laparoscopy for a suspected ectopic pregnancy resembles that for the ruptured oviduct. At least one large-bore intravenous line is established for rapid fluid infusion should excessive hemorrhage occur. Blood is collected for a hematocrit and a type and screen. The patient is premedicated with sodium citrate prior to general anesthesia. In the operating room oxygen is administered by mask. Minimal monitoring consists of a precordial stethoscope, blood pressure cuff, inspired oxygen monitor, electrocardiogram, and intra-abdominal pressure manometer. Also useful is an end-tidal carbon dioxide monitor if carbon dioxide is used to inflate the abdomen. Additionally, pulse oximetry is advisable to assess oxygen saturation.

Anesthesia for laparoscopy must suit the outpatient situation. Intravenous fentanyl, 1 to 2 μg per kg, may reduce recovery time because of this analgesic's ability to decrease anesthetic requirements.[31] Small doses of intravenous droperidol given prior to induction may control nausea and vomiting, significant problems following laparoscopy. Studies[32,33] indicate that low-dose droperidol (0.25 to 1.0 mg) may be effective without prolonging recovery.

General anesthesia follows the same protocol as that for a ruptured oviduct. Anesthesia maintenance utilizes nitrous oxide, a potent inhalation agent, and a muscle relaxant. Practitioners frequently choose enflurane because it may have a slightly shorter emergence time than halothane or isoflurane;[34] additionally, enflurane may produce fewer anesthesia-related side effects than either halothane or isoflurane.[35] A balanced technique may provide an alternative approach; however, some[36] believe this technique causes a higher incidence of early postoperative morbidity than inhalation agents.

If laparoscopy reveals an ectopic pregnancy, laparotomy and salpingectomy follow. At the conclusion of surgery, tracheal extubation is done once the patient is awake and physiologically stable. If laparotomy proves unnecessary, the patient may be discharged home after recovering in the postanesthetic care unit.

INTERSTITIAL PREGNANCY

The interstitial or cornual pregnancy—the least common and potentially most dangerous type of tubal pregnancy—occurs with implantation of the fertilized ovum into the segment of oviduct penetrating the uterine wall. Rupture appears later in this type of ectopic pregnancy, compared with ampullar or isthmic tubal pregnancy (usually between the 8th and 16th gestational week), due to greater distensibility at the site of implantation. Because of the abundant blood supply adjacent to the implantation site, hemorrhage may lead to rapid death. The large uterine defect following rupture often dictates performing a hysterectomy. Anesthesia resembles that for the ruptured oviduct, with increased probability of hypovolemia from hemorrhage. Unlike the more common types of ectopic pregnancy, interstitial pregnancy generally presents during the second trimester. Hypoxia appears more likely because of increased oxygen consumption with the larger fetus and decreased functional residual capacity, which becomes evident during this trimester. Therefore, preoxygenation of the patient must precede induction of anesthesia. The second trimester also involves a greater risk for inferior vena cava compression in the supine position, and at least until removal of the uterus, left uterine displacement may be required to improve venous return. Regardless of the timing of the last oral intake, one should regard such patients as having full stomachs. Pretreatment with sodium citrate and a cuffed endotracheal tube following rapid-sequence induction with cricoid pressure and awake extubation are mandatory measures to prevent aspiration.

ABDOMINAL PREGNANCY

Almost all cases of abdominal pregnancy follow early rupture or abortion of a tubal pregnancy into the peritoneal cavity. They occur rarely and most fetuses die.[37,38] If the fetus dies after reaching a size too large for absorption, its surgical removal usually follows. The operation for abdominal pregnancy may precipitate massive hemorrhage, relating to the lack of constriction of the hypertrophied opened blood vessels after placental separation. As soon as the diagnosis is made, surgery should proceed because of the risk of hemorrhage following separation of the placenta. Surgery usually consists of delivery of the fetus and, in most cases, leaving the placenta in the abdominal cavity. The maternal mortality with abdominal pregnancy is 6 percent, compared to the overall mortality for ectopic pregnancy which is 0.08 percent.[37,39] Anesthetic considerations include the likelihood of massive hemorrhage. Precautionary measures include establishing adequate intravenous access and having at least four units of compatible blood in the operating room prior to skin incision. In the second trimester, left uterine displacement facilitates resuscitation of the hemorrhaging patient.

Neoplastic Trophoblastic Diseases

The neoplastic trophoblastic diseases include hydatidiform mole, invasive mole, and choriocarcinoma. Hydatidiform moles are characterized by abnormalities of the chorionic villi with proliferation of the trophoblast and edema of the villous stroma. Invasion of the uterus and adjacent structures by chorionic villi constitutes an invasive mole. Proliferation of the trophoblast without stroma, spreading locally and disseminating to distant organs, characterizes choriocarcinoma.

HYDATIDIFORM MOLE

Hydatidiform moles, occurring once in every 1500 to 2000 pregnancies in the United States,[40] can be complete or incomplete (partial). A complete hydatidiform mole occupies the entire uterine cavity and has a greater propensity to become a malignant choriocarcinoma than the incomplete hydatidiform mole (characterized by focal or less advanced trophoblastic proliferation). The recurrence of a hydatidiform mole is uncommon (2 percent of cases).[41]

Symptoms

Even though the very early stage of development of a hydatidiform mole remains almost indistinguishable from a normal pregnancy, later in the first trimester noticeable changes appear. Uterine bleeding and unexpected uterine enlargement usually occur, the latter producing some apparent physiologic changes. For example, reduced functional residual capacity may predispose the patient to hypoxia; aortocaval compression may appear more prominent than anticipated from the gestational age; and gastric pressure may increase, predisposing to a greater risk of aspiration. Because pregnancy-induced hypertension frequently associates with molar pregnancies, hypertension in early pregnancy suggests the diagnosis of molar pregnancy, and any patient with a molar pregnancy and hypertension should be evaluated for a coagulopathy, especially if regional anesthesia is anticipated.

Diagnosis and Treatment

A history of persistent bleeding and a larger-than-expected uterus may denote the presence of a hydatidiform mole. Sonography usually confirms the diagnosis. Also useful is amniography with transabdominal intrauterine instillation of radiopaque contrast material. Many clinicians continue to measure chorionic gonadotrophin levels, which should be substantially increased.

Treatment of a hydatidiform mole consists of immediate evacuation of the uterus and follow-up for the detection of malignant change.

Anesthetic Management

Preoperative evaluation involves a thorough history and physical examination. Maternal hypertension, possibly indicating pregnancy-induced hypertension, mandates evaluation of a patient's coagulation status, especially if the physician anticipates using regional anesthesia (see Chap. 21). Blood is sent for typing and cross-matching and a hematocrit, since anemia commonly occurs. At least one large-bone intravenous line is established for possible rapid fluid administration. Because of the possibility of aspiration, a nonparticulate oral antacid is administered. Either regional or general anesthesia may be used (keeping in mind that these women are frequently outpatients). For regional anesthesia, the dose of local anesthetic is lowered to avoid high blocks, and hypotension is reduced with fluid pretreatment and perhaps uterine displacement. When using general anesthesia, these patients are considered as having full stomachs. A rapid-sequence induction with cricoid pressure, using sodium thiopental and succinylcholine followed by tracheal intubation with a cuffed endotracheal tube is mandatory. To decrease uterine bleeding and reduce the risk of perforation, oxytocin is infused throughout the procedure. Because potent inhalational agents can induce uterine relaxation, a balanced technique may be a safer alternative. The threat of uncontrolled hemorrhage or uterine trauma warrants use of facilities and personnel equipped for immediate laparotomy. Surgery for hydatidiform moles usually consists of vacuum aspiration; however, the patient and physician may opt for hysterectomy if no more pregnancies are desired.

CHORIOCARCINOMA

Choriocarcinoma, an extremely malignant disease, may develop during or after a normal or abnormal pregnancy (hydatidiform mole, abortion, ectopic, or term). Choriocarcinoma exaggerates the predisposition of the normal trophoblast for invasive growth and erosion of blood vessels, and metastases occur early and often. The lungs are the most common site of metastasis, followed by the vagina. In many cases, the vulva, kidneys, liver, ovaries, and brain also contain metastases.

Choriocarcinoma presents with irregular uterine bleeding after the termination of pregnancy. The bleeding may be intermittent or continuous, sometimes with massive hemorrhage. Perforation of the uterus can result in intraperitoneal hemorrhage. The first indication of choriocarcinoma may be metastatic disease. If not treated, the course rapidly progresses, death occurring in a few months, usually from hemorrhage. Chemotherapy has successfully replaced hysterectomy as treatment; however, a perforated uterus calls for surgery. The overall cure rate for choriocarcinoma is 90 percent.[42]

INVASIVE MOLE

Invasive mole occupies an intermediate position between hydatidiform mole and choriocarcinoma. This condition, like choriocarcinoma, is rare. Invasive moles, although capable of spreading locally, generally lack the tendency for widespread metastasis. Treatment may consist of chemotherapy, but the patient may require hysterectomy if uterine perforation by tumor occurs. One should anticipate massive hemorrhage.

Abortions

Abortion describes the termination of pregnancy by any means before the fetus attains viability. Abortions fall into three groups: spontaneous, therapeutic, and voluntary.

SPONTANEOUS ABORTIONS

An estimated 10 percent of all pregnancies end in spontaneous abortion.[43] During early pregnancy death of embryo fetus nearly always precedes spontaneous abortion. Abnormalities of the fetus or the maternal reproductive tract as well as systemic diseases of the mother (and rarely the father) may contribute to fetal death. Developmental abnormalities of the embryo, fetus, or placenta represent the most common morphologic findings in early spontaneous abortions.[44]

Spontaneous abortion subclassifications include: threatened, inevitable, incomplete, missed, and habitual abortions. Threatened abortion, which occurs when any bloody vaginal discharge or vaginal bleeding appears during the first half of pregnancy, calls for conservative management, since bleeding ceases in some patients. Continued bleeding with resulting severe anemia may indicate evacuation of the products of conception by curettage. Gross rupture of the membranes in the presence of cervical dilation signals an inevitable abortion. Uterine contractions often begin spontaneously, resulting in expulsion of the products of conception; otherwise the uterus is emptied surgically. An incomplete abortion involves retention of the placenta in the uterus. Missed abortion refers to prolonged retention of a fetus who died during the first half of pregnancy. Occasionally, after prolonged retention of the dead products of conception, serious coagulation defects develop, especially if gestation reaches the second trimester before the fetus dies. Coagulation studies may be helpful, especially when regional anesthesia is anticipated. Habitual abortions correspond to repeated spontaneous abortions, usually three or more occurring consecutively.

THERAPEUTIC AND VOLUNTARY ABORTIONS

A therapeutic abortion terminates pregnancy before the time of fetal viability for the purpose of safeguarding the health of the mother. Voluntary or elective abortion interrupts pregnancy before viability at the request of the woman, but for reasons other than impaired maternal health or fetal disease.

ABORTION TECHNIQUES

Surgical Techniques

These include cervical dilation and evacuation of the uterine contents by curettage or vacuum aspiration (suction curettage) or both, hysterotomy, or hysterectomy.

The complications of curettage and vacuum aspiration are uterine perforation, cervical laceration, hemorrhage, incomplete removal of the fetus and placenta, and infection. Generally, uterine perforation is easily recognized, and observation may prove sufficient therapy for small perforations, since such small defects often heal readily without complication. However, considerable intra-abdominal damage may necessitate performing a laparoscopy to examine the intra-abdominal contents. For the most part, obstetricians prefer vacuum aspiration to mechanical curettage for abortion, since the latter is quicker, has a lower perforation rate, induces less blood loss during surgery, and produces fewer infections.

Medical Techniques

Medical techniques include intravenous oxytocin, intravaginal prostaglandins and prostaglandin analogs, and intra-amniotic hyperosmotic fluids (20-percent sodium chloride or 30-percent urea).

When the cervix is favorable, oxytocin can effectively induce abortion; but, because of its antidiuretic properties, oxytocin may elicit water intoxication when combined with large volumes of electrolyte-free solutions. Other risks include oxytocin-induced rupture of the uterus during the first half of pregnancy in women of high parity[45] and hypotension elicited by a large intravenous bolus of oxytocin, a vasodilator. Prostaglandins, widely used to terminate pregnancies, especially in the second trimester, are placed either adjacent to or into the cervical canal or are injected into the amniotic sac. Some clinicians administer vaginal prostaglandins in combination with intravenous oxytocin or prior to curettage. Disseminated intravascular coagulation may follow the use of prostaglandins. Intra-amniotic hyperosmotic solutions of sodium chloride and urea induce abortion during the second trimester. Serious complications of hypertonic saline include death, hyperosmolar crisis, cardiac failure, septic shock, peritonitis, hemorrhage, disseminated intravascular coagulation, water intoxication, and myometrial damage.

PREOPERATIVE MANAGEMENT

Most patients receive treatment as outpatients. The anesthesiologist should evaluate the patient preoperatively with a thorough history and physical examination, taking care to ascertain the duration of the pregnancy, since this affects not only the physiology of the patient, but also, in the case of second-trimester abortions, the possibility of severe hemorrhage and coagulopathy. In addition, evaluation of the patient's intravascular fluid volume is essential, since significant hemorrhage could have already occurred.

As for other early pregnancy complications, arrange for intravenous fluid delivery and determine pertinent blood data. The latter should include preoperative hematocrit and blood compatibility studies for the bleeding or severely anemic patient or for the patient in her second trimester. The woman should undergo coagulation studies if the fetus has been dead for more than 1 week, especially during the second trimester, although maternal coagulation problems rarely develop less than 1 month after fetal demise.[46]

Because these patients commonly experience emotional trauma and anxiety, premedication with fentanyl (1 to 2 μg per kg) or midazolam (0.08 mg per kg) is acceptable,[31,47] regardless of the type of anesthesia subsequently given. The judicious use of preoperative sedatives and analgesics in outpatients helps to relieve anxiety and pain without prolonging recovery. Nonparticulate antacids reduce the risk of aspiration,[48] and low-dose droperidol can prevent nausea and vomiting without prolonging recovery.[32,33] Premedication can include cimetidine and metoclopramide at admission.

ANESTHETIC MANAGEMENT

Anesthetic considerations can be complex, due in part to the outpatient status of most abortion patients.

Local and General Anesthesia

A large retrospective study[49] evaluated the safety of local and general anesthesia for first-trimester voluntary abortions. "Local anesthesia" was any paracervical anesthetic with or without sedatives or analgesics, and "general anesthesia" included a wide variety of techniques. The investigators noted significant differences between the two groups for certain complications. Patients who received local anesthesia ran a higher risk for convulsions and postoperative fever while those who had general anesthesia were at greater risk for uterine hemorrhage, uterine perforation, and cervical injury. Both groups experienced the same rates for major complications. The authors concluded that local anesthesia and general anesthesia demonstrate the same overall safety for first-trimester voluntary abortions.

A similar study[50] evaluated the safety of local and general anesthesia for the more risky voluntary second-trimester abortions, which have greater morbidity and mortality. Dilation and evacuation under local anesthesia was associated with more instances of retained products of conception, postoperative hemorrhage, and repeat curettage; general anesthesia, with increased intraoperative hemorrhage and postoperative fever. Overall, the risk of serious complications ranked higher with general than with local anesthesia. The authors concluded that local anesthesia appeared safer than general anesthesia for women undergoing dilation and evacuation for voluntary second-trimester abortions. However, more and more clinicians are using dilation and evacuation rather than amniotic infusion of hypertonic saline or urea, since the former yields lower risks for mortality and morbidity than amniotic infusions.

Both of these studies revealed more hemorrhaging, which required transfusion in patients receiving general anesthesia. However, the type of general anesthesia has a tremendous affect on blood loss. Comparing various general anesthetic techniques with paracervical block for blood loss in first-trimester voluntary abortions, Cullen and colleagues,[51] concluded that blood loss was greatest with halothane and least with paracervical block. Interestingly, general anesthesia with nitrous oxide, sodium thiopental, and meperidine did not increase hemorrhage significantly. Others[52,53] have demonstrated that potent inhalational agents are potent uterine relaxants and require caution during abortions.

Peterson and coworkers[54] have retrospectively investigated the risk of death from voluntary first-trimester abortions performed with local and general anesthesia. Death associated with general anesthesia was 0.37 per 100,000 and 0.15 per 100,000 with local anesthesia. These authors concluded that the risk of death from anesthesia-related complications was greater with general anesthesia than with local anesthesia, and the risk of death from all causes was greater with general anesthesia. Drug overdose and hypoxia represented the leading causes of death with general anesthesia, whereas the primary reason for death from local anesthesia was systemic local anesthetic toxicity. The former may relate to the physiologic changes affecting women during early pregnancy. Increased alveolar ventilation, decreased functional residual capacity, and reduced minimal alveolar concentration all contribute to easier anesthetic overdose. The reduction in functional residual capacity, increased oxygen consumption, and airway difficulties make the pregnant patient more susceptible to hypoxia. In addition, the risk of aspiration increases during pregnancy.

If the team chooses general anesthesia for an abortion, a balanced technique with sodium thiopental, nitrous oxide, and a narcotic appears preferable to a potent inhalational agent. The patient is preoxygenated and anesthesia is induced with intravenous sodium thiopental or ketamine (if significant hemorrhage has occurred). If the patient has recently eaten or in any second-trimester patient anesthesia is induced in a rapid-sequence fashion with cricoid pressure followed by tracheal intubation with a cuffed endoctracheal tube. The patient may not necessarily need tracheal intubation for an electively scheduled abortion during the first trimester. Intravenous oxytocin administered during the procedure contracts the uterus and reduces hemorrhage.

Abortions may prove safer when performed using local anesthesia. In addition, local anesthesia provides the most rapid recovery.[55] Paracervical block combined with intravenous sedation and analgesia may be appropriate for some patients but not all. In fact, abortions done under paracervical blockade are not without risks since paracervical block may produce systemic local anesthetic toxicity and, occasionally, preventable death.[56] Thus the clinician must take care to limit total local anesthetic dose, and avoid intravenous injections, and must possess the skills and equipment necessary to treat toxic reactions (see Chap. 7).

Regional Anesthesia

Spinal and epidural anesthesia are attractive alternatives to general and local anesthesia, minimizing both the side effects of general anesthesia (e.g., blood loss) and postoperative analgesia requirements (due to the residual effects of regional blocks). Spinal anesthesia is fast and reliable, and the high incidence of post–lumbar puncture headache in this patient population can be minimized by using a 25- or 26-gauge spinal needle.[57] Epidural anesthesia reduces the incidence of spinal headache and is associated with shorter discharge times and fewer side effects than general anesthesia.[58] The increased local anesthetic spread occurring even during early pregnancy calls for reducing doses of local anesthetics for these patients. Intravenous sedatives and analgesics can supplement regional anesthesia. These patients should not be discharged from the postanesthetic care unit until they demonstrate full recovery of motor and sensory function; any outpatient who has received sedation, analgesia, or general anesthesia should be cautioned to defer important decisions and activities requiring special skills for 48 to 72 hours.[59]

SEPTIC ABORTION

Pathogenic organisms of the bowel or vaginal flora are primarily responsible for abortion-related sepsis. Infection most commonly stays confined to the uterus but parametritis, peritonitis, and septicemia may occur, and endotoxemia and exotoxemia can cause severe and even fatal shock; septic shock is now rare. The physiologic changes induced by septic shock include damage to vascular endothelium, vasodilation, and decreased myocardial function. Therapy for septic abortion consists of closely monitoring blood pressure and urinary output, control of infection with antibiotics, and prompt removal of infected products of conception by curettage. Hysterectomy rarely proves necessary unless the uterus has been lacerated or is intensely infected. Septic shock therapy includes oxygenation, fluid replacement, blood transfusions, steroids, pressor agents, and control of disseminated intravascular coagulation. Renal failure represents a serious complication of septic abortion, stemming from infection and hypovolemia. The use of a radial artery cannula and pulmonary artery catheter aids in the evaluation of cardiovascular sequelae and assists in fluid therapy.

Incompetent Cervix

Painless dilation of the cervix, prolapse of membranes through the cervix, and ballooning of the membranes into the vagina characterize the incompetent cervix. Effective treatment averts rupture of the membranes and expulsion of the fetus. This condition, typically occurring in the second trimester or early in the third trimester, tends to recur with subsequent pregnancies.

Treatment, consisting of surgical reinforcement of the weak cervix with a purse-string suture, is usually performed after the first trimester but before cervical dilation reaches 4 cm. Bleeding and uterine contractions contraindicate surgery.

ANESTHETIC MANAGEMENT

Procedures for cervical incompetence are usually performed in the second or third trimester. Thus, anesthetic considerations for patients with cervical incompetence resemble those for anesthesia during second-trimester abortions but involve numerous complexities. In addition to the profound physiologic alterations in the respiratory, cardiovascular, and gastrointestinal systems associated with the second trimester, fetal well-being now demands consideration. Thus anesthesia should not stimulate uterine contractions or precipitate premature labor, should maintain uteroplacental perfusion, and should have a low potential for teratogenicity and abortion (see Chap. 27).

Toxicity to the Fetus

Almost all commonly used anesthetics have some teratogenicity in various animal species.[60] However extrapolating animal data to humans requires caution. In humans, anesthetic exposure during pregnancy does not seem to increase the incidence of fetal anomalies, but acute and chronic exposure to the operating room environment may increase the incidence of spontaneous abortions.[61,62]

In addition to drug exposure, other factors influencing teratogenicity may include variations in individual sensitivities and stage of development. The most critical time for drug exposure is the period of organogenesis, which takes place in the first trimester (15 to 56 days), although central nervous system sensitivity to exposure may exist later during gestation. The vulnerable period for brain development may extend from the 7th intrauterine month to the first few months after birth.

Effects on Uteroplacental Perfusion

Maternal oxygenation and uteroplacental perfusion, major determinants of fetal well-being, may be significantly altered during anesthesia and surgery. Many factors decrease uteroplacental perfusion. Excessive positive-pressure ventilation may decrease uterine blood flow resulting in fetal hypoxia and acidosis,[63,64] and maternal hyperventilation can reduce umbilical blood flow.[65] Maternal hypotension may follow sympathetic blockade, hypovolemia, aortocaval compression, or deep general anesthesia and compromise uterine blood flow.[66] Finally, uterine artery vasoconstriction from endogenous or exogenous catecholamines can decrease uterine blood flow, thus jeopardizing fetal well-being.[67,68]

Preoperative Management

Patients with cervical incompetence receive premedication with sodium citrate prior to anesthetic induction. Reassurance may avoid the need for preoperative analgesics and sedatives. To decrease the incidence of aortocaval compression, patients are transported to and from the operating room in the lateral decubitus position, and uterine displacement is maintained during the surgical procedure.

Perioperative Management

Regardless of the anesthetic technique, the patient should receive supplemental oxygen, since maternal hyperoxia improves fetal oxygenation.[69,70] Maternal oxygenation should be assessed during surgery with a pulse oximeter.

Spinal anesthesia remains the method of choice for the patient with an incompetent cervix, providing ideal surgical conditions, limiting drug exposure to one agent, and minimizing the chance of acid aspiration. The anesthesiologist may use epidural anesthesia but must take great care to avoid intravenous injection of toxic amounts of local anesthetic, since these can trigger fetal hypoxia by producing maternal convulsions and hypoxia, and cause uterine hypertonus with resultant decreased uterine blood flow.[71] Researchers[72] have not reported teratogenicity with local anesthetics in animals or humans. One should avoid hypotension in these patients by adequate intravenous fluid administration, uterine displacement, reduction of local anesthetic dose, and intravenous ephedrine if necessary.

If general anesthesia is selected, thorough preoxygenation minimizes hypoxia during induction. The increased risk of aspiration necessitates the following measures: rapid-sequence induction with cricoid pressure followed by tracheal intubation with a cuffed endotracheal tube, awake extubation, and preoperative sodium citrate administration. A generous dose of succinylcholine and a peripheral nerve stimulator help to prevent coughing and bucking, which can lead to rupture, especially in those with bulging membranes. To reduce the fetal hazards of drug exposure, patients should receive only those drugs with a long history of safety such as sodium thiopental, morphine sulfate, meperidine, succinylcholine, halothane, and perhaps nitrous oxide. Nitrous oxide reduces the concentration of inspired oxygen and is believed by some[73,74] to be contraindicated because of its effects on DNA synthesis. Halothane, well known as a potent myometrial depressant, in theory may reduce the incidence of premature delivery, although the effect is short-lived postoperatively. Hyperventilation reduces uterine blood flow and must be avoided, and end-tidal carbon dioxide levels should be monitored with a capnograph. Fetal heart rate (FHR), an important monitor indicating fetal homeostasis, should be monitored if possible. Using a Doppler, FHR can be monitored from the 16th week of gestation.

Postoperative Management

Careful patient monitoring is essential in the recovery room, where hypoxia and hypotension may occur. The threat of premature labor calls for postoperative uterine activity monitoring and possible administration of tocolytic agents.

Summary

The problems of early pregnancy include ectopic pregnancy, neoplastic trophoblastic disease, abortion, and cervical incompetence. Anesthesia for the early obstetric patient must take into account the profound physiologic adaptations that accompany early pregnancy. In addition, anesthesia for cervical incompetence must include anesthetic considerations for the well-being of the fetus. Only with this knowledge can these patients be approached in an intelligent and competent manner.

References

1. Albright, GA, et al: Anesthesia in Obstetrics: Maternal, Fetal, and Neonatal Aspects. Butterworth, Woburn, MA, 1986, p 49.
2. Weinberger, SE, et al: Pregnancy and the lung. Am Rev Respir Dis 121:559, 1980.
3. Tyler, JM: The effect of progesterone on the respiration of patients with emphysema and hypercapnia. J Clin Invest 39:34, 1960.
4. Widlung, G: Cardio-pulmonary function during pregnancy: A clinical experimental study with particular respect to ventilation and oxygen consumption among normal cases in rest and after work tests. Acta Obstet Gynaecol Scand 25:1, 1945.
5. Cugell, DW, et al: Pulmonary function in pregnancy. I: Serial observations in normal women. Am Rev Tuberc 67:568, 1953.
6. Archer, GW, Jr and Marx, GF: Arterial oxygen tension during apnoea in parturient women. Br J Anaesth 46:358, 1974.
7. Palahniuk, RJ, Shnider, SM and Eger, EI II: Pregnancy decreases the requirements for inhaled anesthetic agents. Anesthesiology 41:82, 1974.
8. Goland, RS, et al: Human plasma beta-endorphin during pregnancy, labor, and delivery. J Clin Endocrinol Metab 52:74, 1981.
9. Lund, CT and Donovan, JC: Blood volume during pregnancy: Significance of plasma and red cell volumes. Am J Obstet Gynecol 98:393, 1967.
10. Metcalfe, J and Ueland, K: Maternal cardiovascular adjustments to pregnancy. Prog Cardiovasc Dis 16:363, 1974.
11. Ueland, K and Hansen, JM: Maternal cardiovascular

dynamics. II: Posture and uterine contractions. Am J Obstet Gynecol 103:1, 1969.
12. Bieniarz, J, et al: Aortocaval compression by the uterus in late human pregnancy. II: An arteriographic study. Am J Obstet Gynecol 100:203, 1968.
13. Bromage, PL: Continuous lumbar epidural analgesia for obstetrics. Can Med Assoc J 85:1136, 1961.
14. Fragraeus, L, Urban, BJ and Bromage, PR: Spread of epidural analgesia in early pregnancy. Anesthesiology 58:184, 1983.
15. Datta, S, et al: Differential sensitivities of mammalian nerve fibers during pregnancy. Anesth Analg 62:1070, 1983.
16. Christofides, ND, et al: Decreased plasma motilin concentrations in pregnancy. Br Med J 285:1453, 1982.
17. Davison, JS, Davison, MC and Hay, DM: Gastric emptying time in late pregnancy and labour. J Obstet Gynaecol Br Commonw 77:37, 1970.
18. Brock-Utne, JG, et al: Gastric and lower oesophageal sphincter (LOS) pressures in early pregnancy. Br J Anaesth 53:381, 1981.
19. Attia, RR, et al: Maternal, fetal and placental gastrin concentrations. Anaesthesia 37:18, 1982.
20. Roberts, RB and Shirley, MA: Reducing the risk of acid aspiration during cesarean section. Anesth Analg 53:859, 1974.
21. Wyner, J and Cohen, SE: Gastric volume in early pregnancy. Anesthesiology 57:209, 1982.
22. Rubin, GL, et al: Ectopic pregnancy in the United States: 1970 through 1978. JAMA 249:1725, 1983.
23. Prichard, JA, MacDonald, PC and Gant, NF: Williams Obstetrics. Appleton-Century-Crofts, Norwalk, CT, 1985, p 424.
24. Pritchard, JA and Adams, RH: The fate of blood in the peritoneal cavity. Surg Gynecol Obstet 105:621, 1957.
25. Fishburn, JI: Anesthesia for laparoscopy: Considerations, complications and techniques. J Reprod Med 21:37, 1978.
26. Magno, R, et al: Acid-base balance during laparoscopy: The effects of intraperitoneal insufflation of carbon dioxide and nitrous oxide on acid-base balance during controlled ventilation. Acta Obstet Gynaecol Scand 58:81, 1979.
27. Baratz RA and Karis, JH: Blood gas studies during laparoscopy under general anesthesia. Anesthesiology 30:463, 1969.
28. Drummond, GB and Martin, LVH: Pressure-volume relationships in the lung during laparoscopy. Br J Anaesth 50:261, 1978.
29. Marshall, RL, et al: Circulatory effects of carbon dioxide insufflation of the peritoneal cavity for laparoscopy. Br J Anaesth 44:680, 1972.
30. Ivankovich, AD, et al: Cardiovascular effects of intraperitoneal insufflation with carbon dioxide and nitrous oxide in the dog. Anesthesiology 42:281, 1975.
31. Horrigan, RW, et al: Etomidate vs. thiopental with and without fentanyl: A comparative study of awakening in man. Anesthesiology 52:362, 1980.
32. Valanne, J and Korttila, K: Effect of a small dose of droperidol on nausea, vomiting and recovery after outpatient enflurane anaesthesia. Acta Anaesth Scand 29:359, 1985.
33. O'Donovan, N and Shaw, J: Nausea and vomiting in day-case dental anaesthesia. Anaesthesia 39:1172, 1984.
34. Fisher, MD, et al: Comparison of enflurane, halothane, and isoflurane for diagnostic and therapeutic procedures in children with malignancies. Anesthesiology 63:647, 1985.
35. Carter, JA, Dye, AM and Cooper, GM: Recovery from day-case anaesthesia: The effect of different inhalational anaesthetic agents. Anaesthesia 40:545, 1983.
36. Heneghan, C, et al: Morbidity after outpatient anaesthesia: A comparison of two techniques of endotracheal anaesthesia for dental surgery. Anaesthesia 36:4, 1981.
37. Strafford, JC and Ragan, WD: Abdominal pregnancy: Review of current management. Obstet Gynecol 50:548, 1977.
38. Beacham, WD, et al: Abdominal pregnancy at Charity Hospital in New Orleans. Am J Obstet Gynecol 84:1257, 1962.
39. Dorfman, SF: Deaths from ectopic pregnancy: United States 1979 to 1980. Obstet Gynecol 62:344, 1983.
40. Pritchard, JA, MacDonald, PC and Gant, NF: Williams Obstetrics. Appleton-Century-Crofts, Norwalk, CT, 1985, p 447.
41. Wu, FY: Recurrent hydatidiform mole: A case report of nine consecutive molar pregnancies. Obstet Gynecol 41:2000, 1973.
42. Lewis, JR, Jr: Treatment of metastatic gestational trophoblastic neoplasms. Am J Obstet Gynecol 136:163, 1980.
43. Pritchard, JA, MacDonald, PC and Gant, NF: Williams Obstetrics. Appleton-Century-Crofts, Norwalk, CT, 1985. p 467.
44. Hertig, AT and Sheldon, WH: Minimal criteria required to prove prima facie case of traumatic abortion or miscarriage: An analysis of 1,000 spontaneous abortions. Ann Surg 117:596, 1943.
45. Peyser, MR and Toaff, R: Rupture of uterus in the first trimester caused by high-concentration oxytocin drip. Obstet Gynecol 40:371, 1972.
46. Pritchard, JA: Haematological problems associated with delivery, placental abruption, retained dead fetus, and amniotic fluid embolism. Clin Haematol 2:563, 1973.
47. Rita, L, et al: Intramuscular midazolam for pediatric preanesthetic sedation: A double-blind controlled study with morphine. Anesthesiology 63:528, 1985.
48. Ong, BY, Palanhniuk, RJ and Cumming, M: Gastric volume and pH in out-patients. Can Anaesth Soc J 25:36, 1978.
49. Grimes, DA, et al: Local versus general anesthesia: Which is safer for performing suction curettage abortions? Am J Obstet Gynecol 135:1030, 1979.
50. Mackay, HT, Schulz, KF and Grimes, DA: Safety of local versus general anesthesia for second-trimester dilatation and evacuation abortion. Obstet Gynecol 66:661, 1985.
51. Cullen, BF, Margolis, AJ and Eger, EI II: The effects of anesthesia and pulmonary ventilation on blood loss

during elective therapeutic abortion. Anesthesiology 32:108, 1970.
52. Naftalin, NJ, Phear, WPC and Goldberg, AH: Halothane and isometric contractions of isolated pregnant rat myometrium. Anesthesiology 42:458, 1975.
53. Munson, ES and Embro, WJ: Enflurane, isoflurane, and halothane and isolated human uterine muscle. Anesthesiology 46:11, 1977.
54. Peterson, HB, et al: Comparative risk of death from induced abortion at less than 12 weeks' gestation performed with local versus general anesthesia. Am J Obstet Gynecol 141:763, 1981.
55. Meridy, HW: Criteria for selection of ambulatory surgical patients and guidelines for anesthetic management: A retrospective study of 1553 cases. Anesth Analg 61:921, 1982.
56. Grimes, DA and Cates, W Jr: Deaths from paracervical anesthesia used for first-trimester abortion: 1972–1975. N Engl J Med 295:1394, 1976.
57. Flaaten, H and Raeder, J: Spinal anaesthesia for outpatient surgery. Anaesthesia 40:1108, 1985.
58. Bridenbaugh, LD: Regional anesthesia for outpatient surgery: A summary of 12 years experience. Can Anaesth Soc J 30:548, 1983.
59. Herbert, M, et al: Profile of recovery after general anaesthesia. Br Med J 286:1539, 1983.
60. Smith, BE: Teratology in anesthesia. Clin Obstet Gynecol 17:145, 1974.
61. Duncan, PG, et al: Fetal risk of anesthesia and surgery during pregnancy. Anesthesiology 64:790, 1986.
62. Buring, JE, et al: Health experiences of operating room personnel. Anesthesiology 62:325, 1985.
63. Levinson, G, et al: Effects of maternal hyperventilation on uterine blood flow and fetal oxygenation and acid-base status. Anesthesiology 40:340, 1974.
64. Moya, F, et al: Influence of maternal hyperventilation on the newborn infant. Am J Obstet Gynecol 91:76, 1965.
65. Motoyama, EK, et al: Adverse effect of maternal hyperventilation on the foetus. Lancet 1:286, 1966.
66. Greiss, FC Jr: Pressure-flow relationship in the gravid uterine vascular bed. Am J Obstet Gynecol 96:41, 1966.
67. Shnider, SM, et al: Uterine blood flow and plasma norepinephrine changes during maternal stress in the pregnant ewe. Anesthesiology 50:524, 1979.
68. Adamsons, K, Mueller-Heubach, E and Myers, RE: Production of fetal asphyxsia in the rhesus monkey by administration of catecholamines to the mother. Am J Obstet Gynecol 109:248, 1971.
69. Marx, GF and Mateo, CV: Effects of different oxygen concentrations during general anesthesia for elective caesarean section. Can Anaesth Soc J 18:587, 1971.
70. Ramanathan, S, et al: Oxygen transfer from mother to fetus during cesarean section under epidural anesthesia. Anesth Analg 61:576, 1982.
71. Greiss, FC Jr, Still, JG and Anderson, SG: Effects of local anesthetic agents on the uterine vasculatures and myometrium. Am J Obstet Gynecol 124:889, 1976.
72. Fujinaga, M and Mazze, RE: Reproductive and teratogenic effects of lidocaine in Sprague-Dawley rats. Anesthesiology 65:626, 1986.
73. O'Sullivan, H, et al: Human bone marrow biochemical function and megaloblastic hematopoiesis after nitrous oxide anesthesia. Anesthesiology 55:645, 1981.
74. Baden, JM, et al: Thymidine and methionine syntheses in pregnant rats exposed to nitrous oxide. Anesth Analg 62:738, 1983.

PART 2

ANESTHESIA FOR THE UNCOMPLICATED PATIENT

CHAPTER 6

ANESTHETIC ALTERNATIVES FOR OBSTETRICS

GRAHAM H. MCMORLAND, M.B., Ch.B., D.A., F.R.C.P.C.

Women have sought relief from pain during childbirth throughout recorded history. However, modern obstetric anesthesia began when James Simpson[1] and John Snow[2] in Britain and Walter Channing[3] in the United States used open-drop administration of ether and chloroform. Other inhalation agents, such as nitrous oxide, methoxyflurane, trichlorethylene, and cyclopropane, have all subsequently served to provide analgesia and anesthesia. In recent years, obstetric anesthesiologists have added halothane, enflurane, and isoflurane to the armamentarium.

Systemic analgesics for labor came into popular use in the early part of this century when morphine was combined with scopolamine to produce a state known as "twilight sleep." The synthetic narcotics have now supplanted morphine for use during labor, but the depressant effect of these drugs on both mother and fetus has become recognized with consequent reduction in frequency of administration.

Although clinicians practiced subarachnoid and epidural anesthesia in the early part of this century, the rational basis for their use awaited Cleland's identification of the sensory innervation of the birth canal in 1933.[4]

The multitude of studies that have contributed to a greater understanding of the effects of drugs on the fetus, neonate, and progress of labor have profoundly influenced the current practice of obstetric analgesia and anesthesia. The recent emphasis on prenatal preparation for childbirth has resulted in well-informed parturients who demand minimal exposure to depressant drugs during childbirth and an increased emphasis on psychoprophylactic techniques for coping with labor pain. Many obstetric units now observe a decrease in demand for chemical analgesia during labor, particularly of systemic narcotics. However, Melzack[5] has shown that even after careful prenatal preparation, most women experience labor pain. The true value of prenatal preparation lies in the increased ability to cope with, rather than to suppress, this pain.

The "ideal" obstetric analgesic remains to be discovered. It should provide pain relief for the parturient while avoiding fetal depression and adverse effects on the progress of labor. Additionally, maternal analgesia should be safe; free from toxic side effects; predictable in onset time, analgesic potency, and duration of action; easy to administer; and freely available. Until such a perfect analgesic becomes evident, the known effects of existing techniques on mother, fetus, and neonate govern the choice of analgesia or anesthesia.

Labor and Vaginal Delivery

PHYSIOLOGY OF LABOR AND DELIVERY

Pain Pathways

Sensory fibers that travel with sympathetic fibers to the spinal cord transmit the pain of labor. Those from the body of the uterus, which transmit painful impulses during the first stage of labor, enter the neuraxis at the 10th, 11th and 12th thoracic and first lumbar spinal segments. During the second stage of labor, sensory fibers from the lower birth canal travel via the pudendal nerves to the second, third, and fourth sacral segments of the spinal cord. The sensory function, if any, of the pelvic parasympathetic nerves, which travel to the S2, S3, and S4 segments (nervi erigentes), remains controversial, but may explain the persistent backache noted in some labors which persists despite segmental lumbar epidural blockade of the lower thoracic and upper lumbar segments.

Endocrine Changes in Labor

Maternal plasma catecholamine levels rise during normal labor to levels significantly higher than those seen in late pregnancy.[6] Studies in primates,[7,8] and sheep[9] demonstrate that the psychological stress associated with painful labor may produce fetal hypoxia and acidosis. This probably results from decreased uterine blood flow and placental hypoperfusion secondary to the vasoconstrictive effects of high maternal plasma catecholamine levels. Studies on human parturients[10,11] show that women who have severe pain or who experience anxiety and exhaustion have higher plasma levels of epinephrine and, consequently, decreased uterine activity and longer labor. These women manifest an increased incidence of abnormal fetal heart rate patterns, and their babies tend to have lower Apgar scores.[8] Increased maternal plasma catecholamine levels additionally augment the already increased cardiac output associated with pregnancy.

Shnider and coworkers[12] demonstrated that lumbar epidural analgesia during labor decreases maternal plasma epinephrine by 56 percent and also abolishes the rise in plasma catecholamine levels occurring at the height of each contraction. Another study by Hagerdal[13] showed that epidural analgesia will prevent the significant increases in maternal oxygen consumption and minute ventilation that normally occur during uterine contraction. Together these studies suggest that, when nonpharmacologic techniques of pain management during labor prove ineffective or inadequate, well-managed chemical analgesia reduces stress and benefits mother, fetus, and neonate.

Plasma levels of β-endorphin and β-lipotropin are higher in pregnant than in nonpregnant women and increase further during labor.[14–18] Epidural analgesia during labor significantly lowers plasma β-endorphin levels,[17,18] suggesting that pain and psychological stress, rather than labor itself, stimulate the increased secretion of β-endorphin. However, Steinbrook and others[19] reported that CSF β-endorphin levels do not increase significantly during labor. This finding causes some doubt over inferences regarding behavioral changes during parturition based on plasma endorphin measurements.

Mechanism of Labor

Although the mechanism for the onset of labor remains unknown, a number of factors are probably involved. Prostaglandins $F_{2\alpha}$ and $E_{2\alpha}$, present in maternal blood and in amniotic fluid throughout pregnancy, increase significantly during normal labor and will stimulate uterine contraction.[20–22] Fuchs[23] has suggested that prostanoids released from maternal decidua and amniotic membranes may initiate labor.

OBSTETRIC CONSIDERATIONS

An ideal analgesic technique employed during labor should have minimal effect on the quality and duration of labor. As suggested above, the judicious use of pharmacologic techniques of pain relief may reduce (or prevent) maternal exhaustion and the concomitant adverse effects on labor and fetal well-being. Obstetricians and anesthesiologists frequently disagree on the effect of analgesia on uterine activity, duration of labor, and maternal ability to push in the second stage. Obstetricians expect maternal relaxation during the first stage of labor, with no inhibition of uterine activity or adverse effect on fetal well-being. They also expect anesthesiologists to avoid any inhibition of motor function, in order to maintain maternal expulsive efforts in the second stage.

CHOICE OF ANESTHESIA

Systemic Medication

In spite of the rise in popularity of regional analgesia during labor, many parturients still depend on intramuscular or intravenous drugs for relief of labor pain. This section briefly considers the use of systemically administered drugs. (Refer to Chapter 2 for a detailed discussion of the placental transfer of these drugs and their fetal and neonatal effects.)

Narcotics. Narcotic drugs, used widely to provide labor analgesia, all produce dose-related respiratory depression and peripheral vasodilation. Indeed, the doses required to produce complete analgesia will produce maternal and neonatal hypoventilation, orthostatic hypotension, and sedation. Additionally, large doses may obtund protective laryngeal reflexes and inhibit uterine activity. These drugs may cause severe nausea and vomiting in some parturients and inhibit gastric motility and delay stomach emptying.[24,25]

Meperidine. The peak effect of meperidine, the most frequently used narcotic in parturients, occurs 40 to 50 min after intramuscular injection and 5 to 10 min after intravenous administration. Analgesic action lasts for 3 to 4 hours. Placental transmission rapidly follows maternal intravenous injection, with the agent reaching the fetal circulation within 90 sec.[26,27] Shnider and Moya[28] recorded an increase in the number of depressed infants 2 hours after maternal intramuscular injection of meperidine. Recently, Kuhnert and coworkers[29,30] demonstrated that neonatal levels of meperidine metabolites (notably normeperidine) increase with longer administration of drug-to-delivery intervals. Although neurobehavioral changes have been observed for 60 to 72 hours after birth in infants whose mothers received meperidine during labor,[31] Kuhnert[30] noted that the less-than-optimal neurobehavioral scores relate to longer drug-to-delivery intervals. Kuhnert[32,33] also reported that an increased effect of meperidine (and normeperidine) on the neonate follows multiple maternal doses during labor and attributed this to continuing mother-to-fetus concentration gradients. The maximal neonatal effect comes about upon combination of a longer drug-to-delivery interval with administration of multiple doses.

Meperidine usage during labor may also proceed by continuous intravenous infusion or by means of a patient-controlled demand apparatus. The latter consists of a prefilled syringe attached to an infusion pump. The patient activates the pump to receive a predetermined dose of intravenous meperidine, but a timing mechanism ensures that the pump can be activated no more frequently than a preset interval. Use of this technique requires further study before it can be recommended for common use during labor.

Morphine. The obstetric team rarely employs this long-acting narcotic. In equianalgesic doses, it produces approximately 10 times more neonatal respiratory depression than meperidine, possibly because morphine has a greater ability to penetrate the infant's brain.[34]

Fentanyl. This potent narcotic (100 μg is equianalgesic to 10 mg morphine) has a rapid onset and short duration of action. Redistribution, rather than metabolism, accounts for the short duration of action, and repeated doses result in drug accumulation.

Agonist-Antagonist Drugs. These agents, which combine potent analgesic effects with minimal respiratory depression, have recently generated interest. Butorphanol and nalbuphine appear to provide good analgesia without the psychotomimetic effects associated with pentazocine. Butorphanol (2 mg intramuscularly or 1 mg intravenously) and meperidine have proved equally effective and safe for labor analgesia.[35] Nalbuphine, in a dose of 10 to 15 mg intramuscularly, is equipotent to morphine. It produces some respiratory depression, comparable with that produced by morphine and meperidine. However, a "ceiling" for respiratory depression exists, and doses above 20 mg produce less respiratory depression than equipotent doses of meperidine.[36]

Sedatives and Tranquilizers. Psychological preparation for labor can allay fear and anxiety, but, whether owing to inadequate preparation or inherent emotional instability, some women require medication to reduce anxiety. Parturients should not routinely receive any depressant drug, even in early labor, as these agents increase the risk of neonatal depression. When sedation becomes necessary, carefully titrated doses of phenothiazines, hydroxyzine, or lorazepam are less depressant to the fetus than barbiturates.

Ketamine. Intense analgesia and amnesia with only mild sedation characterize the intramuscular or intravenous injection of ketamine. Although ketamine is not used during labor, Akamatsu and associates[37] recommend its use in low doses (0.2 to 1.4 mg per kg intravenously) for vaginal delivery. Analgesia develops rapidly (<30 sec), and recovery begins approximately 4 min after administration. This technique merits consideration for difficult vaginal delivery and low forceps extraction or when regional analgesia is contraindicated or proves inadequate. Disadvantages include profound maternal amnesia and possible psychotomimetic effects. The mother's airway must be monitored continuously, even with small doses of ketamine, and equipment for endotracheal intubation must be immediately available.

Inhalation Analgesia

This term describes the administration of inhalation anesthetic agents in subanesthetic concentrations to provide analgesia during labor or delivery. Ideally the mother remains fully conscious and cooperative, while maintaining her protective laryngeal reflexes. The degree of analgesia provided is not comparable with that obtained with regional analgesia, but it is adequate for many parturients. Anesthesiologists are not always available in obstetric units, and inhalation analgesia is a technique that may be used by nurse anesthetists and (in some countries) midwives or even by the parturient through self-administration.

The reduction in functional residual capacity and increased alveolar ventilation in pregnant women, combined with the decrease in minimum alveolar concentration (MAC) for inspired anesthetic agents, will increase the risk of accidental anesthetic overdose. Even during self-administration, the patient requires constant supervision and observation because of the serious consequences of acid aspiration.

Almost all known inhalation agents have been used to provide analgesia during labor. Nitrous oxide (50 percent), isoflurane (0.5 to 0.7 percent) and enflurane (0.3 to 0.8 percent) currently are the most commonly used agents. Methoxyflurane, now obsolete, once enjoyed a period of popularity as a self-administered agent. A study in the United Kingdom[38] showed loss of consciousness in a significant number of parturients who inhaled 70-percent nitrous oxide. Intermittent administration of 50-percent nitrous oxide during uterine contraction produces peak analgesia about 45 sec after inhalation commences. Thus the patient should begin inhalation at the onset of each contraction, rather than waiting for contraction pain to become intense. No apparent fetal depression develops during intermittent inhalation of nitrous oxide. In fact, because 50-percent oxygen accompanies nitrous oxide administration, the fetus may benefit from this method. Older demand-flow devices for the delivery of nitrous oxide–oxygen mixtures (Fig. 6–1) allowed significant environmental pollution by the exhaled gas. A fixed-concentration nitrous-oxide apparatus for self-administration that is currently available (Fig. 6–2) provides for scavenging of waste gases.

Several types of hand-held vaporizers can deliver volatile anesthetic agents and allow for a predetermined vapor concentration to be set and locked (Fig. 6–3). Some patients may prefer commercially available disposable mouthpieces to the usual face mask. Methoxyflurane is no longer used in most countries because of concerns about nephrotoxicity. Additionally, many patients object to its pungent odor. Halothane, which provides no analgesia, is not suitable as an inhalation analgesic during labor. Isoflurane and enflurane do provide analgesia, and both are being evaluated for this purpose.

Regional Analgesia

Lumbar Epidural Analgesia. In most centers lumbar epidural block has become the most popular technique for providing analgesia for labor and delivery. Insertion of an indwelling

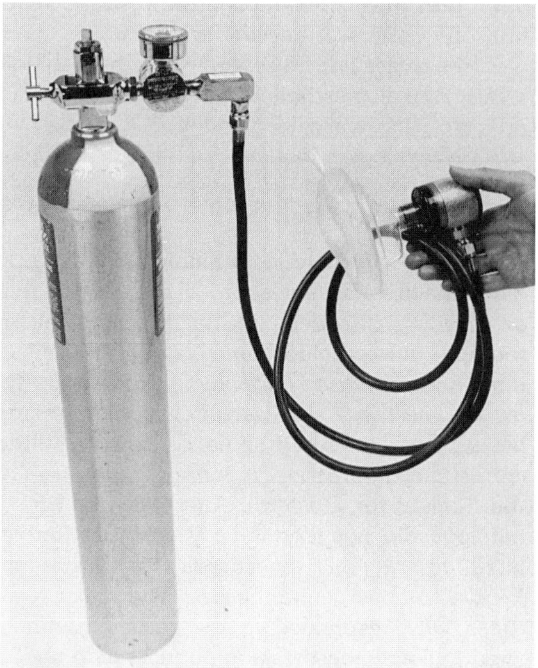

Figure 6–1. Self-administered inhalation apparatus (Entonox) with cylinder containing 50-percent nitrous oxide with oxygen.

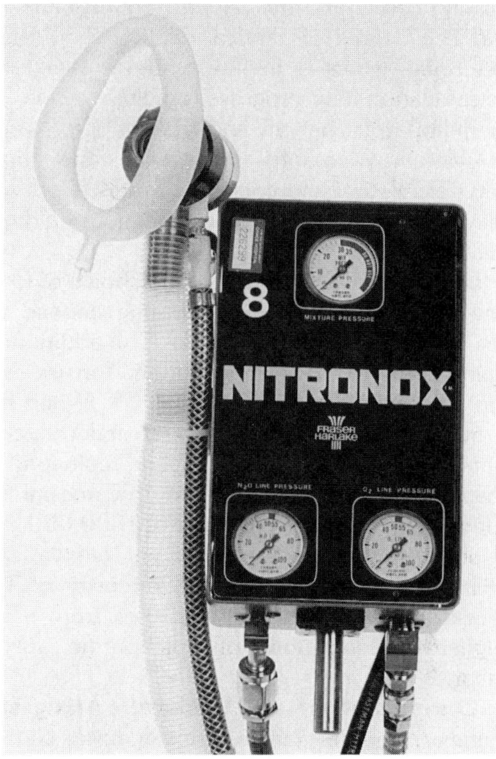

Figure 6–2. Nitrous oxide-oxygen inhalation apparatus for self-administration. Note the large-bore tube for waste gas scavenging.

lumbar epidural catheter makes it possible to provide segmental levels of analgesia that selectively block pain impulses from the contracting uterus during labor while maintaining sensation in the perineum and avoiding motor blockade. Intermittent injections or continuous infusions of a local anesthetic agent through the epidural catheter maintain analgesia. Appropriately chosen local anesthetic doses and careful monitoring generally avoid significant effects on the progress of labor and the expulsive powers in the second stage. Perineal analgesia established too early in labor may delay rotation of the descending fetal head and increase the incidence of transverse arrest or peristent occipitoposterior position. Conversely, slow uncoordinated labor patterns caused by maternal anxiety, pain, and exhaustion often improve or accelerate following establishment of good epidural analgesia and relaxation of the parturient, because adequate pain relief results in a reduction in maternal plasma catecholamine level.[12]

The epidural catheter is inserted when regular and efficient uterine contractions produce a

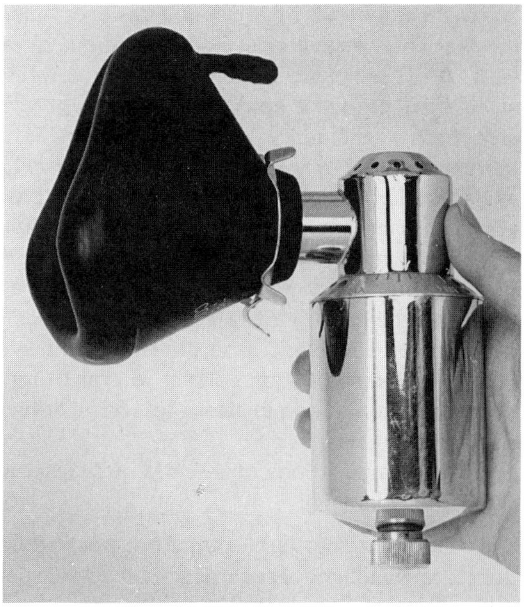

Figure 6–3. Cyprane inhaler for volatile anesthetic agents.

dilating cervix and the patient requests analgesia. The degree of cervical dilation should not determine when to initiate epidural analgesia, since dilation may progress rapidly in a relaxed or multiparous patient and may be slow when the woman is anxious and in pain. More rapid cervical dilation and coordinate uterine activity may follow establishment of adequate epidural analgesia.

Local Anesthetic Doses. The choice of local anesthetic drugs and their dosage depend on the desired effect (Table 6–1). The addition of epinephrine to the local anesthetic for use during labor remains controversial.[39,40] While improving the quality of analgesia and reducing uptake of local anesthetic agent, epinephrine may also reduce uterine blood flow and inhibit uterine contractility. The use of 1 : 800,000 epinephrine added to 0.125-percent bupivacaine will consistently increase the intensity of the block, and little advantage derives from using higher concentrations of epinephrine during labor.

Complications of Epidural Analgesia. Lumbar epidural analgesia exaggerates the effects of aortocaval compression. The associated sympathetic block causes vasodilation and a resultant relative hypovolemia and also inhibits the vasoconstrictor response to hypotension. The increased risk of hypotension necessitates establishing an intravenous infusion line prior to commencement of regional analgesia or anesthesia. The intravenous administration of at least 1000 ml of an isotonic solution prior to establishment of the epidural block can greatly reduce the incidence of hypotension. The uterus should be displaced laterally by putting a wedge under the patient's right hip or by positioning her on her side. In addition to carefully monitoring maternal blood pressure, the anesthesia team should monitor the uterine contractions and the fetal heart rate. Should significant hypotension occur, increase the rate of intravenous infusion, verify or correct lateral uterine displacement and administer 5 to 15 mg ephedrine intravenously.

Other complications of epidural analgesia include the following:

1. Unintentional dural puncture; post–dural puncture headache develops in 50 to 70 percent of cases if untreated.
2. Total spinal anesthesia if the accidental dural puncture is not recognized prior to injection of larger local anesthetic doses.
3. Intravascular injection, with high blood levels of local anesthetic causing acute CNS and possibly cardiovascular toxicity.
4. Neurologic sequelae, although uncommon, may follow direct trauma to nerve roots by needle or catheter.

The few absolute contraindications to epidural analgesia during labor include coagulation- or bleeding disorders (including anticoagulant therapy), uncorrected hypovolemia, local infection, and increased intracranial pressure. Regional anesthesia for parturients with genital herpes has generated some concern but little consistency in practice. A survey of members of the Society for Obstetric Anesthesia and Perinatology did not identify any complication related to regional anesthesia in parturients known to have genital herpes. The majority of those who responded to the survey routinely used regional anesthesia in patients who underwent cesarean section in order to prevent herpes infection in the neonate. Ramanathan[41] reported uncomplicated administration of epidural anesthesia for cesarean section to 43 parturients with herpes genitalis lesions. Ravindran[42] described the safe use of this technique in 30 pregnant women with HSV-2 infection. Although many anesthesiologists refuse to administer epidural anesthesia to patients with known herpes genitalis, it is probable that many regional blocks have been performed on patients who had the disease but either neglected to inform the anesthesiologist or concealed the fact. I and my colleagues provide epidural analgesia or anesthesia to asymptomatic parturients with a history of recurrent herpes genitalis, with or without visible lesions. A possible exception to this rule may be a patient with active lesions over the sacral or lumbar region. Patients with primary infection, or recurrent infection with systemic symptoms (fever, arthralgia, headache, photophobia, and other signs of meningeal irritation), do not qualify for epidural block, unless an absolute contraindication to general anesthesia arises.

Caudal Block. This form of epidural analgesia[43] has become less popular for use during labor. It requires a 15- to 20-ml volume of local anesthetic to reach the T10 level and subsequent, slightly smaller top-up doses. This tech-

Table 6-1. LOCAL ANESTHETICS AND DOSES* RECOMMENDED FOR LUMBAR EPIDURAL ANALGESIA FOR LABOR AND DELIVERY

	Initial Dose	Top-up	Forceps
Intermittent			
Bupivacaine 0.5%	—	—	10–15 ml
Bupivacaine 0.25%	6–10 ml	6–8 ml	—
Bupivacaine 0.125% with 1:800,000 epinephrine	—	8–12 ml	—
Lidocaine 2%	—	—	10–15 ml
Lidocaine 1%	8–10 ml	8–10 ml	—
2-Chloroprocaine 2%	6–10 ml	6–8 ml	—
2-Chloroprocaine 3%	—	—	10–15 ml
	Initial Dose	**Maintenance**	
Continuous Infusion			
Bupivacaine 0.25%	6–10 ml	4–8 ml/hr	
Bupivacaine 0.125%	—	8–12 ml/hr	
2-Chloroprocaine 0.5%	—	20–30 ml/hr	
2-Chloroprocaine 2%	6–10 ml	—	
Lidocaine 0.5%	—	10–12 ml/hr	
Lidocaine 1%	6–10 ml	—	

*These doses serve as basic guidelines only and should be adjusted as necessary for each parturient.

nique nearly always blocks the sacral spinal cord segments, which may inhibit proper rotation of the fetal head causing a subsequent delay in the second stage. In comparison with lumbar epidural blockade, the degree of analgesia in labor is more extensive, and larger local anesthetic doses are required. Cleland[44] described a double catheter technique in which a lumbar epidural catheter provided analgesia for the first stage and a caudal catheter for the second stage of labor. This technique has never gained popularity and is rarely used. Caudal epidural analgesia is technically more difficult to perform than lumbar epidural blockade. Anatomic variations in the sacral hiatus occur frequently, and its diameter may be as small as 2 mm. In obese patients, the hiatus may be difficult to identify because of a subcutaneous fat pad. The needle may pass anterior to the sacrum and puncture the rectum or the fetal scalp.[45] The physician should perform a rectal examination before injecting the drug. The close proximity of the sacral hiatus to the rectum increases the risk of infection entering the site of needle puncture.

Lumbar Sympathetic Block. Bilateral lumbar sympathetic block provides reliable analgesia for the first stage of labor.[46] It is more difficult to perform than lumbar epidural blockade, and perineal analgesia in the second stage requires a different technique. Hunter[47] reported increased uterine activity after lumbar sympathetic block, and it may even be followed by tumultuous labor or uterine tetany. This technique, seldom used for obstetric analgesia, is contraindicated in mothers with fetal distress, breech presentation, or placental abruption.

Paracervical Block. This simple procedure, generally performed by the obstetrician, entails injection of local anesthetic through each lateral fornix of the vagina, adjacent to the cervix.[48] Although it was once used frequently, the popularity of the technique waned as reports of fetal bradycardia and occasional fetal death appeared in the literature. The etiology of the bradycardia remains uncertain but may relate to high fetal blood levels of the local anesthetic or to decreased uterine blood flow resulting from local anesthesia–induced constriction of uterine arteries. The current status of paracervical block in obstetric practice remains controversial. Shnider and associates[49] reported an increased incidence of bradycardia in the presence of pre-existing fetal distress or prematurity.

Bupivacaine is probably contraindicated for this procedure because of its greater vasoconstrictive and cardiotoxic effects. The local anesthetic of choice is 2-chloroprocaine, which has a short plasma half-life and low toxicity, although its action persists for only about 40 min. Fetal demise has followed accidental injection of local anesthetic into the fetal scalp, and caution should be exercised if cervical dilation exceeds 8 cm.

Pudendal Block. This provides perineal anesthesia for low forceps delivery and episiotomy.[50] The obstetrician usually administers the block transvaginally, with the local anesthetic injected just posterior to the ischial spines, beneath the sacrospinous ligaments. Ten milliliters of lidocaine (1-percent), mepivacaine (1-percent), or 2-chloroprocaine (2-percent) is injected on each side, usually with the patient in the lithotomy position. The method is safe and generally reliable. Intravascular injection may cause acute drug toxicity, and it is possible to perforate the rectum with a misplaced needle.

Subarachnoid Block. Although not used during labor, subarachnoid injection of local anesthetics frequently provides anesthesia for forceps delivery. Easier to perform than lumbar epidural analgesia in the second stage of labor, subarachnoid block develops rapidly and provides profound anesthesia. A small dose of hyperbaric local anesthetic, injected with the patient in a sitting position, provides anesthesia of the sacral segments. In practice, the block generally extends to the T10 dermatome, which provides good anesthesia for instrument delivery or manual exploration of the uterine cavity. Tetracaine (5 mg) or 5-percent lidocaine (30 to 40 mg) are the most commonly used agents. Bupivacaine (7.5 mg) provides longer lasting anesthesia. Lidocaine 1.5-percent (22.5 to 30 mg) offers excellent analgesia and preserves motor power, thus facilitating expulsive efforts. The use of a 25- or 26-gauge needle decreases the incidence of post–dural puncture headache[51] in comparison with needles of a larger diameter. Hypotension can occur and is treated by additional uterine displacement, rapid intravenous fluid infusion, and possibly intravenous ephedrine.

Intraspinal (Subarachnoid or Epidural) Narcotics. Subarachnoid injections of morphine in doses of 0.5 to 2 mg can provide prolonged analgesia for the first stage of labor but not enough analgesia for delivery.[52,53] There is a high incidence of side effects (pruritus, nausea and vomiting, somnolence, post–dural puncture headache), and onset of analgesia develops slowly. Patients with heart disease, some of whom may be considered unsuitable for epidural analgesia, may benefit from this technique because it avoids sympathetic block and hypotension.

Experience with epidural morphine during labor has been discouraging. Hughes and others[54] reported that a dose of 7.5 mg provides adequate analgesia for the first stage of labor in most patients, but does not produce perineal anesthesia for episiotomy or instrumentation at delivery. Smaller doses of morphine (2 mg and 5 mg) in the epidural space were ineffective.

Other narcotics, such as meperidine and fentanyl, have been administered epidurally during labor. Since they have greater lipid solubility, these drugs have a more rapid onset of action than morphine but provide limited analgesia. The combination of fentanyl (50 to 100 μg) and bupivacaine provides good epidural analgesia for labor, with a rapid onset of action and a longer duration than bupivacaine alone.[55]

Psychologic Techniques

Hypnosis. This technique, used occasionally to provide pain relief in labor, requires a lot of preparation time prior to onset of labor as well as a skilled hypnotherapist. Some authors[56] suggest that hypnosis shortens labor and may result in a lower incidence of operative deliveries. However, this form of analgesia may cause complications and may provoke an acute anxiety state or even frank psychosis in some subjects.[57]

Psychoprophylaxis. "Prepared childbirth" has gained popularity as an approach to management of the pain of labor and delivery. The unrealistic claims and expectations of the recent past gradually are being replaced by the recognition that prenatal education, controlled breathing and relaxation during labor, and the assistance of a labor "coach" enhance the ability of the parturient to cope with the pain of uterine contraction and reduce the need for chemical analgesia. Many women who receive careful psychoprophylactic (Lamaze) training request additional analgesia during labor, and Melzack[5] has suggested that their preparation aims at coping with, rather than preventing, pain. Saling and Ligidas[58] demonstrated that hyperventilation, occurring commonly in parturients wishing to avoid chemical analgesia, produces acidotic neonates.

Transcutaneous Electrical Nerve Stimulation (TENS)

The use of transcutaneous electrical nerve stimulation for relief of pain has been advocated for many years,[59,60] initially for treatment of chronic pain and later to relieve postoperative and labor pain.[61,62] Melzack and Wall's[63] gate theory of pain provoked interest in producing analgesia by electrical stimulation of afferent nerves. Solomon[64] suggested that TENS works by stimulating endogenous opioid production, although others dispute this theory.[65]

During labor, two pairs of electrodes are placed on the parturient's back, the upper pair over the dermatomes of the posterior rami of T10-L1 on each side of the spine, and the lower pair on each side of the sacrum. The electrodes connect to the TENS unit, which has a patient-operated switch to allow for a change of output from a preset low amplitude during each contraction. The parturient activates the upper pair of electrodes during the first stage of labor and employs the sacral electrodes late in the first stage, when pain is felt in the lower back. Attendants adjust the amplitude of the unit to produce a tingling sensation between contractions and a higher level during contractions. The degree of stimulation required varies with the need and tolerance of each patient. The range of amplitude is generally from 1 to 40 MA, with a frequency range of 40 to 150 Hz and pulse duration of 30 to 250 microseconds.

Analgesia with TENS is safe, noninvasive, and easily administered by nurses and midwives. Some patients find the sensation unpleasant and ask for the machine to be removed. Most reports are anecdotal, and there are few controlled studies of the analgesic value of this technique. One study from Europe[66] reported that 44 percent (of 147 patients) judged pain relief good to very good, and 12 percent considered that TENS had no beneficial effect.

Electrical interference with electronic fetal heart rate monitoring is the one major disadvantage of this technique. Reportedly TENS does not affect fetal heart rate, but its use in labor will remain limited until filters become available to block interference with monitoring equipment.

Acupuncture

Although acupuncture has been practiced in China for over a thousand years, Chinese women have, by tradition, delivered vaginally without analgesia. Thus no traditional acupuncture points for labor and vaginal delivery have evolved. Two North American studies[67,68] used the acupuncture points described for hysterectomy and dysmenorrhea to provide labor analgesia. Wallis and coworkers[67] reported that 19 of 21 patients experienced inadequate analgesia and 16 requested alternative forms of analgesia. Abouleish and Depp[68] assessed the effect of acupuncture on 12 parturients and noted poor and inconsistent analgesia. It does not presently appear to offer much advantage in the management of labor pain.

Anesthesia for Assisted Vaginal Delivery

Forceps Delivery or Vacuum Extraction. High forceps deliveries are no longer considered good practice, and parturients formerly requiring their use now generally deliver by cesarean section. Mid-forceps delivery has become somewhat controversial,[69,70] the need for the procedure often resulting from malrotation of the fetal head. Low (or outlet) forceps delivery implies that the bony fetal head has reached the perineum and is visible during uterine contractions, or the forceps may be indicated for delivery of the head in a breech presentation.

Mid-forceps delivery, with or without rotation of the fetal head, requires anesthesia of the sacral segments and good pelvic muscle relaxation. When an epidural catheter is in place and has been successfully used for labor analgesia, extension of the block to the sacral segments using chloroprocaine, lidocaine, or bupivacaine (see Table 6–1) should provide optimal conditions for the procedure. In the absence of a preplaced epidural catheter, it may be possible to institute an epidural block for the mid-forceps delivery or to establish a low subarachnoid (spinal) block. Occasionally, general anesthesia is indicated by acute fetal distress or other contraindication to regional anesthesia (Table 6–2). One should take the usual precautions to prevent regurgitation and pulmonary aspiration of gastric contents (antacid therapy, preoxygen-

Table 6–2. CONTRAINDICATIONS TO REGIONAL ANESTHESIA

Acute fetal distress, when rapid delivery is required
Uncorrected maternal hypovolemia
Maternal blood coagulopathies
Local infection
Patient refusal

ation, cricoid pressure, and rapid endotracheal intubation). The lithotomy position increases the danger of regurgitation and aspiration. Unless there is an overriding obstetric indication for the lithotomy position, the woman's legs are lowered prior to induction of anesthesia.

Anesthesia for low forceps delivery may be provided by extension of an existing epidural block, low spinal anesthesia, or pudendal block. Incomplete pudendal analgesia may be supplemented by inhalation analgesia (nitrous oxide, isoflurane, or enflurane) or low-dose ketamine (0.25 mg per kg).

Vacuum extraction, popular in many countries, consists of a metal suction cup applied to the fetal scalp, with steady, gentle traction applied during each contraction. This technique permits rotation of the head to occur in an almost physiologic manner. Anesthetic considerations are the same as for forceps delivery.

Obstetricians employ a "trial of forceps" when uncertain of a successful vaginal delivery and when planning to proceed to immediate cesarean section in case of failure. This procedure should take place in an operating room, and an anesthetic technique must be chosen that can also be used for cesarean section, if necessary. Lumbar epidural anesthesia for forceps delivery, which can be readily extended upward to T4, is the recommended technique.

Breech Delivery and Multiple Pregnancy. Consult Chapter 18 for a discussion of anesthetic management of these complications of vaginal birth. In general I prefer to employ epidural analgesia, which can be rapidly extended to provide anesthesia for operative delivery.

Retained Placenta. This occurs in about 1 percent of parturients and usually requires manual exploration of the uterus, which is painful for the mother. Occasionally inhalation analgesia (50-percent nitrous oxide or 0.5- to 0.75-percent isoflurane) will permit gentle manual removal of the placenta, especially in a multiparous patient. Low-dose ketamine (0.25 mg per kg intravenously) provides more profound analgesia for the procedure. A pre-existing epidural block may be extended if significant hemorrhage has not occurred, but the sympathetic block produced may make resuscitation difficult should severe bleeding subsequently develop. Rapid induction of general anesthesia after the patient's legs have been lowered from the lithotomy position is the safest course in most cases. Ketamine may be the induction agent of choice if the patient has hemorrhaged severely. Severe hemorrhage usually accompanies placenta accreta and, because the diagnosis is made only during attempts to separate the placenta from the uterine wall, this hemorrhage may develop unexpectedly and suddenly. Volume resuscitation becomes necessary as described in Chapter 15.

Cesarean Section

INDICATIONS FOR CESAREAN SECTION

The incidence of cesarean births has risen in recent years and may commonly exceed 20 percent of all deliveries. The reasons for this higher incidence include the increasing number of repeat cesarean sections, the trend to abdominal delivery of breech and premature babies, improved methods for detection of acute fetal distress, the ubiquitous "failure to progress," and the current concern over potential litigation. As more women gain the support of their obstetricians in choosing a "trial of labor" and vaginal birth following previous cesarean delivery, the rate of cesarean section may stabilize.

Electronic, biochemical, and other fetal monitoring techniques provide better understanding of fetal distress and may influence decisions to perform cesarean delivery.

OBSTETRIC CONSIDERATIONS

Optimal Operating Conditions

The obstetrician, as a surgeon, expects the anesthesiologist to provide a quiet patient with adequate muscle relaxation for surgery. The increased use of regional anesthesia for cesarean section requires careful attention to the comfort and emotional state of the patient. Thorough preanesthetic preparation for regional anesthesia is essential to allay anxiety and decrease restlessness. The current trend toward admitting the father to the operating room requires that he, too, should prepare for the procedure and have a clear understanding of his role.

Maternal Cardiopulmonary Support

The successful outcome of the cesarean section depends to a large degree on the effect of the anesthetic procedure on both mother and fetus. Placental perfusion is maintained by avoiding hypotension and drugs that reduce uterine blood flow. Avoid aortocaval compression by left uterine displacement. We place an inflatable wedge under the right hip that can be deflated after delivery of the baby (Fig. 6–4); or, the operating table may be tilted to the patient's left.

Maternal tissue perfusion must be maintained by avoiding hypotension and cardiac dysrhythmias. Provision of normal respiratory gas exchange and acid-base status require careful attention, particularly when hypovolemia has developed prior to the anesthetic. Oxygen administered by mask prior to induction of anesthesia and use of an oxygen-enriched mixture during maintenance reduce the risk of maternal hypoxemia and improve fetal oxygenation.

Choice of Drugs

All anesthetic drugs cross the placenta and may cause fetal and neonatal depression. The choice of drugs and dosage should be planned to minimize this effect.

CHOICE OF ANESTHESIA

Both general and regional (subarachnoid or epidural block) anesthetics are regularly and safely administered for cesarean section. Local anesthesia, or field block, generally proves unsatisfactory and is seldom employed. The current emphasis on family-oriented childbirth has been partially responsible for the increased use of regional anesthesia, often with the father present in the operating room.

The choice of anesthetic technique for cesarean section depends on careful evaluation of a number of factors, such as the degree of urgency, the reason for the operation, the maternal and fetal condition, the desire of the mother to be awake or asleep, and the anesthesiolo-

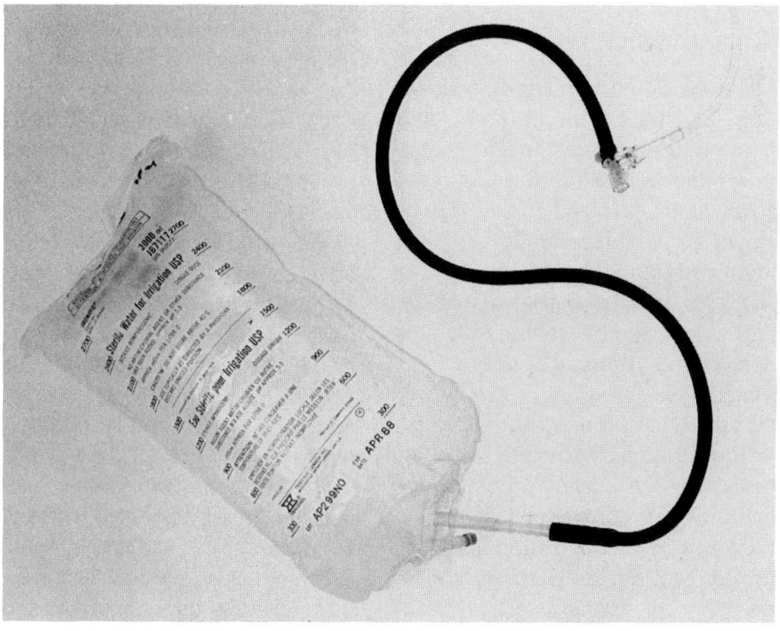

Figure 6–4. Inflatable wedge for uterine displacement.

gist's skill and experience. Maternal safety and comfort, fetoneonatal safety, and the presence of contraindications to a specific technique also warrant consideration.

Studies have shown that, provided aortocaval compression is avoided, fetal acid-base status varies little with anesthetic technique, in the absence of pre-existing fetal distress or anesthetic complications.[71-73] Regardless of anesthetic technique, a prolonged uterine incision-to-delivery time relates directly to fetal hypoxia and acidosis.[74,75] Hysterotomy and prolonged manipulation of the uterus adversely affect placental perfusion, and uterine incision-to-delivery times in excess of 3 min are associated with lower Apgar scores and decreased cord blood pH.

Local Anesthesia

Local field blocks are rarely performed for cesarean section. They frequently prove unsuccessful and present the danger of exceeding toxic doses of local anesthetics. Supplementation with excessive doses of sedatives and narcotics often becomes necessary. Obstetricians with considerable experience in this technique can employ it successfully and safely, but currently there are few such obstetricians in North America.

Regional Anesthesia

Both epidural and spinal (subarachnoid) blocks provide excellent anesthesia for cesarean section; the latter method offers easier administration and more rapid and profound anesthesia. Because epidural block evolves more slowly, hypotension develops less frequently and less precipitously than with spinal block. Injection of incremental doses of local anesthetic through the epidural catheter makes it easier to obtain an appropriate level and intensity of nerve block with epidural anesthesia.

Advantages and Disadvantages. Table 6–3 lists the advantages and disadvantages of regional anesthesia for cesarean section, and Table 6–2 identifies the contraindications.

Table 6–3. REGIONAL ANESTHESIA FOR CESAREAN SECTION

Advantages	Disadvantages
Conscious patient: Early-infant-mother bonding, father present, minimal risk of aspiration	Risk of hypotension
Generally reliable and predictable anesthesia level	Post–dural puncture headache
Reduced risk of fetal drug exposure and neonatal depression	Possible neurotoxic drug effects or overdose toxicity
Generally good operating conditions	Risk of unintentional "total spinal" block
Able to administer epidural narcotics following epidural anesthesia	

Principles. Prior to administration of anesthesia for cesarean section, all patients should be regarded as being at increased risk for pulmonary aspiration of acid gastric contents and, consequently, should receive a nonparticulate antacid prior to induction. Sodium citrate rapidly neutralizes gastric acid and may be given when the patient leaves for the operating room or, in emergency cases, following the decision to proceed with cesarean section.

Venous access is established by inserting a large-bore indwelling cannula and infusing 1000 to 2000 ml of dextrose-free isotonic crystalloid solution prior to initiating the regional block. Left uterine displacement prevents aortocaval compression. A syringe containing ephedrine is prepared to treat hypotension, which sometimes occurs in spite of adequate fluid "preload" and uterine displacement.

Epidural Anesthesia. Induction of lumbar epidural anesthesia commences with insertion of an epidural catheter at L2-3 or L3-4. Lidocaine (2-percent), 2-chloroprocaine (3-percent), or bupivacaine (0.5 percent), with 1:400,000 to 1:200,000 epinephrine, will provide adequate anesthesia and good operating conditions. A test dose of 3 ml of local anesthetic containing 15 μg epinephrine is recommended. This dose will produce anesthesia in the event of unintentional subarachnoid placement of the catheter. In many cases it will also reveal unintentional intravascular injection of the drug, as the epinephrine causes tachycardia. This effect is often transient, and an electronic cardiac monitor should always serve to detect transient change in maternal heart rate. Aspiration of the epidural catheter for CSF or blood will often, but not invariably, indicate subarachnoid or intravascular catheter placement, and a careful test dose is advised. Even after the test dose, avoid injection of a large bolus of local anesthetic. Incremental injections of 5-ml doses obviate the danger of large intravascular or subarachnoid doses and also afford more careful observation of the proximal spread of the block to approximately the T4 level.

Maternal blood pressure and ECG monitoring should continue throughout the procedure, and the fetal heart should be electronically monitored while the block develops. Constant verbal contact with the patient enhances her composure and will also give early warning of somnolence or agitation. One should be prepared to treat complications instantly and have equipment for endotracheal intubation immediately available (Chap. 7).

Spinal Anesthesia. This technique, easier to perform than epidural anesthesia, has a rapid onset of action and produces profound sensory and motor blockade. However hypotension occurs commonly and develops rapidly. Adequate intravenous fluid preload and careful attention to uterine displacement reduce the incidence and severity of hypotension. I do not administer ephedrine prophylactically but inject 5 to 10 mg intravenously at the first sign of hypotension; additional doses are given as required.

Either the sitting or lateral position may be used for insertion of the spinal needle. The sitting position makes identification of the lumbar spinous processes easier in obese patients and also reduces the time required for cerebrospinal fluid to appear at the hub of 25- or 26-gauge needles. The spinal cord terminates at the lower border of L1 or the upper border of L2 and, to avoid trauma of the cord, the spinal needle should not be inserted above the L2–3 interspace. Local anesthetics used for spinal anesthesia include 5-percent lidocaine with 7.5-percent dextrose (60 to 80 mg), 1-percent tetracaine with 10-percent dextrose (7 to 10 mg), and 0.75-percent bupivacaine (8 to 12 mg).

General Anesthesia

Properly administered general anesthesia for cesarean section (Table 6–4) includes rapid induction, reliable anesthesia, good operating conditions, less cardiovascular depression than regional anesthesia, and adequate control of respiratory function. It does, however, present an increased risk of pulmonary aspiration of gastric contents, frequently secondary to the hazards associated with rapid endotracheal intubation. Table 6–5 lists the advantages and disadvantages of general anesthesia. Chapter 2 discusses the effects of anesthetic drugs on the neonate.

Indications. The indications for general anesthesia include:

1. Maternal desire to be unconscious; some

Table 6–4. SUGGESTED METHOD OF GENERAL ANESTHESIA FOR CESAREAN SECTION

1. Preoperative administration of clear antacid, within 1 hour of operation, possibly H_2 blockers and metoclopramide.
2. Avoidance of aortocaval compression by uterine displacement.
3. Intravenous infusion of crystalloid via large-bore cannula.
4. Preoxygenation.
5. Induction after abdominal preparation and draping: thiopentone, 4 mg/kg, and succinylcholine, 1.5 mg/kg.
6. Cricoid pressure by assistant, maintained until endotracheal tube cuff is inflated.
7. Rapid endotracheal intubation.
8. Maintenance of anesthesia: N_2O with 50% oxygen and volatile agent (0.5% halothane, 0.75–1% enflurane, or 0.5–0.75% isoflurane).
9. Avoid hyperventilation.
10. Muscle relaxants as required: vecuronium, atracurium, or succinylcholine 0.1% drip.
11. Narcotic supplements after delivery to deepen anesthesia; the volatile agent may be continued at low concentration, if desired.
12. Extubation with mother on side and after protective laryngeal reflexes are regained.

Table 6–5. GENERAL ANESTHESIA FOR CESAREAN SECTION

Advantages	Disadvantages
Rapid induction (e.g., fetal distress, cord prolapse)	Danger of aspiration
Reliability:	Fetal and neonatal effects
Total pain relief, ease of maintenance, control of recovery	Possible maternal awareness and recall
Cardiovascular stability (usually)	Hypertension during induction
Less hypotension	Hazards of rapid endotracheal intubation
Unconscious patient	Patient unable to "participate" in delivery, father not present
Good surgical conditions	Greater blood loss

women fear having a needle inserted in the back or being awake for a surgical procedure.

2. Maternal coagulopathies or bleeding disorders that contraindicate regional anesthesia (Chap. 15).

3. Some believe that acute fetal distress, warranting rapid delivery and maintenance of normal maternal hemodynamics, indicates general rather than regional anesthesia, however Marx and coworkers,[76] comparing regional and general anesthesia administered for cesarean sections for fetal distress, found that both groups had similar umbilical vein and artery pH and blood gas values, while the 1-min Apgar scores were significantly better in the regional anesthesia group. The determining factor in cases of fetal distress appears to be the degree of urgency of the procedure, provided maternal hypotension can be avoided.

4. Uncorrected maternal hypovolemia generally contraindicates regional anesthesia because of the danger of severe hypotension secondary to sympathetic block and vasodilation. However, it seldom becomes necessary to proceed with an operative delivery prior to correction of hypovolemia.

5. Lack of skill in administration and management of regional anesthesia on the part of the anesthesiologist, obstetrician, or nursing team.

6. Some anesthesiologists prefer general anesthesia in the presence of a pre-existing neurologic disorder.

Principles. For cesarean section, these include measures to prevent pulmonary aspiration of gastric contents, intravenous infusion of crystalloid solution, preoxygenation, and prevention of aortocaval compression.

Aspiration. Pulmonary aspiration of gastric contents remains a major cause of maternal morbidity and mortality (Chap. 4). Methods to prevent aspiration include administration of clear antacids, metoclopramide, histamine-receptor antagonists, and rapid-sequence induction technique utilizing cricoid pressure (Chap. 7). Differences of opinion exist regarding effectiveness and dose requirements of chemical prophylaxis. When the decision is made to perform emergency cesarean section, I administer 30-ml 0.3 molar sodium citrate. Preparation for elective cesarean section under general anesthesia includes ranitidine, 80 mg orally the previous night and 90 min prior to induction of anesthesia. Metoclopramide, 10 mg, is administered orally with the second dose of ranitidine to obese patients and others in whom difficult endotracheal intubation is anticipated.

Intravenous Fluids. A large-bore (18-gauge or larger) intravenous cannula is inserted prior to either general or regional anesthesia, to rapidly infuse induction agents, oxytocic drugs, and fluids. I advocate prehydration with at least 1000 ml of dextrose-free crystalloid solution prior to induction.

Preoxygenation. Thorough maternal denitrogenation should precede induction to ensure adequate maternal and fetal oxygen delivery. This may be accomplished by allowing the patient either to breathe 100-percent oxygen by mask for 3 to 5 min or to take four maximally deep inspirations of pure oxygen.[77] This helps prevent the precipitous fall in PaO_2 which can occur during the apnea associated with laryngoscopy and endotracheal intubation.[13] Chapter 1 discusses the physical changes responsible for rapid maternal desaturation.

Precurarization. Many anesthesiologists no longer routinely use precurarization to prevent muscle fasciculations and the rise in intragastric pressure that follow succinylcholine injection. Pregnant women do not experience the severe fasciculations seen in nonpregnant patients,[78] and precurarization may inhibit the relaxation produced by succinylcholine, making rapid endotracheal intubation difficult.

Rapid-Sequence Induction. Thiopentone, 4 mg per kg, immediately followed by succinylcholine, 1.5 mg per kg, achieves a rapid-sequence induction, following draping of the patient's abdomen and preoxygenation. Ketamine, 1 mg per kg, may be preferred if the maternal hemodynamic state is unstable, but it often causes unpleasant dreams and restlessness during the recovery period. Pressure over the cricoid cartilage, as described by Sellick,[79] occludes the esophagus and prevents regurgitation of gastric contents as the patient loses consciousness and the cricopharyngeal sphincter relaxes. An assistant initiates cricoid pressure as the anesthesiologist injects induction drugs and maintains it until the endotracheal tube is in proper position and the cuff inflated. The anesthesiologist ventilates with pure oxygen while verifying the position of the endotracheal tube.

Failed or Difficult Intubation. Occasionally endotracheal intubation proves difficult or even impossible. This promotes maternal and fetal hypoxia and is often associated with regurgitation of stomach contents and pulmonary aspiration. This serious problem (frequently leading to significant morbidity and mortality) mandates careful preanesthetic evaluation of the patient to rule out obesity, short neck, receding chin, prominent teeth, and limitation of movement of neck or temporomandibular joints. Upper airway congestion in late pregnancy often significantly narrows the laryngeal opening and trachea indicating the use of a relatively small endotracheal tube (6.5 or 7 mm). Successful resolution of the difficult or failed intubation requires ready availability of necessary equipment and a sound plan of management (Chap. 7). Figure 6–5 summarizes the plan I use in such instances.

Maintenance of Anesthesia. Prior to delivery of the infant, anesthesia is maintained with 50-percent nitrous oxide with oxygen and muscle relaxant. Patient awareness sometimes occurs at this concentration of nitrous oxide and may be prevented by addition of 0.5-percent halothane, 0.7-percent isoflurane, or 0.8-percent enflurane (Chap. 7). Halogenated agents decrease uterine muscle tone and increase postpartum blood loss. This effect is dose related,[80,81] and the low concentrations recommended do not cause increased blood loss.[82] Exceeding the recommended concentration of halogenated agents may produce fetal depression.[82]

Uterine Displacement. Tilting the operating table to the left or placing a wedge under the right hip of the patient displaces the uterus to prevent aortocaval compression. I prefer an inflatable wedge that can be readily deflated after delivery of the infant. One can be devised cheaply from a disposable 3-liter plastic bag (used for bladder irrigation), a length of tubing, and a stopcock. Oxygen from the wall outlet or anesthesia machine inflates the bag, which easily deflates by opening the stopcock (Fig. 6–4).

Maternal Monitoring. Recommended maternal monitoring methods, during general anesthesia include ECG, blood pressure, capnography (detects esophageal intubation and hyperventilation), plus oximetry (demonstrates hypoxia, especially during intubation apnea), and peripheral nerve stimulator.

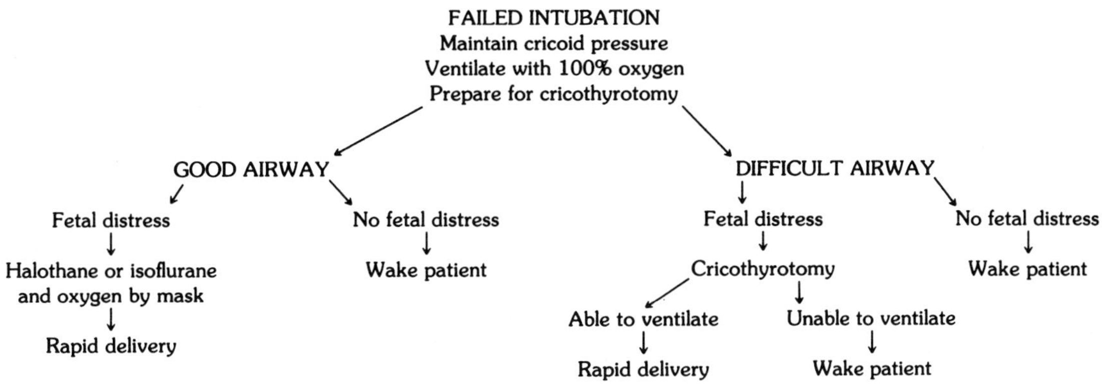

Figure 6–5. Management of failed intubation.

Uteroplacental Perfusion and Anesthesia

Both general and regional anesthesia can significantly influence the maintenance of adequate uterine artery blood flow and placental perfusion. They may, by their effect on blood pressure, cardiac output, and peripheral resistance, cause a reduction in uteroplacental perfusion or, conversely, prevent the adverse effects of stress and pain during labor.

General Anesthesia. Jouppila and others[83] using radioactive xenon demonstrated a 35-percent decrease in placental intervillous perfusion in humans after induction of general anesthesia. Maintenance of anesthesia with 50-percent nitrous oxide, oxygen, and 0.5-percent halothane or isoflurane, causes a 22-percent increase in uterine blood flow in resting pregnant ewes.[84] Endotracheal intubation followed by light anesthesia results in increased endogenous catecholamine release, with increased maternal blood pressure and heart rate. Shnider and coworkers[85] demonstrated that such stress, sufficient to cause hypertension in pregnant ewes, caused a significant decrease in uterine blood flow.

Regional Anesthesia. The effect of epidural anesthesia on uteroplacental blood flow during labor and cesarean section has been extensively studied in both humans[86-88] and animals.[89] Provided uterine displacement, adequate intravenous fluid preload, and/or ephedrine prevent hypotension, regional anesthesia does not reduce placental perfusion. In fact, Jouppila and others[90] have reported that epidural block improves intervillous blood flow in women with pre-eclampsia.

Epinephrine. The use of epinephrine in epidural analgesia remains controversial. High blood levels, produced by large doses or accidental intravascular injection, will manifest predominantly the α-adrenergic effects —hypertension, vasoconstriction, increased uterine activity, and reduced uterine artery blood flow. In contrast, the low plasma levels seen after epidural administration of local anesthetics containing 1:800,000 to 1:200,000 epinephrine primarily produce β-adrenergic effects. Albright and coworkers[40] reported that epidural administration of 10 ml of 2-chloroprocaine with 1:200,000 epinephrine during labor produced no reduction in intervillous blood flow. Thus the clinical doses of epinephrine used in obstetric epidural anesthesia appear to have little effect on labor or fetal well-being. In the presence of a compromised fetus, when any decrease in placental perfusion might have a deleterious effect, it may be wise to avoid epinephrine altogether. The same logic applies in pregnancy-induced hypertension with arteriolar vasoconstriction and reduced uterine blood flow.

Father in the Operating Room

Many parents approach labor with carefully prepared birth plans which are unfulfilled if cesarean section becomes necessary. In the absence of any medical contraindications, most parents request regional anesthesia and the father's presence in the operating room. Those institutions that routinely follow this practice have reported few problems. In our institution, the father enters the operating room after the epidural block has been established. He sits next to his partner's head, and the couple receive the baby after the pediatrician judges that the infant is stable and vigorous. If the father wants to be present for purposes of parent-infant bonding during general anesthesia, he enters the operating room after anesthesia has been induced and stays with the pediatrician, well out of the way of the anesthesiologist.

Summary

In my practice, the improvement in the quality of prenatal preparation for labor and the desire of many paturients for unmedicated labor has resulted in a reduction in the number of requests for pharmacologic analgesia. There is still considerable ignorance and much prejudice about available techniques, even on the part of some obstetricians. The lay public and even physicians who do not spend much time in the delivery suite often fail to appreciate the rapidity with which a "low-risk" parturient can unexpectedly come to be at high risk. Fortunately the valuable contributions the skilled obstetric anesthesiologist makes to the obstetric team are becoming better recognized and, at least in my institution, obstetricians are coming to regard their anesthesiologist colleagues as their primary critical-care consultants.

Many patients are poorly informed about the effects of pain and stress on the progress of labor and fetal well-being. A prenatal education program that addresses the patient's fears about the possible effect of analgesics on the baby is crucial. Not every parturient requires pharmacologic analgesia. A woman with a high pain threshold and uncomplicated labor may deliver her baby safely without requiring pain relief. However, when pain and maternal stress become evident, provision of analgesia benefits both mother and baby. Adverse effects of analgesic drugs are generally dose related, and careful attention must be paid to the specific needs of each patient. A number of alternative analgesic methods exist for labor and delivery. The choice depends upon the skills of the anesthesiologist, the mother's wishes, the stage of labor, presence of maternal or fetal complications, available facilities, and availability of skilled nursing assistance. Obstetric complications may develop rapidly and the obstetric anesthesia personnel must pay careful attention to detail, to avoid causing or contributing to such complications.

References

1. Simpson, JY: Account of a New Anaesthetic Agent as a Substitute for Sulphuric Ether in Surgery and Midwifery. Sutherland & Knox, Edinburgh, 1847, p 12.
2. Snow, J: On Chloroform and Other Anaesthetics: Their Action and Administration. John Churchill, London, 1858.
3. Channing, W: A Treatise on Etherization in Childbirth. William D. Ticknor & Co., Boston, 1848, p 21.
4. Cleland, JGP: Paravertebral anesthesia in obstetrics. Surg Gynecol Obstet 57:51, 1933.
5. Melzack, R, et al: Labour is still painful after prepared childbirth training. Can Med Assoc J 125:357, 1981.
6. Lederman, RP, et al: Endogenous plasma epinephrine and norepinephrine in last-trimester pregnancy and labor. Am J Obstet Gynecol 129:5, 1977.
7. Morishima, HO, Yeh, MN and James, LS: Reduced uterine blood flow and fetal hypoxemia with acute maternal stress: Experimental observation in pregnant baboons. Am J Obstet Gynecol 134:270, 1979.
8. Myers, RE: Maternal psychological stress and fetal asphyxia: A study in the monkey. Am J Obstet Gynecol 122:47, 1975.
9. Shnider, SM, et al: Uterine blood flow and plasma norephinephrine changes during maternal stress in the pregnant ewe. Anesthesiology 50:524, 1979.
10. Lederman, RP, et al: The relationship of maternal anxiety, plasma catecholamines and plasma cortisol to progess in labor. Am J Obstet Gynecol 132:495, 1978.
11. Lederman, E, et al: Maternal psychological and physiological correlates of fetal-newborn health status. Am J Obstet Gynecol 139:956, 1981.
12. Shnider, SM, et al: Maternal catecholamines decrease during labor after lumbar epidural anesthesia. Am J Obstet Gynecol 147:13, 1983.
13. Hagerdal, M, et al: Minute ventilation and oxygen consumption during labor with epidural analgesia. Anesthesiology 59:425, 1983.
14. Genazzani, AR, Facchinetti, F and Parrini, D: β-lipotropin and β-endorphin plasma levels during pregnancy. Clin Endocrinol 14:409, 1981.
15. Goland, RS, et al: Human plasma β-endorphin during pregnancy, labor and delivery. J Clin Endocrinol Metab 52:74, 1981.
16. Fletcher, JE, Thomas, TA and Hill, RG: β-endorphin and parturition. Lancet 1:310, 1980.
17. Hoffman, DI, et al: Plasma β-endorphin concentrations prior to and during pregnancy, in labor and after delivery. Am J Obstet Gynecol 150:492, 1984.
18. Raisanen, I, et al: Pain and plasma β-endorphin level during labor. Obstet Gynecol 64:783, 1984.
19. Steinbrook, RA, et al: Dissociation of plasma and cerebrospinal fluid beta-endorphin-like immunoactivity levels during pregnancy and parturition. Anesth Analg 61:893, 1982.
20. Karim, SMM: Appearance of prostaglandin $F_{2\alpha}$ in human blood during labor. Br Med J 4:618, 1968.
21. Brennecke, SP, et al: Maternal plasma prostaglandin E_2 metabolite levels during human pregnancy and parturition. Br J Obstet Gynaecol 92:345, 1985.
22. Mitchell, MD, et al: Plasma concentrations of prostaglandins during late human pregnancy: Influence of normal and preterm labor. J Clin Endocrinol Metab 46:947, 1978.
23. Fuchs, AR: Oxytocin and the initiation of human parturition. II: Stimulation of prostaglandin production in human decidua by oxytocin. Am J Obstet Gynecol 141:694, 1981.
24. Nimmo, WS, Wilson, J and Prescott, LF: Narcotic analgesics and delayed gastric emptying during labor. Lancet 1:890, 1975.
25. LaSalvia, LA and Steffan, EA: Delayed gastric emptying time in labor. Am J Obstet Gynecol 50:1075, 1950.
26. Crawford, JS and Rudofsky S: Placental transmission of pethidine. Br J Anaesth 37:929, 1965.
27. Shnider, SM, Way, EL and Lord MJ: Rate of appearance and disappearance of meperidine in fetal blood after administration of narcotic to the mother. Anesthesiology 27:227, 1966.
28. Shnider, SM and Moya, F: Effects of meperidine on the newborn infant. Am J Obstet Gynecol 89:1009, 1964.
29. Kuhnert, BR, et al: Meperidine and normeperidine levels following meperidine administration during labor. II: Fetus and neonate. Am J Obstet Gynecol 133:907, 1979.
30. Kuhnert, BR, et al: Effects of low doses of meperidine on neonatal behavior. Anesth Analg 64:335, 1985.
31. Hodgkinson, R and Farkhanda, JH: The duration of

effect of maternally administered meperidine on neonatal neurobehavior. Anesthesiology 56:51, 1982.
32. Kuhnert, BR, et al: Disposition of meperidine and normeperidine following multiple doses during labor. I: Mother. Am J Obstet Gynecol 151:406, 1985.
33. Kuhnert, BR, et al: Disposition of meperidine and normeperidine following multiple doses during labor. II: Fetus and neonate. Am J Obstet Gynecol 151:410, 1985.
34. Way, WL, Costley, EC and Way, EL: Respiratory sensitivity of the newborn infant to meperidine and morphine. Clin Pharmacol Ther 6:454, 1965.
35. Maduska, AL and Hajghassemali, M: A double-blind comparison of butorphanol and meperidine in labor: Maternal pain relief and effect on the newborn. Can Anaesth Soc J 25:398, 1978.
36. Romagnoli, A and Keats, AS: Ceiling effect for respiratory depression by nalbuphine. Clin Pharmacol Ther 27:478, 1980.
37. Akamatsu, TJ, et al: Experiences with the use of ketamine for parturition. I: Primary anesthetic for vaginal delivery. Anesth Analg 53:284, 1974.
38. Committee on Nitrous Oxide Analgesia in Midwifery. Clinical trials of different concentrations of oxygen and nitrous oxide for obstetric analgesia. Br Med J 1:709, 1970.
39. Wallis, KL, et al: Epidural anesthesia in the normotensive pregnant ewe: Effects on uterine blood flow and fetal acid-base status. Anesthesiology 44:481, 1976.
40. Albright, GA, et al: Epinephrine does not alter human intervillous blood flow during epidural anesthesia. Anesthesiology 54:131, 1981.
41. Ramanathan, S, Sheth, R and Tumdorf, H: Anesthesia for cesarean section in patients with genital herpes infections: A retrospective study. Anesthesiology 64:807, 1986.
42. Ravindran, RS, Gupta, CD and Stoops, CA.: Epidural analgesia in the presence of herpes simplex virus (type 2) infection. Anesth Analg 61:714, 1982.
43. Bonica, JJ: Principles and Practice of Obstetric Analgesia and Anesthesia. Vol 1, FA Davis, Philadelphia, 1967, p 588.
44. Cleland, GP: Continuous epidural and caudal block in obstetrics and surgery with postoperative analgesia. Anesth Analg 31:289, 1952.
45. Sinclair, JC, et al: Intoxication of the fetus by a local anesthetic. A newly recognized complication of maternal caudal analgesia. N Engl J Med 273:1173, 1965.
46. Meguiar, RV and Wheeler, AS: Lumbar sympathetic block with bupivacaine: Analgesia for labor. Anesth Analg 57:486:1978.
47. Hunter, CA: Uterine motility studies during labor. Am J Obstet Gynecol 85:781, 1963.
48. Asling, JH, et al: Paracervical block anesthesia in obstetrics. Am J Obstet Gynecol 107:626, 1970.
49. Shnider, SM, et al: Paracervical block anesthesia in obstetrics. I: Fetal complications and neonatal morbidity. Am J Obstet Gynecol 107:619, 1970.
50. Kobak, AJ, Evans, EF and Johnson, GR: Transvaginal pudendal nerve block. Am J Obstet Gynecol 71:981, 1956.
51. Greene, BA: A 26-gauge lumbar puncture needle. Its value in the prophylaxis of headache following spinal analgesia for vaginal delivery. Anesthesiology 11:464, 1950.
52. Abboud, TK, et al: Intrathecal administration of hyperbaric morphine for the relief of pain in labor. Br J Anaesth 56:1351, 1984.
53. Scott, PV, et al: Intrathecal morphine as sole analgesic during labor. Br Med J 281:351, 1980.
54. Hughes, SC, et al: Maternal and neonatal effects of epidural morphine for labor and delivery. Anaesth Analg 63:319, 1984.
55. Justins, DM, et al: A controlled trial of epidural fentanyl in labor. Br J Anaesth 54:409, 1982.
56. Flowers, CE, Littlejohn, TW and Wells, HB: Pharmacologic and hypnoid analgesia. Obstet Gynecol 16:210, 1960.
57. Wahl, CW: Contraindications and limitations of hypnosis in obstetric analgesia. Am J Obstet Gynecol 84:1869, 1962.
58. Saling, E and Ligidas, P: The effect on the fetus of maternal hyperventilation during labour. Br J Obstet Gynaecol 76:877, 1969.
59. Shealy, CH, Mortimer, JT and Reswick, JB: Electrical inhibition of pain by stimulation of the dorsal columns. Anesth Analg Curr Res 46:489, 1967.
60. Long, DM: External electrical stimulation as a treatment of chronic pain. Minn Med 57:195, 1974.
61. Erkkola, R, Pikkola, P and Kanto, J: Transcutaneous nerve stimulation for pain relief during labour: A controlled study. Ann Chir Gynaecol 69:273, 1980.
62. Bundsen, P, et al: Pain relief in labor by transcutaneous electrical nerve stimulation. Acta Obstet Gynecol Scand 61:129, 1982.
63. Melzack, R and Wall, PD: Pain mechanisms: A new theory. Science 150:971, 1965.
64. Solomon, RA, Viemstein, MC and Long, DM: Reduction of postoperative pain and narcotic use by transcutaneous electrical nerve stimulation. Surgery 87:142, 1980.
65. Abram, SE, Reynolds, AC and Cusick, JF: Failure of naloxone to reverse analgesia from transcutaneous electrical stimulation in patients with chronic pain. Anesth Analg 60:81, 1984.
66. Augustinsson, LE, et al: Pain relief during delivery by transcutaneous electrical nerve stimulation. Pain 4:59, 1977.
67. Wallis, L, et al: An evaluation of acupuncture analgesia in obstetrics. Anesthesiology 41:596, 1974.
68. Abouleish, E and Depp, R: Acupuncture in obstetrics. Anesth Analg 54:83, 1975.
69. Bowes, WA and Bowes, C: Current role of the midforceps operation. Clin Obstet Gynecol 23:549, 1980.
70. Richardson, DA, Evans, MI and Cibils, LA: Midforceps delivery: A critical review. Am J Obstet Gynecol 145:621, 1983.
71. James, FM, et al: A comparison of general anesthesia and lumbar epidural analgesia for elective cesarean section. Anesth Analg 56:228, 1977.
72. Fox, GS, et al: Anesthesia for cesarean section: Further studies. Am J Obstet Gynecol 133:15, 1979.
73. Datta, S and Brown, WU: Acid-base status in diabetic mothers and their infants following general or spinal anesthesia for cesarean section. Anesthesiology 47:272, 1977.

74. Crawford, JS and Davies, P: A return to trichlorethylene for obstetric anaesthesia. Br J Anaesth 47:482, 1975.
75. Datta, S, et al: Neonatal effect of prolonged anesthetic induction for cesarean section. Obstet Gynecol 58:331, 1981.
76. Marx, GF, Luykx, WM and Cohen, S: Fetal-neonatal status following caesarean section for fetal distress. Br J Anaesth 56:1009, 1984.
77. Norris, MC and Dewan, DM: Preoxygenation for cesarean section: A comparison of two techniques. Anesthesiology 62:827, 1985.
78. Thind, GS and Bryson, THL: SIngle dose suxemethonium and muscle pain in pregnancy. Br J Anaesth 55:743, 1983.
79. Sellick, BA: Cricoid pressure to control regurgitation of stomach contents during induction of anaesthesia. Lancet 2:404, 1961.
80. Marx, GF, et al: Postpartum uterine pressures under halothane or enflurane anesthesia. Obstet Gynecol 51:695, 1978.
81. Munson, ES and Embro, WJ: Enflurane, isoflurane, and halothane and isolated human uterine muscle. Anesthesiology 46:11, 1977.
82. Warren, TM, 'et al: Comparison of the maternal and neonatal effects of halothane, enflurane and isoflurane for cesarean delivery. Anesth Analg 62:516, 1983.
83. Jouppila, P, et al: Effect of induction of general anesthesia for cesarean section on intervillous blood flow. Acta Obstet Gynecol Scand 58:249, 1979.
84. Palahniuk, RJ and Shnider, SM: Maternal and fetal cardiovascular and acid-base changes during halothane and isoflurane anesthesia in the pregnant ewe. Anesthesiology 41:462, 1974.
85. Shnider, SM, et al: Uterine blood flow and plasma norepinephrine changes during maternal stress in the pregnant ewe. Anesthesiology 50:524, 1979.
86. Jouppila, R, et al: Placental blood flow during caesarean section under lumbar extradural analgesia. Br J Anaesth 50:275, 1978.
87. Jouppila, R, et al: Effect of segmental extradural analgesia on placental blood flow during normal labour. Br J Anaesth 50:563, 1978.
88. Jouppila, P, et al: Placental blood flow during caesarean section performed under subarachnoid blockade. Br J Anaesth 56:1379, 1984.
89. Wallis, KL, et al: Epidural anesthesia in the normotensive pregnant ewe: Effects on uterine blood flow and fetal acid-base status. Anesthesiology 44:481, 1976.
90. Jouppila, P, et al: Lumbar epidural analgesia to improve intervillous blood flow during labor in severe pre-eclampsia. Obstet Gynecol 59:158, 1982.

CHAPTER 7

COMPLICATIONS OF OBSTETRIC ANESTHESIA

BARRY C. CORKE, M.B., Ch.B., F.F.A.R.C.S.

The complications that sometimes arise during surgical anesthesia can also appear in obstetric patients. Rather than presenting an encyclopedic list of such complications, this chapter concentrates on those problems prone to emerge in parturients. The involvement of both mother and fetus magnifies the seriousness of anesthetic complications since the combined life expectancy of the mother and her unborn child exceeds a century. Additionally, the recent trend toward litigation following a complication during pregnancy has had a significant impact upon the medical profession. As a result, obstetric practice is now shaped, in numerous instances, to conform with what has become termed as "the prevailing standard of care." Reliable evidence suggests that the recent rise in the cesarean section rate relates at least in part to fears of litigation.[1]

All physicians who administer anesthesia to parturients must be aware of changes in maternal physiology that may influence the type of anesthesia being administered (Chap. 1). Obstetric anesthesia is the province of well-trained, experienced practitioners, not unaided novices.

This chapter describes potential complications in the obstetric patient, and more important discusses how one can anticipate these complications and manage them should they occur.

Maternal Complications

GENERAL ANESTHESIA

Despite a significant increase in the use of regional anesthesia for both vaginal delivery and cesarean section, a large percentage of parturients still require general anesthesia. Fortunately the use of general anesthesia for vaginal delivery has declined almost to zero. However, the mother may require general anesthesia immediately postpartum for complications such as manual removal of a retained placenta. Most factors that increase the pregnant patient's anesthetic risk still remain in the postpartum period.

Aspiration Pneumonitis

Mendelson[2] originally described the pulmonary pathophysiology produced by the aspiration of stomach contents. This complication is still a potentially lethal problem for the pregnant patient who receives general anesthesia. It is difficult to accurately assess the incidence of death following aspiration pneumonitis. In 1951 Merrill and Hingson[3] estimated that aspiration produced 100 deaths annually in the United States. Figures from the United Kingdom[4] (more easily obtainable) show an aspiration-related death rate of 1 in 5000 to 1 in 6000 cesarean sections during the period from 1976 to 1978. In the pregnant patient the incidence of death following aspiration approximates 10 to 25 percent. Significantly higher mortality occurs when severe pulmonary symptoms develop. Surprisingly the incidence of death cited in Mendelson's[2] original paper was much lower. Despite enormous advances in medical treatment aspiration pneumonitis remains relatively unaffected by modern therapy. Therefore, the emphasis toward prevention must continue. An understanding of factors that increase the risk of aspiration will facilitate formulation of the most effective means of prevention.

Volume and pH of Gastric Fluid. Several factors increase the volume of gastric contents in the parturient. Impairment of gastric emptying during the third trimester has been attributed to a combination of mechanical and hormonal factors. The enlarging uterus distorts the pylorus, producing mechanical impairment to gastric emptying. Increased levels of progesterone[5] coupled with decreased levels of motilin[6] account for the decline in gastric motility and prolonged gastric emptying. When labor commences, gastric motility decreases even more, although some gastric emptying still continues during labor. The administration of narcotics during labor significantly impedes gastric function.[7]

The increased amounts of the hormone gastrin secreted during pregnancy[8] probably originate in the placenta. Gastrin stimulates increased secretion of gastric acid. For these multiple reasons, the stomach of the parturient likely contains large volumes of fluid with a low pH.

It is difficult to accurately predict the amount of gastric aspirate required to produce pulmonary damage. Animal studies suggest that the volume needed to produce pulmonary damage approaches 25 ml in the normal-size adult human. Fluid with a pH of lower than 2.5 usually produces pulmonary damage if aspirated.[9,10] The parturient with increased acid production and delayed gastric emptying in all probability has both a gastric volume exceeding 25 ml and a pH below 2.5 and, so, is at high risk for aspiration of gastric contents and its sequelae.

Intragastric Pressure. Passive regurgitation and active vomiting differ significantly. Careful anesthetic technique can usually prevent the latter, particularly by avoiding instrumentation of the pharynx until the full effect of induction occurs. Passive regurgitation relies upon a pressure differential between intragastric contents and atmospheric pressure at the mouth. A greater pressure differential increases the likelihood of regurgitation. During the third trimester the presence of the greatly enlarged uterus increases intragastric pressure. The lithotomy position and use of fundal pressure exaggerate this effect.

Decreased Patency of the Lower Esophageal Sphincter. The junction between the distal esophagus and the stomach forms a functional sphincter, which, in the absence of other factors, including hiatal hernia, can prevent passive regurgitation. During pregnancy, the muscle relaxant effect of progesterone and the anatomic derangement caused by the gravid uterus can interfere with sphincter function. Many women complain of heartburn during pregnancy, indicating decreased patency of the lower esophageal sphincter and an increased risk of regurgitation.[6] Both the increase in intragastric pressure and the decrease in lower esophageal sphincter tone place the mother at greater risk for passive regurgitation and, consequently, acid aspiration.

Prevention. Since the parturient runs an increased risk for acid aspiration and treatment remains so ineffective, prevention is the means for minimizing morbidity.

The increased use of regional anesthesia and the abandonment of routine general anesthesia for vaginal delivery have significantly reduced the problem of acid aspiration. Regional anesthesia provides excellent analgesia and relaxation for instrument delivery. Its use for cesarean section does not totally eliminate the possibility of aspiration but significantly reduces its likelihood. Aspiration may occur when a regional block rises to an inappropriately high level, as in a total spinal. Aspiration may also occur if the patient becomes hypotensive, loses consciousness, and cannot protect her airway. In either case, it is important to make an early decision as to whether the airway requires protection by means of a cuffed endotracheal tube. Rapid treatment of hypotension by intravenous fluid administration, increasing lateral tilt, and administration of ephedrine restore consciousness.

With education of all personnel involved in the management of pregnant women and thorough prenatal counseling of the parturient, it is hoped that the increased use of regional analgesia will continue. Administering regional analgesia in an optimal manner ensures that the benefits of the technique outweigh the side effects.

Despite the increased awareness of the advantages of regional analgesia, a significant percentage of parturients either require or request general anesthesia. General anesthetic techniques can significantly influence the likelihood of aspiration.

Premedication. In 1966, Taylor and Pryse-Davies[11] demonstrated that the administration of a particulate antacid such as magnesium trisilicate, every 4 hours, could maintain gastric pH above 2.5. This became a routine practice during labor, and many expected it to significantly decrease the likelihood of acid pneumonitis, should aspiration occur. Recent evidence, however, indicates that this practice has not met expectations. Patients still die from pulmonary damage following aspiration, despite having received what was thought to be adequate prophylaxis with antacids.[4,12] Furthermore, intrapulmonary particulate antacids produce severe respiratory damage in animals[13] almost as severe as acid injury.

Therapy with nonparticulate antacids may prove more efficacious. Thirty milliliters of 0.3-M sodium citrate effectively neutralizes gastric acid and elevates pH above 2.5.[14–16] The main disadvantages of sodium citrate include its unpalatability, nausea, vomiting, and diarrhea with repeated doses and, more important, short duration of action. Effective gastric acid neutralization lasts less than 1 hour in many patients. Therefore, sodium citrate has greater effect when administered just prior to induction.

The histamine-receptor antagonists cimetidine and ranitidine reportedly are suitable alternatives to antacids. Both reduce gastric volume and elevate gastric pH.[17–19] However, because they do not alter the pH of stomach contents already present, antacid administration (e.g., sodium citrate) should still precede induction of anesthesia. Both drugs require time for good effect and prove suitable only when given well in advance of induction.

Another agent, metaclopramide, speeds gastric emptying. Its effectiveness in reducing the risk of acid aspiration remains less well known;[20] however, metaclopramide probably will not overcome narcotic-induced gastric stasis.

There is a great deal of debate over which prophylactic medications most effectively reduce the parturient's risk of acid aspiration. Future studies should clarify the situation. For now, most authorities accept the following regimen, since it produces negligible maternal and fetal sequelae:

1. Sodium citrate, 30 ml of 0.3-M solution, Bicitra, or Alka-Seltzer Gold, 30 ml, orally immediately prior to induction.
2. When appropriate, a histamine receptor–antagonist serves as a valuable adjunct: ranitidine in a dose of 150 mg orally the night before surgery followed by 50 mg intravenously 1 to 2 hours prior to surgery. The intravenous dose is used for emergency surgery, provided a 1-hour period has elapsed between administration and induction of anesthesia.

   As an alternative, cimetidine, 300 mg orally is used the night before surgery, followed by 300 mg intramuscularly 1 hour prior to surgery. The intramuscular dose also proves suitable for emergency surgery, provided that a period of at least 1 hour transpires between administration and induction of anesthesia.
3. Metaclopramide, 10 mg intravenously prior to induction, may increase gastric emptying. Provided injection occurs over a 1- to 2-min period, side effects are rare.

Side effects appear to be less likely with ranitidine than with cimetidine.[21] Ranitidine crosses the blood-brain barrier less easily and binds less avidly to hepatic microsomal P450 enzymes. For this reason, ranitidine, unlike cimetidine, does not delay the breakdown of some drugs, including amide local anesthetics, which rely on hepatic metabolism.

Induction of Anesthesia. Despite premedication, one should still assume that all parturients have full stomachs and treat them accordingly.

In the past there was controversy over whether the patient's position might influence the risk of aspiration. For example, induction of anesthesia in the full sitting position might raise the amount of hydrostatic pressure required for regurgitation.[22] In contrast, the head-down, lateral position promotes drainage away from the trachea. In general, most authorities now advocate adopting the position most advantageous for rapid endotracheal intubation, namely, the supine position with left uterine displacement and the head in the "sniffing position."

Cricoid pressure during induction has become routine for obstetric patients.[23] Downward pressure applied directly to the cricoid cartilage effectively obliterates the esophageal lumen and usually prevents regurgitation. The person applying cricoid pressure should become familiar with the maneuver and must continue to apply pressure until completion of tracheal intubation and attainment of adequate cuff inflation.

Other important factors are adequate preoxygenation prior to induction and the avoidance of positive-pressure ventilation by mask unless required to overcome hypoxia. Mask ventilation increases the intragastric pressure by allowing some gas to enter the stomach.

Extubation. The patient remains at risk for aspiration at the completion of surgery and must be awake before the endotracheal tube is removed. Positive pressure is applied during extubation to prevent material that has collected above the cuff from entering the lungs.

Management of Pulmonary Aspiration. Initial clinical presentation of the aspiration of gastric contents depends upon whether the aspirate is solid or liquid. Solid material causes asphyxia, and immediate resolution is imperative. Any means available must be used to clear the airway and reoxygenate the patient. Initial clearing of the airway may require manual removal of foreign material using gauze and fingers followed by vigorous suction to remove the remaining material. Bronchoscopy should follow if symptoms suggest the presence of intratracheal or intrabronchial material.

Aspiration of gastric fluid may interfere with ventilation, but problems usually are more insidious. Bronchospasm but not tachypnea often accompanies the chemical pneumonitis that follows acid aspiration in the anesthetized, ventilated patient. Difficulty in maintaining adequate oxygenation despite a high inspired oxygen concentration represents another early sign, as does a frothy pulmonary exudate. Although the signs and symptoms may not appear for a period of 6 to 12 hours, manifestations usually become evident within 1 to 3 hours. Chest films have proven unreliable for the initial diagnosis of acid aspiration. Arterial blood gas measurements provide the best initial assessment of the extent of pulmonary damage.

Positive-pressure ventilation is the mainstay of treatment for acid aspiration. Early initiation of mechanical ventilation increases survival rates after acid aspiration in animal models.[24] A 24-hour delay in ventilation reduces survival from 100 to 40 percent.[24] Aspiration therapy depends upon the ability of the patient to maintain oxygenation and frequently requires the use of positive end-expiratory pressure (PEEP) as well as mechanical ventilation. A drop in the PaO_2 to less than 50 mmHg on room air calls for initiating PEEP.[25] Adjustments in oxygen (FIO_2) should maintain a PaO_2 of at least 70 mmHg. PEEP should be instituted when a high FIO_2 (>50 percent) fails to provide an adequate arterial oxygen level.

Apart from providing pulmonary support with controlled ventilation and pharmacologic management of cardiac problems, little else can be done for the patient with severe aspiration pneumonitis. Invasive hemodynamic monitoring provides valuable information regarding the progress of the condition. Steroids are avoided[26,27] since studies in animal models and, more recently, in humans, have not substantiated the claim that the anti-inflammatory and vascular-stabilizing effects of steroids help to resolve aspiration pneumonitis.

Acid aspiration is an extremely dangerous condition that responds poorly to treatment. For these reasons, when conditions mandate general anesthesia, management should remain in the hands of well-trained practitioners working in an environment with anesthesia equipment and monitoring comparable to those available in modern operating suites. More experience with newer drugs capable of suppressing acid secretion and gastric emptying may lead to greater safety.

Hypoxia

Although specialists generally agree that inhalation of gastric contents represents the most important cause of anesthesia-related maternal mortality, the 1976 to 1978 Confidential Enquiry into Maternal Deaths in England and Wales[4] indicates that hypoxia constitutes an equally lethal hazard to the parturient.

Pathophysiology. The gravida experiences significant physiologic changes (Chap. 1). Many of the pulmonary changes occur at an early stage in pregnancy. The decrease in functional residual capacity (FRC), which declines by 20 to 25 percent below the nonpregnant state, is quite significant. Reductions occur in both components of the FRC, the residual volume and the expiratory reserve volume.

At the same time, increased cardiac and respiratory workloads, coupled with fetal and placental oxygen consumption, increase maternal oxygen use by 20 to 30 percent over the nonpregnant state.

Both the decline in FRC and increased oxygen consumption accelerate the fall in arterial PO_2 during apnea in the pregnant female. In the nonpregnant state, PO_2 falls approximately 50 mmHg per min during apnea (150 mmHg per min during pregnancy).[28] Obviously proficient airway management is critical in the parturient during rapid-sequence induction of general anesthesia. Avoiding manual ventilation prior to endotracheal inhalation should prevent aspiration. Preoxygenate the patient to raise the maternal PO_2 maximally prior to induction. Following injection of thiopental and succinylcholine, delay intubation for 45 to 60 sec. This decreases the chance of active vomiting. Provided intubation is accomplished rapidly, hypoxia rarely ensues; if it is delayed, hypoxia develops quickly. Cardiac arrhythmias and subsequent cardiac arrest are the most likely sequelae of uncorrected hypoxia. The rapid onset of hypoxia explains most of the deaths described in the Confidential Enquiry into Maternal Deaths in England and Wales of 1976 to 1978.[4] In this survey death followed repeated attempts to pass an endotracheal tube without maintaining adequate oxygenation. This also indicates that only experienced personnel should administer obstetric anesthesia. Reliable monitors which continuously measure peripheral oxygen saturation accurately identify the onset of hypoxia. When it occurs, attempts at intubation should be abandoned in favor of mask ventilation; cricoid pressure is maintained; and no further attempts at intubation are made until oxygenation reaches adequate levels. Pulse oximetry comes highly recommended for all obstetric patients who receive both general and regional anesthesia.

When intubation fails, it is vital to follow a clear-cut plan, as this may prevent unnecessary hypoxia deaths.

The Difficult Intubation. Regardless of experience, availability of adequate equipment, and patient evaluation, failure to intubate can still occur and the situation demands a deliberate method of management (Table 7–1).

A favorable outcome depends on effective communication between the obstetrician and anesthesiologist. Good fetal status may allow awakening the mother and use of a regional block. Alternatively, fiberoptic intubation may be performed on an awake patient. Fetal distress mandates continuation and rapid completion of surgery, and every effort is made to avoid any unnecessary abdominal pressure. Ox-

Table 7–1. FAILED INTUBATION DRILL

1. Ventilate by face mask with 100-percent O_2, maintaining cricoid pressure.
2. If no element of fetal distress is present, allow patient to awaken:
   a. If not contraindicated, use a regional technique.
   b. May attempt intubation using fiberoptic bronchoscope.
3. If surgery continues:
   a. Maintain mask ventilation with O_2 and 0.5 MAC halothane or isoflurane, continuing to apply cricoid pressure. Intravenous ketamine may also be administered.
   b. Decide whether to use further relaxants or to allow spontaneous ventilation to return.
   c. Following delivery of neonate, decide whether to make further attempts to intubate.
4. If mask ventilation fails:
   a. Perform cricothyrotomy using a cricothyrotomy cannula.
   b. A 12-gauge intravenous cannula with a 4.5-mm endotracheal tube adaptor suffices if specific cricothyrotomy cannulas are not available.

ygen is administered together with a low concentration of a volatile agent (0.5 MAC) by face mask. Low-dose intravenous ketamine (<1 mg per kg) also effectively reduces maternal awareness. Finally, cricoid pressure must be maintained to prevent aspiration.

The anesthesiologist must decide whether to allow the return of spontaneous ventilation or to continue paralysis and to control ventilation.

During difficult or failed intubation, preventing hypoxia — the most serious maternal and fetal life-threatening sequela — becomes the first priority. The second is minimizing the likelihood of aspiration. Ideally, one should accomplish both of these goals without the mother's awareness, undue fetal depression, or uterine relaxation.

Esophageal Intubation. Hypoxia rapidly follows misplacement of an endotracheal tube into the esophagus. Methods of verification of correct placement include: observing the tube pass between the cords, hearing bilateral breath sounds on auscultation, observing equal chest expansion, noting that the patient remains pink, absence of gas entry sounds on auscultation over the stomach, and normal oxygen saturation on the pulse oximeter. Occasionally, however, correct placement of the endotracheal tube may not be obvious, particularly in the obese patient or when visualization of the cords proves difficult. Breath sounds may be difficult to hear owing to excessive adipose tissue. The anesthesiologist must decide quickly whether to continue with the tube in place or to repeat laryngoscopy and intubation following ventilation. Capnography, which detects expired carbon dioxide, offers valuable information in this situation, since carbon dioxide in expired gases provides insurmountable evidence of tube placement in the trachea. In contrast, a falling oxygen saturation, as measured by pulse oximetry, usually indicates esophageal placement.

Failure to detect esophageal intubation at an early stage places the patient in extreme danger and accounts for many maternal deaths. Unfortunately, not all operating suites come equipped with sophisticated monitoring, and clinical judgment still remains the mainstay for making a decision as to tube placement; this further emphasizes the need for experienced personnel to administer anesthesia to pregnant patients.

Maternal Awareness

Because of the desire to avoid fetal depression and to achieve optimal oxygenation, the depth of general anesthesia during cesarean section barely prevents the parturient from being aware during surgery. Prior to the realization that small concentrations of halogenated inhalation agents offered safe analgesia before delivery, mothers were frequently aware of the procedure. The incidence varied from 5 to 20 percent when 50-percent nitrous oxide was used as the sole maintenance agent.[29,30] Since the introduction of volatile agents in low concentrations, usually on the order of 0.5 MAC, the incidence of maternal awareness has fallen to nearly zero.[31,32]

Although awareness does not threaten life, caution dictates avoiding it. In addition to experiencing severe psychological upset, possibly sufficient to require therapy, the patient faces the prospect that future deliveries may require a cesarean section. Should awareness occur, the anesthesiologist must discuss the events surrounding awareness with the mother, stressing that it resulted from attempts to avoid fetal depression, and should inform her about how future surgery can avoid awareness.

Usually good anesthetic technique and attention to detail prevent awareness. Obviously, one must ensure that the anesthesia machine actually delivers the correct concentration of the agents used. Gas analysis systems achieve this goal but are not standard in all operating suites. Exhaustion of the nitrous oxide supply has accounted for many incidents of awareness in the past. Adequate supplies of nitrous oxide and volatile agents in the vaporizer must be assured prior to commencing anesthesia.

INHALATION ANALGESIA

Americans use inhalation analgesia infrequently, whereas in Europe it is one of the mainstays of obstetric analgesia,[33] being administered during the late first and second stages of labor instead of further doses of narcotic. Analgesia proceeds by self-administration with a hand-held device, under the supervision of a trained observer. The main agents include nitrous oxide in a 50-percent mixture with oxygen[33] and, alternatively, 0.35-percent methoxyflurane in air.[34]

Self-administered inhalation analgesia occasionally leads to overdose. Most devices administer nitrous oxide from a cylinder containing 50-percent oxygen. The patient holds the mask and connector, which has a large thumb hole. Patient drowsiness or loss of consciousness causes release of pressure on the thumb hole, with no further delivery of inhalation agent. Methoxyflurane administration uses either an air draw-over vaporizer or a disposable whistle device[35] with similar built-in safety features.

Potential complications of inhalation analgesia include the risk of loss of consciousness and protective laryngeal reflexes. The use of appropriate equipment and adequate briefing of both the mother and nursing attendant regarding its use should obviate this. Although the metabolic products of methoxyflurane can cause renal damage, no reports exist of high-output renal failure in either mother or neonate following the use of methoxyflurane for this purpose.

Inhalation analgesia represents an extremely safe technique. The only real complication involves inadequate analgesia secondary to suboptimal utilization. Uptake of analgesic agents requires time, and inhalation must begin prior to the onset of contractions so that adequate blood levels develop prior to the onset of pain. When correctly administered, this method shows a degree of analgesia comparable to that provided by narcotics.[36]

KETAMINE

Ketamine, a rapidly acting intravenous anesthetic with a short duration of action, produces intense analgesia and an anesthetic state described as "dissociative anesthesia." Unlike most other intravenous agents it does not depress cardiovascular function, and anesthesia personnel frequently use it in emergency situations (e.g., hemorrhage) in which drugs such as thiopental are contraindicated. Because ketamine increases maternal blood pressure by approximately 20 percent, its use requires caution in hypertensive states such as pre-eclampsia.

In doses of 0.25 to 0.5 mg per kg, intravenous ketamine produces profound analgesia for delivery without loss of consciousness or laryngeal reflexes. Low-dose ketamine proves especially useful for the patient who requires immediate analgesia during a difficult delivery when there is not enough time to initiate a regional block.[37] Complications rarely appear, provided one does not exceed these smaller doses. Ketamine may lead to airway problems by increasing pharyngeal secretions. It also causes extremely unpleasant dreams and hallucinations. However, psychotomimetic phenomena usually do not surface with the low-dose technique. Despite original claims to the contrary, ketamine can depress laryngeal reflexes following administration of larger doses (>0.5 to 1.0 mg per kg). To prevent aspiration, high-dose ketamine (>1 mg per kg) is used only in situations involving safe control of the airway via endotracheal intubation. Fetal depression also becomes a concern when the dose exceeds 1 mg per kg.[37]

REGIONAL ANESTHESIA

The increased use of regional analgesia and the declining use of general anesthesia have resulted in a lower incidence of serious maternal complications, including aspiration. However, regional analgesia presents its own set of complications, some of which threaten life. Good technique can avert the majority of these sequelae, although some may occur despite optimal administration. Personnel involved in administration of regional blocks for obstetrics must understand the nature of these complications and know how to manage them.

Hypotension

Hypotension is the most common complication following the administration of a regional block. Hypotension usually responds rapidly to proper therapy, but if ignored, it can place the patient at mortal risk. Sympathetic blockade and vascular dilation accompany major regional block. Rapid onset of sympathetic blockade increases the likelihood of hypotension. The higher the dermatomal spread of sympathetic blockade, the greater the likelihood of hypotension.

Lumbar Epidural Analgesia: Vaginal Delivery. Epidural blockade usually provides adequate analgesia for vaginal delivery when the level of block extends from T10 to S4. Hypotension rarely occurs with this extent of blockade unless the following occur: rapid onset of blockade (e.g., use of 2-chloroprocaine), blockade extending above T10, dehydration, pregnancy-induced hypertension, or supine position.

Prior to initiating a regional block approximately 500 ml of a balanced salt solution such as lactated Ringer's is infused intravenously. Dehydration or significant pre-eclampsia requires a larger volume. Fluids should not contain dextrose since this can trigger neonatal hypoglycemia and acidosis.[38]

Parturients require approximately 30 percent less local anesthetic for epidural analgesia than nonpregnant females. Failure to adjust doses accordingly produces unnecessarily high levels of anesthesia. In the parturient epidural analgesia is initiated using 10 to 12 ml of 0.25-percent bupivacaine or 10 to 12 ml of 2-percent 2-chloroprocaine. These doses normally relieve the pain of labor without producing significant hypotension.

Because of the gravid uterus, the supine position impedes venous return via compression of the patient's inferior vena cava.[39,40] The vascular physiology of the unmedicated parturient usually adequately compensates for this reduction in vena caval flow by returning blood to the heart via collateral channels, including vertebral veins, and by peripheral vasoconstriction. These mechanisms usually maintain normal blood pressure. Unfortunately, compensation may reduce placental perfusion and fetal oxygenation. During epidural blockade, vena caval occlusion exacerbates hypotension, thus increasing the risk of severe placental hypoperfusion. Therefore, no patient should labor in the supine position, especially after receiving epidural analgesia.

Lumbar Epidural Analgesia: Cesarean Section. The same general principles regarding hypotension apply to an epidural block placed for a cesarean section. However, cesarean section requires analgesia to the fourth thoracic dermatome, and hypotension occurs more frequently. Because prehydration is essential a volume of 1500 to 2000 ml of lactated Ringer's is infused prior to the onset of maximum sympathetic blockade, and the parturient is kept in a 15-degree left lateral tilt to avoid vena caval occlusion. Local anesthetic should be infused in small increments, to reduce the likelihood of local anesthetic toxicity and to provide a slower onset of sympathetic blockade, allowing compensation by peripheral vascular reflexes.

Treatment. Significant hypotension, defined as a 25- to 30-percent decrease in systolic blood pressure or a fall to below 100 torr systolic pressure while the parturient is in the lateral position, requires prompt and effective treatment (Table 7–2). Treatment effectiveness is monitored with frequent (every 60 sec) blood pressure measurements. Fluids should be infused rapidly while turning the mother to the full left lateral position. If, as occasionally happens, this increases the severity of hypotension, the mother is turned to the right lateral position, which is better for some parturients. Some women need intravenous ephedrine and supplemental oxygen, specifically when blood pressure remains depressed for more than 2 or 3 min.

Subarachnoid Block: Vaginal Delivery. A low spinal (or saddle block) provides excellent analgesia for delivery. It is usually administered with the mother in the sitting position, and a hyperbaric local anesthetic solution is used to limit the extent of spread to below lower thoracic dermatomes. Although this technique infrequently produces significant hypotension, monitoring should continue nonetheless as for other regional blocks, and the patient should avoid the supine position.

Table 7–2. MANAGEMENT OF SIGNIFICANT HYPOTENSION ASSOCIATED WITH REGIONAL ANESTHESIA

1. Intravenous Fluids	Infuse bolus of 200–300 ml; maintain infusion at higher rate.
2. Position	Provide full left lateral. Occasionally right lateral decubitus may be advantageous. 10–15 degrees Trendelenburg may help.
3. Pressors	Give intravenous ephedrine in 5–10-mg increments, if fluids and position fail to correct hypotension.
4. Oxygen	If hypotension persists, administer O_2 by face mask.

Subarachnoid Block: Cesarean Section. As with an epidural block, subarachnoid blocks for a cesarean section require sensory anesthesia to the level of the fourth thoracic dermatome. Autonomic block during spinal analgesia extends four to six dermatomes above sensory block.[41] Recent studies[42] using heat-sensitive imaging techniques suggest the difference may be as great as 10 dermatomes. High levels of sympathetic blockade obliterate most of the sympathetic control of peripheral blood vessels.

The extremely rapid onset of spinal block further increases the likelihood of hypotension. Therefore, hypotension commonly follows subarachnoid block for cesarean section, but prophylaxis may reduce its occurrence: prehydration with 1500 to 2000 ml of lactated Ringer's administered in a 20-min period prior to the subarachnoid block; avoidance of the supine position at all times; monitoring blood pressure every minute for the first 15 to 20 min and every 5 min thereafter.

In the event of hypotension the intravenous fluid infusion rate is increased, as is the degree of left lateral tilt. If blood pressure does not respond within 60 sec, 5 to 10 mg of ephedrine is injected intravenously. Administering intramuscular ephedrine prior to administration of subarachnoid block may reduce the incidence of hypotension. Many authorities do not consider this necessary. Persistent hypotension necessitates administration of additional ephedrine and oxygen by face mask (Table 7–2).

In general, hypotension following regional blockade is short lived and responds well to the described therapeutic measures. Adequate prophylactic measures and prompt treatment usually suffice, so that brief periods of maternal hypotension do not change Apgar scores or the neurobehavioral status of the neonate.[43] This lack of effect upon the newborn should not lead to complacency regarding maternal hypotension. Minimal changes in blood gas parameters do occur, and a discernible decline in neonatal outcome will follow longer periods of significant hypotension.

Headache After Dural Puncture

Although not a life-threatening complication headache after dural puncture proves sufficiently troublesome to prevent the postpartum patient from managing a demanding neonate, and may prevent her discharge at the appropriate time. Therefore, thorough and rapid management should follow. As with most complications in medical practice, prevention is the most important measure.

Spinal headaches result from leakage of CSF through the dural puncture hole, with subsequent shifts in cranial structures putting tension on the brain and meninges.

Symptoms. Dural puncture headache has typical features that make diagnosis relatively easy (Table 7–3). The headache locates occipitally and/or frontally and may involve the neck. It worsens when the patient sits or stands and

Table 7–3. POSTDURAL PUNCTURE HEADACHE

Symptoms	Headache, usually occipital and/or frontal Always relieved or partially relieved by supine position Onset immediately following to several days after dural puncture
Prevention	Incidence declines with reducing diameter of needle: 18-g: 10 to 50% 22-g: approximately 10% 25-g: approximately 1% Avoidance of accidental dural puncture with large-gauge epidural needle; appropriate training of anesthesiologists Assumption of supine position immediately after dural puncture does not influence incidence of headache. Avoidance of dehydration Limitation of bearing down in laboring patient
Treatment	
Initial	Symptomatic or conservative, including analgesics, bed rest, adequate hydration, abdominal binders; intravenous caffeine occasionally helps.
24 to 48 hours	Epidural blood patch is definitive. Treatment 95 to 98% successful but depends on diameter of dural puncture

significantly improves when she lies down, which differentiates it from other causes of headache, such as pre-eclampsia or intracranial hemorrhage. Nausea and vomiting, temporary cranial nerve deficits, and photophobia may accompany severe spinal headache.

Prevention. One should use the smallest-gauge needle for dural puncture. For example, a 1-percent incidence of headache occurs following use of a 25-gauge needle,[44] but the incidence is 5- to 26 percent with a 22-gauge needle.[45,46] Puncture of the dura with a 17-gauge needle is associated with a very high incidence of headache.[47] This necessitates careful training of anesthesiologists in the technique of epidural analgesia.

In the past many clinicians advocated maintenance of the supine position for 8 to 24 hours after dural puncture. Recent studies[48,49] demonstrate no difference in the incidence of headache whether patients remain flat or sit up.

When accidental dural puncture occurs during attempted epidural analgesia for labor, bearing down in the second stage should be limited as much as possible. If a catheter is placed at another interspace local anesthetic solution should be given in reduced dose and over a longer period, since rate of spread may increase and the block may extend higher than was anticipated. In the postpartum period, instillation of preservative-free sterile saline into the epidural space has some value in reducing the incidence of headache.[50,51]

There is no evidence that postpartum hydration increases CSF production. Prevention of dehydration which might occur because of nausea and vomiting is extremely important, since dehydration decreases CSF production, clearly an undesirable effect.

Treatment. Initial treatment remains conservative and consists of maintaining fluid intake, oral analgesics, and abdominal binders, and administering caffeine, 0.5 to 1.0 mg, which can help in some cases. If an incapacitating headache persists after 24 hours, an epidural blood patch offers relief in 90 to 98 percent of cases (Table 7–4).[52,53] Ten to 20 ml of autologous blood injected into the epidural space at the site of dural puncture acts as a gelatinous seal to prevent further CSF leakage. Occasional recurring headaches require a repeat blood patch.

Remarkably few complications follow epidural blood patch, and the technique provides safe, effective treatment.[54] Minor sequelae include transient back pain at the site of injection, which is easily relieved by administration of analgesics or by use of a heating pad.

Table 7–4. EPIDURAL BLOOD PATCH

Indications	Headache for 24–48 hours following dural puncture headache unrelieved by conservative management; patient detained in hospital or unable to manage newborn
	Pain should have typical characteristics of headache after dural puncture.
Procedure	Use lateral position; sitting position is uncomfortable for patient.
	Prep and drape as for any epidural.
	Locate epidural space with 17-gauge needle.
	Obtain 20 ml blood under sterile conditions, usually from antecubital vein.
	Slowly inject blood into epidural space. Stop if patient complains of discomfort. Recommence injection after 30–60 sec. If pain recurs cease injection and withdraw needle.
	Attempt to inject at least 10–15 ml of blood.
	Allow patient to remain supine for 15–20 min.
	Slowly elevate head until fully upright.
	Allow to ambulate.
	Discharge, if appropriate.

Sterile technique is very important when blood is injected epidurally. Failure to take precautions may produce an epidural abscess, which has serious neurologic implications. Prophylactic epidural blood patch (prior to 24 hours) is inadvisable since not all patients develop dural-puncture headache and the success rate decreases considerably.[55] Previous exposure to a blood patch does not affect epidural analgesia; studies[52,56] report successful epidural analgesia in subsequent pregnancies.

Accidental Intravenous Injection

Systemic toxicity can occur following any local anesthetic technique. Regional analgesia with the correct drug in the appropriate dose and in the correct site produces an extremely low incidence of toxicity. Accidental injection of local anesthetic directly into the vascular compartment, however, introduces the potential for significant systemic toxicity. Accidental intravenous injection is most likely to occur when drug injection involves a catheter inserted into the epidural space. The physiologic changes associated with pregnancy induce marked dilation of the epidural veins and increase the risk of intravenous cannulation and subsequent injection of local anesthetic.

Local Anesthetic Toxicity. Local anesthetic toxicity is predictable and dose dependent. Local anesthetic compounds lower the excitability of biologic membranes, leading eventually to both neurologic and cardiac effects. With most local anesthetics, cardiac toxicity rarely occurs in the presence of CNS toxicity if the patient receives no more drug. Recently, reports describe maternal death following the administration of large boluses of bupivacaine through an unsuspected intravenous epidural catheter.[57] Subsequent studies demonstrated that bupivacaine cardiotoxicity and CNS toxicity appear at very similar blood levels. A number of the reported incidents ended in cardiac arrest and death.

Prevention. The epidural catheter is aspirated prior to each drug dose; the presence of blood indicates an intravascular catheter and contraindicates injection of drug. Aspiration identifies the majority of intravascular catheters prior to injection, but occasionally it fails to produce blood return when the catheter is indeed in a vessel because the catheter orifice lies against the vessel wall or the vein collapses. Since negative aspiration does not guarantee safe placement, other means of verification must be used. The initial dose (a test dose) should consist of 2 to 3 ml. Prodromal signs of CNS toxicity include tinnitus, metallic taste, and lightheadedness. Signs of subarachnoid placement of drug should also be sought. After 5 min, provided no evidence of toxicity or subarachnoid placement develops the remainder of the drug may be injected. The drug is administered in 3- to 5-ml increments, allowing 45 to 60 sec between doses.[58] Each incremental injection serves as another test dose. If the original test dose fails to produce signs of intravenous injection when the needle does lie in a vessel, early CNS toxicity will become evident on subsequent injections, before the whole dose has been administered. Incremental dosing is mandatory to avoid severe CNS and cardiovascular toxicity.

Some authors[59] advocate using an anesthetic solution containing epinephrine to detect intravenous catheter placement, since it will produce a brief period of tachycardia that indicates misplacement. Pre-eclamptic patients cannot receive epinephrine, for an intravenous injection could produce severe hypertension. Because many patients experience only a brief period of tachycardia that the clinician can overlook, it is extremely important to use small incremental doses, with a period of observation between increments.

Owing to the possible cardiotoxicity induced by bupivacaine, the FDA has banned the use of the 0.75-percent concentration in parturients.[60]

Treatment. Local anesthetic toxicity calls for prompt and effective treatment. Seizure activity follows prodromal CNS signs with larger doses given in a short period of time. As with any seizure, muscle spasm, soft-tissue obstruction, or the presence of vomiting may compromise the airway. Following rapid provision of a good airway oxygenation and ventilation by mask or endotracheal tube is begun. Some dispute the correct drug therapy for generalized convulsion. Moore and Bridenbaugh[61] recommend neuromuscular blocking drugs because a large component of the problem relates to cerebral depression. Ausinch and coworkers[62] also propose intravenous diazepam to reduce the electrical activity in the brain. Doses should remain small (2.5 to 5.0 mg) to avoid further cerebral depression. Small doses (50 to 100 mg) of thiopental achieve the same result and may be more readily available.

Significant cardiovascular toxicity following incremental injection of local anesthetic drug requires treatment of symptoms, using appropriate monitors to assess the progress of treatment. Arterial blood sampling will assess the adequacy of ventilation and whether acid-base abnormalities require correction.

Total Spinal. A total spinal follows injection of an inappropriately large mass of local anesthetic into the subarachnoid space. This may occur during the progress of a subarachnoid block when the anesthesiologist administers too large a dose for the patient, or during an attempted epidural block, with accidental drug injection into the subarachnoid space. Total spinal may also follow introduction of an apparently appropriate dose of local anesthetic into the subarachnoid space. Either situation yields similar results, both requiring immediate measures to prevent serious complications.

The initial presenting sign is hypotension, usually perceived by the patient as lightheadedness and/or nausea. Difficulty in swallowing and breathing rapidly follow. Since most patients maintain adequate resting ventilation when the intercostal muscles become paralyzed, only when the block reaches the cervical dermatomes, C3, C4, C5, do significant ventilatory problems arise. At this stage, marked hypotension and difficulties in swallowing increase the risk of aspiration.

The occurrence of a total spinal requires rapid management to prevent hypotension and hypoxia. (Treatment of hypotension was described in Table 7–2.) One should rapidly assess the adequacy of ventilation by adding oxygen with a face mask. Ventilation frequently proves inadequate and requires immediate intubation, which one can accomplish in most cases without further medication. A patient who remains conscious may require thiopental and succinylcholine for intubation. Cricoid pressure is maintained during attempts at intubation.

This complication further underlines the principle that the practice of obstetric anesthesia should include only those practitioners with considerable experience who perform such anesthesia on a regular basis. Whenever performing major blocks, ensure the availability of emergency equipment for maintainance of ventilation.

Neurologic Sequelae

Nerve Damage. Neurologic sequelae related directly to spinal anesthesia rarely appear,[63,64] and those that occur originate either from poor technique or improper positioning. Since neurologic disorders develop rather commonly following pregnancy and delivery, it is important to make a realistic assessment of the relationship between major regional anesthesia and nerve damage.[65]

Spinal Anesthesia. Local anesthetic drug injected intraneurally or intraspinally can damage nerves. Intraneural or intraspinal injection involves considerable resistance to injection and produces acute pain. Both represent immediate signals to cease all attempts at injection and to withdraw the needle. The neurologic damage from intraneuronal injection is usually permanent, since neurolysis occurs. The resulting deficit will depend upon the site of neurolysis and may consist of both motor and sensory effects.

Chronic adhesive arachnoiditis can result when irritants enter the subarachnoid space. Although the local anesthetics available for subarachnoid injection have no toxic or irritant effects when used in the appropriate concentrations, adhesive arachnoiditis may occur upon injection of contaminants, including substances used for skin preparation and substances entering ampules during sterilization. Chronic adhesive arachnoiditis following spinal anesthesia most frequently leads to cauda equina damage (syndrome) and produces lower limb motor loss and loss of sphincter control.

Patients with pre-existing neurologic disease should have the extent of their disease assessed and documented prior to consideration for conduction anesthesia. The presence of nerve root symptoms calls for evaluating the patient's ability to flex the hips prior to anesthesia, so that the patient care team does not attempt hyperflexion under anesthesia when the patient would not perceive pain, which normally limits flexion. Should one fail to take this precaution, exacerbations of pain might occur in the postpartum period, with the clinician wrongfully attributing this to the spinal anesthetic.

Epidural Anesthesia. Neurologic sequelae rarely follow correctly administered epidural analgesia.[66] Severe pain during placement of an epidural warns of nerve root damage. Small epidural hematomas probably occur frequently but do not appear to have clinical significance in most cases. In patients with impaired coagulation due either to disease or to concurrent medication, bleeding in the epidural space may cause pressure on the spinal cord and require surgical intervention. Therefore, patients with coagulation abnormalities should not receive epidural or spinal blocks. Caution dictates avoiding epidural analgesia in patients receiving low-dose heparin, since its role in this group has not yet been fully elucidated.

Epidural hematomas also form a nidus for abscess formation if bacteremia develops. When considering epidural anesthesia in patients with known bacterial infection the risks and the benefits of the procedure should be carefully weighed. In general, epidural analgesia may proceed, provided the infection remains localized and the patient has adequate antibiotic management (see Chap. 22). An epidural abscess is an acute surgical emergency. Symptoms of neurologic involvement, including both motor and sensory deficit, follow. The patient frequently loses sphincter function, and there is acute pain at the site of infection and accompanying fever.

The presence of a space-occupying lesion in the epidural space, including both hematoma and abscess, requires immediate surgical resolution. Otherwise, permanent neurologic deficit will likely occur. The use of modern imaging techniques (CT scan) simplifies the proper diagnosis of such complications. When such a complication is suspected, a full neurologic work-up and roentgenographic studies such as a CT scan are ordered. Diagnosis of a lesion calls for immediate surgical drainage of blood or infected material to prevent neurologic damage.

Secondary genital herpes does not contraindicate epidural or spinal analgesia (Chap. 22). This author believes, however, that either a severe primary infection with marked viremia or the presence of herpetic lesions on the back in close proximity to the needle insertion site contraindicates epidural analgesia.

Chloroprocaine Toxicity. Within the recent past, a group of reports related permanent neurologic damage to the use of 2-chloroprocaine during epidural analgesia.[67–70] Initially many considered 2-chloroprocaine neurotoxic, perhaps because of its low pH (3.1). Further investigation revealed that most, if not all, cases involved the accidental subarachnoid injection of large amounts of 2-chloroprocaine. Commercially available 2-chloroprocaine also contains the antioxidant sodium bisulfite, a neurotoxin in some animal studies. The overall picture of chloroprocaine toxicity remains quite unclear, since various animal studies reveal conflicting results. Most of the clinical cases involved a high level of sympathetic blockade with the probability of hypotension and hypoperfusion of the spinal cord, combined with markedly increased intradural pressures as a result of the large volume of drug injected. Increased intradural pressure further reducing spinal cord perfusion and, thus, leading to spinal cord ischemia, could account for neurologic damage.[71] Some have also attributed neurotoxicity to the production of sulphur dioxide from sodium bisulphite at a low pH. Newer commercial preparations have either significantly reduced concentrations of sodium bisulphite or no preservative, in an attempt to decrease the likelihood of neurotoxicity.[72]

Most workers now agree that 2-chloroprocaine is safe and efficacious when used appropriately in the epidural space. One must test carefully for subarachnoid placement by catheter aspiration and should test dose with caution. In case of accidental subarachnoid injection of larger volumes of 2-chloroprocaine, a needle is inserted into the CSF and as much fluid as possible is removed; it is replaced with preservative-free sterile saline. The lavage is repeated several times to reduce the amount of drug deposited in the CSF. It is more important, however, to deal with the hemodynamic consequences that usually accompany total spinal, in an effort to maintain spinal cord blood flow. The majority of reported cases of neurologic damage following the subarachnoid injection of large volumes of 2-chloroprocaine described a cauda equina syndrome, characterized by retention or incontinence of urine and feces, loss of perineal sensation, and loss of sexual function. Motor weakness followed.

Bladder Dysfunction

Because urinary retention is a relatively common complication of delivery, irrespective of whether the patient undergoes a regional block,[73] determining the etiology of bladder dysfunction proves difficult. Epidural anesthesia may make the patient unaware of bladder distention, which would normally be a signal to void. If bladder distention continues, the detrusor muscle becomes partially paralyzed and urinary retention follows. During labor with an epidural block, make frequent checks to determine if bladder filling has become excessive. Unsuccessful spontaneous voiding necessitates catheterization.

Low Back Pain

As with bladder dysfunction, this is also a common complication of vaginal delivery (30 to 40 percent).[73] Regional analgesia does not increase the incidence of low back pain. Treatment should be conservative, and further investigation is undertaken only for prolonged or severe back pain.

Failed Regional Analgesia

Despite the extremely high success rate for regional analgesia in the parturient, failures do occur and deserve recognition. Whenever a block is unsuccessful it is repeated or another acceptable form of analgesia is substituted.

Spinal Analgesia. Spinal analgesia proves extremely reliable as long as one obtains CSF and administers the correct drug dose. Occasionally, despite an apparently adequate dermatome level, the patient still complains of pain on peritoneal traction during cesarean section. Intravenous ketamine, inhalation analgesia, or intravenous narcotics after delivery may provide relief. In the event of an inadequate dermatome level prior to incision, the block is repeated or general anesthesia is chosen. The latter necessitates rapid-sequence induction and endotracheal intubation. For repeated subarachnoid blocks, the dose of local anesthetic injected is reduced, depending on the degree of inadequacy of the original block. A second dural puncture increases the incidence of headache after spinal injection.

Epidural Analgesia. More bizarre complications can occur with epidural analgesia, including unilateral blocks and blocks which develop bilaterally but miss one segment unilaterally, usually L1. Further increments of local anesthetic drug administered with the patient in a lateral position and with the unblocked area dependent may alleviate the problem. For catheter insertion of more than 2 to 3 cm, withdraw the catheter 1 cm and give a further dose. If these procedures do not provide relief the block is repeated or other analgesics are used.

Broken Needles and Catheters

Needle breakage during regional analgesia rarely occurs as most modern spinal and epidural needles are well manufactured and do not break. If breakage does occur, it usually results from faulty technique and undue stress placed upon the needle. Rarely, some part of the needle may contain faulty material, allowing it to break during normal use, most frequently at the junction between the shaft and hub. When this occurs, one can extract the needle easily. An unexposed broken needle requires surgical removal.

Epidural catheters consist of soft, pliant materials that easily withstand the stresses of correct normal use. Breakage most commonly results from withdrawal of a catheter already advanced through the needle. Should a situation call for withdrawal, needle and catheter are pulled out as a unit. Occasionally, catheters become knotted inside the epidural space and attempts at withdrawal end in breakage or tissue damage. After a catheter is withdrawn the tip is inspected to ensure removal of the entire catheter. Most catheters have a radiopaque mark at the tip.

If the physician is unable to remove the catheter tip the patient must be informed. Since epidural catheters are made of inert nontoxic materials, surgical removal is not required, and attempts at removal prove unnecessary unless root symptoms develop or the patient insists.

Fetal and Neonatal Complications

Maternal anesthesia and analgesia may adversely affect the fetus and neonate in one of two ways: either from the direct effect of drugs crossing the placenta from mother to fetus, or indirectly, secondary to changes in maternal physiologic status, arising from effects of a drug or anesthetic technique.

DIRECT DRUG EFFECTS

Since the placenta's ability to limit the transfer of some drugs from mother to fetus remains incomplete, many drugs that provide anesthesia and analgesia traverse it quite freely, resulting in a maternal-fetal concentration ratio of close to 1:1. In general, lipid-soluble and un-ionized drugs transfer most rapidly (Chap. 2). Safe administration of anesthetics and analgesics during labor and delivery partly depends on dose adjustment, which takes into account placental transfer. Most anesthetic and analgesic agents act on the mother's CNS and, to do so, must pass through the blood-brain barrier. The ability of a drug to reach the maternal brain usually signifies a similar degree of placental transport to the fetus. The most obvious neonatal response to drugs transferred from the mother is respiratory depression. This usually needs conservative management and, only occasionally, specific intervention, such as mechanical ventilation.

Paracervical Block

The technique of paracervical block produces analgesia for the first stage of labor (Chap. 6). However, it produces an unacceptably high incidence of fetal bradycardia, which relates to fetal hypoxia (and occasionally, fetal death).[74] Many authorities correlate the fetal bradycardia with a high level of local anesthetic in fetal blood: this occurs secondarily to drug injection adjacent to the uterine blood supply, with subsequent rapid absorption. Some cases revealed higher levels in the fetus than in maternal blood.[75,76]

Most local anesthetics produce increased myometrial muscle tone. The blood levels that occur locally in the area of the myometrium during the course of a paracervical block are sufficient in many cases to produce such an effect. An intrauterine pressure monitor detects an increase in uterine tone, which lasts for as long as 15 to 20 min following paracervical block and may decrease uterine blood flow. Consequently, fetal hypoxia may develop and it represents an additional factor in the etiology of bradycardia associated with paracervical block.

Ketamine

Most drugs which produce a vasopressor response also reduce uterine blood flow. Administration of ketamine, a pressor, in an animal model did not decrease uterine blood flow, despite an oxytocic effect on uterine tone.[77] The parturient can safely receive ketamine, provided the dose does not exceed 1 mg per kg. Doses greater than 1 mg per kg can result in placental transfer of sufficient drug to produce neonatal depression.

INDIRECT EFFECTS

Intravascular Injection of Local Anesthetics

As described previously, pregnancy increases the risk of accidental injection of local anesthetic drug during an epidural block. When this occurs, high levels of drug in maternal blood often increase myometrial tone, which may in turn produce fetal hypoxia. Furthermore, blood levels of local anesthetic in the neonate following placental transfer may reach levels sufficient to cause direct cardiac depression.

Maternal Respiratory Changes

Although narcotics can cause maternal respiratory depression, leading to fetal hypoxia, this rarely happens in modern obstetric practice, since most limit the total dose given to the mother. Hypoxia usually results from prolonged maternal apnea or failed intubation during general anesthesia.

Controlled hyperventilation during general anesthesia may lead to fetal hypoxia. A maternal oxygen inspired concentration between 50 and 60 percent produces optimal oxygenation of the neonate at delivery. Ventilation should maintain a maternal $PaCO_2$ in the physiologic range for pregnancy (30 to 35 mmHg). Lowering the $PaCO_2$ to a level significantly below this will reduce uterine blood flow, as part of the vasoconstrictor response to hypocarbia.[78] Hypocarbia also impairs fetal oxygenation by decreasing placental oxygen transport (Bohr effect).

Maternal Cardiovascular Changes

Placental blood flow is very sensitive to changes in maternal hemodynamic status. Administering anesthesia, either regional or general, to a parturient must involve efforts to avoid fetal compromise secondary to hypotension or intense uterine vasoconstriction.

The supine position is avoided at all times, especially during anesthesia. Maternal compensation for the effects of vena caval compression that normally occur in the absence of anesthesia can be significantly impaired when anesthesia depresses vascular reflex mechanisms. Laboring patients with epidural analgesia require nursing in a full or semilateral position at all times. General anesthesia is induced with the patient in a 15-degree left lateral tilt. Additionally, sudden alterations of blood pressure are avoided. Hypotension is treated as previously described. Failure to treat hypotension will rapidly produce changes in the fetal heart rate tracing suggestive of hypoxia.

Severe hypertension secondary to induction of general anesthesia may also harm the fetus as well as the mother. Intense vasoconstriction during hypertension includes the placental circulation. When anticipating significant hypertension, as in a pre-eclamptic mother, both mother and fetus benefit from maintaining pressure at a reasonable level using an infusion of a vasodilator agent during the induction period. The pressure is carefully monitored by inserting an intra-arterial catheter (Chap. 21).

NEONATAL NEUROBEHAVIORIAL ASSESSMENT

Once the realm of the pediatrician, the study of newborn neurobehavior has now entered into the anesthesiologist's domain. An early study[79] demonstrated that epidurally administered lidocaine and mepivacaine produce detectable changes in the neonate. The finding of decreased muscle tone lead to the description of the babies as being "floppy but alert." The same studies completed on babies born to mothers receiving epidural bupivacaine demonstrated muscle tone preservation.[80,81] Unfortunately, the true significance of neurobehavioral studies remains unknown and may not have any bearing upon long-term outcome. Nevertheless, the F.D.A. now screens new drugs for possible neurobehavioral effects prior to their approval for use in pregnancy. Since studies have been confined to full-term deliveries devoid of obstetric complications, one cannot accurately project the effect of drugs to abnormal situations such as prematurity. Accomplishing this would require a large number of additional studies using rather large patient groups. Since many other factors influence neurobehavioral performance, proper selection of patients would complicate completion of studies in high-risk pregnancies, especially those examining effects of drugs. A further problem results from the standardization of testing. One cannot compare results from one study with those from another. Upon repeating the original studies with lidocaine, researchers[82,83] could not demonstrate the changes reported in the initial studies. Thus, lidocaine once again qualifies as acceptable for obstetric anesthesia, particularly since the recent awareness of problems with 2-chloroprocaine and bupivacaine.

A great deal of confusion surrounds neurobehavioral studies. They do however give the anesthesiologist a guide as to which drugs or techniques are least likely to produce neonatal complications.

Summary

This chapter identifies some of the more important complications that may occur when administering anesthesia to the parturient and emphasizes those which predominate. As a general rule, any form of management that benefits the mother equally benefits the newborn.

This chapter has repeatedly emphasized the following general guidelines since complications from obstetric anesthesia will continue to occur. These guidelines may reduce the number and severity of complications:

1. Only practitioners who are experienced in the management of anesthetic complications should administer or supervise others giving anesthesia.
2. These practitioners should have a firm understanding of the physiologic changes of pregnancy and their relevance to anesthesia. Understanding the principles of placental transfer is essential.
3. Anesthesia for parturients is undertaken only in the presence of equipment capable of dealing with any emergency *and* staff experienced in the initial management of anesthetic complications. Qualified help is indispensable.
4. Obstetric anesthesia is administered only in institutions that regularly perform these procedures; in other words, the occasional or inexperienced practitioner should not attempt to deliver anesthesia to the parturient.

These guidelines will minimize the incidence of dangerous complications and will assure as safe a practice as possible.

References

1. Shiono, PH, et al: Recent trends in cesarean birth and trial of labor rates in the United States. JAMA 257:494, 1987.
2. Mendelson, CL: Aspiration of stomach contents into lungs during obstetric anesthesia. Am J Obstet Gynecol 52:191, 1946.

3. Merrill, RB and Hingson, RA: Studies of the incidence of maternal mortality from the aspiration of vomitus during anesthesia occurring in major obstetric hospitals in the United States. Anesth Analg 30:121, 1951.
4. Tomkins, J, et al: Report on confidential enquiries into maternal deaths in England and Wales 1976–78. Department of Health and Social Security. Her Majesty's Stationery Office, London, 1982.
5. Csapo, A: Progesterone block. Am J Anat 98:279, 1956.
6. Christofides, ND, et al: Decreased plasma motilin concentrations in pregnancy. Br Med J 285:1453, 1982.
7. Nimmo, WS, Wilson, J, and Prescott, LF: Narcotic analgesics and delayed gastric emptying during labor. Lancet 1:890, 1975.
8. Attia, RR, et al: Maternal, fetal and placental gastrin concentrations. Anesthesia 37:18, 1982.
9. Roberts, RB and Shirley, MA: Reducing the risk of acid aspiration during cesarean section. Anesth Analg 53:859, 1974.
10. Roberts, RB and Shirley, MA: The obstetrician's role in reducing the risk of aspiration pneumonitis with particular reference to the use of oral antacids. Am J Obstet Gynecol 124:611, 1976.
11. Taylor, G and Pryse-Davies, J: The prophylactic use of antacids in the prevention of the acid–pulmonary aspiration syndrome (Mendelson's syndrome). Lancet 1:288, 1966.
12. Whittington, RM, Robinson, JS, and Thompson, JM: Fatal aspiration (Mendelson's) syndrome despite antacids and cricoid pressure. Lancet 2:228, 1979.
13. Gibbs, CP, et al: Antacid pulmonary aspiration in the dog. Anesthesiology 51:380, 1979.
14. Gibbs, CP, Sophu, L, and Schmidt, D: The effectiveness of sodium citrate as an antacid. Anesthesiology 57:44, 1982.
15. Dewan, DM, et al: Sodium citrate premedication for elective cesarean section. Anesth Analg 63:205, 1984.
16. Chen, CT, et al: Evaluation of Alka-Seltzer effervescent in gastric acid neutralization. Anesth Analg 63:325, 1984.
17. Pickering, BG, Palahniuk, RJ, and Cumming, M: Cimetidine premedication in elective cesarean section. Can Anaesth Soc J 27:33, 1980.
18. Hodgkinson, R, et al: Comparison of cimetidine (Tagamet) with acidity before elective cesarean section. Anesthesiology 59:86, 1983.
19. Maile, CJD and Francis, PN: Pre-operative ranitidine. Anesthesia 38:324, 1983.
20. Cohen, S and Barrier, G: Does metaclopramide decrease gastric volume in cesarean section patients? Anesthesiology 59A:403, 1983.
21. Zeldis, JB, Friedman, LS, and Isselbacher, KJ: Ranitidine: A new H2–receptor antagonist. N Engl J Med 309:1368, 1983.
22. Snow, RG and Nunn, JF: Induction of anaesthesia in the foot-down position for patients with a full stomach. Br J Anaesth 31:493, 1959.
23. Sellick, BA: Cricoid pressure to control regurgitation of stomach contents during induction of anesthesia. Lancet 2:404, 1961.
24. Cameron, JL, et al: Aspiration pneumonia: Results of treatment by positive-pressure ventilation in drugs. J Surg Res 8:447, 1968.
25. Chapman, RL: Treatment of aspiration pneumonitis. Int Anesthesiol Clin 15:85, 1977.
26. Giesecke, AH Jr.: Anesthesia for trauma surgery. In Miller, RD (ed): Anesthesia. Churchill Livingstone, New York, 1981, p 1253.
27. Modell, JH: Aspiration pneumonitis. In Annual Refresher Course Lectures, ASA. JB Lippincott, Philadelphia, 1983, p 163.
28. Archer, GW Jr. and Marx, GR: Arterial oxygen tension during apnoea in parturient women. Br J Anaesth 46:358, 1974.
29. Crawford, JS: Awareness during operative obstetrics under general anaesthesia. Br J Anaesth 43:179, 1971.
30. Palahnuik, RJ, et al: Maternal and neonatal effects of methoxyflurane, nitrous oxide and lumbar epidural anaesthesia for cesarean section. Anesth Analg 51:701, 1972.
31. Moir, DD: Anaesthesia for cesarean section: An evaluation of a method using low concentration of halothane and 50 percent of oxygen. Br J Anaesth 42:136, 1970.
32. Warren, TM, et al: Comparison of the maternal and neonatal effects of halothane, enflurane and isoflurane for cesarean delivery. Anesth Analg 62:516, 1983.
33. Committee on Nitrous Oxide Analgesia in Midwifery, Sir Douglas Baird, Chairman, Clinical trials of different concentrations of oxygen and nitrous oxide for obstetric analgesia. Br Med J 1:709, 1970.
34. Major, V, Rosen, M, and Mushin, WW: Methoxyflurane as an obstetric analgesic: A comparison with trichlorethylene. Br Med J 2:1554, 1966.
35. Marx, GF, Chen, LK and Tabora, JA: Experiences with a disposable inhaler for methoxyflurane analgesia during labor: Clinical and biochemical results. Can Anaesth Soc J 16:66, 1969.
36. Rosen, M, et al: Field trial of methoxyflurane, nitrous oxide and trichloroethylene as obstetric analgesia. Br Med J 3:263, 1969.
37. Janeczko, GF, et al: Low dose ketamine anesthesia for obstetrical delivery. Anesth Analg 53:828, 1974.
38. Kenepp, NB, et al: Dextrose hydration in cesarean section patients. Anesthesiology 53:S304, 1981.
39. Kerr, MG: Cardiovascular dynamics in pregnancy and labour. Br Med Bull 24:19, 1968.
40. Bieniarz, J, et al: Aorto-caval compression by the uterus in late human pregnancy. Am J Obstet Gynecol 100:203, 1978.
41. Greene, NM: The area of differential block during spinal anesthesia with hyperbaric tetracaine. Anesthesiology 19:45, 1958.
42. Chamberlain, DP and Chamberlain, BD: Changes in the skin temperature of the trunk and their relationship to sympathetic blockade during spinal anesthesia. Anesthesiology 65:139, 1986.
43. Corke, BC, et al: Spinal anaesthesia for cesarean section: The influence of hypotension on neonatal outcome. Anaesthesia 37:658, 1982.
44. Ebner, H: An evaluation of spinal anesthesia in obstetrics. Anesth Analg 38:378, 1959.
45. Arner, O: Complications following spinal anesthesia:

Their significance and technic to reduce their incidence. Acta Chir Scand (Suppl) 167:7, 1952.
46. Green, BA: A 26 gauge lumbar puncture needle: Its value in the prophylaxis of headache following spinal anesthesia for vaginal delivery. Anesthesiology 11:464, 1950.
47. Harris, LM and Harmel, MH: The comparative incidence of post lumbar puncture headache following spinal anesthesia administered through 20 and 24 gauge needles. Anesthesiology 14:390, 1953.
48. Jones, RL: The role of recumbency in the prevention and treatment of post spinal headache. Anesth Analg 53:788, 1974.
49. Carboat, P and Van Crevel, H: Lumbar puncture headache. Controlled study on the preventive effect of 24 hours' bed rest. Lancet 2:1133, 1981.
50. Crawford, JS: Headache after lumbar puncture: correspondence. Lancet 2:418, 1981.
51. Craft, JB, et al: Prophylaxis of dural-puncture headache with epidural saline. Anesth Analg 52:228, 1977.
52. Abouleish, ES, et al: Long term follow up of epidural blood patch. Anesth Analg 54:459, 1975.
53. Ostheimer, GS, et al: Epidural blood patch for post–lumbar puncture headache. Anesthesiology 41:307, 1974.
54. Crawford, JS: Experience with epidural blood patch. Anesthesiology 35:513, 1980.
55. Loeser, EA, et al: Time vs. success for epidural blood patch. Anesthesiology 49:147, 1978.
56. Abouleish, ES, et al: Regional analgesia following epidural blood patch. Anesth Analg 54:634, 1975.
57. Albright, GA: Cardiac arrest following regional anesthesia with etidocaine or bupivacaine. Anesthesiology 51:285, 1979.
58. Corke, BC and Spielman, FJ: Problems associated with epidural anesthesia in obstetrics. Obstet Gynecol 65:837, 1985.
59. Albright, GA: Epinephrine should be used with the therapeutic dose of bupivacaine, correspondence. Anesthesiology 61:217, 1984.
60. FDA Drug Bulletin: Adverse Reactions with Bupivacaine. U.S. Department of Health and Human Services publications, Rockville, MD, 1983, vol. 13, p 23.
61. Moore, DC and Bridenbaugh, LD: Oxygen: The antidote for systemic toxic reactions from local anesthetic drugs. JAMA 174:842, 1960.
62. Ausinsch, B, Mazagodi, MH and Munson, ES: Diazepam in the prophylaxis of lignocaine seizures. Br J Anaesth 48:309, 1976.
63. Moore, DC and Bridenbaugh, LD: Spinal (subarachnoid) block: A review of 11,574 cases. JAMA 195:123, 1966.
64. Greene, NM: Neurological sequelae of spinal anesthesia. Anesthesiology 22:682, 1961.
65. Aminoff, MJ: Neurological disorders and pregnancy. Am J Obstet Gynecol 132:325, 1978.
66. Usubiaga, JE: Neurological complications following epidural anesthesia. Int Anesthesiol Clin 13(2):1, 1975.
67. Reisner, LS, et al: Persistent neurologic deficit and adhesive arachnoiditis following intrathecal 2-chloroprocaine. Anesth Analg 59:452, 1980.
68. Ravindran, RS, et al: Prolonged neural blockade following regional analgesia with 2 chloroprocaine. Anesth Analg 59:447, 1980.
69. Moore, DC, et al: Chloroprocaine neurotoxicity. Four additional cases. Anesth Analg 61:155, 1982.
70. Sheskey, MC and Mallampati, SR: Prolonged neural blockade following caudal block with 2-chloroprocaine. Reg Anesth 10:28, 1985.
71. Gissen, AJ, Datta, S and Lambert, D: The chloroprocaine controversy: I. An hypothesis to explain the neural complications of chloroprocaine epidural. Reg Anesth 9:124, 1984.
72. Gissen, AJ, Datta, S and Lambert, D: The chloroprocaine controversy: II. Is chloroprocaine neurotoxic? Reg Anesth 9:135, 1984.
73. Grove, LH: Backache, headache and bladder dysfunction after delivery. Br J Anaesth 45:1147, 1973.
74. Rosefsky, JB and Petersil, ME: Perinatal deaths associated with mepivacaine paracervical block anesthesia in labor. N Engl J Med 278:530, 1968.
75. Theiry, M and Vroman, S: Paracervical block analgesia during labor. Am J Obstet Gynecol 113:988, 1971.
76. Petrie, RH, et al: Placental transfer of lidocaine following paracervical block. Am J Obstet Gynecol 120:793, 1974.
77. Levinson, G, et al: Maternal and foetal cardiovascular and acid base changes during ketamine anesthesia in pregnant ewes. Br J Anaesth 45:1111, 1973.
78. Morishima, HO, et al: Effects of positive pressure ventilation of the mother upon the acid base status of the fetus. Am J Obstet Gynecol 93:269, 1965.
79. Scanlon, JW, et al: Neurobehavioral responses of newborn infants after maternal epidural anesthesia. Anesthesiology 40:121, 1974.
80. Corke, BC: Neurobehavioural responses of the newborn: Effects of different forms of maternal analgesia. Anaesthesia 32:539, 1977.
81. Scanlon, JW, et al: Neurobehavioral responses and drug concentrations in newborn after maternal epidural anesthesia with bupivacaine. Anesthesiology 45:400, 1976.
82. Kileff, ME, et al: Neonatal neurobehavioral responses after epidural anesthesia for cesarean section using lidocaine and bupivacaine. Anesth Analg 63:413, 1984.
83. Abboud, TK, et al: Lack of adverse neonatal neurobehavioral effects of lidocaine. Anesth Analg 62:473, 1983.

PART 3

MATERNAL PROBLEMS BY SYSTEM

CHAPTER 8

NEUROLOGIC DISEASE

EZZAT ABOULEISH, M.B., Ch.B., D.A., D.M., M.D.

Neurologic diseases occur infrequently during the childbearing years, making it unlikely that one anesthesiologist will have extensive experience in the management of all these disorders. Scant information appears in the anesthesia literature regarding neurologic diseases in pregnancy. Therefore, I have based the data and opinions presented in this chapter on a paucity of published information and my experience. Table 8–1 presents the various groups of neurologic diseases. Examples of these groups are discussed and serve as models to facilitate understanding in approaching, comprehending, and managing related disorders.

Neurofibromatosis

In 1882, Von Recklinghausen described neurofibromatosis. The disease occurs in 1 in 2500 to 3000 births and is transmitted by an autosomal-dominant gene.[1] Increased skin pigmentation (café-au-lait spots) combined with multiple neurofibromas characterize the disease. The tumors arise from the neurilemmal sheath (Schwann cells) and the fibroblasts of peripheral nerves.[2] They are usually multiple and vary in size from minute lesions to large tumors. The nodules, as well as the pigmentation, increase in size and number during pregnancy and regress after delivery.

The parturient with neurofibromatosis presents special problems. The disease process itself can alter her reaction to muscle relaxants.[3–5] Magbagbeola[4] reported prolonged apnea in one patient following succinylcholine (12 min instead of 4 to 5 min) and pancuronium (117 min instead of 45 min). Manser[3] reported the outcome of two women with Recklinghausen's disease having general anesthesia for cesarean section at term. The first patient had an exaggerated response to d-tubocurarine while the second experienced prolonged apnea following succinylcholine administration. Baraka[5] described a patient resistant to succinylcholine and unduly sensitive to d-tubocurarine. The reason for the altered response to muscle relaxant remains unclear. It may be due to denervation of the motor end-plate produced by the generalized neurofibromatosis.[5] Denervation sensitizes the striated muscle both to the chemical transmitter acetylcholine and to other depolarizers such as succinylcholine. This increased sensitiv-

Table 8-1. ORGANIC NEUROLOGIC DISEASES

Congenital
Neurofibromatosis*
Acquired
Infectious: present or past history of:*
Meningitis
Encephalitis
Poliomyelitis
Syphilis
Traumatic: paraplegia*
Vascular: cerebrovascular disorders
Cerebral aneurysm
Cerebral embolism
Degenerative
Multiple sclerosis*
Neoplastic
Brain tumors*
Benign intracranial hypertension*
Spinal cord tumor
Brain activity disorders
Epilepsy*
Hydrocephalus and extracranial shunts*
Skeletomuscular disease
Muscular dystrophy*
Myotonic congenita*
Myotonic dystrophy*
Severe scoliosis
Prolapsed disc and back surgery
Myoneural junction disease
Myasthenia gravis*

*These subjects are discussed in detail.

ity for depolarization has been attributed to the spread of the chemoreceptive area from the end-plate region to cover most of the muscle membrane.[6] Thus, the administration of succinylcholine may lead to contracture rather than relaxation. The increased sensitivity to nondepolarizing relaxant may represent a myasthenic reaction.[5] Therefore, when using a muscle relaxant, employ the more controllable relaxants rather than depolarizing drugs. Because of the possibility of an abnormal response to muscle relaxants, regional analgesia is preferable to general anesthesia.

Laryngeal and pharyngeal neurofibromas may occur leading to airway obstruction, so the airway must be carefully examined before anesthesia.

The neurofibromas increase in size during pregnancy; thus, they may cause pressure manifestations, and hemorrhage may occur in these masses.[7] Pelvic neurofibromas may lead to obstructed labor necessitating abdominal delivery.[8]

Neurofibromatosis may be associated with impaired general physical development, and most patients show some osseous changes (e.g., pathologic fracture, scoliosis).[9] The disease may also be associated with spina bifida, rendering epidural and caudal analgesia inadvisable but spinal block relatively easy. Interstitial lung disease may occur leading to hypoxemia and cor pulmonale.

The incidence of pheochromocytoma increases with Recklinghausen's disease.[10,11] Both neurofibromas and the adrenal medulla originate from the embryonic neural crest. Neurofibromatosis occurs in approximately 5 to 25 percent of patients with pheochromocytomas.[10] Even in the absence of pheochromocytoma, known vascular changes accompany neurofibromatosis (e.g., intimal and subintimal proliferation and renal artery stenosis).[1,12] These changes increase during pregnancy and may cause hypertension. With neurofibromatosis, the normal increase in maternal blood volume during pregnancy may contribute to the hypertension because of the limited elasticity of the blood vessels. Therefore, the patient with neurofibromatosis is more liable to become hypertensive during pregnancy and may be mistakenly diagnosed as being pre-eclamptic.

Neurofibromatosis may be associated with increased intracranial pressure due either to an intracranial tumor such as an acoustic neuroma, meningioma, or glioma, or to obstruction of cerebrospinal fluid (CSF) flow as a result of stenosis of the aqueduct of Sylvius.[2] Such cases contraindicate spinal analgesia, while inadvertent dural puncture must be avoided during lumbar epidural block. Therefore, pudendal nerve block represents a safer method of pain relief for vaginal delivery.

Infectious Diseases

Active inflammatory disease in the spinal canal, such as acute meningitis or infection of the skin at the necessary puncture site, contraindicates an intravertebral block. However, when the inflammatory condition has completely subsided (for instance, childhood poliomyelitis), an intravertebral block can be used when indicated. No evidence reveals that such a block can aggravate her condition or exacerbate the old inflammatory problems. The numbness and paralysis may remind the parturient of her original attack of poliomyelitis. This feeling should be explained to her before the block with assurance that the changes will last only a few hours. When possible, one should administer epidural rather than spinal anesthesia using the minimal local drug concentration to achieve pain relief in order to preserve as much motor function as possible.

Paraplegia

The patient with paraplegia or quadriplegia presents an anesthetic challenge. The lesion can be due to trauma or to spinal cord disease.

EFFECT OF PREGNANCY ON THE DISEASE

Paraplegic or quadriplegic patients may experience a peculiar phenomenon called "autonomic hyperreflexia" (mass reflex), first described in 1917 by Head and Reddoch.[13] The syndrome consists of pilomotor erection, sweating, facial flushing, severe headache, bradycardia, and severe hypertension leading to loss of consciousness, convulsions, and possibly subarachnoid or cerebral hemorrhage.[14,15] The syndrome does not develop in lesions below T7 and, for unknown reasons, occurs in only 85 percent of patients with lesions about T7. Autonomic hyperreflexia results from afferent impulses reaching the isolated spinal cord. The response, uninhibited or modulated by the higher centers, is massive rather than specific. Stimulation of the skin below the level of the lesion or distention and contraction of a hollow viscus, such as the urinary bladder, uterus, or gut, precipitate massive stimulation of the sympathetic nervous system and the isolated adrenal glands, which derive their sympathetic nerve supply from the greater splanchnic nerve (T5–T9). In addition, the denervated blood vessels are extra sensitive to catecholamines, thus the precipitous elevation of blood pressure can be quite dangerous.[16] Since spinal cord transection does not interfere with afferent connections of the baroreceptors and slowing of the heart via reflex vagal response to hypertension, an associated bradycardia results. Heart block may also cause bradycardia, rendering ECG monitoring essential. Temperature regulation may be impaired. Thus, careful body temperature monitoring is important. Attention to respiratory functions should continue during the peripartum period because of the possible impairment of the muscles of respiration. Every effort should be made to avoid decubitus ulcers by moving the patient gently from one side to the other and caring for the skin at the pressure points.

Autonomic reflexia causes severe hypertension during parturition in about 11 percent of paraplegic patients.[17]

COURSE OF LABOR

When spinal cord injury resulting in paraplegia occurs during the course of an established pregnancy, spontaneous abortion or stillbirth may follow.[18] Premature labor occurs more often in paraplegic than in normal patients. With lesions above T10, patients may be unaware of labor, and premature delivery may occur under unfavorable conditions. Therefore, paraplegic patients should be examined regularly. More frequent examinations are necessary after 28 weeks, and the patient should be hospitalized at 32 weeks' gestation unless cervical dilation occurs earlier. Surveillance for urinary tract infection, anemia, and skin ulcers is recommended.[19]

Paraplegia does not increase the incidence of pre-eclampsia.[17] Parturients with traumatic paraplegia above T10 experience spontaneous labor with strong and painless uterine contractions.[17] Patients with paraplegia due to spinal cord disease may perceive pain sensations during uterine contractions; in addition, marked muscle spasm and ankle clonus can make labor unpleasant and distressing. Vaginal delivery usually occurs. Obstetricians perform cesarean section only for obstetrical indications. In a report of 39 deliveries, only three patients had cesarean section, a rate of about 8 percent.[17] During vaginal delivery, weak expulsive efforts may necessitate the use of forceps to shorten the second stage of labor.

EFFECTS ON THE FETUS AND NEONATE

A high stillbirth rate (78 per 1000 births compared with 13 per 1000 in the general population) accompanies paraplegia.[17] Congenital anomalies or neonatal deaths do not occur more frequently to paraplegics than to normal women.

Anesthesia

During the 3 to 6 weeks following an upper-motor-neuron lesion that produces paraplegia or hemiplegia, administration of succinylcholine can be dangerous because of the resulting hyperkalemia.[19] A similar situation can occur in neuromuscular diseases such as muscular dystrophies, multiple sclerosis, and amyotrophic lateral sclerosis.[20] A denervated or degenerating muscle leaks potassium and is especially sensitive to chemical stimulation of acetylcholine or succinylcholine.[21] Therefore, the administration of succinylcholine produces hyperkalemia, which can lead to cardiac arrhythmias and even ventricular fibrillation. The parturient with paraplegia or quadriplegia requires little or no anesthesia, depending on the level and extent of the lesion. If anesthesia is required, regional anesthesia proves safer than general anesthesia. Moreover, regional anesthesia provides an important tool for controlling autonomic hyperreflexia during labor, especially if the patient's history indicates the presence of mass reflexia, for instance due to distention of the urinary bladder. In one reported case, continuous epidural technique successfully blocked the reflex arc for autonomic hyperreflexia, thus preventing excessive hypertension.[22] Spinal anesthesia reportedly prevents autonomic hyperreflexia in quadriplegic patients undergoing various surgical procedures.[23] During labor, spinal block may cause a precipitous fall in blood pressure. Labor may last longer than the block unless the anesthesiologist employs a continuous spinal technique. Continuous epidural infusion provides pain relief for the duration of labor, and I prefer it to intermittent injection techniques. A concentration of 0.25 to 0.125 percent bupivacaine adequately blocks the reflex arc causing hypertension.

Epidural meperidine, recently used during labor, controlled autonomic hyperreflexia while sparing the resting sympathetic tone which cord transection had already compromised.[24] Arterial blood pressure and heart rate remain more stable than with epidural or spinal anesthesia. One hundred milligrams of preservative-free meperidine diluted in 10-ml preservative-free normal saline is an appropriate dose for epidural injection. Experimental studies showing blocking by opiates of nociceptive impulses in the spinal cords of transected cats formed the basis for trying epidural narcotics in paraplegics.[25]

ARTERIAL THROMBOSIS

The incidence of an arterial thrombosis in pregnancy and the puerperium is 1 in 20,000.[26] The mortality is more than double that of males of the same age group and triple that of nonpregnant females of the same age group. During pregnancy, thrombosis occurs most commonly in the middle cerebral artery; during the puerperium, the internal carotid artery is the main site. The pathologic basis of occlusion of major arteries remains uncertain. Since oral contraceptive therapy also increases the incidence of arterial occlusion by three- to fourfold, a hormonal cause probably exists. The changes in blood coagulation associated with pregnancy could play a role. Once an occlusion of a major cerebral artery has occurred, treatment proves ineffective.

VENOUS THROMBOSIS

Venous thrombosis develops most commonly between the second and fourth week postpartum.[27] The main symptoms include the development of progressive paresis and seizures over a period of a few hours. Arteriography confirms the diagnosis. Treatment of venous thrombosis consists mainly of anticonvulsants, anticoagulants, and antibiotics (on the assumption that an associated infection may exist). A special syndrome, cortical vein thrombosis, may occur during pregnancy with a clinical picture similar to eclampsia.[28,29] The progress of the disease reflects its diagnosis (e.g., repeated convulsions with associated focal neurologic signs such as paralysis). Since disseminated intravascular coagulopathy (DIC) and thromboembolic phenomena may accompany this syndrome, the presence of these clinical manifestations dictates obtaining a computed tomogram (CT) of the head and performing angiography for confirmation. The anesthetic management depends on the blood coagulation. If the patient has DIC, general anesthesia is the method of choice for cesarean section; otherwise, a properly administered regional block suffices, unless intracranial pressure has increased excessively or an asymmetric mass lesion such as a hematoma complicates the picture.

PRIMARY INTRACEREBRAL HEMORRHAGE

Apart from hemorrhage associated with eclampsia, primary intracerebral hemorrhage rarely occurs. Pre-eclampsia, by causing hypertension and cerebrovascular changes, can lead to cerebral hemorrhage. In a review of 533 deaths due to eclampsia and pre-eclampsia, cerebral dysfunction accounted for 180 fatalities, in 89 of which gross evidence of intracranial hemorrhage existed.[30] Hypertension and cerebral hemorrhage may also develop intra- or postpartum following the administration of ergot drugs or vasopressors.[31]

SUBARACHNOID HEMORRHAGE

Subarachnoid hemorrhage, appearing in less than 1 in 10,000 pregnancies,[32] originates from a leaking aneurysm or arteriovenous malformation, the former representing the most common cause. Of 27 patients who experienced subarachnoid hemorrhage during pregnancy, 25 had a demonstrable cause—11 arteriovenous anomalies and 14 intracranial aneurysms.[33] An arteriovenous anomaly may bleed at any time during pregnancy, and the incidence increases as pregnancy progresses. Surprisingly, only 3 percent bleed during labor.

Physicians identify cardiovascular stresses of pregnancy as an obvious reason for subarachnoid hemorrhage. Cardiac output increases during the first trimester, even more so during labor, and exceeds 100 percent of normal nonpregnant levels immediately after delivery.[34] The rise in cardiac output during the first stage of labor cannot be prevented, and some rise in blood pressure accompanies it. During the second stage of labor, the blood pressure rises, and the Valsalva maneuver increases the CSF pressure, thus supporting the intracranial vessels against the increased intramural pressure.[35,36] However, at the end of the Valsalva maneuver, the CSF pressure falls more rapidly than the arterial, causing peak vascular stress at that time. Postpartum subarachnoid hemorrhage may actually start during the second stage of labor.

Diagnosis

Symptoms are severe headache, often occipital, nuchal rigidity, nausea and vomiting, loss of consciousness, hemiplegia, and involvement of cranial nerves (in descending order of frequency). Grossly bloody CSF at lumbar puncture indicates subarachnoid hemorrhage. Xanthochromia in the supernant fluid after lumbar puncture and CSF collection indicates subarachnoid hemorrhage and differentiates it from traumatic lumbar puncture. Clinical neurologic examination fails to differentiate an aneurysm from an arteriovenous malformation. Cerebral angiography and CT scanning prove indispensable in the diagnosis of intracranial bleeds.[27,37] Pregnancy should not delay angiography since the risks of the aneurysm or malformations to rebleed are greater than those of fetal exposure.

Neurosurgical Management

The neurosurgical management of a subarachnoid hemorrhage during pregnancy consists of finding the cause and then treating it surgically when feasible. This offers the best chance for a satisfactory outcome for mother and baby. The fetus should receive extra protection during roentgenographic investigations. Without surgery, the maternal mortality rate reaches 50 percent over the ensuing 8 weeks.[37] Causes of death include massive brain laceration from the initial hemorrhage, recurrent hemorrhage, the formation of intracerebral or subdural hematomas, softening of the brain tissue from arterial spasm or thrombosis, and obstruction of the CSF circulation. Bleeding occurs most frequently during the second and third week following hemorrhage. Surgical treatment offers a favorable prognosis: all patients in all reported series of surgical treatment survived.[32,37]

Preparation for surgery usually takes a few days to correct cerebral edema by bed rest, sedation with phenobarbital or diazepam, and administration of corticosteroids.[32]

Obstetric Management

Several recent reports have described delivery by cesarean section immediately followed by clipping of a cerebral aneurysm during the same anesthetic.[38,39] However, the ideal management allows pregnancy to continue after surgical treatment and labor to occur at full term. Obstetricians strive for vaginal delivery whenever possible, for the abdominal route usually offers no special advantage.[40] Elective induction of labor employing an oxytocic agent is also possible.

Anesthetic Management

The bleeding intracranial vessel, as well as the delivery process itself, complicates the anesthetic management of these patients. Controlled hypotension is the anesthetic method of choice for the surgical treatment of cerebral aneurysm.[41] By decreasing the tension in the aneurysm wall, it minimizes the chances of rupture during surgical manipulation and clipping. Controlled hypotension facilitates the surgical procedure and decreases the operative time by reducing intracranial pressure and diminishing bleeding. Pregnancy influences the choice of hypotensive drug as well as the degree and duration of hypotension. I prefer trimethaphan because its relatively high molecular weight (597) impedes placental transfer,[42] as does its rapid hydrolysis by plasma cholinesterase. No harmful effect to fetus or neonate followed the administration of trimethaphan,[32,43] even in large doses (1700 mg) over 2 hours.[44] In comparison, trinitroglycerin (MW 227) readily crosses the placenta, possibly decreasing fetal blood pressure. Sodium nitroprusside has been used for controlling maternal blood pressure. However in ewes nitroprusside readily reaches the fetus. In ewes that were resistant to the hypotensive effect of the drug and, so, received large doses, toxic levels of cyanide appearing in the fetal blood led to death in utero.[45] This fetal effect might be a species difference—nitroprusside has been successfully used in humans. Therefore, although nitroprusside has been used without incident for controlling the blood pressure in pregnant women,[32] trimethaphan appears to be a safer drug.

Maternal hypotension decreases uterine blood flow and intervillous perfusion, possibly causing fetal asphyxia. Therefore, it is essential to monitor the fetus by continuous fetal heart rate (FHR) recording throughout the surgical procedure. In two cases out of seven, the FHR showed transient bradycardia with maternal hypotension and recovery with termination of hypotension.[32] On the whole, the fetus tolerates well-controlled hypotension. For example, in a pregnant woman in the third trimester, mean blood pressure remained at 50 mmHg without fetal bradycardia.[43] Three minutes after aneurysmal sac rupture and a fall in mean blood pressure to 20 mmHg, FHR decreased from 120 to 60 beats per min. When maternal mean blood pressure returned to 35 mmHg, the FHR rose to 120 and remained at that level while the maternal mean blood pressure was maintained at 40 mmHg. The fetus seems to tolerate decreases in maternal blood pressure during controlled hypotension better than during other causes of maternal hypotension such as hemorrhage.[46] Perhaps ganglionic blockade prevents the uterine artery constriction that accompanies maternal hypotension from other causes, thereby maintaining better uterine blood flow. Also, general anesthesia may reduce the oxygen requirement of the fetus and/or ameliorate his response to reduced intervillous circulation. With general anesthesia, beat-to-beat variability disappears even before controlled hypotension.[46] During anesthesia, only the FHR, which should measure between 140 and 160 beats per min, indicates fetal well-being. No congenital anomalies have been found in those babies whose mothers underwent controlled hypotension to facilitate surgical correction of cerebral aneurysm during the third trimester.[32]

Despite the favorable reports on deliberate hypotension, I feel its duration should be as short as possible and the degree of hypotension should be as minimal as possible. No absolute level of blood pressure should be sought; the state of the surgical field during operation and the opinion of the neurosurgeon determine the level of hypotension.

If the patient has bled recently and has labile hypertension, instrumentation of the upper airway produces a brief but sometimes severe rise in blood pressure. This may cause rebleeding, with catastrophic results.[43] Induction of anesthesia using thiopental and inhalation anesthetics to a reasonably deep level before administering the muscle relaxant helps blunt the hypertensive response. Alternatively, an intravenous antihypertensive agent may provide blood pressure control during laryngoscopy and tracheal intubation.

The principles of anesthesia and controlled hypotension in these cases include measures to (1) prevent increased intracranial pressure: smooth induction, unobstructed airway, hyperventilation, no hypoxia, no bucking on the endotracheal tube, and elevation of the operative field; and (2) reduce the intracranial pressure (administration of a diuretic such as furosemide [Lasix] 40-mg or 40-gm mannitol intravenously as the surgeon elevates the skull flap, cerebrospinal fluid drainage by lumbar puncture as he opens the dura, and controlled hypotension). Because diuretics in excessive doses may cause the fluid to shift from the fetus to the mother,[47] their use may be reserved as a last resort.

The details of controlled hypotension vary with the anesthesiologist's preference. I find the following technique to be satisfactory. The patient receives diazepam, 0.10 mg per kg, and meperidine, 1 mg per kg, intramuscularly, 1 hour before surgery. Anesthesia induction includes thiopental, 5 mg per kg, followed by succinylcholine, 1.5 mg per kg, after which the patient is ventilated with oxygen, the larynx is exposed, and the trachea, larynx, and pharynx are well sprayed with 4-percent lidocaine. Intubation follows using the largest possible tube, which should be cuffed and made of a material that does not kink. Anesthetic maintenance consists of nitrous oxide and oxygen, 3:2, and 1- to 2-percent isoflurane. When signs of recovery from succinylcholine occur, d-tubocurarine, 0.5 mg per kg, is injected intravenously. The head of the table is elevated. An accurate method (e.g., intra-arterial line) continuously monitors the blood pressure. The central venous pressure is also monitored and the body temperature and arterial blood gases are measured to maintain PaO_2 above 100 mmHg and PCO_2 around 30 mmHg. These measures usually suffice to provide a good operative field until the surgeon reaches the aneurysm. At this stage, trimethaphan may be infused intravenously, if needed, to further reduce the blood pressure until the surgeon clips the aneurysm. Thereafter, trimethaphan is terminated and the blood pressure is controlled using the previous methods. Before closing the dura, the concentration of isoflurane can be reduced or it can be terminated to allow the blood pressure to rise gradually. Secure all bleeding points before closing the dura and replacing the flap.

For labor and delivery, the double-catheter technique is ideal for patients who have an intracranial vascular defect. The parturient receives local anesthesia via the lumbar epidural catheter for the first stage of labor to prevent increases in cardiac output, and through the caudal catheter to prevent the Valsalva maneuver in the second stage. The use of forceps for delivery shortens the second stage and avoids the risk of bearing down.[33] In the postpartum period, use of the epidural technique can prevent increased cardiac output.

For cesarean section, epidural analgesia qualifies as the method of choice. If a contraindication to epidural block exists, such as acute fetal distress, general anesthesia should proceed with a rapid-sequence technique employing all the usual precautions to prevent the aspiration of gastric contents. Measures to prevent or correct the hypertensive response to endotracheal intubation may be necessary.

Multiple Sclerosis

Multiple sclerosis (MS) is a demyelinating disease characterized by remissions and exacerbations and progressive deterioration of the central nervous system. The disease shows a hereditary tendency, but its cause remains unknown. An increasingly compelling, albeit indirect, case can be made for autoimmune/viral processes in which humoral and cellular responses damage both myelin components and normal immunoregulatory effector cells, such as the suppressor T lymphocytes.[48] In the most intense forms of the disease, all nerve tissue elements may be destroyed.

INTERACTION BETWEEN MULTIPLE SCLEROSIS AND PREGNANCY

Whether a patient with multiple sclerosis should become pregnant remains controversial. If she does, how does the disease affect pregnancy and what effect does pregnancy have on the disease? The disease, or the pregnancy per se or the number of pregnancies, do not directly affect each other.[49] The use of corticosteroids during pregnancy does not adversely affect the human fetus except for a small reduction in weight.[134] Thus there is no contraindication to the use of corticosteroids to control MS, if required. The mother should rest as much as possible during the puerperium because of the greater chance that her condition may worsen during that period.[26] Obstetric indications should determine the method of delivery.

ANESTHESIA

Several authors find no correlation between the progress of MS and general anesthesia or surgery.[49–52] When indicated on their own merits, little justification arises to avoid surgery and anesthesia. Only 1 out of 88 general anesthetics in 42 patients contributed to deterioration beginning in the first postoperative month.[53] This incidence of 0.14 relapse per patient per year is less than the expected incidence of spontaneous relapses (0.27 per patient per year).

Can spinal anesthesia aggravate multiple sclerosis? Bamford and coworkers state, "We do not encourage the use of spinal anesthesia in multiple sclerosis or in any patient who has pre-existing myelopathy or neurologic disease, if there is a reasonably safe and convenient alternative. We base this opinion on a review of the medical literature, rather than on our limited experience."[37] In one of their cases, the patient developed weakness of the left leg a few weeks following spinal anesthesia at childbirth. Three years later, spinal block was given for another delivery without deterioration of her condition. They also stated that 98 patients probably received more than 1000 local anesthetics while having MS. I believe the deterioration following the first spinal block was coincidental and not caused by the block. Four patients experienced aggravation of MS symptoms in the postanesthetic month, an incidence consistent with the coincidental occurrence of relapses characteristic of the natural history of the disease. This shows that local anesthetic drugs per se do not aggravate MS. Could it be the lumbar puncture? Schapira[54] found that lumbar puncture has little effect on the course of MS. Moreover, 5 out of 250 patients with MS had been subjected to myelography. In no instance did this procedure perceptibly alter the patient's condition.[54] In my experience, the loss of sensory and especially motor function during a spinal block distresses some patients by reminding them of exacerbations of their disease. Therefore, they should be assured of the temporary nature of the spinal block.

Epidural analgesia with low concentrations of local anesthetics having only analgesic effects (0.125 to 0.25 percent bupivacaine) is the method of choice for labor and delivery. After the first edition of this book, I was delighted to learn that eminent anesthesiologists across the world share my view that patients with multiple sclerosis or other chronic neurologic diseases should not be denied regional anesthesia because scientific proof has not demonstrated that their condition deteriorates as a result of these techniques, and the fear of litigation is unfair and unfounded.[55]

General anesthesia can be used for cesarean section. However, if the mother wishes to remain awake during the operation, epidural or spinal blocks serve as alternatives, depending on the circumstances, including the preference of the anesthesiologist and the degree of limitation of the patient's ventilation.

General anesthesia procedures for either vaginal or abdominal delivery in patients with MS usually include thiopental, succinylcholine, intubation, followed by nitrous oxide and oxygen and muscle relaxants. Baskett and Armstrong[56] suspect aggravation of the disease by thiopental and methoxyflurane, an effect not seen following nitrous oxide and halothane. However, a small number of patients and a variable response to anesthesia on different occasions make it difficult to interpret their results. Siemkowicz[57] used thiopental without problems. Careful attention is necessary to prevent elevation of body temperature since exacerbations of MS symptoms occur with pyrexia. Patients receiving steroids require continuation of the therapy to prevent a relapse.

Brain Tumors

The cause and the frequency of various subtypes of intracranial tumors continue unknown.[27] The coexistence of brain tumors and pregnancy appears to be coincidental.[58] The incidence and subtypes of brain tumors in a pregnant population do not differ from those in a nonpregnant population. Seventy-five percent of intracranial tumors in women of reproductive age produce their signs and symptoms during pregnancy, probably because they enlarge. The mechanism of this enlargement can follow increase in size of the tumor cells and/or vascularity. The diagnosis of brain tumors does not differ during pregnancy. No specific guidelines exist for the management of brain tumors during pregnancy. Tumors with high mortality require immediate surgical intervention. Severe uncontrolled rise in intracranial pressure and rapid deterioration of vision that do not respond to medical therapy are some of the relative indications for termination of pregnancy after 32 weeks' gestation. Patients with benign tumor at a favorable location can have their surgery postponed until spontaneous delivery occurs or until the fetus becomes viable. Some authors recommend a 2- to 3-week delay after delivery to allow for regression of the tumor.[59] Cerebral edema caused by brain tumor during either the surgical treatment or course of pregnancy should receive aggressive treatment with corticosteroids which are relatively harmless to the fetus. Experimental data suggest that mannitol is inadvisable during pregnancy because it shifts water from the fetus to the mother. Bellur[27] has employed hypothermia and/or hyperventilation during surgery to reduce intracranial pressure with relative safety to the fetus.

Obstetric indications dictate the method of delivery. Vaginal delivery is acceptable if the medical team provides pain relief and obtunds the bearing-down reflex, thereby preventing further elevation of intracranial pressure. The fear of respiratory depression contraindicates the use of narcotics. To obtund the perineal reflex and provide adequate analgesia for forceps delivery, the alternatives include subarachnoid, lumbar epidural, caudal, and pudendal nerve block. When brain tumors increase intracranial pressure, lumbar puncture becomes dangerous; thus, subarachnoid block is contraindicated. Epidural injection of fluid can produce a significant rise in intracranial pressure due to decreased intracranial compliance.[60,61] The possibility of unintentional dural puncture and the further rise in intracranial pressure contraindicate epidural anesthesia in patients with an intracranial space-occupying lesion or increased intracranial pressure other than the benign form (discussed below). Caudal anesthesia may seem safer because the dural sac ends 5 cm from the sacral hiatus, thus the possibility of dural puncture and transmitted rise of pressure to the subarachnoid space is remote.[61,62] However, with increased CSF pressure, the subarachnoid space may extend further caudad than it does normally. This technique, therefore, requires extreme caution. Sudden injection of a drug into the caudal canal has caused apnea.[63,64] The dose should be administered in 3-ml increments over 5 to 10 min. To avoid unintentional dural puncture, a needle-cannula catheter is used to perforate the posterior sacrococcygeal ligament, and only the cannula is advanced after perforating the ligament.[61] All things considered, pudendal nerve block qualifies as the safest technique for vaginal delivery.

For cesarean section, general anesthesia with a smooth induction, maintenance, and recovery is the best anesthetic technique. Precautions should be taken to prevent further increases in intracranial pressure (e.g., hypoxia, hypercarbia, or straining). Means to lower the intracranial pressure may be necessary.

Benign Intracranial Hypertension

Benign intracranial hypertension (BIH), also called "pseudotumor cerebri," is a syndrome of elevated intracranial pressure without clinical, laboratory, or roentgenographic evidence of a focal lesion or hydrocephalus.[65] The four criteria of BIH are: elevated intracranial pressure (CSF $>$ 200 mm water), normal CSF composition, no alteration in the state of consciousness, and no focal intracranial lesion.

Treatment of BIH aims at control of the intracranial pressure to preserve the patient's vision through repeated lumbar puncture, the method of choice. In Weisberg's series,[66] 28 patients had lumbar puncture as the sole form of therapy. Most of his patients had an opening pressure of 300 mm water. Generally, up to 30 ml of fluid is withdrawn to lower the intracranial pressure to normal. CSF normally forms at a rate of 20 ml per hour. This means that 30 ml is reproduced in 90 min. Surprisingly, patients often notice improvement of symptoms for several days after a single lumbar puncture. The explanations include: production of a persistent CSF leak that closes after several days and/or the transient relief of the elevated pressure may allow compressed intracranial structures to reassume their normal shapes.

In some patients with BIH, repeated lumbar puncture fails to control the increased intracranial pressure. In these refractory cases, a course of steroids for a week often results in clinical improvement, presumably because of reduction of brain swelling. Acetazolamide (Diamox), a carbonic anhydrase inhibitor, reduces CSF production. This drug may serve in some cases either as an alternative to or in combination with steroids. Only lack of success of medical treatment accompanied by rapidly failing vision call for surgery to create a shunt between the CSF compartment and the peritoneal cavity. Lumboperitoneal shunt represents the most common operation because the small ventricles render ventricular shunts difficult to perform.

With pregnancy, the symptoms of increased intracranial pressure, mainly headaches and visual deterioration, worsen in 50 percent of the cases and invariably resolve after abortion or delivery.[67] Therefore, a woman with active disease should be advised to delay pregnancy until all signs and symptoms have abated. Worsening of the condition during pregnancy rarely requires termination of pregnancy, provided the patient receives adequate therapy. Vaginal delivery may proceed, despite pressure elevation during uterine contractions.

A lumbar puncture is unsafe for a patient with increased intracranial tension caused by a space-occupying lesion. A sudden decrease in CSF pressure due to lumbar puncture may cause considerable herniation of the cerebellar tonsils, leading to pressure on the medulla oblongata. With BIH, the brain tissue as a whole swells. Such a uniform swelling and the natural position of the cerebellar tonsils prevent herniation and compression of the brain stem. Thus, lumbar puncture in these patients is safe, and spinal anesthesia is the method of choice for cesarean section.[68] One of the main objections to spinal anesthesia, namely post – lumbar puncture headache, has no relevance in this case, as the leakage of CSF benefits the patient. Epidural analgesia, of course, provides an alternative to spinal block in a patient with BIH, and it has been used.[69]

For a patient with lumboperitoneal shunt, general anesthesia is preferable to spinal analgesia for two reasons. Before a spinal block, a roentgenogram is required to localize the site of entry and position of the lumboperitoneal tube in the subarachnoid space. General anesthesia avoids this necessity and the associated risk of fetal exposure to irradiation. Second, with spinal analgesia, the local anesthetic injected into the subarachnoid space may partially escape into the peritoneal cavity through the shunt, leading to inadequate anesthesia.

Epilepsy

The prevalence (the number of cases occurring at any one time) of epilepsy in the general population is 0.5 percent or one in two hundred.[26] Idiopathic or primary epilepsy is the most common type. Epilepsy may occur at any age; however, 75 percent of those afflicted present before the age of twenty. Thirty percent of epilepsy patients have a positive family history.

DRUG THERAPY

Bromide, introduced in the last century, was the first drug used to treat epilepsy. Phenobarbital was introduced in 1912, and phenytoin, in 1938. The number of anticonvulsants has increased during the last decade; over 20 preparations are now in use. The drugs most commonly employed include phenobarbital, phenytoin, and primidone or a combination thereof. Side effects, usually dose dependent, relate to intolerance, and appear especially with long-term therapy. They include blood dyscrasias, cutaneous manifestations (dermatitis or hirsutism), osteomalacia, and gingivitis.

Metabolism of the common anticonvulsants occurs mainly in the liver through parahydroxylation, with only about 10 percent of the drugs being excreted unchanged in the bile. Since parahydroxylation represents an important pathway for many other drugs, significant interactions may result. In the presence of hepatic dysfunction due to liver disease or reduced hepatic flow, metabolism of these drugs is compromised and a relative overdose occurs, manifested by drowsiness and dizziness progressing to diplopia, dysarthria, ataxia, or nystagmus and, ultimately, confusion and coma. If these symptoms are not recognized in advance, general anesthesia may confuse the picture, especially if complicated by hypoxia, hypotension, or hypocarbia leading to prolonged unconsciousness.[70]

Effects on the metabolic degradation pathway include enzyme induction and inhibition, and protein binding. In enzyme induction, long-term administration of certain drugs like phenobarbital can induce an increase in the microsomal enzyme activity concerned with their own metabolism (augmented hepatic hydroxylation) as well as the metabolism of other drugs that share the same enzyme pathway, such as phenytoin, digoxin, and certain anticoagulants. The simultaneous administration of phenobarbital can lead to increased breakdown of these drugs, with a consequent fall in their plasma concentration. Conversely, following phenobarbital withdrawal during treatment with any of the above drugs, enzyme stimulation ceases and the plasma concentration of the drug rises, possibly to toxic levels.

Phenobarbital-enzyme induction speeds metabolism of methoxyflurane,[71] halothane, and fluroxene,[72] producing increased fluoride levels in the liver and kidney, and possibly leading to an increased likelihood of hepatic and renal toxicity.

In enzyme inhibition, certain drugs may compete with phenytoin for a common metabolic degradation pathway; this may result in a rise in plasma phenytoin levels. Such drugs include chlorpromazine, diazepam, chlordiazepoxide, chloramphenicol, isoniazid, and aminosalicylic acid.

Interactions may also result when drugs compete for protein binding sites in the plasma. For example, salicylic acid can raise phenytoin plasma levels by displacing it from the plasma proteins. Metabolic interaction may also occur between nondepolarizing relaxants and phenytoin. Phenytoin, acting on the prejunctional membrane, has an additive effect to the neuromuscular blocking property of d-tubocurarine.[73]

TYPES OF EPILEPSY

True Gestational Epilepsy

In this rare condition, a grand mal seizure occurs only during pregnancy. It is usually limited to one pregnancy, rarely recurring during subsequent ones. It may happen anytime during pregnancy, labor, or the puerperium. The EEG may be normal.

Idiopathic Epilepsy

This is the most common form of epilepsy (75 percent). The frequency of seizures during pregnancy increases in 45 percent of patients, remains unchanged in 50 percent, and decreases in 5 percent. Following pregnancy, the frequency of seizures usually reverts to the pregestational pattern. Idiopathic epilepsy may occur for the first time during pregnancy and continue thereafter.

Symptomatic Epilepsy

This form may follow a localized brain lesion such as a brain tumor, meningitis, or brain injury. The course of the disease during pregnancy resembles that of the idiopathic type.

Status Epilepticus

This condition will be discussed later in more detail because of its seriousness and the role of the anesthesiologist in its management.

EFFECT OF EPILEPSY ON PREGNANCY

Since both pregnancy and epilepsy are common (63 percent of epileptic women experience their first convulsion between the ages of 11 and 35 years), the occasional coincidental occurrence of the first seizure during pregnancy is not surprising. Obstetric complications happen more frequently to epileptic than to nonepileptic patients.[74] For example, toxemia and vaginal hemorrhage develop more often in epileptic patients. Parturients with epilepsy have a higher incidence of premature rupture of membranes, premature labor, cesarean sections, and fetal anomalies. Prematurity, intrauterine growth retardation, surgical intervention, and congenital malformations account for the higher perinatal mortality rates in epilepsy. Therefore, these women should be considered a high-risk group who need special attention during pregnancy and special care during labor.[75] Epilepsy per se does not necessitate the termination of pregnancy. Even status epilepticus, in contrast to eclampsia, does not indicate pregnancy termination. Modern therapeutic regimens usually achieve seizure control, the paramount objective. Pregnancy may then be allowed to continue to term with careful anticonvulsant therapy and good supervision.

EFFECT OF PREGNANCY ON EPILEPSY

The course of epilepsy during pregnancy varies. Patients with a high frequency of convulsions in the pregestational state (one or more per month) often have an increased number when pregnant. In subsequent pregnancies, no specific pattern of epilepsy ensues. Many factors can ameliorate or exaggerate the epileptic condition during pregnancy. Moreover, fluctuations in the frequency of clinical attacks characterize epilepsy itself. Thus, if epileptic patients were studied during a randomly selected 9-month period, a certain proportion would experience more convulsions, some less, and others would show no change. The reasons for the unpredictability of the course of epilepsy during pregnancy are discussed below.

Anticonvulsant Therapy

Anticonvulsant drug use may vary during pregnancy. For example, the patient may be more diligent in the regular use of the drug. Her physician may also deliberately attempt to control her seizures more energetically. On the other hand, the patient or her doctor may reduce therapy in order to lessen the risk of teratogenicity. Vomiting in early pregnancy, delayed absorption due to gastrointestinal stasis, a change in gastric pH, increased clearance by the liver, and the dilutional effect of weight gain and extracellular fluid expansion may all work against achieving adequate levels of anticonvulsant. On the whole, plasma concentration of epileptic drugs falls during pregnancy and increases during the puerperium.[76] If the patient has been compliant with her medication and seizure activity does not increase, this decrease in anticonvulsant drug levels should not worry the treating physician, and an increase in dosage of the anticonvulsant drugs is not warranted.[27]

Water Retention During Pregnancy

This may cause some brain edema, lowering the brain's threshold to seizure. Water loading followed by pitressin produces seizures in about one third of nonpregnant patients with EEG dysrhythmia.[77] Fluid retention causes over one third of the weight gain during pregnancy. Moreover, some investigators have shown rapid and excessive weight gain preceding more frequent convulsions. The same mechanism may underlie so-called menstrual epilepsy. Rapid gains in weight should certainly be discouraged. Water retention can dilute serum electrolytes (sodium, potassium, calcium, and magnesium), precipitating seizures in nonpregnant dysrhythmic persons.[78]

Alkalosis

Respiratory alkalosis produced by hyperventilation regularly accentuates dysrhythmia during EEG recording and may provoke actual seizure. During pregnancy, alveolar carbon dioxide tension decreases and, although compensation is usually adequate, concurrent vomiting may contribute to the production of true alkalosis. Pain during labor and delivery may produce both vomiting and hyperventilation. Such an increase in pH may provoke an epileptic seizure.

Strong Emotional Stress

This occasionally precipitates convulsions. Pregnancy, labor, or the puerperium may each provide opportunity for emotional factors to influence epilepsy.

Summary

Multiple factors, both beneficial and adverse, and mostly unpredictable, will dictate the course of epilepsy during pregnancy. Severe epilepsy is likely to be adversely affected. Rapid gain in weight may herald an increased frequency of seizures. The unpredictable factors include the usual fluctuation of epilepsy itself, the patient's attitude to anticonvulsant therapy, and the metabolic and hormonal changes of pregnancy. This composite adequately explains the variation of response among individuals and in successive pregnancies in the same patient. On the whole, gestation proves more harmful than beneficial to epileptic women. Thus, the majority of reported series shows that the number of epileptics having more seizures during pregnancy exceeds those having fewer seizures.

EFFECTS ON FETUS AND NEWBORN

Epileptic patients under treatment have infants with a higher incidence of congenital anomalies, especially cleft lip, palate, or both, congenital heart disease, malformations of the urogenital tract, and spina bifida.[78] The 4.5 percent[75] incidence exceeds that of nonepileptic patients by 4 to 10 times.[79] Antiepileptic drugs, especially valproic acid,[78] seem to have a teratogenic effect, because the incidence of congenital malformations increases twofold in treated epileptics compared with those not on medication. However, the slight teratogenic properties of anticonvulsant drugs must be accepted in view of the far graver consequences of status epilepticus affecting both mother and fetus, which may occur upon indiscriminate withdrawal of therapy.[80,81]

Anticonvulsants freely cross the placenta. One must closely observe the neonate for withdrawal symptoms consisting of irritability; occasional seizures may ensue. Special cases may require 3 to 5 mg per kg per 24 hours of phenobarbital. Anticonvulsant drugs depress vitamin K–dependent clotting factors. Thus neonates of anticonvulsant-treated mothers should routinely receive vitamin K. For these reasons, all infants born to mothers with epilepsy require close observation in an intensive care nursery for at least 24 hours.[82]

MANAGEMENT DURING PREGNANCY

The epileptic gravida must have monthly antepartum visits, should continue adequate drug therapy, and should receive folic acid to reduce drug toxicity.[79] Any woman who experiences epilepsy for the first time during pregnancy needs a thorough evaluation to exclude an underlying focal disease, which appears as a common cause.[79] Withhold anticonvulsants in such patients unless a second seizure occurs, since cases of true gestational epilepsy usually involve a single seizure and recurrences are uncommon in subsequent pregnancies.

ANESTHESIA AND ANALGESIA

On admission to the labor and delivery suite, the epileptic patient's chart should be clearly identified. The anesthesiologist and nursing staff should know the anticonvulsant drugs used and their dosage as early as possible following admission. This prevents confusion and possibly dangerous treatment which could occur when a patient with unknown history convulses during labor or delivery. It also identifies the presence of enzyme-inducing drugs which modify the therapeutic and toxic effects of anesthetic drugs.

Local Anesthesia

Epileptic patients do not have a greater susceptibility to local anesthetics than normal individuals.[83] Lidocaine has even been successfully used to terminate seizures during status epilepticus.[84] Therefore, local anesthetic techniques such as epidural or spinal should not be denied to epileptic patients.[85] As in any patient, avoid intravascular injection of local anesthetic drugs or a gross overdose.

General Anesthesia

Avoid anesthetic drugs which have convulsive potential such as enflurane,[70] ketamine, methohexital, and Althesin. Thiopental induction followed by succinylcholine and nitrous oxide and oxygen maintenance supplemented by a muscle relaxant can be used. Avoid hypoxia and marked variation in $PaCO_2$ levels. Halothane or a narcotic-diazepam combination may supplement nitrous oxide to reduce maternal awareness or allow an increase of the FIO_2. For example nitrous oxide and oxygen, 1:2, plus a muscle relaxant can be used until after delivery, when morphine, 0.2 mg per kg, and diazepam, 0.1 mg per kg, are injected intravenously.[86] Diazepam is an antiepileptic drug.[87] Morphine, like most opioids, has a convulsant effect only at dose levels far above those mentioned here, more than 100 times the usual analgesic dosage.[88] Therefore, the supplementary use of a diazepam-morphine mixture as described above produces an anticonvulsing rather than a convulsing effect.

STATUS EPILEPTICUS

Status epilepticus, a continuous seizure lasting at least 30 min, threatens the life of both mother and fetus. Because of the seriousness of the situation, the patients require special attention to management, monitoring, and treatment. A central venous line and an arterial line facilitate management. Blood samples serve to determine the anticonvulsant levels, glucose, blood urea nitrogen, creatinine, electrolytes and CBC, blood gases, and acid-base status.[27] The patient receives continuous monitoring for respiration, heart rate, arterial blood pressure, and electrocardiogram. Continuous EEG may be used. Depending on the gestational age, the FHR is also continuously recorded.

Treatment basically consists of correcting any underlying precipitating factor and stopping the convulsions. Diazepam and phenytoin represent the drugs employed most commonly to stop the convulsions. Intravenous diazepam stops convulsions within 3 to 5 min in 80 percent of the patients. However, since diazepam redistributes quickly and widely to various tissues and organs, seizures may recur in 10 to 20 min after the cessation of diazepam administration. Phenytoin given simultaneously in another line prevents such a recurrence. The anticonvulsant effects of phenytoin become evident 10 to 20 min after the start of infusion. Infuse diazepam no faster than 2 mg per min until seizures stop or until a total dose of 20 mg has been administered. Infuse phenytoin at a rate of 50 mg per min to a total dose of 18 mg per kg body weight.[89] If seizures persist, aggressive treatment consists of continuous administration of intravenous phenobarbital or diazepam and controlled respiration after intubation. Continuous intravenous phenobarbital usually requires a dose of 50 mg per min with a maximum of 100 mg per min until seizures stop or a total dose of 20 mg per kg body weight. Continuous intravenous diazepam consists of the infusion of 50 to 100 mg diluted in 500 ml of 5-percent dextrose solution and run at a rate of 40 ml per hour. This ensures a serum diazepam level of 0.2 to 0.4 μg per ml. If such a regimen fails, general anesthesia with a nondepolarizing muscle relaxant may be used.[89] All these CNS depressant drugs abolish fetal beat-to-beat variability which returns belatedly after cessation of administration of these drugs.

Hydrocephalus

Increased sophistication in the techniques and methods of cerebrospinal fluid diversion has improved the prognosis for persons with hydrocephalus of nonneoplastic origin. The most common techniques used involve extracranial shunting such as ventriculoatrial and ventriculoperitoneal shunts. Extracranial shunting catheters utilize a valve system, usually allowing the drainage of cerebrospinal fluid at a pressure between 60 and 80 mm water.[90] During pregnancy and particularly during labor, intra-abdominal pressure increases and may cause temporary impedance of CSF flow in patients with ventriculoperitoneal shunts. This transitory impedance usually does not pose a serious hazard. Adequate analgesia and avoidance of excessive Valsalva maneuvers can minimize increases in intra-abdominal and intracranial pressure. Monfared and coworkers[90] recommend shortening the second stage of labor by using low forceps delivery under epidural analgesia. Continuous epidural block appears ideal for providing analgesia for both stages of labor; however, narcotic analgesia for the first stage and pudendal nerve block for the second stage can prove satisfactory.[90]

A functional extracranial shunt system connected to cerebral ventricles does not contraindicate spinal anesthesia and nearly eliminates the risk of "coning" and tentorial herniation. As in patients with valvular heart disease, prophylactic antibiotic therapy seems appropriate in view of the possible bacteremia associated with parturition. The mere presence of an extracranial shunt does not necessitate cesarean section. Abdominal delivery carries the additional risk of intra-abdominal sepsis which should be avoided, particularly in women with ventriculoperitoneal shunts.

Muscular Dystrophy

Muscular dystrophy is an inherited disorder of the muscle characterized by progressive loss of its functions, resulting in weakness.[91] These disorders are of seven major categories:

1. Severe X-linked recessive (Duchenne) progressive muscular dystrophy (PMD)
2. Milder X-linked recessive (Becker variety)
3. Limb-girdle muscular dystrophy
4. Fascioscapulohumeral dystrophy
5. Ocular and oculopharyngeal dystrophy
6. Distal muscular dystrophy
7. Myotonia atrophica (to be discussed separately)

Most types, especially Duchenne PMD, are sex-linked to males, but some females clinically manifest muscular dystrophy in their child-bearing years.

Patients with muscular dystrophy have weak

muscles, with atrophy and pseudohypertrophy due to infiltration by fatty and fibrous tissues. Contractures occur, leading to deformities including scoliosis, kyphosis, lordosis, or contractions. Their fragile bones can fracture easily in advanced cases and require gentle handling. Myocardial myopathy may be present but can be masked by the limited activities caused by the skeletal myopathy.[92-94] However, the cardiac involvement can be so serious as to lead to cardiac arrest during or after anesthesia. Respiratory muscles progressively weaken during the course of the disease. Respiratory failure commonly causes death. Respiratory failure for no apparent reason may occur after an uneventful anesthetic recovery. Those patients with advanced disease may have difficulty in swallowing. Patients can aspirate accumulated secretions, and this, combined with weak muscles for coughing, leads to pneumonitis. Because of the progressive destruction of muscle fibers, certain serum enzymes such as aldolase, creatinine phosphokinase (CPK), and serum glutamic oxaloacetic transaminase (SGOT) rise. The administration of succinylcholine leads to excessive elevation of these enzymes, hyperkalemia, and elevation of the body temperature. This mimics malignant hyperpyrexia (MH). Although some of these patients are susceptible to MH, such a clinical picture does not always indicate the development of MH. The diagnosis of MH susceptibility should include a muscle biopsy and in vitro contracture studies.[93] Muscular dystrophy contraindicates both halothane and succinylcholine because either may precipitate cardiac problems or MH. Keep dantrolene readily available in case a need for general anesthesia arises. Titrate the anesthetics and narcotics to meet these patients' needs because of the weakness of their respiratory muscles. Postoperative ventilatory support may prove necessary. The above problems demand careful attention to the airway during and after anesthesia, as does the delayed gestric emptying due to the hypomotility of the gastrointestinal tract. Place a nasogastric tube and evacuate the stomach contents, preferably prior to general anesthesia.[93] Where possible, use regional anesthesia or analgesia for vaginal delivery or cesarean section. For limited respiratory capacity, epidural anesthesia represents a better choice than spinal anesthesia.

Myotonia

The myotonic syndromes consist of a group of autosomal-dominant diseases that primarily affect skeletal muscles. Myotonia, characterized by difficulty in initiating a movement followed by delayed relaxation, represents a common feature of these syndromes. The myotonia is usually most severe following rest, and decreases with exercise. These syndromes have a characteristic electromyographic pattern.[95]

MYOTONIA CONGENITA (THOMSEN'S DISEASE)

Myotonia congenita includes myotonia and sometimes pseudohypertrophy of specific voluntary muscles such as the glutei and calf muscles. Dystrophic changes do not occur and, in the classic case, smooth and cardiac muscle are spared. Though it is usually considered to be an autosomal-dominant disease, recently an autosomal-recessive form has been described.[96] The disease appears in childhood, usually at 6 to 8 years of age. Usually it does not progress in severity nor decrease life expectancy. Quinine has been used for treatment, but procainamide, 250 to 500 mg orally 3 times per day, qualifies as the drug of choice. Pregnancy may aggravate the myotonia, especially in the latter half of the gestational period, and improvement occurs after delivery.[18]

PARAMYOTONIA CONGENITA

Paramyotonia congenita represents the rarest of the myotonic syndromes with symptoms and signs identical to those of myotonia congenita but initiated by exposure to cold.

MYOTONIA ATROPHICA (MYOTONIA DYSTROPHICA; STEINERT'S DISEASE)

This most severe and most common form of myotonia is an autosomal-dominant, multisystem disease. It usually appears later in life than myotonia congenita. Associated wasting of skeletal muscles, involvement of the cardiac and smooth muscles, endocrine dysfunction, and disturbances of other organ systems characterize myotonia atrophica. During the course of the disease, the patient may suffer from recurrent attacks of pulmonary infections, resulting from difficulty in swallowing, aspiration, and weak respiratory muscles. Death usually occurs in about the sixth decade of life owing to bulbar involvement, cardiac failure, or aspiration pneumonitis. Ovarian insufficiency associated with this disease leads to amenorrhea, infertility, and a high incidence of early abortion in those who become pregnant. Involvement of the adrenal glands may produce adrenocortical insufficiency.

Myotonia may influence the course of labor and increase the anesthetic risk. The following discussion applies mainly to myotonia atrophica.

Effect of Pregnancy

The symptoms may worsen during pregnancy or remain unchanged, but they do not improve. The increase in weakness relates to the effect of progesterone on the muscle membrane potential and on the intracellular-to-extracellular potassium ratio.[97]

Effect on Parturition

With myotonia atrophica, hydramnios frequently accompanies pregnancy, probably due to inability of the fetus to swallow.[98] The major reported obstetric complications of myotonia atrophica include threatened, spontaneous, and habitual abortion.[18] Premature labor may occur because of hydramnios or uterine myotonia. Researchers[99] describe a prolonged first stage of labor as a consistent complication. Evidence does not justify this conclusion, for some patients have a shorter course than normal, and others respond favorably to oxytocin stimulation or rupture of membranes.[100] Muscle weakness may prolong the second stage, and forceps may be needed to assist delivery.

Effect on the Fetus and Neonate

A high rate of fetal loss follows spontaneous abortion, prematurity, and neonatal involvement with the disease. Ultrasonographic features of pregnancies with affected fetuses include hydramnios and decreased fetal movement, breathing motion, and swallowing.[101] Although many neonates with myotonic dystrophy remain asymptomatic, severely affected newborns have a recognizable disorder unrelated to the extent of the maternal disease. Arthrogryposis involving predominantly the lower extremities, generalized hypotonia and weakness, and impaired swallowing and sucking reflexes comprise the most common neonatal manifestations.[100] Less frequent features include facial diplegia, diaphragmatic paralysis, respiratory failure, congenital cataracts, and electrocardiographic abnormalities. Aspiration pneumonitis most commonly causes their demise.

Anesthesia

Preanesthetic Evaluation. The patient should undergo pulmonary function tests. Physiotherapy should be started during pregnancy to minimize pulmonary complications. Some patients with myotonia atrophica have arrhythmias and various degrees of heart block secondary to myocardial involvement, which necessitates electrocardiography. The anesthesiologist should review the medications used for the treatment of the disease. For example, quinine therapy potentiates d-tubocurarine. Some of the patients may be taking steroids, which should be increased or at least continued to cope with the stress of labor and delivery. Endocrine dysfunction is tested by glucose tolerance test and protein-bound iodine determination; creatinine phosphokinase, which often rises, should be assayed.

General Anesthesia. Myotonic patients are highly susceptible to the development of apnea in response to thiopental,[102] but the duration of action of the drug remains unchanged.[103] Apnea also occurs with other CNS depressants, such as narcotics, diazepam, and halothane.[104] Therefore, use these drugs cautiously and assist or control respiration when necessary.

Do not use succinylcholine in myotonic patients for, after its administration, a contracture proportional to dose develops.[49,104,105] Succinylcholine does not cause fasciculations, but generalized contracture associated with apnea and difficulty in maintaining the airway and ventilating the patient may occur.[106]

The patient with myotonia responds normally to d-tubocurarine, which has been used safely in such patients.[104,107] In patients receiving quinine, the dose of d-tubocurarine should be reduced by one third. Although Kauffman[108] advocates avoiding neostigmine, suggesting that it precipitates myotonic crisis (generalized contracture) by reversing nondepolarizing muscle relaxants, Mitchell and associates[104] used neostigmine safely in myotonic patients and noted a normal response to the drug. Therefore, the action of nondepolarizing drugs is terminated either by administering neostigmine or by artificially ventilating the patient until elimination of the muscle relaxant occurs. Atracurium has been successfully used in a patient with myotonia atrophica.[109] The rapid breakdown of atracurium by "Hofmann" elimination leads to a predictable recovery and eliminates the need for neostigmine.

Volatile anesthetics have minimal effect on myotonia; however, marked shivering should be avoided because it may precipitate a generalized contracture.[105] The low incidence of shivering qualifies enflurane as a suitable anesthetic.[109] The operating room should be warm to help maintain normal body temperature.

In any patient with myotonia, a contracture may be elicited in a skeletal muscle group by voluntary contraction, mechanical stimulation, electrical stimulation of the nerve or muscle, or chemical stimulation by agonist drugs such as acetylcholine or succinylcholine. Once contracture develops, spinal anesthesia, any other regional block technique, or the use of nondepolarizing muscle relaxants cannot terminate it. Therefore, the initiation of generalized contracture must be avoided during anesthesia. Retraction during surgery can elicit localized contracture. Only infiltration of the muscle with a local anesthetic can remedy this. Acute myotonic crisis characterized by generalized contracture during or after anesthesia rarely occurs. Intravenous quinidine (300 to 600 mg) and larger doses of steroids (1 g or more) can counter such a crisis.[108] Dentrolene decreases intracellular calcium ion activity and has successfully treated malignant hyperthermia. It may be of value in terminating a myotonic crisis. Because of the associated cardiomyopathy, cardiac depressants should be avoided in myotonia atrophica. With myotonia atrophica, delayed gastric emptying and weak intestinal motility predispose the patient to aspiration pneumonitis.[110] She may require preoperative cimetidine and metoclopramide plus proper cricoid pressure to minimize the risk of aspiration.

Although myotonia atrophica is one of the degenerative muscle diseases that have been associated with the development of malignant hyperpyrexia, data currently fail to prove a definite relationship between the two diseases.[19]

Regional Anesthesia. The problems associated with the administration of general anesthesia in myotonic patients make regional anesthesia the method of choice when feasible.[111] Spinal or epidural blocks can provide analgesia for either vaginal delivery or cesarean section. Significantly compromised respiratory capacity contraindicates spinal anesthesia for cesarean section. A high incidence of shivering, which may precipitate generalized contracture, represents a theoretical disadvantage to epidural analgesia. In my experience, epidural analgesia is a safe technique if the patient is kept warm. Pudendal nerve block offers an alternative to intravertebral blocks for vaginal delivery.

Postpartum Care

The neonate may have difficulty breathing, so personnel and equipment for neonatal resuscitation should be present at the delivery. Physiotherapy of the mother should continue postpartum to prevent atelectasis.

Local analgesia can be used for postpartum tubal ligation. Wheeler and James[112] reported the safety of using local analgesia for laparoscopic tubal ligation in a patient with myotonia atrophica. Intravenous fentanyl provided analgesia, while skin, fascia, and peritoneum were infiltrated with 0.5-percent bupivacaine. To provide analgesia for subsequent cauterization, 5 ml of 0.5-percent bupivacaine were dripped on each fallopian tube. These investigators encountered no problems during or after surgery.

Myasthenia Gravis

Thomas Willis first described myasthenia gravis (MG) in 1672.[2] The condition appears twice as often in females and has an overall incidence of 1 in 15,000 to 1 in 40,000. MG usually first occurs at about 20 years of age.[113] It rarely develops in more than one member of a family. Genetic and environmental factors, although not definitely related to the etiology, may play a role.[113] It most frequently affects the oculomotor, facial, laryngeal, and respiratory muscles.

Partial recovery follows rest and the administration of anticholinesterase drugs.

PATHOGENESIS

The motor end-plates are abnormally thin and unbranched. The surface area of the nerve terminal diminishes by 30 to 40 percent, the width of the synaptic clefts increases, the postsynaptic folds become shallower, and their number declines. The proposition that MG represents an autoimmune disease originates from indirect evidence, such as the high incidence of thymic abnormalities, remissions after thymectomy, and association of autoimmune diseases with myasthenic patients. However, the presence of receptor antibody in the serum of 87 percent of MG patients serves as direct evidence.[114] This antibody blocks the receptor sites and accelerates their degradation, thus reducing the available acetylcholine receptors by 70 to 89 percent.[115] An experimental model of MG has been developed in rats by injecting a certain amount of a specific neuromuscular blocking agent, α-cobra toxin.[116] This permanently blocks a certain number of receptors. The animal model reproduces all the typical features of human MG. The weakened animals show decremental responses on repetitive nerve stimulation, sensitivity to curare, improvement with anticholinesterase agents, the certain posttetanic changes considered particularly characteristic of MG. These findings support the hypothesis that a decrease of available acetylcholine receptors per se can account for the clinical and physiologic defects of myasthenia gravis. Another animal model was produced by immunizing rabbits with acetylcholine receptors from electric eels.

Recently, cells that resemble muscle cells (called "myoid cells") have been found in the thymus gland. Tissue cultures produce cells that act like muscle and have acetylcholine receptors which interact with receptor antibody.[115] The high association of thymus gland abnormalities with MG and the discovery of these cells point to the gland as the source of the autoimmune response of the disease. What initiates the response, however, remains unclear, but infection by an unknown virus is a probable cause.[2]

Simpson has recently speculated that the normal thymus may play a role in promoting regeneration of acetylcholine receptors.[117] Thus, isolation of this specific factor could lead to an ultimate cure for MG.

EFFECT OF PREGNANCY

Pregnancy may influence the course of the disease; conversely, the disease and drug therapy may affect labor, delivery, and the newborn.[118] Improvement of the myasthenic condition usually follows spontaneous abortion, but induced abortion does not alter the course of the disease. Hence, exacerbation of symptoms does not call for termination of pregnancy.[113] The course of MG during a previous pregnancy may differ from that in future pregnancies.

Whether pregnant or not, a myasthenic patient may present with marked muscle weakness and respiratory insufficiency, which can be due to myasthenia or overtreatment (cholinergic crisis). The latter produces nausea, abdominal cramps, diarrhea, excessive salivation, miosis, and bradycardia. However, differentiation between a myasthenic and a cholinergic crisis may be difficult. Edrophonium helps. First, vital capacity, grip strength, and the presence of ptosis objectively assess the patient's strength. Muscle strength is reassessed 30 to 90 sec after an intravenous test dose of 2- to 10-mg edrophonium. Keeping the dose of edrophonium on the low side prevents severe bradycardia.[119,120] Equivocal results with edrophonium call for a placebo injection of saline. Since the effect of edrophonium dissipates rapidly, the test can be repeated in 10 minutes. In inadequately medicated patients, muscle strength improves dramatically. In overmedicated patients, muscle strength does not change or may deteriorate. The edrophonium test has replaced the neostigmine and curare tests in the diagnosis of MG. Anticholinesterases improve the muscle strength to a certain extent, but further increases in medication only intensify the weakness.[121]

The use of anticholinesterase drugs in MG carries a theoretic risk of increasing uterine tone and inducing abortion. Nevertheless, anticholinesterases have not been implicated as harmful to the course of pregnancy. Despite its sensitivity to acetylcholine, neostigmine (and other anticholinesterases) have little effect on the uterus,[113] probably because the uterus does not continuously release acetylcholine. The administration of anticholinesterase will not significantly increase the acetylcholine level in this organ. However, since spontaneous abortion tends to occur in MG and since edrophonium may have a direct effect on cholinergic receptor sites, the edrophonium test should be applied with small doses and only when absolutely necessary during the early months of pregnancy.

Emotional stress or infection may precipitate a myasthenic crisis. Antibiotics require careful selection since many — neomycin, streptomycin, gentamicin, kanamycin, polymixin, colistin, tetracycline, lincomycin, penicillin V, and erythromycin among others — have muscle-relaxing properties. The only antibiotics devoid of neuromuscular blocking properties are penicillin G, cephradine, and cephaloridine.[122]

LABOR AND DELIVERY

Myasthenia gravis neither affects the course of labor nor necessitates delivery by cesarean section. Outlet forceps frequently serve to shorten the second stage of labor, thereby minimizing muscle fatigue associated with expulsive efforts.[121] Cesarean section should proceed according to usual obstetric indications. The combination of MG and pregnancy carries a high maternal and fetal mortality[74] because of prolonged labor, especially in the second stage,[51] postpartum pulmonary complications caused by respiratory muscle weakness, the need for obstetric intervention, the danger of anesthesia, and the possibility of neonatal MG.

The patient should not receive magnesium sulfate, as it increases muscle weakness by decreasing acetylcholine release from the motor nerve terminal and by reducing the excitability of the postjunctional membrane.[122]

Anticholinesterase therapy must continue during labor. Maximum effect of an oral dose peaks at 1 hour. Neostigmine remains active for 2 to 3 hours after an oral dose, while pyridostigmine's effects persist for 3 to 4 hours. Because of the unreliable gastric uptake of all drugs during parturition, intramuscular equivalents should supplant oral administration at the onset of labor (Table 8–2).

Table 8–2. DOSES OF COMMONLY USED ANTICHOLINESTERASES

Drug	IV Dose (mg)	IM Dose (mg)	Oral Dose (mg)
Neostigmine (Prostigmin)	0.25–0.75	0.5–1.5	10–20
Pyridostigmine (Mestinon)	1–3	3–5	50–70

THE POSTPARTUM PERIOD

The first 10 days postpartum may be especially hazardous. Plauche[123] reported that symptoms worsened in 57 percent of patients and 2.4 percent died of myasthenic crisis during the puerperium. The patient should resume her normal oral medication as soon as possible, and her disease status should be monitored carefully for 10 days, preferably in the hospital. It remains unclear whether breast feeding exacerbates symptoms. Anticholinesterase therapy does not contraindicate breast feeding, for these drugs do not enter breast milk in detectable amounts. However, mother and/or physician may opt for bottle feeding if breast feeding interferes with the mother's rest.

FETAL AND NEONATAL EFFECTS

Maternal MG may adversely affect the offspring by producing congenital or neonatal MG. Congenital MG may also appear at birth in the newborns of normal mothers,[124] its course is similar to that observed in adults. Neonatal MG emerges transiently in 20 to 30 percent of babies born to mothers with MG, usually presenting any time within the first 24 hours after delivery, although the latent period may extend up to 3 days. Drachman[125] recently attributed the cause to the transplacental transfer of the small-molecular-weight immunoglobulin G that includes antibody to the receptor substance. This hypothesis has merit, for antibodies to acetylcholine receptor have been detected in a myasthenic mother and her clinically affected newborn twins.[119] The neonate has an expressionless face and a weak cry. Sucking, swallowing, and breathing may be impaired. Inadequate respiratory efforts call for intubating and ventilating the newborn before conducting diagnostic tests. Rapid clinical improvement following 0.5 to 1 mg of intramuscular edrophonium may confirm neonatal myasthenia.

Infants born of myasthenic mothers who show evidence of transient MG usually recover in a few weeks. They require anticholinesterase therapy for about 21 days (maximum 47 days). One case of neonatal MG resolved completely after an exchange transfusion for hyperbilirubinemia on the second day of life.[126] In one reported case, a baby manifesting neonatal MG developed MG at the age of 2 years.[127]

During delivery, the anesthesiologist must anticipate resuscitation of the newborn delivered of a myasthenic mother. Anesthesiologists can meet the task only if they have prepared themselves well ahead for these responsibilities.

ANESTHETIC CONSIDERATIONS

Preanesthetic Assessment

Preanesthetic assessment of neuromuscular diseases in general does apply to MG. In addition to determining the degree of functional derangement of locomotion, pulmonary ventilation, and cardiac function, the anesthesiologist should strive to predict the likelihood of anesthesia-induced complications.[20] Personal and family histories of anesthetic exposure and reaction are important. The patient should undergo a normal clinical evaluation. Electrocardiography will help to determine cardiomyopathy and susceptibility of the patient to arrhythmias. Blood chemistry should include electrolytes and determination of creatinine phosphokinase, aldolase, lactic dehydrogenase, and transaminase levels, all of which may increase in muscle disease. Elevated serum enzymes indicate active muscle breakdown. Chest roentgenography detects cardiomegaly and pulmonary changes such as infiltration. Pulmonary function tests, such as spirometry and peak expiratory flow rate, may help to determine the degree of restrictive respiratory inadequacy. In patients with restricted ventilation, baseline arterial blood gases should be determined. Electromyography and nerve conduction studies indicate whether the disease is neurologic or primarily muscular, and myotonic conditions can be specifically identified. Muscle biopsy helps to provide a definite diagnosis and prognosis and may indicate the severity of the disease. In patients possibly susceptible to malignant hyperpyrexia, muscle testing in vitro can confirm and give some indication of overall and specific drug sensitivity. Although dantrolene is safe to use in MG, such patients require careful monitoring because of possible decreases in their respiratory functions 1 to 3 hours after administration of the drug.[128]

More specific to MG, the anesthesiologist should evaluate the patient's condition and obtain information regarding drug therapy. Respiratory function tests and ECG should be performed because MG may produce focal necrosis of the myocardium, as evidenced by alterations in the T wave and ST segment. Myasthenia gravis may also be associated with hyperthyroidism; therefore, any clinical suspicion of thyroid dysfunction calls for thyroid function studies. Approximately 75 percent of patients with MG have thymic abnormalities of which 85 percent show hyperplasia; the remaining 15 percent have gross or microscopic thymomas. Thymemectomy relieves the myasthenic symptoms in 40 percent of cases.

Bronchogenic carcinoma, especially small-cell carcinoma, may lead to muscle weakness, a condition called the myasthenic syndrome (Eaton-Lambert syndrome). Electromyography differentiates this syndrome from MG. With tetanic contractions, the muscle power improves, as it does not in MG. Patients with myasthenic syndrome respond poorly to anticholinesterases, but guanidine produces marked improvement. They demonstrate extreme sensitivity to both depolarizing and nondepolarizing muscle relaxants. However, both groups experience the same perioperative problems.

The myasthenic parturient should be acquainted with the nurses and the physicians who will eventually take care of her during and after delivery. Her well-being demands this psychological and emotional preparation, which should start during prenatal visits. A woman with MG frequently fears that no one will understand her myasthenia and that some may consider her lazy because of her inability to carry out routine personal care while, in reality, the disease itself or overtreatment has weakened her.

Anesthesia for Vaginal Delivery

The danger of respiratory depression necessitates judicious use of tranquilizers and narcotics. Moreover, anticholinesterases potentiate narcotics. Regional anesthetic techniques provide a better choice. Spinal or epidural analgesia to the T10 level will decrease the requirements for systemic medications, prevent fatigue, and facilitate the use of outlet forceps. In theory, large doses of local anesthetics may interfere with neuromuscular transmission.[98] They decrease the release of acetylcholine and reduce the amplitude of end-plate potential by interfering with sodium conductance across the cell membrane.[129] However, only toxic doses would have any significant effect on the myoneural junction of myasthenic patients to local anesthetic drugs. Myasthenic patients have received safe epidural analgesia on several occasions.[63,121,126,130]

Cholinesterase hydrolyzes chloroprocaine and tetracaine. Anticholinesterase drugs may impair their hydrolysis, thus enhancing maternal and fetal drug toxicity. On this theoretic basis, one should exclude large doses of ester-type local anesthetics from conduction of anesthesia. However, for spinal anesthesia, the small dose employed avoids a prolonged effect; therefore, tetracaine is used. There is no evidence that MG or anticholinesterase drugs alter the metabolism of amide-type drugs. Therefore, the amide local anesthetics are preferable for regional blocks, including epidural analgesia. Local infiltration of the perineum or pudendal nerve block, with or without nitrous oxide and oxygen analgesia, offers an alternative to spinal or epidural analgesia.

During labor vital capacity should be evaluated frequently to detect early development of respiratory insufficiency. Progressive decrements in a series of three consecutive vital capacities indicate muscle fatigue. Anticholinesterase therapy may require adjustment during labor because of varying physical exertion and emotional status. The delayed gastric emptying during labor recommends the intramuscular route. An intramuscular dose should be given 30 min before delivery to assure maximum maternal strength needed for the pushing efforts.

If regional anesthesia is contraindicated, general anesthesia may be used. Thiopentone has a weak action on the myoneural junction since its infusion increases the neuromuscular block produced by curare and gallamine in cats.[129] Halothane and other potent inhalation anesthetics mainly act centrally by depressing the evoked motor-nerve activity, thereby decreasing the release of acetylcholine from the nerve endings. In contrast, ether and, to a lesser extent, enflurane and isoflurane have a curare-like action at the myoneural junction. Nitrous oxide does not potentiate muscle relaxants or increase the paresis in the myasthenic patient.[129] Although many anesthesiologists recommend inducing anesthesia with nitrous oxide and oxygen and halothane by mask for MG, this technique proves unsuitable in the obstetric patient with a potentially full stomach. Either awake endotracheal intubation or rapid thiopental induction with cricoid pressure and immediate intubation is suitable. Awake intubation can be unpleasant while rapid thiopental induction is often easily accomplished in patients with MG without additional agents. However, muscle relaxants may be required to facilitate rapid intubation, especially in mild MG. Precurarization before succinylcholine is avoided because patients with MG are sensitive to curare. In MG, a small dose of curare will have a rapid onset and an exaggerated response; 2 to 3 mg of curare may suffice for intubation. Since redistribution and excretion of curare follow as in normal persons, duration of action in MG is the same as for equipotent doses in normal patients.

Succinylcholine has an unpredictable effect in MG, since uninvolved muscles are resistant and involved muscles are more sensitive. A dose of 30 to 50 mg usually provides suitable conditions for tracheal intubation;[131] however, the duration of paralysis may persist up to 90 min due to anticholinesterase therapy.[118] The predictability and reversibility of a small dose of a nondepolarizing muscle relaxant makes it preferable to succinylcholine. When uterine relaxation is necessary, halothane may be used. The anesthesiologist must intubate the patient and control her ventilation during general anesthesia, irrespective of the agent or agents used. Considering the potential hazards of general anesthesia in the myasthenic patient, pudendal nerve block or local infiltration combined with nitrous oxide analgesia are good alternatives when contraindications to spinal or epidural blocks arise.

Anesthesia for Cesarean Section

With the higher level of conduction analgesia required for cesarean section, the danger of impairment of respiratory or swallowing muscles increases. This holds true especially for subarachnoid block. Therefore, if a patient has bulbar or respiratory muscle involvement, general anesthesia with tracheal intubation is preferable; otherwise, epidural or spinal techniques can be successful alternatives.[121]

Myoneural junction response must be monitored whenever one administers a muscle relaxant or general anesthetic. Myasthenia gravis rarely requires a muscle relaxant for abdominal relaxation during general anesthesia. If required, increments of 0.5- to 1-mg curare suffice; the response is monitored by a nerve stimulator.[132] Reversal of nondepolarizing relaxants is accomplished with 0.5-mg increments of neostigmine, and twitch height and the response to tetanic stimulation are monitored lest a cholinergic crisis be precipitated. Indeed, some advise against reversing the neuromuscular block, preferring to ventilate the patient until neuromuscular function recovers spontaneously. Usually the anesthesiologist can reverse the muscle blockade and extubate patients who have stable and well-controlled MG preoperatively.

Postoperative Care

Postoperative mortality and morbidity frequently follow overzealous anticholinesterase therapy.[131,133] Anticholinesterase requirements vary widely in the immediate postpartum period and must be assessed by repeated measurements of the vital capacity and by response to edrophonium. Meticulous respiratory care includes adequate ventilatory support and, if necessary, endotracheal suction and chest physical therapy. Most patients who have a vital capacity less than 2 liters, who have had the disease for more than 6 years and who have had recurrent respiratory infections need respiratory support in the postoperative period. Patients having circulatory instability from associated myocarditis require intensive care for at least 48 hours postoperatively.

Summary

The parturient with a neurologic disorder may qualify as a high-risk patient requiring utmost care and a special caliber of experience. Cooperative teamwork by obstetrician, neurologist, and anesthesiologist cannot be overstressed.

References

1. Swapp, GH and Main, RA: Neurofibromatosis in pregnancy. Br J Dermatol 80:431, 1973.
2. Isselbacher, JK, et al: Harrison's Principles of Internal Medicine, ed 10. McGraw Hill, New York, 1980.
3. Manser, J: Abnormal responses in Von Recklinghausen's disease. Br J Anaesth 42:183, 1970.
4. Magbagbeola, JAO: Abnormal responses to muscle relaxants in a patient with Von Recklinghausen's disease (multiple neurofibromatosis) (correspondence). Br J Anaesth 42:710, 1970.
5. Baraka, A: Myasthenic response to muscle relaxants in Von Recklinghausen's disease. Br J Anaesth 46:701, 1974.
6. Miledi, R: The acetylcholine sensitivity of frog muscle fibres after complete or partial denervation. J Physiol (Lond) 1551:1, 1960.
7. Fisher, MM: Anesthetic difficulties in neurofibromatosis. Anaesthesia 30:648, 1975.
8. Griffiths, ML and Theron, EJ: Obstructed labor from pelvic neurofibroma. S Afr Med J 53:781, 1978.
9. Crowe, FW, Schull, WJ and Neel, JV: A Clinical, Pathological, and Genetic Study of Multiple Neurofibromatosis. Charles C Thomas, Springfield, IL, 1956.
10. Chapman, CR, Kemp, EV and Taliaferro, I: Pheochromocytoma associated with multiple neurofibromatosis and intracranial hemorrhage. N Engl J Med 26:833, 1959.
11. Healey, FM and Mekelatos, G: Vascular lesions causing hypertension in neurofibromatosis. N Engl J Med 258:540, 1958.
12. Bourke, E and Gatenby, PBB: Renal artery dysplasia with hypertension in neurofibromatosis. Br Med J 3:681, 1971.
13. Head, H and Reddoch, G: The automatic bladder, excessive sweating and some other reflex conditions in gross injury of the spinal cord. Brain 40:188, 1917.
14. Kurnick NB: Autonomic hyperreflexia and its control in patients with spinal cord lesions. Ann Intern Med 44:678, 1956.
15. Abouleish, E: Hypertension in a paraplegic parturient. Anesthesiology 53:348, 1980.
16. Debarge, O, et al: Plasma catecholamines in tetraplegics. Paraplegia 12:44, 1974.
17. Robertson, DNS: Pregnancy and labour in the paraplegic. Paraplegia 10:209, 1972.
18. Aminoff, MJ: Maternal neurologic disorders. In Creasy, RK and Resnik, R (eds): Maternal-Fetal Medicine. WB Saunders, Philadelphia, 1984.
19. Cooperman, LH, Strobel, GE and Kennel, EM: Massive hyperkalemia after administration of succinylcholine. Anesthesiology 32:161, 1970.
20. Ellis, FR: Neuromuscular disease and anaesthesia. Br J Anaesth 46:603, 1974.
21. Axelsson, J and Thesleff, S: A study of supersensitivity in denervated mammalian skeletal muscle. J Physiol (Lond) 147:178, 1959.
22. Stirt, JA, Marco, A and Conklin, KA: Obstetric anesthesia for a quadriplegic patient with autonomic hyperreflexia. Anesthesiology 51:560, 1979.

23. Ciliberti, BJ, Goldfein, J and Rovenstine, EA: Hypertension during anesthesia in patients with spinal cord injuries. Anesthesiology 15:273, 1954.
24. Baraka, A: Epidural meperidine for control of autonomic hyperreflexia in a paraplegic parturient. Anesthesiology 62:688, 1985.
25. Kitahata, LJ and Collins, JG: Spinal action of narcotic analgesics. Anesthesiology 54:153, 1981.
26. Hopkins, A: Neurological disorders. Clin Obstet Gynaecol 4:419, 1977.
27. Bellur, S: Neurologic disorders in pregnancy. In Gleicher, N (ed): Principles of Medical Therapy in Pregnancy. Plenum, New York, 1985.
28. Younker, D, et al: Maternal cortical vein thrombosis and the obstetric anesthesiologist. Anesth Analg 56:1007, 1986.
29. Dunn, R, Lee, W and Cotton, DB: Evaluation by computerized axial tomography of eclamptic women with seizures refractory to magnesium sulfate therapy. Am J Obstet Gynecol 155:267, 1986.
30. Donnelly, JF and Lock, FR: Causes of death in 533 fatal cases of toxemia of pregnancy. Am J Obstet Gynecol 68:184, 1954.
31. Abouleish, E: Postpartum hypertension and convulsion after oxytocic drugs. Anesth Analg (Cleve) 55:813, 1976.
32. Minielly, R, Yuzpe, AA and Drake, CG: Subarachnoid hemorrhage secondary to ruptured cerebral aneurysm in pregnancy. Obstet Gynecol 53:64, 1979.
33. Robinson, JL, Hall, CJ and Sedzimir, CB: Subarachnoid hemorrhage in pregnancy. J Neurosurg 36:27, 1972.
34. Edelstone, D: Changes in maternal physiology during pregnancy, parturition, and the puerperium. In Abouleish, E (ed): Pain Control in Obstetrics. JB Lippincott, Philadelphia, 1977.
35. Hamilton, WF, Woodbury, RA and Harper, HT: Physiologic relationships between intrathoracic, intraspinal and arterial pressures. JAMA 107:853, 1936.
36. McCausland, AM and Holmes, F: Spinal fluid pressure during labor; preliminary report West J. Surg 65:220, 1957.
37. Cannel, DE and Botterell, EH: Subarachnoid hemorrhage and pregnancy. Am J Obstet Gynecol 72:844, 1956.
38. Conklin, KA, Herr, G and Fung, D: Anesthesia for cesarean section and cerebral aneurysm clipping. Can Anaesth Soc J 34:451, 1984.
39. Lennon, RL, Sundt, TM Jr and Gronert, GA: Combined cesarean section and clipping of intracerebral aneurysm. Anesthesiology 60:240, 1984.
40. Pool, JL and Pott, DG: Aneurysms and Arteriovenous Anomalies of the Brain: Diagnosis and Treatment. Harper & Row, New York, 1965.
41. Willoughby, JS: Sodium nitroprusside, pregnancy and multiple intercranial aneurysms. Anaesth Intensive Care 12:351, 1984.
42. Diaz, SF and Marx, GF: Placental transfer of nitroglycerin. Anesthesiology 51:475, 1979.
43. Aitken, RR and Drake, CG: A technique of anesthesia with induced hypotension for surgical correction of intracranial aneurysms. Clin Neurosurg 21:107, 1974.
44. Poulton, TJ, James, FM III and Lockridge, O: Prolonged apnea following trimethaphan and succinylcholine. Anesthesiology 50:54, 1979.
45. Lewis, PE, et al: Placental transfer and fetal toxicity of sodium nitroprusside. Gynecol Obstet Invest 8:46, 1977.
46. Newman, B and Lam, AM: Induced hypotension for clipping of a cerebral aneurysm during pregnancy: A case report brief review. Anesth Analg 65:675, 1986.
47. Bruns, PD, et al: The placental transfer of water from fetus to mother following the intravenous infusion of hypertonic mannitol to the maternal rabbit. Am J Obstet Gynecol 86:160, 1963.
48. Arnason, BGW: Multiple sclerosis: Current concepts and management. Hosp Pract [off] 17:81, 1982.
49. Paterson RA, Tousignant, M and Skene, DS: Caesarean section for twins in a patient with myotonic dystrophy. Can Anaesth Soc J 32:418, 1985.
50. RIdley, A and Schapira, K: Influence of surgical procedures on the course of multiple sclerosis. Neurology 2:81, 1961.
51. Miller, H: Aetiological factors in disseminated sclerosis. Proc R Soc Med 54:7, 1961.
52. Keschner, M: The effects of injuries and illness on the course of multiple sclerosis. Res Publ Assoc Res Nerv Ment Dis 28:533, 1950.
53. Bamford, C, Sibley, W and Laguna, J: Anesthesia in multiple sclerosis. Can J Neurol Sci 5:41, 1978.
54. Schapira, K: Is lumbar puncture harmful in multiple sclerosis? J Neurol Neurosurg Psychiatry 22:238, 1959.
55. Crawford, JS, et al: Regional analgesia for patients with chronic neurological disease and similar conditions. Anaesthesia 36:821, 1981.
56. Baskett, PJF and Armstrong, R: Anesthetic problems in multiple sclerosis: Are certain agents contraindicated? Anesthesiology 25:397, 1970.
57. Siemkowicz, E: Multiple sclerosis and surgery. Anaesthesia 31:1211, 1976.
58. Haas, JF, Janisch, W and Stanczek, W: Newly diagnosed primary intracranial neoplasms in pregnant women: A population-based assessment. J Neurol Neurosurg Psychiatry 49:874, 1986.
59. Donaldson, JO: Neurology of Pregnancy (Major Problems in Neurology, Vol 7). WB Saunders, Philadelphia, 1982.
60. Wildsmith, JAW: Extradural blockade and intracranial pressure. Br J Anaesth 58:579, 1986.
61. Hilt, H, Gramm, H-J and Link, J: Changes in intracranial pressure associated with extradural anaesthesia. Br J Anaesth 58:676, 1986.
62. Crawford, JS: Principles and Practice of Obstetric Anesthesia, ed 4. Blackwell Scientific Publications, Oxford, 1978.
63. Usubiaga, JE, et al: Effect of saline injections on epidural and subarachnoid space pressures and relation to post spinal anesthesia headache. Anesth Analg 46:293, 1967.
64. Abouleish, E: Intracranial hypertension and caudal anaesthesia. Br J Anaesth 59:1478, 1987.
65. Ahlskog, JE and O'Neill, BP: Pseudotumor cerebri. Ann Intern Med 97:249, 1982.

66. Weisberg, LA: Benign intracranial hypertension. Medicine (Baltimore) 54:197, 1975.
67. Koontz, WL, Herbert, WNP and Cefalo, RC: Pseudotumor cerebri in pregnancy. Obstet Gynecol 62:324, 1983.
68. Abouleish, E, Ali, V and Tang, RA: Benign intracranial hypertension and anesthesia for cesarean section. Anesthesiology 63:705, 1985.
69. Palop, R, Choed-Amphai, E and Miller, R: Epidural anesthesia for delivery complicated by benign intracranial hypertension. Anesthesiology 50:159, 1979.
70. Evans, DE: Anaesthesia and the epileptic patient: A review. Anaesthesia 30:34, 1975.
71. Van Dyke, RA: Metabolism of volatile anesthetics. 3. Induction of microsomal dechlorinating and ether-cleaving enzymes. J Pharmacol Exp Ther 154:364, 1966.
72. Blake, DA, et al: Biotransformation of fluroxene: 1. Metabolism in mice and dogs in vivo. Biochem Pharmacol 16:1237, 1967.
73. Harrah, MD, Way, WL and Katzung, BG: The interaction of d-tubocurarine with antiarrhythmic drugs. Anesthesiology 33:406, 1970.
74. Hansson, U, Irestedt, L and Moberg, PJ: Delivery complicated by myasthenia gravis and epilepsy. Acta Obstet Gynecol Scand 57:183, 1978.
75. Bjerkedal, T and Bahna, IL: The course and outcome of pregnancy in women with epilepsy. Acta Obstet Gynecol Scand 52:245, 1973.
76. Philbert, A and Dam, J: Antiepileptic drug disposition during pregnancy: Review of the literature. In Jand, D, Bossi, L and Dam, J (eds): Epilepsy, Pregnancy and the Child. Raven Press, New York, 1982.
77. Burnett, CWF: A survey of the relation between epilepsy and pregnancy. J Obstet Gynaecol Br Commonw 53:539, 1946.
78. Bertollini, R, Mastroiacovo, P, and Segni, G: Maternal epilepsy and birth defects: A case-control study in the Italian Multicentric Registry of Birth Defects. Eur J Epidemiol 1:67, 1985.
79. Knight, AH and Rhind, EG: Epilepsy and pregnancy: A study of 153 pregnancies in 59 patients. Epilepsia 16:99, 1975.
80. Robertson, IG: Prescribing in pregnancy: Epilepsy in pregnancy. Clin Obstet Gynaecol 13:365, 1986.
81. Hiilesmaa, VK, Bardy, A and Teramo, K: Obstetric outcome in women with epilepsy. Am J Obstet Gynecol 152:499, 1985.
82. Davies, SM: Epilepsy and pregnancy. Am Fam Physician 34:179, 1986.
83. deJong, RH and Walts, LF: Lidocaine-induced psychomotor seizures in man. Acta Anaesth Scand (suppl) 23:257, 1952.
84. Bohm, E, Flodmark, S and Petersen, I: Effect of lidocaine (Xylocaine) on seizure and interseizure electroencephalograms in epileptics. A.M.A. Arch Neurol Psychiat 81:550, 1959.
85. Abouleish, E: Local anesthetic drugs. In Abouleish, E (ed): Pain Control in Obstetrics. JB Lippincott, Philadelphia, 1977.
86. Abouleish, E and Taylor, FH: Effect of morphine-diazepam on signs of anesthesia, awareness and dreams of patients under N_2O for cesarean section. Anesth Analg 55:702, 1976.
87. Browne, TR and Penry, JK: Penzodiazepine in the treatment of epilepsy: A review. Epilepsia 14:277, 1973.
88. Goodman, LS and Gilman, A: The Pharmacological Basis of Therapeutics, ed 5. Macmillan, New York, 1975.
89. Delgado-Escueta, AV and Ernile-Bascal, F: Combination therapy of status epilepticus: Intravenous diazepam and phenytoin. In Delgado-Escueta, AV, Wasterlain, C and Trieman, DM (eds): Status Epilepticus: Mechanism of Brain Damage and Treatment. Advances in Neurology, vol 34. Raven Press, New York, 1982.
90. Monfared, AH, et al: Obstetric management of pregnant women with extracranial shunts. Can Med Assoc J 120:563, 1979.
91. Bellur, SN: Diseases of the striated muscles in pregnancy. In Gleicher, N (ed): Principles of Medical Therapy in Pregnancy. Plenum, New York, 1985.
92. Hunsaker, RH, et al: Cardiac function in Duchenne's muscular dystrophy. Am J Med 42:179, 1982.
93. Smith, CL and Bush, GH: Anesthesia and progressive muscular dystrophy. Br J Anaesth 57:1113, 1985.
94. Smith, CL and Bush, GH: Anaesthesia and progressive muscular dystrophy. Br J Anaesth 57:1113, 1985.
95. Sokoll, MD and Gergis, SD: Anesthesia and neuromuscular disease. Anesth Rev 2:20, 1975.
96. Becker, PE: Genetic approaches to the nosology of muscle diseases: Myotonias and similar diseases. Birth Defects 7:52, 1971.
97. Hopkins, A and Wray, S: The effect of pregnancy on dystrophica myotonia. Neurology 17:166, 1967.
98. Dunn, LJ and Dierker, LJ: Hydramnios associated with myotonia dystrophica. Obstet Gynecol 42:104, 1973.
99. Sciarra, JJ and Steir, CM: Uterine contractions during labor in muscular dystrophy. Am J Obstet Gynecol 82:612, 1961.
100. Sarnat, HB, O'Connor, T and Byrne, PA: Clinical effects of myotonic dystrophy on pregnancy and the neonate. Arch Neurol 33:459, 1976.
101. Fox, GN and Garvett, MG: Neonatal myotonic dystrophy associated with prenatal ventriculomegaly: A case report. J Reprod Med 31:729, 1986.
102. Bourke, TD and Zuck, D: Thiopentone in dystrophica myotonica. Br J Anaesth 29:35, 1957.
103. Dundee, JW: Thiopentone in dystrophica myotonica. Anesth Analg 31:257, 1952.
104. Mitchell, MM, Ali, HH and Savarese, JJ: Myotonia and neuromuscular blocking agents. Anesthesiology 49:44, 1978.
105. Thiel, RE: The myotonic response to suxamethonium. Br J Anaesth 39:815, 1967.
106. Paterson, IS: Generalized myotonia following suxamethonium: Case report. Br J Anaesth 34:340, 1962.
107. Hook, R, Anderson, EF and Note, P: Anesthetic management of a parturient with myotonia atrophica. Anesthesiology 43:689, 1975.
108. Kaufman, L: Anaesthesia in dystrophia myotonica. Proc Roy Soc Med 53:183, 1960.
109. Nightingale, P, Healy, TEJ and McGuinness, K: Dys-

trophica myotonica and atracurium: A case report. Br J Anaesth 57:1131, 1985.
110. Ishizawa, Y, et al: A serious complication due to gastrointestinal malfunction with myotonic dystrophy. Anesth Analg 65:1066, 1986.
111. Cope, DK and Miller, JN: Local and spinal anesthesia for cesarean section in a patient with myotonic dystrophy. Anesth Analg 65:687, 1986.
112. Wheeler, AS and James, FM III: Local anesthesia for laparoscopy in a case of myotonia dystrophica. Anesthesiology 50:169, 1979.
113. Foldes, FF and McNall, PG: Myasthenia gravis: A guide for anesthesiologists. Anesthesiology 23:837, 1962.
114. Lindstrom, JM, et al: Antibody to acetylcholine receptor in myasthenia gravis: Prevalence, clinical correlates, and diagnostic value. Neurology (Minneap) 26:1054, 1976.
115. Drachman, DB: Myasthenia gravis: Part 1. N Engl J Med 298:136, 1978.
116. Satyamuri, S, Drachman, DB and Stone, F: Blockade of acetylcholine receptors: A model of myasthenia gravis. Science 187:955, 1975.
117. Simpson, JA: Myasthenia gravis: A personal view of pathogenesis and mechanism: Part 2. Muscle Nerve 1:151, 1978.
118. Rolbin, SH, et al: Anesthetic considerations for myasthenia gravis and pregnancy. Anesth Analg 57:44, 1978.
119. Ludwig, S and Bristow, G: Hazards of edrophonium. Anesthesiology 52:567, 1979.
120. Youngberg, JA: Cardiac arrest following treatment of paroxysmal atrial tachycardia with edrophonium. Anesthesiology 50:234, 1979.
121. McNall, PG and Jafarnia, MR: Management of myasthenia gravis in the obstetrical patient. Am J Obstet Gynecol 92:518, 1965.
122. Ham, J: Factors affecting administration of neuromuscular blocking agents. Annual refresher course lectures, American Society of Anesthesiologists, 1979.
123. Plauche, WC: Myasthenia gravis in pregnancy. Am J Obstet Gynecol 88:404, 1964.
124. Vincent, O, et al: Myasthenia gravis and pregnancy. Exerpta Med 296:79, 1973.
125. Drachman, DB: Myasthenia gravis: Part 2. N Engl J Med 298:186, 1978.
126. Dunn, JM: Neonatal myasthenia. Am J Obstet Gynecol 125:265, 1976.
127. Osserman, EK: Myasthenia Gravis. Grune & Stratton, New York, 1958.
128. Mora, CT, Eisenkraft, JB and Paptestras, AE: Intravenous dentrolene in a patient with myasthenia gravis. Anesthesiology 64:371, 1986.
129. Churchill-Davidson, HC: A Practice of Anaesthesia, ed 4. WB Saunders, Philadelphia, 1978.
130. Perry, CP, et al: Myasthenia gravis in pregnancy. Ala J Med Sci 12:219, 1975.
131. Perry, AE and Livesley, B: Puerperal respiratory failure due to acute myasthenia gravis. J Obstet Gynaecol Commonw 74:773, 1967.
132. Azar, I: The response of patients with neuromuscular disorders to muscle relaxants: A review. Anesthesiology 61:173, 1984.
133. Miller, JH, Sellmann, AH and Mickal, A: Myasthenia gravis of pregnancy at Charity Hospital. J La State Med Soc 120:231, 1968.
134. Burrow, GN and Serris, TF: Medical Complications During Pregnancy, ed 2. WB Saunders, Philadelphia, 1982, p 485.

CHAPTER 9

CARDIAC DISEASE

THOMAS H. JOYCE, III, M.D.
QUISQUEYA T. PALACIOS, M.D.

Heart disease occurs in approximately 0.5 to 2 percent of obstetric patients in the United States and still remains one of the leading nonobstetric causes of maternal mortality.[1] Although rheumatic heart disease is the predominant type associated with pregnancy, preventive measures and improved pharmacologic treatment of rheumatic fever have produced a decline in the relative incidence of rheumatic heart disease during the past 25 years. In addition, concomitant advances in noninvasive diagnostic techniques, better, more aggressive medical management, and successful surgical correction of specific cardiac lesions have given rise to a relatively new and growing category of patients with congenital heart disease who now reach child-bearing age and attempt pregnancy. Smoking and the postponement of child bearing to later life contribute to an increasing number of gravidas with ischemic heart disease. Table 9–1 delineates the incidence of heart disease in pregnancy and the cardiovascular lesions associated with significant maternal and fetal mortality.

Cardiac disease in pregnancy often presents an ultimate challenge to the anesthesiologist. The pregnant woman usually tolerates asymptomatic mitral stenosis, mitral insufficiency, aortic stenosis, aortic insufficiency, and less severe congenital lesions with left-to-right shunts relatively well. However, symptomatic mitral stenosis, congenital right-to-left cardiac shunts, primary pulmonary hypertension, coarctation of the aorta, peripartal cardiomyopathy, and myocardial infarction are poorly tolerated, contributing to significant maternal mortality and fetal loss. In such cases, the risk of cardiac decompensation peaks during the third trimester of pregnancy, parturition, and the immediate puerperium, when the cardiovascular changes of pregnancy impose maximal stress on an already compromised heart.

Thus, the anesthesiologist who undertakes to anesthetize a pregnant cardiac patient without a thorough knowledge of the anatomy of the disease, its pathophysiology, and the normally altered cardiovascular dynamics of pregnancy, truly sets sail with neither course nor tiller.

Table 9–1. INCIDENCE AND MORTALITY OF RHEUMATIC AND CONGENITAL HEART DISEASE IN PREGNANCY

Disease	Distribution (%)	Maternal Mortality (%)	Fetal Mortality (%)
Rheumatic heart disease (75%)			
Mitral stenosis	90	1–17	3.5
Mitral insufficiency	6.5		
Aortic insufficiency	2.5		
Aortic stenosis	1.0		
	100		
Congenital heart disease (25%)			
Ventricular septal defect	7–26	7–40	2–16
Atrial septal defect	8–38	1–12	1–12
Patent ductus arteriosus	6–20	5–6	17
Tetralogy of Fallot	2–15	4–12	36–59
Eisenmenger's syndrome	2–4	12–33	30–54
Coarctation of the aorta	4–18	3–9	10–20
Aortic stenosis	2–10		22
Pulmonic stenosis	8–16		4
Primary pulmonary hypertension	1–2	53	7

(From Shnider, SM and Levinson, G (eds): Anesthesia for Obstetrics. Williams & Wilkins, Baltimore, © 1987, with permission.)

Physiology: Cardiopulmonary

Pregnancy represents a hyperdynamic cardiovascular state. Significant hemodynamic changes occurring as early as the end of the first trimester (Fig. 9–1), have been ascribed to numerous factors, most significantly, increasing plasma levels of progesterone and prostaglandins. Stimulation of the renin-angiotensin system during pregnancy may further contribute to some cardiovascular changes. During the first 24 to 28 weeks of gestation, total blood volume increases by 40 percent then remains relatively stable until term (see Chap. 1). Decreased availability and utilization of iron further aggravate the dilutional anemia of pregnancy. Maternal heart rate increases 10 to 15 beats per min, stroke volume increases by 30 percent until week 28 to week 30 then slowly declines, and cardiac output progressively increases until 28 to 32 weeks, remaining relatively stable to term when the mother is in the lateral position.[2] However, in the supine position, aortocaval compression markedly alters cardiac output so that 10 percent of women in the third trimester develop the supine hypotension syndrome associated with decreased venous return, decreased cardiac output, and syncope (Chap. 1). Near

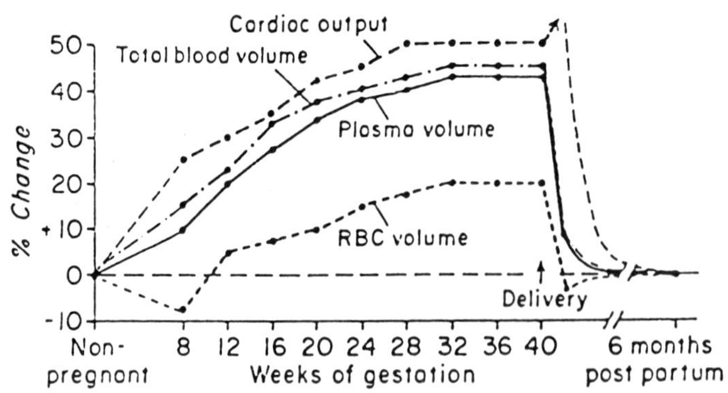

Figure 9–1. Changes in blood volume, plasma volume, red cell volume, and cardiac output during pregnancy and the puerperium. The curves represent trends in percentage change rather than absolute values. (From changes in blood volume, plasma volume, red cell volume, and cardiac output during pregnancy and the puerperium. Dr. Bonica's Obstetric Analgesia and Anesthesia, World Federation of Societies of Anesthesiologists, Amsterdam, 1980, with permission.)

term, cardiac output may increase as much as 30 percent when the mother shifts from the supine to the lateral position (Fig. 9–2), which has important implications for the pregnant cardiac patient. Blood pressure tends to remain relatively stable, declining by 15 mmHg despite an increase in stroke volume and cardiac output; this reflects a concomitant decrease in total peripheral resistance.[1,3] A slightly greater decrease in diastolic pressure than systolic pressure takes place, resulting in a widened pulse pressure.

Compression of the inferior vena cava by the gravid uterus combined with the increased total body sodium contribute to a 50- to 80-percent incidence of peripheral edema in healthy gravidas. The incidence increases with maternal age and reflects an increase of 1 to 5 liters of water in the extracellular spaces. Pregnancy alters other determinants of ventricular work and oxygen consumption. Preload increases due to elevated central venous pressure and left ventricular end-diastolic pressure. On the other hand, afterload decreases because of a decrease in peripheral vascular resistance.[4] Myocardial contractility appears to increase during pregnancy, while a decreased pre-ejection time and an increased velocity of circumferential shortening suggest improved ventricular work.[5] Thus, the combination of increased preload, decreased afterload, and positive chronotropism improve ventricular performance. Resting oxygen consumption increases progressively by 20 to 30 percent near term, requiring increased oxygen transport and delivery to tissues. In early pregnancy, arterial-venous oxygen differences are small, but they gradually increase throughout pregnancy, reaching nonpregnant levels near term.[6]

Many signs and symptoms frequently associated with cardiac disease in nonpregnant patients may be considered common findings in healthy gravidas and are related to the normal cardiovascular and anatomic changes of pregnancy.[7] The heart is displaced cephalad and anterolaterally and rotated transversely, result-

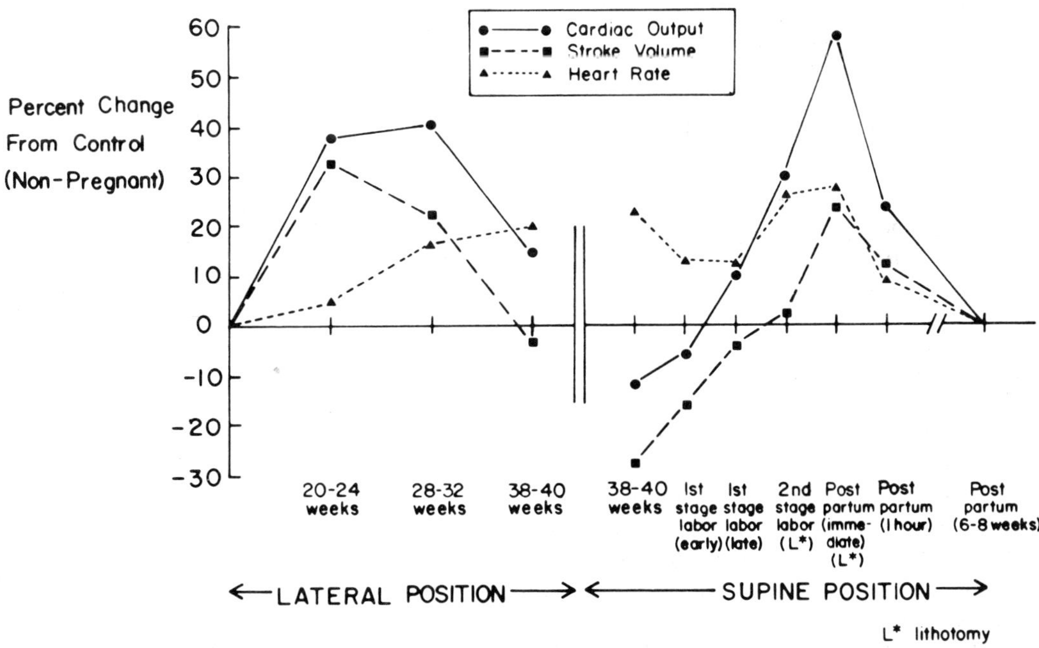

Figure 9–2. Maternal cardiovascular changes during pregnancy and labor from studies on patients in the lateral and supine positions. (From Shnider and Levinson (eds): Anesthesia for Obstetrics. Williams & Wilkins, Baltimore, 1979, with permission. Based on data reported by Ueland K and Hansen J: Maternal cardiovascular dynamics: II. Posture and uterine contractions. Am J Obstet Gynecol 103:1–7, 1969; Ueland K, Hansen J: Maternal cardiovascular dynamics: III. Labor and delivery under local and caudal analgesia. Am J Obstet Gynecol 103:8–18, 1969; and Ueland K, Novy M, Peterson E, Metcalf J: Maternal cardiovascular dynamics: IV. The influence of gestational age on the maternal cardiovascular response to posture and exercise. Am J Obstet Gynecol 104: 156–164, 1969.)

ing in a tendency toward left axis deviation and lateral displacement of the apical impulse. The ECG often reveals large Q waves and inverted T waves in leads III, V_1, V_2, and aV_F, and occasional depression of the ST−T segment suggests inferior ischemia. Notably louder heart sounds result from increased stroke volume and cardiac output. This hyperdynamic state causes a grade I to grade II systolic functional murmur, usually heard best along the left sternal border. Functional murmurs appear in 96 percent of pregnant patients, while a third heart sound occurs in 84 percent. Venous engorgement and flow through the mammary artery may also produce a continuous precordial murmur. Developing between the 12th and 20th week of pregnancy, most murmurs disappear 1 week postpartum.[3]

Most pregnant patients experience varying degrees of dyspnea and orthopnea. By 30 weeks' gestation, 75 percent develop dyspnea, and paroxysmal nocturnal dyspnea is not uncommon. Maternal hyperventilation, secondary to increased progesterone levels, appears to contribute to this presentation.[8] In addition, weight gain commonly produces fatigue and decreased exercise tolerance. Syncope rarely occurs, and usually results from the supine hypotension syndrome. As stated previously, peripheral edema is a common finding.

Signs of Heart Disease During Pregnancy

About 50 percent of patients are unaware of cardiac problems existing prior to pregnancy. Although many of the physical findings seen in heart disease occur normally during pregnancy, some findings definitely imply cardiac pathology: diastolic murmur; abnormal rhythm, such as atrial fibrillation, paroxysmal atrial tachycardia, and complete heart block; grade III or greater systolic murmur; and cardiomegaly and congestive heart failure (CHF) as depicted by chest films.[9] Presumptive symptoms include anginal chest pain and severe progressive dyspnea associated with cyanosis.[10] In the presence of these signs and/or symptoms, diagnosis should be confirmed with appropriate noninvasive modalities.

Functional Classification

The successful management of the pregnant cardiac patient requires close interaction between anesthesiologist, obstetrician, cardiologist, and neonatologist. The patient must be evaluated early during pregnancy, with particular attention to her ability to progressively adapt to increasing blood volume and cardiac output. A detailed exercise history and physical examination facilitate detection of early cardiac decompensation. Furthermore, the New York Heart Association's (NYHA) classification of functional impairment is valuable for assessing disability and severity of cardiac disease during pregnancy.

CLASSIFICATION OF THE PATIENT WITH HEART DISEASE

Class I. Patients with Class I disease have no limitation of physical activity. Ordinary physical activity does not cause undue fatigue, palpitation, dyspnea, or anginal pain.

Class II. Patients with slight limitation of physical activity have Class II disease; they are comfortable at rest. Ordinary physical activity results in fatigue, palpitation, dyspnea, or anginal pain.

Class III. Patients with marked limitation of physical activity, but who remain comfortable at rest have Class III disease. Less than ordinary activity causes fatigue, palpitation, dyspnea, or anginal pain.

Class IV. Patients with Class IV disease are unable to carry on any physical activity without discomfort. Symptoms of cardiac insufficiency or angina may occur even at rest. Any physical activity produces increased discomfort.

The majority of pregnant cardiac patients fall into functional Class I or II. They are minimally impaired, tolerate pregnancy, and have a low incidence of morbidity and mortality. However, approximately 5 to 10 percent of pregnant cardiac patients fall into NYHA Class III or IV, frequently experiencing severe cardiac disability, which produces a 75- to 90-percent incidence of maternal mortality and a high incidence of fetal loss.[11] Therefore, these patients must be managed in high-risk obstetric centers which also have comprehensive cardiology support services for close observation.

Diagnosis of Heart Disease

Functional classification of heart disease, relying heavily on subjective signs and symptoms, may associate with a range of errors.[12] Serial measurements of more specific and objective cardiopulmonary parameters utilizing noninvasive methods provide accurate assessment of progressive cardiac decompensation during pregnancy while avoiding risk to either mother or fetus (Table 9–2). The vital capacity normally does not change during pregnancy, but patients with increased pulmonary capillary wedge and pulmonary artery pressures, leading to pulmonary vascular engorgement, will exhibit decreased vital capacities. Serial determination of this parameter serves as a reliable, inexpensive screening method for cardiac failure. Additionally, intermittent measurements of peripheral oxygen saturation with a pulse oximeter provide another inexpensive screening method for cardiac failure. Prenatal laboratory tests should include an initial chest roentgenograph which exposes the patient to a maximum of 80 mrad for both lateral and posteroanterior (PA) views. Repeated chest films confirm progressive CHF associated with cardiomegaly, abnormal prominence of the pulmonary vasculature, and pleural or pericardial effusions. Electrocardiography usually detects myocardial ischemia, conduction defects, cor pulmonale, and axis deviation. Holter monitoring for 24 hours establishes the presence of arrhythmias, suggested clinically by palpitations and syncope.

Radionuclide techniques often provide useful information on cardiac function, myocardial perfusion, and intracardiac shunts; however, one must consider the risk-benefit ratios associated with the various methods. A first-pass radionuclide ventriculogram exposes the mother to 500 to 800 mrad, but fetal exposure is less than 1 mrad.[13] This small dose of radiation is unlikely to cause congenital abnormalities or cancer. In contrast, cardiac catheterization results in exposure to as much as 28,000 mrad. Although adverse effects of radiation remain proportional to the total dose of absorbed radiation, indicating potential harm to the fetus, complete evaluation may necessitate cardiac catheterization during pregnancy when other methods cannot provide adequate information, particularly when surgery is contemplated.[12] More recently, two-dimensional contrast echocardiography provides assessment of cardiac valve function during pregnancy with minimal exposure to ionizing radiation,[14] thus offering an alternative to cardiac catheterization. One can also perform right heart catheterization without fluoroscopy and radiation exposure, using a flow-directed pulmonary artery catheter.[15] A Swan-Ganz catheter may be reliably passed into the pulmonary artery percutaneously. Connecting the catheter to a transducer and pressure monitor with an oscilloscope allows observation of characteristic pressure tracings as the catheter progresses from the right atrium, through the right ventricle, and into the pulmonary artery, until the balloon tip wedges in a distal segment.

Although it provides valuable information on cardiac output, systemic and pulmonary vascular resistance, and left ventricular function, pulmonary artery catheterization may cause several complications, including premature ventricular contractions, pulmonary artery rupture, intracardiac knotting, infection, and pneumothorax.[16] However, investigators[17] do report beneficial uses of the Swan-Ganz catheter, particularly in gravidas with NYHA Class III and IV cardiac disease (Table 9–3). Additionally, measurement of mixed venous oxygen saturation allows quantitation of peripheral oxygen extraction and intrapulmonary shunting.[18]

Echocardiography, another reliable, safe, and noninvasive method of evaluating cardiac function during pregnancy, utilizes two-dimensional and M-mode systems to generate high-frequency sound waves and records signals reflected from the blood-tissue interfaces. The re-

Table 9–2. NONINVASIVE TESTS FOR CARDIAC EVALUATION IN THE PREGNANT CARDIAC PATIENT

Physical exam with auscultation and percussion
Exercise tolerance test
Chest film, repeated as necessary
Serial vital capacities
Peripheral oxygen saturation determination
Electrocardiography
Holter monitoring
Echocardiography
2-dimensional
M-mode
Doppler

Table 9–3. INDICATIONS FOR PULMONARY ARTERY CATHETERIZATION OF OBSTETRIC PATIENTS

Indication	Number of Patients
Severe pre-eclampsia or eclampsia and oliguria or pulmonary edema	13
Class III or IV rheumatic or congenital cardiac disease in labor	13
Class II or III rheumatic or congenital cardiac disease and severe pre-eclampsia in labor	3
Septic shock	10
Adult respiratory distress syndrome	2
Amniotic fluid embolism	2
Hypovolemic shock unresponsive to fluid replacement	1
Other*	3
Total	47

*One case with each of the following indications: pulmonary hypertension and respiratory failure secondary to end-stage tuberculosis, not in labor; cesarean section with thyroid storm; congestive heart failure with atrial flutter, not in labor.

(From Clark, SL, et al: Experience with the pulmonary artery catheter in obstetrics and gynecology. Am J Obstet Gynecol 152:374, 1985, with permission.)

flected signals depict the anatomy and the motion of the four cardiac chambers, permitting diagnosis of wall motion abnormalities. The method includes three basic imaging planes: the four-chamber view, the long-axis view, and the short-axis view. Myocardial contractility and the ejection fraction can be determined by measuring the mean velocity of ventricular circumferential fiber shortening in addition to left ventricular ejection time.

Doppler echocardiography, a new noninvasive ultrasound technique,[5] detects the change in frequency of the sound waves reflected from moving targets such as red blood cells. The Doppler shift is proportional to the velocity of movement and provides information about abnormal blood flow, transvalvular pressure gradients, valve area, and cardiac output. Excellent correlation exists between cardiac output measurements made by pulsed Doppler ultrasound and by thermal dilution via a Swan-Ganz catheter, minimizing the need for the invasive techniques.[19]

Management During Pregnancy

GENERAL MEASURES

Prevention and early detection of cardiac dysfunction are of paramount importance in pregnancy. General measures to decrease cardiac stress and work include bed rest, limited physical activity, and avoidance of rapid weight gain and aortocaval compression. Oral iron supplementation helps to prevent anemia which, if severe, should be treated by transfusion to improve oxygen-carrying capacity. The American Heart Association recommends antibiotic administration for subacute bacterial endocarditis (SBE) prophylaxis, as well as to treat active infections (Table 9–4). In parturients, antibiotic

Table 9–4. GUIDELINES FOR SBE PROPHYLAXIS IN PATIENTS WHO HAVE CARDIAC DISEASE*

Endocarditis prophylaxis recommended
- Prosthetic cardiac valves (including biosynthetic valves)
- Most congenital cardiac malformations
- Surgically constructed systemic pulmonary shunts
- Rheumatic and other acquired valvular dysfunction
- Idiopathic hypertrophic subaortic stenosis
- Previous history of bacterial endocarditis
- Mitral valve prolapse with insufficiency*

Other cases in which prophylaxis may be indicated
- Presence of transvenous pacemakers
- Renal dialysis patients with arteriovenous shunts
- Patients with ventriculoatrial shunts

Endocarditis prophylaxis not recommended
- Isolated secundum atrial-septal defect
- Secundum atrial-septal defect repaired without a patch six or more months earlier
- Patent ductus arteriosus ligated and divided 6 or more months earlier
- Postoperative coronary artery bypass graft surgery

*Standard regimen: Ampicillin 2.0 g IM or IV plus gentamicin 1.5 mg/kg IM or IV. Given ½ to 1 hour before procedure or at the start of labor and continued for 2 days after delivery.

Table 9–5. INDICATIONS FOR ANTICOAGULANT THERAPY

Phlebitis, phlebothrombosis, and pulmonary embolism
Atherosclerotic heart disease
Congestive cardiac failure
Cerebrovascular disease
Rheumatic heart disease
Prosthetic cardiac valves
Disseminated intravascular coagulation
Chronic atrial fibrillation
Eisenmenger's syndrome

prophylaxis should begin at the start of labor or 1 hour prior to elective cesarean section and continue for 2 days after delivery.[20,21]

ANTICOAGULATION

Some conditions—chronic atrial fibrillation, a history of previous thromboembolism, and the presence of prosthetic valves—require prophylactic anticoagulation during pregnancy to prevent thromboembolism (Table 9–5). When used early in pregnancy, coumadin may produce congenital malformations as well as abortion, stillbirth, and fetal death secondary to hemorrhage. Because heparin does not cross the placenta, it is the preferred anticoagulant following conception, throughout pregnancy, or at least during the first and second trimester to avoid anomalies. Coumadin can be resumed in midpregnancy. At term, most clinicians substitute heparin until labor begins, at which time anticoagulant therapy ceases until after delivery. The anesthetist may employ regional analgesia during this window in anticoagulant therapy; if required, protamine quickly reverses the effects of heparin. Anticoagulation usually resumes 24 hours after regional blockade or 4 hours after delivery in mothers who do not receive regional blockade.

Management of the cardiac patient should also minimize therapeutic hazard to the fetus. Major cardiac complications require aggressive management with antiarrhythmic drugs, inotropes, diuretics, and β-adrenergic blockers. Vasodilators, vasopressors, and calcium channel blockers may be used when necessary, provided the physician is mindful of their potential to produce deleterious effects on uterine perfusion and contractility. Failure of pharmacologic therapy to control ventricular response to supraventricular tachyarrhythmias calls for cardioversion. The mother and fetus usually tolerate synchronized cardioversion to 100 watt-sec relatively well.[22]

During gestation, fetal growth should be monitored frequently. Weekly biophysical profiles and nonstress tests to assess fetal wellbeing prove especially important in the third trimester (see Chap. 3). Patients at risk for developing CHF and those exhibiting progressive cardiac decompensation require hospitalization for close surveillance of mother and fetus. Furthermore, vaginal or cesarean delivery should be planned for a time of day when the obstetric and anesthesia team have access to maximal consultant services and laboratory facilities.

CONGESTIVE HEART FAILURE

Congestive heart failure represents a major complication of heart disease in pregnancy. The overall incidence of heart failure during pregnancy associated with rheumatic heart disease is 12 percent.[23] Mitral stenosis associated with arrhythmias, cardiomegaly, and advanced age places patients at particular risk. However, Sugrue[23] reported that approximately 40 percent of patients who eventually develop failure initially have Class I status. Heart failure occurs with an overall incidence of 7 percent during pregnancy in patients with congenital heart disease. The risk increases substantially in those with tetralogy of Fallot and congenital aortic stenosis. Physical exertion, toxemia, emotional distress, embolism, transfusions, and threatened abortion may also precipitate CHF.[20] Four percent of cardiac patients develop CHF in the first trimester; 20 percent, in the second trimester; up to 32 percent, in the third trimester; and 9 percent, immediately postpartum.[24]

TERMINATION OF PREGNANCY

Termination of pregnancy prior to 12 weeks' gestation is recommended for patients with Eisenmenger's syndrome, primary pulmonary hypertension, or any condition associated with a functional Class IV status, since significant maternal and fetal mortality occur with these problems. Additionally, one must consider termination of pregnancy for any severe uncorrected cyanotic heart lesion. Conradsson and Werko[25] state, "the decision to recommend termination requires the careful study and assessment of a number of factors, including the severity of heart disease, hazard to the mother, history of previous heart failure, other coexisting disease, religious and moral beliefs, economic and family burdens." Some authorities also recommend sterilization for women with severe cardiac disease, following assessment of these same factors.

Effects of Various Therapeutic Modalities

In pregnant patients, mitral stenosis calls for digoxin to prevent atrial fibrillation and to treat pulmonary edema by increasing myocardial contractility and decreasing the ventricular rate. Although digoxin crosses the placenta, no toxic effects occur in the fetus if doses are within therapeutic levels. Maternal gastrointestinal disturbances commonly develop; otherwise, digoxin appears safe during pregnancy.

Lidocaine serves as a safe and effective antiarrhythmic for acute treatment of digoxin toxicity and controls ventricular extrasystoles. Quinidine and procainamide are also relatively safe for use in pregnancy. However, they may produce oxytocic effects and premature labor.

While diuretics facilitate the treatment of congestive heart failure by decreasing intravascular volume, they potentially reduce placental perfusion. Fetal electrolyte imbalance, neonatal jaundice, thrombocytopenia, liver damage, and fetal death rarely occur. β-adrenergic blockers manage hypertension, tachyarrhythmias, aortic stenosis, and hypertrophic cardiomyopathy. Propranolol crosses the placenta and may cause fetal bradycardia, hypoglycemia, and intrauterine growth retardation. Increased uterine activity can occur, possibly resulting in premature labor and accompanying neonatal respiratory distress syndrome.

Labor and Delivery

CARDIOVASCULAR EFFECTS

With the onset of labor, apprehension and pain contribute to marked elevations of stroke volume, cardiac output, and cardiac work. Between contractions, stroke volume and cardiac output increase by 30 to 40 percent above prelabor values (Chap. 1). Each uterine contraction acutely augments central blood volume by 10 to 25 percent, and cardiac output increases by an additional 15 percent. Elevations in blood pressure and heart rate increase myocardial oxygen consumption. These acute increases in cardiac preload and myocardial work can undermine a previously compromised heart. Additionally, a prolonged second stage of labor should be avoided, since excessive Valsalva maneuvers produce a fall in blood pressure at the time of release, while continued bearing-down efforts progressively increase central venous pressure as well as systolic and diastolic blood pressures.[26]

The most striking changes that promote rapid cardiovascular decompensation occur in the immediate postpartum period, when cardiac output and stroke volume may increase by as much as 60 to 80 percent (Table 9–6).

The pregnant cardiac patient is extremely prone to develop cardiac decompensation during labor, delivery, and the immediate postpartum period. Successful management necessitates a thorough preanesthetic evaluation, detailing the mother's history of progressive exercise intolerance, with determination of the NYHA classification of her functional disability. A baseline physical examination is imperative, followed by necessary laboratory studies: complete blood count, serum electrolytes, blood urea nitrogen, creatinine, arterial blood gas and oxygen saturation measurements, 12-lead ECG, and, if readily available, noninvasive determination of cardiac output by echocardiography to rapidly assess cardiac function. Cardiac medications used during pregnancy should be continued throughout labor and delivery. Plasma levels of cardiac medications such as digoxin are measured at the time of admission. The use of heparin warrants pertinent coagulation tests.

MONITORING

General Measures

All pregnant cardiac patients deserve continuous electrocardiographic monitoring during labor, delivery, and the immediate postpartum period. Portable monitoring units with auto-

Table 9–6. CHANGE IN CARDIOVASCULAR PARAMETERS DURING PREGNANCY AND IMMEDIATELY AFTER DELIVERY

Parameter	Change With Pregnancy (%)	Change After Delivery (%)
Heart rate	+10–15	−15–20
Stroke volume	+20–30	+60–80
Cardiac output	+30–50	+60–80
Blood volume	+20–100	−10–20
Plasma volume	+70–80	−80
Red cell volume	+20–30	−10
Oxygen consumption	+20	−10–15

mated heart rate counters triggered by the ECG signal and easily visualized readouts prove useful for the patient care team, especially when following patients with valvular heart disease. Lead II of the standard ECG reveals cardiac arrhythmias most readily while precordial lead V_5 provides the best means for detecting anterolateral myocardial ischemia. Automated blood pressure monitoring (e.g., Dinamap), pulse oximetry, continuous monitoring of uterine contractions and fetal heart tones, in addition to strict measurement of input and output constitute the minimum standard of care for these patients.

Central Venous Pressure

Routinely, NYHA Class I and II patients do not require invasive hemodynamic monitoring. However, patients with Class III and IV status, especially those having a history of significant pulmonary hypertension or bidirectional or right-to-left shunting, deserve an intra-arterial line for continuous blood pressure monitoring and serial arterial blood gas determinations. Assessment of central venous pressure (CVP) is useful in parturients with moderately severe cardiac disease. CVP values do not always correlate with left ventricular filling pressures. CVP values will indicate changes in filling pressures in the right atrium (venous return) and right ventricle. In patients with normal cardiac function, CVP correlates relatively well with pressures in the left atrium and ventricle and serves as a guide to fluid management.

Pulmonary Artery Pressure

In comparison to CVP determinations, pulmonary capillary wedge pressure (PCWP) monitoring allows better assessment of left ventricular filling pressures and provides better information in management of patients with poor left ventricular function. Recent studies[18] show that the procedure carries no greater risk for pregnant than for nonpregnant persons. In addition to providing PCWP values a Swan-Ganz catheter offers other benefits, most notably thermodilution cardiac output measurements, which allow calculation of systemic and pulmonary vascular resistance. This information helps the patient-care team to provide therapy specifically aimed at favorable manipulation of preload, afterload, myocardial contractility, or combinations of these functions. However, the use of a Swan-Ganz catheter has been associated with significant morbidity and mortality. Dewitt and coworkers[27] reported a death caused by a pulmonary catheter in a patient with Eisenmenger's syndrome. The risk of thromboembolic phenomena increases with maintenance of the catheter for more than 3 days. Prolonged pulmonary hypertension and the resulting irreversible vascular changes may obscure the benefits. The potential risks should always be considered prior to placement.[27]

Cardiovascular Effects of Various Anesthetic Techniques

PREPARED CHILDBIRTH

Prepared childbirth and psychoprophylaxis during labor may be appropriate for NYHA Class I and II cardiac patients who have tolerated the physiologic changes and stresses of pregnancy. However, the method may be inadvisable for gravidas with cardiac decompensation, considering the previously mentioned changes during labor.

PARENTERAL MEDICATION

Tranquilizers

Small doses of phenothiazines used alone or in conjunction with narcotics to relieve anxiety during labor may produce orthostatic hypotension, readily cross the placenta, and affect thermoregulation in the newborn. Thus, caution dictates careful titration of small doses.

Narcotics

In moderate doses, narcotics produce analgesia and relieve anxiety but they may also cause peripheral vasodilation, hypotension, and respiratory depression. Meperidine induces tachycardia and should not be given to patients with severe mitral stenosis.

INHALATION ANALGESIA

Judicious use of subanesthetic concentrations of various inhalational agents during labor and delivery often proves unsatisfactory. Depth and quality of anesthesia may be unpredictable, and there is the possibility of overdose and loss of protective laryngeal reflexes which could lead to aspiration of gastric contents.

LUMBAR EPIDURAL ANALGESIA

Following epidural injection of local anesthetics, significant hemodynamic alterations can occur.[28] Vasodilation secondary to sympathetic blockade leads to decreased venous return, decreased cardiac output, and hypotension. In addition, significant vascular absorption may cause cardiac depression and decreased cardiac output. Patients with abnormally high sympathetic tone may experience greater hemodynamic changes. Solutions containing epinephrine stimulate beta receptors, leading to tachycardia, increased myocardial contractility and decreased peripheral vascular resistance, and should be avoided. Blockade of the upper thoracic (T1 – T4) cardiac sympathetic fibers may promote bradycardia and negative inotropy. Thus, epidural analgesia is the technique of choice for cardiac patients who would benefit from peripheral vasodilation and afterload reduction. Patients who have received narcotics and intravenous anesthetics may have dampened vascular reflex mechanisms and less ability to compensate for sympathetic blockade. In addition, decreases in systemic vascular resistance during epidural analgesia may lead to worsening of a right-to-left cardiac shunt in patients with cyanotic heart disease or septal defects.

Patients who have cardiovascular compromise tolerate epidural narcotics nicely. Fentanyl given alone in early labor or in combination with dilute bupivacaine (6 to 10 ml of 0.125-percent) during late labor does not cause significant hemodynamic change. Intrathecal injection of morphine, 0.5 to 1.0 mg of preservative-free drug in 1 to 2 ml of normal saline, also provides good pain relief during labor without producing significant blockade of autonomic fibers. Epidural and intrathecal opiates offer reasonable alternatives in patients with severe mitral stenosis, primary pulmonary hypertension, or Eisenmenger's syndrome.

The most common side effects include pruritus, nausea, vomiting, somnolence, urinary retention, and most important, respiratory depression which may be easily reversed with naloxone, 0.04 to 0.08 mg intravenously, followed by continuous infusion of 0.04 mg per hour if necessary.

SUBARACHNOID BLOCKADE

The intrathecal placement of local anesthetics, producing profound sympathetic, sensory, and motor blockade, may lead to severe hypotension and cardiovascular collapse in the pregnant cardiac patient, especially when used for cesarean section, despite thorough hydration and proper positioning. Thus, we recommend avoiding it in parturients with significant cardiovascular impairment.

GENERAL ANESTHESIA

General anesthesia utilizing a balanced technique, with intravenous induction agent, tracheal intubation, and maintenance with anesthetic gases, supplemental narcotics, and muscle relaxants, appears to be the technique of choice for cesarean section (see Chap. 6).

After preoxygenation for 5 min and a rapid-sequence induction with thiopental and succinylcholine to facilitate tracheal intubation, maintenance anesthesia, consisting of nitrous oxide, oxygen, and fentanyl, is begun. The anesthesia team must avoid cardiac depression (with deep levels of volatile agents), hypotension, hypoxia, tachycardia (in mitral stenosis), or reversal of cardiac shunts.

Laryngoscopy causes an adrenergic-mediated response. Increases in systemic vascular resistance, blood pressure, and cardiac output may be blunted by utilizing a modified rapid-sequence technique and intravenous lidocaine. The use of concomitant β-adrenergic blocker and/or supplemental narcotics will minimize the cardiovascular effects of tracheal intubation.[29]

Esmolol, a new short-acting beta blocker, reduces the adrenergic response to intubation and surgical stimulation, but has not currently received approval for obstetric use. The slightly longer-acting mixed alpha and beta blocker labetalol may be administered in slow incremental doses of 10 to 15 mg prior to intubation, although it too remains unapproved for obstetric use. Labetalol decreases heart rate, peripheral vascular resistance, and blood pressure while maintaining cardiac output and slightly improving uteroplacental blood flow.[30]

Alfentanil, an ultra–short-acting narcotic, may serve as an induction agent, but because it must be given in large doses, it may lead to neonatal respiratory depression. Etomidate, an alternate induction agent that spares the cardiovascular system and maintains cardiovascular stability during tracheal intubation, may be used for parturients with poor ventricular function. Induction with ketamine can produce sympathetic stimulation, hypertension, and tachycardia and should be avoided, particularly in gravidas with hypertrophic cardiomyopathy.

Specific Cardiac Lesions

ACQUIRED HEART DISEASE

Mitral Stenosis

Mitral stenosis represents the most common cardiac lesion seen by the anesthesiologist in pregnant women. A thorough history that elicits symptoms of fatigue and dyspnea, progressive decrease in activity, paroxysmal nocturnal dyspnea, orthopnea, and hemoptysis, should alert the anesthesiologist. When severe mitral stenosis exists (i.e., valvular pressure gradients >25 mmHg) acute cardiac decompensation may associate with atrial fibrillation and paroxysmal tachycardia, and pulmonary embolism, congestion, and infarction. During pregnancy, increases in heart rate, blood volume, cardiac output, and pulmonary blood volume aggravate mitral stenosis. Cardiac decompensation most likely occurs at 28 to 32 weeks (when blood volume is maximally increased), during the onset of labor, or early in the postpartum period. Serial determinations of vital capacity at 28 to 40 weeks' gestation assess the patient's adaptation to the physiologic changes of pregnancy and reflect cardiac decompensation during the last trimester of pregnancy. Some authorities suggest administering prophylactic digitalis, since loss of atrial kick associated with atrial fibrillation severely compromises left ventricular filling, stroke volume, and cardiac output. The finding of left ventricular dysfunction in gravidas with mitral stenosis suggests the presence of mitral insufficiency, aortic valve involvement, or inadequate coronary perfusion.

Anesthesia Considerations. Regardless of anesthetic method employed, the anesthesiologist must adhere to the following principles:

Prevent Rapid Ventricular Rates. The pregnant woman tolerates heart rates above 100 beats per min poorly, because the short diastolic interval impairs left ventricular filling and decreases cardiac output, leading to increased pulmonary artery pressures, pulmonary edema, and right heart failure. Therefore, drugs such as atropine, scopolamine, meperidine, ketamine, and pancuronium must be avoided. Additionally, increased anxiety levels or pain associated with labor increases maternal plasma catecholamine levels, resulting in tachycardia. Possible treatment of maternal tachycardia includes: cardioversion with 25 to 100 watt-sec;[22] propranolol, 0.2 to 0.5 mg intravenously every 3 min until the rate falls below 110 beats per min; and digoxin, 0.5 mg intravenously over 10 min followed by 0.25 mg intravenously every 2 hours to achieve complete digitalization, or small doses of verapamil or edrophonium.

Fluid Management. Rapid infusions of intravenous fluids or increases in central blood volume are to be avoided, since these may produce pulmonary hypertension, pulmonary edema, right heart failure, or atrial fibrillation. These may occur during acute volume preloading, overhydration, overtransfusion, or the Trendelenburg position. Appropriate monitoring of CVP and PCWP is necessary to assess increases in right and left atrial filling pressures.

Afterload Reduction. A rapid fall in systemic vascular resistance may produce reflex tachycardia as a homeostatic compensatory mechanism in the patient with severe mitral stenosis, possibly leading to heart failure. The judicious use of an intravenous infusion of an alpha agonist, such as metaraminol (10 mg in 250 ml of saline), re-establishes systemic vascular resistance and blood pressure but may simultaneously decrease uterine blood flow.[31] Metaraminol preserves uterine blood flow more effectively than neosynephrine or methoxamine and yet, like them, maintains systemic vascular resistance. Ephedrine may cause more rapid heart rates than the α-adrenergic vasopressors.

Pulmonary Vascular Considerations. Hypercarbia, hypoxia, acidosis, and hyperinflation of the lungs will increase pulmonary vascular resistance and pulmonary artery pressures, placing an increased work load on the right ventricle. The patient with right ventricular failure can receive inotropic support with dopamine (3 to 8 μg per kg per min) and pulmonary vasodilation with trimethaphan (1 mg per min) intravenously. Avoidance of high doses of sodium nitroprusside minimizes the possibility of fetal cyanide toxicity.[32]

Anesthesia for Vaginal Delivery. In consideration of the pathophysiology of mitral stenosis, the physiologic changes of pregnancy, and the events occurring at parturition, the ideal anesthetic technique would prevent maternal pain and tachycardia, dampen the cardiovascular changes associated with the urge to push, and prevent maternal fatigue and acidosis. Judicious administration of segmental lumbar epidural analgesia for labor and vaginal delivery produces all these desired effects.[33] To avoid the effects of the Valsalva maneuver, we recommend early introduction of perineal anesthesia with fetal descent accomplished by uterine contraction and delivery facilitated with vacuum extraction or outlet forceps. Local anesthetic solutions used for epidural block should not include epinephrine, because of the potential for tachycardia and peripheral vasodilation. Avoid aortocaval compression, which will enhance the cardiovascular changes associated with sympathetic blockade. Treat maternal hypotension with judicious infusions of balanced salt solution, using CVP and PCWP monitoring as a guide, as well as with additional left lateral displacement of the uterus.[34]

Anesthesia for Cesarean Section. Either regional or general anesthesia can be utilized. Most clinicians prefer continuous lumbar epidural block to spinal anesthesia because it provides a slower, more controllable onset of sympathetic blockade, especially when established gradually with small doses of local anesthetic. A CVP or Swan-Ganz catheter measures patient responses to a gradual fluid preload and sympathetic blockade. Spinal anesthesia may cause sudden maternal hypotension, resulting in maternal tachycardia and imposing the risks associated with excessive hydration and the use of vasopressors. If general anesthesia is selected for cesarean section, the technique must prevent maternal tachycardia. Therefore, glycopyrrolate is preferred over atropine when an anticholinergic agent is necessary. For muscle relaxation, succinylcholine—in a bolus dose or by continuous infusion—or vecuronium should supplant pancuronium. Anesthetic induction with 4 to 5 mg per kg thiopental is preferable to ketamine. A dose of 1.0 to 1.5 mg per kg intravenous lidocaine prior to induction, followed by 0.5-percent halothane, or 1.0-percent enflurane, nitrous oxide (40- to 50-percent), and oxygen (50- to 60-percent) for maintenance, may modify the sympathetic responses to surgical stimulation. Severe mitral stenosis may indicate an inhalation induction with a halothane, nitrous oxide-oxygen technique, possibly including a beta blocker to avoid postintubation tachycardia. The attendant risks of maternal gastric aspiration are modified by preanesthetic administration of oral antacids, a histamine blocker such as ranitidine (50 mg) or cimetidine (300 mg) intravenously or intramuscularly, metoclopramide (10 mg), and maintenance of cricoid pressure until tracheal tube placement and cuff inflation have been completed. The addition of an oral dose of ranitidine or climetidine the night before elective surgery provides even greater protection against aspiration pneumonitis.

Mitral Insufficiency

In contrast to those of mitral stenosis, the pathologic hemodynamic patterns in mitral insufficiency include diastolic volume overloading of the left ventricle, a decrease in effective forward stroke volume, and, thus, a decrease in left ventricular stroke ejection fraction. The regurgitated blood raises left atrial pressure and may produce increased PCWP values, pulmonary vascular congestion, and pulmonary edema. Additionally, advanced disease leads to left ventricular enlargement, hypertrophy, and failure, further promoting pulmonary hypertension and right ventricular compromise. By decreasing systemic vascular resistance, afterload reduction reduces pressure gradients across the aortic valve, increasing forward flow and decreasing mitral regurgitation.

Anesthesia Considerations. Generally speaking, physiologic responses or pharmacologic therapy, which increase systemic vascular resistance, compromise the patient with mitral insufficiency because of increased regurgitation of blood through the mitral valve. Depending on the patient's functional heart classification, appropriate invasive monitoring is recommended, especially the use of PCWP and continuous blood pressure recordings in severe disease. Additionally, as left ventricular work progressively increases to maintain adequate cardiac output, patients show poor tolerance for agents that acutely depress the myocardium or produce bradycardia, due to the decreases in stroke volume seen in severe cases. Mangano[1] recommends continuous monitoring of murmur intensity because changes in intensity correlate well with fluctuations in flow through the mitral valve.

Lumbar epidural analgesia is the method of choice for labor and vaginal delivery. By producing profound analgesia, it minimizes the release of catecholamines and the accompanying increased myocardial work. Sympathetic blockade also decreases peripheral vascular resistance and improves left ventricular performance through afterload reduction. Pulmonary congestion associated with this valvular lesion may also be reduced by means of lower left atrial pressures. These features of lumbar epidural block make it preferable to balanced general anesthesia for cesarean section, because the latter allows catecholamine release, thereby increasing peripheral vascular resistance.[1]

Mitral Valve Prolapse (Barlow's Syndrome)

Barlow and coworkers[35] have described mitral valve prolapse, a phenomenon characterized by either local hoodlike protrusion or a generalized ballooning of the mitral leaflet into the left atrium during left ventricular systole. This defect occurs as an isolated abnormality or presents secondarily in patients with mitral regurgitation, resulting from papillary muscle rupture or infarction. The lesion produces minimal degrees of mitral regurgitation, especially in women, so significant sequelae are relatively uncommon. The overall incidence remains unknown, although it occurs more commonly in women from the third to fifth decades of life. Interestingly, localized abnormalities of left ventricular contraction or relaxation frequently coexist with mitral valve prolapse but have little effect on ejection fraction or left ventricular diastolic pressure-volume relationships. However, severe mitral regurgitation may develop in 5 to 10 percent of patients, and ventricular arrhythmias have been reported.[35] In addition to arrhythmias, rupture of mitral chordae tendinae, platelet dysfunction, and endocarditis are the most common complications. Krantz and associates[36] recently associated coronary artery spasm as the cause of sudden death in patients with mitral valve prolapse.

Anesthesia Considerations. Our experience with five patients during parturition, all having NYHA Class I status, showed no untoward sequelae. Therefore, anesthetic management for vaginal delivery or cesarean section usually includes any of the regional or general anesthetic techniques. In patients who have sequelae, regional anesthesia should avoid excessive vasodilation, which facilitates prolapse, whereas during general anesthesia the sympathetic response to intubation and surgical stimulation must be circumvented. Intravenous narcotics may be necessary, and one should have a beta blocker ready. If severe mitral regurgitation coexists, the anesthetic considerations presented in the section on mitral regurgitation apply. The presence of regurgitation indicates administration of prophylactic antibiotics, especially in women undergoing complicated deliveries.

Aortic Stenosis

The basic hemodynamic problem of aortic stenosis is obstruction of outflow leading to left ventricular systolic pressure overloading. As valvular stenosis increases, the mean left ventricular to aortic pressure gradient increases along with the left ventricular ejection time. In advanced stages, the stroke volume falls, requiring an increase in left ventricular systolic pressure, which ultimately produces hypertrophy of the left ventricular wall. Left ventricular thickening, in conjunction with the high ventricular chamber pressures during systole, reduces subendocardial blood flow and subsequently produces ischemia. Significant tachycardia produces insufficient time for ejection of stroke volume through the narrowed valve while additionally increasing myocardial work. Vasodilation decreases mean aortic pressure, coronary artery perfusion pressure, and, hence, blood flow to the thickened myocardium.

Anesthesia Considerations. During parturition, these patients generally tolerate the increased catecholamine levels associated with labor and stress (unlike patients with mitral stenosis). Because acute changes in systemic vascular resistance can produce myocardial ischemia, the anesthesia team does best to avoid sympathetic blockade. Lumbar epidural analgesia has been used for labor but requires judicious administration with incremental injections of local anesthetics. Furthermore, the possibility of hypotension indicates continuous intra-arterial blood pressure monitoring. Aortocaval compression must be avoided by the use of left uterine displacement. One best manages hypotension with intravenous fluids and, when necessary, carefully titrated doses of intravenous vasopressors such as ephedrine.

Generally speaking, the use of parenteral analgesia for labor and pudendal blockade combined with inhalational analgesia for delivery provide safer maternal conditions than regional anesthesia. For cesarean section, we recommend general endotracheal anesthesia with thiopental, nitrous oxide, oxygen, and a muscle relaxant. Supplementation with halogenated agents requires extreme caution owing to possible effects on blood pressure and myocardial contractility. Continuous monitoring of lead V_5 usually detects signs of ventricular ischemia. When ST-segment changes occur, the systemic vascular resistance should be increased or maintained at previous levels with an infusion of metaraminol or phenylephrine.[37]

Hypertrophic Cardiomyopathy

Idiopathic hypertrophic subaortic stenosis (IHSS) is now considered to be an extreme manifestation of asymptomatic septal hypertrophy (ASH). In this relatively uncommon autosomal-dominant inherited disorder disproportionate hypertrophy of the intraventricular septum results in a variety of clinical and hemodynamic effects, although most patients are asymptomatic. The best known symptomatic subgroup, IHSS, involves substantial septal hypertrophy with bizarre-shaped myocardial cells. Bulging into the left ventricular cavity, this abnormal muscle contracts during ventricular systole in a manner which obstructs the ventricular outflow tract in mid- to late systole. Increases in myocardial contractility heighten the degree of outflow obstruction. Therefore, the administration of propranolol is the mainstay of current therapy, since it decreases myocardial contractility. Despite potential fetal hazards of chronic maternal propranolol therapy, the use of the drug should continue throughout pregnancy for control of maternal symptoms.

Generally, symptoms of IHSS increase during exercise, stress, or any condition that causes increased catecholamine secretion, such as labor and delivery. Therapy that decreases left atrial pressure and left ventricular end-diastolic volume (vasodilator agents) or increases left ventricular ejection velocity (β-adrenergic agonists) worsens the outflow gradient in IHSS, possibly causing severe arterial hypotension. Conversely, manipulations that increase arterial pressure (α-adrenergic agonists), and maintain left ventricular ejection velocity (propranolol), decrease transvalvular gradients and help to treat hypotension.

Anesthesia Considerations. Anesthesia for labor and delivery follows the principles formulated for severe aortic stenosis. Therefore, the use of systemic medication, inhalational analgesia, and paracervical and pudendal blocks is the safest methods for these patients. Conduction techniques such as spinal and epidural block may reduce systemic vascular resistance, thereby increasing the outflow obstruction. For cesarean section, we recommend general endotracheal anesthesia with the addition of a halogenated hydrocarbon (halothane 0.5-percent or enflurane 0.75-percent) due to the negative inotropic and chronotropic effects provided by these agents.

Aortic Insufficiency

The pathophysiology of aortic regurgitation consists of a decrease in net forward stroke volume because of diastolic regurgitation of blood from the aorta into the left ventricle. This retrograde flow produces both systolic and diastolic volume overloading. High systemic vascular resistance and bradycardia increase retrograde flow. The decrease in systemic vascular resistance and the increase in pulse rate normally associated with pregnancy can be beneficial in this condition. On the other hand, the hypervolemia of pregnancy, coupled with the pain and stress of labor (increased systemic vascular resistance) can produce left ventricular dysfunction and failure.

Anesthesia Considerations. Anesthesia for labor and vaginal delivery should resemble that for other procedures on patients who have mitral insufficiency. The sympathetic blockade of lumbar epidural analgesia prevents increases in peripheral systemic vascular resistance associated with pain, making the method well suited for those with significant regurgitation. One must be careful to prevent bradycardia; heart rates should be maintained between 80 and 100 beats per min. For cesarean section, the patient may receive either regional or general anesthesia, as previously described for mitral insufficiency.[1]

Cardiac Surgery During Pregnancy

Occasionally medical management of the pregnant cardiac patient with mitral stenosis fails, and progressive cardiac dysfunction severely compromises maternal and fetal well-being. This situation calls for cardiac surgery, ideally performed prior to 20 weeks' gestation but after the time of fetal organogenesis (12 to 14 weeks). Both mother and fetus usually tolerate mitral valvulotomy, which most often entails short cardiopulmonary bypass times and the use of normothermic perfusion. In contrast, mitral valve replacement necessitates open heart surgery with significant bypass times. The severity of symptoms requiring surgery presupposes a significant degree of residual disease involving the pulmonary artery, the presence of right heart failure, and possible left ventricular failure, in both the intraoperative and postoperative periods. The presence of atrial fibrillation increases the likelihood of pulmonary edema and the risk of systemic embolization. Generally, the use of fetal monitoring, maintenance of left lateral tilt position, and provision of normal perfusion pressures are recommended throughout surgery and the postoperative period.[38] Extensive cardiopulmonary bypass time correlates with significant fetal mortality,[39] and the following principles should be followed:

Precautions During Extensive Cardiopulmonary Bypass:

1. Fetal heart rate (FHR) monitoring roughly indicates satisfactory mean arterial pressure, regarding uterine blood flow and the condition of the fetus. During nonpulsatile flow on bypass, higher mean pressures generate higher rates of placental perfusion.
2. Maternal PaO_2 is kept around 200 torr. Temporary hyperoxia does not associate with deleterious maternal or fetal effects.
3. Although mild hypothermia (32°C to 34°C) has been reported with good fetal outcome, one should avoid profound hypothermia.
4. Pure α-adrenergic agonists should be used cautiously and only when required for maternal stability, for they diminish uterine blood flow. Consider dopamine, dobutamine, or metaraminol as alternative choices to methoxamine and phenylephrine.[40]
5. Heparinization does not initiate spontaneous bleeding into the placenta or fetus and does not cross the placenta.

Considerations After Valve Replacement. Fetal risks during mitral valve replacement relate to the effects of cardiopulmonary bypass, to the type of prosthesis used, and to the higher risk of thromboembolism which requires anticoagulation. Postoperatively, these patients may have a relatively fixed cardiac output and a greater degree of myocardial dysfunction.[41]

Conversely, patients receiving aortic valve replacement fare better following surgery, frequently demonstrating little cardiovascular impairment and, thus, a NYHA Class I status. They generally have normal cardiac output at rest and a normal response to both exercise and stresses related to pregnancy; residual pulmonary hypertension and ventricular compromise are less likely postoperatively. Frequently, these patients require no anticoagulation, since the risk of thromboembolism remains low. Antibiotic prophylaxis is recommended during parturition.

As stated previously, patients are best maintained on heparin near the time of delivery, since it does not cross the placenta and can be easily reversed. The use of regional anesthesia depends on consultation with members of the obstetric and cardiology teams to determine whether and when anticoagulants can be discontinued during labor and delivery. The anesthesia team should verify normal coagulation parameters before proceeding with regional anesthetic techniques.[41]

CONGENITAL HEART DISEASE

Congenital heart lesions account for less than 10 percent of heart disease in pregnant women. However, with improved methods of diagnosis and corrective surgery, many of these patients approach their reproductive years with a partially or fully corrected congenital heart lesion. The pathophysiology of congenital heart disease primarily entails a left-to-right or a right-to-left shunt. A left-to-right shunt occurs in the presence of a ventricular or atrial septal defect. The anesthesiologist must evaluate the cardiovascular status of such patients in consultation with a knowledgeable cardiologist. When available, data from cardiac catherization must be reviewed, especially if the congenital defect has not been completely corrected. In this way, the anesthesiologist will be well versed in the pathophysiology of the patient's particular lesion.

Ventricular Septal Defect

In most circumstances, ventricular septal defects are surgically corrected by the time a woman reaches her reproductive years, especially if lesions are large enough to create symptoms during childhood. However, an occasional patient achieves conception and still has an uncorrected symptomatic defect; the following physiologic parameters generally apply. Increased systemic vascular resistance intensifies the degree of left-to-right shunt, producing pulmonary hypertension and increased right ventricular work. These women also poorly tolerate marked increases in heart rate. In the presence of pulmonary hypertension and increased right ventricular pressure, substantial decreases in systemic vascular resistance may acutely produce a right-to-left shunt, leading to hypoxemia. Factors that further increase pulmonary vascular resistance, such as hypoxia, hypercarbia, or excessive pulmonary (inflation) pressures, should be avoided when there is pre-existing pulmonary hypertension and right ventricular compromise.

Atrial Septal Defect

Atrial septal defects infrequently produce symptoms unless pulmonary hypertension develops. Patients tolerate supraventricular arrhythmias and tachycardia poorly, since these conditions may increase systemic vascular resistance and decrease pulmonary vascular resistance, thus facilitating the degree of left-to-right shunting. Any factor that increases a left-to-right shunt will decrease left ventricular output and cause systemic hypotension. Increases in pulmonary vascular resistance will exacerbate pre-existing pulmonary hypertension, potentiate the development of right ventricular failure, and promote acute right-to-left shunts.

Anesthesia Considerations. For patients with ventricular or atrial septal defects, continuous segmental lumbar epidural block provides suitable anesthesia for vaginal delivery or cesarean section. This method avoids the hazards of increased systemic vascular resistance. One must take care, however, to prevent an imbalance between pulmonary and systemic vascular resistance, which may reverse shunt flow toward the left (manifested by peripheral cyanosis). This can be treated by increasing systemic vascular resistance, either by decreasing anesthetic dose or by giving small doses of vasopressors. Poor ventricular function calls for enriching the oxygen atmosphere, withdrawing anesthesia, and using inotropes such as dopamine. Patients with a history of significant pulmonary hypertension require continuous measurements of systemic blood pressure (by arterial cannula) and central venous pressure.

Tetralogy of Fallot

Tetralogy of Fallot and Eisenmenger's syndrome most commonly produce right-to-left shunt. Obstruction to outflow from the right ventricle (infundibular stenosis), right ventricular hypertrophy, ventricular septal defect, and an overriding aorta characterize tetralogy of Fallot. Survival to reproductive age necessitates corrective surgery, which usually includes closure of the ventricular septal defect and pulmonary valvulotomy (resection of the infundibular stenosis). Pregnancy does not contraindicate pulmonary valvulotomy.[42] Patients with corrected tetralogy of Fallot may exhibit right ventricular failure and require special care as in primary pulmonary hypertension. During anesthesia, inspired oxygen concentrations should be maximized while decreases in systemic vascular resistance, blood volume, venous return, and myocardial contractility must be avoided.

Anesthesia Considerations. Anesthesia for vaginal delivery can include inhalational analgesia, paracervical-pudendal block, or major regional anesthetic techniques, if extreme caution is observed. For cesarean section, general anesthesia with the judicious use of inhalation agents such as halothane or enflurane is preferable to regional anesthesia. In patients with significant infundibular stenosis, an increased right-to-left shunt with peripheral cyanosis may occur in association with tachycardia, hypoxia, hypercarbia, increased myocardial contractility, increased inflation pressures, or decreased right ventricular volume. Therefore, general anesthesia must be maintained at a level which maintains venous return. Significant increases in myocardial contractility and heart rate can be treated by intravenous propranolol.

Eisenmenger's Syndrome

Eisenmenger's syndrome represents an extreme form of cyanotic congenital heart disease. Although the incidence during pregnancy is low (2 to 4 percent), the syndrome produces maternal and fetal mortality of 33 percent and 50 percent, respectively. Long-standing atrial or ventricular septal defect, with the development of progressive pulmonary hypertension characterizes this syndrome.[43] The degree and direction of shunting depends on the severity of pulmonary hypertension; the shunt may be right-to-left or bidirectional. Women with advanced medial and intimal pulmonary vascular thickening and plexiform lesions have an exceptionally poor prognosis.[44] Pregnancy should be terminated prior to 12 weeks' gestation, if oxygen desaturation fails to respond to oxygen therapy.[25] Pregnancy aggravates the syndrome because pulmonary vascular resistance remains fixed while systemic vascular resistance decreases, thereby increasing the degree of right-to-left shunting, hypoxemia, and peripheral cyanosis. Progressive failure of the right ventricle further decreases pulmonary blood flow, functionally increasing the shunt.

Although patients with Eisenmenger's syndrome may be asymptomatic, the New York Heart classification is not a good prognosticator of outcome. All patients should be invasively monitored with a radial arterial line (for assessment of blood pressure and blood gas tensions) and a central venous pressure catheter. Pulmonary artery catheters present many risks but may be beneficial, particularly when using an oximetric Swan-Ganz catheter.[27] Most patients receive anticoagulants and deliver during a window in heparin therapy. The reversibility of the shunt must be assessed with oxygen, since death frequently results from acute increases in pulmonary vascular resistance, which may be successfully treated with 100-percent oxygen.[45]

Anesthesia Considerations. The anesthetic techniques employed in Eisenmenger's syndrome should maximize pulmonary blood flow and minimize increases in the right-to-left shunt. One must avoid decreases in systemic vascular resistance and venous return, as well as all factors that increase pulmonary vascular resistance (hypoxia, hypercarbia, increased inflation pressures, etc.).

Vaginal delivery utilizing epidural analgesia with minimal doses of local anesthetics, possibly combined with narcotics is the preferred method. Maternal mortality associated with vaginal delivery approaches 35 percent, whereas cesarean section confers a higher maternal mortality (60 percent). Some authorities recommend general anesthesia with fentanyl, ketamine, pure oxygen, and a relaxant for cesarean section. Cardiac depression and the theoretical increase in pulmonary vascular resistance associated with the use of inhalational agents and nitrous oxide, respectively, should be avoided.[46] Epidural anesthesia also has been used successfully despite the theoretical possibility of unwanted changes in preload and afterload.[47] Several investigators[48,49] failed to note increased shunt flow during epidural anesthesia to a T7 level for cesarean section.

Despite successful delivery utilizing a variety of anesthetic techniques, sudden death may occur any time during the first 2 weeks of the postpartum period; this has been attributed to pulmonary thromboembolism, hypotension, or a sudden increase in pulmonary vascular resistance. Therefore, these patients should be carefully monitored postoperatively in an intensive care setting. Hypovolemia and hypoxemia must be avoided. The duration of indwelling PA catheters should not exceed 3 days, since prolonged use may promote embolus formation, which presumably contributed to sudden death in one patient.[27]

OTHER HEART CONDITIONS

Primary Pulmonary Hypertension

By definition pulmonary hypertension exists when pulmonary artery pressures exceed 30/15 mmHg or mean pulmonary artery pressure exceeds 25 mmHg. Secondary to fixed, relatively nonreactive pulmonary vasculature, progressive pulmonary hypertension increases right ventricular work, leading to right ventricular hypertrophy and, eventually, to failure.

Also referred to as "idiopathic pulmonary hypertension," the disorder occurs most often in young women in whom progressive involvement produces death within 2 years of onset of symptoms. Secondary pulmonary hypertension may relate to mitral stenosis, pulmonary venous stenosis, intravenous drug abuse, interstitial fibrosis, and chronic obstructive pulmonary disease.

Pulmonary hypertension begets more pulmonary hypertension unless the underlying cause is identified and corrected early. Progressive right ventricular hypertrophy occurs subsequent to increasing pulmonary vascular resistance. A relatively fixed and low cardiac output leads to increased systemic vascular resistance. Eventually, cardiac failure occurs. Symptoms include dyspnea on exertion, dizziness, syncope, fatigue, hemoptysis, and chest pain. Physical examination reveals right ventricular heave, a loud second heart sound, peripheral cyanosis, and clubbing.

Pregnancy, labor, and delivery exacerbate pulmonary hypertension which is associated with maternal mortality of 50 percent. Most deaths occur immediately postpartum or within the first 7 days, from intractable cardiac failure or thromboembolism. Often, the cause of death is unknown. Fetal wastage occurs more commonly since pulmonary hypertension produces a very high rate of spontaneous abortion and prematurity. Continuous monitoring of radial artery and pulmonary artery pressures is mandatory in these patients.

Anesthesia Considerations. Successful management of patients with primary pulmonary hypertension requires careful attention to the following principles:

1. Preanesthetic evaluation must include determination of severity of pulmonary hypertension and reactivity of the pulmonary vasculature to vasodilators (nitroprusside, tolazoline, and phentolamine). Oxygen, however, is the pulmonary vasodilator of choice. The presence of congestive heart failure must be ascertained.
2. When possible, the anesthesia team should avoid increased pulmonary vascular resistance, which occurs with hypercarbia, hypoxia, acidosis, large ventilatory (tidal) volumes, vasopressors, and stress. Mothers should receive supplemental oxygen at all times, including in the puerperium.
3. Marked increases or decreases in preload which affect right ventricular volume and pressures are poorly tolerated.
4. Acute increases in myocardial oxygen consumption and systemic hypotension should

be avoided since the fixed ventricular output limits cardiac output. Thus, the anesthesiologist attempts to maintain systemic vascular resistance and to avoid myocardial depression.

Anesthesia for labor and vaginal delivery should include only those drugs and techniques that produce minimal cardiovascular effects, namely intravenous narcotics, inhalational analgesia, and paracervical and/or pudendal nerve blocks. Sufficient doses of intravenous sedatives and narcotics allay apprehension and reduce discomfort but necessitate close attention to maternal ventilation and the possibility of drug depression in the neonate. Intermittent measurement of arterial blood gas tensions helps to assess the degree of hypoventilation (hypercarbia) as well as oxygen requirements. Sorenson[47] describes the successful use of selective, segmental epidural analgesia during labor combined with bilateral pudendal block for delivery. Complications associated with epidural or spinal anesthesia arise from decreased systemic vascular resistance and reduction in venous return. Intrathecal morphine avoids these effects. Subarachnoid injection of hyperbaric morphine provides excellent analgesia during early labor without any significant autonomic or motor effects. Abboud[50] reported on the method in two patients with pulmonary hypertension, noting good analgesia and an uneventful immediate postpartum course, although both patients succumbed 7 to 9 days following delivery. Death in this group of patients could relate to increased venous return (autotransfusion) after delivery, right heart failure, or increased pulmonary resistance.

For cesarean section, these patients probably tolerate general anesthesia better than conduction techniques, due to the possibility of decreased preload and hypotension frequently occurring with regional blocks. Controlled ventilation, with tidal volumes of 5 to 10 ml per kg, should prevent increases in pulmonary vascular resistance and overinflation of the lungs. The use of an end-tidal carbon dioxide monitor assures prevention of hypoventilation and hypercarbia. Pulse oximetry provides important information regarding adequacy of arterial oxygenation and necessary adjustments in FIO_2. To avoid cardiovascular depression, we prefer induction with ketamine (1 mg per kg) or etomidate, with small doses of fentanyl or alfentanil; we avoid nitrous oxide due to its effect on the pulmonary vasculature. Halogenated agents are used very cautiously.

Myocardial Infarction

Hankins and Wendel[51] recently reviewed the anesthetic considerations of myocardial infarction during pregnancy. As a result of the increased incidence of smoking, postponement of child bearing, and the pervasiveness of ischemic heart disease in the United States, myocardial infarction occurs more frequently during pregnancy now than in past decades. While it is still quite uncommon, the problem relates to a maternal mortality of 30 to 40 percent.[52] Better maternal survival occurs following myocardial infarction in the first and second trimester than in the third trimester and postpartum period. The majority of parturients with a history of myocardial infarction also have a history of hyperlipidemia.

The presence of severe coronary artery disease indicates continual surveillance of cardiac status during the second and third trimesters. Appropriate therapy to provide optimal cardiac function is instituted and maintained to facilitate uncomplicated parturition. During labor and delivery, arterial and PCWP measurements and ECG lead V_5 are monitored continuously.

Timing of delivery with respect to the infarction is critical. Delivery within 2 weeks of infarction is associated with a maternal mortality of 50 percent.[51] However, if one can postpone delivery more than 2 weeks postinfarction, the incidence of death becomes zero. Fetal mortality appears to associate primarily with maternal outcome, generally occurring at the time of infarction. Following infarction, vaginal delivery correlates with a more stable course and a significantly lower maternal mortality rate (14 percent) as compared to delivery by cesarean section (23 percent).[51]

Anesthesia Considerations. For vaginal delivery, regional techniques generally provide the best conditions for parturients with severe coronary artery disease. The reductions in afterload resulting from spinal or epidural blocks benefit the patient, decreasing left ventricular work and myocardial oxygen consumption. Regardless of anesthetic method used, nitroglycerin in the form of sublingual tablets, cutaneous paste, or intravenous infusion should be immediately available and initiated when ECG (lead V_5) monitoring detects myocardial ischemia. Significant hypotension and myocardial hypoperfusion can be avoided by uterine displacement, thorough prehydration, and vasopressor, if necessary. During general anesthesia, efforts should proceed to prevent maternal hypertension and tachycardia by using intravenous nitroglycerin and propranolol, respectively, especially during laryngoscopy and tracheal intubation.

The principles of management of pregnancy following a previous myocardial infarction and aortocoronary artery bypass grafting have recently been outlined by Chestnut.[53] Cardiac function should be assessed by serial ECGs, echocardiography, and exercise tolerance tests. Propranolol should be continued during pregnancy to reduce myocardial oxygen demand and decrease anginal episodes. Abrupt withdrawal of beta blockers will lead to rebound β-adrenergic receptor stimulation. Maintenance of lateral uterine displacement, administration of supplemental oxygen, and early institution of regional anesthesia are emphasized for uncomplicated vaginal delivery. Anesthetic considerations are similar for the patient with recent myocardial infarction; however, patients with good cardiovascular function and no angina can receive treatment with any technique.

Summary

The occasionally formidable obstacles in anesthesia for the pregnant cardiac patient during labor and delivery can be safely surmounted with judicious use of drugs, conscientious induction of anesthesia, and careful invasive monitoring of hemodynamic and biochemical performance. The beneficial effects of epidural analgesia on preload and afterload, the lack of interference with myocardial contractility, the minimal effects on sensorium, and persistence of analgesia into the postoperative period often make this method particularly valuable for pregnant cardiac patients.

Regardless of anesthetic method used, one should prevent an imbalance between myocardial oxygen demand and blood supply.[54] Myocardial contractility and blood flow must be maintained at levels sufficient to sustain both mother and fetus. The hemodynamic alterations during labor, especially tachycardia, hypotension, hypertension or increased left ventricular filling pressures, should be recognized and treated promptly. The massive sympathetic stimulation associated with laryngoscopy and endotracheal intubation under light general anesthesia is a major concern in this area. The hemodynamic alterations associated with remission of anesthetic effect should be recognized and treated promptly, necessitating intensive care in the postpartum as well as the intrapartum period.

References

1. Mangano, DT: Anesthesia for the cardiac patient. In Shnider, SM and Levinson, G (eds): Anesthesia for Obstetrics. Williams & Wilkins, Baltimore, 1987.
2. Ueland, K, et al: Maternal cardiovascular dynamics: IV. The influence of gestational age on the maternal cardiovascular response to posture and exercise. Am J Obstet Gynecol 104:856, 1969.
3. Kahler, RL: Cardiac Disease. In Burrow, GN and Ferris, TF (eds): Medical Complications During Pregnancy. WB Saunders, Philadelphia, 1975, p 105.
4. Ueland, K, Metcalfe, J and Novy, MJ: Hemodynamic responses of patients with heart disease to pregnancy and exercise. Am J Obstet Gynecol 113:47, 1972.
5. Rubler, S, et al: Cardiac size and performance during pregnancy estimated with echocardiography. Am J Cardiol 40:534, 1977.
6. Elkayam, U and Gleicher, N (ed): Cardiovascular physiology of pregnancy. In Cardiac Problems in Pregnancy. Alan R Liss, New York, 1982.
7. Elkayam, U and Gleicher, N: Cardiac problems in pregnancy. JAMA 251:2838, 1984.
8. Metcalfe, J and Ueland, K: Maternal cardiovascular adjustments to pregnancy. Prog Cardiovasc Dis 16:363, 1974.
9. Burwell, CS and Metcalfe, J: Heart Disease and Pregnancy. Little, Brown & Co, Boston, 1958.
10. McAnulty, JH, et al: General guidelines in the management of cardiac disease. Clin Obstet Gynecol 24:773, 1981.
11. Ostheimer, GW and Alper, MH: Intrapartum anesthetic management of the pregnant patient with heart disease. Clin Obstet Gynecol 18:81, 1975.
12. Rahimtoola, SH: The need for cardiac catheterization and angiography if valvular heart disease is not disproven. Ann Intern Med 97:433, 1982.
13. Elkayam, U, et al: Contrast echocardiography to reduce ionizing radiation associated with cardiac catheterization during pregnancy. Am J Cardiol 52:213, 1983.
14. Sullivan, JM and Ramanathan, KB: Management of medical problems in pregnancy: Severe cardiac disease. N Engl J Med 313:304, 1985.
15. Berkowitz, RL and Rafferty, TD: Pulmonary artery flow-directed catheter use in the obstetric patient. Obstet Gynecol 55:507, 1980.

16. Boyd, KD, et al: A prospective study of complications of pulmonary artery catheterizations. Chest 84:245, 1983.
17. Clark, SL, Horenstein, JM and Phelan, JP: Experience with the pulmonary artery catheter in obstetrics and gynecology. Am J Obstet Gynecol 152:374, 1985.
18. Cotton, DB and Benedetti, TJ: Use of the Swan-Ganz catheter in obstetrics and gynecology. Obstet Gynecol 56:641, 1980.
19. Smith, MD, et al: Value and limitations of continuous-wave Doppler echocardiography in estimating severity of valvular stenosis. JAMA 255:3145, 1986.
20. Mason, SJ: Cardiac failure and arrhythmias during pregnancy. In Berkowitz, RL (ed): Critical Care of the Obstetric Patient. Churchill Livingstone, New York, 1983.
21. Ueland, K: The pregnant cardiac patient. In Queenan, JT (ed): Management of High-Risk Pregnancy. Medical Economics, Oradel, 1980.
22. Schroeder, JS and Harrison, DC: Repeated cardioversion during pregnancy: Treatment of refractory paroxysmal atrial tachycardia during three successive pregnancies. Am J Cardiol 27:445, 1971.
23. Sugrue, D, et al: Pregnancy complicated by maternal heart disease at the National Maternity Hospital, Dublin, Ireland, 1969–1978. Am J Obstet Gynecol 139:1, 1981.
24. Berkowitz, RL: Critical Care of the Obstetric Patient. Churchill Livingstone, New York, 1983
25. Conradsson, TB and Werko, L: Management of heart disease in pregnancy. Prog Cardiovasc Dis 16:407, 1974.
26. Hansen, JM and Ueland, K: Maternal cardiovascular dynamics during pregnancy and parturition. In Marx, GF (ed): Parturition and Perinatology. FA Davis, Philadelphia, 1974.
27. Dewitt, JH, Noble, WH and Byrick, RJ: A Swan-Ganz catheter related complication in a patient with Eisenmenger's syndrome. Anesthesiology 57:335, 1982.
28. Bonica, JJ, et al: Circulatory effects of peridural block: I. Effects of level of analgesia and dose of lidocaine. Anesthesiology 33:619, 1970.
29. Datta, S and Alper, MH: Anesthesia for cesarean section. Anesthesiology 53:142, 1980.
30. Kanto, JH: Current status of labetalol, the first alpha- and beta-blocking agent. Int J Clin Pharmacol Ther Toxicol 23:617, 1985.
31. Ralston, DH, Shnider, SM and deLorimier, AA: Effects of equipotent ephedrine, metaraminol, mephentermine, and methoxamine, on uterine blood flow in the pregnant ewe. Anesthesiology 40:354, 1974.
32. Naulty, J, Cefalo, R and Lewis, PE: Fetal toxicity of nitroprusside in the pregnant ewe. Am J Obstet Gynecol 139:708, 1981.
33. Bromage, PR: Epidural Analgesia. WB Saunders, Philadelphia, 1978, p 513.
34. Marx, GF: Aortocaval compression: Incidence and prevention. Bull NY Acad Med 50:443, 1974.
35. Barlow, JB, et al: The significance of late systolic murmurs. Am Heart J 66:443, 1963.
36. Krantz, EM, et al: Mitral valve prolapse. Anesth Analg 59:379, 1980.
37. Laver, M and Lowenstein, E: Anesthesia and the patient with heart disease. In Johnson, RQ, Haber, E and Austen, WG (eds): The Practice of Cardiology. Little, Brown & Co, Boston, 1980, p 1103.
38. Levy, DL, Warriner, RA and Burgess, GE: Fetal response to cardiopulmonary bypass. Obstet Gynecol 56:112, 1980.
39. Becker, RM: Intracardiac surgery in pregnant women. Ann Thorac Surg 36:453, 1983.
40. Fishburne, JI, et al: Vascular and uterine responses to dobutamine and dopamine in the gravid ewe. Am J Obstet Gynecol 137:944, 1980.
41. Saka, DM and Marx, GF: Management of a parturient with cardiac valve prosthesis. Anesth Analg 55:214, 1976.
42. Baker, JL, et al: Closed pulmonary valvotomy in the management of Fallot's tetralogy complicated by pregnancy. J Obstet Gynaecol Br Commonw 70:154, 1963.
43. Piolo, AK and Herren, AL: Eisenmenger's syndrome and pregnancy. Anesthesiol Rev 6:9, 1979.
44. Alpert, JS: Physiopathology of the Cardiovascular System. Little, Brown & Co, Boston, 1984.
45. Midwall, J and Taffin, H: Shunt flow and pulmonary hemodynamics during labor and delivery in the Eisenmenger syndrome. Am J Cardiol 42:299, 1978.
46. Schulte-Sasse, U: Pulmonary vascular response to nitrous oxide in patients with normal and high vascular resistance. Anesthesiology 57:9, 1982.
47. Sorensen, MD and Korshin, JD: The use of epidural analgesia for delivery in a patient with pulmonary hypertension. Acta Anesth Scand 26:180, 1982.
48. Spinnato, JA, et al: Eisenmenger's syndrome in pregnancy: Epidural anesthesia for elective cesarean section. N Engl J Med 304:1215, 1981.
49. Asling, JH and Fung, DL: Epidural anesthesia in Eisenmenger's syndrome: A case report. Anesth Analg 53:965, 1974.
50. Abboud, TK, Raya, J and Noueihed, R: Intrathecal morphine for relief of labor pain in a parturient with severe pulmonary hypertension. Anesthesiology 59:477, 1983.
51. Hankins, GD and Wendel, GD: Myocardial infarction during pregnancy: A review. Obstet Gynecol 65:139, 1985.
52. Abboud, TK, et al: Anesthetic management of the parturient with a recent myocardial infarction. Anesth Rev 12:17, 1980.
53. Chestnut, DH, et al: Pregnancy in a patient with a history of myocardial infarction and coronary artery bypass grafting. Am J Obstet Gynecol 155:372, 1986.
54. Curtris, J: The effects of painful uterine contractions, position, and epidural anesthesia on maternal transcutaneous oxygen tension (+cPO2). Anesthesiology 53: S315, 1980.

Bibliography

Berkowitz, RL: Critical Care of the Obstetric Patient. Churchill Livingstone, New York, 1983.

Bonica, JJ: Obstetric analgesia and anesthesia. World Federation of Societies of Anesthesiologists, Amsterdam, 1980.

Hurst, JW: The Heart, ed 4. McGraw-Hill, New York, 1978.
Johnson, RA, Haber, E and Austen, WG: The Practice of Cardiology. Little, Brown & Co, Boston, 1980.
Joyce, TH: Cardiac disease. In James, FM and Wheeler, AS (eds): Obstetric Anesthesia: The Complicated Patient. FA Davis, Philadelphia, 1982, p 87.
Kahler, RL: Cardiac disease. In Burrow, GN and Ferris, TF (eds): Medical Complications During Pregnancy. WB Saunders, Philadelphia, 1975, p 105.
Mangano, DT: Anesthesia for the cardiac patient. In Shnider, SM and Levinson, G (eds): Anesthesia for Obstetrics. Williams & Wilkins, Baltimore, 1986.
Mendelson, CL: Cardiac Disease in Pregnancy. FA Davis, Philadelphia, 1960.

CHAPTER 10

RESPIRATORY DISEASE

MARK C. NORRIS, M.D.

Pregnancy produces considerable changes in the pulmonary physiology of the mother. In the presence of respiratory disease pulmonary function can be further taxed; altered pulmonary function may adversely affect fetal growth and development. Fortunately, in most cases, women with respiratory dysfunction tolerate their pregnancies well. However, among severely affected patients with chronic hypoxemia and borderline respiratory status there can be significant maternal and fetal morbidity. In this chapter, I shall review the pathophysiology of several respiratory diseases and develop an understanding of how these diseases "interact" physiologically with pregnancy. I shall review the therapies for these diseases and the special concerns of managing patients with respiratory disease during parturition. Finally, I shall explore how pregnancy and pulmonary disease affect the anesthetic management of these women, beginning with asthma, the most common serious respiratory ailment in pregnancy. I shall also consider other types of obstructive diseases including: emphysema, bronchitis, bronchiectasis, cigarette smoking, and cystic fibrosis. Then I shall review infectious diseases, sarcoidosis, and pulmonary malignancy. Finally I shall discuss acute respiratory distress syndrome (ARDS) and the management of ventilatory failure in the parturient.

Physiology of Pregnancy and Respiratory Disease

Pregnancy requires extra efforts from the respiratory system. Oxygen consumption and minute ventilation increase significantly, the latter more than the former, and in normal patients, relative hyperventilation occurs.[1,2] In contrast, patients with respiratory disease may have smaller increases in minute ventilation, and those with severe disease may increase their ventilation only to match (but not exceed) their rising oxygen demand (Fig. 10–1).[1]

Asthma

Asthma, a multifactorial disease of uncertain etiology, is characterized by intermittent bronchospasm in response to a variety of stimuli. Its severity changes either spontaneously or with

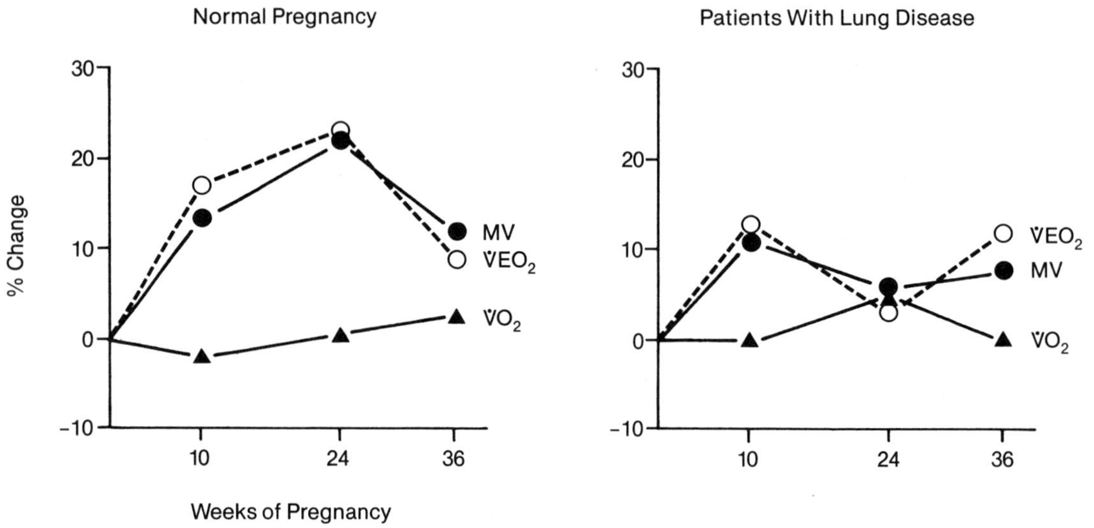

Figure 10 – 1. Changes in minute ventilation (MV) oxygen uptake ($\dot{V}O_2$), and ventilatory equivalent for oxygen ($\dot{V}EO_2$) throughout pregnancy. (Adapted from Gazioglu K, et al,[1] p 445, with permission.)

treatment. It has been posited that "Asthma is actually a collection of poorly understood inflammatory events of the airways that is not well subdivided into etiologic or mechanistic events."[3] However, bronchial hyperactivity is a common denominator of all types of asthma. Inciting factors vary from individual to individual, but a classification according to the etiologic factors may aid in guiding appropriate therapy.[4] A simple classification divides causes into extrinsic (allergy to inhalants and irritants) and intrinsic ("The cause lies within the patient's body"[5]). Inviting as this classification may seem, tremendous heterogeneity exists among asthmatics and the potential settings and stimulants for each patient's asthma should be sought.[6] Common inciting factors include: IgE-mediated immediate hypersensitivity, acute respiratory tract infections, non – IgE mediated reactions to inhaled irritants (smoke, dust, air pollution), aspirin intolerance, bronchodilator abuse, exercise, atmospheric change (cold air), and emotional upset.[4,6] In many, the specific inciting factors are unknown (idiopathic).[4,6] In an individual patient, one or several elements may predominate, but others may have contributing influence and should not be neglected.

PATHOPHYSIOLOGY

The pathophysiology of asthma is extremely complex and only poorly understood. For a more detailed discussion, the reader should refer to the admirably detailed text by Weiss, Segal, and Stein.[7] The process begins with IgE molecules binding to special receptors on mast cell membranes (Fig. 10 – 2). This binding initiates a series of enzymatic reactions resulting in a change in membrane fluidity, influx of calcium ions, release of preformed mediators, and synthesis and release of other mediators. In addition to histamine, these mediators include the products from the cyclo-oxygenase and lipo-oxygenase pathways of arachidonic acid metabolism: prostaglandins E_2 and D_2 and the leukotrienes LTC_4, LTD_4 (Tables 10 – 1, 10 – 2). Other mediators involved include platelet-activating factors, bradykinin, products of the complement cascade (C3a and C5a), and eosinophilic chemotactic factor.[4,8–11] In addition to inciting contraction of bronchial smooth muscle, these compounds increase vascular permeability and chemically attract a variety of inflammatory cells. These actions produce the other hallmarks of bronchial asthma: mucosal edema, epithelial damage, and increased mucus production. Cell damage, possibly caused by eosinophil products, exposes sensory receptors located immediately beneath the epithelium. Stimulation of these axons may result in recurrent local reflex[12] or vagally mediated[13] bronchoconstriction, tissue edema, and mucus secretion (Fig. 10 – 3).

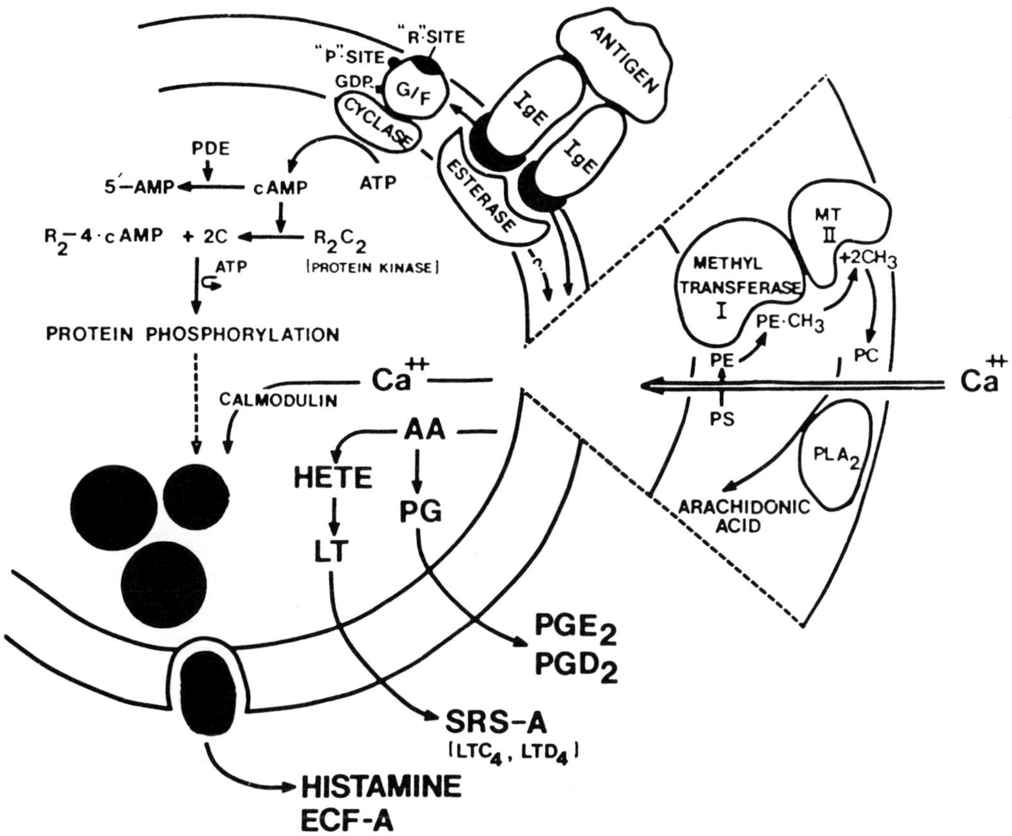

Figure 10–2. Mast cell schematic of the biochemical events of mediator release. PDE = phosphodiesterase; G/F = GTP binding, fluoride-activated regulatory protein "R"-site = adenosine-binding site activated by analogs containing an unaltered ribose moiety; "P"-site = adenosine-binding site activated by adenosine analogs containing an intact purine ring; R_2C_2 = inactive protein kinase tetramer containing two catalytic (C) and two regulatory (R) proteins; AA = arachidonic acid; HETE = hydroxyeicosatetraenoic acid; PG = phosphatidylserine; PE = phosphatidylethanolamine; $PE \cdot CH_3$ = monomethylphosphatidylethanolamine; $+2CH_3$ = addition of two methyl groups forming phosphatidylcholine (PC); PLA_2 = phospholipase A_2. (From Weiss EB, Segal MS and Stein,[7] with permission.)

Diffuse bronchial smooth muscle hypertrophy is one of the most prominent pathologic changes seen in asthmatics. In addition, hyperplastic goblet cells and enlarged mucus glands produce copious amounts of thick tenacious secretions, resulting in widespread bronchial plugging. Microscopic examination reveals extensive exudative inflammation, marked edema of the airway walls, eosinophilic infiltration, epithelial shedding and destruction, and a thickened basement membrane with evidence of increased epithelial cell turnover.[14]

Smooth muscle contraction, mucus plugging, and airway narrowing and obstruction involve both large and small airways. As resistance to air flow increases, forced expiratory volume (FEV_1) and peak expiratory flow rate (PEFR) decrease.[15] Incomplete exhalation with air trapping increases functional residual capacity (FRC) and residual volume (RV). As lung volumes increase, dynamic compliance improves initially but then worsens as hyperinflation stretches lung tissues more and more (Fig. 10–4). These changes in airway resistance and compliance increase the work of breathing, recruit accessory muscles of respiration, and increase oxygen consumption.[16]

Hypoxia commonly occurs during asthma attacks. When a person breathes room air hypoxemia can be expected when FEV_1 falls below 30 to 60 percent of predicted values. Maldistribution of ventilation and perfusion usually cause this hypoxia. Ventilation scans in asthmatics are grossly abnormal with segmental and lobar

Table 10-1. CYCLO-OXYGENASE AND LIPOXYGENASE PRODUCTS THAT HAVE A ROLE IN ASTHMA AND ALLERGY

Cyclo-oxygenase Products

Compound	*Tissue Source*	*Action*
PGD_2	Mast cells	Inhibits platelet aggregation, possibly prevents release of PAF Constricts pulmonary artery and airways
PGE_2	Many cells, macrophages	Relaxes smooth muscle of airways and microvasculature Potentiates vascular actions of LTB_4 and LTD_4. Immunosuppressant
$PGF_{2\alpha}$	Many cells	Contracts smooth muscle of airways and microvasculature
PGI_2 (prostacyclin)	Vascular endothelium, brain, lung parenchyma, kidney	Relaxes arterioles; dilates pulmonary vessels Reverses platelet aggregation Minimal effects on airways
Thromboxane	Platelets, lung parenchyma	Aggregates platelets Constricts arterioles, pulmonary vessels, and airways

Lipoxygenase Products

Compound	*Tissue Source*	*Action*
5-HETE	Granulocytes	Chemotaxis* granulocytes Chemokinesis† granulocytes, T lymphocytes Augments histamine release
12-HETE	Platelets	Chemotaxis,* chemokinesis†
15-HETE	T lymphocytes, lungs	Inhibits 5-lipoxygenase WBC, 12-lipoxygenase platelets Major arachidonic acid product in lung
5,12-diHETE	Granulocytes	Chemotaxis,* chemokinesis†
LTB_4	Granulocytes	Potent chemotactant for neutrophils, eosinophils
	Macrophages, eosinophils	Causes adhesion of leukocytes to endothelium and migration of white blood cells into extravascular space Constricts airways
LTC_4	Mast cells	Constricts peripheral and central airways
LTD_4, SRS	Macrophages	Constricts coronary arteries, pulmonary vessels
LTE_4	Eosinophils Basophils	Increases vascular permeability → edema Increases bronchial mucus, slows transport

*Chemotactic potency: LTB_4 >> 5-HETE > 5,12–diHETE > 12–HETE
†Chemokinesis refers to random migration leukocytes.
(From Weiss EB, Segal MS and Stein M,[7] p 164, with permission.)

areas of reduced ventilation[17] and areas of ventilation and perfusion mismatching.[18] Hyperventilation and hypocarbia ($PaCO_2$ 25 to 35 mmHg) usually accompany the hypoxemia. A rise of $PaCO_2$ to normal or higher signifies the onset of ventilatory failure, an indication for mechanical ventilation and a poor prognostic sign.

PREGNANCY AND ASTHMA

Theoretical Considerations

Several of the physiologic changes associated with pregnancy potentially interact with maternal asthma. Minute ventilation increases with resultant respiratory alkalosis.[19] Normal blood gases in a parturient include $PaCO_2$ between 27

Table 10–2. SELECTED MAST CELL MEDIATORS AND THEIR PROPOSED PHYSIOLOGIC FUNCTION IN ASTHMA

Mediator	Proposed Role in Asthma
Preformed rapidly released mediators	
Histamine	Bronchoconstrictor
Eosinophil chemotactic factor of anaphylaxis	Eosinophil infiltration
Neutrophil chemotactic factors	Neutrophil infiltration
Superoxide anions	Thickening of basement membrane
Kininogenase	Production of bradykinin, a bronchoconstrictor
Newly synthesized mediators	
Prostaglandins $F_{2\alpha}$, D_2	Bronchoconstriction
Thromboxane A_2	Bronchoconstriction
Prostaglandin E_2, I_2	Bronchodilation
Leukotrienes C_4, D_4, E_4	Bronchoconstriction
Leukotriene B_4	Chemotaxis of neutrophils and eosinophils
Acetyl glyceryl ether phosphorylcholine (PAF)	Bronchoconstriction (PAF is a potent bronchoconstrictor in monkeys.)

(From Greenberger PA,[4] p 578, with permission.)

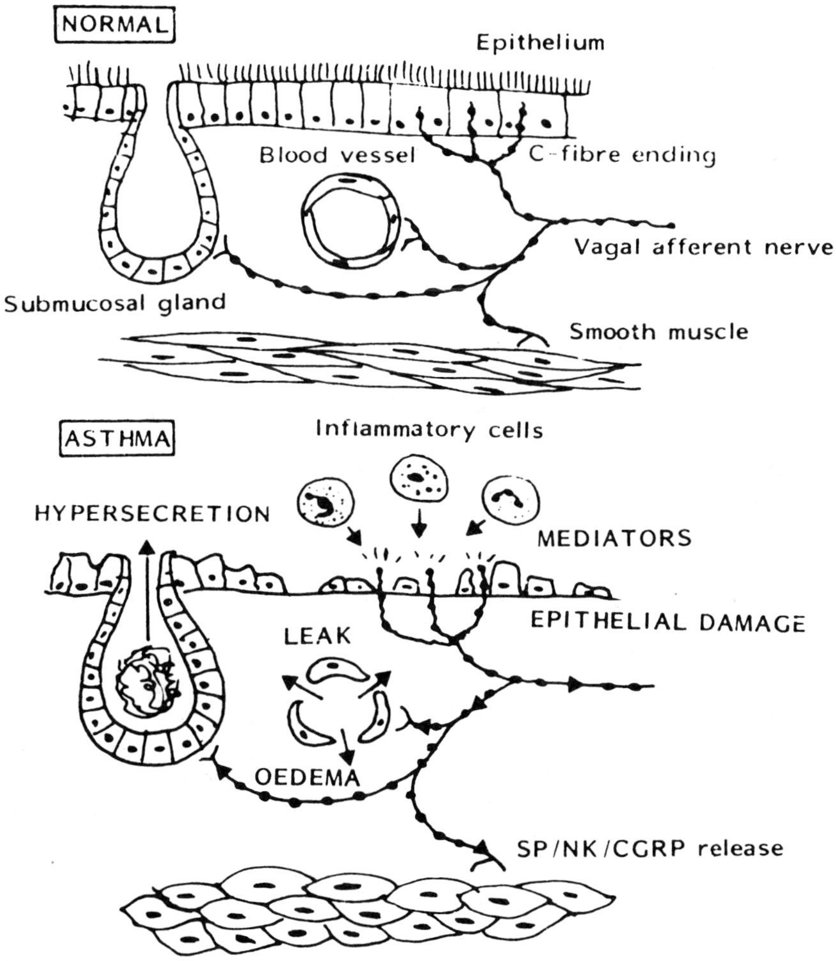

Figure 10–3. Axon reflex mechanisms in asthma. Damage to airway epithelium, possibly by eosinophil products, exposes C-fiber nerve endings. Stimulation results in a local (axon) reflex with antidromic conduction down afferent nerve collaterals and release of sensory neuropeptides including, substance P (SP), neurokinin A (NA), and calcitonin gene-related protein (CGRP). These peptides are potent airway constrictors and induce bronchial edema, mucous hypersecretion and inflammatory cell infiltration. (From Barnes PJ,[12] with permission.)

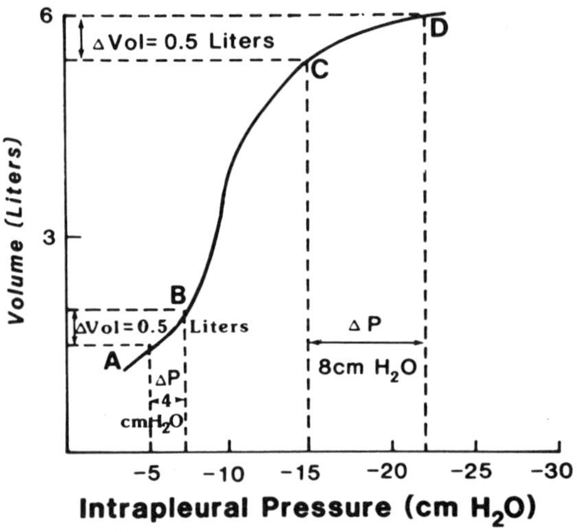

Figure 10–4. A compliance curve showing change in lung volume on y-axis and change in intrapleural pressure on the x-axis. Normal ventilation occurs on the lower, flattened part of the curve (A-B) as FRC increases. During an episode of bronchospasm, compliance initially improves (D-C), but eventually the lung becomes hyperinflated and progressively greater changes in intrapleural pressure are required to generate adequate tidal volumes (C-D). (From Kingston HGG, Hirshman CA,[16] with permission.)

and 32 mmHg and pH between 7.40 and 7.45. Consequently, a pregnant asthmatic with a $PaCO_2$ over 35 and a pH under 7.40 faces a greater risk of respiratory failure than her nonpregnant counterpart.[20] In addition, maternal pH and $PaCO_2$ significantly influence uterine blood flow and fetal oxygenation.[21–24] The hyperventilation and hypoxemia that occur during an asthma attack can thus combine to limit fetal oxygen delivery.[25]

During pregnancy multiple hormonal changes occur that have the potential to affect airway tone and asthma. Serum progesterone levels increase throughout pregnancy. This change appears important in stimulating the hyperventilation of pregnancy,[19] and may also decrease pulmonary resistance and increase airway conductance in normal pregnant women.[26] Free cortisol levels increase during pregnancy, as do prostaglandins E and $F_{2\alpha}$, a potent bronchodilator and a bronchoconstrictor, respectively.[19,24] Plasma cyclic nucleotide concentrations, which mediate the balance between contraction and relaxation of bronchial smooth muscle, also change throughout pregnancy.[19] What effect, if any, these hormonal changes have on pulmonary function in the asthmatic parturient remains unknown.

Some lung volumes change with pregnancy. Expiratory reserve volume and residual volume decrease, resulting in a 9.5- to 25-percent reduction in functional residual capacity (FRC).[19] Airway closure is also affected; the difference between FRC and closing capacity decreases so that airway closure occurs more readily in the parturient during tidal breathing.[27–30] This predisposes even the normal parturient to ventilation/perfusion (V/Q) mismatch and hypoxemia.[31] The asthmatic, subject to V/Q mismatch and hypoxemia even when asymptomatic,[17,18] may face even greater risk during pregnancy.

Despite these various physiologic changes in respiratory function, pregnancy has no consistently measurable effect on asthma, and most women with pre-existing asthma tolerate pregnancy without undue difficulty. However, one cannot predict the course of asthma in a given patient during pregnancy. Review of the many clinical studies of asthma and pregnancy suggests that in about half of pregnancies the disease remains unchanged while in some (22 percent) asthma worsens and in others (29 percent) it improves.[25] Rarely, do patients have severe worsening of their asthmatic condition during gestation, but when they do, it resolves promptly with termination of pregnancy.[32,33] Some authors feel that the course of asthma with one pregnancy predicts the course in future pregnancies.[20] Examination of the limited case reports that often lead to these conclusions reveals that women with severe asthma in one pregnancy may be just as likely to have a subsequent pregnancy without disease as a subsequent pregnancy with recurrent severe disease.[32] Most likely, factors other than pregnancy itself, such as seasonal variation and the occurrence of upper respiratory tract infection, primarily determine the course of asthma during pregnancy.[20,25] In addition, women with severe disease appear more likely to have exacerbations during pregnancy than those with mild disease.[20,34,35]

Data on maternal morbidity and mortality in pregnant asthmatics are inconsistent. One retrospective study[36] found an increased incidence of hyperemesis, hemorrhage, and toxemia in pregnant asthmatics. In another study,[37] women with severe, inadequately treated[25] asthma were at very high risk of death. These two studies suggest that untreated or marginally treated asthmatic parturients face increased risks. In subsequent studies of well-controlled, steroid-dependent asthmatics during pregnancy there was no increase in maternal morbidity or mortality.[38,39]

Maternal asthma may also affect fetal outcome. Fetal oxygen in the normal state is borderline. Poorly controlled maternal respiratory disease can produce fetal hypoxia, decrease birth weight,[35] and increase perinatal mortality.[36,37] However, with good control of maternal disease and avoidance of hypoxemia and alkalosis,[38] neonatal outcome can be normal, even for the infants of mothers with severe asthma.

Practical Considerations

The goals in treating the pregnant asthmatic are the same as those for the nonpregnant patient. Prevention and aggressive treatment of bronchospasm can prevent both maternal and fetal morbidity and mortality. However, the need for good control of maternal disease must be weighed against the teratogenic potential of antiasthmatic drugs. In this section, we shall review the therapeutic use and possible teratogenic effects of the currently used antiasthmatic drugs.

Theophylline. Theophylline compounds have been the mainstay of asthma therapy for many years. The drug is available in oral form. However, its water solubility is quite low, and the intravenous preparation, aminophylline, is the ethylenediamine salt of theophylline. Aminophylline solutions are 85 percent theophylline by weight.

Theophylline's mechanism of action remains unknown. Inhibition of the enzyme phosphodiesterase blocks the degradation of cAMP, a potent bronchodilator. In vitro, theophylline is a phosphodiesterase inhibitor but only in concentrations that would prove toxic in vivo. In addition, other phosphodiesterase inhibitors (i.e., dipyridamole and papaverine) do not produce bronchodilation. Though it was once thought that the mechanism of action of theophylline was phosphodiesterase inhibition, this explanation is no longer accepted.[40] Theophylline also stimulates adrenal catecholamine release and may cause bronchodilation by increasing the amount of catecholamines in the bloodstream.[41] Effects on prostaglandins, effects on intracellular calcium kinetics, and increasing the efficacy of cAMP may also explain theophylline's bronchodilation.[40]

Widely used in the management of pregnant asthmatics, theophylline seems free of teratogenic effects.[20,24,42] Its pharmacokinetics in pregnancy need additional study; preliminary data show an increased volume of distribution with unchanged clearance,[43] suggesting that pregnancy may increase the dose requirement.[20] However, Mintz[44] reports the clinical impression that clearance decreases with pregnancy and expresses concern about possible toxicity in the parturient. In general, however, it seems safe and effective to continue with previously well-tolerated doses of theophylline during pregnancy. When in doubt, monitor therapy by measuring serum theophylline concentrations.[40] Theophylline, a potent uterine relaxant,[45] may prolong labor.[20,44] However, the benefits of maintaining the mother free of bronchospasm far outweigh the risk of any possible prolongation of labor, and theophylline should be continued throughout gestation.[25]

Theophylline freely crosses the placenta, and neonatal effects may be observed. About 10 percent of neonates exhibit transient jitteriness and tachycardia,[46–48] and rarely, an infant may vomit initially.[48] Interestingly, these signs of toxicity occur when maternal and neonatal theophylline concentrations are in the "therapeutic" range. Contributing factors may include decreased protein binding and increased red-cell uptake of theophylline in the infant.[46] Newborns exhibit a markedly prolonged elimination half-life, up to 30 hours in the premature infant.[49] In addition, premature newborns metabolize theophylline to caffeine (term neonates and adults do not), thus increasing total methylxanthine exposure.[50] Irrespective of mechanism all neonates exposed to theophylline in utero should be monitored for signs of toxicity.[47]

Beta Sympathomimetics. Stimulation of beta adrenoreceptors activates the enzyme adenyl cyclase which catalyzes the formation of cAMP. Cyclic AMP, the "second messenger" interacts with cAMP–dependent protein kinase to initiate a variety of cellular processes. In the asthmatic, the most important result of β-adrenergic stimulation is bronchial smooth muscle relaxation.

There are two types of beta adrenoreceptors. Heart and fat contain predominantly β_1 receptors, and stimulation causes tachycardia and lipolysis. Bronchial and vascular smooth muscle, skeletal muscle, and liver contain predominantly β_2 receptors. Stimulation of these receptors causes smooth muscle relaxation, muscle tremor, glycogenolysis, and at times, reflex tachycardia from vasodilation. Receptor specificity varies widely among beta-sympathomimetic drugs (Table 10–3). Isoproterenol stimulates β_1 and β_2 receptors equally, while isoetherine and methaproterenol produce predominantly β_2 stimulation with some β_1 activity. Terbutaline and albuterol (salbutamol) are almost exclusively β_2 agonists. The route of administration can significantly affect apparent receptor specificity; aerosol administration greatly enhances the β_2 specificity.[51]

Considerable controversy surrounds the use of β-sympathomimetic agents during pregnancy. There is little data on the possible human teratogenic effects of these drugs.[20] In addition, they are potent uterine relaxants.[52,53] High-dose

Table 10–3. USEFUL DRUGS FOR ASTHMA

Name	Action	Dose	Comment
Epinephrine	alpha, nonselective beta stimulation	0.2–0.5 mg SC q 20–30 min 3 times Onset: 5–15 min Peak: 30–120 min Duration: 2–3 hr	May decrease uterine blood flow and cause fetal distress[76–78]
Isoproterenol	Potent, nonselective beta stimulation	Meter: 0.125 mg/puff, 2 puffs q 4–6 hr Aerosol: 1.25–2.5 mg q 3–6 hr (q 20 min 3 times for acute symptoms[82]) Onset: 2–5 min Peak: 5–30 min Duration: 1–3 hr	Short duration; high incidence of tachycardia; fewer systemic side effects when inhaled
Isoethrine	Slightly β_2-selective	Meter: 0.35 mg/puff, 1–2 puffs q 3–4 hr Aerosol: 1% solution, 2.5–10 mg q 3–6 hr Onset: 5 min Peak: 15–60 min Duration: 1.5–3 hr	Less potent than isoproterenol
Metaproterenol	β_2-selective sympathomimetic	PO: 10–20 mg q 6–8 hr Metered: 650 μg/puff Aerosol: 5% solution, 10–15 mg q 3–6 hr (15 mg q 1 hr for acute symptoms[83]) Onset: 2–10 min (inhaled) Peak: 30–40 min Duration: 1–5 hr	Longer duration than isoproterenol; effective orally; β_2 selectivity greatest when inhaled[51]
Terbutaline	β_2-selective sympathomimetic	PO: 2.5–5.0 mg q 6–8 hr SC: 0.25–0.5 mg q 15–30 min 3 times Metered: 0.25 mg/puff q 4–6 hr	Long acting; can cause tachycardia; secondary vasodilation[51]; potent tocolytic; as effective as SC epinephrine[51,80]

Table 10–3. USEFUL DRUGS FOR ASTHMA *(continued)*

Name	Action	Dose	Comment
		Onset: 5–15 min (SC) Peak: 30–60 min Duration: 1–7 hr	
Albuterol (Salbutamol)	β_2-selective sympathomimetic	PO: 2–4 mg q 6–8 hr Metered: 90 μg/puff, 2 puffs q 4–6 hr Aerosol: 0.5% solution 5–10 mg q 4 hr Onset: 1–5 min (aerosol) Peak: 45–90 min Duration: 4–6 hr	Long acting; most β_2-selective; fewest cardiac side effects.[81] Can cause postpartum hemorrhage secondary uterine atony.[54]
Theophylline[85]	Uncertain (see text)	PO: 50–500 mg q 6–12 hr IV[101] loading dose: 1 mg/kg for each 2-μg/ml increase in serum concentration desired Healthy smokers: 0.7 mg/kg/hr Healthy nonsmokers: 0.4 mg/kg/hr In presence of cardiac or liver decompensation: 0.2 mg/kg/hr	Infusion rates of theophylline (aminophylline = theophylline/0.85) target steady state concentration: 10 μg/ml; measure theophylline within 12–24 hr of infusion and adjust rate accordingly
Corticosteroids uncertain (see text)			
Prednisone		PO: 5–60 mg qd	Can cause adrenal suppression; taper to lowest effective dose
Methylprednisolone		IV: 125 mg q 4–6 hr	
Beclamethasone		Inhaler: 50 μg/puff, 2–5 puffs qid	Minimal systemic effects

β_2-sympathomimetic therapy for premature labor may cause significant maternal morbidity, including pulmonary edema. Albuterol (salbutamol) has been reported to cause uterine hemorrhage at spontaneous abortion.[54] Citing these risks, some authors feel that β-sympathomimetic drugs should be avoided during pregnancy if possible.[20,24] However, others citing clinical experience find these drugs, especially the β_2-selective agents metoproterenol terbutaline and albuterol, very useful and effective in the management of the pregnant asthmatic.[19,42,44,55]

Corticosteroids. The use of corticosteroids to treat asthma in the parturient proves even more controversial than use of beta sympathomimetics. Corticosteroids affect asthma via several mechanisms.[56,57] The steroid molecule enters the cell and binds to a specific steroid receptor. The receptor-steroid complex then enters the nucleus, binds with chromatin, and initiates DNA synthesis. The proteins synthesized actively mediate many of the delayed corticosteroid effects. Steroids also act immediately and directly on previously synthesized proteins and nonspecifically by insertion into cell membranes. Many of these immediate effects involve changes in calcium ion flux, enhancing or inhibiting its entry into different cells. Beneficial steroid actions include direct dilation of large and small bronchi, anti-inflammatory effects, and blockade of the synthesis, release, and activity of many biochemical mediators of asthma. They also cause redistribution of pulmonary blood flow to better match ventilation and improve oxygenation. A very important effect of corticosteroids is their ability to restore cellular responsiveness to β-sympathomimetic stimulation, a combination of an immediate increase in the affinity of cellular receptors for beta-agonists with improved intracellular coupling to adenylate cyclase as well as a delayed increase in synthesis of beta receptors. The beneficial effects of steroids begin within an hour but do not peak until 4 to 24 hours after administration.[56,57]

Data on the safety of corticosteroids in pregnancy are conflicting. While earlier studies[25,58] attributed an increase in stillbirths and cleft palate to maternal corticosteroid use, subsequent studies[25,38,39] have found no increase in fetal or maternal complications. The numbers of patients and the methods used in these studies make it impossible to state with certainty that no harm will come from the use of corticosteroids in pregnancy.[59] As with other antiasthmatic drugs, the risks of fetal hypoxia from uncontrolled asthma outweigh the potential risks of therapy, and steroids should be used if needed to control the mother's symptoms.[38,39,42,44,55] The potential risks and benefits should be discussed with patients before making therapeutic decisions.[59] Other potential side effects of corticosteroid use during pregnancy include fetal and maternal adrenal suppression. Prednisone and prednisolone enter the fetal circulation only poorly, and documented neonatal adrenal suppression is rare.[44] Inhaled beclamethasone can effectively limit systemic exposure to steroids and decrease maternal side effects.[39]

Cromolyn. Cromolyn sodium does not cause bronchodilation but is a useful prophylactic against mediator-induced and reflex bronchospasm.[60] Although the manufacturers do not recommend its use in pregnancy, it has nevertheless been widely used and no significant problems have been reported.[4,23,42,61] If cromolyn sodium has been effective for a woman before pregnancy it probably should be continued.

Immunotherapy. Immunotherapy, widely used in the treatment of allergic disease, seems safe in pregnancy according to both a recent study[62] and long clinical experience.[44] Effective hyposensitization should be continued throughout pregnancy.[25,44,59,62] The greater risk of anaphylaxis early in treatment and lack of substantial benefits in the first months of treatment contraindicate the initiation of therapy during pregnancy.[44] Similarly, conservative increases in dose limit the risk of anaphylaxis.[25]

Antihistamines. Antihistamines, often used during seasonal exacerbations and upper respiratory infections, have been extensively utilized with apparent safety in pregnancy.[20,40,63] However, a recent large retrospective study of premature infants found an unanticipated association between retrolental fibroplasia and maternal antihistamine use during the last 2 weeks of pregnancy.[64,65] These data suggest that parturients, especially those at high risk for premature delivery, should avoid antihistamines beginning late in the second trimester.

Antibiotics. Respiratory tract infections require aggressive antibiotic therapy. Penicillin and cephalosporin class drugs appear safe,[44,63] as does erythromycin.[20,44] Tetracyclines (tooth discoloration, damage to growing bone) and choramphenicol (gray-baby syndrome) should be avoided altogether. Sulfonamides are safe except near term (kernicterus).[44]

Other Drug Therapy. Asthmatic parturients should completely avoid several classes of drugs. Some over-the-counter expectorant preparations contain iodine. Maternal iodide ingestion during pregnancy can cause fetal goiter and hypothyroidism. Mental retardation or neonatal death from respiratory obstruction may ensue.[66] Prostaglandins E_2 and $F_{2\alpha}$ often serve to induce labor either at term or for second trimester abortions. Prostaglandin $F_{2\alpha}$ is an extremely potent bronchoconstrictor in asthmatics.[67] Both prostaglandins $F_{2\alpha}$ and E_2 increase lung resistance when given by intravenous,[68] intramuscular, or intra-amniotic[69] injection to nonasthmatic parturients. Bronchospasm can occur when asthmatic parturients receive those drugs.[70]

Summary. Several basic guidelines determine therapy in the pregnant asthmatic. Maternal hypoxia associated with undertreated asthma can increase maternal and fetal morbidity.[36] The therapeutic agents discussed above should be used as needed to control maternal symptoms. Multiple approaches have been successful.[4,20,24,42,44,55] Some experts attempt to wean beta sympathomimetics and control asthma with theophylline, steroids, and cromolyn,[4] while others use beta sympathomimetics as the first line of treatment.[20,44] Regardless of the therapy chosen, careful discussion with the patient of risks and benefits and close monitoring of effectiveness are essential.

ACUTE ASTHMA

Assessment

Acute worsening of airway obstruction in the asthmatic is a medical emergency. Careful assessment of the patient's condition and close monitoring of responses to treatment determine and guide therapy. The history is the initial step in assessing acute asthma. An adequate history may alert the physician to precipitating factors such as exposure to allergens and irritants, respiratory infection, emotional stress, exercise, inadequate maintenance therapy, overuse of inhaled bronchodilators, or abrupt withdrawal of corticosteroids.[71-73] History can also identify patients at increased risk for hospitalization, mechanical ventilation, or death. High-risk factors include increased frequency of attacks, previous need for hospitalization or mechanical ventilation, long delay in seeking medical attention, and current high-dose steroid use.[71,73] The patient's own assessment (Table 10–4) of the severity of her asthma can sometimes[72,74] be useful in evaluating the severity of the attack and the response to therapy.

Table 10–4. EMERGENCY ROOM EVALUATION OF ACUTE ASTHMA

- History
  - Identification of major precipitating factors
    - Exposure to allergens or irritants
    - Respiratory tract infections
    - Overuse of aerosol bronchodilators
    - Abrupt withdrawal of corticosteroids
    - Inadequate maintenance treatment
    - Emotional stress
  - Features that identify the high-risk patient
    - Frequency of attacks
    - Last attack or hospitalization
    - Long delay by the patient before seeking attention
    - Prior need for intensive care treatment or intubation
    - Current use of high-dose corticosteroids
- Physical examination: evaluation of general appearance
  - Anxiety, fatigue, cyanosis, diaphoresis, flushing
  - Vital signs
  - Pulsus paradoxus
  - Accessory muscle use
  - Evidence of hyperinflation (hyperresonance to percussion, decreased diaphragmatic exertion, or a quiet chest)
  - Evidence of bronchopneumonia, pneumothorax, or pneumomediastinum
  - Determination of vital capacity, forced expiratory volume in 1 sec, or peak expiratory flow rate

(From Weiss EB, Segal MS and Stein M,[7] p 805, with permission.)

The common presenting symptoms of acute asthma include dyspnea, chest tightness, wheezing, and cough.[73] Wheezing, the classic physical finding of asthma, may be scattered and occur at the beginning or end of expiration in mild attacks or progress to holoexpiratory and then inspiratory and expiratory wheezing as bronchoconstriction becomes more severe.[73,75] Some patients with severe airway obstruction may have few or no breath sounds, an ominous sign of impending respiratory failure.[73,74] Hypertension and tachycardia are common. Heart rates greater than 120 to 130 beats per min and respiratory rates greater than 30 per min often signify worsening obstruction and hypoxemia.[73-75] Pulsus paradoxus can be a reliable indicator of severe obstruction; a decrease in systolic blood pressure of more than 18 mmHg with inspiration indicates severe air flow obstruction.[73,74] However, pulsus paradoxus is highly effort dependent and may not be present in the tiring patient with impending respiratory failure.[73] Recruitment of the sternocleidomastoid and scalene muscles, retraction of intercostals, and use of abdominal muscles during exhalation all occur in moderate to severe asthmatic episodes.[71-73] Other physical findings indicative of severe obstruction include diaphoresis, orthopnea, and altered mental status (see Table 10–4).[73]

Arterial hypoxemia develops commonly with acute bronchoconstriction as does respiratory alkalosis with hypocarbia. A normal or elevated $PaCO_2$ signifies impending respiratory failure.[73,75] Normal $PaCO_2$ in the parturient ranges from 30 to 35 mmHg, and a $PaCO_2$ greater than 35 mmHg in an asthmatic parturient is cause for serious concern.[20,55]

Treatment

Upon completion of diagnosis and assessment of acute asthma, intensive appropriate therapy becomes essential for good maternal and fetal outcome. Supplemental oxygen is a necessity. Many recommend subcutaneous epinephrine, 0.3 ml of a 1:1000 solution (300 μg) as the first line of treatment of mild to moderate asthma in the parturient.[24,55] However, even small doses of epinephrine can decrease uterine blood flow in animals.[76,77] This effect is transient; yet, even apparently healthy fetuses may develop signs of fetal distress lasting up to 20 min after the mother receives an epinephrine injection.[78] The stressed fetus of a mother with acute asthma may have an even worse response to epinephrine. Fortunately, terbutaline, 0.25 mg subcutaneously[79] or 5 mg by inhalation,[80] is as effective a bronchodilator as subcutaneous epinephrine. Other β-sympathomimetic agents including metaproterenol and albuterol also effectively counter acute asthma (see Table 10–3).[81] These drugs may be given by metered aerosol every 20 to 30 min in mild attacks. In moderate to severe attacks, a nebulizer works more effectively.[75] Patients who do not respond to inhaled beta sympathomimetics usually receive aminophylline as well.[55,75] However, several studies indicate that addition of aminophylline to β-sympathomimetic therapy does not significantly increase air flow when compared to continued β-sympathomimetic therapy (Fig. 10–5).[82,83] However, the addition of theophylline does increase the frequency of side effects, including tremor, nausea, anxiety, and palpitations.[83] When theophylline is used in an acute setting, overdose can occur easily. The widely quoted dosage regimen—a loading dose of 5.6 mg per kg followed by a continuous infusion of 0.9 mg per kg per hr[84]—may produce serious toxicity. Table 10–3 illustrates the currently recommended lower dose.[85]

Corticosteroids play an important role in the treatment of severe acute asthma. Typically, physicians consider corticosteroids too slow-acting for routine use and withhold them until patients fail to respond to methylxanthine and β-sympathomimetic therapy.[75] However, a recent double-blind study has shown that intravenous administration of 125 mg methylprednisolone upon presentation in the Emergency Room improved air flow and resulted in significantly

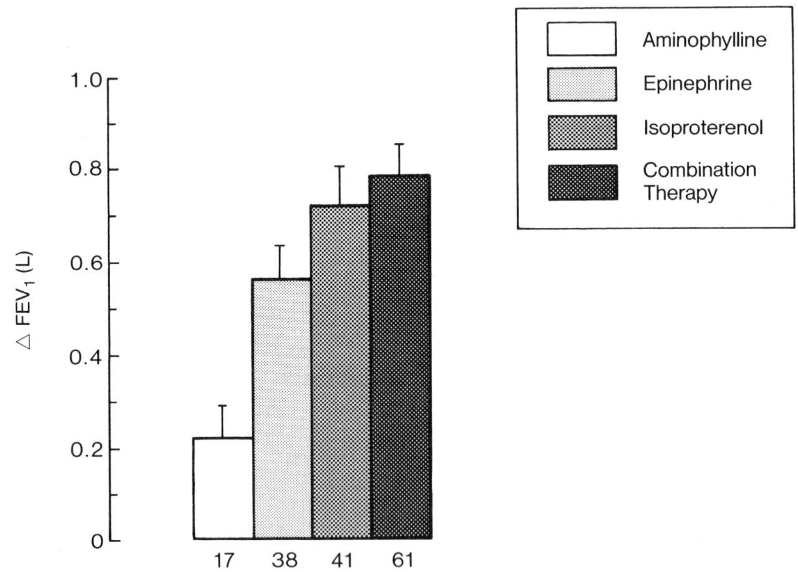

Figure 10–5. Response to treatment, single-drug versus two-drug regimens (mean ± SEM). The numbers at the bases of the vertical bars indicate number of patients. ΔFEV_1 = change in FEV_1 after 1 hour of treatment. (From Fanta, CH, Rossing TH and McFadden, ER,[82] p 5, with permission.)

fewer hospital admissions (Table 10–5).[86] Others[73,74] also recommend early steroid administration in acute asthma.

Additional supportive measures include adequate hydration and antibiotics if indicated.[74] Sedation can be fetal and should be avoided.[74,75] Some workers recommend anticholinergics such as atropine.[74,75] Nebulized atropine, 1 to 3 mg, may produce bronchodilation in patients who do not respond to β-sympathomimetic therapy.[75]

Status asthmaticus occurs when the above therapies do not significantly improve the patient's condition.[79] These patients require hospitalization and may need endotracheal intubation and mechanical ventilation. Progressive deterioration with an increasing $PaCO_2$, a persistent tachycardia, loss of consciousness, and onset of arrhythmias or metabolic acidosis strongly indicate intubation and ventilation (Table 10–6).[74] The above therapies should be continued. Careful intravenous administration of beta sympathomimetics with continuous ECG monitoring may be needed.[79] Inhalation anesthesia with halothane, enflurane, or isoflurane has been used in patients with severe refractory status asthmaticus.[87,88] Finally, emergency termination of pregnancy has also been employed as an effective last resort.[32,33]

Table 10–6. SUGGESTED CRITERIA FOR VENTILATION BASED ON SEQUENTIAL OBSERVATIONS*

Deterioration in pulmonary function
Falling PaO_2, rising $PaCO_2$
Danger levels: PaO_2 <40 mmHg, $PaCO_2$ >50 mmHg
Onset cardiac dysfunction
Persistent tachycardia (>140 beats/min)
Cardiac dysrhythmias
General deterioration
Somnolence
Oliguria
Metabolic acidosis
Emergency indications
Drug-induced respiratory depression
Acute pneumothorax or pneumomediastinum
Cardiovascular collapse

*Each patient must be assessed individually. It is difficult to define absolute values for ventilation.

(Adapted from Tatham, ME and Gellert, AR,[74] p 603, with permission.)

Labor and Delivery

Medical and Obstetric Management. Asthmatic patients do not require special obstetric considerations for the management of labor and delivery. Pitocin may be used safely[75] for induction or augmentation of labor, but prostaglandins should be avoided.[67–70]

Labor is emotionally and physically stressful. Minute ventilation may increase to as much as 300 percent above nonpregnant values.[89] Such stress may induce bronchospasm in the asthmatic. Conversely, antiasthmatic medications can decrease the parturient's uterine contractility and slow labor.[49,52] Consequently, although regular antiasthmatic medications should be continued throughout the puerperium, maternal drug therapy should be optimized in the last weeks before delivery with the lowest effective doses of methylxanthines and beta sympathomimetics.[24] Should wheezing occur during labor, several issues must be considered. Beta sympathomimetics, even when inhaled, can be potent uterine relaxants[52,53,54] and may slow labor[52] or predispose to increased blood loss at delivery.[54] Intravenous aminophylline, a less potent uterine relaxant,[45] may be preferred for initial therapy but is less effective as the sole therapeutic agent (see Fig. 10–5).[82] Theophyl-

Table 10–5. METHYLPREDNISOLONE IN ACUTE ASTHMA: EMERGENCY ROOM DISCHARGE RESULTS

	Control Group (n = 49)	Methylprednisolone Group (n = 48)	P
Hospital admission rate (%)	46.9	18.8	0.003
FVC (mean % predicted)	66.0	73.0	0.08
FEV_1 (mean % predicted)	57.7	65.0	0.07

(Adapted from Littenberg, B and Gluck EH,[86] pp 150–152, 1980, with permission.)

line crosses the placenta readily,[47] and neonatal toxicity may occur even with "therapeutic" maternal levels.[48] Patients receiving chronic corticosteroid therapy during gestation require supplementation with hydrocortisone 100 mg intramuscularly every 8 hours during labor and delivery.[20,24,25,44] Adrenal insufficiency rarely occurs in infants of mothers receiving chronic corticosteroid therapy; these infants warrant careful observation but not prophylactic treatment.[20]

Labor Analgesia. Epidural analgesia can be useful during labor and delivery in the asthmatic parturient. Adequate pain relief serves to decrease maternal anxiety and hyperventilation, thus diminishing the risk of exacerbating her asthma. In this setting, continuous infusion analgesia can effectively avoid the recurrence of pain between redoses common with the intermittent bolus technique. Epidural infusion of 0.125-percent bupivacaine also provides good relief during the second stage of labor. In the primagravida, continuous epidural infusion weakens maternal expulsive efforts and prolongs the second stage of labor. However, this effect does not adversely effect neonatal outcome.[90] In multiparous patients, continuous analgesia has little if any effect on the second stage of labor. Epidural analgesia is the best, but not the only, available alternative. Psychoprophylaxis, if effective, can reduce maternal anxiety and minimize maternal hyperventilation. Small doses of narcotics may be used early in labor, provided there is no evidence of respiratory compromise.[91] Inhalation analgesia with enflurane or low doses of ketamine can also be safe and effective,[91] provided the anesthetist has adequate experience with these techniques. For vaginal delivery, local infiltration, pudendal block, and low spinal anesthesia may all be used alone or with nitrous oxide, ketamine, or potent inhalational agent supplementation. Active wheezing contraindicates sedatives and other respiratory depressants.

Cesarean Section. The choice of anesthesia depends on the indication for surgery and the patient's condition at the time of surgery. Elective cesarean section should not be performed on a patient who is actively wheezing.

Regional Anesthesia. For most cesarean sections, regional anesthesia represents the technique of choice. However, high levels of sympathetic blockade leave the lung with unopposed parasympathetic tone, which may cause bronchospasm; even lower levels (T10 to L1) of blockade may diminish adrenal epinephrine output and may contribute to the development of bronchospasm.[92] On the other hand, thoracic sympathetic blockade reportedly relieves severe bronchospasm.[93] Other problems can arise with regional anesthesia for cesarean section. Asthmatic mothers may be uncomfortable lying supine; blockade of chest wall sensation may cause a feeling of dyspnea and contribute to this discomfort. High levels of blockade also decrease expiratory reserve volume and the mother's ability to cough. Spinal anesthesia produces a two- to three-segment higher motor block than do similar levels of epidural blockade[94] and therefore has a more profound effect on coughing and forced expiration. However, epidural analgesia results in less dense blockade than subarachnoid analgesia, and patients may experience more discomfort during uterine and peritoneal manipulation. Epidural fentanyl, 50 to 100 μg, can effectively relieve this pain.[95] This dose of epidural fentanyl also provides analgesia for 3 to 4 hours after delivery with minimal sedation[96] and little or no risk of respiratory depression.

General Anesthesia. Should general anesthesia be required, only a rapid-sequence induction with cricoid pressure and endotracheal intubation safely secures the mother's airway and protects her against aspiration of gastric contents. Placement of an endotracheal tube in any patient produces measurable diffuse airway constriction.[97] In the asthmatic, airway stimulation provokes a more marked response, and significant bronchospasm and wheezing may result.[98] Several strategies can help reduce or prevent the airway response to endotracheal intubation. Thiopental neither causes[16,95] nor prevents[99] bronchospasm. When used clinically, ketamine reportedly prevents or reverses bronchospasm,[100] leading some workers to consider it the best induction agent for asthmatic patients.[16] Studies in dogs show that ketamine effectively prevents antigen-induced increases in lung resistance.[99] In anesthetized humans, however, ketamine does not prevent increases in respiratory resistance following aerosol challenge.[101] Ketamine probably[99] exerts its effect via a centrally mediated increase in circulating catecholamines.[102] Pre-existing central nervous system (CNS) depression (i.e., anesthesia) blunts this stimulation[103] and thus would be expected to mask the bronchodilating effect of ketamine. Both laboratory evidence and clinical experience suggest ketamine as the agent of choice for rapid-sequence induction of anesthesia in the asthmatic.[16] Coadministration of ketamine and aminophylline lowers the seizure threshold in mice,[104] and seizure activity may occasionally occur during ketamine induction in an asthmatic patient receiving oral or intravenous aminophylline.[104]

Lidocaine blunts the cough reflex,[105] and both aerosol and intravenous lidocaine prevent irritant but not antigen-induced increases in airway reflexes.[106,107] Therefore, some[16] suggest lidocaine be used as an adjunct for induction in the asthmatic patient. However, topical lidocaine may itself produce irritant-induced bronchoconstriction,[16,106] and intravenous lidocaine may cause uterine hypertonus, uterine artery constriction, and fetal compromise.[108] Therefore, one should not administer intravenous or topical lidocaine during induction of general anesthesia in the parturient.

Preoperative administration of H_2 receptor–blocking drugs decreases maternal gastric acid secretion and protects against acid pneumonitis.[109] However, blockade of smooth muscle–relaxing H_2 receptor leaves the constricting H_1 receptors unopposed and enhances the bronchoconstriction response to histamines.[110,111] The newer more potent H_2 receptor antagonists ranitidine and famotidine may be less likely than cimetidine to augment bronchoconstriction and may be preferred if one considers these drugs essential to a patient with asthma.[112]

For maintenance of anesthesia, a potent inhalation agent should be used. Although halothane is still the most frequently mentioned bronchodilator, both enflurane and isoflurane prove equally effective in preventing or reversing antigen-induced bronchoconstriction.[113,114] Since halothane sensitizes the myocardium to catecholamine-induced arrhythmias[115] it may be best avoided in patients receiving β-sympathomimetic drugs. All of the potent inhalation agents and many antiasthmatic drugs relax the uterus.[45,52,53,116] The combination of potent inhalation agent and beta sympathomimetic may predispose to increased blood loss at delivery.[59]

Succinylcholine safely provides rapid onset of muscle relaxation.[98] Pancuronium or vecuronium is the agent of choice for maintaining adequate neuromuscular blockade. Curare, which can cause histamine release, markedly increases respiratory resistance, even in nonasthmatic patients.[117] Metocurine and atracurium, though less likely than curare to cause histamine release, are nonetheless probably best avoided.

Ventilation should be controlled intraoperatively: large tidal volumes, slow inspiratory rates, and low inspiratory: expiratory (I:E) ratios should be maintained to minimize peak inspiratory pressure and allow adequate time for exhalation, preventing air trapping, and increased intrathoracic pressure. After delivery, narcotic analgesics can be added. Morphine, which causes histamine release,[118] should be avoided.

Extubation should be delayed until the patient awakens and demonstrates intact airway reflexes, yet excessive coughing and bucking should be avoided. Adequate doses of narcotics (at least 5 μg per kg fentanyl after delivery) help at the end of surgery to prevent coughing and bronchospasm during extubation. As an alternative to narcotics, intravenous lidocaine in a 75- to 100-mg bolus followed by a 1- to 4-mg per minute infusion has been recommended.[91] Fortunately, airway smooth muscle responsiveness appears to be depressed for up to 24 hours after anesthesia,[119] and reflex bronchospasm causes fewer problems during emergence than induction.

Intraoperative Wheezing. Bronchospasm most often explains intraoperative wheezing in the asthmatic. However, the anesthetist must eliminate other possible sources of wheezing, including kinking or obstruction of the endoctracheal tube, pulmonary edema, anaphylaxis, amniotic fluid embolism, aspiration of gastric contents, and pneumothorax. The treatment for intraoperative bronchospasm resembles the treatment of acute asthma in any setting. Beta sympathomimetics can be administered by aerosol directly into the anesthesia circuit.[16] In addition, a potent inhalation agent may be administered. Acute administration of aminophylline during halothane[120–122] (but not enflurane[123] or isoflurane[124]) anesthesia may predispose to ventricular dysrhythmias. Chronic administration of aminophylline appears less dysrhythmogenic.[125] The combination of potent inhalation agent, beta sympathomimetic, and aminophylline may increase uterine bleeding by causing uterine relaxation.[54] Less inhalation agent, extra pitocin, and methylergometrine may be necessary for good hemostasis. Ergotrate given intravenously can cause marked hypertension which, in the presence of vasopressor therapy, can reach dangerous levels.[126] Prostaglandins, potent bronchoconstrictors, should be avoided.[67–70]

Cigarette Smoking and Chronic Bronchitis

PATHOPHYSIOLOGY

Cigarette smoking during pregnancy has multiple harmful effects on mother and fetus. Prolonged irritation of the bronchi by tobacco smoke produces most of the maternal effects. Submucosal glands enlarge and hypersecrete mucus. Airways become edematous and ciliary function deteriorates, rendering the smoker susceptible to pulmonary infection.[127] Acute and then chronic bronchitis may result. ("Chronic bronchitis" is defined as the occurrence of symptoms most days for at least 3 months per year for 2 consecutive years.) With prolonged smoking, damage can progress to severe obstructive pulmonary disease and emphysema. Fortunately, even women with severe chronic obstructive pulmonary disease appear to tolerate pregnancy without worsening pulmonary status.[1] However, pregnant smokers may have an increased risk of placentia previa, placental abruption, and premature rupture of membranes.[128]

Epidemiologic evidence also points to a wide variety of deleterious fetal effects of maternal tobacco abuse. Intrauterine growth retardation is the best-documented effect. Birth weight decreases in direct proportion to the number of cigarettes smoked.[128] Indeed, smoking even less than 20 cigarettes per day results in a 52-percent increase in the incidence of birth weight below 2500 g. Smokers of more than 20 cigarettes daily increase the risk of low birth weight by 130 percent.[128] The mechanisms involved may include nicotine-mediated uteroplacental vasoconstriction, a direct, nicotine-mediated growth-inhibiting effect on fetal tissue, carbon monoxide-induced increases in fetal carboxyhemoglobin concentrations with resultant fetal tissue hypoxia, and thiocyanate toxicity.[129] In addition, a 30- to 70-percent increase occurs in the rate of spontaneous abortion and perinatal mortality.[128] Tobacco abuse may increase the rate of congenital malformations.[128,129] The increased risks do not stop at birth; children of smokers have lower IQs, slower physical growth, and higher rates of morbidity and mortality than do children of nonsmokers.[128]

TREATMENT

Therapy for these women begins with strong encouragement to quit smoking. Antibiotics may be needed for acute pulmonary infections. Patients with chronic bronchitis and wheezing may require bronchodilators, although they respond less dramatically than the asthmatics.

ANESTHESIA

Anesthetic management of heavy smokers and patients with chronic bronchitis resembles that of asthma patients. Careful attention is paid to oxygenation and the management of secretions. Regional anesthesia is usually preferred. The decrease in expiratory reserve volume[99] (and, consequently, the inability to cough that accompanies the high level of blockade required for cesarean section) may distress some parturients. Persistent attempts to clear secretions by coughing can make abdominal closure more difficult. Small doses of intravenous narcotics sometimes effectively diminish the cough reflex and can facilitate surgery. Postoperatively, early mobilization and aggressive pulmonary toilet may diminish respiratory morbidity.

Emphysematous Blebs

Rupture of an emphysematous bleb is the most common cause of spontaneous pneumothorax. Blebs, a manifestation of interstitial emphysema, usually form at the apex of the lung and may accompany chronic bronchitis.[127]

Rupture of a bleb, with the development of pneumothorax, may occur any time throughout pregnancy, but most commonly happens with maternal expulsive efforts during the second stage of labor.[127]

Tension pneumothorax, whereby a ball-valve

mechanism results in ever-increasing amounts of extrapleural air, occurs in 3 to 5 percent of patients who experience spontaneous pneumothorax. Increasing intrathoracic pressure progressively impedes venous return, and cardiovascular collapse may ensue. The signs and symptoms of pneumothorax include cough, chest pain (often referred to the shoulder), dyspnea, diminished breath sounds, and hyperresonance on percussion. The anesthetized, mechanically ventilated patient may initially manifest only tachycardia and hypotension. Eventually, increased airway pressure, tracheal deviation, and subcutaneous emphysema develop.[130]

A small asymptomatic pneumothorax generally requires no treatment. Larger, persistent air leaks call for insertion of a chest tube and suction. Tension pneumothorax may necessitate immediate needle aspiration and subsequent chest tube insertion.[127,130]

The parturient with a history of recurrent pneumothorax must avoid pushing, and her obstetrician should shorten the second stage of labor with outlet forceps. I recommend regional anesthesia for both vaginal and cesarean delivery.

Bronchiectasis

Patients with recurrent pulmonary infections may develop bronchiectasis, permanent abnormal dilation of the bronchi. If severe, hypoxemia may result. Treatment includes physiotherapy, prophylactic antibiotics, and surgical resection of localized disease.[131] Little has been reported concerning pregnancy in patients with bronchiectasis. An association with intrauterine growth retardation has been suggested,[132] although others report no significant maternal or fetal complications.[133]

Cystic Fibrosis

Cystic fibrosis (CF), the most common lethal genetic disease of Caucasians, is transmitted as an autosomal-recessive trait. The gene occurs in as many as one in 20 persons, and the disease, in about one in 1000 live births. The cause of this disease, characterized by systemic abnormalities in exocrine gland function, remains unknown. Patients experience recurrent respiratory infections secondary to impaired ciliary function and thick, tenacious sputum. Although the respiratory system usually manifests the most serious clinical problems, CF patients can also have abnormal pancreatic function. Pancreatic enzyme insufficiency frequently leads to malabsorption and steatorrhea. Portal hypertension and cirrhosis may also develop. Abnormal sweat gland function increases excretion of sodium chloride.

Cystic fibrosis is most commonly diagnosed in children at a mean age of 3.7 years.[134] However, milder forms of the disease occur, and women who survive to child-bearing age are often not diagnosed until later in life,[134] occasionally not until they become pregnant.[135] Characteristic clinical findings, including recurrent respiratory infection, chronic cough, and production of copious, thick sputum suggest the diagnosis. Hemoptysis, pneumothorax, or bronchiectasis may also be seen. Nasal polyposis, malabsorption, and steatorrhea are common. These patients can be chronically hypoxemic and their digits develop clubbing. Salt depletion can take place due to poor gastrointestinal absorption and excess excretion. An elevated level of chloride in the sweat confirms the diagnosis. Chest films show prominent vascular markings, pulmonary infections, hyperinflation, fibrosis, cystic changes, and persistent atelectasis.[136] Management guidelines include prophylactic antibiotics, daily chest physiotherapy, and a low-fat diet, often with pancreatic enzyme supplements.[136] Careful follow-up is essential.

CYSTIC FIBROSIS AND PREGNANCY

With improved diagnosis and treatment, more women with CF are surviving into the reproductive years. Although patients with moderate to severe disease may decompensate during or immediately after pregnancy, parturition does not increase the overall death rate.[134] Women with mild disease and good gravid clinical condition usually do well.[134,137,138] Children with mild disease maintain fairly normal activity levels (good school attendance), and fairly good nutritional status (growth to at least the 15th percentile level), fair muscle tone, and only moderate symptoms of steatorrhea. They may cough but on physical exam should have normal vital signs, clear chests, and no clubbing. Chest films should also show only minimal changes.[137] However, patients with moderate to severe disease, including those with restricted activity, poor growth and muscle tone, moderate to severe steatorrhea, frequent cough with rales, clubbing, and abnormal chest films (emphysema, atelectasis, bronchiectasis)[137] do poorly, deteriorate, and may die when pregnant or in the 6 months postpartum.[134] The disease of these sicker women usually does not return to the prepregnant status.[134,135]

The fetal effects of maternal CF result mostly from chronic maternal hypoxemia and malnutrition. Perinatal morbidity and mortality increase, with a greater incidence of growth retardation, premature delivery, and perinatal death.[137] This increased morbidity correlates with the mother's clinical condition. Good clinical condition with good maternal weight can improve perinatal outcome.[134]

Medical Management

Management of CF during pregnancy focuses primarily on pulmonary function, with the objectives of maintaining open airways and avoiding infection. Vigorous pulmonary toilet is essential. Antibiotics may be given continuously[136] or as needed following frequent sputum cultures.[135] Patients must also maintain good nutritional status with vitamins[135,137] and pancreatic enzyme supplements (if needed).[138] Patients with severe disease or deteriorating clinical status may elect therapeutic abortion.[134,138]

Obstetric Anesthetic Management

CF has little effect on obstetric management. Patients are at high risk for premature labor[134] and may receive appropriate tocolytic therapy.[135] Optimal maternal and fetal condition during labor require adequate hydration, supplemental oxygen, and avoidance of respiratory depressants. It may be useful to minimize maternal exertion and to use forceps to shorten the second stage of labor. Only obstetric indications call for cesarean section. Regional anesthesia with local anesthetics can be used safely for labor and vaginal or cesarean delivery. Hyde and Harrison recommend intrathecal morphine for labor analgesia, with pudendal block for delivery.[139] Pulse oximetry helps ensure adequate maternal oxygenation during both general and regional anesthesia.

In conclusion, pregnancy can prove dangerous for the woman with cystic fibrosis. However, with thorough, aggressive medical therapy, outcome for mother and fetus can be salutary.

Pulmonary Infection During Pregnancy

VIRAL PNEUMONIA

Influenza is the most thoroughly studied of the respiratory viral infections that occur during pregnancy. Although it is generally well tolerated by healthy women, those with underlying chronic disease may do poorly and should be vaccinated.[17] The possible teratogenetic effect of maternal influenza and questions about subsequent childhood malignancy are of more concern. Studies of the teratogenicity of maternal influenza yield conflicting data, and any increased risk is small.[19] Data about subsequent childhood malignancy prove even less conclusive and many feel the correlation between maternal influenza and childhood malignancy is nonexistent.[17]

Varicella pneumonia occurs rarely but carries a high maternal mortality and an increased incidence of abortion, prematurity, stillbirth, or neonatal infection. Treatment with intravenous acyclovir markedly improves the mother's prognosis.

BACTERIAL PNEUMONIA

Bacterial pneumonia frequently caused maternal morbidity in the preantibiotic era; 20 to 30 percent of infected parturients succumbed.[140] With the introduction of antibiotics maternal mortality declined to 3 to 9 percent in the 1950s and 1960s.[141] No fatalities occurred in a series of cases occurring in the 1970s.[142] Pneumonia most frequently occurs in women with other significant disease.[141,142] While *Streptococcus pneumoniae* is the most common pathogen, *Hemophilus influenzae, Staphylococcus aureus,* and hospital-acquired pneumonias are also seen.[141,142] Appropriate therapy depends on isolating the causative organism from sputum or blood cultures and treating with effective antibiotics.[142] In addition the mother may experience hypoxemia during the acute phase; supplemental oxygen may be needed to prevent fetal hypoxia. With appropriate diagnosis and therapy, the fetus should not suffer harm.[142]

Bacteremia can occur during the acute phase of pneumonia and may contraindicate regional anesthesia, especially continuous epidural. Clinicians often hesitate to administer spinal anesthesia to bacteremic patients for fear of seeding the CSF with pathogens.[143] However, physicians routinely perform lumbar puncture during work-up of the septic medical patient without any apparent increase in the risk of causing meningitis.[144] Thus, subarachnoid morphine may be useful for labor analgesia in these patients, while spinal anesthesia can be used for cesarean section. Alternatives for providing labor analgesia are limited since systemic narcotics and respiratory depressants should be avoided in these patients.[144] Inhalational analgesia with nitrous oxide in oxygen or enflurane may provide some relief. When using general anesthesia for abdominal delivery the anesthesiologist must preoxygenate the patient prior to induction and monitor oxygenation by sampling arterial blood gases or employing pulse oximetry. Pulse oximetry monitoring should continue during the postoperative period as well.

FUNGAL PNEUMONIA

Fungal pneumonias during pregnancy are rare. Coccidioidomycosis, the most common, is endemic in the southwestern United States.[145] Although it is usually a benign, nondisseminated disease, disseminated systemic disease can be fatal. Dissemination can occur during pregnancy, especially if the primary infection arises during the second or third trimester.[145] If untreated, maternal mortality approaches 100 percent.[145] Fortunately, amphotericin B effectively treats coccidioidomycosis.[146] Disseminated disease also poses severe risks to the fetus; placental (but not fetal) infection takes place. Premature delivery and fetal death are a frequent happening.[145] Therapy also significantly improves fetal prognosis.[146]

Not uncommonly asthma patients develop allergic bronchopulmonary aspergillosis.[41,47,122] Asthma which acutely worsens or a patient who presents with wheezing and eosinophilia should arouse suspicion. A skin reaction to *Aspergillus fumigatus* antigen, culture of *A.fumigatus* from sputum, or elevated serum levels of specific IgE confirm the diagnosis.[147] Untreated disease can cause progressive fibrosis, irreversible lung disease, and bronchiectasis. Treatment with corticosteroids works effectively.[147] Experience with aspergillosis in pregnancy remains limited, but obvious deterioration does not seem to occur.[4] Other fungal diseases develop primarily in immunosuppressed patients.[148]

TUBERCULOSIS

Despite remarkable advances in therapy, tuberculosis still poses a significant public health problem in the United States.[149] The incidence of inactive tuberculosis varies from population to population but approaches 5 percent in certain high-risk groups.[149] Only 3 to 4 percent of all parturients with tuberculosis have active disease.[149] WIth adequately treated disease, good maternal and fetal outcome occurs,[19,149] and even mothers treated with pneumonectomy or therapeutic pneumothorax do well.[2] However, delayed diagnosis or advanced disease can cause significant maternal and fetal morbidity.[149] While Shaffer[149] recommends a screening chest film for all parturients, a screening tuberculin test (chest film being reserved for new converters or patients with suspicious symptoms or physical findings) probably suffices for most patient populations.[19,150] Treatment varies with the stage of the mother's disease. Shaffer[149] feels that recent converters should receive 1 year of isoniazid prophylaxis, regardless of pregnancy status. Others,[19] citing small but significant possible risks of teratogenesis, suggest withholding prophylaxis until after delivery. Active disease, however, must be treated. Physicians most commonly combine isoniazid and ethambutal therapy to eliminate possible resistant bacteria.[19,149] Rifampin has been used safely in pregnancy, but concerns about its DNA–dependent RNA polymerase–inhibiting activity and its ability to cross the placenta limit its use.[19,149] Because streptomycin in high doses can cause fetal ototoxicity it should be avoided.[19,149]

Although congenital tuberculosis is extremely rare,[149] the infant of a woman with active tuberculosis runs a high risk of acquiring the disease in the first year of life.[19] Bacille Calmette Guerin (BCG) vaccination, frequent skin testing, or prophylactic isoniazid are all options to counteract this problem.[19,149]

Patients with active tuberculosis (3 weeks' adequate chemotherapy[151]) remain infectious and can contaminate anesthesia equipment. To minimize this risk, use disposable equipment when possible and place filters between the patient and the anesthesia machine. Heat or gas sterilize nondisposable equipment before reuse. Alcohol, phenol, or iodophor solutions adequately disinfect nonsterilizable articles such as carts and anesthesia machines.[19]

Sarcoidosis

A systemic granulomatous disease of unknown etiology, sarcoidosis frequently involves the lung. Demonstration of the characteristic noncaseating granuloma makes the diagnosis. Remissions and exacerbations characterize this disease which often requires no treatment. However, in its severe form, sarcoidosis can cause restrictive pulmonary disease with marked decreases in total lung capacity and forced expiratory volumes.[1] Hypoxemia may occur. Severe extrapulmonary and rapidly progressing forms of sarcoidosis may be treated with corticosteroids.[151] Patients with sarcoidosis seem to do well when pregnant. The inactive disease usually remains quiescent, and active disease often improves.[1] Increased maternal corticosteroids probably produce remission of sarcoidosis,[19,151] but exacerbations can follow delivery. Anesthetic management of patients with sarcoidosis usually presents no problems. However, severe disease can impair oxygenation and cause cardiac, hepatic, or renal dysfunction. About 2 percent of patients with sarcoidosis have granulomas in the larynx, necessitating careful examination of the airway.[151] In addition, postintubation edema may predispose to respiratory obstruction for up to 36 hours postoperatively.[152] In general, these patients tolerate regional and general anesthesia well, but the anesthesiologist must monitor oxygenation carefully.

Malignancy

Rarely does a patient with malignant disease become pregnant. Primary pulmonary or metastatic malignancy embarrasses pulmonary function in several ways. Direct interstitial involvement can limit pulmonary function and gas exchange. Pleural effusions may prevent expansion of one or both lungs. Severe ascites or massive abdominal tumor can diminish descent of the diaphragm. In addition, CNS disease may affect the respiratory center. Management of these patients is primarily symptomatic; special attention is given to patient comfort and the adequacy of respiration. If the mother's disease becomes life threatening, cesarean section may be necessary to deliver a viable fetus from a moribund mother.

Adult Respiratory Distress Syndrome and Ventilatory Failure

Increased pulmonary capillary permeability plus alveolar flooding and collapse with shunting of venous blood through the lung characterize the adult respiratory distress syndrome (ARDS), a potentially fatal pulmonary disease. Increased pulmonary shunting produces hypoxemia, which cannot be corrected simply by increasing inspired oxygen concentration. The disease may be seen following many types of severe systemic or pulmonary insult. In obstetric patients, ARDS has occurred in association with pre-eclampsia and eclampsia, amniotic fluid embolism, abruptio placentae, the dead fetus syndrome, pneumonia and sepsis, aspiration of gastric contents, and following severe trauma or in association with severe systemic disease.[153-157] We recently encountered ARDS in a young woman following treatment of premature labor with terbutaline, magnesium, and indomethecin. The exact pathophysiology of ARDS remains poorly understood. Progressive hypoxemia, diffuse patchy infiltrates on chest films, and pulmonary edema associated with low left-sided cardiac filling pressures suggest the diagnosis.[153,154,157] The primarily supportive therapy involves treating the underlying cause, if possible, and maintaining adequate oxygenation (oxygen saturation >90 percent) at nontoxic oxygen concentrations (<60 percent). Patients with ARDS often require mechanical ventilation with positive end-expiratory pressure (PEEP).[157]

RESPIRATORY FAILURE

A wide variety of other pulmonary, cardiac, neuromuscular, and central nervous system derangements also cause respiratory failure. The etiologies fall into two broad categories: failure to oxygenate (oxygen saturation <90 percent) and failure to ventilate (eliminate carbon dioxide). In addition to treating the underlying cause of respiratory failure (e.g., drug overdose, cardiac failure, bronchospasm) the respiratory system may be addressed directly. Failure to oxygenate (oxygen saturation <90 percent while breathing room air) should first be treated by administering supplemental oxygen. If administration of 50- to 70-percent oxygen by face mask does not increase oxygen saturation above 90 percent, significant intrapulmonary shunting (perfusion of unventilated alveoli) exists. Re-expansion of these alveoli with continuous positive airway pressure can significantly improve oxygenation. Intubation with mechanical ventilation and PEEP is often needed at this point. Failure to ventilate usually occurs when fatigue or depression of the muscles of respiration prevents adequate elimination of carbon dioxide. Causes include central nervous system depression (drug overdose) or peripheral muscle failure (residual neuromuscular blockade). An acute rise in $PaCO_2$ to greater than 45 mmHg and a fall in pH to less than 7.35 suggest the diagnosis. Therapy consists of supportive mechanical ventilation to maintain normal pH and $PaCO_2$ while determining and treating the underlying etiology.

Summary

Despite significant physiologic changes in the respiratory system, most women with respiratory disease do well during pregnancy. Most often, gestation does not exacerbate respiratory illness, and, in the absence of maternal hypoxemia, mother and baby do well. However, with severe disease, maternal hypoxemia or inadequate therapy, morbidity and mortality increase for both mother and fetus. Fortunately, most therapeutic regimens appear to be safe and can be continued throughout pregnancy and parturition. Labor and delivery should be managed primarily according to obstetric considerations. Anesthetic planning requires assessment of the patient's pathology and the efficacy of therapy. Regional anesthesia techniques are appropriate for most patients with respiratory disease. General anesthesia should be reserved for emergencies, especially in patients with bronchospastic conditions, but can be safely accomplished if necessary with careful attention to maternal oxygenation. Monitoring maternal oxygen saturation with a pulse oximeter can be extremely helpful with these patients.

References

1. Gazioglu, K, et al: Pulmonary function during pregnancy in normal women and in patients with cardiopulmonary disease. Thorax 25:445, 1970.
2. Gaensler, EA, et al: Pulmonary function in pregnancy: III. Serial observations in patients with pulmonary insufficiency. Am Rev Tuberc Pulmon Dis 57:779, 1953.
3. Rocklin, RE and Findlay, SR: Immunologic mechanisms and recent advances in asthma. In Weiss, EB, Segal, MS and Stein, M (eds): Bronchial Asthma: Mechanisms and Therapeutics, ed 2. Little, Brown & Co, Boston, 1985, p 41.
4. Greenberger PA: Asthma in pregnancy. Clin Perinatol 12:571, 1985.
5. Rackemann, FM: A clinical study of one hundred and fifty cases of bronchial asthma. Arch Intern Med 22(Oct):517, 1918.
6. Dawson, A and Simon, RA: Bronchospastic disorders: An overview. In Dawson, A and Simon, RA (eds): The Practical Management of Asthma. Grune & Stratton, New York, 1984, p 3.
7. Weiss, EB, Segal, MS and Stein, M (eds): Bronchial Asthma: Mechanisms and Therapeutics. Little, Brown & Co, Boston, 1985.
8. Lewis, RA: A presumptive role for leukotrienes in obstructive airway diseases. Chest 88:98S, 1985.
9. Samuelsson, B, et al: Leukotrienes and slow reacting substance of anaphylaxis (SRS-A). Allergy 35:375, 1980.
10. Anderson, WH: Biochemical mediators: Release chemistry and function. In Weiss, EB, Segal, MS and Stein, M (eds): Bronchial Asthma: Mechanisms and Therapeutics, ed 2. Little, Brown & Co, Boston, 1985, p 57.
11. Ahmed, T and Abraham, WM: Role of calcium-channel blockers in obstructive airway disease. Chest 88:142S, 1985.

12. Barnes, PJ: Asthma as an axon reflex. Lancet 1:242, 1986.
13. Nadel, JA and Sheppard, D: Mechanisms of bronchial hyperreactivity in asthma. In Weiss, EB, Segal, MS and Stein, M (eds): Bronchial Asthma: Mechanisms and Therapeutics, ed 2. Little, Brown & Co, Boston, 1985, p 30.
14. Hogg, JC: The pathology of asthma. In Weiss, EB, Segal MS and Stein, M (eds): Bronchial Asthma: Mechanisms and Therapeutics, ed 2. Little, Brown & Co, Boston, 1985, p 209.
15. Woolcock, AJ: The pathophysiology of asthma. In Weiss, EB, Segal, MS and Stein, M (eds): Bronchial Asthma: Mechanisms and Therapeutics, ed 2. Little, Brown & Co, Boston, 1985, p 180.
16. Kingston, HGG and Hirshman, CA: Perioperative management of the patient with asthma. Anesth Analg 63:844, 1984.
17. Fazio, F, et al: Studies of regional ventilation in asthma using ^{81m}Kr. Lung 156:185, 1979.
18. Wagner, PD, et al: Ventilation-perfusion inequality in asymptomatic asthma. Am Rev Respir Dis 118:511, 1978.
19. Weinberger, SE, et al: Pregnancy and the lung. Am Rev Respir Dis 121:559, 1980.
20. Schatz, M: Asthma and pregnancy. In Dawson, A and Simon RA (eds): The Practical Management of Asthma. Grune & Stratton, New York, 1984, p 195.
21. Moya, F, et al: Influence of maternal hyperventilation on the newborn infant. Am J Obstet Gynecol 91:76, 1965.
22. Motoyama, EK, et al: The effect of changes in maternal pH and $PaCO_2$ on the PO_2 of fetal lambs. Anesthesiology 28:891, 1967.
23. Levinson, G, et al: Effects of maternal hyperventilation on uterine blood flow and fetal oxygenation and acid-base status. Anesthesiology 40:340, 1974.
24. Greenberger, PA and Patterson, R: Management of asthma during pregnancy. N Engl J Med 312:897, 1985.
25. Turner, ES, Greenberger, PA and Patterson, R: Management of the pregnant asthmatic patient. Ann Intern Med 6:905, 1980.
26. Gee, JBL, et al: Pulmonary mechanics during pregnancy. J Clin Invest 46:945, 1967.
27. Bevan, DR, et al: Closing volume in pregnancy. Br Med J 1:13, 1974.
28. Craig, DB and Toole, A: Airway closure in pregnancy. Can Anaesth Soc J 22:665, 1975.
29. Holdcroft, A, et al: Airway closure and pregnancy. Anaesthesia 32:517, 1977.
30. Garrard, GS, Littler, WA and Redman, CWG: Closing volume during normal pregnancy. Thorax 33:488, 1978.
31. Awe, RJ, et al: Arterial oxygenation and alveolar-arterial gradients in term pregnancy. Obstet Gynecol 53:182, 1979.
32. Gelber, M, et al: Uncontrollable life-threatening status asthmaticus: An indicator for termination of pregnancy by cesarean section. Respiration 46:320, 1984.
33. Topilsky, M, et al: Status asthmaticus in pregnancy: A case report. Ann Allergy 32:151, 1974.
34. Gluck, JC and Gluck, PA: The effects of pregnancy on asthma: A prospective study. Ann Allergy 37:164, 1976.
35. Sims, CD, Chamberlain, DVP and DeSwiet, M: Lung function tests in bronchial asthma during and after pregnancy. Br J Obstet Gynaecol 83:434, 1976.
36. Bahna, SL and Bjerkedal, T: The course and outcome of pregnancy in women with bronchial asthma. Acta Allergol 27:397, 1972.
37. Gordon, M, et al: Fetal morbidity following potential anoxigenic obstetric conditions. VII. Bronchial asthma. Am J Obstet Gynecol 106:421, 1970.
38. Schatz, M, et al: Corticosteroid therapy for the pregnant asthmatic patient. JAMA 233:844, 1975.
39. Greenberger, PA and Patterson R: Beclomethasone diproprionate for severe asthma during pregnancy. Ann Intern Med 98:478, 1983.
40. Hendeles, L, Massanari, M and Weinberger, M: Update on the pharmacodynamics and pharmacokinetics of theophylline. Chest 88:103S, 1985.
41. Stirt, JA and Sullivan, SF: Aminophylline. Anesth Analg 60:587, 1981.
42. Spector, SL: The treatment of the asthmatic mother during pregnancy and lactation. Ann Allergy 51:173, 1983.
43. Sutton, PL, et al: The pharmacokinetics of theophylline in pregnancy (abstract). J Allergy Clin Immunol 61:174, 1978.
44. Mintz, S: Pregnancy and asthma. In Weiss, EB, Segal, MS and Stein, M (eds): Bronchial Asthma: Mechanisms and Therapeutics, ed 2. Little, Brown & Co, Boston, 1985, p 878.
45. Lipshitz, J: Uterine and cardiovascular effects of aminophylline. Am J Obstet Gynecol 131:716, 1978.
46. Labovitz, E and Spector S: Placental theophylline transfer in pregnant asthmatics. JAMA 247:786, 1982.
47. Arwood, LL, Dasta, JF and Friedman C: Placental transfer of theophylline: Two case reports. Pediatrics 63:844, 1979.
48. Yeh, TF and Pildes, RS: Transplacental aminophylline toxicity in a neonate (letter). Lancet 1:910, 1977.
49. Aranda, JV, et al: Pharmacokinetic aspects in theophylline in premature newborns. N Engl J Med 295:413, 1976.
50. Bory, C, et al: Metabolism of theophylline to caffeine to premature infants. J Pediatrics 94:988, 1979.
51. Tashkin, DP and Venne, JW: Alpha and beta adenergic agents. In Weiss, EB, Segal, MS, and Stein, M (eds): Bronchial Asthma: Mechanisms and Therapeutics, ed 2. Little, Brown & Co, Boston, 1985, p 604.
52. Anderson, K-E, et al: The relaxing effect of terbutaline in the human uterus during term labor. Am J Obstet Gynecol 121:602, 1975.
53. Lipshitz, J and Baillie, P: The effects of the fenoterol hydrobromide (Partusisten) aerosol on uterine activity in the cardiovascular system. Br J Obstet Gynaecol 83:864, 1976.
54. Vinall, PS and Jenkins, DM (letter): Salbutamol and haemorrhage at spontaneous abortion. Lancet 2:1355, 1977.

55. Hernandez, E, Angell, CS and Johnson, JWC: Asthma in pregnancy: Current concepts. Obstet Gynecol 55:739, 1980.
56. Collins, J, McAllister, WAC and Morley, J: Corticosteroids: Mechanisms and dosage schedules. In Weiss, EB, Segal, MS and Stein, M (eds): Bronchial Asthma: Mechanisms and Therapeutics, ed 2. Little, Brown & Co, Boston, 1985, p 675.
57. Morris, HG: Mechanisms of glucocorticoid action in pulmonary disease. Chest 88:133S, 1985.
58. Warrell, DW and Taylor, R: Outcome for the foetus of mothers receiving prednisolone during pregnancy. Lancet 1:117, 1968.
59. Greenberg, F: The potential teratogenicity of allergy and asthma treatment in pregnancy. Immunol Allergy Pract 7:15, 1985.
60. Bernstein, IL: Cromolyn sodium and cromolyn-like drugs. In Weiss, EB, Segal MS and Stein, M (eds): Bronchial Asthma: Mechanisms and Therapeutics, ed 2. Little, Brown & Co, Boston, 1985, p 724.
61. Wilson, J: Use of sodium cromoglycate during pregnancy. J Pharm Med 8:45, 1982.
62. Metzger, WJ, Turner, E and Patterson, R: The safety of immunotherapy during pregnancy. J Allergy Clin Immunol 61:268, 1978.
63. Greenberger, P and Patterson, R: Safety of therapy for allergic symptoms during pregnancy. Ann Intern Med 89:234, 1978.
64. Zierler, S and Purohit, D: Prenatal antihistamine exposure as a potential cause of retrolental fibroplasia (RLF) (abstr). Pediatr Res 18:1566A, 1984.
65. Purohit, DM, et al: Risk factors for retrolental fibroplasia: Experience with 3,025 premature infants. Pediatrics 76:339, 1985.
66. Carswell, F, Kerr, MM and Hutchison, H: Congenital goitre and hypothyroidism produced by maternal ingestion of iodides. Lancet 1:7659, 1970.
67. Mathe, A, et al: Bronchial hyperreactivity to prostaglandin F_2 alpha and histamine in patients with asthma. Br Med J 1:193, 1973.
68. Smith, AP: The effects of intravenous infusion of graded doses of prostaglandins F_2 alpha and E_2 on lung resistance in patients undergoing termination of pregnancy. Clin Sci 44:17, 1973.
69. Kreisman, H, Van De Weil, W and Mitchell, CA: Respiratory function during prostaglandin-induced labor. Am Rev Respir Dis 111:564, 1975.
70. Fishburne, JI, et al: Bronchospasm complicating intravenous prostaglandin F_2 alpha for therapeutic abortion. Obstet Gynecol 39:892, 1972.
71. Edelson, JD and Rebuck, AS: The clinical assessment of severe asthma. Arch Intern Med 145:321, 1985.
72. Williams, MH and Shim, CS: Clinical evaluation of asthma. In Weiss, EB, Segal, MS and Stein, M (eds): Bronchial Asthma: Mechanisms and Therapeutics, ed 2. Little, Brown & Co, Boston, 1985, p 310.
73. Fischl, MA: Approach to acute asthma in the emergency room. In Weiss, EB, Segal, MS and Stein, M (eds): Bronchial Asthma: Mechanisms and Therapeutics, ed 2. Little, Brown & Co, Boston, 1985, p 802.
74. Tatham, ME and Gellert, AR: The management of acute severe asthma. Postgrad Med J 61:599, 1985.
75. Stibolt, TB: Asthma. Med Clin North Am 70:909, 1986.
76. Misenhimer, MR, et al: Effects of vasoconstrictive drugs on the placental circulation of rhesus monkey. Invest Radiol 7:496, 1972.
77. Hood, DD, Dewan, DM and James, FM III: Maternal and fetal effects of epinephrine in gravid ewes. Anesthesiology 64:610, 1986.
78. Leighton, BL, et al: Limitations of epinephrine as a marker of intravascular injection in laboring women. Anesthesiology 66:688, 1987.
79. Syber, TA and Weiss, EB: Status asthmaticus. In Weiss, EB, Segal, MS and Stein, M (eds): Bronchial Asthma: Mechanisms and Therapeutics, ed 2. Little, Brown & Co, Boston, 1985, p 808.
80. Tinkelman, BG, et al: Comparison of nebulized terbutaline and subcutaneous epinephrine in the treatment of acute asthma. Ann Allergy 50:398, 1983.
81. Stiell, IG and Rivington, RM: Adrenergic agents in acute asthma: Valuable new alternatives. Ann Emerg Med 12:493, 1983.
82. Fanta, CH, Rossing, TH and McFadden, ER: Treatment of acute asthma: Is combined therapy with sympathomimetics and methylxanthines indicated? Am J Med 80:5, 1986.
83. Siegel, D, et al: Aminophylline increases the toxicity but not the efficacy of an inhaled beta-adrenergic agonist in the treatment of acute exacerbations of asthma. Am Rev Respir Dis 132:283, 1985.
84. Mitenko, PA and Ogilvie, RI: Rational intravenous doses of theophylline. N Engl J Med 289:600, 1973.
85. Hendeles, L and Weinberger, M: Guidelines for avoiding theophylline overdose (letter). N Engl J Med 300:1217, 1979.
86. Littenberg, GB and Gluck, EH: A controlled trial of methylprednisolone in the emergency treatment of acute asthma. N Engl J Med 314:150, 1986.
87. Schwartz, SH: Treatment of status asthmaticus with halothane. JAMA 251:2688, 1984.
88. Parnass, SM, et al: Status asthmaticus treated with isoflurane and enflurane. Anesth Analg 66:193, 1987.
89. Albright, GA, et al: Physiology and pharmacology. In Albright, GA, et al (eds): Anesthesia in Obstetrics, Maternal, Fetal and Neonatal Aspects. Butterworth & Co, Boston, 1986, p 55.
90. Chestnut, TH, et al: The influence of continuous epidural bupivacaine analgesia on progress of the second stage of labor: A randomized, double-blind, placebo controlled study (abstr). Anesth 66:774, 1987.
91. Eisler, EA: Anesthesia for the pregnant patient with asthma. In Shnider, SM and Levinson, G (eds): Anesthesia for Obstetrics. Williams & Wilkins, Baltimore, 1987, p 382.
92. Mallampati, SR: Bronchospasm during spinal anesthesia. Anesth Analg 60:839, 1981.
93. Bromage, PR: Epidural Analgesia. WB Saunders, Philadelphia, 1978, p 638.
94. Freund, FG, et al: Ventilatory reserve and level of motor block during high spinal and epidural anesthesia. Anesthesiology 28:834, 1967.
95. Gaffud, MP, et al: Surgical analgesia for cesarean

delivery with epidural bupivacaine and fentanyl. Anesthesiology 65:331, 1986.

96. Naulty, JS, et al: Epidural fentanyl for post cesarean delivery pain management. Anesthesiology 63:694, 1985.
97. Gal, TJ: Pulmonary mechanics in normal subjects following endotracheal intubation. Anesthesiology 52:27, 1980.
98. Shnider, SH and Papper, EM: Anesthesia for the asthmatic patient. Anesthesiology 22:886, 1961.
99. Hirshman, CA, et al: Ketamine block of bronchospasm in experimental canine asthma. Br J Anaesth 51:713, 1979.
100. Corssen, G, et al: Ketamine in the anesthetic management of asthmatic patients. Anesth Analg 51:588, 1972.
101. Waltemath, CL and Bergman, NA: Effects of ketamine and halothane on increased respiratory resistance provoked by ultrasonic aerosols. Anesthesiology 41:473, 1974.
102. Kumar, SM, Kothary, SP and Zsigmond, K: Plasma free norepinephrine and epinephrine concentrations following diazepam-ketamine induction in patients undergoing cardiac surgery. Acta Anaesth Scand 22:593, 1978.
103. White, PF, Way, WL and Trevor, AJ: Ketamine: Its pharmacology and therapeutic uses. Anesthesiology 56:119, 1982.
104. Hirshman, CA, et al: Ketamine-aminophylline-induced decrease in seizure threshold. Anesthesiology 56:464, 1982.
105. Steinhaus, JE and Gaskin, L: A study of intravenous lidocaine as a suppressant of cough reflex. Anesthesiology 24:285, 1963.
106. Downes, H and Hirshman, CA: Lidocaine aerosols do not prevent allergic bronchoconstriction. Anesth Analg 60:28, 1981.
107. Downes, H, Gerber, N and Hirshman, CA: IV lignocaine in reflex and allergic bronchoconstriction. Br J Anaesth 52:873, 1980.
108. Greiss, FC, Jr, Still, JG and Anderson, SG: Effects of local anesthetic agents on uterine vasculatures and myometrium. Am J Obstet Gynecol 124:889, 1976.
109. Ostheimer, GW: Effects of maternally administered drugs on the fetus/newborn. In Ostheimer, GW (ed): Manual of Obstetric Anesthesia. Churchill Livingstone, New York, 1984, p 81.
110. Nathan, RA, et al: The effects of H_1 and H_2 antihistamines on histamine inhalation challenges in asthmatic patients. Am Rev Respir Dis 120:1251, 1979.
111. Nathan, RA, Segall, N and Schocket, AL: A comparison of the actions of H_1 and H_2 antihistamines on histamine-induced bronchoconstriction and cutaneous wheal response in asthmatic patients. J Allergy Clin Immunol 67:171, 1981.
112. Koga, Y, Iwatsuki, N and Hashimoto, Y: Direct effects of H_2-receptor antagonists on airway smooth muscle on responses mediated by H_1- and H_2-receptors. Anesthesiology 66:181, 1987.
113. Hirshman, CA and Bergman, NA: Halothane and enflurane protect against bronchospasm in an asthma dog model. Anesth Analg 57:629, 1978.
114. Hirshman, CA, et al: Mechanism of action of inhalation anesthesia on airways. Anesthesiology 57:107, 1982.
115. Hall, KD and Norris, FH, Jr: Fluothane sensitization of dog heart to action of epinephrine. Anesthesiology 19:631, 1958.
116. Munson, ES and Embro, WJ: Enflurane, isoflurane, and halothane and isolated human myometrium. Anesthesiology 46:11, 1977.
117. Crago, RR, et al: Respiratory flow resistance after curare and pancuronium measured by forced oscillations. Can Anaesth Soc J 19:607, 1972.
118. Rosow, CE, et al: Histamine release during morphine and fentanyl anesthesia. Anesthesiology 56:93, 1982.
119. Amyot, R, et al: Prolonged hyporesponsiveness of airway smooth muscle to histamine following general anesthesia. Anesthesiology 64:758, 1986.
120. Roizen, MF and Stevens, WC: Multiformed ventricular tachycardia due to interaction of aminophylline and halothane. Anesth Analg 57:738, 1978.
121. Stirt, JA, et al: Arrhythmogenic effects of aminophylline during halothane anesthesia in experimental animals. Anesth Analg 59:410, 1980.
122. Stirt, JA, et al: Halothane-induced cardiac arrhythmias following administration of aminophylline in experimental animals. Anesth Analg 60:517, 1981.
123. Stirt, JA, et al: Safety of enflurane following administration of aminophylline in experimental animals. Anesth Analg 60:871, 1983.
124. Stirt, JA, Berger, JM and Sullivan, SF: Lack of arrhythmogenicity of isoflurane following administration of aminophylline in dogs. Anesth Analg 62:568, 1983.
125. Prokocimer, PG, et al: Epinephrine arrhythmogenicity is enhanced by acute but not chronic aminophylline administration during halothane anesthesia in dogs. Anesthesiology 65:13, 1986.
126. Casady, JN, Moore, DC and Bridenbaugh, LD: Postpartum hypertension after use of vasoconstrictor and oxytocic drugs. JAMA 172:1011, 1960.
127. Brown, WU, Jr: Respiratory problems. In James, FM III and Wheeler, AS, (eds): Obstetric Anesthesia: The Complicated Patient. FA Davis, Philadelphia, 1982, p 103.
128. Longo, LD: Some health consequences of maternal smoking: Issues without answers. Birth Defects 18:13, 1982.
129. Werler, MM, Pober, BR and Holmes, LB: Smoking and pregnancy. Teratology 32:473, 1985.
130. Denlinger, JK: Pneumothorax. In Orkin, FK and Cooperman, RH (eds): Complications in Anesthesia. JB Lippincott, Philadelphia, 1983, p 173.
131. LoSasso, AM, Gibbs, PS and Moorthy, SS: Obstructive pulmonary disease. In Stoelting, RK and Dierdorf, SF (eds): Anesthesia and Co-existing Disease. Churchill Livingstone, New York, 1983, p 171.
132. Templeton, A: Intrauterine growth retardation associated with hypoxia due to bronchiectasis. Br J Obstet Gynaecol 84:389, 1977.
133. Howie, AD and Milne, JA: Pregnancy in patients with bronchiectasis. Br J Obstet Gynaecol 85:197, 1978.
134. Cohen, LF, diSant'Agnese, PA and Friedlander, J:

Cystic fibrosis and pregnancy: A national survey. Lancet 2:842, 1980.
135. Johnson, SR, et al: Diagnosis of maternal cystic fibrosis during pregnancy. Obstet Gynecol 61:2S, 1983.
136. Shwachman, H, Kowalski, M and Chaw, K-T: Cystic fibrosis: A new outlook. Medicine 56:129, 1977.
137. Palmer, J, et al: Pregnancy in patients with cystic fibrosis. Ann Intern Med 99:596, 1983.
138. Corkey, CWB, et al: Pregnancy in cystic fibrosis: A better prognosis in patients with pancreatic function? Am J Obstet Gynecol 140:737, 1981.
139. Hyde, NH and Harrison, BM: Intrathecal morphine in a parturient with cystic fibrosis. Anesth Analg 65:1357, 1986.
140. Oxorn, H: The changing aspects of pneumonia complicating pregnancy. Am J Obstet Gynecol 70:1057, 1955.
141. Hopwood, HG: Pneumonia in pregnancy. Obstet Gynecol 25:875, 1965.
142. Benedetti, TJ, Valle, R and Ledger, WJ: Antepartum pneumonia in pregnancy. Am J Obstet Gynecol 144:413, 1982.
143. Shelley, WC and Gutsche, BB: Anesthesia for the febrile parturient. In James, JM, III and Wheeler, AS (eds): Obstetric Anesthesia: The Complicated Patient. FA Davis, Philadelphia, 1982, p 297.
144. Eng, RHK and Saligman, SJ: Lumbar puncture-induced meningitis. JAMA 245:1456, 1981.
145. Harris, RE: Coccidioidomycosis complicating pregnancy. Obstet Gynecol 28:401, 1966.
146. Smale, LE and Waechter, KG: Dissemination of coccidioidomycosis in pregnancy. Am J Obstet Gynecol 107:356, 1970.
147. Ricketti, AJ, et al: Allergic bronchopulmonary aspergillosis. Arch Intern Med 143:1553, 1983.
148. Purtilo, DT: Opportunistic mycotic infection in pregnant women. Am J Obstet Gynecol 122:607, 1975.
149. Schaefer, G, et al: Pregnancy and pulmonary tuberculosis. Obstet Gynecol 46:706, 1975.
150. Fishburne, JI: Physiology and disease of the respiratory system in pregnancy. J Reprod Med 22:177, 1979.
151. Alfery, DD and Benumof, JL: Pulmonary diseases. In Katz, J, Benumof, JL and Kadis, JB (eds): Anesthesia and Uncommon Diseases, ed 2. WB Saunders, Philadelphia, 1981, p 221.
152. Wills, MH and Harris, MH: An unusual airway complication with sarcoidosis. Anesthesiology 66:554, 1987.
153. Anderson, HF, Lynch, JP and Johnson, TRB, Jr: Adult respiratory distress syndrome in obstetrics and gynecology. Obstet Gynecol 55:291, 1980.
154. Keefer, JR, et al: Noncardiogenic pulmonary edema and invasive cardiovascular monitoring. Obstet Gynecol 58:46, 1981.
155. Boucher, M, et al: Adult respiratory distress syndrome: A rare manifestation of listeria monocytogenes infection in pregnancy. Am J Obstet Gynecol 149:686, 1984.
156. Feldman, JM: Adult respiratory distress syndrome in a pregnant patient with pheochromocytoma. J Surg Oncol 29:5, 1985.
157. Gallagher, TJ: Etiology in treatment of respiratory failure. In Kaplan, JA (ed): Thoracic Anesthesia. Churchill Livingstone, New York, 1983, p 665.

CHAPTER 11
RENAL DISEASE

SIVAM RAMANATHAN, M.D.
HERMAN TURNDORF, M.D.

Recent advances in medical care have enabled patients with serious renal disease to become pregnant. Renal disease affects the course of pregnancy in many ways. In addition to frequent hypertension, patients with kidney disease experience a significant reduction in renal function following each pregnancy due to enormous demands imposed on the kidneys. A hostile intrauterine environment increases the risk of intrauterine fetal growth retardation and premature delivery. Diminished renal function prolongs the excretion of many drugs. Further, in systemic disorders such as lupus erythematosus and diabetes mellitus, the kidney is only one of the many target organs that sustain damage. Finally, the threat of acute renal failure is ever present in patients with chronic renal disease.

To formulate safe anesthesia management for the obstetric patient the anesthesiologist must have a basic knowledge of 1) pregnancy-induced changes in renal function, 2) the pathologic conditions leading to renal compromise, and 3) the tests available for evaluating renal function.

Applied Physiology

The ability of the nephron to maintain positive sodium balance represents perhaps the most important change in renal function produced by pregnancy. Unlike Chapter 1, which discussed renal function changes in pregnancy, this chapter will review only changes in the tubular mechanisms. These mechanisms are vital to water, acid-base, and electrolyte homeostasis. In its journey through the different segments of the nephron the glomerular filtrate undergoes a series of changes in its osmolarity. Most filtered sodium and water reabsorption takes place primarily in the tubules (Fig. 11–1).[1,2] Except for some active transport in the pars recta sodium reabsorption takes place passively in the proximal tubule, producing an isosmotic filtrate.

Normally, only one third of the glomerular filtrate enters the descending limb. Removal of solutes in the proximal tubule makes the fluid entering the descending limb hyposmotic. The descending limb reabsorbs water but not sodium, with the result that the tubular fluid becomes hyperosmotic in the loop of Henle. The next section of the tubule, the ascending limb, however, allows passage of sodium but not

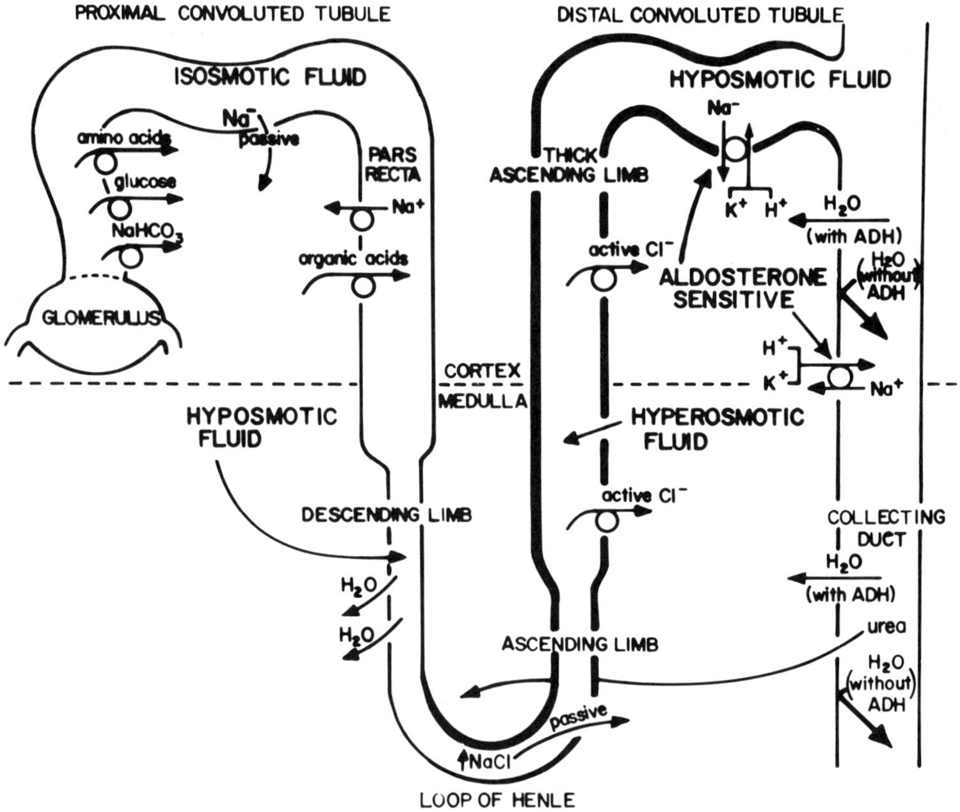

Figure 11–1. Transport function of the various segments of the nephron. For details, see text. (Modified from Brenner, BM;[1] reproduced with permission.)

water. Active electrogenic chloride transport also occurs in the ascending limb while sodium follows passively. Thus the fluid reaching the distal convoluted tubule becomes hyposmotic, and the medullary interstitium becomes hypertonic.

Aldosterone mediates sodium reabsorption in the distal convoluted tubule and in the collecting system, causing exchange of potassium and hydrogen for sodium. Most of the distal convoluted tubule is impermeable to water. The antidiuretic hormone (ADH) acts mainly at the cortical and papillary portions of the collecting duct. In the presence of ADH, avid water reabsorption produces a hypertonic urine.

The lateral decubitus position mobilizes large volumes of fluid in pregnant subjects, leading to increased urine formation. However, the upright and supine postures have an antidiuretic effect independent of changes in renal plasma flow,[3] possibly due to increased ureteral pressure, which makes the proximal nephron absorb water more readily.

Evaluation of Renal Function

BASIC CONCEPTS

The kidney eliminates different metabolic waste products via different excretory mechanisms which include glomerular filtration and tubular secretion. In addition, some substances may undergo tubular reabsorption. During renal failure the rate of rise of plasma concentrations of these waste products depends on the most seriously affected aspect of renal function (Fig. 11–2).[2] Since urea and creatinine depend entirely on glomerular filtration for their elimination, a

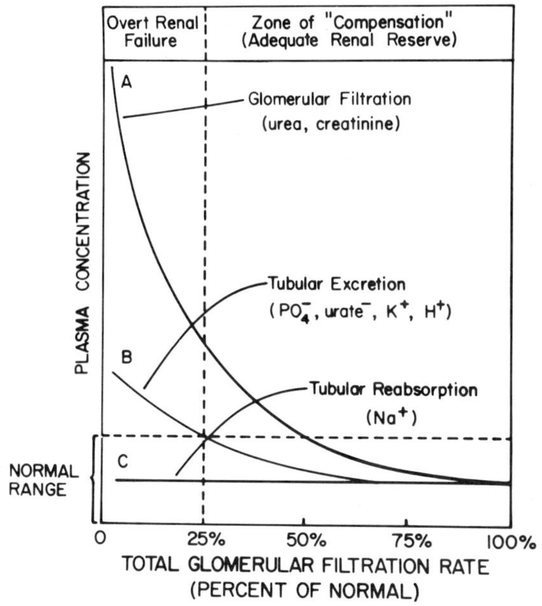

Figure 11–2. The rate of rise of plasma concentrations of three classes of substances as a function of decreased GFR. *(Curve A)* Substances that depend for elimination on glomerular filtration. *(Curve B)* Substances that depend on tubule transport mechanisms. *(Curve C)* Reabsorbed substances. (From Brenner BM[1] with permission.)

50-percent decrease in glomerular function causes a rapid increase in the plasma concentrations of these two substances. Substances that depend on tubular excretion (phosphate, urate, potassium and hydrogen) remain less affected, unless kidney function substantially decreases. A third class of substances such as sodium undergo both glomerular filtration and extensive tubular reabsorption. When filtration fails, the nephron can maintain sodium balance by decreasing reabsorption; this achieves a constant level of elimination. In other words, sodium balance continues by slow modification of the reabsorptive process in the remaining nephrons. Figure 11–1 describes the sites of normal sodium reabsorption. Thus, whereas plasma sodium concentration may remain unaffected until renal disease reaches the terminal stage, blood urea nitrogen (BUN) and creatinine change earlier in the course of the disease and represent sensitive indices of early renal dysfunction. Severe electrolyte abnormalities usually indicate advanced renal disease.

RENAL FUNCTION TESTS

Routine Assessment

The anesthesiologist can perform a battery of tests to assess several aspects of renal function. The anesthesiologist must correctly interpret these tests, for they often enable him or her not only to pinpoint the extent of renal dysfunction but to tailor fluid and electrolyte therapy suitably in the perioperative period. In patients with minor impairment, BUN and serum creatinine measurements prove adequate for assessing renal function. However, in the presence of severe impairment, clearance tests have greater value because they measure the glomerular filtration rate (GFR).[4] The creatinine clearance represents a simple test that requires only urine collection and a plasma creatinine measurement. Clearance tests at best reflect only the overall elimination of a substance by the kidney and offer little help in evaluating the individual segment of the nephron. (A summary of clinically useful renal function tests appears in Table 11–1.)

In normal pregnancy, increased renal blood flow (RBF) reduces the plasma concentrations of BUN and increases plasma creatinine clearance. Although acceptable in nonpregnant subjects, a BUN value of 15 mg per dl and a serum creatinine value of 0.85 mg per dl should arouse a high degree of suspicion in pregnant patients.[5]

Glomerular Filtration Rate and Renal Plasma Flow

Inulin clearance and para-aminohippuric acid (PAH) clearance measure GFR and renal plasma flow (RPF), respectively. The Fick equation provides the basis for measuring RPF. Inulin is ideal for measuring GFR, for the kidney neither reabsorbs nor excretes it. The major problem with PAH is that 10 to 15 percent of the RPF supplies areas of the kidney that cannot remove the drug. Thus, the renal vein concentration of PAH is *not* zero, and consequently the PAH clearance measures not the total RPF but the effective RPF to those portions of the kidney which do remove the drug.[6] The same considerations apply to iodohippurate.[6]

Table 11–1. RENAL FUNCTION TESTS

Test	Normal Values
Tests of Glomerular Function	
Clinical tests	
BUN	10–20 mg/dl (nonpregnant) 5–8 mg/dl (pregnant)
Serum creatinine	0.6–1 mg/dl (nonpregnant) 0.58 mg/dl (pregnant)
Creatinine clearance	85–125 ml/min (nonpregnant) 120–180 ml/min (pregnant)
Investigational tests	
Insulin clearance (C_{In}) (GFR)	110 ml/min/1.73 m^2 (nonpregnant)
PAH clearance* (effective RPF)	660 ml/min/1.73m^2
Effective RBF (=RPF/(1-hematocrit))	1200 ml/min/1.73m^2
Filtration fraction (GFR/RPF or C_{In}/C_{PAH})	0.2
Tests of Tubular Function	
Fractional sodium excretion	<1% in prerenal azotemia >1% in acute tubular necrosis
Free water clearance	Negative in prerenal azotemia; zero or positive in ARF

Fractional excretion of sodium = urine sodium concentration/urine creatinine concentration × plasma creatinine concentration/plasma sodium concentration × 100%

Free water clearance = urine volume − osmolar clearance

Osmolar clearance = urine osmolarity × urine volume per min/plasma osmolarity

*See text for inaccuracies associated with PAH clearance.

Glomerular Function

Fractional excretion and fractional reabsorption tests evaluate global glomerular function. These tests help distinguish prerenal azotemia from acute tubular necrosis (ATN).

$$\text{Fractional excretion of a substance X} = \frac{\text{concentration X in urine/concentration in plasma}}{\text{concentration inulin in urine/inulin concentration in plasma}}$$

For an approximate calculation, the corresponding creatinine concentration may substitute for inulin concentration.

$$\text{Fractional reabsorption} = 1 - \text{fractional excretion}$$

Concentrating Ability of Kidney

Free water clearance measures the ability of the tubule to concentrate or dilute the urine. When the amount of water excreted exceeds osmolar clearance, the quantity of water inappropriately matches the amount of solute present in the urine, signifying defective tubular function. For instance, a patient with polyuric renal failure may have a positive free water clearance because the volume of water excreted exceeds that volume needed for producing isosmotic urine. A negative free water clearance indicates prerenal azotemia.[7]

Pregnancy and Renal Disease

The serum creatinine level reflects the severity of renal disease in pregnancy.[5] In mild disease, serum creatinine remains below 1.4 mg per dl. In moderate impairment, the level rises to between 1.5 and 3 mg per dl. In severe impairment the creatinine level exceeds 3 mg per dl and BUN, 30 mg per dl. Although many women with severe impairment become infertile, an occasional patient may conceive.

Using six studies as their sources, Davison and associates[5] summarized the effects of renal disease on pregnancy. Hypertension, proteinuria, and declining renal function may complicate the antenatal course. Early diagnosis of pre-eclampsia often proves difficult in patients with renal disease.[8] The frequency of preterm deliveries, intrauterine growth retardation, stillbirths, and neonatal deaths is higher for these patients compared with normal patients.[9–13] Long-term follow-up shows that a significant percentage of patients may develop hypertension and permanent deterioration of renal function. Because of the threat of further deterioration in renal function, perinatologists advise patients with severe renal impairment to avoid pregnancy.[5] The development of *hypertension* represents the single most important factor that determines pregnancy outcome. In the absence of hypertension, many patients with mild disease can expect a normal outcome. When hypertension complicates pregnancy, the prognosis for the mother and the fetus is poor (Fig. 11–3).[8]

TYPES OF RENAL DISEASES IN PREGNANCY

Except for pre-eclamptic nephropathy, the etiology of renal disease in a pregnant patient resembles the causes found in the general population. The type of renal disease not only influences the pregnancy outcome but determines to what extent pregnancy affects renal function.[1,4] Table 11–2 summarizes the types of lesions typically seen in pregnant patients.

Chronic Pyelonephritis

The disease involves the tubulointerstitial renal tissue. Exacerbations commonly appear during pregnancy because of the increased tendency to bacteriuria and dehydration. Generally, these patients tend to have a more benign antenatal

Table 11–2. TYPES OF RENAL DISEASE IN PREGNANCY

Chronic pyelonephritis
Chronic glomerulonephritis
Lupus nephropathy
Diabetic nephropathy
Urinary calculi
Transplanted kidney
Permanent urinary diversion
Nephrotic syndrome
Hemodialysis
Polycystic kidney
Solitary kidney
Periarteritis nodosa
Scleroderma
Acute renal failure

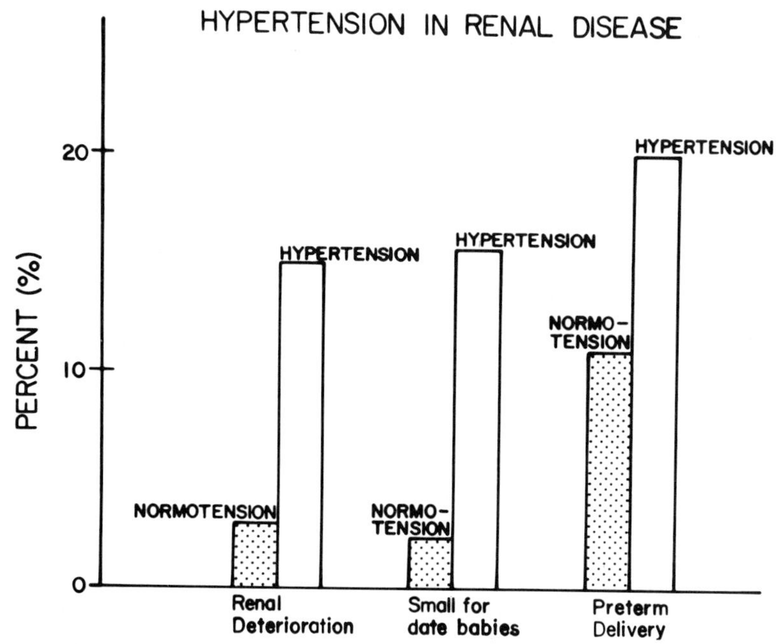

Figure 11–3. Hypertension in renal disease. (Data from Surian, M, et al,[8] with permission.)

course than those with glomerular involvement.[5]

Chronic Glomerulonephritis

This condition presents histopathologically as focal, diffuse, proliferative, or lupus type. Pre-eclampsia occurs more frequently in these patients. Chronic glomerulonephritis may lead to nephrotic syndrome. The perinatal mortality can reach 18 percent.[15] A bleeding diathesis due to platelet abnormalities is associated with a rare form of this condition, the hereditary nephritis.[5]

Systemic Lupus Erythematosus

In addition to renal involvement, systemic lupus erythematosus (SLE) has protean manifestations. Endocarditis (Libman-Sacks) and coronary artery narrowing occur in some individuals. The disease will worsen in 50 percent of patients who experience exacerbations in the 6 months preceding conception.[16] Among those in remission, a smaller percentage of patients will have a relapse. Abortion, perinatal mortality, and premature delivery occur with increased frequency.[16–22] In addition to clinical exacerbations, some will undergo a transient or permanent deterioration of renal function. Proteinuria and reduced creatinine clearance indicate poor prognosis.

Many serologic tests define the severity and help diagnose exacerbations of SLE. The serum factors include complements (total complements and CH50, C4, and C3 fractions), antibody to nuclear antigens (ANA), and the lupus anticoagulant. Reduced concentrations of CH50 and C4 reportedly represent early indicators of renal exacerbations. The antibody to the soluble DNA (anti–RO[SS-A]) may cross the placenta and cause neonatal lupus erythematosus which resembles the adult condition. Congenital anomalies, particularly heart block and endocardial fibroelastosis, appear more frequently in babies born of women who have SLE than in the general population. Antibody deposition in the developing fetal heart probably plays a role in the pathogenesis of the heart block.[14,23] Some workers speculate that the lupus anticoagulant binds with platelet membranes, thus causing platelet aggregation and an increased incidence of spontaneous arterial and venous thrombosis. This probably explains the extensive thrombotic changes in the placenta and the increased abortion rate. The anticoagulant only rarely causes a bleeding diathesis. Treatment with low-dose aspirin and/or corticosteroids may prove beneficial when thrombotic complications occur.[24]

Patients with SLE should receive corticosteroids and/or immunosuppressants such as azathioprine. Suspicion exists that these two drugs cause fetal malformations such as cleft palate and intrauterine growth retardation. However, the risk appears small and therefore one should use the drugs, especially for severe maternal disease.[16] The administration of corticosteroids must continue for at least 2 months following delivery. A subsequent section of this chapter discusses problems associated with azathioprine use.

Diabetic Nephropathy

Diabetic nephropathy often causes death in juvenile diabetics. The onset of proteinuria usually signals a life expectancy of less than 5 years. The nephropathy mainly affects the glomeruli. Two types of lesions develop: localized nodular glomerulosclerosis (Kimmelstiel-Wilson syndrome) and the diffuse type,[25] in which thickening of the glomerular basement membrane occurs throughout the kidney. Pregnancy per se may not worsen renal function, but moderate to heavy proteinuria occurs in 50 percent of pregnant women with diabetic nephropathy. The incidence of pre-eclampsia rises considerably, and the perinatal mortality reaches 25 percent in severe cases.[5] For these reasons, many authorities feel that patients with severe nephropathy must avoid pregnancy. In many patients with diabetic nephropathy, retinopathy may also coexist.[25] Severe retinopathy may require photocoagulation for the treatment of retinal detachment. Patients with retinopathy must often undergo a cesarean section to avoid possible straining during vaginal birth. Patients with diabetic nephropathy often qualify for future renal transplantation.[15]

Urinary Calculi

Urinary calculi appear in less than 1 percent of all pregnancies. They often produce alarming symptoms necessitating surgical removal. Lumbar epidural analgesia extending between T11 and L2 segments can relieve ureteric colic. Because of its antispasmodic effect, epidural analgesia could even cause spontaneous passage of the stone.[26]

Transplanted Kidney

Although earlier studies report successful pregnancies,[27] patients with a transplanted kidney have an increased incidence of complications during pregnancy. Excluding therapeutic abortions, 71 percent can expect a normal pregnancy outcome. Nine percent of women, however, experience serious rejection episodes during pregnancy.[28] Table 11–3 summarizes other serious maternal and fetal problems associated with kidney transplantation. Although azathioprine and/or corticosteroids, the two immunosuppressants, produce congenital anomalies in animal fetuses, they do not appear to be risky for humans. Both azathioprine and its active metabolite 6-mercaptopurine undergo only limited placental transfer. The administration of these two drugs must continue throughout pregnancy.[28]

Azathioprine structurally resembles aminophylline, a phosphodiesterase inhibitor. Injected intra-arterially, azathioprine increases the excitability of the skeletal musculature, thus producing a dose-related increase in the force of muscle contraction. Because of this property, it reverses the effects of nondepolarizing relaxants and potentiates those of succinylcholine. Any patient receiving this drug needs close monitoring of the neuromuscular transmission.[29]

Table 11–3. PREGNANCY OUTCOME IN PATIENTS WITH TRANSPLANTED KIDNEY

Outcome	Occurrence (%)
Mother	
Full-term delivery	71
Rejection episodes	9
Pre-eclampsia	30
Mechanical obstruction*	5–10
Ureteral obstruction	
Ileal loop obstruction	
Dystocia (mechanical obstruction)	
Fetus	
Prematurity	20
Neonatal deaths (prematurity)	3

*Mechanical obstruction is due to the pelvic location of the transplanted kidney.

Permanent Urinary Diversion

Women with congenital anomalies of the lower urinary tract require surgical urinary diversion, which predisposes to urinary tract infection, acute pyelonephritis, and renal dysfunction during pregnancy. The gravid uterus may obstruct the ileal conduit or the ureterocolic anastomosis. The cesarean section rate rises due to coincidental lower genitourinary tract abnormality. Urinary diversion does not preclude vaginal delivery. Since patients with ureterosigmoid anastomosis need an intact anal sphincter for urinary continence,[14] one must avoid damage to the perineum. Blocking the second, third, and the fourth sacral segments with a lumbar epidural anesthetic may avoid a precipitate delivery, thus preventing anal sphincter damage. Physicians rarely perform ureterosigmoidoscopy nowadays because of the risk of hyperchloremic acidosis secondary to intestinal exchange of chloride ion for bicarbonate.

Nephrotic Syndrome

The condition involves albuminuria (>3.5 g per 24 hr), hypoalbuminemia, hyperlipidemia, and edema.[30] The edema results from reduced plasma oncotic pressure (POP). The serum concentrations of low-density lipoproteins and cholesterol often rise. Urinary loss of thyroglobulin and immunoglobulin results in a hypothyroid state and IgG deficiency, respectively.

The nephrotic syndrome frequently appears in the third trimester[5] secondary to pre-eclampsia. Other causes of nephrotic syndrome resemble those of nonpregnant subjects. Nephrotic syndrome predisposes patients to bilateral or unilateral renal vein thrombosis[31] characterized by fever, severe flank pain, and rapid deterioration of renal function. The hypercoagulable state of pregnancy increases the risk of renal vein thrombosis, even in pregnant women with normal kidney function. Thus, these patients require anticoagulation therapy to treat renal vein thrombosis effectively, especially in the presence of pulmonary embolism.

Nephrologists do not recommend diuretics for the treatment of nephrotic edema, because these agents can precipitate hypovolemic renal failure. Nor does salt-poor albumin therapy prove effective (except in cases of severe hypoalbuminemia), because most of the albumin is excreted with the urine.[30] Serum albumin decreases approximately 1 g per dl in normal pregnancy, a fact worth remembering when using serum albumin as an index of renal dysfunction.[5]

Chronic Hemodialysis

Women on chronic hemodialysis usually become infertile. When serum creatinine and BUN levels remain elevated above 3 mg per dl and 30 mg per dl, respectively, conception rarely occurs. However, one out of every 200 women on dialysis does become pregnant. Spontaneous abortions occur frequently, and these women must often undergo therapeutic abortions to spare their lives. Fetal problems include low birth weight and prematurity. During or immediately following hemodialysis, premature labor, vaginal bleeding, and systemic hypotension reportedly occur.[15]

Hemodialysis may contribute to low platelet count, the possibility of rebound or residual heparinization, and hypovolemia (Table 11–4). Thrombocytopenia often follows retention of platelets on the dialysis membranes. Even with full heparinization, thrombocytopenia can occur because heparin does not decrease the surface activity of platelets and reportedly augments adenosine disphosphate (ADP)–induced platelet aggregation.[32] The newer dialysis membranes do not cause a reduction in plasma pseudocholinesterase activity as did the older ones.[33]

Polycystic Kidney Disease

An unaffected kidney functioning normally generally indicates a favorable outcome. However, patients with this condition do have a higher incidence of hypertension and pre-eclampsia. In one study, 40 percent of such patients experienced hypertension.[34]

Solitary Kidney

This condition results from a previous nephrectomy or congenital absence of one kidney. Infection in the solitary kidney that does not respond to antibiotics may dictate pregnancy termination. The ectopic solitary kidney seems more vulnerable to infection than a normally situated one.[5]

Polyarteritis Nodosa

Renal involvement, usually affecting medium and small arteries, occurs in 80 percent of patients with this condition. Some have proposed immunologic etiology, and many studies have implicated hepatitis B virus as the antigen.[35] A syndrome indistinguishable from polyarteritis nodosa occurs in drug addicts.[35] Malignant hypertension, common in patients with polyarteritis nodosa, often necessitates therapeutic termination of pregnancy.

Scleroderma

Diffuse fibrosis of the skin and of internal organs, including the lung, gastrointestinal tract, heart, and the kidney occurs. Cardiac fibrosis leads to heart blocks and arrhythmias. Dilatation of the lower two thirds of the esophagus increases the risk of regurgitation of gastric contents. Acute onset of fibrinoid necrosis of the wall of the afferent glomerular arteriole may lead to malignant hypertension, acute renal failure, and death. A more benign variant with proteinuria exists without hypertension.[36] Renal

Table 11–4. PROBLEMS DUE TO DIALYSIS

Complication	Manifestation (Mechanism)
Hypoxia	Excessive HCO_3^- removal
Hypoventilation	Same as above
Hypovolemia	Hypotension (excessive fluid removal)
Acetate toxicity	Hypotension (acetate in dialysate)
Thrombocytopenia	Bleeding (surface adhesion of platelets)
Rebound heparinization	Bleeding (vaginal bleeding)
Disequilibrium syndrome	Headache, nausea (elevated CVP)
Dialysis encephalopathy	Slurred speech, death (aluminum toxicity)
Digitalis toxicity	Cardiac arrhythmias (hypokalemia)

Table 11–5. CAUSES OF ACUTE RENAL FAILURE IN PREGNANCY

Condition	Probable Causes
Antepartum hemorrhage	Abortion, placenta previa, abruptio placentae
Postpartum hemorrhage	Uterine atony, retained placenta
Pre-eclampsia	
Disseminated intravascular coagulation	Amniotic fluid embolism, fetal demise, abruptio placentae
Septic shock	Pyelonephritis, chorioamnionitis, septic abortion
Transfusion reactions	
Nephrotoxins	X-ray contrast media, antibiotics (aminoglycosides, cephalosporin, amphotericin B), nonsteroidal anti-inflammatory drugs* (acetaminophen, phenbutazone, salicylates, indomethacin)

*Nonsteroidal anti-inflammatory drugs prevent prostaglandin synthesis in the kidney, thereby leading to renal vasoconstriction and renal failure.

blood flow decreases in cold ambient temperatures, thus explaining the increased number of deaths from renal failure in fall and winter. Therefore, intravenous fluids should be warmed before they are infused.

Acute Renal Failure

Acute renal failure (ARF) in pregnancy accounts for 50 percent of all ARF in young women (Table 11–5).[37] Prerenal, renal, or postrenal complications contribute to ARF. In early pregnancy, ARF usually is associated with septic abortion and in late pregnancy, with abruptio placentae, obstetric hemorrhage, and/or pre-eclampsia. Disagreement exists as to the exact pathophysiologic mechanisms underlying ARF.[38,39] Oliguric renal failure appears to be related to intense outer cortical vasoconstriction and a marked increase in preglomerular vascular resistance, leading to filtration failure.[39]

In obstetric patients, the most common cause of oliguric renal failure remains systemic hypotension due to hemorrhage or hyperemesis. Persistent hypovolemia results in reduced cortical blood flow and acute tubular necrosis (ATN). One can differentiate between prerenal oliguria and ATN by infusing 500 ml of saline rapidly, followed by administration of furosemide (100 to 120 mg; see also Table 11–6). Failure of urinary output to improve within 2 hours calls for the insertion of a central venous pressure (CVP) catheter and administration of a further 500 ml of saline and additional doses of furosemide. If urinary output does not improve (despite a normal CVP), the oliguria most likely represents a response to ATN.

Pre-eclampsia. ARF occurs more frequently in multiparous women and probably relates to increased renal vascular resistance.

Major Transfusion Reaction. Obstetric patients who face the threat of severe hemorrhage run the greatest risk.

Renal Cortical Necrosis (RCN). The limited number of cases of RCN reported in the literature relate primarily to pregnancy complications such as abruptio placentae or pre-eclampsia. RCN produces permanent deterioration in renal function. While total anuria rarely accompanies ATN it commonly lasts several days in RCN. In most cases, RCN remains an irreversible condition. When renal necrosis shows confluence, the mortality rate reaches 100 percent if dialysis does not begin early in the course of the disease.[37]

Obstructive Uropathy. The gravid uterus can obstruct the ectopic kidney, transplanted kidney, ileal conduit, and ureterosigmoid anastomosis.

Postpartum Hemolytic Uremic Syndrome. This rare condition, characterized by fibrinoid necrosis in the renal vessels, starts with an influenza-like prodrome and results in acute ARF. Hemodialysis and correction of hemolytic anemia represent the only hopes for survival.[37] The etiology of the condition remains unknown. An autoimmune mechanism has been proposed.[40]

PRINCIPLES OF MANAGEMENT OF RENAL FAILURE

Since hypovolemia significantly contributes to AFR in the obstetric-patient population, one must correct circulating volume deficits without

Table 11–6. DIFFERENCES BETWEEN PRERENAL AZOTEMIA AND ACUTE TUBULAR NECROSIS

Test	Prerenal	Oliguric ARF
Urine osmolarity (mOsm/kg H_2O)	>500	<350
Urine sodium (mEq/liter)	<20	>40
Urine/plasma urea nitrogen	>8	<3
Urine/plasma creatinine	>40	<20
Renal failure index	<1	>1
Fractional excretion of filtered sodium	<1	>1
Urine sediment	Not remarkable	Brown granular casts

$$\text{Renal failure index} = \frac{\text{urinary sodium concentration}}{\text{urine/plasma creatinine ratio}}$$

delay. The obstetrician must attempt to identify whether renal or prerenal factors are causing ARF (Table 11–6). Monitoring right heart filling pressures proves helpful. Administration of mannitol or a loop diuretic such as furosemide in high doses early in the course of renal failure may help to re-establish urine flow.[41] However, the effect of diuretic therapy on the long-term outcome and mortality remains unknown. Some workers advocate the use of mannitol for the management of transfusion reaction.[37]

In the oliguric phase of ARF, limit fluid intake to the output volume plus 400 ml per day for insensible loss. The diet should consist of 40 g of protein and 100 g of carbohydrates per day. The patient in a catabolic state may require parenteral hyperalimentation. Acid-base and electrolyte imbalances and infection demand immediate control. Mild metabolic acidosis does not require correction, and the patient needs $NaHCO_3$ only when the serum HCO_3^- concentration falls below 10 mEq per liter. Treatment of hyperkalemia, a cause of life-threatening cardiac arrhythmias, should aim at 1) antagonizing the cardiac effects of potassium with calcium ions, 2) producing redistribution of potassium with $NaHCO_3$ and/or glucose-insulin infusion, and 3) producing increased excretion of the potassium with potassium exchange resin or with hemodialysis (Table 11–7).

Failure to institute hemodialysis in a pregnant patient could result in premature labor due to fluid and electrolyte abnormalities associated with ARF. The following represent indications for instituting dialysis: 1) serum potassium greater than 6.5 mEq per liter, 2) severe volume overload, 3) uremic encephalopathy, 4) pericardial effusion with circulatory compromise, 5) BUN over 120 mg per dl, 6) severe metabolic acidosis, and 7) the presence of a dialyzable nephrotoxin.[37]

PREANESTHETIC EVALUATION OF PATIENTS WITH RENAL DISEASE

Evaluation of the Mother

Severe renal disease affects almost every system in the body (Table 11–8). The preoperative evaluation must focus on the possible presence of hypertension, pericardial effusion, uremic lung, anemia, renal osteodystrophy, hepatic dysfunction (in severe cases, hepatorenal syndrome), and acid-base and electrolyte disorders. Patients on hemodialysis often carry hepatitis B virus. The physician must evaluate

Table 11–7. TREATMENT OF HYPERKALEMIA

Treatment	Mechanism	Onset	Duration
Calcium gluconate IV 10–30 ml (1–3 ampules)	Direct antagonism	Immediate	Brief
$NaHCO_3$ (45–135 mEq) IV	Redistribution	Minutes	Hours
Glucose 10% (500 ml) + Regular insulin 10 U	Redistribution	Minutes	Hours
Potassium-exchange resin + Sorbitol 70% (20 ml oral, 50 ml rectal)	Elimination	Hours	Hours
Hemodialysis	Elimination	Hours	Hours

Note: If serum K^+ increases above 6.5 mEq/liter and if ECG signs are present, institute therapy immediately. Redistribution causes K^+ to enter the intracellular medium.

Table 11–8. MULTISYSTEM INVOLVEMENT IN RENAL FAILURE

Cardiovascular Hypertension Pericarditis Cardiac tamponade Cardiomyopathy	Musculoskeletal Renal osteodystrophy Low back pain Compression fracture Soft-tissue calcification
Respiratory Bat-wing infiltrates (uremic lung) Mild restrictive lung disease Reduced CO diffusion Infection Pulmonary calcification Pleural effusion	Endocrine Secondary hyperparathyroidism Adrenal insufficiency Glucose intolerance (decreased tissue sensitivity to insulin) Spontaneous hypoglycemia
Neurologic Autonomic neuropathy (decreased baroceptor action) Uremic encephalopathy Peripheral neuropathy (affects lower limbs)	Gastrointestinal Hepatic dysfunction Mouth ulcers Delayed gastric emptying Hiccough Nausea, vomiting Hyperacidity
Hemopoietic Anemia Thrombocytopenia Bleeding tendency Hypoproteinemia Hemolysis	Metabolic Acid-base disorders Electrolyte disorders Immunologic Hepatitis Immunosuppression

antihypertensive therapy and immunosuppressant therapy with azathioprine and corticosteroids. Pre-eclampsia and diabetes mellitus (if present) require careful evaluation.

Evaluation of the Fetus

The severe intrauterine growth retardation associated with renal disease mandates antenatal surveillance of the fetus. The fetal biophysical profile, which includes nonstress testing and ultrasound examination of fetal breathing motion, fetal body motion, fetal tone, and amniotic fluid volume fulfills this purpose. Urinary estriol measurements yield misleading results in patients with renal disease because 1) estriol elimination depends on glomerular filtration,[15] 2) estriols do not predict fetal well-being in growth-retarded fetuses,[42] and 3) corticosteroid therapy alters estriol production. Many authorities favor delivery of a severely growth-retarded fetus with an estimated body weight of 1500 g, regardless of the gestational age, because his or her chance of survival improves in a neonatal intensive care unit as compared with a hostile intrauterine environment.[5]

LABORATORY EVALUATION

Patients with mild renal impairment require only routine testing. Severe impairment calls for multiple tests to more comprehensively evaluate the patient (Tables 11–1, 11–9). Complete

Table 11–9. LABORATORY TESTS FOR PREANESTHETIC EVALUATION OF THE PARTURIENT WHO HAS RENAL DISEASE

Complete blood count
Platelet count
Bleeding, clotting, prothrombin, and partial thromboplastin times
BUN, uric acid, serum cholesterol
Serum creatinine
Creatinine clearance
Serum electrolytes: Na^+, K^+, Ca^{2+}, PO_4^{2-}, Mg^{2+}, HCO_3^-
Complete liver function tests (including blood glucose and serum albumin)
ECG (hypertensive cardiovascular disease, hyperkalemia)
Urinalysis (casts, osmolarity, proteinuria, hematuria, specific gravity, 24-hour protein excretion)
Arterial blood pH and gas tensions
Chest film

blood count, platelet count, urinalysis and measurement of serum creatinine, BUN, serum electrolytes, and arterial blood pH and gas tensions usually provide sufficient information. Examination of urinary sediment yields valuable information as to the type of renal disease.[15] Any increase in proteinuria usually suggests deteriorating renal function. In addition, one should evaluate the coagulation system using partial thromboplastin and prothrombin times. An ECG may show signs of uremic pericarditis, hypertensive cardiomegaly, and hyperkalemia.

Effects of Anesthesia on the Kidney

Anesthesia and surgery profoundly affect renal function. Difficulty often arises in distinguishing the renal effects of anesthetics from those of perioperative stress, which also diminishes renal function. Anesthesia may affect the kidneys immediately, or conversely, a delayed response may follow.[6] The immediate effects can be either indirect or direct. Anesthetics act indirectly by influencing hemodynamics, sympathetic system activity, and/or endocrine function. Some anesthetics also directly inhibit certain aspects of tubular function. Nephrotoxicity caused by methoxyflurane represents a delayed effect.

INDIRECT EFFECTS

In surgical patients with normal renal function, anesthetics depress GFR, RBF, and sodium excretion. Renal vasoconstriction occurring secondary to systemic hypotension may cause a 25- to 35-percent reduction in RBF and GFR.[6] Agents that produce sympathetic stimulation (diethyl ether or cyclopropane) cause more renal vasoconstriction than do substances such as halothane that do not activate the sympathetic system. Berne[43] demonstrated the role of the sympathetic system in anesthesia-induced reduction of GFR and RBF, showing that RBF and GFR decreased after induction of anesthesia only in the nondenervated kidney. In the denervated kidney, RBF and GFR remained unchanged. Thus, anesthetics seem to increase renal vascular resistance by increasing sympathetic activity. Spinal and epidural anesthesia extending to the T5 level interfere only minimally with RPF and GFR provided that the circulating blood volume and blood pressure remain normal. An ability to produce afferent denervation of the kidney explains their minimal interference with renal function.[6]

Controversy exists regarding the effects of anesthetics on renal autoregulation. In isolated preparations, anesthesia with 1 minimum alveolar concentration (MAC) halothane has no effect on renal autoregulation, but in intact animals, halothane significantly interferes with this regulatory mechanism.[44] Autoregulation enables the kidney to maintain a relatively constant RPF over a wide range of mean arterial pressures (MAP) (80 to 150 mmHg). When the MAP exceeds normal values, the afferent arterioles of the glomerulus act as step-down transformers to reduce the hydrostatic pressure in the glomerular capillary thus maintaining a constant RPF (Fig. 11–4).[4] Since 80 mmHg represents the lower limit of MAP at which autoregulation fails (50 mmHg for cerebral autoregulation), the anesthesiologist must maintain a normal perfusion pressure and a normal renal vascular resistance in the perioperative period.

The effects of anesthetics or RBF and GFR relate to their drug dosages.[45,46] Extracellular volume contraction exaggerates the renal effects of anesthetics. Fluid infusion may reverse some of the depressant effects of anesthetics on renal function. Even balanced anesthesia with nitrous oxide and curare reduces GFR.[47] Spinal anesthesia produces only minimal changes in renal function.[48,49]

Anesthesia and surgery alter renal function indirectly through neuroendocrine mechansims. Surgical stress releases ADH and catecholamines. Labor pains often produce stress and anxiety. Other potent stimuli for ADH release include hypovolemia and both parenteral and epidural use of morphine. ADH secretions increase tubular reabsorption of water, resulting in oliguria. Both adrenaline and noradrenaline produce marked renal vasoconstriction, especially of the afferent arteriole, leading to depressed RBF, GFR, and renal electrolyte excretion.[6] Catecholamines also shunt the blood away from the renal cortex, thereby reducing cortical perfusion.[50] Agents with α-adrenergic activity (droperidol) diminish the catecholamine-induced redistribution of RBF.[51]

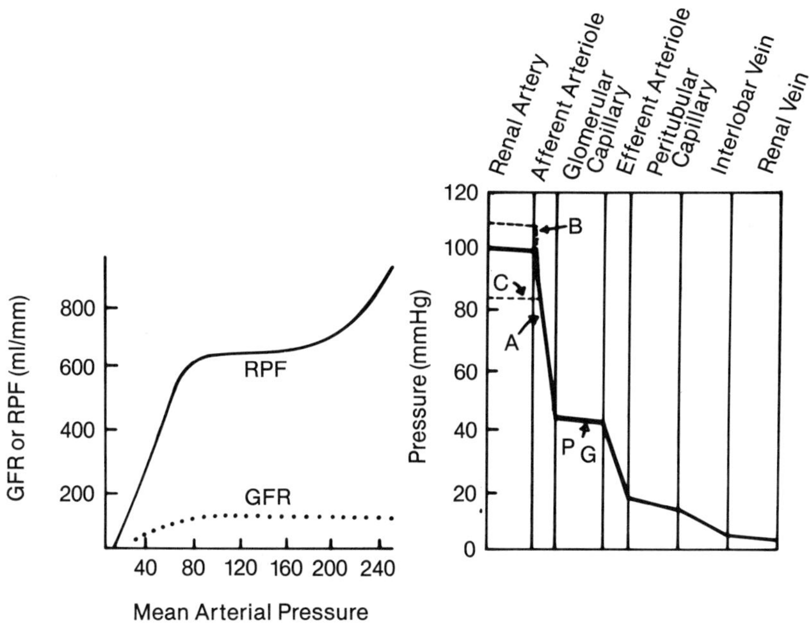

Figure 11–4. Autoregulation by the kidney. *(Left panel)* At mean blood pressure 80 to 180 mmHg the renal plasma flow and glomerular filtration rate change only minimally. *(Right panel)* A change in the caliber of the glomerular afferent arteriole prevents changes in perfusion pressure, thus maintaining GFR at a relatively constant level. *(A)* Normal mean pressure; *(B)* hypertension; and *(C)* less than normal mean pressure; P_G, glomerular capillary hydrostatic pressure.

DIRECT EFFECTS

Anesthetics also directly inhibit renal function. However, the indirect effects overshadow the direct effects. Experiments on isolated toad bladder provide evidence concerning the direct effects. Anesthetics inhibit transport of sodium across the toad bladder, a response that could also occur in the renal tubules.[52] Anesthetics also depress organic acid transfer in the renal tubules.[53] In vitro studies have shown that anesthetics cause diminished uptake of para-aminohippuric acid by kidney slices.[54]

DELAYED EFFECTS

Many volatile anesthetic agents undergo biotransformation, releasing by-products that can affect renal function. Methoxyflurane and enflurane metabolism release inorganic fluoride ion. Serum levels of fluoride peak earlier with enflurane than with methoxyflurane, although the fluoride reaches much lower peaks and returns to preanesthesia values faster with enflurane than with methoxyflurane.[55] Halothane and isoflurane do not release significant amounts of fluoride. Nephrotoxicity may occur when serum fluoride levels exceed 35 μM and when serum concentrations remain above 20 μM for 18 hours or longer.[56]

Overt nephrotoxicity sometimes follows methoxyflurane anesthesia that lasts longer than 7 MAC hours. Shorter exposure produces subclinical toxicity. Nephrotoxic symptoms include vasopressin-resistant polyuria, increased serum osmolarity, increased uric acid levels, and a diluting-concentrating defect in the renal tubules. Nephrotoxicity appears most often in obese patients and in patients receiving enzyme-inducing drugs (phenobarbital) or other nephrotoxic drugs (aminoglycoside antibiotics). Because of its analgesic properties, methoxyflurane once served as a popular agent for obstetric use. It provided inhalational analgesia during labor and anesthesia for vaginal and abdominal deliveries. Although serum fluoride concentrations measured in obstetric patients receiving methoxyflurane[57] were not alarmingly high, one patient did have a value that approached nephrotoxic levels. Methoxyflurane should be avoided in patients with renal disease, since no data document its safety in obstetric patients with renal disease. The anesthesiologist can choose from safer anesthetic agents for obstetric purposes.

Some case reports describe acute renal failure following administration of enflurane.[58] Mazze and associates[59] reported that the use of enflurane in patients with pre-existing renal disease does not cause further deterioration of renal function. However, no studies examine this issue in obstetric patients. In patients with renal disease, pregnancy per se may cause further deterioration of renal function. Postpartum renal dysfunction represents a leading cause of ARF in young women. For these reasons, one must use enflurane with caution in pregnant patients with renal disease. When hypertension in a pre-eclamptic patient or bronchial spasm in an asthmatic patient calls for a potent volatile agent, isoflurane and halothane offer safe alternatives. Table 11–10 summarizes the renal effects of anesthesia and surgery.

Anesthesia Guidelines

GENERAL PREPARATION

Pre-existing diabetes mellitus controlled with insulin infusion. Administration of immunosuppressants, corticosteroids, and antihypertensive medications must continue. Hydrocortisone hemisuccinate can provide additional supplementation during labor or before cesarean section.

Table 11–10. RENAL EFFECTS OF GENERAL ANESTHESIA AND SURGERY

Immediate Effects
- Indirect effects
  - Reduction in GFR, RBF, and Na^+ excretion
  - Renal vasoconstriction
  - Impaired renal autoregulation
  - Stress: ADH release
  - Stress: catecholamine release:
    - Increased renal vascular resistance
    - Redistribution of renal blood flow
- Direct effects
  - Inhibition of electrolyte and organic acid transport in the tubules
  - Inhibition of PAH uptake by kidney slices

Delayed Effects
- Inorganic fluoride nephrotoxicity

MONITORING

Patients with mild impairment require only routine monitoring. However, severe renal compromise calls for central venous pressure (CVP) monitoring. Patients with cardiovascular compromise may additionally need a pulmonary artery (PA) catheter. Monitoring of CVP or PA pressures helps not only to detect pre-existing hypovolemia (chronic hemodialysis) but to avoid overhydration in the anephric patient. Individuals with severe hypertension also require an indwelling arterial line. Avoid insertion of peripheral intravenous cannulas into the forearm veins as they may serve as portals for an arteriovenous fistula for hemodialysis. A Doppler flow probe will verify the patency of a pre-existing fistula. Extra precautions must be taken to protect the fistula from accidental injury during labor and surgery.

A modified V5 lead may reveal possible myocardial ischemia in those with hypertensive cardiovascular disease or lupus coronary artery disease. An indwelling Foley catheter assists in monitoring urinary output, which requires maintenance of more than 0.5 ml per kg per hour.

TRANSFUSIONS

Until recently, physicians avoided giving transfusions to patients with renal failure for fear that transfusions could lead to the formation of antileukocyte antibodies that would threaten the survival of a subsequent kidney transplant. Those who required transfusions received only frozen red blood cells free of antileukocyte antibodies. However, Opelz and Teraski[60] reported a higher percentage of graft survival in anemic patients who received routinely cross-matched packed red blood cells. They also found that the use of frozen red blood cells did not relate to increased graft survival. Since maternal anemia may interfere with fetal oxygenation, hemoglobin concentration of less than 7 g per dl requires packed cell transfusion.

Patients with impaired renal function reportedly benefit from cryoprecipitate transfusion.[61] Cryoprecipitate contains opsonic α-2 glycoprotein, which stimulates removal of blood-borne waste products by the reticuloendothelial system. Cryoprecipitate transfusion proves especially useful when coagulation abnormalities accompany renal failure.

INTRAVENOUS FLUIDS

In anephric patients, replace insensible water loss with 5-percent dextrose in water, 500 ml per day. Administer saline, 0.45 percent, to replenish urine volume, and restore with packed cells. Treat third-space loss produced by major abdominal surgery by administering 0.9 percent saline or salt-poor albumin solutions at 2 to 5 ml per kg per hour. When available, CVP or PA pressure measurements serve as reliable guidelines, especially before rapid administration of intravenous fluids prior to performing regional blocks.[33]

Labor Analgesia

SYSTEMIC MEDICATION

The pain of uterine contractions produces significant maternal stress, which causes norepinephrine and epinephrine release from storage sites. Catecholamines decrease uterine blood flow, produce renal vasoconstriction, and shunt blood flow away from the renal cortex.[62,50] Prolonged painful labor will result in accumulation of lactate in both the mother and fetus.[63,64] Expulsive efforts produce further deterioration in the maternal condition. Although inconsequential in healthy parturients, these changes in RBF and acid-base status contribute to an adverse outcome in patients with renal impairment. Therefore, one must avoid painful and prolonged labor in patients with renal disease.

NARCOTIC ANALGESICS

Parenteral administration of narcotic analgesics alone or in combination with an anxiolytic agent produces pain relief during labor. In choosing a narcotic for labor analgesia, the following factors require consideration: renal failure may modify its elimination; decreased plasma protein concentrations may reduce its protein binding, thus intensifying their action; the agent itself may affect renal function directly or indirectly through an ADH mechanism; and the growth-retarded fetus has greater vulnerability to the narcotic depressant effects of the narcotic.

Meperidine. Meperidine, commonly used for relieving labor pain, becomes 60-percent bound to plasma proteins. In some patients with severe renal impairment normeperidine (a metabolite of meperidine) accumulates, leading to excitation or CNS irritability.[65] Because normeperidine has a half-life of 15 to 20 hours, administer it sparingly in those patients with severe renal impairment.

Morphine. In normal individuals, the action of morphine lasts 4 to 6 hours. Detoxification primarily involves conjugation of morphine with glucuronic acid, following which it undergoes renal elimination. In those with reduced urinary output it acts longer.[66] Since morphine depresses the respiratory center of the newborn more than meperidine[67]—especially the growth-retarded fetus—patients with severe renal dysfunction should not receive it.

Fentanyl. Fentanyl offers a suitable alternative to long-acting narcotics. Clinicians administer fentanyl intramuscularly or intravenously in 25- to 50-μg increments. A single intramuscular injection will produce peak effect in 15 min, and analgesia will last 30 to 60 min. After intravenous injection analgesia begins in 7 to 8 min and lasts 1 to 2 hours. Rapid hepatic metabolism of fentanyl ensues, and only 10 percent appears in the urine.[68] Thus, unlike meperidine, fentanyl possesses little potential for producing cumulative toxicity. Even high doses of fentanyl do not appreciably affect kidney function.[69] Fentanyl readily crosses the placenta, but small doses affect the fetus only minimally.[70]

The long-held belief that narcotics like morphine produce antidiuresis by releasing ADH has recently come under scrutiny.[71] Recent reports have suggested that chronic administration of morphine actually results in diuresis.[72] The antidiuresis, which occurs independently of ADH release, relates partly to the hypotensive action of morphine.[73] The effect of surgical stress and stimulation on ADH release remains unclear. The activation of different opioid receptors may account for these conflicting findings. Whereas the stimulation of mu receptors produces antidiuresis, stimulation of kappa receptors results in diuresis.[72]

Narcotic-Anxiolytic Combination. Production of labor analgesia by combining a narcotic with an anxiolytic agent such as diazepam or a phenothiazine is standard practice. Diazepam metabolism, occurring primarily in the liver, generates the pharmacologically active metabolite desmethyldiazepam. Both diazepam and its metabolite bind extensively to protein. Ochs and coworkers[74,75] studied the pharmacokinetics of diazepam and its metabolite in patients with advanced renal disease. Renal disease diminished protein binding of diazepam and its metabolite. Although the clearance rate of unbound diazepam did not change significantly, the clearance rate of the metabolite slowed 50 percent in patients with renal disease. One may combine small intravenous doses of diazepam (2.5 mg) with fentanyl to produce safe and effective systemic analgesia. Since desmethyldiazepam accumulates these patients should not receive repeated doses of diazepam. Phenothiazine derivatives reportedly cause psychotic reactions in patients receiving hemodialysis.[76] An additional problem with phenothiazines concerns their ability to produce systemic hypotension. Thus, patients with renal insufficiency must use small amounts of phenothiazine derivatives or none at all.

CONDUCTION BLOCKS

Epidural Block

Epidural block provides unsurpassed analgesia and minimizes the stress caused by labor pains. The liver metabolizes amide local anesthetics. Used in appropriate amounts, their volume of distribution and clearance rate remain unaltered by renal disease (Table 11–11).[77] Ester-type local anesthetics such as 2-chloroprocaine undergo hydrolysis by plasma cholinesterase. Thus, lumbar epidural analgesia (LEA) with an amide or an ester derivative proves suitable for these patients.

Sodium bisulfite, the antioxidant contained in 2-chloroprocaine solution, allegedly produces chronic neurologic damage.[78] In patients with uremic polyneuropathy, one must choose a preparation of 2-chloroprocaine that contains the least amount of the antioxidant. A preparation of 2-chloroprocaine without sodium bisulfite has become available commercially (Astra Pharmaceuticals).

Certain precautions warrant practice before inducing an epidural block. Assess the adequacy of circulating fluid volume status using CVP or PA pressures, especially in women on chronic hemodialysis. Close monitoring of CVP or PA pressures is critical in anephric patients who cannot tolerate even the slightest fluid overload. Proceed carefully when delivering epidural anesthesia to severly hypertensive patients because of the risk of sudden reduction in blood pressure.[33] Patients with uremic coagulopathy should not receive epidural anesthesia. Although no evidence exists that epidural anesthesia worsens neuropathy, this issue should be discussed with patients who have uremic polyneuritis.

Sensory anesthesia extending to T10 level will not affect renal function, if one avoids the supine position and systemic hypotension. It may increase renal blood flow by diminishing catecholamine response to labor pains. Lidocaine, 1.5 percent (4 to 6 ml), bupivacaine, 0.25 percent (6 to 8 ml), or 2-chloroprocaine, 2 percent (4 to 6 ml in selected cases) produces effective analgesia when injected through an epidural catheter inserted through the L3–4 intervertebral space.

Ephedrine administered in 5-mg increments effectively treats systemic hypotension due to epidural anesthesia. Although dopamine appears to represent a logical choice for patients with renal disease (because of its beneficial effects on renal function), it may reduce uterine blood flow when administered in quantities sufficient to maintain perfusion pressure. There-

Table 11–11. LIDOCAINE PHARMACOKINETICS IN VARIOUS DISEASE STATES

	Volume of Distribution at Steady State (liters/kg)	Clearance (ml/min/kg^{-1})	Termination Elimination Half-Life
Normal	1.32	10.0	1.8
Cardiac failure	0.88	6.3	1.9
Hepatic disease*	2.31	6.0	4.9
Renal disease*	1.20	13.7	1.3

*Note the difference between hepatic and renal disease.
(From Thomson, PD, et al,[77] with permission.)

fore, some authorities[79] do not recommend its routine use for treating maternal hypotension. This chapter previously discussed potential beneficial effects of segmental epidural anesthesia in patients with renal colic and urinary diversion.

Paracervical Block

Paracervical block produces fetal bradycardia in a significant number of patients. Since patients with renal disease appear likely to have a growth-retarded fetus, they should not receive paracervical block.

Anesthesia for Vaginal Births

When continuous epidural anesthesia is used for labor analgesia, additional injection of local anesthetics with the patient in the sitting position suffices for normal or low forceps delivery. If labor proceeded without any conduction analgesia, a bilateral pudendal block offers a suitable alternative for performing episiotomy. Inhalation of 40 percent nitrous oxide in oxygen provides supplementation. Usually patients receiving 50 percent nitrous oxide do not require endotracheal intubation since very few will become unconscious during its inhalation.[80] A subarachnoid block often provides excellent conditions for forceps delivery. The next section discusses the effect of renal disease on the onset and duration of spinal anesthesia. Also see below for guidelines to general anesthesia for vaginal birth.

Anesthesia for Cesarean Section

REGIONAL ANESTHESIA

Obstetric indications or acute or chronic fetal distress sometimes call for cesarean section. Since patients with renal disease often have gastric hyperacidity, oral administration of antacids such as sodium citrate is necessary to raise the gastric fluid pH[33,81] before proceeding with the block. Women who complain of heartburn may benefit from cimetidine, an H-2 blocker. Renal impairment does not affect cimetidine metabolism.[81] Patients with renal disease and those on chronic hemodialysis often abuse antacids containing magnesium. In addition, hypermagnesemia may occur in renal disease, so these patients should not receive antacids containing magnesium.[33]

Regional anesthesia remains preferable to general anesthesia. Since a decreased circulating volume stimulates renal vasoconstriction, the obstetric team must optimize the circulating fluid volume. Spinal anesthesia remains appropriate in the absence of severe hypertension or coagulopathy. However, in the presence of preeclampsia, it may cause severe hypotension (because of rapid onset). Spinal anesthesia affects renal function minimally as long as the anesthesiologist can avoid systemic hypotension and maintain an adequate circulating fluid volume (Table 11–12).[44,48,49] Even with high spinal anesthesia, renal blood flow, renal clearance, and elimination of indicators remain relatively unaffected. However, general anesthesia markedly interferes with these parameters. In addition general anesthesia reduces the renal fraction of the cardiac output and may interfere with renal autoregulation[48] (see Table 11–10). High spinal anesthesia in a patient with inadequate circulating volume severely diminishes the RBF and GFR.

Chronic renal disease modifies spinal anesthesia by causing a more rapid spread of the anesthetic, slightly increasing sensory levels, and by shortening the duration of action. Uremic demyelination of the neurons may contribute to the faster spread of spinal anesthesia.[82] The hyperdynamic circulation increases the clearance of the local anesthetic from the subarachnoid space, thus shortening the duration of anesthesia.[82]

For cesarean section under lumbar epidural anesthesia, the anesthesiologist can choose lidocaine or bupivacaine. Acidosis decreases the threshold for local anesthetic-induced seizure.[33] Following a regional block, blood levels of local anesthetics increase more rapidly in patients with renal disease than in healthy patients, probably due to the hyperdynamic circulation.[83] Therefore, the anesthesiologist must increase the sensory level gradually using small increments of local anesthetics. Epinephrine is inappropriate for prolonging the duration of local anesthetics because of its ability to induce car-

Table 11–12. RENAL FUNCTION WITH GENERAL AND SPINAL ANESTHESIA

Parameter	Control*		General		Control*		Spinal	
	Mean	(SD)	Mean	(SD)	Mean	(SD)	Mean	(SD)
Cardiac output: liters/min	4.5	(0.3)	3.4	(0.1)	5.0	(0.5)	6.3	(1.0)
Renal blood flow: liters/min	0.59	(0.02)	0.37	(0.02)	0.69	(0.06)	0.61	(0.08)
Iodohippurate extraction ratio	0.6	(0.01)	0.4	(0.03)	0.76	(0.01)	0.75	(0.03)
Iodohippurate clearance: ml/min	355	(9)	146	(5)	525	(40)	457	(47)
Cefoxitin extraction ratio	0.58	(0.05)	0.3	(0.05)	0.77	(0.02)	0.78	(0.05)
Cefoxitin clearance: ml/min	344	(29)	110	(27)	528	(42)	478	(74)

*Control measurements were done in basal awake state.
(Data from Mather, LE, et al[44] and Runciman, WB, et al.[26]

diac arrhythmias and/or pulmonary edema, especially in the presence of metabolic acidosis and hyperkalemia.[33]

GENERAL ANESTHESIA

Patients about to undergo general anesthesia must ingest an antacid preparation, preferably sodium citrate, to raise the intragastric fluid pH. Thiopental is suitable for induction of anesthesia, but patients with renal disease must receive smaller-than-usual doses because of the decreased protein-binding capacity and defective blood-brain barrier for barbiturates in uremic patients.[84] Although succinylcholine does not produce complications in normokalemic patients with chronic renal disease,[85] it may lead to serious hyperkalemia and cardiac arrest in those with hyperkalemia.[81,86] Patients with a serum potassium exceeding 5.5 mmol should not receive succinylcholine.[81,87] An exaggerated hyperkalemic response can also occur in patients with severe uremic polyneuritis.[33] Because the duration of action of the nondepolarizing relaxants atracurium and vecuronium remains unaffected in renal failure, these agents represent the relaxants of choice.[85] Pancuronium and gallamine, which undergo significant renal excretion, have a longer duration of action in patients with renal disease.[85] Figures 11–5 and 11–6, respectively, show the elimination half-lives and clearance rates of common muscle relaxants and the anticholinesterase drugs used to reverse their actions. Anticholinesterases have prolonged action in renal-failure patients, too, because they also undergo renal elimination.[88,89] Thus patients receiving adequate doses of reversal agents at the end of the surgical procedure rarely experience postoperative recurarization. When the patient receives mag-

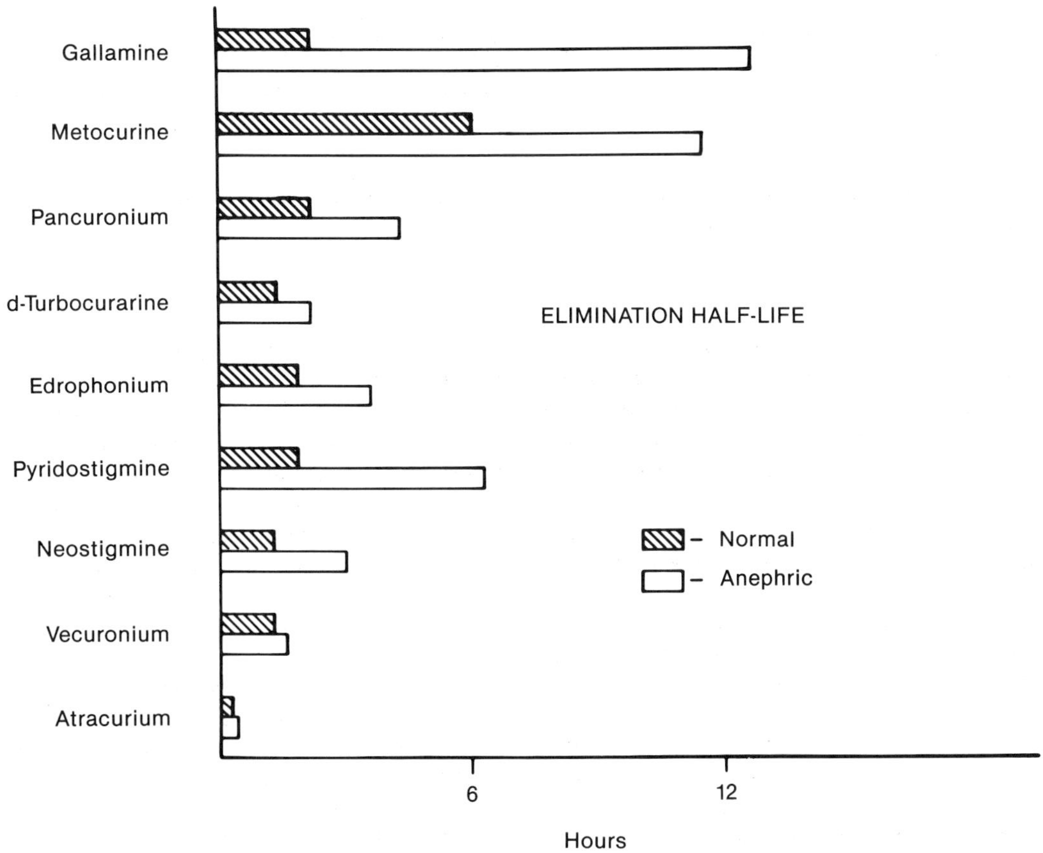

Figure 11–5. Elimination half-life of different muscle relaxants and reversal agents in subjects with normal renal function and in anephric subjects. The half-life of vecuronium and atracurium remain unaffected in anephric subjects. (Data from Mazze, RI.[89])

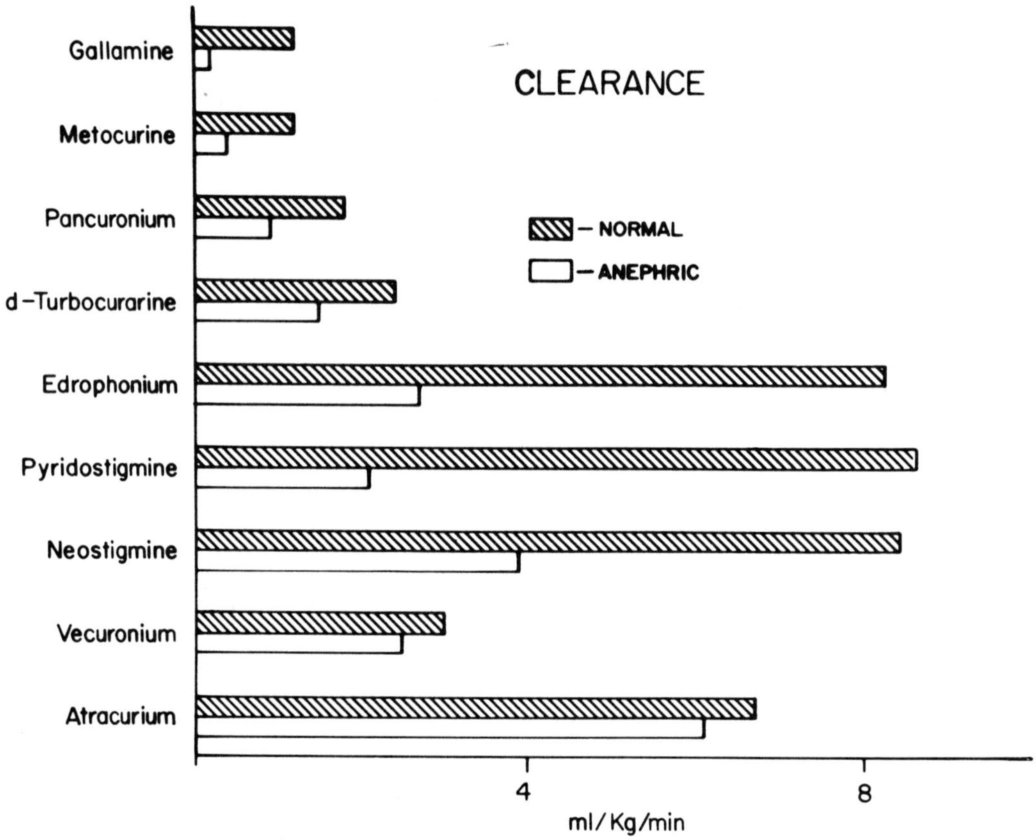

Figure 11–6. Clearance rates of muscle relaxants and the reversal agents. The clearance rates of vecuronium and atracurium remain unaffected in anephric subjects. (Data from Mazze, RI.[89])

nesium therapy for pre-eclampsia the anesthesiologist must use a nerve stimulator to titrate the dose of the muscle relaxant. A previous section of this chapter described the interaction between muscle relaxants and azathioprine.

For maintenance of general anesthesia, a balanced technique with fentanyl proves preferable to inhalational agents because it undergoes rapid nonrenal elimination. However, the anesthesiologist may use small concentrations of halothane or isoflurane to control intraoperative hypertension. Small doses of droperidol (2.5 to 5 mg) also effectively control hypertension[81] without appreciably affecting renal function. Other agents that treat hypertension include diazoxide, hydralazine, and sodium nitroprusside. Because diazoxide and hydralazine undergo renal elimination, suitable dose reductions are necessary. Because of the potential risk of fluoride-induced nephrotoxicity, the anesthesiologist must use enflurane cautiously, and avoid methoxyflurane in patients with renal impairment. Maintenance of intraoperative circulating blood volume is vital to prevent deterioration in renal function. Blood loss calls for transfusion of adequate amounts of packed red blood cells without delay. Measurement of arterial blood pH and gas tensions and suitable adjustments of FIO_2 are essential to prevent arterial hypoxemia.

General anesthesia causes increased ADH release, probably owing to inadequate suppression of surgical stimuli (Fig. 11–7). Plasma ADH levels increase soon after induction of anesthesia. Although the use of LEA causes no rise in ADH levels intraoperatively, ADH levels start climbing in the postoperative period.[90] Postoperative pain may also cause the release of ADH.[91] Effective analgesia eliminates ADH

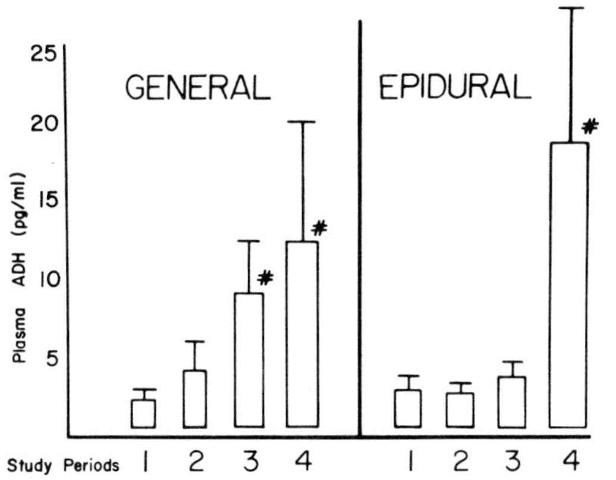

Figure 11–7. Plasma ADH concentration changes with general and epidural anesthesia. Study periods: 1, control; 2, induction of anesthesia; 3, skin incision; and 4, 4 hr after operation. (# = significantly different from control.) Note the lack of changes in ADH intraoperatively with epidural anesthesia. Postoperatively, similar changes occur with epidural and general anesthesia. (From Bonnet, F,[90] with permission.)

release caused by postoperative pain. Since intermittent parenteral injections of narcotic do not produce uninterrupted analgesia, they do not control ADH release in the postoperative period (Fig. 11–8).[91] However, epidural administration of narcotics such as fentanyl controls postoperative pain adequately, thus preventing ADH release. Because fentanyl has little potential for rostral spread due to its high lipid solubility, it therefore lacks direct ADH-releasing action from the posterior hypophysis (Fig. 11–8). In contrast, narcotics with little lipid solubility, such as morphine, reach the posterior hypophysis via cerebrospinal fluid and cause ADH release.[92]

Postoperative Care

Postoperative hypertension requires treatment with sodium nitroprusside or hydralazine. In the postoperative period, patients may stay in the high-risk unit (if available) or in the ICU. Postoperative oliguria requires immediate attention. Nephrotoxins (aminoglycoside antibiotics, cephalosporins, nonsteroidal anti-inflammatory drugs) can further impair renal function.

Summary

Pregnancy worsens renal disease, and renal disease compromises pregnancy outcome. Hypertension and pre-eclampsia offer a poor prognosis for the mother and fetus. Since many systemic illnesses cause renal disease, the preoperative assessment must elucidate the exact etiology of the renal disorder. Concentrations of BUN and serum creatinine serve as reliable indices of functional impairment. Tests to assess intrauterine fetal well-being also prove necessary. Preoperative preparation of these patients includes optimization of circulating volume and normalization of electrolyte and acid-base abnormalities. General anesthesia decreases GFR

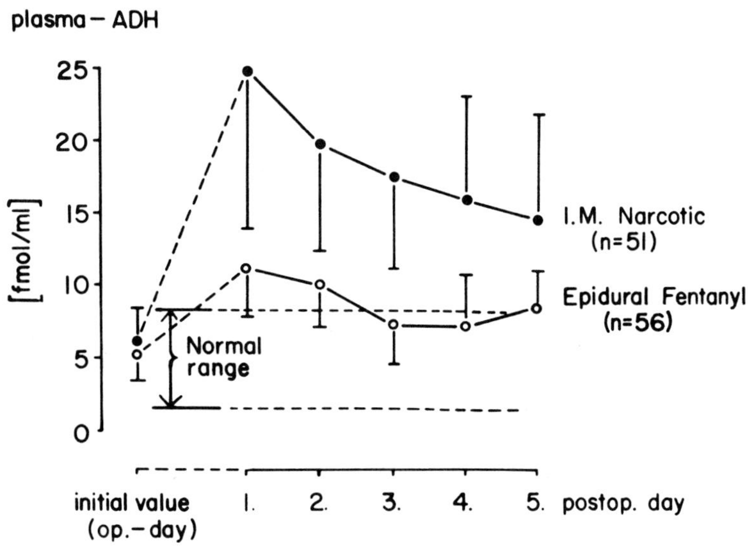

Figure 11–8. Plasma levels of ADH in patients receiving intramuscular narcotic or epidural fentanyl for postoperative pain relief. (From Bormann, BV,[91] with permission.)

and RBF, a problem less likely to occur with regional anesthesia so long as systemic pressure remains normal. Epidural block provides optimal labor analgesia. One should consider using meperidine or fentanyl in moderate amounts for systemic analgesia when conduction block proves difficult. Epidural, subarachnoid, or pudendal block provides adequate anesthesia for vaginal delivery. Epidural or subarachnoid block stands preferable to general anesthesia for cesarean section. General anesthesia, when used, should include a balanced technique using nitrous oxide, fentanyl, and muscle relaxants (atracurium or vecuronium) rather than inhalational agents. Hypertension requires prompt treatment in the postoperative period.

References

1. Brenner, BM and Hostetter, TH: Disturbances of renal function. In Petersdorf, RG, et al (eds): Harrison's Principles of Internal Medicine, ed 10. McGraw-Hill, New York, 1983, p 1599.
2. Bricker, NS: On the pathogenesis of the uremic state: An exposition of the "trade-off" hypothesis. N Engl J Med 286:1093, 1972.
3. Barron, WM and Lindheimer, MD: Renal sodium and water handling in pregnancy. In Wynn, R (ed): Obstet Gynecol Manual. Appleton-Century-Crofts, Norwalk, CT, 1984, p 36.
4. Laiken, N and Fanestil, DD: Body fluids and renal function. In West, JB (ed): Best and Taylor's Physiologic Basis of Medical Practice. Williams & Wilkins, Baltimore, 1985, p 438.
5. Davison, JM, Katz, AI and Lindheimer, MD: Kidney disease and pregnancy: Obstetric outcome and long-term renal prognosis. Clin Perinatol 12:497, 1985.
6. Cousins, MJ, Skowronski, G and Plummer, JL: Anesthesia and the kidney. Anaesth Intensive Care 11:292, 1983
7. Sladen, RN: Renal function and critical care. Seminars in Anesthesia 1:323, 1982.
8. Surian, M, Imbascuiti, E and Cosci, P: Glomerular disease and pregnancy: A study of 123 pregnancies in patients with primary and secondary glomerular diseases. Nephron 36:101, 1984.
9. Katz, AI: Pregnancy in women with kidney disease. Kidney Int 18:192, 1980.
10. Barcelo, P and Lopez, J: Glomerulonefritis y embarazo. Proceedings of 15 Curso de Nefrologia para post graduados sobre Rinon y Embarazo. Fundacion Puigvert. Reuniones y Congresos S.A, Madrid, 1984, p 89.
11. Jungers, P, et al: Chronic kidney disease and pregnancy. Adv Nephrol 15:103, 1986.
12. Hou, SH, Grossman, SD and Madias NE: Pregnancy in women with renal disease and moderate renal insufficiency. Am J Med 78:185, 1985.
13. Imbasciati, E, et al: Pregnancy in women with chronic renal failure. Proceedings of 4th World Congress of the International Society for the Study of Hypertension in Pregnancy, 1984, p 79.
14. Davison, JM and Lindheimer, MD: Chronic renal disease. Clin Obstet Gynecol 27:891, 1984.
15. Gabert, HA and Miller, JM, Jr: Renal disease in pregnancy. Obstet Gynecol Surg 40:449, 1985.
16. Burkett, G: Lupus nephropathy and pregnancy. Clin Obstet Gynecol 28:311, 1985.
17. Hayslett, JP and Lynn, RI: Effect of pregnancy in patients with lupus nephropathy. Kidney Int 18:207, 1980.
18. Houser, MT, et al: Pregnancy and systemic lupus erythematosus. Am J Obstet Gynecol 138:409, 1980.
19. Jungers, P, et al: Lupus nephropathy and pregnancy. Arch Intern Med 142:771, 1982.
20. Fine, LG, et al: Systemic lupus erythematosus in pregnancy. Ann Intern Med 94:667, 1981.
21. Imbasciati, E: Lupus nephropathy and pregnancy: A study of 26 pregnancies in patients with systemic lupus erythematosus and nephritis. Nephron 36:46, 1984.
22. Gimovsky, ML, Montoro, M and Paul, RH: Pregnancy outcome in women with systemic lupus erythematosus. Obstet Gynecol 63:686, 1984.
23. Scott, JS, et al: Connective-tissue disease, antibodies to ribonucleo-protein and congenital heart block. N Engl J Med 309:209, 1983.
24. Anticardiolipin antibodies: A risk factor for venous and arterial thrombosis. Lancet 1:912, 1985.
25. Glassock, RJ and Brenner, BM: Glomerulopathies associated with multisystem disease. In Petersdorf, RG, et al (eds): Harrison's Principles of Internal Medicine, ed 10. McGraw-Hill, New York, 1983, p 1642.
26. Ready, BL and Johnson, ES: Epidural block for the treatment of renal colic. Can Anaesth Soc J 28:77, 1981.
27. Merrill, LK, Board, JA and Lee, HM: Complications of pregnancy after renal transplantation including a report of spontaneous uterine rupture. Obstet Gynecol 41:270, 1973.
28. Rudolph, JE, Schweizer, RT and Bartus, SA: Pregnancy in renal transplant patients. Transplantation 27:26, 1979.
29. Drechen, KL, et al: Azathioprine: Effects on neuromuscular transmission. Anesthesiology 45:604, 1976.
30. Glassock, RJ and Brenner, BM: The major glomerulopathies. In Petersdorf, RG, et al (eds): Harrison's Principles of Internal Medicine, ed 10. McGraw-Hill, New York, 1983, p 1632.
31. Rubens, D, Sterns, RH and Segal, AJ: Postpartum renal vein thrombosis. Urol Radiol 7:80, 1985.
32. Lindsay, RM and Clark, WF: Platelet destruction in renal disease. Semin Thromb Haemost 8:138, 1982.
33. Weir, PHC and Chung, FF: Anaesthesia for patients with chronic renal disease. Can Anaesth Soc J 31:468, 1984.
34. Milatinovic, J, et al: Fertility and pregnancy complications in women with autosomal dominant polycystic kidney disease. Obstet Gynecol 61:566, 1973.
35. Hollenberg, NK: Vascular injury to the kidney. In Petersdorf, RG, et al (eds): Harrison's Principles of Internal Medicine, ed 10. McGraw-Hill, New York, 1983, p 1661.

36. Gilliland, BC and Mannik, M: Progressive systemic sclerosis (diffuse scleroderma). In Petersdorf, RG, et al (eds): Harrison's Principles of Internal Medicine, ed 10. McGraw-Hill, New York, 1983, p 2002.
37. Knuppel, RA, Montenegro, R and O'Brien, WF: Acute renal failure in pregnancy. Clin Obstet Gynecol 28:288, 1985.
38. Myers, BD and Moran, SM: Hemodynamically medicated acute renal failure. N Engl J Med 314:97, 1986.
39. Oken, DE: Hemodynamic basis for human acute renal failure (vasomotor nephropathy). Am J Med 76:702, 1984.
40. Donadio, JV, Jr and Holley, KE: Postpartum acute renal failure: Recovery after heparin therapy. Am J Obstet Gynecol 118:510, 1974.
41. Brown, CB, Ogg, CS and Cameron, JS: High-dose furosemide in acute renal failure: A controlled trial. Clin Nephrol 15:90, 1981.
42. Polin, JI and Frangippane, L: Current concepts in the management of obstetric problems for pediatricians. I: Monitoring the high risk fetus. Pediatr Clin North Am 33:621, 1986.
43. Berne, RM: Haemodynamics and sodium excretion of denervated kidney in anesthetized and unanesthetized dogs. Am J Physiol 171:148, 1952.
44. Mather, LE, Runciman, WB and Isley, AH: Anesthesia-induced changes in regional blood flow. Implications for drug disposition. Reg Anesth 7:S24, 1982.
45. Halperin, BD and Feeley, TW: The effect of anesthesia and surgery on renal function. Int Anesthesiol Clin 22:157, 1984.
46. Mazze, RI, et al: Renal function during anesthesia. Anesthesiology 24:279, 1963.
47. Deutch, S, et al: The effects of neuromuscular blocking drugs on renal function in normal man. Br J Anaesth 41:807, 1969.
48. Runciman, WB, et al: A sheep preparation for studying interactions between blood and drug disposition. IV: The effects of general and spinal anaesthesia on blood flow and cefoxin disposition. Br J Anaesth 57:1239, 1985.
49. Mather, LE, et al: A sheep preparation for studying interactions between blood flow and drug disposition. V: The effects of general and subarachnoid anaesthesia on blood flow and pethidine disposition. Br J Anaesth 58:888, 1986.
50. Truniger, B, et al: Redistribution of renal blood flow in haemorrhagic hypotension: Role of renal nerves and catecholamines. Eur J Clin Invest 1:277, 1971.
51. Gorman, HM and Graythorne, NWB: The effects of a new neurolept analgesic agent (Innovar) on renal function in man. Acta Anaesthesiol Scand (Suppl) 24:111, 1966.
52. Andersen, NB: Synergistic effect of cyclopropane and epinephrine on sodium transport in toad bladder. Anesthesiology 28:438, 1967.
53. Dedrick, DR and Greene, NM: Effect of anesthetics on the organic acid transport system of renal tubules. Experientia 27:252, 1971.
54. Bastron, RD and Kaloyanides, GJ: Effects of methoxyflurane (MOF) on PAH uptake by rabbit kidney tissue slices. Am J Physiol 227:460, 1974.
55. Cousins, MJ, et al: Metabolism and renal effects of enflurane in man. Anesthesiology 44:44, 1976.
56. Mazze, RI, Calverley, RK and Smith NT: Inorganic fluoride toxicity: Prolonged enflurane and halothane anesthesia in volunteers. Anesthesiology 46:265, 1977.
57. Palahniuk, RJ and Cumming, M: Plasma fluoride levels following obstetrical use of methoxyflurane. Can Anaesth Soc J 22:291, 1975.
58. Loehning, RW and Mazze, RI: Possible nephrotoxicity from enflurane in a patient with severe renal disease. Anesthesiology 40:203, 1974.
59. Mazze, RI, Sievenpiper, TS and Stevenson, J: Renal effects of enflurane and halothane in patients with abnormal renal function. Anesthesiology 60:161, 1984.
60. Opelz, G and Terasaki, PI: Dominant effects on transfusions on kidney graft survival. Transplantation 29:153, 1980.
61. Annest, SJ, et al: Increased creatinine clearance following cryoprecipitate infusion in trauma and surgical patients with decreased renal function. J Trauma 20:726, 1980.
62. Shnider, SM, et al: Uterine blood flow and plasma norepinephrine changes during maternal stress in the pregnant ewe. Anesthesiology 50:524, 1979.
63. Marx, GF and Greene, NM: Maternal lactate, pyruvate and excess lactate production during labor and delivery. Am J Obstet Gynecol 90:786, 1964.
64. Zador, G and Nilsson, BA: Continuous drip lumbar epidural anesthesia with lidocaine for vaginal delivery: Effects on maternal and fetal acid-base status. Acta Obstet Gynaecol Scand (Suppl)34:41, 1974.
65. Drayes, DE: Active drug metabolites and renal failure. Am J Med 62:486, 1977.
66. Don, HF, Dieppa, RA and Taylor, P: Narcotic analgesics in anuric patients. Anesthesiology 42:745, 1975.
67. Way, WL, Costley, EC and Way, EL: Respiratory sensitivity of the newborn infant to meperidine and morphine. Clin Pharmacol Ther 6:454, 1965.
68. Monks, PS and Lumley, J: Anesthetic aspects of renal transplantation. Ann Coll Surg Engl 50:354, 1972.
69. Morgan, M and Lumley, J: Anesthetic considerations in chronic renal failure. Anaesth Intensive Care 3:218, 1975.
70. Eisele, JH, Wright, R and Rogge, P: Newborn and maternal fentanyl levels at cesarean section. Anesth Analg 61:179, 1982.
71. Jaffe, JH and Martin, WR: Opioid analgesics and antagonists. In Gilman, AG, et al (eds): Goodman and Gilman's The Pharmacological Basis of Therapeutics, ed 7. Macmillan, New York, 1985, p 491.
72. Leander, JD: A kappa opioid effect: Increased urination in the rat. J Pharmacol Exp Ther 224:89, 1983.
73. Wilson N and Ngsee, J: Antidiuretic effect of acute morphine administration in the conscious rat. Can J Physiol Pharmacol 60:201, 1982.
74. Ochs, HR, et al: Diazepam kinetics in patients with renal insufficiency or hyperthyroidism. Br J Clin Pharmacol 12:829, 1981
75. Ochs, HR, et al: Clorazepate dipotassium and diazepam in renal insufficiency: Serum concentrations and protein binding of diazepam and desmethyldiazepam. Nephron 37:100, 1984.
76. McAllister, CJ, Scoeden, EB and Stone WJ: Toxic psychoses induced by phenothiazine administration in

patients with chronic renal failure. Clin Nephrol 10:191, 1978.
77. Thomson, PD, et al: Lidocaine pharmacokinetics in advanced heart failure, liver disease and renal failure in humans. Ann Intern Med 78:499, 1973.
78. Wang, PC, et al: Chronic neurological damage and Nesacaine CE: An effect of the anesthetic, 2-chloroprocaine, or the antioxidant sodium busulfite? Anesth Analg 63:445, 1984.
79. Rolbin, SH, et al: Dopamine treatment of spinal hypotension decreases uterine blood flow in the pregnant ewe. Anesthesiology 51:36, 1978.
80. Committee on Nitrous Oxide Analgesia in Midwifery. Sir Douglas Bird, Chairman: Clinical trials of different concentrations of nitrous oxide for obstetrical anesthesia. Br Med J 1:709, 1970.
81. Maddern, PJ: Anaesthesia for the patient with impaired renal function. Anesth Intens Care 11:321, 1983.
82. Orko, R, Pitkanen, M, and Rosenberg, PH: Subarachnoid anesthesia with 0.75% bupivacaine in patients with chronic renal failure. Br J Anaesth 58:605, 1986.
83. Strasser, K, et al: Plasma level of etidocaine within the first two hours after axillary plexus block in healthy adults and patients with renal insufficiency. Anaesthetist 30:14, 1981.
84. Hilgenberg, JC: Renal Disease. In Stoelting, RK and Dierdorf, SF (eds): Anesthesia and Co-existing Disease. Churchill Livingstone, New York, 1983, p 377.
85. Shanks, CA: Muscle relaxants in renal failure patients. In Katz RL (ed): Muscle Relaxants: Basic Clinical Aspects. Grune & Stratton, New York, 1985, p 171.
86. Roth, F and Wuthrich, H: The clinical importance of hyperkalemia following suxamethonium administration. Br J Anaesth 41:311, 1969.
87. Miller, RD, et al: Succinylcholine induced hyperkalemia in patients with renal failure. Anesthesiology 36:138, 1972.
88. Cronnelly, R: Muscle relaxant antagonists. In Katz, RL (ed): Muscle Relaxants: Basic Clinical Aspects. Grune & Stratton, New York, 1985, p 197.
89. Mazze, RL: Anesthesia for patients with abnormal renal function and genitourinary operations. In Miller, RD (ed): Textbook of Anesthesia, ed 2. Churchill Livingstone, New York, 1986, p 1651.
90. Bonnet, F, et al: Suppression of antidiuretic hormone hypersecretion during surgery by extradural anaesthesia. Br J Anaesth 54:29, 1982.
91. Bormann, VB, et al: Influence of epidural fentanyl on stress induced elevation of plasma vasopressin (ADH) after surgery. Anesth Analg 62:727, 1983.
92. Korinek, AM, et al: Effect of postoperative extradural morphine on ADH secretion. Br J Anaesth 57:4, 1985.

CHAPTER 12

ORTHOPEDIC DISEASE

JAMES C. EISENACH, M.S., M.D.

Pregnancy may produce orthopedic pathology. Back pain, pelvic pain, and carpal syndrome are common in pregnancy, and hormonal changes may produce joint instability and osteopenia. Pregnancy may also affect pre-existing orthopedic pathology. Remission of rheumatoid arthritis occurs, and spondylolisthesis, severe scoliosis, and ankylosing spondylitis frequently progress during pregnancy. This chapter reviews the pathophysiology of orthopedic disease in pregnancy and provides guidelines for anesthetic management of pregnant women with orthopedic problems. Specific entities to be discussed are listed in Table 12–1.

Pathophysiology

A variety of mechanical and hormonal changes occurring during pregnancy may affect or produce orthopedic disease (Table 12–2).

MECHANICAL CHANGES

The pathologic mechanical effect of the enlarging uterus on the lumbosacral spine can be understood by examining the anatomy of the pelvic girdle.[1] The sacrum, which supports the weight of the vertebral column and upper trunk, is suspended from the iliac bones by the dense posterior sacroiliac ligaments. In the normal standing posture the line of gravity is posterior to the acetabula, and the sacrum rotates downward posteriorly. This creates a pelvic tilt and lessens the degree of lumbar lordosis (Fig. 12–1*A*). Obesity, stooped posture, and pregnancy shift the line of gravity anterior to the acetabula. The pelvis rotates anteriorly and downward, increasing lumbar lordosis and stretching the thin anterior sacroiliac ligaments and joint capsule, producing acute pain (Fig. 12–1*B*). The stretched abdominal muscles provide less anterior support during pregnancy and exacerbate the anterior rotation.

Edema also produces orthopedic pathology during pregnancy. In a recent review,[2] carpal tunnel syndrome occurred in 25 percent of 1000 pregnancies, usually during pre-eclampsia. Most women had bilateral involvement, became symptomatic in the third trimester, and had experienced carpal tunnel syndrome in previous pregnancies.

Table 12-1. ORTHOPEDIC DISEASES DURING PREGNANCY

Mechanical backache and herniated lumbar disc
Scoliosis
Rheumatic diseases
Rheumatoid arthritis
Ankylosing spondylitis
Neural tube defects
Myelomeningocele, meningocele
Spina bifida
Primary bone disorders
Osteogenesis imperfecta
Achondroplasia
Miscellaneous disorders
Spondylolisthesis
Phantom limb pain
Autonomic hyperreflexia

Hormonal Changes

Hormonal changes during pregnancy also affect the orthopedic system. Relaxin, a peptide hormone similar in structure to insulin, is synthesized and released by the corpus luteum.[3] Although the role of relaxin in human pregnancy is not certain, in animals it produces myometrial relaxation, pelvic ligament laxity, and cervical dilatation. In humans, serum relaxin concentrations increase 10-fold during pregnancy, and pelvic[4] and peripheral[5] joint laxity occur concomitantly. Ligamentous laxity may exacerbate the previously discussed mechanical factors and produce instability of the symphysis pubis and the sacroiliac joints leading to severe pelvic pain. MacLennan and associates[6] report significantly higher serum relaxin concentrations in 35 pregnant women with severe pelvic pain compared with pregnant controls without pain. The highest relaxin concentrations occur in patients who are the most incapacitated, which implies a causal relationship between relaxin secretion and back and pelvic pain.

Table 12-2. PREGNANCY-INDUCED CHANGES THAT AFFECT ORTHOPEDIC DISEASE

Mechanical
Enhanced lumbar lordosis (backache)
Anterior rotation of sacroiliac joints (backache)
Edema (carpal tunnel syndrome)
Trauma (subluxation of pubic symphysis)
Hormonal
Relaxin (backache, may result in progression of disease)
Parathyroid hormone (osteopenia, pathologic fractures)
Cellular immunity (remission of rheumatoid arthritis)

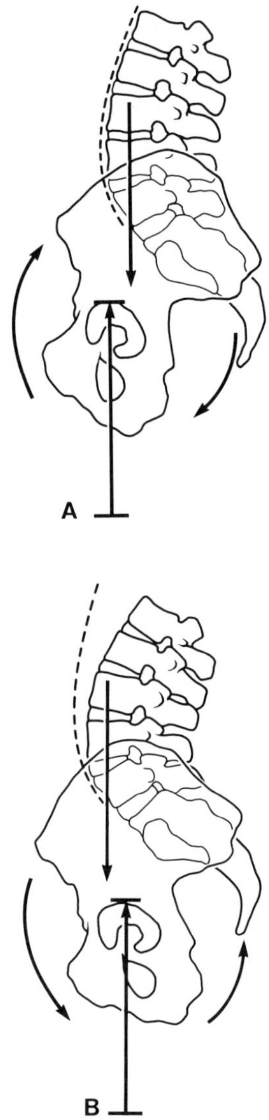

Figure 12-1. Effect of pregnancy on pelvic mechanics. *(A)* Nonpregnant: note line of gravity is posterior to acetabulum. *(B)* Pregnant: line of gravity is anterior to acetabulum, producing anterior rotation of sacroiliac joints and enhanced lordosis. (From DonTigny, RL,[1] with permission.)

Some authors[7] suggest that pregnancy is a state of relative hyperparathyroidism, since parathyroid hormone levels increase and serum 25-OH, Vitamin D, and calcium decrease.

During pregnancy and lactation increased movement of calcium from the gut and skeleton may produce osteoporosis which, if severe, leads to vertebral[8] or peripheral[9] bone fractures. In addition, this metabolic alteration could make previously undetected skeletal abnormalities more extensive, provoking symptoms.

Backache and Herniated Lumbar Disc

Backache occurs commonly in pregnancy, usually due to anterior sacroiliac joint dysfunction. In a survey[10] of 180 women, 48 percent experienced backache in pregnancy. For one third of these, severe back discomfort limited activity and was frequently associated with pain radiating down one or both legs. Exacerbation of back pain occurs with positions producing anterior rotation of the pelvis (bending, lifting, making beds, ironing). Surprisingly, pain is not aggravated by weight, weight gain, or obesity.

In contrast, pain due to herniated lumbar disc is rare in pregnancy. In two large series[11,12] totaling 75,760 patients the incidence of acute herniated lumbar disc disease during pregnancy approximated 1 in 10,000. This evaluating physician distinguishes herniated lumbar disc from mechanical causes of backache in pregnancy by noting the presence of aggravating factors (e.g., sneezing, coughing, turning in bed) and specific neurologic findings (altered lower extremity reflexes, pain produced by straight leg raising and pressure on the sciatic notch, and motor disturbances).

OBSTETRIC CONSIDERATIONS

Back pain of mechanical origin is treated with bedrest, physiotherapy, and, in severe cases, trials of lidocaine-steroid injections in the sacroiliac joints. Mechanical backache does not affect the mode of delivery.

The radiologic diagnosis of herniated lumbar disc may be delayed until after delivery[11] due to concern about fetal radiation exposure.[13] Lumbar disc disease may be treated with pelvic traction and has been successfully treated with transcutaneous neurostimulation.[11] Nonsteroidal anti-inflammatory analgesics, especially acetylsalicylic acid, can be considered and are discussed in the section on rheumatoid arthritis.

ANESTHESIA CONSIDERATIONS

Neither epidural nor spinal anesthesia is contraindicated for women who experience backache during pregnancy. Some anesthesiologists would avoid these techniques, citing recent data[14] that postpartum paresthesia or motor dysfunction unrelated to anesthesia can occur and could erroneously be attributed to epidural or spinal anesthesia. This assumption is wrong for two reasons. First, the incidence of such problems is rare (19 in 10,000) and, in all cases reported, resolved with 72 hours.[14] Second, mechanically induced backache of pregnancy is transient and is not worsened by epidural anesthesia. The incidence of backache following delivery with epidural or spinal anesthesia is not higher than that following pudendal[15] or general[16] anesthesia. Careful patient positioning before and after institution of the block avoids twisting the back. Prior to placement of epidural or spinal needles, injection of 1.0 ml of 0.5-percent bupivacaine bilaterally into the interspinous space near the lamina may decrease the incidence of backache, resulting from the procedure itself by blocking the recurrent spinal nerves.[17]

No evidence shows that epidural or spinal anesthesia contributes to exacerbation or progression of herniated lumbar disc. However, technical problems may occur. Benzon and coworkers[18] compared the speed of onset and completeness of anesthesia following epidural mepivacaine injections in 15 patients with back pain and ten patients without back pain. Onset of action was delayed (35 to 90 min) in those with pain. When delay occurred, the nerve roots affected by disc disease were blocked 10 to 70 min after the contralateral unaffected roots. Shachner and Abram[19] inserted an epidural catheter into the L2–3 interspace in a woman with a history of damage to the L4–5 intervertebral disc and chronic right L5 radiculopathy. They could not produce anesthesia below the right L4 dermatome or alleviate the pain of uterine contractions on the right side. A second epidural catheter subsequently placed at L4–5 successfully provided complete right-sided anesthesia. Epidural adhesions or scarring resulting from the healing process following intervertebral disc injury may limit the spread of epidurally injected solutions and explain these reports. Review of 600 epidurograms in patients with suspected disc injury reveals that contrast material fails to rise in the epidural space above the affected disc in 4.9 percent of cases and does not reach the encroached nerve root in 33 percent.[20] Catheter malposition accounts for most cases of unilateral or patchy blocks. However, the rare patient with lumbar disc disease and a unilateral epidural block may benefit from a double-catheter technique or subarachnoid block (morphine for labor and local anesthetic for cesarean section).

Scoliosis

Nicholas Andre coined the term *orthopedics* ("straight child") in 1742,[21] and much of modern orthopedic practice is concerned with the treatment of scoliosis, or lateral curvature of the spine. Scoliosis is described by the location and degree of lateral curvature and can be thought of as a final common pathway from a variety of disease processes (Table 12–3).[22,23]

Table 12–3. CLASSIFICATION OF SCOLIOSIS

- Idiopathic
  - Infantile (<4 years, boys > girls, thoracic curve)
  - Juvenile (4–9 years)
  - Adolescent (>10 years, girls > boys, thoracic curve)
- Congenital
  - Vertebral abnormalities
  - Abnormal spinal cord development
  - Congenital rib fusions
- Neuromuscular
  - Lower motor neuron lesion (e.g., poliomyelitis)
  - Upper motor neuron lesion (e.g., cerebral palsy)
- Myopathic
  - Muscular dystrophy
  - Myotonic dystrophy
  - Others (e.g., Friedreich's ataxia)
- Neurofibromatosis
- Connective-tissue disorders
  - Marfan's syndrome, Ehlers-Danlos syndrome
  - Osteogenesis imperfecta
  - Acquired (e.g., rheumatoid arthritis, ankylosing spondylitis)
- Trauma
  - Vertebral
  - Extravertebral
- Secondary to irritative phenomenon (e.g., spinal cord tumor)

(From Kafer, ER,[42] with permission.)

The affected vertebrae and spinous processes rotate toward the concavity of the curve, and the disks, vertebral bodies, and vertebral canal are narrower on the concave side of the curve. The orthopedic management of scoliosis depends on the degree of curvature: expectant management for curves less than 20 degrees, external braces for curves of 20 to 40 degrees, and surgical stabilization of curves greater than 40 degrees.[24]

Idiopathic scoliosis accounts for 75 percent of all cases and is five times more common in females than in males. Although the incidence of mild scoliosis (<10 degrees) is high (40 in 10,000),[25] severe scoliosis during pregnancy affecting obstetric or anesthetic management is rare (1 to 5 in 10,000).[26] In some cases scoliosis may be due to hypoestrogenism,[27] while, in others, it may result from abnormal processing of vestibular signals within the CNS.[28] According to this model, nonerect vertical alignment between intervertebral structures is interpreted at a subconscious level as "erect" or "straight," leading to altered axial muscle control and progressive lateral strain and curvature.

Untreated idiopathic scoliosis of the thoracic spine produces progressive respiratory compromise, usually causing death secondary to respiratory and right heart failure by age 45.[29] Pulmonary function testing shows a restrictive pattern. Vital capacity, total lung capacity, and functional residual capacity decrease with increased thoracic curvature.[30] Ventilation-perfusion maldistribution promotes arterial hypoxemia.[31] Increased dead space ventilation may produce alveolar hypoventilation, leading to chronic carbon dioxide retention with reliance on hypoxic ventilatory drive. Scoliosis secondary to neuromuscular disease can be associated with inadequate airway reflexes and chronic and acute pulmonary aspiration.

In some patients, idiopathic scoliosis coexists with coarctation of the aorta and cyanotic heart disease[32] and potentiates the development of right heart failure. Interestingly, mitral valve prolapse occurs in 25 percent of patients with scoliosis.[33] Pulmonary vascular resistance increases, since fewer alveoli and arteries than normal are present and may atrophy due to distortion.[34] Compression of lung by the ribcage deformity produces hypoxic lung regions with associated hypoxic pulmonary vasoconstriction. Oxygen therapy ameliorates the latter. Electrocardiographic abnormalities such as right atrial and right ventricular hypertrophy occur late in the course of increased pulmonary vascular resistance and right heart strain.[35] Echocardiography provides earlier diagnosis.

Pregnancy may accentuate both the bony and cardiorespiratory abnormalities of scoliosis. Larger untreated curves (>25 degrees) may progress during pregnancy[36] due to mechanical and hormonal effects. Cardiac output, metabolic demand, and minute ventilation increase while functional residual capacity decreases during pregnancy. Additionally, plasma volume and cardiac output increase during labor and delivery and these changes, coupled with the encroachment of the enlarging uterus on the noncompliant thorax, heighten the possibility of cardiorespiratory failure in parturients with severe scoliosis. Maternal morbidity and mortality from cardiorespiratory failure relates to the site of the curvature (thoracic) and degree of pulmonary restriction before pregnancy. Mortality increases if vital capacity is less than 1.25 liters, but pregnancy is well tolerated if antenatal lung volumes exceed 50 percent of predicted.[37,38]

OBSTETRIC CONSIDERATIONS

Women with uncorrected curves greater than 25 degrees or lung volumes less than 50 percent of predicted should be counseled concerning the risks of further progression of scoliosis and respiratory failure. In general, the complications are primarily medical with thoracic curves and obstetric with lumbar curves. In cases of severe thoracic scoliosis, pulmonary function testing including arterial blood gas analysis is performed serially during pregnancy. Since early right heart failure may lead to peripheral edema, increased sympathetic activity and hypertension, the diagnosis of pre-eclampsia is made only after exclusion of cardiorespiratory failure.

Premature labor may occur more frequently in women with scoliosis.[39] Malposition at delivery is uncommon,[26] and in patients without cephalopelvic disproportion, vaginal delivery occurs uneventfully without excessive blood loss, suggesting normal uterine function.[26] When scoliosis distorts pelvic anatomy, instrumented deliveries, perineal tears, and uterine prolapse occur with greater frequency,[40] and maternal and neonatal morbidities increase.[41] Cesarean delivery becomes necessary in more than 75 percent of patients and may be technically difficult due to the acute anteflexion of the uterus caused by approximation of the xiphisternum and symphysis pubis.[40]

ANESTHESIA CONSIDERATIONS

General reviews[32,42] recently described the anesthetic management of patients with scoliosis. Anesthetic assessment should stress etiology, severity, and surgical history of the scoliosis as well as the presence of associated respiratory, cardiovascular, neuromuscular, and other disorders (Table 12–4).

Epidural analgesia minimizes muscular and respiratory fatigue associated with labor and avoids the risk of respiratory depression resulting from systemic opiates. In cases of respiratory compromise, supplemental oxygen, arterial cannulation for serial assessment of arterial

Table 12–4. PREANESTHETIC ASSESSMENT IN SEVERE SCOLIOSIS

History
Scoliosis (etiology, duration, surgical correction)
Respiratory disease (restriction worsened in pregnancy?)
Cardiac disease (cor pulmonale, mitral valve prolapse, congenital heart disease)
Neuromuscular disease (muscular dystrophy, myotonia, ataxia)
Physical examination
Scoliosis (degree, location, landmarks for regional technique)
Respiratory (rate, pattern, cyanosis, thoracic expansion, auscultation)
Cardiac (rate, regularity, S_4, jugular venous distension)
Neuromuscular (muscle tone, bulk, myotonia, deficits)
Laboratory
Complete blood count (polycythemia, platelets)
Pulmonary function tests
Vital capacity, total lung capacity >50%
Resting arterial blood gas tensions
Electrocardiogram
Echocardiogram
Pulmonary artery pressure (in severe cases)

blood gas tensions, and the sitting position may be helpful.

Technical difficulties during epidural catheter insertion should be anticipated in the presence of scoliosis. Previous roentgenograms may help to identify the degree of vertebral rotation. Unilateral blockade may occur due to malposition of the catheter secondary to vertebral rotation or to maldistribution of local anesthetic resulting from postoperative adhesions in the epidural space. Poor landmarks and distortion of ligamentous anatomy often impair localization of the epidural space. Despite these considerations, lumbar epidural catheter insertion has been reported[43] without difficulty for anesthesia for cesarean section in a woman with severe uncorrected scoliosis and for labor and delivery in women following extensive posterior spinal fusion.[44] When technical difficulties or unilateral block occurs, intrathecal injection of opiates and local anesthetics provides analgesia for labor and cesarean section, respectively. In women with advanced pulmonary disease and/or possible pulmonary hypertension, spinal morphine provides analgesia without hypotension, requiring less intravenous fluid than epidural analgesia with local anesthetics.[45]

For cesarean section, epidural anesthesia usually maintains respiratory function, minimizes risk of aspiration, and avoids respiratory depressants. However, women with cardiorespiratory failure may not tolerate lying supine, and cesarean section may be technically difficult with the patient in the sitting position. Many anesthesiologists prefer general anesthesia, which provides control of the airway, assures adequate ventilation, and does not require operation in the sitting position.[44] Supplemental oxygen, pulse oximetry, continuous ECG monitoring, and, in many cases, direct arterial blood pressure monitoring should be used throughout surgery. Special considerations for associated diseases are listed in Table 12–5.

Adequate postoperative pulmonary toilet requires good postoperative analgesia. Pulmonary function returns to normal more rapidly following abdominal surgery when patients use controlled intravenous analgesia or epidural morphine than when patients undergo traditional methods for postoperative analgesia. Adequate monitoring must be available in either case because of potential respiratory depression.

Table 12–5. ANESTHETIC CONCERNS IN PATIENTS WITH SCOLIOSIS

General anesthesia
Difficult intubation (e.g., rheumatoid arthritis)
Reactions to succinylcholine
Malignant hyperthermia (e.g., scoliosis, muscular dystrophy)
Myotonia (e.g., myotonic dystrophy)
Hyperkalemia (e.g., muscular dystrophy, lower motor neuron lesion)
Increased sensitivity to nondepolarizing muscle relaxants (e.g., muscular dystrophy, myotonic dystrophy)
Epidural and spinal anesthesia
Technical difficulties in needle placement
Sitting position required (in patients with severe orthopnea)
Sensitivity to decreases in cardiac preload and/or afterload (e.g., associated aortic and mitral valve abnormalities, pulmonary hypertension)
General and regional anesthesia
Pulmonary
Ventilation-perfusion maldistribution—hypoxemia
Chronic CO_2 retention and reliance on hypoxic drive
Acute and chronic aspiration (e.g., muscular dystrophy, polio)
Cardiac
Right heart failure
Associated valvular and cyanotic cardiac disorders
Intraoperative dysrhythmias (e.g., mitral valve prolapse)
Subacute bacterial endocarditis prophylaxis

Rheumatic Diseases

RHEUMATOID ARTHRITIS

Rheumatoid arthritis is a chronic systemic inflammatory disease in which proliferation of the synovial membrane leads to destruction of joint cartilage and subsequent deformities. The incidence of clinically important rheumatoid arthritis is 0.35 percent,[46] with women affected three times more often than men. In regard to etiology, authorities[47] propose an immune response to an unidentified antigen in synovial tissue that is not held in check because of an inadequate population of suppressor T cells.[47]

Clinical improvement in rheumatoid arthritis occurs in 75 percent of women during pregnancy, usually beginning late in the first trimester.[48] Elevated levels of IgG and IgM are predictive of gestational remissions.[49] During pregnancy, an unknown factor in serum blocks the sensitization of monocytes to synovial components that occurs in this disease, which may explain clinical remission.[50] Although the source of this factor is unknown, soluble factors produced by activated fetal suppressor cells have been postulated.[47]

Obstetric Considerations

Rheumatoid arthritis probably has no effect on pregnancy or the fetus.[48] Acetylsalicylic acid (ASA) is the preferred drug for treatment of symptoms during pregnancy because of the large experience with this compound and the fetal toxicity associated with other drugs used in rheumatoid arthritis. However, prolonged use of maximal therapeutic doses of ASA may be associated with prolonged gestation, longer labor, greater blood loss at delivery, and increased prevalence of anemia, perinatal mortality, and antepartum and postpartum hemorrhage.[47] Mechanical problems rarely occur at delivery, but they can present when severe hip involvement produces limited abduction. In such cases no stirrups or modified stirrups are recommended for delivery.[47] Patients with significant pulmonary dysfunction will have reduced ability to push effectively in stage II, necessitating use of forceps.

Anesthetic Considerations

The extra-articular features of rheumatoid arthritis may affect anesthetic management. Rheumatoid nodules occur in about 20 percent of patients.[51] Pulmonary granulomas are more frequent in patients who smoke, and may lead to infections, or may cavitate, rupture, and cause pneumothorax. Granulomas occurring in the coronary arteries may give rise to angina, while granulomas in the root of the aorta or aortic or mitral valvular rings may lead to valvular dysfunction. Finally, myocardial granulomas may produce conduction system disorders. Although they rarely have symptomatic disease, approximately 50 percent of patients with rheumatoid arthritis demonstrate old adhesive pleurisy or pericarditis at autopsy.[47]

Rheumatoid arthritis may also compromise lung and airway function. Costochondral junction involvement restricts rib cage movement and produces restrictive pulmonary disease, which can worsen during pregnancy (see previous discussion of scoliosis). Acute cricoarytenoid involvement limits vocal fold movement and produces edema, leading to airway obstruction that is often mistaken for asthma. Chronic inflammation may distort laryngeal anatomy and decrease laryngeal diameter. Intubation may be difficult due to limitation of neck extension from cervical spine involvement and distorted laryngeal anatomy, or hazardous due to possible atlantoaxial subluxation and spinal cord damage during neck extension.

Anesthetic management should be tailored to the degree and type of extra-articular pathology. For a discussion of the management of patients with valvular or conduction system dysfunction, see Chapter 9. Epidural anesthesia avoids the risks of intubation and respiratory depression, but it should be used with caution in patients with certain cardiac pathology. For example, Sachs and associates[52] successfully used epidural anesthesia for labor in a woman with rheumatoid arthritis and constrictive pericarditis.[52] They instituted radial artery and pulmonary artery pressure monitoring prior to the block and carefully titrated intravenous fluids during epidural injection to minimize a decrease in the preload required to maintain cardiac output. If general anesthesia is chosen, airway assessment, including neck range of motion, lateral neck roentgenograms, and careful history regarding previous attacks of wheezing are important. A fiberoptic laryngoscope and/or jet ventilation system for transtracheal ventilation should be readily available when airway evaluation indicates difficult intubation.

ANKYLOSING SPONDYLITIS

Ankylosing spondylitis is a chronic rheumatic disease that affects primarily the sacroiliac, apophyseal, and costovertebral joints. Chondritis of the upper anterior vertebral margins leads to anterior spondylitis, calcification of paraspinal ligaments, and, eventually, bony bridges between vertebrae. Progressive limitation of lumbar flexion, thoracic and cervical extension, and chest expansion occurs. Rib cage fixation causes a greater reliance on diaphragmatic breathing. Neurologic impairment may come about with cord damage from atlantoaxial subluxation, fracture of cervical vertebrae, or from the cauda equina syndrome.[53] Proximal aortitis leading to aortic insufficiency and complete heart block presents in some patients.

Obstetric Considerations

Although ankylosing spondylitis had been thought to be rare in women, recent reports[54] reveal an equal distribution in both sexes, but often with a slower and more benign course in women.[54] A large series[55] indicated that ankylosing spondylitis does not detrimentally affect pregnancy or the fetus and is not associated with an increased incidence of cesarean section. However, restrictive lung disease from costovertebral involvement would be expected to worsen during pregnancy (see previous discussion of Scoliosis). Unlike rheumatoid arthritis, the symptoms of ankylosing spondylitis often progress during pregnancy.[56]

Anesthetic Considerations

Although they avoid the hazards of endotracheal intubation, epidural and spinal anesthesia may be technically difficult in women with ankylosing spondylitis because of restricted lumbar spine motion and calcified ligaments. Use of a paramedian approach may obviate some of these difficulties. Considerations for general anesthesia are similar to those for women with rheumatoid arthritis and include the possibility of difficult or hazardous intubation. Aortic, aortic-valve, and conduction-system disease are complications of long-standing ankylosing spondylitis[57] and are rare in young pregnant women.[55]

Neural Tube Defects

Failure of closure of the caudal end of the neural tube produces spina bifida, a bone abnormality in which the vertebral arch fails to close, and meningoceles and meningomyeloceles, which are saclike dilatations containing meninges and neural tissue, respectively. Most neural tube defects are dorsal, and diagnosis is usually made in the neonatal period. Nonbony abnormalities are corrected early in life. Distortion of normal paraspinous musculature in all three disorders frequently leads to scoliosis.

OBSTETRIC CONSIDERATIONS

Obstetric management of patients with spina bifida or corrected meningocele or meningomyelocele entails routine practice. In contrast, *anterior* meningocele or meningomyelocele occur rarely, but can present with neurologic symptoms during pregnancy, due to the pressure of the enlarging uterus on the sac. In such cases, cesarean section is preferred for delivery to avoid further pressure on neural tissue. If scoliosis is severe, worsening of restrictive lung disease likely develops during pregnancy (see previous discussion of Scoliosis).

ANESTHESIA CONSIDERATIONS

Use of epidural anesthesia for pain relief during labor in a woman with spina bifida has been reported.[58] Because there are no normal ligaments over the defect (usually at L5–S1 but spanning multiple lumbar interspaces in some cases) it may be difficult to identify the epidural space, increasing the likelihood of accidental dural puncture. Occult intrasacral meningocele is rare,[50] but could theoretically result in dilution of spinally administered local anesthetic and, consequently, inadequate anesthesia.

Primary Bone Disorders

OSTEOGENESIS IMPERFECTA

Osteogenesis imperfecta is a rare connective tissue disorder associated with heart disease that results from lack of normal ossification of endochondral bone. There are two clinical forms—osteogenesis imperfecta congenita, which is usually fatal in the neonatal period, and osteogenesis imperfecta tarda, which appears in childhood. The latter leads to dwarfism, kyphoscoliosis, pectus excavatum, and pathologic fractures. Late manifestations include otosclerosis and deafness.

Obstetric Considerations

The incidence of osteogenesis imperfecta in pregnancy approximates 4 in 100,000.[60] Abdominal delivery is preferred because of the risks of cephalopelvic disproportion, pelvic fractures, uterine rupture, and intra- and postpartum hemorrhage.[61,62] Respiratory insufficiency secondary to pectus excavatum and scoliotic deformities may progress during pregnancy (see previous discussion of Scoliosis).

Anesthetic Considerations

Use of epidural anesthesia for cesarean delivery has been reported[63] in a patient with osteogenesis imperfecta. Since platelet dysfunction (i.e., decreased platelet adhesiveness, decreased platelet aggregation to adenosine diphosphate, and impaired release of platelet factor 3)[64] occurs in this disease, laboratory studies should include a bleeding time. Special care should be taken in positioning the patient both before and after epidural injection to avoid pathologic fractures due to minimal trauma.

If general anesthesia is chosen, difficult endotracheal intubation should be anticipated, due to a short mandible, possible old mandibular fractures, decreased cervical spine movement, and brittle teeth. In addition, these patients may have abnormal cellular metabolism and temperature regulation, and may develop intraoperative hyperthermia similar in severity to malignant hyperthermia.[65] Thus, careful temperature monitoring should be employed, with cold fluids and cooling blankets immediately available.[65] As with epidural anesthesia patient positioning during general anesthesia requires special efforts to avoid pathologic fractures.

ACHONDROPLASIA

Achondroplasia occurs in 4 in 100,000 live births and is the most common cause of dwarfism; females are affected more frequently than males. Decreased rates of endochondral ossification produce shorter bones,[66] resulting in various orthopedic problems including severe lumbar lordosis, kyphoscoliosis, spinal stenosis, and a decreased symphysis pubis-to-xiphoid distance.[67] Premature fusion of the bones at the base of the skull may produce a small foramen magnum, which requires surgical correction if neurologic symptoms develop.

Obstetric Considerations

Low fertility rates are observed[68] in achondroplastic dwarfs. When successful conception achieves the third trimester, the obstetrician chooses abdominal delivery because of the small pelvis and enhanced lumbar lordosis.[67] The enlarging uterus may restrict diaphragmatic movement, decrease functional residual capacity, and produce respiratory distress.

Anesthetic Considerations

Epidural,[68] general, and spinal[69] anesthesia have been used successfully for cesarean section in achondroplastic women. Airway difficulties include difficulty in neck extension[70,71] and possible cervical cord trauma during neck extension. The anesthesia team, anticipating a difficult intubation, should have available a variety of endotracheal tubes (5.0- to 7.0-mm) and laryngoscope blades. A fiberoptic laryngoscope should be readily available. Epidural or spinal needle placement may be technically difficult due to the severe lumbar lordosis. Spinal stenosis, deformed vertebral bodies, and osteophytes[72] may impede insertion of epidural catheters and limit CSF flow during dural puncture.[68] General anesthesia requires careful manipulation of the head and neck during laryngoscopy and intubation.

Miscellaneous Disorders

Pain produced by spondylolisthesis may increase during pregnancy, although progressive slipping during pregnancy has not been reported. Labor progresses normally.[73] Anesthetic considerations are similar to those in patients with herniated lumbar disc disease.

Patients with previous amputations may experience phantom-limb pain, which spinal anesthesia may exacerbate.[74,75] Carrie and Glynn[76] successfully used lumbar epidural anesthesia for cesarean section in a woman with a previous amputation and phantom-limb pain. Although epidural anesthesia did not initially provoke phantom-limb pain, symptoms appeared during regression of the block. They used epidural fentanyl to relieve the pain, and suggest that epidural narcotics specifically relieve this type of deafferentation pain.

Autonomic hyperreflexia can develop in patients with orthopedic trauma with spinal cord damage above T6,[77] and presents during labor in up to two thirds of women with such cord lesions.[78] Acute hypertension and bradycardia can be severe, introducing the possibility of intraventricular hemorrhage.[78] Blood pressure recordings between contractions do not reflect the condition. Uterine contractions, vaginal and rectal examinations, urinary catheter insertion, and abdominal belts for fetal monitoring may trigger the reflex.[78] Stirt and colleagues[79] used epidural injections of bupivacaine, while Baraka gave epidural meperidine[80] to successfully suppress autonomic hyperreflexia during labor. Epidural narcotics have the advantage of not producing further motor, sensory, or sympathetic blockade.

Summary

The salient points from this chapter follow:

- The most common orthopedic complaint during pregnancy is backache, which is rarely due to herniated lumbar disc and is not a contraindication to regional anesthesia.
- Restrictive lung disease produced by orthopedic pathology (thoracic scoliosis, rheumatoid arthritis, ankylosing spondylitis, osteogenesis imperfecta, achondroplasia) may worsen dramatically during pregnancy, leading to respiratory failure or cor pulmonale.
- The choice of anesthetic in patients with restrictive lung disease depends on the degree of respiratory failure and associated cardiac pathology. Anesthesia concerns in these diseases include (with spinal and epidural anesthesia) risks of hypotension and intravenous fluid administration and (with general anesthesia) difficult and hazardous endotracheal intubation.
- Although regional anesthesia may be technically difficult to perform in women with orthopedic disease, spinal and epidural anesthesia have been used in pregnancies complicated by all the conditions described in this chapter.
- Following epidural injection unilateral or incomplete anesthesia, due to adhesions in the epidural space, may occur. In such cases anesthesia can be achieved by spinal injection of morphine for labor or of local anesthetic for cesarean delivery.

References

1. DonTigny, RL: Function and pathomechanics of the sacroiliac joint: A review. Phys Ther 65:35, 1985.
2. Voitk, AJ, et al: Carpal tunnel syndrome in pregnancy. Can Med Assoc J 128:277, 1983.
3. Byant-Greenwood, GD: Relaxin as a new hormone. Endo Rev 3:62, 1982.
4. Abramson, D, Roberts, SM and Wilson, PD: Relaxation of the pelvic joints in pregnancy. Surg Gynecol Obstet 58:595, 1934.
5. Calguneri, M, Bird, HA and Wright, V: Changes in joint laxity occurring during pregnancy. Ann Rheum Dis 41:126, 1982.
6. MacLennan, AH, et al: Serum relaxin and pelvic pain of pregnancy. Lancet 2:243, 1986.
7. Reitz, RE, et al: Calcium magnesium, phosphorus and parathyroid hormone interrelationships in pregnancy and newborn infants. Obstet Gynecol 50:701, 1977.
8. Smith, R, et al: Osteoporosis of pregnancy. Lancet 1:1178, 1985.
9. Dandona, P, Okonofua, F and Clements, RV: Osteomalacia presenting as pathological fractures during pregnancy in Asian women of high socioeconomic class. Br Med J 290:837, 1985.
10. Mantle, MJ, Greenwood, RM and Currey, HLF: Backache in pregnancy. Rheumatol Rehabil 16:95, 1977.
11. LaBan, MM, Perrin, JCS and Latimer, FR: Pregnancy and the herniated lumbar disc. Arch Phys Med Rehabil 64:319, 1983.
12. Crawford, JS: Some maternal complications of epidural analgesia for labour. Anaesthesia 40:1219, 1985.
13. Harvey, EB, et al: Prenatal x-ray exposure and childhood cancer in twins. N Engl J Med 312:541, 1985.
14. Ong, BY, et al: Paresthesias and motor dysfunction after labor and delivery. Anesth Analg (Cleve) 66:18, 1987.
15. Moir, DD, and Davidson, S: Postpartum complications of forceps delivery performed under epidural and pudendal nerve block. Br J Anaesth 44:1197, 1972.
16. Bonica, JJ: Principles and Practice of Obstetric Anesthesia and Analgesia. FA Davis, Philadelphia, 1967.
17. Peng, ATC, Behar, S, and Blancato, LS: Reduction of postlumbar puncture backache by the use of field block anesthesia prior to lumbar puncture. Letter to the editor. Anesthesiology 63:227, 1985.
18. Benzon, HT, Braunschweig, R and Molloy, RE: Delayed onset of epidural anesthesia in patients with back pain. Anesth Analg (Cleve) 60:874, 1981.
19. Schachner, SM and Abram, SE: Use of two epidural catheters to provide analgesia of unblocked segments in a patient with lumbar disc disease. Anesthesiology 56:150, 1982.
20. Luyendijk, W and van Voorthuisen, AE: Contrast examination of the spinal epidural space. Acta Radiol (Diagn) (Stockh) 5:1051, 1966.
21. Garcia, A: The spine: Where it all started. Orthopaed Rev 13:555, 1984.

22. Beals, RK: Nosologic and genetic aspects of scoliosis. Clin Orthop 93:23, 1973.
23. Goldstein, LA and Waugh, TR: Classification and terminology of scoliosis. Clin Orthop 93:10, 1973.
24. Winter, RB: Adolescent idiopathic scoliosis. Letter to the editor. N Engl J Med 314:1379, 1986.
25. Shands, AR and Eisberg, HB: The incidence of scoliosis in the state of Delaware. J Bone Joint Surg 37A:1243, 1955.
26. Kopenhager, T: A review of 50 pregnant patients with kyphoscoliosis. Br J Obstet Gynaecol 84:585, 1977.
27. Warren, MP, et al: Scoliosis and fractures in young ballet dancers: Relation to delayed menarche and secondary amenorrhea. N Engl J Med 314:1348, 1986.
28. Herman, R, et al: Idiopathic scoliosis and the central nervous system: A motor control problem. Spine 10:1, 1985.
29. Freyschuss, U, Nilsonne, U and Lundgren, KD: Idiopathic scoliosis in old age. I: Respiratory function. Acta Med Scand 184:365, 1968.
30. Kafer, ER: Idiopathic scoliosis: Mechanical properties of the respiratory system and ventilatory response to carbon dioxide. J Clin Invest 55:1153, 1975.
31. Kafer, ER: Idiopathic scoliosis: Gas exchange and the age-dependence of arterial blood gases. J Clin Invest 58:825, 1976.
32. Gibbons, PA and Lee, IS: Scoliosis and anesthesia. Int Anesthesiol Clin 23:149, 1985.
33. Hirschfeld, SS, et al: Incidence of mitral valve prolapse in adolescent scoliosis and thoracic hypokyphosis. Pediatrics 70:451, 1982.
34. Davies G and Reid, L: Effect of scoliosis on growth of alveoli and pulmonary arteries and on right ventricle. Arch Dis Child 46:623, 1971.
35. Turino, GM, Goldring, RM and Rishman, AP: Cor pulmonale in musculoskeletal abnormalities of the thorax. Bull NY Acad Med 41:959, 1965.
36. Shneerson, JM, Venco, A and Prime, FJ: A study of pulmonary artery pressure, electrocardiography and mechanocardiography in thoracic scoliosis. Thorax 32:700, 1977.
37. Berman, AT, Cohen, DL and Schwentker, EP: The effects of pregnancy on idiopathic scoliosis: A preliminary report on eight cases and a review of the literature. Spine 7:76, 1982.
38. Sawicka, EH, Spencer, GT and Branthwaite, MA: Management of respiratory failure complicating pregnancy in severe kyphoscoliosis: A new use for an old technique? Br J Dis Chest 80:191, 1986.
39. Manning, CW, Prime, FJ and Zorab, PA: Pregnancy and scoliosis. Lancet 2:792, 1967.
40. Jones, DH: Kyphoscoliosis complicating pregnancy. Lancet 1:517, 1964.
41. Phelan, JP, Dainer, MJ and Cowherd, DW: Pregnancy complicated by thoracolumbar scoliosis. South Med J 71:76, 1978.
42. Kafer, ER: Respiratory and cardiovascular functions in scoliosis and the principles of anesthetic management. Anesthesiology 52:339, 1980.
43. Feldstein, G and Ramanathan, S: Obstetrical lumbar epidural anesthesia in patients with previous posterior spinal fusion for kyphoscoliosis. Anesth Analg 64:83, 1985.
44. Carlson, DW, Engelman, DR and Bart, AJ: Epidural anesthesia for cesarean section in kyphoscoliosis. Anesth Analg 57:125, 1978.
45. Hyde, NH and Harrison, DM: Intrathecal morphine in a parturient with cystic fibrosis. Anesth Analg 65:1357, 1986.
46. O'Sullivan, JB and Cathcart, ES: The prevalence of rheumatoid arthritis: Follow-up evaluation of the effect of criteria on rates in Sudbury, Massachusetts. Ann Intern Med 76:573, 1972.
47. Thurnau, GR: Rheumatoid arthritis. Clin Obstet Gynecol 26:558, 1983.
48. Cecere, FA and Persellin, RH: The interaction of pregnancy and the rheumatic diseases. Clin Rheum Dis 7:747, 1981.
49. Ostensen, M: The influence of pregnancy on blood parameters in patients with rheumatic disease. Scand J Rheum 13:203, 1984.
50. Appelboom, T and Persellin, RH: Leukocyte sensitization against synovial components in rheumatoid arthritis: Blocking by pregnancy serum. Int Arch Allergy Appl Immunol 74:200, 1984.
51. Holligsworth, JW and Saykaly, RJ: Systemic complications of rheumatoid arthritis. Med Clin North Am 61:217, 1977.
52. Sachs, BP, et al: Constrictive pericarditis and pregnancy. Am J Obstet Gynecol 154:156, 1986.
53. Pirlo, AF and Herren, AL: Ankylosing spondylitis. Case report and review of literature. Anes Rev 5:13, 1978.
54. Calin, A and Fries, JF: Striking prevalence of ankylosing spondylitis in "healthy" W27-positive males and females. N Engl J Med 293:835, 1975.
55. Ostensen, M, Romberg, O and Husby, G: Ankylosing spondylitis and motherhood. Arthritis Rheum 25:140, 1982.
56. Ostensen, M and Husby, G: A prospective clinical study of the effect of pregnancy on rheumatoid arthritis and ankylosing spondylitis. Arthritis Rheum 26:1155, 1983.
57. Graham, DC and Smythe, HA: The carditis and aortitis of ankylosing spondylitis. Bull Rheum Dis 9:171, 1958.
58. Vaagenes, P and Fjaerestad, I: Epidural block during labour in a patient with spina bifida cystica. Anaesthesia 36:299, 1981.
59. Joseph, RA and McKenzie, T: Occult intrasacral meningocoele. J Neurol Neurosurg Psychiatry 33:493, 1970.
60. Graffeo, LW, Tisdall, LH and de Vita, JR: Osteogenesis imperfecta. Am J Obstet Gynecol 66:1333, 1953.
61. Roberts, JM and Solomons, CC: Management of pregnancy in osteogenesis imperfecta: New perspectives. Obstet Gynecol 45:168, 1975.
62. Key, TC and Horger, EO: Osteogenesis imperfecta as a complication of pregnancy. Obstet Gynecol 51:67, 1978.
63. Cunningham, AJ, Donnelly, M and Comerford, J: Osteogenesis imperfecta: Anesthetic management of a patient for cesarean section: A case report. Anesthesiology 61:91, 1984.
64. Hathaway, WE, Solomons, CC and Ott, JE: Platelet

function and pyrophosphates in osteogenesis imperfecta. Blood 39:500, 1972.
65. Solomons, CC and Myers, DN: Hyperthermia of osteogenesis imperfecta and its relationship to malignant hyperthermia. In Gordon, RA, Britt, BA and Kalow, W (eds): Malignant Hyperthermia. Charles C Thomas, Springfield, 1973, p 319.
66. Mayhew, JF, et al: Anaesthesia for the achondroplastic dwarf. Can Anaesth Soc J 33:216, 1986.
67. Tyson, JE, et al: Obstetric and gynecologic considerations of dwarfism. Am J Obstet Gynecol 108:688,1970.
68. Cohen SE: Anesthesia for cesarean section in achondroplastic dwarfs. Anesthesiology 52:264, 1980.
69. Kalla, GN, Fening, E and Obiaya, MO: Anaesthetic management of achondroplasia. Br J Anaesth 58:117, 1986.
70. Walts, LF, Finerman, G and Wyatt, GM: Anesthesia for dwarfs and other patients of pathological small stature. Can Anaesth Soc J 22:703, 1975.
71. Mather, JS: Impossible direct laryngoscopy in achondroplasia. Anaesthesia 21:244, 1966.
72. Vogl, A and Osborne, RL: Lesions of the spinal cord (transverse myelopathy) in achondroplasia. Arch Neurol 61:644, 1949.
73. Vebostad, A: Spondylolisthesis. Acta Orthop Scand 45:711, 1974.
74. Mackenzie, N: Phantom limb pain during spinal anaesthesia: Recurrence in amputees. Anaesthesia 38:886, 1983.
75. Murphy, JP and Anandaciva, S: Phantom limb pain and spinal anaesthesia. Anaesthesia 39:188, 1984.
76. Carrie, LES and Glynn, CJ: Phantom limb pain and epidural anesthesia for cesarean section. Anesthesiology 65:220, 1986.
77. Kurnick, NB: Autonomic hyperreflexia and its control in patients with spinal cord lesions. Ann Intern Med 44:678, 1956.
78. McGregor, JA and Meeuwsen, J: Autonomic hyperreflexia: A mortal danger for spinal cord–damaged women in labor. Am J Obstet Gynecol 151:330, 1985.
79. Stirt, JA, Marco, A and Conklin, KA: Obstetric anesthesia for a quadriplegic patient with autonomic hyperreflexia. Anesthesiology 51:560, 1979.
80. Baraka, A: Epidural meperidine for control of autonomic hyperreflexia in a paraplegic parturient. Anesthesiology 62:688, 1985.

CHAPTER 13

ENDOCRINE DISEASE

SHEILA E. COHEN, M.B., Ch.B., F.F.A.R.C.S.
WILLIAM G. BROSE, M.D.

Many endocrine disorders result in reduced fertility, with the result that they present relatively infrequently in pregnant women. However, with improved diagnosis and treatment, more women with endocrine disease are becoming pregnant. This chapter discusses the changes in endocrine physiology that occur in normal pregnancy, the abnormalities associated with pathologic states of hypersecretion or hyposecretion, and the anesthetic considerations of caring for these patients during labor and delivery or surgical removal of an endocrine gland during pregnancy. As the anesthesia literature relating to management of pregnant patients with these disorders is confined to relatively few anecdotal reports, most of our recommendations are based on known pathophysiologic principles and management of nonpregnant patients with similar conditions.

Adrenal Gland

Although adrenocortical dysfunction is usually associated with infertility, improved endocrine therapy has increased the incidence of pregnancy in affected women. Hyperfunction of the *adrenal cortex* can produce Cushing's syndrome, hyperaldosteronism, or the adrenogenital syndrome, each with its own clinical characteristics. Adrenocortical hyposecretion leads to one clinical syndrome which may be iatrogenic (following steroid therapy) or be caused by Addison's disease or hypopituitarism. Hyperfunction of the *adrenal medulla* results from tumors known as pheochromocytomas.

ADRENAL CORTEX

Physiology

The adrenal cortex secretes three groups of hormones: *glucocorticoids* (mainly cortisol), which have a catabolic influence on carbohydrate, protein, and lipid metabolism and stimulate gluconeogenesis in the liver; *mineralocorticoids* (mainly aldosterone), which promote sodium retention by the kidney; and *sex steroids* (mainly androgens), which regulate protein anabolism. All steroid hormones are initially synthesized from cholesterol, the particular steroid produced depending on the presence or absence of specific enzymes located in the three zones of the gland. The outermost layer, the zona glomerulosa, contains the necessary enzymes to elaborate aldosterone and some corticosterone, while the zona fasciculata and -reticularis produce both glucocorticoids and sex hormones.[1]

Cortisol secretion is controlled by a negative feedback mechanism whereby low plasma cortisol levels (Fig. 13–1) stimulate release of pituitary adrenocorticotropic hormone (ACTH). Also, in response to a variety of stimuli, the hypothalamus secretes corticotropin-releasing hormone (CRH) into the hypophyseal-portal circulation, stimulating ACTH secretion and, thus, cortisol production. Stressful situations enhance ACTH secretion.[2]

A number of factors act independently or synergistically to control aldosterone levels. A negative feedback mechanism involving the renin-angiotensin system responds to hypotension or hypovolemia by means of increased renin secretion; this results in increased production of angiotensin II, which stimulates aldosterone release (Fig. 13–2). Changes in electrolyte balance such as hyperkalemia or hyponatremia cause increased aldosterone release. Finally, ACTH stimulates aldosterone production.

Changes in Pregnancy

During pregnancy, enlarged adrenal glands are associated with augmented adrenocortical function.[1] In response to an increase in circulating estrogen, levels of transcortin, a binding protein, increase. Secretion of melanocyte-stimulating hormone (MSH) and ACTH is enhanced, resulting in the commonly observed pigmentation of pregnancy. Plasma 17-hydroxycorticosteroids increase progressively throughout pregnancy, reaching levels almost four times those of normal, nonpregnant women. Urinary glucocorticoids remain within normal limits, although levels may rise as pregnancy progresses. During vaginal delivery, plasma cortisol levels rise even further, exceeding the more modest increases found during elective cesarean section. Increased aldosterone secretion also occurs during pregnancy, perhaps due to high levels of circulating progesterone. The secretion of sex hormones by the adrenal gland remains

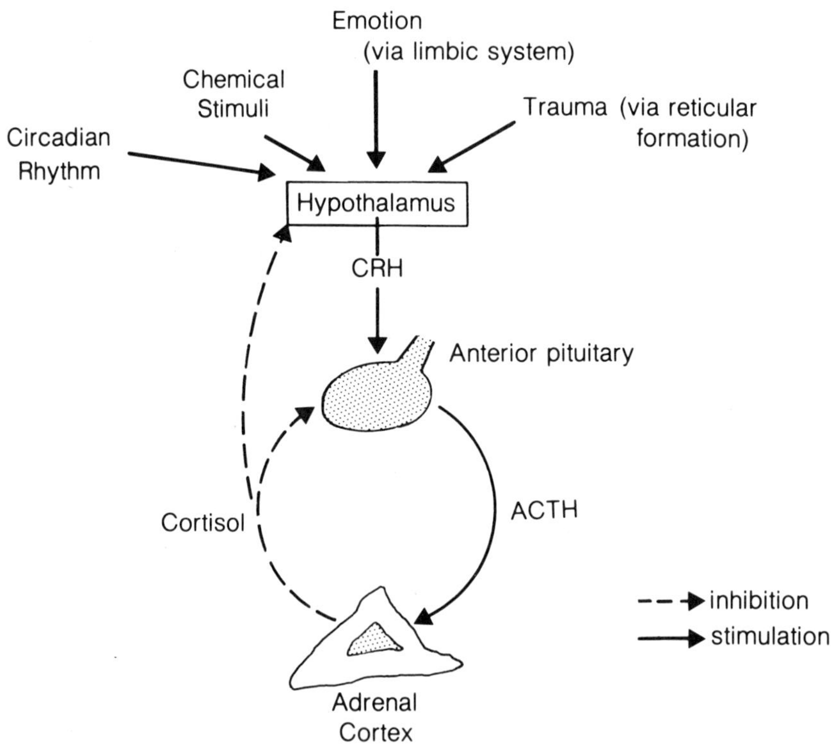

Figure 13–1. Negative feedback mechanism that controls ACTH secretion.

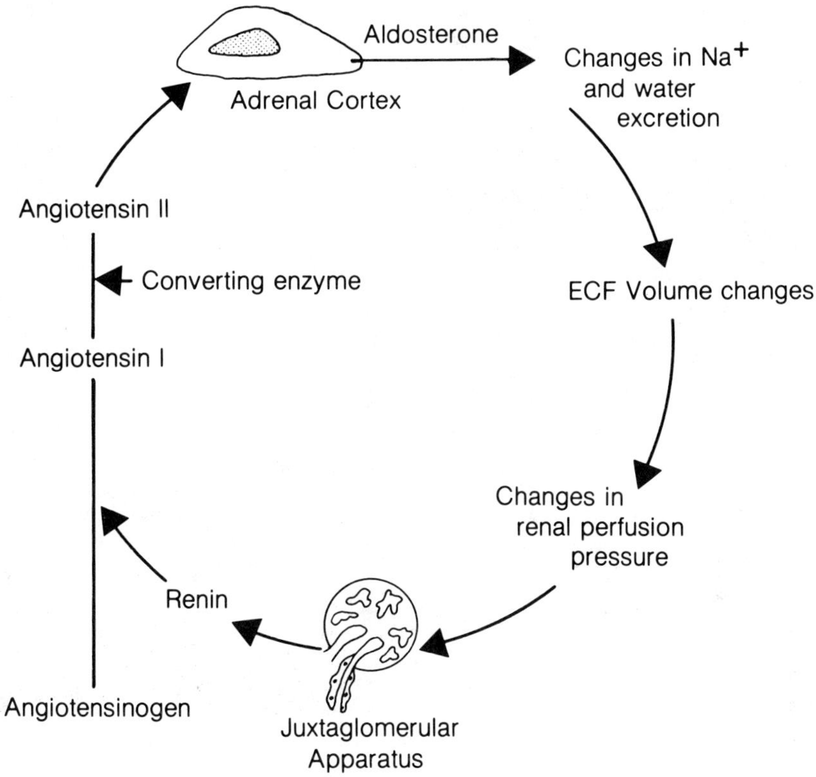

Figure 13–2. Negative feedback mechanism that controls aldosterone secretion.

within normal limits as the placenta assumes this function as pregnancy progresses.

Cushing's Syndrome

Clinical Features. Cushing's syndrome (excessive circulating glucocorticoid levels) has several causes (Table 13–1). Patients present with a variety of clinical signs and symptoms that reflect the multiple effects of glucocorticoid hormones.[3,4] Typically they are hirsute, with central obesity, a "buffalo hump," and a moon-shaped face (Fig. 13–3). Purple abdominal striae and ecchymoses due to capillary fragility occur frequently, and diabetes, hypertension, and even frank psychosis may be present. Infertility and menstrual disorders commonly occur, and ovulation and pregnancy are rare.[5–7] Most pregnancies end in abortion, prematurity, or stillbirth, the latter sometimes being associated with adrenal atrophy in the fetus. Pregnancy frequently exacerbates Cushing's syndrome, which may first become manifest during gestation. Spontaneous remission also has been reported following termination of pregnancy.[8]

Diagnosis. Symptoms of pregnancy or preeclampsia such as weight gain, abdominal striae, hypertension, and edema can mimic Cushing's syndrome and make diagnosis difficult. Twenty-four-hour urinary free cortisol levels rise above those normal for gestation,

Table 13–1. CAUSES OF CUSHING'S SYNDROME

Adrenal adenoma: most common cause in pregnancy
Adrenal carcinoma
Bilateral adrenal hyperplasia
Hypothalamic dysfunction
Pituitary tumors: basophilic adenoma (Cushing's disease)
ACTH–producing tumors
Nonendocrine tumors: oat-cell carcinoma of the lung
Iatrogenic: prolonged use of glucocorticoids or ACTH

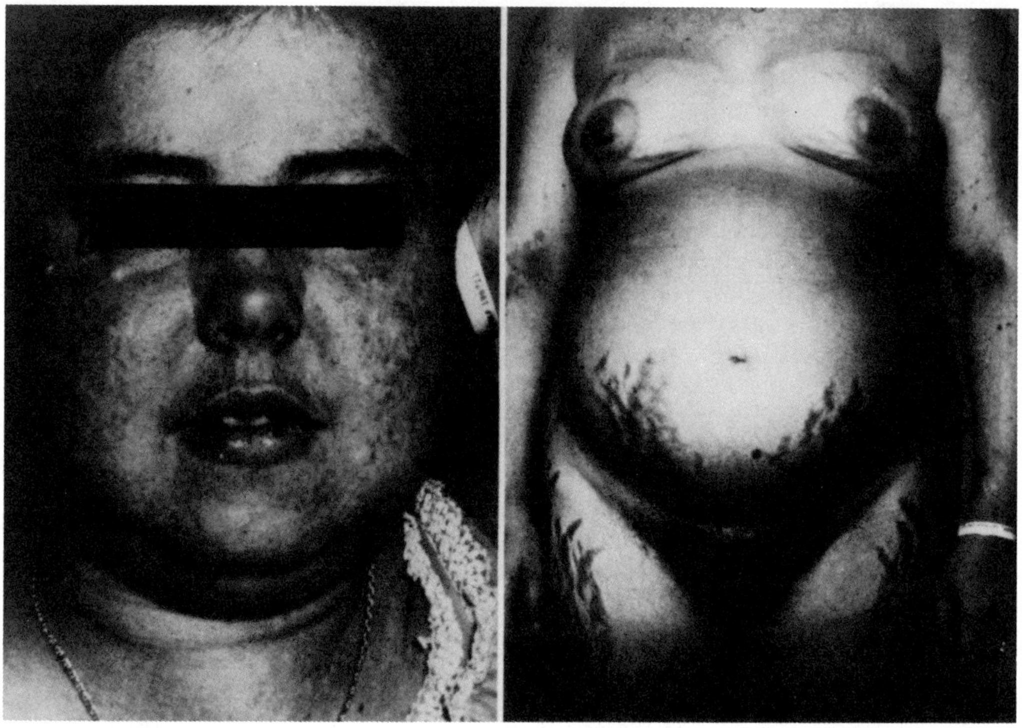

Figure 13–3. Cushing's disease in pregnancy. (From Grimes, et al,[3] with permission.)

with loss of the normal circadian rhythm. Plasma ACTH assay proves helpful in determining whether the disease is of adrenal or pituitary origin. High ACTH levels suggest a pituitary problem (or an ectopic source of ACTH), whereas low or undetectable levels suggest feedback suppression secondary to increased cortisol production by an adrenal tumor.[4] Cushing's syndrome in pregnancy most often is associated with an adrenal adenoma or carcinoma, perhaps because pregnancy occurs more often in these conditions than when the disease originates in the pituitary or in another site.[1]

Exposure to diagnostic x-rays should be kept to a minimum until after delivery if the neonate is to be salvaged. A plain abdominal film may show a tissue shadow with kidney displacement, which may be due to an adrenal carcinoma. Ultrasound may also be helpful in diagnosis if the tumor is of adequate size. Although computed tomography of the adrenals and sella turcica may delineate small lesions, the ionizing radiation limits its usefulness during pregnancy. Magnetic resonance imaging, which does not employ ionizing radiation, may be an excellent diagnostic tool in this circumstance.

Management. Factors such as the severity of the mother's disease and the gestational age and well-being of the fetus influence whether patients with Cushing's syndrome should receive medical or surgical treatment. An increased incidence of placental insufficiency and *abruptio placentae* is associated with the coincident diabetes and hypertension, and can lead to fetal death. Inhibition of the fetal adrenal gland by maternal glucocorticoids can result in low maternal estrogen levels, since the fetal adrenal gland contributes to the synthesis of this hormone. Many experts[1,3,9] recommend surgical removal of adenomas that present during pregnancy.

Preoperative Preparation. Patients with Cushing's syndrome must be prepared carefully for anesthesia, whether for surgical intervention or for vaginal or cesarean delivery. Glassford and associates[10] recently drew attention to a number of problems that merit attention from the anesthesiologist. Hyperglycemia, due to increased gluconeogenesis and suppression of peripheral utilization of glucose, may require insulin therapy for adequate perioperative control. Hypertension also may require treatment, and diuretics may be necessary if congestive cardiac failure develops in response to the increased blood volume of pregnancy. Pulmonary edema has occurred during pregnancy or around the time of delivery in almost half the reported cases of Cushing's syndrome.[7]

An increased susceptibility to infection from high cortisol levels and the presence of diabetes necessitate meticulous attention to sterile technique when performing invasive procedures. Increased excretion of potassium causes hypokalemia, which should be corrected before surgery. Diuretics, when necessary, must be administered carefully to these patients. Muscle weakness resulting from electrolyte imbalance and increased protein catabolism can attenuate pulmonary ventilation and coughing. This may predispose the mother to respiratory infection and increase her sensitivity to the respiratory depressant effects of anesthetic drugs. Finally, osteoporosis, which occurs commonly, demands care in moving the patient in order to avoid pathologic fractures.

The normal endocrine response to surgical stress includes significant increases in levels of cortisol and other hormones of the pituitary-adrenal axis. Cushing's syndrome often impairs the pituitary adrenal stress response and thus requires preoperative steroid coverage in spite of elevated cortisol levels. Roizen[11] recently reviewed the issue of perioperative steroid supplementation and found few objective data to support one regimen over another. Plumpton and associates[12] administer intravenous hydrocortisone, 100 mg every 6 hours for 3 days, while Symreng and colleagues[13] administer only 25 mg intravenously shortly after induction of anesthesia, followed by an additional 100 mg infused slowly over the next 24 hours. Although the latter method produces plasma cortisol levels close to those normally seen with surgery, it does not supply steroids in the quantities secreted during a maximal stress response (approximately 300 mg per day). Therefore, we recommend following a regimen similar to that outlined in Table 13–2.

Anesthesia. Whether anesthetic agents or techniques that suppress pituitary-adrenal function offer any advantages or present any risks in this condition remains unknown. Ether and cycloprane, the only agents that stimulate adrenal function, are no longer in use. In general, low doses of inhalation or intravenous agents do not modify the surgical response to stress, and high doses do so only as long as high concentrations are maintained in the blood and tissues.[14] Etomidate inhibits corticosteroid synthesis in a reversible, dose-dependent manner, impairing the cortisol response to both surgical stress and exogenously administered ACTH (endogenous ACTH levels rise in this circumstance).[15] This response probably contraindicates the use of etomidate for these patients. Midazolam also suppresses the cortisol response to minor surgery, however the adrenal response to exogenously administered ACTH remains normal.[15] Since midazolam administration depresses endogenous ACTH levels, central depression of the hypothalamic-pituitary-adrenal axis probably occurs. Regional techniques (epidural and spinal blocks) denervate the adrenal glands, preventing the adrenocortical hyperfunction associated with surgery.[16] However, plasma cortisol levels become elevated during prolonged spinal anesthesia and after regression of regional blockade, indicating only transient suppression.[17] The use of epidural opiates in conjunction with local anesthetics delays this rise in plasma cortisol, whereas continued use of epidural local anesthetics for postoperative analgesia prevents it completely.[18]

General Anesthesia. The thick-set neck, obesity, and buffalo hump all limit neck mobility and make airway positioning difficult.[10] Further-

Table 13–2. SUGGESTED REGIMEN FOR STEROID COVER

	Day 1	Days 2 and 3	Day 4
Major surgery (including cesarean section and delivery)	Hydrocortisone phosphate 100 mg IV every 8 hr	Hydrocortisone phosphate 100 mg IV or IM every 8–12 hr	Discontinue, return to maintenance dose or taper off (see text)
Minor surgery	Hydrocortisone 100 mg IV	Discontinue or return to maintenance dose	

more, increased mucosal friability and vessel fragility can lead to bleeding with airway manipulation. Because of these factors and the gastrointestinal changes of pregnancy, careful awake intubation (with or without the aid of fiberoptic laryngoscopy) may be indicated.

Hypotension and cardiac dysrhythmias resulting from electrolyte abnormalities may complicate the induction of general anesthesia. Anesthesia for adrenalectomy can be maintained with a relaxant, nitrous oxide (50- to 60-percent), and a volatile inhalation anesthetic or a narcotic. For cesarean section, nitrous oxide (50-percent), a low concentration of a volatile agent, and a relaxant can be used until delivery, after which an intravenous narcotic can be substituted. In the perioperative period, continuous monitoring of central venous pressure (CVP), arterial blood pressure (with an intra-arterial catheter), and the ECG allows necessary assessment of cardiovascular status.

Regional Anesthesia. The condition of the mother determines whether regional anesthesia is appropriate for labor or cesarean section. Regional anesthesia may be technically difficult because of obesity, osteoporosis, or vertebral compression fractures, but if these problems can be overcome and arterial blood pressure and CVP can be adequately monitored, epidural anesthesia for cesarean section provides controllable anesthesia while avoiding the potential cardiorespiratory risks of general anesthesia.

Primary Hyperaldosteronism

Aldosterone, a mineralocorticoid, causes reabsorption of sodium in exchange for potassium and hydrogen in the distal renal tubule. Primary hyperaldosteronism results from excessive secretion of aldosterone. The condition is usually caused by a benign adrenocortical adenoma (Conn's syndrome) but is occasionally associated with nodular hyperplasia of the adrenal cortex (idiopathic hyperaldosteronism). In secondary hyperaldosteronism, excessive production of aldosterone occurs in response to elevated levels of plasma renin. Urinary aldosterone excretion rises progressively in normal pregnancy then falls rapidly postpartum. As electrolyte imbalance does not usually occur, this appears to be an example of secondary hyperaldosteronism, perhaps occurring in response to the salt-wasting effect of progesterone.[19,20]

Clinical Features. Pregnancy occurs very rarely in primary hyperaldosteronism. Several clinical presentations can occur as a result of the metabolic effects of aldosterone.[2] Hypertension, commonly present, may be difficult to differentiate from pre-eclampsia and renal or essential hypertension. A hypokalemic nephropathy can also develop, with symptoms of polyuria and polydipsia. Finally, low serum potassium levels can lead to intermittent muscle weakness and paralysis.

Diagnosis. Hypokalemia, increased urinary potassium excretion, and elevated urinary and serum aldosterone levels confirm the diagnosis. High aldosterone levels occur in spite of normal or low plasma renin activity.

Management. Hypertension constitutes the most serious feature of this disease, causing deleterious effects on both mother and fetus. If diagnosis occurs early in pregnancy, exploration of the adrenal gland in the second trimester (after the period of organogenesis) has been recommended.[9,21] Diagnosis in late pregnancy calls for conservative management with spironolactone, an aldosterone antagonist, until after delivery, in order to decrease fetal risk.[22] Spironolactone therapy proves more successful in patients with bilateral adrenal hyperplasia than in those with cortical adenomas.

Anesthesia. Preoperative preparation should include correction of the hypokalemic alkalosis with potassium supplements and spironolactone. Inadequate potassium replacement may result in increased susceptibility to cardiac arrhythmias and abnormal sensitivity to muscle relaxants. Hydrocortisone is not usually required, except when both adrenal glands are mobilized or if total adrenalectomy is performed.

In this condition no particular anesthetic agent or technique has been reported to be advantageous.[23] Invasive monitoring of arterial blood pressure and CVP is advisable for any anesthetic intervention. Muscle relaxants have been used in hyperaldosteronism without any complications, despite the theoretical problems associated with electrolyte imbalance.[23] Temporary hypoaldosteronism may follow adrenalectomy, necessitating treatment with maintenance doses of fluorohydrocortisone.

Adrenocortical Insufficiency

Adrenocortical insufficiency, or Addison's disease, represents the most common disorder of the adrenal gland occurring in pregnancy. Because of the low maternal mortality in treated patients who deliver spontaneously at term, this disease no longer contraindicates pregnancy.[1] Adrenal insufficiency can occur when patients who have adrenal atrophy from prolonged corticosteroid therapy experience stressful situations or discontinue their medications (often because of nausea, vomiting, or an acute illness).[4] Other causes include primary atrophy (most often due to an autoimmune process), tuberculosis, metastatic carcinoma, amyloidosis, adrenal infarction, or previous adrenalectomy. Pituitary dysfunction also can produce hypoadrenalism and, in the past, Sheehan's syndrome (hypopituitarism following severe hemorrhagic shock in pregnancy) was a well-recognized cause.

Clinical Features. Adrenal insufficiency can present acutely, with life-threatening cardiovascular collapse, or insidiously, with vague signs and symptoms. The nonspecific symptoms in Addison's disease of malaise, weight loss, nausea and vomiting, constipation, and increased pigmentation strikingly resemble symptoms found in early pregnancy. Even the hypotension, syncope, abdominal pain, and hypoglycemia found in Addison's disease occur commonly enough in normal pregnancy to make diagnosis difficult. However, persistence of nausea and vomiting and continued weight loss should raise the suspicion of Addison's disease.

Patients with untreated Addison's disease tend to tolerate pregnancy without difficulty, perhaps because of hypertrophy of any remaining adrenal tissue and transfer to the mother of corticosteroids secreted by the fetal adrenals.[24] Serious complications such as acute adrenal crisis can first present during labor or delivery in response to stress, or postpartum, probably as a result of the diuresis and dehydration that follow delivery.[25,26]

Diagnosis. In the early stages of the disease, serum and urinary electrolytes may be within normal limits. Subsequently, serum sodium decreases, serum potassium and urea increase, and urinary excretion of sodium rises markedly. Plasma and 24-hour free urinary cortisol levels are low, with loss of circadian rhythm. Occasionally they stand within the normal nonpregnant range, since during pregnancy even in Addison's disease cortical binding globulin and free plasma cortisol levels increase, probably due to alteration of the set-point in the hypothalamic-pituitary-adrenal axis.[1] ACTH assays and ACTH stimulation tests help to distinguish between disease of pituitary and adrenal origin.[4]

Management. Preservation of normal electrolyte balance and an adequate response to the stress of labor and delivery represent the goals of therapy during pregnancy. A recommended maintenance regimen includes cortisol, 25 to 30 mg in the morning, plus 12.5 mg in the evening, and fluorohydrocortisone, 0.1 mg daily.[1] The presence of hypertension or edema often calls for reduced doses of mineralocorticoid.

The majority of parturients with adequate steroid replacement currently are allowed a spontaneous labor and vaginal delivery supported by appropriate hydration with a balanced salt solution and increased glucocorticoid administration. The latter should be continued for several days after vaginal or cesarean delivery as described in Table 13–2. Although some experts recommend gradual postpartum withdrawal of steroids to the preoperative maintenance level, others advocate abrupt cessation of supplemental doses to provide maximal stimulus for normal adrenal function. This, of course, pertains only to patients who have some residual adrenal activity such as those with atrophy secondary to steroid administration. After investigating the adrenal response to stress following steroid therapy, Plumpton and coworkers[12] recommend steroid coverage during surgery and delivery only when these agents have been used within the previous 2 months. Treatment of an Addisonian crisis requires rapid administration of hydrocortisone, 200-mg intravenous bolus, followed by 100 mg in each liter of briskly infused balanced salt solution; the first liter of fluid should also contain 5-percent glucose, to counteract hypoglycemia.[1]

Anesthesia. The presence of anemia, hyperkalemia, hypoglycemia, generalized debilitation, and hypovolemia increase the anesthetic risk to patients with Addison's disease, although adequate preoperative hydration and hydrocortisone supplementation reduce this hazard. During labor and delivery the elevated cortisol levels seen in normal, lightly medicated parturients indicate that requirements for adrenocortical function increase (Fig. 13–4).[27] Since continuous lumbar epidural analgesia significantly attenuates this response, it most likely results from the pain and stress of labor and delivery. Hypovolemia increases the likelihood of profound hypotension during regional block administered for labor or cesarean delivery. Thus, aggressive fluid loading, uterine displacement, and perhaps prophylactic ephedrine should be employed. General anesthesia can be induced with ketamine or reduced doses of thiopental (2 to 4 mg per kg), and maintained with 50-percent nitrous oxide, a relaxant, and a very low concentration of a volatile agent. Caution with anesthetic drug dosage proves necessary as patients with Addison's disease demonstrate greater susceptibility to the depressant effects of barbiturates and narcotics.[17] Because of its effect on adrenal function[15] etomidate should not be used in this condition. As adrenal crises can occur at any time, cardiovascular status must be closely monitored during labor, vaginal or cesarean delivery, and the puerperium.

ADRENAL MEDULLA

The adrenal medulla produces norepinephrine, which is synthesized from tyrosine at postganglionic sympathetic nerve endings, and epinephrine, which is manufactured by methylation of norepinephrine in the medulla. These amines have a half-life in the circulation of less than 1 min, owing partially to their rapid metabolism by monoamine oxidase and catechol-o-methyl transferase to 3-methoxy-4-hydroxymandelic acid (VMA). Pregnancy does not alter adrenal medullary function.

Pheochromocytoma

Pheochromocytomas secrete epinephrine, norepinephrine, or both neurotransmitters in varying proportions. They arise in chromaffin tissue, the commonest site being the adrenal medulla (82 percent of all lesions).[28] However, the tumor can arise anywhere along the neural axis, including the sympathetic chain, para-aortic areas, retroperitoneum, and even the bladder. Although they are usually benign, in one series 14.5 percent were malignant and 9.2 percent were multifocal.[29] Occasionally they are associated with severe neurocutaneous dysplasias, medullary carcinoma of the thyroid, or renal artery stenosis occurring on the same side as the tumor.[30]

Incidence. Pheochromocytoma rarely occurs during pregnancy, but is extremely hazardous to the mother and the fetus. In a study of 89 cases, maternal mortality was 58 percent and fetal mortality 55 percent when the diagnosis was missed prior to delivery.[31] Antepartum

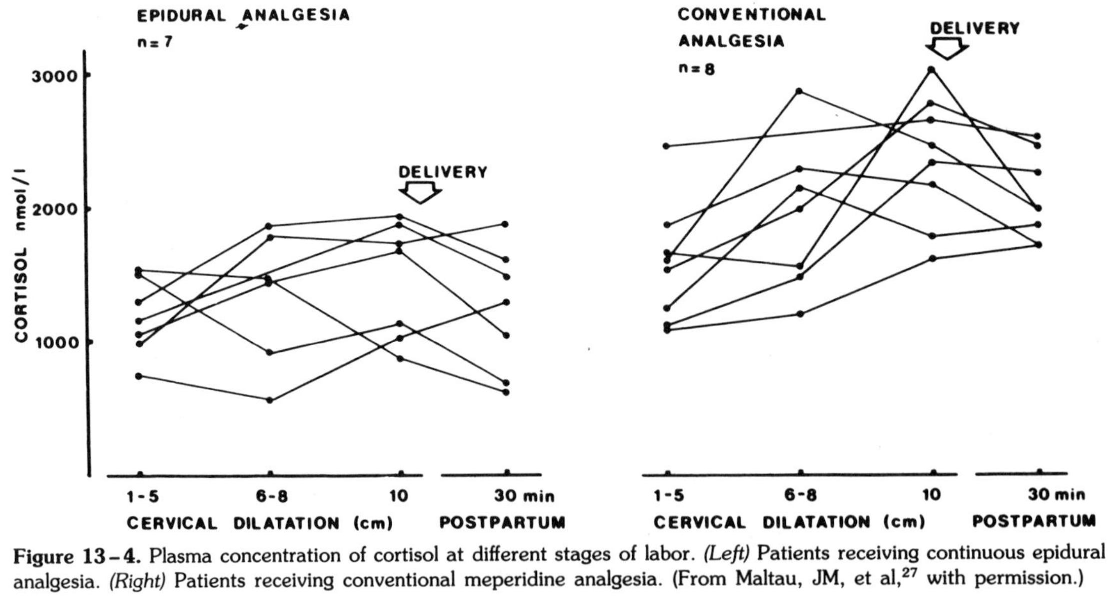

Figure 13–4. Plasma concentration of cortisol at different stages of labor. *(Left)* Patients receiving continuous epidural analgesia. *(Right)* Patients receiving conventional meperidine analgesia. (From Maltau, JM, et al,[27] with permission.)

diagnosis reduced maternal mortality to 18 percent; fetal mortality, however, remained high (50 percent).[31] Maternal death has usually resulted from a hypertensive crisis, cardiac failure, ventricular arrhythmias, or severe hypotension following removal of the tumor. More recently, use of both α- and β-adrenergic blocking drugs has further decreased maternal mortality (to 10.6 percent) and slightly improved fetal mortality (46 percent).[32]

Clinical Features. Elevated catecholamine levels produce both α- and β-adrenergic effects, causing headache, sustained or intermittent hypertension, palpitations, excessive perspiration, blurred vision, heat intolerance, and excessive weight loss. Intermittent tumor secretion accounts for paroxysmal symptoms, the severity of which relate to the amount of catecholamines released. On physical examination, pallor resulting from intense peripheral vasoconstriction may be seen, and cardiomegaly, arrhythmias, and pulmonary edema should be sought. Prolonged α-adrenergic stimulation results in decreased plasma volume, which can cause postural hypotension and a falsely elevated hematocrit. Biochemical abnormalities include a hypermetabolic state with elevated blood sugar and free fatty acid levels, due to the effect of increased catecholamines on hepatic and fat metabolism.

Diagnosis. Pheochromocytoma must be differentiated from pre-eclampsia, malignant hypertension, and hyperthyroidism. Edema or proteinuria seldom accompanies the hypertension associated with pheochromocytoma, while glucosuria often occurs. The familial occurrence of the disease and the coexistence of neurofibromatosis may be helpful in establishing the correct diagnosis.

Provocative tests such as the histamine test, which when positive causes an elevation in blood pressure, and the phentolamine (Regitine) test, which results in hypotension, have been used in the past to aid diagnosis. However, in addition to being potentially dangerous, both false-positive and false-negative results can occur. Currently, diagnosis depends on detection of excessive amounts of free catecholamines or VMA in blood or urine. Measurement of both 24-hour urinary catecholamine secretion and VMA are more reliable than measurement of VMA alone, as excess catechols are secreted continuously, even when symptoms are episodic.[33] The normal values for 24-hour urinary excretion during pregnancy are epinephrine, 0.2 μg; norepinephrine, 20 to 70 μg; and VMA, 2 to 7 mg.[33] The clonidine suppression test has been used in nonpregnant patients with only slightly elevated norepinephrine levels and a suspected diagnosis of pheochromocytoma. Clonidine does not suppress norepinephrine secreted by a pheochromocytoma.[34] Unlike the provocative tests using histamine or phentolamine, this test does not endanger either the mother or fetus.

Following diagnosis of pheochromocytoma, abdominal palpation can locate the tumor in approximately 25 percent of cases. However, this is not recommended since it often precipitates an attack. Very high urine and plasma epinephrine levels strongly suggest an adrenal medullary origin, while symptoms occurring at micturition indicate a bladder lesion. Radiologic methods of tumor localization are relatively contraindicated during pregnancy, making ultrasound particularly useful. Recently, magnetic resonance imaging of pheochromocytoma during pregnancy also has been reported.[35]

Management. The optimal management of pheochromocytoma remains controversial. When the diagnosis takes place in the first two trimesters, many authors recommend the administration of adrenergic antagonists followed by surgical excision, in spite of the risk of spontaneous abortion.[22,32,33,36–40] When diagnosis occurs in the third trimester, most experts[22,38–44] favor the use of α-blocking agents until the fetus reaches maturity, at which time they perform combined elective cesarean section and tumor resection. This strategy is associated with favorable maternal and fetal prognosis. If the tumor cannot be located during this procedure, it can be removed some weeks later with no increase in mortality.[45] Delayed excision may be easier because the vascularity of pregnancy will have regressed, access to the tumor will be improved, and the lesion can be more accurately localized preoperatively. Adrenalectomy after successful vaginal delivery also has been reported.[45,46]

Preoperative Preparation. Preoperative administration of an α-blocking agent is mandatory for control of blood pressure and expansion of intravascular volume.[31] Although gross fetal abnormalities have not been reported following such therapy, its long-term effects are relatively unknown. Phenoxybenzamine, 40 to 100 mg per day by mouth should be administered for at least 3 days prior to operation, although treatment for 10 to 14 days is optimal.[44] Adequacy of alpha blockade can be assessed by noting control of hypertension, presence of postural hypotension, nasal stuffiness, increased frequency of bowel movements, and a fall in hematocrit.

Patients with severe tachycardia or cardiac arrhythmias should receive β-blocking agents such as propranolol, although their use in pregnancy provokes controversy.[47,48] They cross the placenta and have been associated with intrauterine growth retardation.[48] In addition, beta blockade could theoretically increase myometrial irritability and lead to premature labor. Other possible effects include fetal bradycardia, impaired responsiveness to anoxic stress, and neonatal depression and hypoglycemia. Lack of variability of the heart rate makes monitoring of these fetuses particularly difficult. Despite these potential risks, beta blockade may be necessary to control the hyperdynamic myocardium in patients with pheochromocytoma. This need, in conjunction with evidence that fetal status improves in hypertensive patients treated with beta blockers,[48] justifies the use of these agents in patients with pheochromocytoma. When used, beta blockers should be instituted only after achieving alpha blockade in order to avoid unopposed alpha stimulation. The use of metyrosine, a tyrosine analog and competitive inhibitor of tyrosine hydroxylase, may be helpful during preoperative preparation as well as postoperatively if complete surgical resection of a malignant pheochromocytoma proves impossible.[49] Preoperative volume expansion with blood or crystalloid also has been suggested,[44] but gradual alpha blockade and adequate oral hydration usually make it unnecessary.

Anesthetic Management. Although heavy premedication and deep anesthesia are usually advocated for removal of pheochromocytomas in nonpregnant patients, the deleterious neonatal effects of such an approach must be considered when resection is combined with cesarean section. Adequate control of hypertension with alpha blockers and a thorough preoperative visit by the anesthesiologist should minimize the need for premedication. If sedation seems necessary, small doses of diazepam or midazolam can be administered. Avoid anticholinergics because of the resultant tachycardia and central nervous system stimulation.

Almost every anesthetic agent and technique has been recommended for the removal of pheochromocytomas.[11] Regardless of the technique selected, factors provoking catecholamine release, such as hypoxia, hypercarbia, and hypotension, must be avoided. Particularly hazardous periods include induction of anesthesia, intubation, manipulation of the tumor, and the period following tumor excision. These patients must be continuously monitored with intra-arterial and CVP measurements and a pulmonary artery catheter.[50] Blood gas analyses should be performed and urinary output monitored.

Epidural or spinal anesthesia has been advocated for excision of pheochromocytomas,[51–53] but the attendant hypotension, particularly likely in the parturient, may precipitate catecholamine release and a dangerous hypertensive crisis. The successful use of regional anesthesia mandates judicious volume expansion, as determined by invasive cardiovascular monitoring.

General anesthesia seems preferable since it permits better blood pressure control and surgical exposure.[37] An infusion of phentolamine can be started before induction, and nitroprusside should be available to treat severe hypertension during intubation. Although the possibility of fetal cyanide toxicity contraindicates prolonged administration of nitroprusside before delivery, its brief use to treat life-threatening hypertension during laryngoscopy and tracheal intubation appears justified. Beta-adrenergic blockers should similarly blunt the hypertensive response to intubation. A smooth induction with a thiobarbiturate should precede a rapid, gentle intubation. Avoid agents that cause histamine or catecholamine release. Since light anesthesia results in sympathetic stimulation, administration of fentanyl (100 to 250 μg) intravenously prior to delivery is appropriate. Such low doses of narcotic seldom cause neonatal depression, although naloxone therapy and neonatal resuscitation should be available. Anesthesia can be maintained with nitrous oxide (50- to 60-percent), a nondepolarizing muscle relaxant, and enflurane or isoflurane (0.5 to 1 MAC) until delivery. As large amounts of epinephrine and norepinephrine often enter the circulation during tumor resection, halothane may be undesirable because of its arrhythmogenic potential.[54,55] Conversion to a narcotic technique after delivery is usually preferable.

Specific intraoperative problems include severe hypertension before tumor excision and hypotension due to blood loss at delivery or following ligation of the venous drainage of the tumor. Initially, a nitroprusside infusion or phentolamine, 1 to 5 mg intravenously, supplemented as necessary with other hypotensive agents, can serve to treat hypertension. Adequate preoperative restoration of intravascular volume in conjunction with alpha blockade minimizes hypotension. Blood loss during surgery must be carefully monitored and promptly replaced.

In patients with cardiomyopathy, transient cardiac failure occasionally follows sudden removal of catecholamine stimulation.[56] Intraoperative tachycardia and ventricular arrhythmias occur commonly and call for treatment with small doses of propranolol or lidocaine.

Postoperative Course. In the postoperative period troublesome hypotension is initially managed with intravenous fluids and, if necessary, vasopressors such as norepinephrine, neosynephrine, or dopamine. Also consider adrenocortical insufficiency and, if indicated, administer hydrocortisone.

Anesthesia for Vaginal Delivery. Patients adequately controlled by medical treatment may be allowed to deliver vaginally at term. During labor and delivery they should be closely monitored with intra-arterial and central venous catheters, an ECG, and continuous assessment of urine output. Both vasopressor and hypotensive agents should be immediately available. During regional anesthesia, hypotension must be avoided; thus patients require proper intravascular volume expansion prior to blockade and should be placed in the lateral position.

Pituitary Gland

The pituitary gland controls numerous physiologic processes by the secretion of hormones that stimulate target organs and thereby cause release of other hormones. The anterior lobe secretes growth hormone (GH), prolactin, adrenocorticotropic hormone (ACTH), thyroid stimulating hormone (TSH), and the gonadotropic hormones, luteinizing hormone and follicular stimulating hormone (LH, FSH). The posterior lobe, or neurohypophysis, stores vasopressin, or antidiuretic hormone (ADH), and oxytocin. During pregnancy the normal pituitary gland enlarges, probably as a result of elevated estrogen levels, which induce hypertrophy and hyperplasia, particularly of the acidophilic cells involved in prolactin secretion.[57]

HYPERPITUITARISM (PITUITARY TUMORS)

Pregnancy has been uncommon in women with pituitary tumors because normal reproductive pathways are interrupted. However, with improved radiologic techniques for imaging the sellar region, the introduction of radioimmunoassays for prolactin, and greater awareness of the pathophysiology of pituitary tumors, many patients with secondary infertility are being diagnosed as having pituitary microadenomas of the prolactin-secreting type (prolactinomas). In the early stages of the disease these microadenomas may be associated with regular ovulatory cycles, while later they may produce amenorrhea, galactorrhea, and infertility. Tumors formed by other cell types include those that secrete growth hormone (producing acromegaly) and adenomas of basophilic cells (resulting in Cushing's disease). Adenomas of cells that produce gonadotropins and thyrotropins rarely occur.

Pituitary tumors tend to increase in size during pregnancy, often converting a small asymptomatic lesion in the nonpregnant state into a symptomatic condition.[58] Estrogen binding to receptors found in some tumors may cause this growth,[59] and explain why spontaneous remission of pituitary tumors sometimes occurs after delivery.[60] Ideally, ovulation should not be induced in the infertile patient until the diagnosis of pituitary tumor has been excluded. Unfortunately, radiologic techniques cannot always detect microadenomas, which may become obvious only during a subsequent pregnancy.

Clinical Features. The clinical picture depends entirely on the pathophysiologic process present. Manifestations resulting from an expanding pituitary lesion include headache, visual disturbances (bitemporal hemianopia), increased intracranial pressure, and extraocular muscle palsies. A chromophil adenoma or craniopharyngioma can cause pituitary hypofunction by compressing adjacent glandular tissue, whereas hyperplasia of hormone-secreting cells results in one of three clinical syndromes depending on the type of cell affected. Prolactinoma, resulting in reproductive problems, headache, visual loss, and occasionally hypopituitarism, represents the most common lesion. Acromegaly, resulting from tumors of acidophilic cells, produces the classic syndrome of enlarged hands, feet, tongue, and nose, excessive sweating, and hoarseness. Amenorrhea and galactorrhea may also be present if the tumor secretes prolactin. Impaired glucose tolerance constitutes the major metabolic disturbance in acromegaly, and frank diabetes mellitus can develop. The coincidental occurrence of acromegaly during pregnancy may be confused with the syndrome known as transient acromegaly of pregnancy, a problem characterized by nonedematous thickening of facial features and extremities. This benign condition disappears in the puerperium. Basophil adenomas cause bilateral adrenocortical hyperplasia, producing Cushing's disease (described earlier in this chapter).

Diagnosis. Diagnosis of pituitary lesions depends on radiologic examination of the sella turcica and radioimmunoassays that reveal excessive amounts of the relevant hormones. Adequate evaluation of pituitary function not only documents hypersecretion of prolactin, growth hormone, or ACTH, but assesses pituitary reserve of the other hormones.[61]

Management. Controversy exists regarding the choice of therapy for pituitary tumors. Alternatives include radiation therapy, pituitary microsurgery, and, if appropriate, prolactin-lowering drugs such as bromocriptine. Ovulation may occur spontaneously following treatment or may have to be induced with clomiphene citrate, gonadotropins, bromocriptine, or a combination of these agents.[62–64]

Bromocriptine (a dopamine-receptor agonist) reduces mitotic activity and inhibits estrogen-induced proliferation of the pituitary, thereby reducing pituitary tumor size.[65] In patients with prolactin-secreting tumors, bromocriptine therapy results in a return of normal menstrual cycles, so pregnancy may occur during treatment. Considerable controversy exists regarding the advisability of pregnancy in these circumstances, because it may stimulate growth of the tumor. Although continuing bromocriptine therapy remains controversial, it has been used throughout pregnancy without adverse fetal effects and without maternal complications resulting from pituitary enlargement.[66–71] In spite of this, current opinion favors surgical intervention as the primary treatment for tumors diagnosed before pregnancy. When conception occurs before removal of the tumor, close monitoring includes regular evaluation of visual fields, roentgen assessment of sella turcica size, and serial prolactin determinations. Symptoms that recur early in pregnancy or progress rapidly call for surgical intervention or bromocriptine therapy.[70,71]

Anesthesia. The apprehensive patient may require premedication before pituitary surgery. Choice of anesthetic agent for induction and maintenance depends upon the patient's general condition and stage of gestation (see Chapter 27). With extremely large tumors, increased intracranial pressure must be avoided during induction. Use of the semisitting position and the likelihood of blood loss from the adjacent carotid sinuses make hypotension during anesthesia the greatest risk to the fetus. Emergence from anesthesia should be smooth, without straining or bucking on the endotracheal tube. Postoperative care includes careful neurologic evaluation and close monitoring of urinary output to detect the development of diabetes insipidus.[72]

For labor and delivery, continuous epidural anesthesia is recommended to avoid excessive straining. For cesarean section no contraindications exist to either regional or general anesthesia, provided tumor size is controlled and there is no intracranial hypertension.

The acromegalic patient presents special problems to the anesthesiologist. Prior to delivery, the patient's diabetic and cardiovascular status must be assessed and appropriate preoperative therapy instituted. Enlargement of the mandible, tongue, and other soft tissues can make establishing an airway difficult. Although regional anesthesia may be technically difficult, it is not contraindicated and avoids the possibility of airway obstruction with general anesthesia.

HYPOPITUITARISM

Panhypopituitarism, or Sheehan's syndrome, can result from necrosis of the pituitary gland following shock or hemorrhage during delivery. Pituitary hypofunction also may follow surgical removal or irradiation of the pituitary, or compression of functioning tissue by tumor. Hypopituitarism usually develops insidiously and frequently goes unrecognized until periods of stress, when it becomes symptomatic or life threatening. The clinical picture depends on the extent of pituitary damage and results from a deficiency of hormones secreted by the adrenal cortex, thyroid, and ovaries. In the postpartum period, failure to lactate with breast involution, may be the earliest sign. Sheehan's syndrome is best avoided by preventing shock and treating hemorrhage effectively at the time of delivery. Panhypopituitarism mandates replacement therapy with varying combinations of hormones (ACTH, TSH, etc.). The major anesthetic problems associated with this disease are considered under Addison's disease and myxedema.

Thyroid Gland

The significant changes that occur in the thyroid during normal pregnancy confuse the clinical presentation of thyroid disease and complicate the interpretation of thyroid function. As it is one of the commoner endocrine diseases occurring in pregnancy, thyroid disease is considered here in detail.

BIOSYNTHESIS OF THYROID HORMONES

Thyroid hormone is synthesized via a complex sequence of reactions (Fig. 13–5). Inorganic iodine, supplied by a normal dietary intake of approximately 150 to 300 μg per day, appears in the plasma in the ionic form as iodine and is then either taken up by the thyroid gland or excreted by the kidneys. The first step in hormonal synthesis involves trapping of iodide from the serum and storing it in the acinar cells of the thyroid gland. This active process works against a normal thyroid-serum iodide concentration gradient of about 20 to 1; in hyperthyroidism it can be as high as 500 to 1. Activity of this trapping mechanism depends on stimulation by pituitary thyrotropin (TSH) as well as the level of stored intrathyroidal iodide. Following oxidation the trapped iodide combines with tyrosine (which is bound to thyroglobulin) to form monoiodotyrosine (MIT) or di-iodotyrosine (DIT). This step is called *binding*. Coupling of two molecules of DIT then takes place to form tetraiodothyronine (thyroxin); one molecule of MIT condenses with one molecule of DIT to form tri-iodothyronine.

Thyroxin (T_4) and tri-iodothyronine (T_3), the physiologically active thyroid hormones, are stored in the acinar colloid. A negative feedback mechanism acting via the hypothalamic-pituitary axis regulates secretion. Decreasing serum levels of free thyroxin and tri-iodothyronine stimulate the release of thyrotropin-releasing hormone (TRH) from the hypothalamus, which in turn causes the release of TSH from the pituitary. This causes proteolytic hydrolysis of thyroglobin and the release of free thyroid hormones into the circulation where plasma thyroxin-binding globulin (TBG) and thyroxin-binding prealbumin bind them.[73]

THYROID FUNCTION IN PREGNANCY

Maternal Thyroid Function

Alterations in thyroid function occur during pregnancy secondary to a number of physiologic changes. The normal pregnant woman remains euthyroid, although thyroid-binding globulin, protein-bound iodine, radioactive iodine uptake, renal clearance of iodine, and the size of the thyroid gland all increase.[73,74] The usual 20 percent increase in basal metabolic rate (BMR) during gestation results predominantly from increased demands of the fetal-maternal unit and an increase in cardiorespiratory work and not from a change in thyroid status.[75] Levels of TSH rise early in pregnancy, returning to normal at term.[76] In addition, the TSH response to TRH increases.[74]

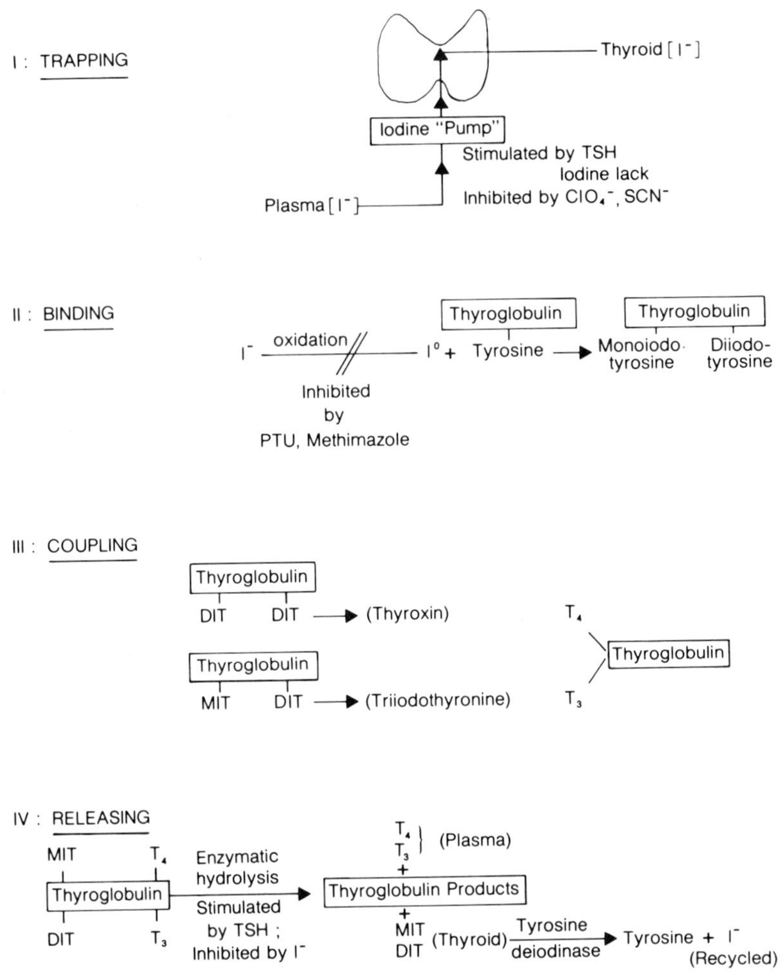

Figure 13–5. Four stages of thyroid hormone synthesis.

Ectopic Thyrotropins. These are produced during pregnancy and in various pathologic conditions. Human chorionic thyrotropin, present in normal trophoblastic tissue, and human chorionic gonadotropin (HCG) have hormonal actions and physicochemical properties similar to those of pituitary TSH. These hormones may cause the increased thyroid stimulating activity observed throughout pregnancy.[4,77,78] In molar pregnancies a thyrotropin of trophoblastic origin probably produces the hypermetabolic state commonly observed.[79]

Thyroid Function Tests in Normal Pregnancy. Thyroid-binding globulin doubles during the first trimester in response to estrogen stimulation of hepatic protein synthesis. This leads to an increase in total serum T_4 and T_3, but the active unbound fraction remains unchanged.[80] Thus, the increase in hormone-binding capacity accounts for the increases in T_4 and T_3 found in pregnancy. The thyroxin-binding capacity can be obtained by the resin tri-iodothyronine uptake (RT_3U) test, which quantitates the unoccupied sites on TBG. As the latter increase during pregnancy, excess sites are available for T_3 and T_4. When labeled T_3 is added to maternal plasma, the excess sites are filled and little T_3 remains to be picked up by the resin, resulting in a low T_3 resin uptake value. However, as levels of T_4 increase during pregnancy, the free thyroxin index (FTI), which is the product of the T_3 resin uptake and T_4 (i.e., $RT_3U \times T_4$), remains in the normal range. An elevated serum thyroxin level, an RT_3U in the hypothyroid range, and an FTI within normal limits are normal laboratory findings during pregnancy.[76]

Fetal Thyroid Function

The fetal thyroid begins to secrete hormones in response to TSH at about 11 to 14 weeks of gestation, suggesting autonomous function of the fetal hypothalamic-pituitary axis.[81] Between 18 and 22 weeks of gestation an abrupt increase in fetal TSH and free T_4 suggests rapid maturation of the system at this time. At term, fetal free T_4 concentration may exceed maternal values.

Placental Transfer

The placenta is relatively impermeable to thyroid hormone, although T_3 crosses more readily than T_4. This may be related to the lesser affinity of T_3 for TBG and the consequent increase in available T_3 for transfer.[82] Long-acting thyroid stimulator (LATS), found in patients with Graves' disease, readily crosses the placenta and can result in neonatal thyrotoxicosis. It is possible to predict this condition antenatally when maternal serum LATS concentrations approach critical levels.[83]

DISEASES OF THE THYROID GLAND

Nontoxic Goiter

A simple nontoxic goiter can increase in size during pregnancy as a result of a relative iodine deficiency. This type of goiter usually remains asymptomatic unless enlargement results in pressure symptoms such as dyspnea, dysphagia, or changes in phonation. All women should receive supplemental iodine throughout pregnancy, particularly if they live in areas endemic for goiter or if they have had goiter in previous pregnancies. Using iodized salt (1 part per 40,000) in cooking and on food easily accomplishes this.

Problems with anesthesia arise only if the gland enlarges significantly or extends retrosternally. The possible development of airway obstruction during general anesthesia makes regional anesthesia preferable for vaginal or abdominal delivery.

Hyperthyroidism

Maternal hyperthyroidism occurs in about 0.2 percent of pregnancies.[73] Pregnancy does not appear to render hyperthyroidism more difficult to control. Mild forms of the disease usually remain stable during gestation and have little effect on maternal or fetal status, although the incidence of low birth weight is higher.[73] In parturients with severe uncontrolled hyperthyrodism, abortion, premature delivery, and abruptio placentae take place with increased frequency. Thyroid storm represents another potential hazard. Graves' disease (diffuse toxic goiter) ranks as the most frequent cause of thyrotoxicosis during pregnancy, whereas Plummer's disease (toxic nodular goiter) occurs less often during child-bearing years. Other causes of hyperthyroidism include toxic multinodular goiter, solitary active nodules, hydatidiform moles, choriocarcinoma, and other diseases associated with ectopic sources of TSH or thyroid hormones.

Diagnosis. The euthyroid parturient may exhibit the classic features of hyperthyroidism, making thyrotoxicosis difficult to diagnose during pregnancy. These features include amenorrhea, tachycardia, systolic flow murmurs, increased cardiac output, increased skin temperature, and heat intolerance. In addition, the weight gain produced by pregnancy may conceal the weight loss usually associated with hyperthyrodism. A resting pulse above 100 beats per minute is a useful diagnostic aid. Pretibial myxedema and ocular signs such as stare, lid lag, and exophthalmos can occur in patients with Graves' disease, even when they are euthyroid. The previously mentioned alterations in thyroid function tests during pregnancy complicate the laboratory diagnosis of hyperthyroidism. However, a serum total T_4 greater than 15 μg per dl or a serum T_3 greater than 220 ng per dl suggests thyrotoxicosis. A normal resin T_3 uptake with an elevated free T_4 or T_3 index is almost diagnostic of the disorder.[84] TSH levels, measured by radioimmunoassay, should be in the normal nonpregnant range. Pregnancy contraindicates other tests of thyroid function such as radioactive iodine uptake and radionucleotide thyroid imaging. Thyroid ultrasonography offers a safe alternative for noninvasive imaging.

Management. Controversy exists regarding the optimal management of thyrotoxicosis during pregnancy. Radioactive iodine therapy has no place in the treatment of the pregnant patient. The decision as to whether treatment should be medical or surgical depends on the physician's judgment and the condition of the patient.

Medical Management. The thiourea compounds, propylthiouracil (PTU) and methimazole (MMI), inhibit the synthesis of thyroid hormone by blocking iodination of the tyrosine molecule. PTU is preferable to MMI because the latter has greater transplacental passage and has been associated with scalp defects in the offspring.[85–87] The usual therapy for hyperthyroidism consists of PTU, 100 to 150 mg every 8 hours. Much larger doses may be necessary to control severe thyrotoxicosis, but once control has been established, dosage should be tapered downward according to maternal T_4 levels.[86] The most common maternal complications of thiourea therapy include purpuric skin rashes, pruritus, drug fever, and nausea. Agranulocytosis occasionally develops and necessitates discontinuing therapy immediately. PTU and MMI dosage should be minimized, as these drugs readily cross the placenta and can produce hypothyroidism and fetal goiter (due to a secondary increase in fetal TSH).[88] Momotami and coworkers[89] recently suggested that monitoring of maternal free T_4 and thyrotropin-inhibiting immunoglobulin should help to optimize neonatal thyroid status. Maintenance of maternal T_4 levels at or just below the thyrotoxic range should minimize the risk of neonatal hypothyroidism.[89] Although several anecdotal reports of goiter, cretinism, and mental retardation following maternal PTU therapy exist, Burrow[90] found the intellectual and physical development of children exposed in utero to PTU to resemble those of nonexposed children.

Propranolol (or a similar β-adrenergic blocker) can also be employed to antagonize the symptoms resulting from increased catecholamine release.[91] Although these agents relieve tachycardia, palpitations, arrhythmias, tremor, restlessness, sweating, and heat intolerance, they do not modify thyroid function. Propranolol proves particularly useful for the rapid control of severe symptoms, allowing thorough diagnostic evaluation in the absence of antithyroid drugs. The controversy regarding the use of beta blockers in pregnancy has been discussed earlier in this chapter.[48]

Surgical Management. Before initiating surgical treatment attempt to optimally control hyperthyroidism with conventional medical therapy. A short preoperative course (10 to 14 days) of iodine enhances the ease of surgical excision by reducing the vascularity of the gland and decreasing thyroid hormone release. Pregnancy mandates cautious administration of iodide, which can produce severe obstructive goiter in the fetus. When possible, surgery should be delayed until the second trimester to avoid the period of maximum organogenesis. The incidence of fetal wastage later in gestation is similar following both medical and surgical therapy. However, if maternal hypothyroidism follows surgery, it results in an increased incidence of fetal loss.[92] Additional risks of thyroid surgery include recurrent laryngeal nerve injury, hypoparathyroidism, and postoperative thyroid storm. In view of these complications and given the relative safety of treatment with PTU, medical therapy would seem preferable.[93]

Anesthetic Management. Ideally, appropriate medical therapy establishes a euthyroid state prior to anesthesia for either thyroid surgery or delivery. However, if emergency surgery becomes necessary in the unprepared patient, the anesthesiologist must avoid situations that exacerbate the disease. The severely hyperthyroid patient requires adequate preoperative sedation (e.g., with a short-acting benzodiazepine such as midazolam), since apprehension will worsen symptomatology by increasing catecholamine release. The thiobarbiturates (thiopental, thiamylal) possess antithyroid activity related to their thiocarbamate structure, and thus may be particularly advantageous for induction of anesthesia.[94] Anticholinergics are contraindicated as they may increase tachycardia and inhibit heat loss.

All patients must be carefully monitored with particular attention to the ECG and temperature. A cooling blanket, refrigerated intravenous solutions, and ice should be readily accessible to treat intraoperative and postoperative hyperthermia. Emergency drugs should include steroids, iodine, hypotensive agents, and propranolol.

For vaginal or cesarean delivery, regional anesthesia supplemented by intravenous sedation is preferred because it attenuates release of catecholamines by the adrenal medulla.[95] If general anesthesia becomes necessary, a technique employing thiopental, nitrous oxide, a relaxant, and a low concentration of a volatile agent can be utilized. Neither general nor regional anesthesia influences the serum thyrotropin level.[96] For subtotal thyroidectomy, general anesthesia is preferable to ensure control of the airway, which already may be compromised by pressure from a very large gland or a retrosternal extension. Almost any combination of anesthetic agents and muscle relaxants can be used, provided the anesthesiologist avoids exacerbating pre-existing symptoms.

In poorly controlled patients, several problems must be anticipated. Cardiac work increases markedly as a result of increased stroke volume, tachycardia, and systolic hypertension; cardiac decompensation and arrhythmias can occur. Surgical manipulation around the carotid sinus can cause hypotension and bradycardia, which can be minimized by infiltration with a local anesthetic to block the carotid sinus reflex. As both normal pregnancy and hyperthyroidism increase oxygen consumption, the use of a pulse oximeter (or frequent arterial blood gas analyses) should help to ensure adequate oxygenation.

The potential for life-threatening complications mandates careful monitoring in the recovery room. The risk of postoperative hematoma, tracheomalacia, or laryngeal edema heighten the possibility of respiratory obstruction. Bilateral recurrent laryngeal nerve injury can necessitate tracheostomy, and sensory loss to the larynx and pyriform sinus resulting from superior laryngeal nerve damage makes aspiration a particular hazard in the parturient. Injury or removal of the parathyroid glands during thyroidectomy can result in hypoparathyroidism. Since the intrinsic laryngeal muscles are extremely sensitive to calcium deficiency, inspiratory stridor may occur before the onset of tetany. Intranveous calcium will ablate all manifestations of hypoparathyroidism.

Thyroid Storm. This term refers to thyrotoxicosis when severe signs and symptoms arise acutely. It occurs most often in untreated or partially treated patients subjected to stress and can be precipitated by labor, infection, ketoacidosis, trauma, or thyroidectomy.[86] Characteristic features include severe tachycardia, atrial fibrillation, hyperpyrexia, and cardiovascular collapse. The high mortality rate associated with untreated or inadequately treated cases makes immediate, aggressive therapy essential.[97] Treatment includes large doses of antithyroid drugs (PTU, 150 to 200 mg every 6 hr) to block further thyroid hormone synthesis; iodine to suppress secretion of stored hormone; intravenous sedation; large doses of intravenous steroids to block the conversion of T_4 to T_3; and β-adrenergic blocking agents.[98,99] Propranolol significantly decreases mortality in this condition. The rapid onset and short duration of action of esmolol may make it ideal for control of the hemodynamic instability associated with thyroid storm. However, it has yet to be evaluated for use in pregnancy. Plasma exchange has also been recommended in severe cases of thyroid storm as an adjunct to the treatment described.[100-102] Other supportive measures include administration of a high inspired oxygen concentration, lowering of body temperature, adequate intravenous hydration, caloric replacement, and antibiotics.

Neonatal Effects. Patients with hyperthyroidism can produce offspring with hyperthyroidism, hypothyroidism, or large goiters. Transplacental passage of LATS from mothers with Graves' disease probably causes neonatal hyperthyroidism.[86] However, the infant metabolizes LATS readily and the problem often remits quickly. Maternally administered antithyroid drugs which cross the placenta and suppress fetal thyroid activity can delay the presentation of neonatal hyperthyroidism. Hypothyroidism (cretinism) occasionally occurs following treatment with PTU, although a direct causal relationship is not well substantiated. The low incidence of cretinism and goiter observed after PTU therapy probably results from sufficient placental transfer of thyroid hormone. This also accounts for the small size of goiters attributable to PTU. In contrast, the much larger goiters induced by iodine therapy, maternal hypothyroidism or hyperthyroidism can produce hyperextension of the fetal head resulting in malpresentation, difficult vaginal delivery, and neonatal respiratory obstruction.

Thyroid Tumors

Pregnancy does not affect the course of thyroid carcinoma, nor does the tumor affect the pregnancy.[103] The diagnosis of thyroid carcinoma does not indicate termination of pregnancy, although radioactive iodine therapy should be withheld until after delivery. Patients with carcinoma are usually euthyroid, but may complain of dyspnea and dysphagia from pressure on the trachea and esophagus.

Hashimoto's Disease

This rarely occurs during pregnancy, although a variant called *chronic lymphocytic thyroiditis* may develop in the postpartum period.

Hypothyroidism (Myxedema)

The rare occurrence of hypothyroidism during pregnancy was previously attributed to reduced fertility. However, current thought incriminates the high incidence of spontaneous abortion among hypothyroid women. Mild to moderate hypothyroidism has little effect on fertility, and uncomplicated term pregnancies have been reported even in untreated patients.[104,105] Hypothyroidism is most commonly iatrogenic, following either thyroid surgery or radioiodine therapy. Less common causes include Hashimoto's disease, hereditary biosynthetic defects, and anterior pituitary insufficiency. During pregnancy, subclinical hypothyroidism may be unmasked by the increased requirements for thyroid function.

Clinical Features. The clinical diagnosis of hypothyroidism is more easily missed during pregnancy as the classic symptoms of constipation, cold intolerance, cool dry skin, coarse hair, periorbital edema, hoarseness, and decreased mental concentration can occur in normal pregnant women. The parturient may present complaining only of more severe fatigue, drier skin, and coarser hair than in previous pregnancies. Careful physical examination (looking for delayed deep tendon reflexes) and noticeable change of voice offer the best chance for diagnosis. Cardiomegaly and, occasionally, congestive heart failure can occur. The ECG shows bradycardia and generalized low-voltage complexes. Pleural and pericardial effusions develop commonly, as do mild anemia and hypercholesterolemia.

A serum T_4 level lower than that expected in pregnancy confirms the diagnosis. Since pregnancy itself results in an increase in unsaturated thyroxin-binding sites, the RT_3U test proves unhelpful. An elevated TSH level is present in primary hypothyroidism, and thyroid antibodies may be helpful in diagnosing Hashimoto's thyroiditis.

Management. Thyroid hormone replacement must be instituted immediately to decrease the possibility of spontaneous abortion, intrauterine death, and the mental and physical abnormalities seen in the offspring of untreated myxedematous mothers.[106,107] Levothyroxine (Synthroid) administered orally produces relatively rapid results and need be given only once daily because of its long half-life. If more rapid control is necessary, administer T_3 intravenously, as its peak effect occurs within hours. This agent must be used cautiously, however, since very rapid administration can cause angina, atrial fibrillation, cardiac failure, ventricular tachycardia, and cardiac arrest.

Anesthesia. The untreated myxedematous parturient may require anesthesia for emergency surgery or delivery. As with hyperthyroidism, complications can occur both intraoperatively and postoperatively.[108] Because cardiac output and cardiac reserve decrease, even minor cardiovascular stress can precipitate congestive failure. Although sodium and water sequester in the interstitial space and result in hyponatremia, particular care must be taken with sodium replacement to prevent fluid overload. These patients tolerate blood loss poorly, yet rapid transfusion may overload an already compromised heart. Pulmonary edema should be suspected if pulmonary compliance and oxygen saturation decrease intraoperatively. Hypotension often resists vasopressors, and the large doses of these agents required for blood pressure control can cause ventricular tachycardia and fibrillation.

Narcotics, sedatives, and tranquilizers cause respiratory depression more readily in myxedematous patients. Ventilation during general anesthesia should be controlled, remembering that increased intrathoracic pressure may further embarrass cardiac output.

Hypothermia presents a particular hazard in myxedema, and further decreases in temperature should be prevented to avoid precipitating coma. Simple methods such as warming intravenous fluids, gas humidification, a heated water mattress, and elevating ambient temperature usually prove adequate. The possibility of local burns or cardiovascular collapse makes vigorous, active rewarming dangerous. Acute adrenocortical insufficiency causes cardiovascular collapse and requires intravenous steroid therapy. As hypoglycemia can develop during treatment with thyroid hormone, blood glucose levels should be measured regularly and treated accordingly.

The increased sensitivity of myxedematous patients to intravenous and inhalation agents makes regional anesthesia preferable for labor and delivery. During epidural or spinal anesthesia, special care must be taken to avoid hypotension by the use of preanesthetic hydration, judicious doses of local anesthetics, and maintenance of a lateral tilt position. The prolonged circulation time caused by low cardiac output can slow the induction of general anesthesia with intravenous agents. This should not be considered an indication to administer higher doses, but rather to proceed more slowly with anesthesia. In contrast, induction of anesthesia with inhalation agents occurs more rapidly because of the decreased cardiac output. Myxedema does not significantly decrease minimum alveolar concentration (MAC).[109] Elimination of fixed agents can be delayed, and those with long half-lives such as morphine and diazepam probably are best avoided. Doses of both intravenous and inhalation agents should be kept to a minimum. Although muscle relaxants are not contraindicated, reduced dosage and careful monitoring with a nerve stimulator are recommended.

During the postoperative period, patients must be observed closely with respect to temperature and the adequacy of ventilation. Recovery from anesthesia often occurs slowly compared with that of euthyroid patients.

Parathyroid Gland

The interaction of parathyroid hormones, vitamin D, and calcitonin regulates calcium metabolism. A decrease in serum calcium concentration causes the release of parathyroid hormone, which increases calcium levels by stimulating bone resorption and increasing both intestinal and renal tubular reabsorption of calcium. Phosphate reabsorption decreases concurrently, resulting in increased urinary phosphate clearance. Vitamin D also increases intestinal absorption of calcium and facilitates the action of parathyroid hormone on bone, and perhaps kidney. Calcitonin, a polypeptide produced in the follicular cells of the thyroid, antagonizes the effect of parathyroid hormone on bone, thus decreasing serum calcium levels.

Serum calcium levels (normally, 9.0 to 10.5 mg per dl) are of major importance in evaluating parathyroid function. Plasma proteins, predominantly albumin, bind approximately 40 percent of the serum calcium. Only the ionized or unbound calcium has metabolic activity. Although total serum calcium decreases with a fall in serum albumin, the ionized fraction remains unchanged. Dietary variation or impairment of renal function renders urinary excretion of calcium unhelpful diagnostically. Although serum phosphate levels also vary considerably with diet, age, and hormonal status, measurement of tubular resorption of phosphate (TRP) can be used in evaluating parathyroid function.[1] Radioimmunoassay of parathyroid hormone provides a useful means for diagnosing pathologic parathyroid states.

PARATHYROID FUNCTION DURING PREGNANCY

Although pregnancy increases calcium requirements, a regular diet usually maintains adequate calcium balance. Total serum calcium concentration begins to decrease at the end of the first trimester (before fetal calcium needs are great) and does so progressively until 28 to 32 weeks. This has been attributed to the hypoalbuminemia of pregnancy, transfer of calcium to the fetus, and increased urinary excretion of calcium as a result of increased glomerular filtration. However, *ionized* calcium values and TRP usually remain unchanged.[1] Parathyroid gland hyperplasia and increased hormone secretion occur during pregnancy, perhaps in an attempt to maintain normal levels of ionized calcium.[110,111]

HYPERPARATHYROIDISM

Benign adenomas, hyperplasia, and carcinomas cause primary hyperparathyroidism. Secondary hyperparathyroidism occurs in conditions in which serum calcium falls, consequently stimulating parathyroid hormone secretion. Females develop hyperparathyroidism more commonly than males, with the disease presenting most frequently between the ages of 20 and 40. Hyperparathyroidism can jeopardize the fetus, yet the mother may remain asymptomatic and undiagnosed.[112] The incidence of spontaneous abortion, stillbirth, premature labor, and neonatal tetany increases, resulting in high neonatal morbidity and mortality.[113] Calcium crosses the placenta by active transport, and high maternal serum calcium levels can suppress fetal parathyroid maturation. A decrease in amniotic fluid parathyroid hormone levels reflects this.[114] Parathyroid hormone does not cross the placenta in significant amounts because of its high molecular weight. In infants born of hyperparathyroid mothers, serum calcium levels fall rapidly in the first few days of life because of the hypofunctioning neonatal parathyroid glands. Calcium levels remain low, resulting in neonatal tetany. Since nonspecific maternal symptoms during pregnancy can mask hyperparathyroidism, the occurrence of neonatal tetany may reveal this diagnosis retrospectively.[115]

Pathophysiology. In pregnancy, a parathyroid adenoma most often causes hyperparathyroidism.[116] Excessive parathyroid secretion results in increases in bone resorption, gastrointestinal absorption of calcium, and renal tubular excretion of phosphate. This produces hypercalcemia, hypercalciuria, phosphaturia, and hypophosphatemia. These changes may eventually produce renal calculi and nephrocalcinosis, leading to a loss of renal concentrating ability. In association with an increased osmotic load, this causes the polyuria and polydipsia typical of this disease. The effect of parathyroid hormone on bone can lead to thinning of bony trabeculae, fractures, and eventually osteitis fibrosa cystica.[1] Hypercalcemia enhances myocardial excitability, resulting in an increased risk of ventricular fibrillation. A shortening of the QT interval, which varies inversely with the serum calcium level, characterizes the ECG. In extreme cases it may be so shortened that the ST segment completely disappears. As hypercalcemia results in an increased release of acetylcholine, a larger dose of muscle relaxant may be required.[117,118]

Clinical Features. Symptoms associated with hypercalcemia include anorexia, nausea, vomiting, lethargy, polyuria, polydipsia, and constipation. In mild cases these can be mistaken for symptoms of normal pregnancy. When serum calcium reaches extremely high levels, hypercalcemic crises occur which are characterized by mental deterioration or coma, renal failure, arrhythmias, and congestive cardiac failure. Other causes of hypercalcemia should be excluded such as neoplastic disease, multiple myeloma, sarcoidosis, milk-alkali syndrome, vitamin D intoxication, thiazide therapy, and hyperthyroidism.

Because of the decrease in serum calcium that occurs in pregnancy, calcium levels may be misleadingly normal in the parturient with hyperparathyroidism. As diagnosis and early treatment result in a significant decrease in maternal and fetal morbidity, serum calcium levels ideally should be determined in every pregnant woman. Normocalcemic hyperparathyroidism should be suspected in the presence of any of the clinical features suggestive of the disease such as repeated abortion, premature labor, and, particularly, neonatal tetany.

Management. Surgical removal of hyperfunctioning tissue represents the treatment of choice to avoid fetal and maternal complications.[119] However, great interpatient variability exists in this condition, and in many cases both mother and fetus readily tolerate the disease. Patients with mild disease initially should be treated conservatively, while those who are symptomatic or who have serum calcium levels greater than 11 mg per dl probably should be treated surgically (ideally in the second trimester). Following removal of the lesion, calculus formation decreases, bone healing occurs, and progression of renal disease usually is halted. The rates of stillbirth and premature labor also should decrease. Regardless of maternal management, the neonate must be carefully observed for signs of tetany. Only selected circumstances, such as advanced renal insufficiency, call for termination of pregnancy.

Anesthesia. Adequate hydration and electrolyte balance should be ensured preoperatively. An attempt should be made to lower serum calcium either by decreasing absorption or by increasing excretion. A low-calcium diet, diuretics, intravenous phosphate, and corticosteroid administration can be employed.

Anesthesia for Parathyroidectomy. No particular anesthetic agent or technique offers special advantages. Patients should be monitored for cardiac arrhythmias, and preparations made to treat hypotension and bradycardia resulting from carotid sinus manipulation. Possible surgical complications include pneumomediastinum, pneumothorax, and postoperative hypoparathyroidism. The first symptoms of hypocalcemia (which are usually transient unless all parathyroid tissue has been removed) include increased neuromuscular irritability and circumoral or extremity paresthesias. Prompt treatment with intravenous calcium chloride prevents the development of generalized convulsions or laryngeal stridor.

Anesthesia for Delivery. In the adequately prepared patient, no specific problems exist and continuous regional anesthesia represents a safe technique for vaginal or cesarean delivery. As hypercalcemia may enhance the effects of local anesthetics,[120] low concentrations of these agents are preferable. If general anesthesia is indicated, a routine technique can be employed.

HYPOPARATHYROIDISM

Hypoparathyroidism rarely occurs during pregnancy, and most often results from damage or removal of the parathyroid glands during thyroid surgery.[121] Idiopathic hypoparathyroidism is extremely rare and occurs mainly in children. Parathyroid hormone deficiency decreases serum and urinary calcium levels and urinary phosphorus excretion, resulting in an elevated serum phosphorus. Neuromuscular irritability increases in proportion to the degree of hypocalcemia, and in extreme cases tetany will occur. In the untreated mother symptoms may be exaggerated because of fetal calcium demands. Alkalosis due to hyperventilation, vomiting, massive transfusion of citrated blood, or uremia can decrease the ionized calcium fraction and should be excluded before considering a diagnosis of hypoparathyroidism.

Clinical Features. Symptoms vary from fatigue, muscle weakness, numbness, and paresthesias to frank tetany with carpopedal spasms, tonic and clonic convulsions, and laryngeal stridor (which can be fatal). Increased neuromuscular irritability can be demonstrated clinically by Chvostek's sign (stimulation of the facial nerve anterior to the ear) and Trousseau's sign (the production of carpopedal spasm by occlusion of the circulation to the arm). Other signs include dry, rough skin, patchy hair distribution, frequent skin infections, cataracts, and mental changes. The ECG shows a prolonged QT interval due to a lengthened ST segment. Myocardial contractility and cardiac output often decrease as calcium normally exerts a positive inotropic effect.

Management. The main objective in treatment is to ensure an adequate supply of calcium by a combination of dietary and drug therapy. The ingestion of aluminum hydroxide gel helps to decrease absorption of dietary phosphate, thereby increasing calcium absorption; vitamin D also increases calcium absorption. In an emergency, slowly administer intravenous calcium chloride or gluconate in the presence of ECG monitoring. Parathyroid hormone has not proven to be a satisfactory therapeutic agent because of its slow onset of action and the alarming frequency with which hypersensitivity occurs.

Anesthesia. Labor and delivery increase the likelihood of tetany because accompanying hyperventilation results in respiratory alkalosis and a decrease in ionized calcium fraction. Continuous epidural anesthesia most effectively prevents hyperventilation, making it the preferred method of pain relief in this condition. If general anesthesia is indicated, no special precautions must be taken other than monitoring the electrocardiogram for signs of hypocalcemia and avoiding hyperventilation. Hypocalcemia may enhance the effect of nondepolarizing muscle relaxants and diminish the ability of neostigmine to antagonize blockade.[112]

References

1. Burrow, GN: Pituitary, adrenal and parathyroid disorders. In Burrow, GN and Ferris, TF (eds): Medical Complications During Pregnancy, ed 2. WB Saunders, Philadelphia, 1982, p 215.
2. Black, GW and Montgomery, DAD: Adrenal disease. In Vickers, MD (ed): Medicine for Anaesthetists, ed 2. Blackwell, Oxford, 1982, p 451.
3. Grimes, EM, Fayez, JA and Miller, GL: Cushing's syndrome and pregnancy. Obstet Gynecol 42:550, 1973.
4. Hollingsworth, DR: Endocrine disorders of pregnancy. In Creasy, RK and Resnik, R (eds): Maternal-

Fetal Medicine. WB Saunders, Philadelphia, 1984, p 897.
5. Blumsohn D, et al: Cushing's syndrome and pregnancy: A case report. S Afr Med J 53:338, 1978.
6. Keegan GT, Grabarits, F and Roland, AS: Pregnancy complicated by Cushing's syndrome. South Med J 69:1207, 1976.
7. Koerten, JM, et al: Cushing's syndrome in pregnancy: A case report and literature review. Am J Obstet Gynecol 154:626, 1986.
8. Reschini, E, et al: Spontaneous remission of Cushing's syndrome after termination of pregnancy. Obstet Gynecol 51:598, 1978.
9. Raut, AJ and Brown, EG: Effects of maternal disease on the fetus and neonate. In Cherry SH, Berkoartz, RL and Kase, NG (eds): Rovisky and Guttmacher's Medical, Surgical and Gynecologic Complications of Pregnancy, ed 3. Williams & Wilkins, Baltimore, 1985, p 379.
10. Glassford, J, Eagle, C and McMorland, GH: Cesarean section in a patient with Cushing's syndrome. Canad Anaesth Soc J 31:447, 1984
11. Roizen, MF: Anesthetic implications of concurrent diseases. In Miller, RD (ed): Anesthesia. Churchill Livingstone, New York, p 255, 1986.
12. Plumpton, FS, Besser, GM and Cole, PV: Corticosteroid treatment and surgery. Anaesthesia 24:2, 1969.
13. Symreng, T, et al: Physiological cortisol substitution of long-term steroid-treated patients undergoing major surgery. Br J Anaesth 53:949, 1981.
14. Kehlet, H: Pain relief and modification of the stress response. In Cousins, MJ and Phillips, SD (eds): Acute Pain Management. Churchill Livingstone, New York, 1986, p 49.
15. Crozier, TA, et al: Endocrinological changes following etomidate, midazolam, or methohexital for minor surgery. Anesthesiology 66:628, 1987.
16. Hagen, C, Brandt, MR and Kehlet, H: Prolactin, LH, FSH, GH, and cortisol response to surgery and the effects of epidural analgesia. Acta Endocrinol 94:151, 1980.
17. Vandam, LD and Moore, FD: Adrenocortical mechanisms related to anesthesia. Anesthesiology 21:531, 1960.
18. Christensen, P, et al: Influence of extradural morphine on the adrenocortical and hyperglycemic response to surgery. Br J Anaesth 54:23, 1982.
19. Kumar, D and Barnes, AC: Aldosterone in normal and abnormal pregnancy. Obstet Gynecol Surv 15:625, 1960.
20. Crane, MG, et al: Primary aldosteronism in pregnancy. Obstet Gynecol 23:200, 1964.
21. Griffen, WO, Dilts, PV and Roddick, JW: Non-obstetric surgery during pregnancy. Curr Prob Surg 1:1, 1969.
22. Geelhoed, GW: Surgery of the endocrine glands in pregnancy. Clin Obstet Gynecol 26:865, 1983.
23. Finch, JS: Primary aldosteronism: Review of the anaesthetic experience in sixty patients. Br J Anaesth 41:880, 1969.
24. Miklovic, K, et al: Maintenance of the plasma corticosterone concentration of adrenalectomized rat by the fetal adrenal glands. Endocrinology 93:115, 1973.
25. Rumfitt, IW: A case of undiagnosed Addison's disease and successful pregnancy. Practitioner 218:553, 1977.
26. Hunt, AB and McConahey, WM: Pregnancy associated with diseases of the adrenal glands. Am J Obstet Gynecol 66:970, 1953.
27. Maltau, JM, Eielsen, OV and Stokke, KT: Effect of stress during labor on the concentration of cortisol and estriol in maternal plasma. Am J Obstet Gynecol 134:681, 1979.
28. Modlin, IM, et al: Pheochromocytomas in 72 patients: Clinical and diagnostic features, treatment and long-term results. Br J Surg 66:456, 1979.
29. Gifford, RW, et al: Clinical features, diagnosis and treatment of pheochromocytoma: A review of 76 cases. Mayo Clin Proc 39:281, 1964.
30. Melicow, MM: One hundred cases of pheochromocytoma (197 tumors) at the Columbia-Presbyterian Medical Center 1926–1976: A clinicopathological analysis. Cancer 40:1987, 1977.
31. Schenker, JG and Chowers I: Pheochromocytoma and pregnancy: Review of 89 cases. Obstet Gynecol Surv 26:739, 1971.
32. Schenker, JG and Granat, M: Phaeochromocytoma and pregnancy: An updated appraisal. Aust NZ J Obstet Gynaec 22:1, 1982.
33. Cryer, PE: Disease of the adrenal medullae and sympathetic nervous system. In Felig, P, et al (eds): Endocrinology and Metabolism. McGraw-Hill, New York, 1981, p 529.
34. Bravo, EL, et al: Clonidine-suppression test: A useful aid in diagnosis of pheochromocytoma. N Engl J Med 305:623, 1981.
35. Greenberg, M, et al: Extraadrenal pheochromocytoma: Detection during pregnancy using MR imaging. Radiology 161:475, 1986.
36. Smith, AM: Pheochromocytoma and pregnancy. J Obstet Gynaecol Br Commonw 80:848, 1973.
37. Mitchell, SZ, et al: Anesthetic management of pheochromocytoma resection during pregnancy. Anesth Analg 66:478, 1987.
38. Fudge, TL, McKinnon, WMP and Geary, WL: Current surgical management of pheochromocytoma during pregnancy. Arch Surg 115:1224, 1980.
39. Chatterjee, TK and Parekh, U: Phaeochromocytoma in pregnancy. Aust NZ J Obstet Gynaecol 25:290, 1985.
40. Pinaud, M, et al: Bilateral phaeochromocytomas in pregnancy: Anesthetic management of combined caesarean section and tumour removal. Eur J Anaesth 2:395, 1985.
41. Burgess, GE: Alpha blockade and surgical intervention of pheochromocytoma in pregnancy. Obstet Gynecol 53:266, 1979.
42. Burgess, GE, et al: Anesthetic management of combined cesarean section and excision of pheochromocytoma. Anesth Analg 57:276, 1978.
43. Ross, EJ, et al: Preoperative and operative management of patients with pheochromocytoma. Br Med J 1:191, 1967.

44. Desmonts, JM and Marty, J: Anaesthetic management of patients with phaeochromocytoma. Br J Anaesth 56:781, 1984.
45. Cleveland, BR, et al: Pheochromocytoma simulating toxemia of pregnancy. Texas Med J 69:70, 1973.
46. Awitti-Sunga, SA and Ursell, W: Phaeochromocytoma in pregnancy: A case report. Br J Obstet Gynaecol 82:426, 1975.
47. Cooperman, LH, Engelman, K and Mann, PEG: Anesthetic management of pheochromocytoma employing halothane and β-adrenergic blockade. Anesthesiology 28:575, 1967.
48. Rubin, PC: Beta blockers in pregnancy. N Engl J Med 305:1323, 1981.
49. Engelman, K, et al: Biochemical and pharmacological effects of alpha-methyl-tyrosine in man. J Clin Invest 47:577, 1968.
50. Mihm, FG: Pulmonary artery pressure monitoring in patients with pheochromocytoma. Anesth Analg 62:1129, 1983.
51. Cousins, MJ and Rubin, RB: The intraoperative management of pheochromocytoma with total epidural sympathetic blockade. Br J Anaesth 46:78, 1974.
52. Bromage, PR and Millar, RA: Epidural blockade and circulating catecholamine levels in a child with pheochromocytoma. Can Anaesth Soc J 5:282, 1958.
53. Stonham, J and Wakefield, C: Phaeochromocytoma in pregnancy: Caesarean section under epidural analgesia. Anaesthesia 38:654, 1983.
54. Kopriva, CJ and Ellingham, R: The use of enflurane during resection of a pheochromocytoma. Anesthesiology 41:399, 1974.
55. Ortiz, FT and Dias, PM: Use of enflurane for pheochromocytoma removal. Anesthesiology 42:495, 1975.
56. Baker, G, et al: Pheochromocytoma without hypertension presenting as cardiomyopathy. Am Heart J 83:688, 1972.
57. Goluboff, LG and Ezrin, C: Effect of pregnancy on the somatatroph and the prolactin cell of the human adenohypophysis. J Clin Endocrinol Metab 29:1533, 1969.
58. Gemzell, C: Induction of ovulation in infertile women with pituitary tumors. Am J Obstet Gynecol 121:311, 1975.
59. Fujimoto, M, et al. Estrogen receptors in brain tumors. Clin Neuropharmacol 7:357, 1984.
60. Fujimoto, M, et al: Spontaneous reduction in size of prolactin-producing adenoma after delivery. J Neurosurg 63:973, 1985.
61. Zeruas, NT and Martin, JB: Management of hormone secreting pituitary adenomas. N Engl J Med 302:210, 1980.
62. Magyar, DM and Marshall, JR: Pituitary tumors and pregnancy. Am J Obstet Gynecol 132:739, 1978.
63. Radwanska, E, et al: Induction of ovulation in women with hyperprolactinemic amenorrhea using clomiphene and human chorionic gonadotropin or bromocriptine. Fertil Steril 32:187, 1979.
64. Tucker, HS, et al: Galactorrhea-amenorrhea syndrome: Follow-up of forty-five patients after pituitary tumor removal. Ann Intern Med 94:302, 1981.
65. MacLeod, RM and Lehmeyer, JE: Suppression of pituitary tumor growth and function by ergot alkaloids. Can Res 33:489, 1973.
66. Griffith, RW, Turkalj, I and Braun, P: Pituitary tumors during pregnancy in mothers treated with bromocriptine. Br J Clin Pharmacol 7:393, 1979.
67. Reichlin, S: The prolactinoma problem. N Engl J Med 300:313, 1979.
68. Turkalj, I, Braun, P and Knapp, P: Surveillance of bromocriptine in pregnancy. JAMA 247:1589, 1982.
69. Corenblum, B: Successful outcome of ergocryptine induced pregnancies in twenty-one women with prolactin-secreting pituitary adenomas. Fertil Steril 32:183, 1979.
70. Bergh, T, Nillius, SJ and Wide, L: Clinical course and outcome of pregnancies in amenorrhoeic women with hyperprolactinaemia and pituitary tumors. Br Med J 1:875, 1978.
71. Lamberts, SWJ, et al: The incidence of complications during pregnancy after treatment of hyperprolactinemia with bromocriptine in patients with radiological evident pituitary tumors. Fertil Steril 31:614, 1979.
72. Messick, JM, Laws, ER and Abboud, CF: Anesthesia for transphenoidal surgery of the hypophyseal region. Anesth Analg 57:206, 1978.
73. Burrow, GN: Thyroid disease. In Burrow, GN and Ferris, TF (eds): Medical Complications During Pregnancy. WB Saunders, Philadelphia, 1982, p 187.
74. Fisher, DA and Burrow, GN: Perinatal thyroid physiology and disease. Raven Press, New York, 1975.
75. Mussei, RD: Thyroid gland and pregnancy. Am J Obstet Gynecol 36:529, 1938.
76. Malkasian, GD and Mayberry, WE: Serum total and free thyroxine and thyrotropin in normal and pregnant women, neonates and women receiving progestogens. Am J Obstet Gynecol 108:1234, 1971.
77. Hennen, G, Pierce, JG and Freychet, P: Human chorionic thyrotropin: Further characterization and study of its secretion during pregnancy. J Clin Endocrinol Metab 29:581, 1969.
78. Carayon, P, Lefort, G and Nisala, B: Interaction of human chorionic gonadotropin and human lutenizing hormone with human thyroid membranes. Endocrin 106:1907, 1980.
79. Anderson, NR, et al: Gestational choriocarcinoma and thyrotoxicosis. Cancer 44:304, 1979.
80. Dowling, JT, Freinkel, N and Ingbar, SH: The effect of estrogens upon the peripheral metabolism of thyroxine. J Clin Invest 39:1119, 1960.
81. Fisher, DA, et al: Thyroid function in the preterm fetus. Pediatrics 46:208, 1970.
82. Fisher, DA, Lehman, H and Lackey, C: Placental transport of thyroxine. J Clin Endocrinol Metab 24:393, 1964.
83. Dirmikis, SM and Munro, DS: Placental transmission of thyroid-stimulating immunoglobulins. Br Med J 2:665, 1975.
84. Mestman, JH: Thyroid disease in pregnancy. Clinics Perinatol 12:3, 1985.

85. Marchant, B, et al: The placental transfer of propylthiouracil, methimazole, and carbimazole. J Clin Endocrinol Metab 45:1187, 1977.
86. Burrow, GN: The management of thyrotoxicosis in pregnancy. N Engl J Med 313:562, 1985.
87. Milham, S and Elledge, W: Maternal methimazole and congenital defects in children. Teratology 5:125, 1972.
88. Mujtaba, O and Burrow, GN: Treatment of hyperthyroidism in pregnancy with propylthiouracil and methimazole. Obstet Gynecol 46:282, 1975.
89. Momotani, N, et al: Antithyroid drug therapy for Graves disease during pregnancy: Optimal regimen for fetal thyroid status. N Engl J Med 315:24, 1986.
90. Burrow, GN, et al: Children exposed in utero to propylthiouracil. Am J Dis Child 116:161, 1968.
91. Langer, A, et al: Adrenergic blockade: A new approach to hyperthyroidism during pregnancy. Obstet Gynecol 44:181, 1974.
92. Talbert, LM, et al: Hyperthyroidism during pregnancy. Obstet Gynecol 36:779, 1970.
93. Worley, RJ and Crosby, WM: Hyperthyroidism during pregnancy. Am J Obstet Gynecol 119:150, 1974.
94. Wase, AW and Foster, WC: Thiopental and thyroid metabolism. Proc Soc Exp Bio Med 91:89, 1956.
95. Pflug, AE and Halter, JB: Effect of spinal anesthesia on adrenergic tone and neuroendocrine response to surgical stress in humans. Anesthesiology 55:120, 1981.
96. Halevy, S, et al: Serum thyroid hormone changes in patients undergoing caesarean section under general or regional anesthesia. Br J Anaesth 50:1053, 1978.
97. Selenkow, HA and Hollander, CS: Physiologic, pharmacologic and therapeutic considerations in surgery for hyperthyroidism. Anesthesiology 24:425, 1963.
98. Stehling, LC: Anesthetic management of the patient with hyperthyroidism. Anesthesiology 41:585, 1974.
99. Ingbar, SH: Management of emergencies: Thyrotoxic storm. N Engl J Med 274:1252, 1966.
100. Derksen, RHWM, et al: Plasma-exchange in the treatment of severe thyrotoxicosis in pregnancy. Europ J Obstet Gynec Reprod Biol 18:139, 1984.
101. Ashkar, FS, et al: Thyroid storm treatment with blood exchange and plasmapheresis. JAMA 214:1275, 1970.
102. Haire, W, Newcomer, J and Hartman, C: Plasmapheresis in the management of thyroid storm. Plasma Ther 2:3, 1981.
103. Rosvoll, RV and Winship, T: Thyroid carcinoma and pregnancy. Surg Gynecol Obstet 121:1039, 1965.
104. Echt, CR and Doss, JF: Myxedema in pregnancy: Report of 3 cases. Obstet Gynecol 22:615, 1963.
105. Kennedy, AL and Montgomery, DAD: Hypothyroidism in pregnancy. Br J Obstet Gynaecol 85:225, 1978.
106. Jones, WS and Man, EB: Thyroid function in human pregnancy. Am J Obstet Gynecol 104:909, 1969.
107. Greenman, GW, et al: Thyroid dysfunction in pregnancy: Fetal loss and follow-up evaluation of surviving infants. N Engl J Med 267:426, 1962.
108. Abbott, TR: Anaesthesia in untreated myxoedema. Br J Anaesth 39:510, 1967.
109. Eger, EI: Anesthetic uptake and distribution. Williams & Wilkins, Baltimore, 1974.
110. Pitkin, RM, et al: Calcium metabolism in human pregnancy. Am J Obstet Gynecol 133:781, 1979.
111. Cushard, WG, et al: Physiologic hyperparathyroidism in pregnancy. J Clin Endocrinol Metab 34:767, 1972.
112. Wagner, G, Transbol, I and Melchior, JC: Hyperparathyroidism and pregnancy. Acta Endocrinol 47:549, 1964.
113. Johnstone, RE II, Kreindler, T and Johnstone, RE: Hyperparathyroidism during pregnancy. Obstet Gynecol 40:580, 1972.
114. Dorey, LG and Gell, JM: Primary hyperparathyroidism during the third trimester of pregnancy. Obstet Gynecol 45:469, 1975.
115. Rosenthal, T, et al: A case of maternal hyperparathyroidism presenting as neonatal tetany. Israel J Med Sci 11:30, 1975.
116. Rossi, RL, ReMine, SG and Clerkin, EP: Hyperparathyroidism. Surg Clin North Am 65:187, 1985.
117. Hutter, OF and Kostial, K: Effect of magnesium and calcium ions on release of acetylcholine. J Physiol 124:234, 1954.
118. Al-Mohaya, S, Naguib, M and Abdelatif, M: Abnormal responses to muscle relaxants in a patient with primary hyperparathyroidism. Anesthesiology 65: 554, 1986.
119. Schenker, JG and Kallner, B: Fetal postpartum hyperparathyroid crises due to primary chief cell hyperplasia of parathyroids. Obstet Gynecol 25:705, 1965.
120. Covino, BG and Vassallo, HG: Local anesthetics: Mechanisms of action and clinical use. In Ditz, RJ and Laver, MB (eds): The Scientific Basis of Clinical Anesthesia. Grune & Stratton, New York, 1976, p 28.
121. Bolen, JW: Hypoparathyroidism in pregnancy. Am J Obstet Gynecol 117:178, 1973.

CHAPTER 14

HEMATOLOGIC DISEASE

W.D.R. WRITER, M.B., Ch.B., F.F.A.R.C.S.(Eng), F.R.C.P.C.

In recent years, major advances have taken place in the management and understanding of hematologic disease. This chapter discusses many blood disorders that may complicate pregnancy (Table 14 – 1), their obstetric significance, and the anesthesia considerations that apply to the parturient.

Normal Physiology

Chapter 1 discusses the major physiologic adjustments in the hematologic system that characterize pregnancy. These changes include increases in plasma volume, red-cell mass and a mild leukocytosis.[1–4] Platelet count generally falls slightly, but mean platelet volume increases by the end of pregnancy. Pregnancy also increases iron and folic acid requirements. Iron transfer to the fetus occurs readily, against a concentration gradient throughout pregnancy.[5] Such placental "trapping" satisfies fetal iron requirements, even in the face of severe maternal iron deficiency. Estimates of the increased folate requirement vary from two to ten times the nonpregnant intake, and the demand increases significantly in multiple pregnancies.[6] Serum vitamin B_{12} (cobalamin) levels fall steadily throughout pregnancy, but fetal transfer has a negligible impact on the large maternal stores.[6]

Anemia in Pregnancy

DEFICIENCY ANEMIAS

Iron Deficiency Anemia

The World Health Organization defines anemia in pregnancy as a hemoglobin concentration of 110 g per liter, or less.[7] Improvements in maternal health and prenatal care, and prophylactic iron administration, have virtually eliminated serious iron deficiency anemia in pregnancy from developed countries, but the condition prevails in poor and underdeveloped communities.[8,9]

In established iron deficiency, the classic hypochromic, microcytic RBCs may not appear until the hematocrit falls well below normal levels. The reticulocyte count falls, platelets frequently increase, and occasional hypersegmented neutrophils appear in peripheral

Table 14–1. CLASSIFICATION OF HEMATOLOGIC DISORDERS

- I. The formed elements
  - A. Erythrocytes
    - 1. The anemias
      - a. Deficiency anemias
        - i. Microcytic, Fe
        - ii. Macrocytic—Folate
          —Vitamin B_{12}
      - b. Aplastic anemias—also affecting leukocytes and platelets
      - c. Hemolytic anemias
        - i. Genetically determined
          - (a) Disorders of hemoglobin
            - (1) Structural variants—the sickling disorders
            - (2) The thalassemias
            - (3) (Other structural variants)
          - (b) Disorders of the red cell membrane
            - (1) Hereditary spherocytosis
            - (2) Hereditary elliptocytosis
          - (c) Disorders of the energy pathways—G6PD deficiency
        - ii. Acquired
          - (a) Due to red cell antibodies
            - (1) Isoimmune hemolytic anemia, e.g., hemolytic disease of the newborn
            - (2) (Autoimmune hemolytic anemia)
            - (3) (Drug induced immune hemolytic anemia)
          - (b) Nonimmune hemolytic anemia (microangiopathic hemolytic anemia)
          - (c) Due to red cell membrane defects (paroxysmal nocturnal hemoglobinuria)
  - B. Leukocytes: leukemia
- II. The coagulation mechanism
  - A. Vascular compartment disorders
    - 1. Inherited
      - a. (Hereditary hemorrhagic telangiectasia: Osler-Weber-Rendu disease)
      - b. Von Willebrand's disease—also affects platelet and coagulation compartments
    - 2. Acquired
      - a. SLE
      - b. Others
  - B. Platelet compartment disorders
    - 1. Inherited—von Willebrand's disease
    - 2. Acquired
      - a. Idiopathic thrombocytopenic purpura
      - b. Thrombotic thrombocytopenic purpura
      - c. (Alloimmune thrombocytopenic purpura)
  - C. Coagulation compartment disorders
    - 1. Inherited
      - a. von Willebrand's disease
      - b. Hemophilia A and B
      - c. Other factor deficiencies
    - 2. Acquired
      - a. (DIC)
      - b. (Drugs e.g., anticoagulants)
      - c. (Hepatic disease)
  - D. Tissue compartment disorders
    - 1. Inherited (Ehlers-Danlos syndrome)
    - 2. Acquired (Cushing's syndrome)
  - E. Thromboembolic disorders

Note: Diseases in parentheses are not discussed in this chapter.

blood.[10] Serum ferritin levels below 12 to 15 ng per ml usually indicate iron deficiency.[11]

Folate Deficiency Anemia

Folate-deficient megaloblastic anemia occurs rarely in North America. In most cases, the diagnosis becomes apparent only in the last 4 weeks of pregnancy or early in the puerperium; anemia presenting at this time should raise the suspicion of folate deficiency. Although nonspecific symptoms such as fatigue predominate, folate-deficient women develop more serious illness than those with iron deficiency. They may experience sore mouth, sore tongue, and even purpura with associated thrombocytopenia. Hemolytic jaundice, edema, proteinuria, and a frank bleeding diathesis may characterize severe cases.[12] The blood film may reveal hypersegmented neutrophils, with five lobes or more, and sometimes leukopenia. Thrombocytopenia may also accompany folate deficiency. Diagnosis ultimately depends on the demonstration of megaloblastic hematopoiesis in the marrow.[13]

Obstetric Considerations in Folate Deficiency. Claims that obstetric complications such as abruptio placentae, pre-eclampsia, and abortion result from folate deficiency, have not been substantiated, and the possible association between folate deficiency and the occurrence of neural tube defects awaits the results of a large-scale controlled trial.[6] A daily folate intake of 200 to 300 μg gives adequate prophylaxis against folate deficiency and should be routinely prescribed for all pregnant women.

Vitamin B_{12} Deficiency

Classical addisonian pernicious anemia occurs infrequently in the reproductive years, and the associated infertility makes pregnancy extremely unlikely except in treated cases. A nutritional B_{12} deficiency may occur in strict vegetarians, but those who develop megaloblastic hematopoiesis invariably have associated infertility. On the rare occasions when pregnancy and vitamin B_{12} deficiency anemia have coexisted, pregnancy has been uncomplicated or, in a few cases, associated with fetal death in utero.[6]

APLASTIC ANEMIA

Knispel and associates[14] reviewed 29 well-documented cases of aplastic anemia in pregnancy, and reports continue to appear in the literature. Cases include pancytopenia, and recurrent, apparently reversible, red-cell aplasia or hypoplasia, but the etiology remains unclear.[15–20] Treatment of pancytopenia usually requires RBCs, granulocytes, and HLA–matched platelets for supportive transfusion therapy, when the disease occurs in late gestation. Granulocyte concentrates increase survival in the presence of sepsis.[21] Platelet transfusions may promote platelet antibodies, which significantly reduce platelet survival. Broad-spectrum antibiotics and corticosteroids constitute the mainstays of drug treatment, and laminar-flow hoods, along with isolation nursing, diminish the risk of infection.

ANESTHETIC CONSIDERATIONS IN ANEMIA OF PREGNANCY

Oxygen Delivery

Hemoglobin binds oxygen reversibly and facilitates its transport from the lungs to body tissues. In anemia, RBCs contain less hemoglobin and consequently have reduced oxygen capacity and content (Table 14–2). However, impor-

Table 14–2. PATHOPHYSIOLOGIC CHANGES IN ANEMIA

Red cells	↓ hemoglobin concentration ↑ 2,3-DPG ↓ O_2 capacity
Arterial blood	↓ PaO_2 ↓ O_2 content ↓ SaO_2
Venous blood	↓ O_2 content ↓↓ S_vO_2
Lungs	↑ A-aDO_2
Cardiovascular system	↑ Qt ↑ Qs/Qt Possible ↑ in tissue vascularity

2,3-DPG = 2,3-diphosphoglycerate; SaO_2 = arterial oxygen saturation; S_vO_2 = oxygen saturation in mixed venous blood; A-aDO_2 = alveolar-arterial oxygen tension difference; Qt = cardiac output; and Qs/Qt = shunt fraction.

(After Gillies, I.D.S.,[22] by permission.)

tant compensatory changes minimize the effect of anemia on oxygen delivery.[22]

Oxygen delivery to the tissues (O_2 flux) depends on the arterial oxygen content (CaO_2) and cardiac output (Q). CaO_2, in turn, depends on the hemoglobin concentration (Hb), binding capacity of hemoglobin (usually estimated as 1.34 ml oxygen per g Hb), and percentage saturation of hemoglobin with oxygen (SaO_2; usually 97 percent). In addition, there is a small amount of dissolved oxygen (P mmHg × .03 ml per liter). With a cardiac output of 5 liters per min and hemoglobin concentration of 150 g per liter, oxygen flux equals:

[(150 × 1.34)	× 0.97 +	100 × .03)]	× 5	~ 1000
Hb	% saturation	PaO_2	Q(LPM)	ml per min

In pregnancy, the 40-percent increase in cardiac output increases oxygen flux, and satisfies the increased maternal and fetal oxygen consumption. Normally, an arteriovenous oxygen saturation difference ($Sa\text{-}vO_2$) of approximately 25 percent provides for basal oxygen consumption (Fig. 14–1, curve B). In anemia, variable increases in red-cell 2,3-DPG shift the oxygen dissociation curve to the right, increasing the P_{50} and favoring oxygen release to the tissues, but at the expense of increased venous desaturation (Fig. 14–1, curve C). This rightward shift alone increases $S(a\text{-}v)O_2$, and helps anemic subjects compensate adequately for hemoglobin levels of 80 to 90 g per liter.[21] While a 50-percent reduction in hemoglobin concentration would theoretically reduce oxygen flux to 500 ml per min, the increased 2,3-DPG results in only a 27-percent decrease in oxygen availability (oxygen flux = ~730 ml).[23,24]

In some severe hemolytic anemias, Heinz bodies (RBC inclusions of denatured hemoglobin) occur. These do not affect hemoglobin estimation, but neither do they combine with oxygen. In these circumstances oxygen capacity may become markedly reduced, despite an apparently normal hemoglobin level. Therefore, hemoglobin level provides only an indication of oxygen delivery, and careful patient assessment becomes all important.

Cardiac Output

Cardiac output, already elevated in pregnancy, must increase further in chronic anemic states, notably sickle-cell anemia. Theoretically, a 50-percent reduction in hemoglobin, to 75 g per liter, should require a doubling of cardiac output. However, in severely anemic, nonpregnant subjects, such as a decrease led to a 36-percent stroke volume increase without change in heart rate.[25] More recent studies show that cardiac

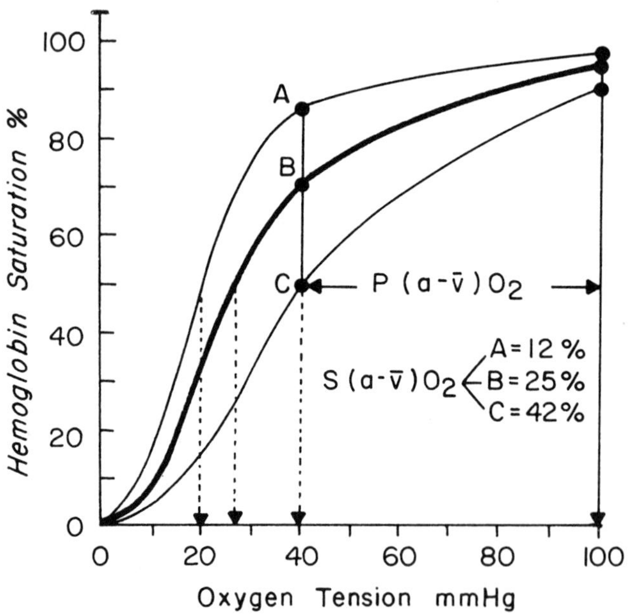

Figure 14–1. Oxygen affinity curves with the same shape to illustrate the effect of different positions (P_{50} shown by the dotted lines) on the ability of hemoglobin to combine with and release oxygen. Curve B is the standard curve. Curve A is an example of displacement to the left (P_{50} decreased) such as might be observed in stored blood. Curve C is an example of a dissociation curve displaced to the right (P_{50} increased) such as might be seen in homozygous sickle cell anemia. Curve C allows the greatest fall in saturation, S (a-v̄) O_2 for the normal arteriovenous oxygen tension difference P (a-v̄) O_2. (Modified from Gillies, IDS,[22] with permission.)

output does not change significantly until hemoglobin levels fall as low as 70 to 90 g per liter, providing P_{50} increases by 5 mmHg. Then, as hemoglobin falls further, cardiac output increases linearly.[26] This major change in cardiac output results from increased stroke volume due almost entirely to afterload reduction secondary to vasodilation and reduced blood viscosity. Anemic subjects also have an exaggerated increase in cardiac output in response to stimuli such as shivering and exercise,[23] and further increases occur with uterine contractions in labor and in the immediate postpartum period.

Arterial desaturation may occur in anemia, because of the rightward shift in the oxygen dissociation curve, increased A-aDO_2[27] and increased venous admixture (Table 14–2).[22] The supine position further impairs respiratory function in late pregnancy, and up to 50 percent of pregnant women, when supine, develop airway closure during normal tidal ventilation.[28,29]

Pathophysiology of Anemia

Harrison[7] discusses the pathophysiology of severe maternal anemia as seen in the underprivileged world. Circulatory changes rarely develop until hemoglobin and hematocrit fall to 65 to 70 g per liter and 0.24, respectively. Heart rate rises, and the skin and mucous membranes, though pale, become warm, suggesting arteriolar dilation. Systemic vascular resistance and diastolic pressure fall. Systolic pressure remains unchanged, and pulse pressure, therefore, rises. Vigorous pulsations of large neck vessels may become visible and associated with a bruit. The percentage utilization of available oxygen increases, and in very severe anemia the $S(a\text{-}v)O_2$ may reach 90 percent. A further drop in hemoglobin and hematocrit levels, to 44 g per liter and 0.14, respectively, causes much more profound circulatory effects. Blood volume now decreases by as much as 40 percent, and right atrial pressure and cardiac output rise. All cardiac chambers dilate, and blood turbulence causes systolic murmurs. In this situation, the mother risks heart failure from myocardial hypoxia, and blood transfusion easily precipitates acute pulmonary edema.

In severe folate deficiency, pancytopenia represents another dangerous complication. When the platelet count in these women falls below 5×10^9 per liter, their hematocrit may be less than 0.12, and women in labor rarely survive, hemorrhage being the immediate cause of death. Severe anemia also impairs cell-mediated immunity,[30,31] leading to flare-up of dormant infections. When anemia coexists with medical and obstetric complications such as hemorrhage, eclampsia, and pre-eclampsia, the prognosis worsens. Anemia also increases placental size and diminishes the amniotic fluid oxygen tension.

Predelivery Assessment

Of the three important variables that affect oxygen flux (hemoglobin, Sa-vO_2, and cardiac output) only the former is easily measured, yet it provides no indication of the mother's adaptation to anemia. Increasing recognition of the hazards of blood transfusion and the knowledge that severely anemic patients tolerate anesthesia well have lessened anesthesiologists' insistence on a "safe" level of preoperative hemoglobin. A 1972 United States survey found that 88 percent of anesthesiologists required a preoperative hemoglobin within 10 percent of the "magic" 100 g per liter.[32] Fifteen years later, most recognize that hemoglobin concentration is only one index of the severity of anemia, and careful clinical evaluation and assessment of her exercise tolerance provide the best indication of the mother's cardiovascular reserve.[21] Although exertional dyspnea often occurs in the third trimester of normal pregnancy, significant breathlessness on minimal exertion in the presence of anemia and without other identifiable cause indicates circulatory decompensation. Other factors to be considered include the severity and chronicity of the anemia, feasibility of its preoperative correction, and the presence of other disease. Pre-existing cardiac disease, for example, may significantly influence preoperative management. Laboratory investigations should include hematocrit, complete blood count and differential, serum ferritin, and red-cell folate.

Blood transfusion must not be undertaken simply to achieve an acceptable preoperative hemoglobin in anemic parturients. Fatalities still occur from hemolytic transfusion reaction, transfusion-associated hepatitis (invariably non-A, non-B), acquired immune deficiency syndrome (AIDS), and anaphylaxis, and the most effective prophylaxis is to use no blood.[33] The remote risks of antibody formation from transfusion of unidentified or irregular antigens should also deter the physician from transfusing women in the child-bearing years, except in absolute emergency. Previous maternal transfusion accounts for 50 percent of cases of non-Rh hemolytic disease of the newborn (HDN).

Preanesthetic deficit correction must be guided by clinical assessment and performed in consultation with the obstetrician and hematologist. While thrombocytopenia below 100×10^9 per liter generally contraindicates regional block, platelet transfusion rarely becomes necessary to secure hemostasis, and mothers with a platelet count in excess of 25×10^9 per liter invariably tolerate labor well. More severe depletion may call for platelet transfusions. All anemic mothers require typing and screening on admission to the labor and delivery area so that blood can be rapidly available if required. Any transfusion in severe anemia must be undertaken slowly, ideally a few days before the surgical procedure, although this may be impractical. Packed cells represent the best product, and in severe anemia their transfusion should be carefully monitored by central venous pressure (CVP) or pulmonary capillary wedge pressure (PCWP).

Analgesia in Labor

A parturient with uncomplicated anemia may choose the labor analgesia. Anemia does not contraindicate narcotic techniques. In more severely anemic mothers, continuous epidural block with appropriate circulatory monitoring offers advantages over other techniques. It helps allay maternal anxiety, avoids narcotic-induced respiratory depression, and improves maternal tissue perfusion by sympatholytic effects on capacitance and resistance vessels.[34] A CVP line inserted before the intravenous preload and induction of epidural block helps monitor maternal response. In severe anemia, and in mothers with class III or IV heart disease, PCWP monitoring gives an indication of left ventricular performance and enables early detection of circulatory overload. Maintenance fluids (normally 1 to 2 ml per kg per hour) should be guided by CVP or PCWP readings. When inducing epidural block, the anesthesiologist must balance sympathetic blockade and fluid infusion to ensure acceptable circulatory pressures (CVP, 5 to 10 mmHg; PCWP, 8 to 15 torr). Direct fetal heart monitoring (scalp electrode) permits continuous fetal evaluation and detects fetal distress from decreased uteroplacental perfusion.

Thrombocytopenia (<80 to 100×10^9 per liter) generally dictates other methods of analgesia than epidural block. Intramuscular narcotics carry a risk of hematoma in thrombocytopenic women. Suitable narcotic techniques include intermittent intravenous meperidine, 25 to 50 mg, and patient-controlled intravenous analgesia (PCA).[35] A number of microcomputer-driven syringe pumps have become available recently for PCA. Upon demand signal, they deliver a programmed dose of meperidine (e.g., 12.5 to 15 mg) after an appropriate "lock-out" interval (12 to 15 min), and obviate the repeated waning of narcotic effect.

Although nitrous oxide, 50-percent, produces mild megaloblastic bone marrow depression after inhalation for 6 hours, this effect has little clinical significance in the labor and delivery area. In parturients with contraindications to regional techniques, inhalation analgesia helps augment narcotics, especially at the time of transition and in the second stage of labor. Techniques such as psychoprophylaxis less reliably provide pain relief for these sick mothers.

Anesthesia for Vaginal Delivery

In nonthrombocytopenic mothers with no epidural block in place, bilateral pudendal block or perineal infiltration of local anesthetic provides acceptable analgesia for spontaneous and low forceps deliveries. Oxygen administration ($FIO_2 = 1.0$) throughout the second stage increases maternal dissolved oxygen levels and improves neonatal umbilical vein and artery PO_2.[36] Alternatively, inhalation analgesia can augment these techniques, while still maintaining an FIO_2 of at least 0.5. Left lateral tilt of the mother throughout delivery maximizes uteroplacental perfusion. For many outlet and uncomplicated forceps deliveries, low-dose intravenous ketamine provides good delivery analgesia, except in hyperdynamic states. After a bolus of 0.25 mg per kg body weight, the parturient receives increments of 10 to 15 mg, to a maximum of 100 mg, or 1 mg per kg.

Operative vaginal deliveries (e.g., mid-forceps rotation) call for epidural analgesia or saddle block. However, in thrombocytopenia, general anesthesia, as described for cesarean section, may become necessary. To minimize airway hematoma, gentle placement of a well-lubricated, sterile tracheal tube should follow a nontraumatic laryngoscopy.

Anesthesia for Cesarean Section

Elective cesarean section permits correction of any preoperative deficits in severely anemic or thrombocytopenic mothers. In chronic anemia this calls for careful maternal surveillance, with CVP or PCWP monitoring in severe cases. Platelet concentrates should be given only prior to surgery or for life-threatening emergencies, and their use invariably requires consultation with a hematologist. Thrombocytopenia below 50×10^9 per liter generally needs preoperative correction, although some hematologists accept values above 25×10^9 per liter.

In severely anemic mothers needing cesarean section, epidural block offers advantages over general anesthesia if no contraindications exist. After insertion of the CVP or PCWP line, the mother receives a monitored intravenous preload approximating 1 liter while in the left lateral tilt position. In my view bupivacaine remains the preferred drug because of its slower action (which permits observation of the mother's response to sympatholysis) and excellent sensory blockade. The anesthesiologist can gradually augment the block with fractionated doses of bupivacaine (5 ml, 0.5-percent). This controlled sympatholysis allows adjustment of the intravenous infusion rate and reduces the need for vasopressors. Small doses of intravenous ephedrine (5 to 10 mg) correct severe hypotension if hydration and uterine displacement fail. Maternal oxygen administration (FIO_2, 1.0) from the onset of the epidural block ensures maternal and neonatal oxygenation.[36] Subarachnoid block produces abrupt onset of sympathetic blockade and hypotension, making it less satisfactory than epidural block in severely anemic, hypervolemic subjects. Thrombocytopenia below 80 to 100×10^9 per liter contraindicates regional techniques because of the increased risk of epidural or intraspinal hematoma. Before inducing regional anesthesia in an anemic patient whose platelet count is between 80 and 100×10^9 per liter, the anesthesiologist should confirm the presence of a normal bleeding time.

Jouppila and Kirkinen[37] studied umbilical vein blood flow (UVBF) in the fetuses of anemic mothers and in cases of Rh-hemolytic fetal anemia. They observed UVBF values above the 90th percentile in approximately 50 percent of the babies from anemic mothers (hemoglobin <100 g per liter). In fetal anemia UVBF values shortly before delivery correlated negatively with the cord hemoglobin level at delivery. Other preliminary studies suggest that epidural block also increases umbilical flow velocity profiles.[38] Whether this increase would occur in fetuses with already elevated UVBF remains speculative, but it seems clear that maternal epidural analgesia has no adverse effects on babies born to anemic mothers.

When the anemic mother requires general anesthesia for emergency cesarean section, hypoxia during induction presents the greatest hazard, and the risk increases in mothers with an increased $A\text{-}aDO_2$.[22] In anemic parturients with an increased P_{50}, hypoxemia lowers the $S(a\text{-}v)O_2$ more than in normal subjects, thus impeding tissue oxygen delivery (Fig. 14–2). When PaO_2 falls to 60 mmHg in a mother with a P_{50} of 30 mmHg, $S(a\text{-}v)O_2$ falls from 28 to 20 percent, diminishing oxygen delivery and causing venous desaturation. Thus, the anemic subject stands at greater risk of hypoxia, and the increased oxygen consumption, decreased FRC, and elevated cardiac output of pregnancy further increase this risk. Thorough and careful preoxygenation, rapid laryngoscopy, reoxygenation following intubation, and a high intraoperative FIO_2 (0.7 to 1.0) become crucial to these women. Pulse oximetry enables continuous monitoring of oxygen saturation and excludes the possibility of significant hypoxemia.

The brisk pressor response that accompanies laryngoscopy and tracheal intubation in lightly anesthetized parturients makes induction agents with prominent cardiovascular effects (e.g., ketamine) undesirable for severely anemic, hypervolemic mothers. Thiopental sodium (3 to 4 mg per kg) has little adverse effect. CVP or PCWP

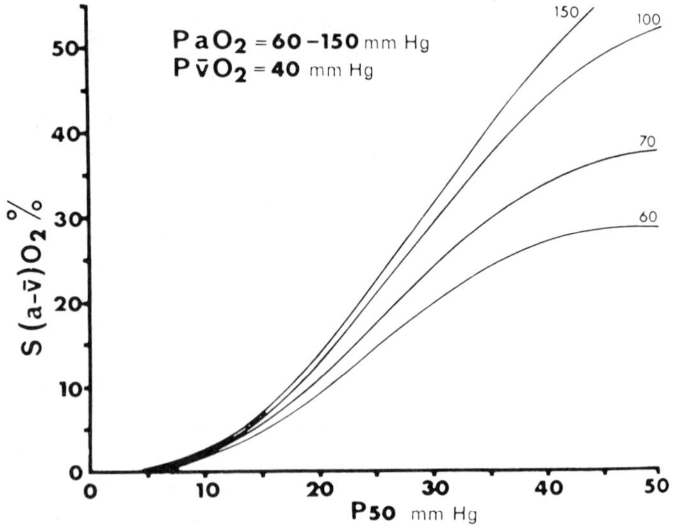

Figure 14–2. Curves showing the relationship between S (a-$\bar{v}$) O_2 and P_{50} at different levels of PaO_2. (From Gillies, IDS,[22] with permission.)

monitoring helps detect adverse changes in right or left ventricular preload and left ventricular performance following induction in more seriously anemic parturients. In thrombocytopenic patients the danger of airway compression and tissue distortion from a neck vein hematoma calls for the peripheral insertion of central monitoring lines. During maintenance of anesthesia, the high FIO_2 ensures maternal and fetal oxygenation, while the addition of halothane (0.5 to 0.7 percent) or enflurane (1 to 1.5 percent) reduces the likelihood of awareness.[39,40] These low concentrations of volatile agents maintain uterine blood flow yet attentuate the sympthetic response to surgical stimulation.[41] Maternal deficiency anemias do not increase the risk of neonatal depression, but the neonatology team should attend the delivery.

Postpartum Considerations

Cardiac output peaks shortly after delivery when the empty uterus involutes and a maternal autotransfusion occurs.[42] Hypervolemic mothers become most vulnerable at this time, and PCWP monitoring gives the best indication of left ventricular performance.

In the postanesthesia recovery room, oxygen administration should continue for 1 to 2 hours, to minimize postoperative hypoxemia. Shivering following epidural or general anesthesia significantly increases cardiac output and oxygen consumption, thus aggravating hypoxemia.[43] A warm environment, close nursing observation, and pulse oximetry of high-risk mothers avert deleterious changes. Small doses of intravenous meperidine (15 to 25 mg) may diminish postoperative shivering.

HEMOLYTIC ANEMIAS DUE TO ABNORMAL HEMOGLOBIN

The hemoglobin molecule comprises four subunits, each with a heme (pigment) portion in a hydrophobic pocket enveloped by a polypeptide (globin) chain.[44,45] The subunits interlock to form a tetrahedron, which folds like a clam shell. In hemoglobin A, each half of the "shell" contains one alpha- and one beta-globin chain —the alpha-beta dimer. Each alpha chain has 141 amino acids, and each beta chain, 146. Together the dimers comprise a tetramer. Three common types of hemoglobin exist:

hemoglobin A: α_2, β_2 (97 percent of normal adult hemoglobin)
hemoglobin A_2: α_2, δ_2 (3 percent of normal adult hemoglobin)
hemoglobin F: α_2, γ_2 (fetal hemoglobin)

Abnormalities of the globin chain that result from deletion, substitution, or inversion of the amino-acid sequence disrupt its stability and have profound effects on hemoglobin behavior.[46,47] A single base mutation in the DNA coding sequence for the amino acid at position six of the beta chain results in the substitution of valine for glutamic acid in the beta chain. This minute change produces hemoglobin S, which polymerizes when deoxygenated making the erythrocyte rigid and nondeformable and distorting it into the sickle shape. In hemoglobin C, lysine substitutes for glutamic acid at position six in the beta chain, and hemoglobin crystallizes but does not sickle.[48]

The Sickling Disorders

The term "sickling disorders" encompasses any disorder in which red blood cells (RBCs) sickle in the deoxygenated state. In this chapter the term "sickle cell disease" connotes those sickling disorders that cause clinical illness: SS, SC, S-β thalassemia, and rare disorders like SD_{PunJab} and SO_{Arab}, but not sickle cell trait (AS). Other mild disorders include SE and S-Lepore.

Classification

Sickle Cell Anemia. HbSS, the homozygous form of the disease with severe clinical symptoms; erythrocytes contain 85 to 95 percent HbS.

Sickle Cell Trait. HbAS, the heterozygous sickling disorder, invariably mild; erythrocytes contain 30 to 50 percent HbS.

Sickle Cell Hemoglobin C Disease. HbSC, heterozygous disease, and a milder variant of HbSS; it occasionally leads to massive, sometimes fatal sickling crises in pregnancy or the puerperium.

Sickle Thalassemia. HbS-β Thal, heterozygous disease with severe symptoms.

Mild Sickle Cell States. Hb SD, Hb SE, HbS-Memphis, heterozygous states with hemoglobin S, where the non-S hemoglobin determines the severity of the illness; clinical symptoms are usually mild.

Generally, sickling hemoglobinopathies follow a classic autosomal-recessive inheritance, and both alleles must be present in order for a homozygous patient (HbSS) to express the clinical symptoms of severe anemia. Sickle cell trait (HbAS), although usually asymptomatic, may exhibit symptoms, which can be severe, when exposed to hypoxia or acidosis.

Pathophysiology. The alpha and beta dimers normally remain apart in deoxyhemoglobin. However, in HbS, the hydrophobic valine residue allows the beta chains of various hemoglobin molecules within the RBCs to interlock, by hydrophobic bonding, with other HbS molecules. The initial aggregation starts slowly, and the tetramers form a helix, which can still revert to normal HbS upon reoxygenation. Later, at some critical point in this polymerization, crystals form and distort the cell into its characteristic sickled shape.[49] The distorted elongated RBC, unable to carry oxygen, passes with difficulty through the microvasculature. Individual RBCs or groups of two or three then become stuck, diminish tissue blood flow, and cause further hypoxia, with increased sickling and tissue infarction. The process is *not* one of thrombosis, and thrombolytic agents cannot undo it.[50] Although reoxygenation reverses polymerization, once the RBCs have sickled they remain permanently deformed (irreversibly sickled cells [ISC]) and must be removed by the reticuloendothelial system.[46] A small number of ISCs normally circulate in all sicklers, especially in mixed venous blood, in the absence of crisis. Acidosis and other conditions that lower oxygen affinity also bring about this irreversible state. Factors such as cell age, HbS or HbF concentration, temperature, and osmotic pressure also influence the process of crystallization and sickling. HbSS erythrocytes begin to sickle when SaO_2 falls below 80 percent (PaO_2, normally, approximately 50 mmHg). HbAS erythrocytes, in contrast, may tolerate a fall in SaO_2 to 25 percent (PaO_2 ~18 mmHg) before sickling. A rightward shift of the oxygen dissociation curve from increased 2,3-DPG further reduces the SaO_2 at which sickling occurs (see Fig. 14–1, curve C).

Detection of Sickling Hemoglobins. Screening tests should detect not only patients with sickle cell disease (HbSS) but also those with HbSC, HbS-Thal, and HbAS genotypes. The commercially available Sickledex (Ortho) rapidly and reliably detects HbS; it has a 5- to 8-percent false-positive rate, with no false-negatives. Definitive diagnosis requires hemoglobin electrophoresis or chromatography to determine the type of sickling hemoglobin present.

Clinical Manifestations of the Sickling Disorders

Eight to nine percent of North American blacks have sickle cell trait (HbAS). Approximately 0.15 percent (1 in 625) have HbSS; 0.1 percent (1 in 850), HbSC; and 0.06 percent (1 in 1650),

HbS-Thal. Survival to adult life with one of these major hemoglobinopathies depends upon medical care, control of infection, and treatment; the disease often becomes less severe with increasing age.[51]

Clinical illness occurs when deoxyhemoglobin polymerizes within the RBC and produces sickling. (Polymers actually exist in RBCs, even at 95-percent oxygen saturation, but are in equilibrium with HbS at this oxygen tension and have no adverse effect.[52]) The major features that occur in patients with HbSS, HbSC, and HbS-Thal genotypes consist of painful recurrent hematologic crises that take three forms.

Vaso-Occlusive Crisis. A sudden significant increase of sickled cells in the bloodstream obstructs the microcirculation, causing pain as the primary symptom. Hypoxia, severe metabolic acidosis, and venous desaturation can provoke vaso-occlusive crisis, but subjects with severe sickling disorders may develop vaso-occlusion in response to nonspecific precipitants such as stress, alcohol, pregnancy, and infection. During a vaso-occlusive crisis the reticuloendothelial system and spleen sequester large numbers of RBCs.[50]

Hemolytic Crisis. Increased destruction of RBCs, elevated indirect bilirubin, and more gradual sickling without significant pain characterize hemolytic crisis.

Aplastic Crisis. This condition is an acute phase of bone marrow aplasia, possibly related to folate deficiency, which produces severe anemia.

The crises associated with sickling disorders and the resultant end-organ damage explain much of the symptomatology, such as severe bone pain and abdominal pain. Most patients with HbSS and HbSC undergo autosplenectomy due to infarction during childhood, and the urinary tract frequently demonstrates renal papillary necrosis and increased susceptibility to infection. The liver shows enlargement (and, rarely, rupture), sclerosis, and sometimes infarction. Subjects not infrequently have congestive heart failure with cardiomegaly and pulmonary infection or embolism. Up to one third of severe sicklers suffer eye changes, and cerebral thrombosis is a major cause of demise in adolescents with the severe disorders.[46] Although such complications cause severe morbidity and shorten the life span, most North American patients survive to the fifth or sixth decade. All young adult HbSS patients demonstrate heart murmurs and jaundice, and many have gall stones. The term "chest syndrome" describes an otherwise unidentified lung infiltrate in a sickler. In this situation PaO_2 requires close monitoring and administration of oxygen may become necessary.

Sickling Disorders and Pregnancy

Concurrent severe sickling disorders jeopardize maternal and fetal outcome. The disease mortality varies widely between countries but now approaches zero in the United States.[10] However there is significant maternal morbidity and, frequently, pregnancy complications occur. Several factors explain the adverse effects of pregnancy, including the increase in coagulation factors, elevated venous pressure in the lower extremities, the increased metabolic demands and CO_2 production, increased likelihood of infection, and the stress of parturition. Pneumonia, pyelonephritis, endometritis, pulmonary embolism, and congestive heart failure are important causes of morbidity. Vaso-occlusive crises complicate up to 40 percent of pregnancies in the major disorders and may occur in association with any of the previously noted complications. Pregnancy-induced hypertension affects up to 15 percent of mothers with severe sickling disorders, and its clinical features may be confused with those of the sickling disorder itself, since proteinuria, nephropathy, and hyperuricemia may accompany HbS. Although pregnancy increases the risk of crisis and other complications, even in mothers who were asymptomatic before pregnancy, contemporary medical and obstetric care continue to diminish morbidity and enhance maternal outcome.[46,47]

Treatment of vaso-occlusive crisis remains supportive. Oral analgesics usually control pain, phenothiazines provide sedation, and some antidepressants (e.g., amitripytyline) give good results.[53] Vigorous rehydration (3 liters per day, at least) prevents hypovolemia, especially in febrile parturients. Martin and Morrison[54] infuse Ringer's lactate, 1 liter over the first 2 hours, then continue fluid replacement at 125 ml per hour. They advocate fresh frozen plasma as an adjunct to fluid therapy in vaso-occlusive crises, to enhance volume expansion, improve tissue perfusion, and stimulate plasma prostacyclin (PGI_2) regeneration, with resultant vasodilation and antiplatelet effects. Alkalinization, magnesium sulfate administration, anticoagulants, hyperbaric oxygenation, transfusions, and chemotherapy, do not attenuate vaso-occlusive crises.[50]

Morrison[47] considers partial exchange transfusion, which decreases the amount of HbS in the patient's circulation, to be the most important therapeutic measure in sickle cell crisis. The procedure aims to increase HbA concentration to at least 40 percent. Transfused blood should be less than 5 days old and preserved in citrate-phosphate-dextrose (CPD) solution to ensure optimal oxygen delivery and normal 2,3-DPG levels. Intrapartum sickle cell crisis demands equally aggressive management, including partial exchange transfusion (if time allows), continuous nasal oxygen, strict maintenance of left lateral tilt throughout labor, frequent assessment of maternal vital signs, and continuous fetal monitoring. Maternal monitoring involves coagulation studies, frequent platelet counts, an arterial line for blood gases, and examination of peripheral blood films for evidence of sickling.

Prophylactic Transfusion Therapy. While there is general agreement that prophylactic transfusion therapy helps prevent crises, Charache[50] believes we lack conclusive proof. Most authorities agree that pregnant sicklers whose disease exacerbates during pregnancy merit transfusion, but controversy surrounds the management of symptom-free anemic patients.[55] Most centers aim to increase the proportion of normal cells to 50 percent or more, and hematocrit to 0.30 to 0.35, but Charache[50] employs prophylactic transfusion only when the patient's course worsens, and the majority of his patients receive no blood. Huehns,[56] in contrast, considers regular transfusions to maintain HbA at 60 to 70 percent the only consistently successful way to reduce complications.

Prenatal Care in Mothers At Risk. The primary obstetric goals are the prevention of crises and maintenance of good maternal and fetal health throughout the prenatal and intrapartum periods. All blacks and other patients at risk undergo screening tests for HbS at the first prenatal visit and examination to exclude evidence of sickle cell crisis and infections. Hemoglobin and hematocrit values, Sequential Multichannel Autoanalyzer with Computer (SMAC), erythrocyte sedimentation rate (ESR), and reticulocyte count also provide useful information. An early ultrasound examination enables determination of fetal biparietal diameter, for later assessment of growth. Mothers then attend every 2 weeks until 24 weeks, to allow for early detection of anemia, recognition of pain, fever, or infection, and evaluation of hematinic therapy.[47] Those who require prophylactic transfusion therapy have hemoglobin electrophoresis twice monthly to quantify the percentage of each hemoglobin fraction. Folic acid deficiency must be excluded since it can lead to superimposed megaloblastic anemia with catastrophic results. After 24 weeks patients attend weekly for full hematologic evaluation and assessment. Some authors advise elective cesarean section at 36 weeks, preceded by exchange transfusion.[13]

Anesthetic Considerations

All black patients and mothers at risk of hemoglobinopathy who present for anesthesia in pregnancy must have an HbS screen before induction of anesthesia. A positive result should be followed by immediate hemoglobin electrophoresis to identify the hemoglobins present.[46] A thorough clinical history should inquire about duration of the disease, previous sickling episodes, and the mother's present status, to elicit symptoms of current problems, such as infection, dehydration, or crisis.[48] A history of cardiopulmonary, hepatic, or renal involvement calls for additional evaluation and investigation. Following a careful physical examination, with particular attention to the possibility of a difficult airway, pertinent laboratory investigations include complete blood count, hemoglobin, hematocrit, hemoglobin electrophoresis for HbS percentage, SMAC, bilirubin, and urinalysis. Anemic mothers also require a reticulocyte count. An HbA concentration below 20 percent, or hematocrit below 0.25, increases risk. Any patient who has HbS can sickle in response to the stress of labor or as a result of hypoxia during anesthesia. However, nonanemic mothers and those with sickle cell trait (HbAS) are generally assumed to be at minimal risk.

Rarely, patients with sickle cell trait have more than 50 percent of HbS, placing them at significant risk; the genotype has been designated HbSA (rather than HbAS) to indicate their increased risk.[57] No randomized, controlled comparisons of perioperative care exist, and every parturient needs individualized care by a team that includes an obstetrician, a hematologist, an anesthesiologist, and a neonatologist.[48] HbSS patients may experience serious problems despite careful management, but prevention and awareness of the possible complications increase the likelihood of an uneventful delivery.

Charache[50] recommends exchange transfusion before patients with sickle cell disease undergo general anesthesia. He aims for a hematocrit of 0.35 to 0.40, with at least 50 percent of normal RBCs. This correct anemia and greatly diminishes the likelihood of sickling in the event of an untoward hypoxic incident. If the mother has no atypical antibodies, rapid exchange transfusion is possible, even in emergency situations. Alternatively, 2 to 4 units of packed RBCs, preferably washed, may help prevent crisis in mothers with a hematocrit below 0.20.[47] The mother needs a warm environment at all times and meticulous attention to hydration, with preoperative electrolyte and dextrose replacement at 1.5 to 2 times normal maintenance requirement, to avoid hypovolemia, hypoperfusion, and metabolic acidosis. Morrison[46] adds sodium bicarbonate, 44.6 mmol, to each liter of intravenous fluid, to prevent metabolic acidosis. Warmed intravenous fluids attenuate hypothermia and shivering. Important measures include left lateral tilt throughout labor and prior to delivery, immediate correction of any hypotension with augmented intravenous fluids, and avoidance of vasopressors because of their vasoconstrictive effect.

Continuous maternal oxygen administration increases maternal and neonatal PaO_2 but does not guarantee adequate capillary PO_2 in areas of circulatory stasis. Pulse oximetry is mandatory during anesthesia in sickle cell states. When possible, CVP lines, Foley catheters, and internal uterine pressure catheters are to be avoided to minimize the risk of maternal infection.[54]

Analgesia in Labor. Epidural block gives excellent analgesia and avoids the sympathetic stimulation and vasoconstriction of pain and anxiety, but it substitutes the risk of hypotension and venous pooling in the lower extremities. A selective epidural technique with bupivacaine (0.125- to 0.25-percent) reduces the chance of hypotension. The use of two epidural catheters (the upper catheter at T12–L1 or L1–2, the lower, at L5–S1 or caudad) provides selective pain relief and reduced risk of hypotension. Bupivacaine, 4 to 6 ml in the upper catheter, will alleviate labor pain without effect on blood pressure, and 8 to 10 ml of bupivacaine (0.5-percent) through the lower catheter provides analgesia for delivery with minimal risk of hypotension. Theoretical considerations suggest epidural narcotics to augment the management of labor pain in sickling parturients. Epidural fentanyl, 50 to 100 μg, reduces local anesthesia requirements (thus reducing the risk of hypotension) and improves analgesia.[58,59] In this dose range maternal respiratory depression from the highly lipophilic epidural narcotic is rare. Although intrathecal morphine (0.5 to 1 mg) provides effective labor analgesia without the risk of hypotension and maintains some sensation,[60] the increased risk of respiratory depression eliminates this option. Moreover, second-stage analgesia usually requires epidural or pudendal anesthesia.

Intravenous narcotics, with or without phenothiazine, offer an alternative to regional analgesia, with the added risk of respiratory depression. Inhalation analgesia with nitrous oxide and oxygen can augment systemic analgesia in late first-stage and in second-stage labor.

Mothers anticipating spontaneous vaginal delivery who require no first-stage analgesia may need a pudendal block. Mid-forceps rotation and difficult vaginal deliveries call for epidural anesthesia or saddle block administered meticulously, to avoid hypotension.

Anesthesia for Cesarean Section. Conduction anesthesia removes the concern about hypoxia, aspiration pneumonitis, and the perioperative pulmonary complications that accompany general anesthesia. However, the anesthesiologist must avoid hypotension and venous pooling in the extremities, and the technique demands thorough prehydration, careful cardiovascular monitoring, and lateral tilt throughout. Harris and colleagues[50] recommend carefully wrapping the patient's legs with elastic bandages and elevating them to minimize the risk of venous pooling and hypotension. (But excessive or non-uniform compression would increase circulatory stasis.) The use of epidural anesthesia with bupivacaine (0.5-percent) in 5-ml increments carries minimal risk of hypotension; however, chloroprocaine or subarachnoid blockade significantly increases this risk.

Balanced general anesthesia probably remains the most frequently used technique, despite the attendant risks of hypoxia, aspiration, and a leftward shift of the oxyhemoglobin dissociation curve due to maternal hyperventilation. In addition to preoperative transfusion, these patients require meticulous attention to all aspects of their anesthesia. The operating room should be appropriately warm, and the patient needs a heating blanket in case of unexpectedly prolonged surgery. Essential intraoperative monitors include an ECG, automated blood pressure cuff, precordial stethoscope, pulse oximeter, in-line oxygen analyzer, temperature probe, and an indwelling Foley catheter. During prehydration (15 to 30 ml per kg body weight) in the left lateral position with pressure points protected, the mother breathes 100-percent oxygen. After monitor placement and immediately before induction, she lies supine, with the operating table in 10 to 15 degrees left lateral tilt. A 5- to 10-degree upward tilt of the trunk above waist level minimizes pressure of the gravid uterus on the diaphragm. After preoxygenation for at least 5 to 7 min induction proceeds with thiopental sodium, 3 to 4 mg per kg, or ketamine, 0.8 to 1 mg per kg. Succinylcholine, 1.5 to 2 mg per kg, facilitates laryngoscopy and tracheal intubation, after which reoxygenation with 100-percent oxygen must be undertaken. Maintenance of an FIO_2 of 1.0 throughout, with enflurane 1- to 1.5-percent, or halothane, 0.5- to 0.7-percent, prevents awareness and maximizes oxygenation. Following delivery, increments of fentanyl, 50 to 75 μg, ensure maternal analgesia and a stable circulation. The anesthetic technique should aim for a PaO_2 exceeding 100 mmHg, fully saturated hemoglobin, and a $PaCO_2$ of approximately 35 mmHg.

Emergence from anesthesia carries risks of hypoxemia from unrecognized aspiration, inadequate ventilation, or excessive shivering. The anesthesiologist must pay particular attention to the mother's body temperature and must extubate her in the left lateral position, in the operating room, when she is fully awake and able to remove her own tracheal tube. Postpartum, mothers require admission to an intensive care area for closer monitoring and continuous oxygen administration. For mothers who received epidural analgesia postoperative epidural morphine improves pain relief. I believe the risk of respiratory depression, which appears to be about 1 in 1000,[61] calls for an attenuated dose (3.5 to 4 mg in the average-sized parturient) and meticulous ICU observation with continuous pulse oximetry. Naloxone infusion may protect against the occurrence of respiratory depression while having little adverse effect on pain relief.[62] Mothers with severe sickle cell disease require perioperative and postpartum antibiotics to combat infection.

Although the careful modern management of mothers with sickle cell disease usually ensures good fetal outcome, the neonatology team must be apprised of the mother's condition and attend for delivery. Prophylactic maternal transfusion reduces the risk of neonatal death to a level comparable with that for all black women, but an increased likelihood of premature or small-for-dates neonates remains.[50] Even homozygous newborns with HbSS genotypes develop no symptoms of sickle cell anemia until 3 months of age because HbF, which cannot sickle, confers protection.

HbAS Disease (Sickle Cell Trait). Sickle cell trait invariably runs a benign course.[46] During pregnancy the mother and fetus fare as do HbAA mothers and, apart from the administration of adequate iron and folic acid, require no special treatment. Although well-conducted anesthesia usually causes no problems, careful attention must be paid to body temperature, perioperative hydration, oxygenation, and blood pressure, to protect against the remote chance of sickling. An unhappy outcome can occur in these mothers,[63,64] and may be related to the SA genotype. Letsky[13] notes that the majority of unexpected deaths associated with HbS have occurred in patients with sickle cell trait in the immediate postoperative or postpartum period.

The Thalassemia Syndromes

The thalassemia syndromes, commonest of the genetic blood disorders, worldwide constitute a vast public health problem. They more frequently affect people of Mediterranean stock (Greek: thalassa = sea) and, to a lesser extent, Far Eastern peoples, but they can occur in persons of many ethnic origins. The basic genetic defect results in suppression or absence of the genes that code for alpha- or beta-globin chain synthesis.[13,48,65]

Alpha-Thalassemia. Alpha-thalassemia has four phenotypes resulting from deletion or reduced expression of one or more of the four alpha-globin genes, and discussed in detail by Weatherall.[66] Affected mothers manifest hypochromic or hemolytic anemia, its severity depending on the number of gene deletions. They require folate supplements throughout pregnancy—as much as 5 mg daily for those women with HbH disease (three-gene deletion). Thalassemic patients have no more iron deficiency than normal subjects, and caution must be exercised in iron administration to avoid overload. Severe anemia in pregnancy or at term may call for blood transfusion if the hemoglobin level appears unacceptably low for delivery, but a history of frequent transfusions in more severely anemic mothers raises concerns about the possibility of iron overload and its sequelae—hepatic dysfunction, glucose intolerance, and cardiomyopathy.[48]

Normal fetal development usually occurs in the presence of maternal α-thalassemia, but mothers may transmit the condition to their infants, and mothers with HbH disease inevitably have thalassemic offspring. Mothers carrying Hb Bart's hydropic infants (a four-gene deletion incompatible with life) demonstrate an increased incidence of anemia, pregnancy-induced hypertension, antepartum hemorrhage, fetal malpresentation, obstructed delivery, and cesarean section. Intrapartum fetal distress, postpartum hemorrhage, and retained placenta also occur more often.[13,67]

Before anesthesia for labor or delivery α-thalassemia mothers, particularly those with HbH disease, may require blood transfusion to correct their anemia. Because HbH has increased oxygen affinity and results in poor tissue oxygen delivery, Gibson[48] recommends subtracting the HbH amount from the total Hb concentration to determine the level of functional hemoglobin. The principles of anesthesia management follow those for parturients with severe anemia as described earlier and include a higher FIO_2, avoidance of hyperventilation (which causes leftward shift of the oxygen dissociation curve), and measures to diminish oxygen demand.[48] The majority of patients with α-thalassemia present no particular difficulties for the anesthesiologist, but in those with HbH disease, drugs known to produce hemolysis in patients with glucose 6-phosphate dehydrogenese deficiency should be avoided.

β-Thalassemia. Two genes, one from each parent, control beta-globin chain production, and β-thalassemia can be classified as: β°-thalassemia (no beta-chain synthesis) or β^{+}-thalassemia (reduced synthesis).[68] Phenotypically β-thalassemia heterozygotes have hypochromic, microcytic RBCs with an increased level of HbA_2 (>3.3 percent). The commonest disorder, heterozygous β^{+}-thalassemia (thalassemia minor), usually presents few problems during pregnancy, although mothers require close surveillance of their hematologic indices. They need oral iron and folate supplements in the prenatal period, but not parenteral iron since it carries the risk of iron overload. Intermediate thalassemia includes patients heterozygous for β-thalassemia (β°, or β^{+}) and other hemoglobin abnormalities or homozygous with a milder disorder. Homozygotes who survive into adult life usually have this milder form of the disease.[69] These mothers manifest more severe anemia and evidence of hemolysis, including scleral icterus and splenic enlargement, and show increased susceptibility to oxidizing agents.[46,70]

Thalassemia major (homozygous β-thalassemia) results from the inheritance of defective beta-globin genes from each parent. Cooley[71] first described this condition in the United States in the 1920s among the children of Greek and Italian immigrants, but the disorder also affects populations in the Middle and Far East.[13] Before the days of routine blood transfusion children born with thalassemia major died in early life from anemia, congestive cardiac failure, and intercurrent infection. Now, with improved medical support, they survive into the teens and early twenties as a result of the introduction of transfusion and chelation progams.[72–74] Thalassemia major almost always delays puberty, and pregnancy is an unsual but increasingly common occurrence.[73,75] Invariably pregnancy takes an extremely complicated course, with severe anemia or pancytopenia, hypervolemia, hyperdynamic circulation, and hepatosplenomegaly. Mothers who have thalassemia major also have a greater likelihood of developing pregnancy cardiomyopathy. Bone deformities, the result of a massive marrow expansion to compensate for the largely ineffective erythropoiesis, also frequently occur in these patients.[13,48]

Mothers with thalassemia minor and -intermedia present no significant anesthetic problems. However, thalassemia major constitutes an anesthetic challenge. In all parturients preoperative investigations include hemoglobin, hematocrit, CBC, and RBC indices. Hemoglobin electrophoresis will identify the proportion of HbA_2 and HbF in peripheral blood. The drug history may include iron chelating agents (e.g., desferrioxamine), antibiotics, diuretics, and, rarely, cardiac glycosides. Preoperative examination should include a thorough cardiovascular evaluation and, where necessary, cardiology consultation in mothers who have cardiomyopathy or are at risk of cardiac failure.

In the absence of thrombocytopenia epidural analgesia in labor provides the best pain relief,[75] but prehydration may need to be guided by CVP or PCWP measurement because of hypervolemia or poor cardiac status. Spinal osteoporosis and deformity may add to the difficulties of regional anesthesia. Intravenous narcotics offer a less satisfactory alternative for labor analgesia when contraindications to epidural block exist.

For cesarean section in parturients with severe β-thalassemia, general anesthesia may be preferable. Many patients require an arterial line, and they may need PCWP monitoring to detect abrupt changes in cardiac preload or afterload if they have significant hypervolemia. Possible maxillary and facial deformities require careful preoperative airway assessment to exclude difficult laryngoscopy.[48] These mothers need thorough preoxygenation and particularly careful induction and tracheal intubation. An FIO_2 of 0.8 to 1.0, with appropriate concentrations of volatile agents to prevent awareness and reduce tissue oxygen demand maximizes oxygenation and favors tissue oxygen delivery. Because they respond adversely to hypo- or hypervolemia, patients with severe β-thalassemia need careful circulatory monitoring intraoperatively and intensive care postpartum. Thrombocytopenic parturients may require corrective platelet transfusion before delivery.

Despite the severity of thalassemia, adverse fetal effects may not occur, but neonatologists must be on hand and fully apprised of the patient's status.[13,69,75]

HEMOLYTIC ANEMIAS THAT DO NOT INVOLVE ABNORMAL HEMOGLOBIN

Hemolytic anemia, characterized by shortened RBC survival due to intrinsic abnormality or extrinsic factors, may first present in pregnancy or may have existed since childhood. Increased erythropoiesis can compensate for decreases in RBC survival to 15 or 20 days, but destruction rates greater than eight times normal (RBC survival $\leq$ 15 days) produce anemia.[12,76] Deficient nutrient or iron supplies during pregnancy may unmask the presence of hemolytic anemia. Increased RBC destruction causes jaundice, with increased levels of indirect bilirubin and urinary urobilinogen and decreased haptoglobin. Splenomegaly, cholelithiasis, characteristic RBC morphologic changes, and increased marrow activity occur to varying degrees. Hemoglobinuria and methemalbuminemia may also accompany acute intravascular hemolysis.

A positive direct antiglobulin (Coombs) test occurs only in extrinsic hemolytic anemias and indicates circulating anti-RBC antibody. When possible, physicians should delay transfusion in mothers with hemolytic anemia until after hematologic evaluation and diagnosis.

Intrinsic Red-Cell Defects (Hereditary Spherocytosis (HS) and Hereditary Elliptocytosis (HE))

Inherited as autosomal-dominant disorders, these abnormalities may exist prenatally or become overt in pregnancy because of excessive iron demands. The RBC membrane defect results from mutation of spectrin, a structural protein, and the cell is more permeable to cations, especially sodium, and more susceptible to lipid loss.[77,78] In HS, the cells become spherical, and in HE, predominantly elliptical forms occur. Symptoms depend on the degree of hemolysis and subsequent anemia and vary from neonatal jaundice, hemolytic episodes, and aplastic crises in childhood to mild pregnancy anemias.

Red-Cell Enzyme Defects

Glucose-6-Phosphate Deficiency (G6PD). The commonest genetically determined disorder of red-cell energy pathways, G6PD affects 1 to 2 percent of black American females.[12,76,79,80] In this X-linked recessive condition female carriers remain generally asymptomatic but affected homozygous females occur in areas where the abnormal gene has a high frequency. Erythrocytes demonstrate decreased survival times, and hemolysis and anemia occur following exposure to oxidizing drugs (Table 14–3), certain disease factors (e.g., infection, diabetic acidosis), or broad beans (favism). The patient experiences an explosive bout of intravascular hemolysis, characterized by shivering, backache, and dark urine. Rapid improvement follows cessation of the offending drug. During hemolytic crises, maintenance of adequate fluid intake and high urine volumes helps avoid renal tubular obstruction.[46] The more severe Mediterranean variant (B^-) is a major cause of neonatal jaundice and kernicterus.

Anesthesia Considerations in Hereditary Red-Cell Defects. Affected mothers need careful preoperative assessment, including CBC, hematocrit, reticulocyte count, indirect bilirubin, and a blood film, to determine the degree of hemolysis and anemia. Transfusion may be necessary in severely anemic parturients, although usually these hemolytic conditions pose little threat to pregnancy. No specific contraindications to regional or general anesthesia exist, other than as previously described for anemic parturients.

Table 14–3. SOME AGENTS WHICH MAY PRODUCE HEMOLYSIS IN G6PD DEFICIENCY

Analgesics
Acetanilid
Acetylsalicylic acid
Antipyrine
Phenacetin
Antibacterial Drugs
Chloramphenicol
Isoniazid
Nitrofurantoin
Para-aminosalicylic acid
Penicillin
Sulfonamides and sulfones
Antimalarials
Chloroquine
Pamaquine
Pentaquine
Primaquine
Quinine
Miscellaneous
Dimercaprol (BAL)
Fava beans
Methylene blue
Naphthalene
Phenylhydrazine
Vitamin K

Leukemia in Pregnancy

Leukemia occurs in approximately 1 in 75 to 1 in 100,000 pregnant women, average onset being at 28 years.[13,81] Several hundred cases have now been reported, but there is no evidence that pregnancy has a deleterious effect on the course of the disease.[13,82,83] All morphologic types (except chronic lymphocytic leukemia) may occur, but the chronic (45 percent) and acute (36 percent) granulocytic forms predominate.[81] Modern therapeutic regimens have improved the prognosis of leukemia, so more women in remission have the opportunity to conceive or to survive the pregnancy-associated disease until the fetus becomes viable. Most frequently, diagnosis is confirmed in the second and third trimester, although the disease may have existed earlier with nonspecific symptoms, such as fatigue and recurrent infections, that were mistakenly attributed to the pregnancy.

ACUTE LEUKEMIA

Acute leukemia usually has an insidious onset and presents symptoms related to bone marrow failure, anemia, leukopenia, and thrombocytopenia. Frequently patients have easy fatigability, perhaps a bleeding diathesis from marrow infiltration, and increased susceptibility to infection by organsims of low virulence or opportunistic strains. Physical examination reveals skin pallor, petechiae or ecchymoses, sternal tenderness and an enlarged liver or spleen. The blood film shows normochromic normocytic anemia and thrombocytopenia; white-cell count can be elevated, normal, or low. Some parturients have reduced fibrinogen levels, increased fibrin degradation products, and disseminated intravascular coagulation.[81]

The problems acute leukemia presents fall into two main groups: those that arise from the disease itself and those that result from its treatment. Acute leukemia in early pregnancy increases the abortion risk, and approximately 35 percent of women experience fetal loss. In addition to hematologic and infective complications, CNS leukemia, characterized by elevated intracranial pressure, cranial nerve involvement, and personality change, may occur. In general, chemotherapy, radiation, and supportive therapy reduce morbidity and improve the outcome. Fetal malformations have followed treatment with cytotoxic drugs in the first trimester, and methotrexate, given early in pregnancy always causes either abortion or congenital malformation. Other cytotoxic drugs can safely be given in the second and third trimesters.[84,85] With supportive therapy only (blood products, antibiotics, or single-agent chemotherapy) 20 to 30 percent of women died during pregnancy, and fetal mortality was approximately 50 percent. Aggressive combination chemotherapy increases maternal and fetal survival. Of 23 reported cases treated with a variety of chemotherapy agents, all mothers survived to delivery, but three fetuses succumbed (13 percent mortality), and 10 to 15 percent had congenital abnormalities.[81]

CHRONIC LEUKEMIA

Chronic myelocytic leukemia (CML) has a similarly insidious onset, with fatigue and abdominal discomfort related to the enlarged spleen. The initial blood film may show only leukocytosis; later the white-cell count rises dramatically, and primitive cells appear. Although the platelet count may be normal or slightly increased, platelets may have a functional abnormality. Pregnancy has no effect on the course of the disease, but untreated CML adversely affects maternal and fetal survival. With modern chemotherapy, more than 90 percent of mothers and 85 percent of fetuses survive to delivery. The chronic stage of CML lasts approximately 7 years, then transforms into an acute blastic state in which survival rarely exceeds 1 year.[81]

ANESTHETIC CONSIDERATIONS

Leukemic mothers need careful evaluation and deserve a sensitive, understanding approach from all their physicians. The emotional implications of the disease may influence the mother's approach to labor and delivery as well as her pain tolerance. Hematologic assessment requires a CBC, hematocrit, blood film, and bleeding time, as an index of platelet function. Some patients have metabolic problems that increase oxygen consumption, and others demonstrate electrolyte abnormalities, including hypo- and hyperkalemia and hyponatremia. In some forms of leukemia, a myasthenia-like syndrome complicates the disease.[24] Previous drug therapy may include steroids, necessitating additional coverage in the intrapartum period. The increased susceptibility to infection calls for special attention to aseptic techniques. Severely anemic mothers may need transfusion before labor and delivery, especially cesarean section.

If the platelet count exceeds 100×10^9 per liter and bleeding time falls within normal limits (usually 8 to 10 min), epidural block diminishes maternal stress and offers the best analgesia for labor and vaginal delivery. Saddle block offers an acceptable alternative for delivery, but CNS leukemia obviously negates this approach. Thrombocytopenia, a consumptive coagulopathy, or prolonged bleeding time contraindicates regional techniques. In this situation, intravenous narcotics, by repeat bolus injection, infusion, or patient-controlled analgesia, provide the best alternative, and inhalation analgesia supplemented by perineal infiltration or pudendal block provides acceptable anesthesia for delivery. However, pudendal block may cause local hematoma formation. Rotational forceps deliveries usually require balanced general anesthesia when circumstances contraindicate a regional techique.

For cesarean section, epidural anesthesia represents the technique of choice for mothers with a normal platelet count and bleeding time. Preoperative assessment must evaluate the anemia to determine the need for transfusion. Significant anemia often implies hypovolemia and may contraindicate regional techniques. Previous drug therapy may call for increased steroid coverage. Although no particular local anesthetic is better, the anesthesiologist should consider longer-acting agents and postoperative epidural narcotics. When general anesthesia is necessary, scrupulous attention to the sterility and cleanliness of anesthesia apparatus becomes imperative. Care must be exercised in airway manipulation in those with thrombocytopenia, to avoid causing bleeding and postoperative respiratory obstruction from hematoma.

The neonatology team should attend the delivery because of the increased risk of fetal abnormality and hematologic sequelae such as pancytopenia resulting from the mother's chemotherapy regimen.

Coagulation Disorders

Chapter 15 describes the process of normal hemostasis, which maintains blood in a fluid state within vessels and prevents blood loss from vessels when damaged.[86] This discussion briefly reviews hemostasis and its mesaurement, as a preface to the description of coagulation disorders.

The bleeding time measures primary hemostasis (formation of a platelet plug at the site of vessel injury); the tests of coagulation measure secondary hemostasis (fibrin clot formation at the site of the platelet plug). Platelet adhesion requires von Willebrand factor (vWf–FVIIIR:Ag), which is deficient in von Willebrand's disease. This phase of the hemostatic mechanism also requires a platelet receptor for vWf (absent in the Bernard-Soulier syndrome). Impaired release of the contents of platelet granules (e.g., ADP) or of thromboxane A_2 (TxA_2) also prolongs bleeding time. Prostacyclin (PGI_2) production by the vessel wall opposes TxA_2 and prevents continuing enlargement of the platelet plug. PGI_2 deficiency increases the risk of thrombosis.

The activated partial thromboplastin time (aPTT) reflects the activity of the intrinsic coagulation pathway, while the prothrombin time (PT) indicates extrinsic system activation. Measurement of individual coagulation factors (e.g., Factor VIII) sheds further light on disorders of the clotting cascade.[86–88]

Hemostatic disorders can conveniently be considered in four compartments:

1. The vascular compartment (impaired vasoconstriction)
2. The platelet compartment (impaired adhesion or aggregation)
3. The coagulation compartment (especially the intrinsic pathway)
4. The tissue compartment, in which rare disorders of the supporting tissues (e.g., Ehlers-Danlos syndrome) cause impaired hemostasis.

EVALUATION OF HEMOSTATIC DISORDERS

A detailed search for a history of bleeding in the patient or her family marks the first step in the evaluation of any hemostatic disorder. Questions should exclude a history of previous bleeding from minor surgery or trauma in the patient or siblings, menorrhagia, previous blood transfusion, and impaired wound healing following surgery or injury. While major coagulation disorders generally manifest themselves early in life, minor hereditary defects may first appear in pregnancy.[89] In disorders of recent onset, the drug history must inquire about the many drugs capable of disturbing platelet function or coagulation[90] (see Drug-Induced Platelet Disorders). The nature of any bleeding may suggest the type of defect. Vascular or platelet compartment abnormalities frequently lead to petechiae and superficial purpura. Patients with coagulation disorders, in contrast, generally have more extensive bleeding characterized by hemorrhage into tissues (ecchymoses) or joint spaces. The physical examination should assess skin and mucous membranes for these abnormalities, for telangiectases, and for the poor elasticity typical of tissue compartment disorders. The presence of joint deformity, effusion, or synovial thickening may indicate prior hemarthroses and a major bleeding disorder. Examination of the optic fundi may reveal retinal hemorrhages.

Routine laboratory screening tests include measurement of the platelet count, PT, aPTT, thrombin clotting time (TCT), and bleeding time. In the 75 years since the introduction of the bleeding time as an indicator of platelet function,[91] hematologists have modified the technique and now recommend the spring-loaded Simplate device, which gives an upper normal limit between 8.5 and 10.5 min.[90,92–94] Aspirin taken within the previous 7 days prolongs bleeding time.

HEMOSTASIS IN NORMAL PREGNANCY

Many coagulation factors increase during normal pregnancy, consistent with the description of pregnancy as a "hypercoagulable state."[95] In the intrinsic pathway the Factor-VIII complex, composed of two proteins, FVIII (measured as FVIII:C [Factor-VIII clotting activity]) and von Willebrand factor, increases significantly. In the extrinsic pathway, Factor VII similarly increases. Factors X and fibrinogen increase in the common pathway. Factors II and V rise early in pregnancy but decrease steadily as pregnancy advances. Antithrombin III (AT III), a glycoprotein inhibitor of thrombin and FX_a, falls slightly. From 11 to 15 weeks' pregnancy, fibrinolytic activity markedly decreases, although fibrin degradation products (FDPs) increase from 21 to 25 weeks onward. This apparent paradox reflects a continuing low level of intravascular coagulation in the placental area, with fibrin digestion, but a systemic reduction in fibrinolytic activity consistent with the hypercoagulable state.

DISORDERS OF THE VASCULAR COMPARTMENT

The Vascular Purpuras

Vascular purpura occurs in several conditions, some inherited (von Willebrand's disease, Osler-Weber-Rendu disease, Ehlers-Danlos syndrome) and others acquired (Henoch-Schönlein purpura, systemic lupus erythematosus [SLE], scurvy).

Henoch-Schönlein Purpura. Generalized vasculitis, skin rash, arthralgia, abdominal pain, and renal involvement characterize this syndrome of unknown etiology which rarely occurs in pregnancy.[96–98] Laboratory investigation reveals a normal aPTT, PT, and platelet count despite the purpura. In patients who exhibit renal involvement, renal biopsy demonstrates a focal proliferative glomerulonephritis, while immunofluorescence studies show strongly positive glomerular staining for IgA and fibrinogen, with variable results for C3 (complement), and IgG. The disease appears to represent an allergic response to infection or drugs and usually subsides spontaneously, but it may progress to cause chronic renal damage.

In the absence of accompanying thrombocytopenia, or a prolonged bleeding time, Henoch-Schönlein purpura does not contraindicate regional anesthesia. In one of only three reported cases in pregnancy the mother received uneventful general anesthesia for cesarean section.[96] Extensive purpura requires extreme caution during laryngoscopy and tracheal intubation, to avoid airway bleeding and subsequent respiratory obstruction.

Systemic Lupus Erythematosus (SLE). This immune complex disorder, with chronic multisystem involvement, shows a predilection for young women, making it not uncommon in pregnancy.[99,100] The American Rheumatism Association lists 11 diagnostic criteria, of which at least four must be present to substantiate the diagnosis.[101] Hematologic abnormalities include thrombocytopenia, vasculitis with resultant purpura, and a potent coagulation inhibitor.[102] In addition, lupus anticoagulant inhibits prostacyclin (PGI_2) production or release, and many subjects show disseminated thrombosis.[103,104] In pregnancy, SLE increases the risk of abortion and fetal loss in late pregnancy (due to hypertension and renal failure) and may cause heart block and other neonatal cardiac defects as a result of transplacental passage of anti – Ro antibody. Exacerbation of SLE is three times more likely in the first half of pregnancy, and at least six times moreso in the puerperium. Drug therapy for these mothers may include steroids and aspirin.[100]

A platelet count below 100×10^9 per liter or a prolonged bleeding time contraindicates conduction anesthesia in the vascular purpuras. The anesthesiologist must also confirm a normal PT and aPTT, to exclude the presence of circulating anticoagulant.[100,102] When the mother has a coagulopathy, intravenous meperidine, by bolus injections or PCA, provides the best labor analgesia. Inhalation analgesia can supplement the intravenous narcotic in the second stage of labor. For spontaneous vaginal delivery perineal local anesthetic infiltration should provide adequate pain relief, but the presence of a coagulopathy may contraindicate procedures such as pudendal block because of the significant risk of hematoma. Uncooperative patients may benefit from intravenous ketamine, 0.25 mg per kg, in increments of 10 to 15 mg to a maximum of 100 mg. Mid-forceps delivery and obstetric procedures requiring vaginal or intrauterine manipulation require general anesthesia.

Mothers undergoing cesarean section who have a coexisting coagulopathy or prolonged bleeding time also require general anesthesia. The anesthesiologist should employ extreme care during laryngoscopy and tracheal intubation, to avoid causing mucous membrane damage and serious airway bleeding. Correction of preoperative deficits such as thrombocytopenia should be considered after consultation with a hematologist. Mothers taking steroid therapy also require increased coverage during labor and delivery.

PLATELET COMPARTMENT DISORDERS

Idiopathic (Immunologic) Thrombocytopenic Purpura (ITP)

In this consumptive disorder, most patients produce IgG–antiplatelet antibodies, identifiable as serum- or platelet-associated antibody (PAIgG).[105–109] The resulting antigen-antibody complex exhances platelet destruction in the reticuloendothelial system and shortens their life span.[105–107] ITP causes particular concern in pregnancy because the placenta has receptors for the Fc portion of the IgG molecule and actively transports IgG antibodies from the maternal into the fetal circulation. Thus neonatal thrombocytopenia associated with significant neonatal morbidity and mortality may complicate the disorder.

Acute ITP typically occurs in children, but the chronic form more often affects adults, especially women of child-bearing age. Thrombocytopenia may be chronic or intermittent, and clinical relapse can occur after long periods of remission so that the disease may first present or become exacerbated in pregnancy.[108,109] Mild cases of chronic ITP may remain unsuspected, and asymptomatic thrombocytopenia has been noted more frequently since the introduction of automated blood platelet counters.[110] Alternatively, the woman may present with bleeding, ranging in severity from minimal to life-threatening, and bruising associated with small petechiae in the early stages of the disease. Later progression to subcutaneous hemorrhages and purpuric lesions may occur, as well as serious bleeding from mucous membranes in the gastrointestinal, respiratory, and genitourinary tracts.[108] The most frequent manifestations in pregnancy include epistaxis, bleeding from the gums, and ecchymoses. Even in the presence of severe thrombocytopenia, intracranial hemorrhage and hemarthroses rarely occur.

A careful medical and obstetric history should exclude other causes of thrombocytopenia, such as pregnancy-induced hypertension, disseminated intravascular coagulation, autoimmune disease, and antiplatelet drugs. In severe cases the platelet count may fall as low as 10×10^9 per liter, but hemoglobin, hematocrit, and white-cell count usually remain within normal limits. Despite thrombocytopenia, bleeding time may remain normal because the larger platelets which characterize the disorder have increased competence (Fig. 14–3). However bleeding time may be prolonged, especially following any significant recent hemorrhage. PT, aPTT, and whole blood coagulation time (WBCT) usually remain within normal limits. The degree of thrombocytopenia depends on the balance between platelet production and destruction and on the type and quantity of antibody coating the platelet. Patients in remission and those who have had splenectomy may still have significantly elevated levels of PAIgG and circulating antiplatelet antibody, and fetal thrombocytopenia can complicate a subsequent pregnancy in nonthrombocytopenic mothers "cured" by splenectomy.[109]

Early case reports suggested that ITP carried serious risks for both mother and fetus. However, prospective studies now indicate significantly less morbidity. Five of 99 fetuses (5 percent) died in utero between 18 and 28 weeks. Forty-eight of 94 (51 percent) live-born infants had thrombocytopenia, but a hemostatic defect occurred in only ten (11 percent), and serious bleeding, in six (7 percent). In most infants the platelet count continues to fall, reaching its low-

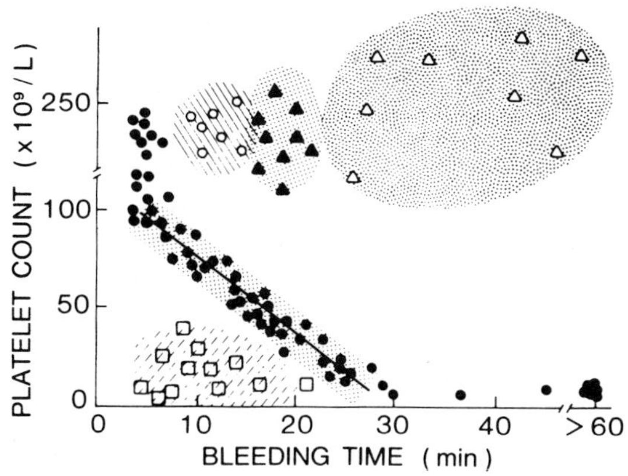

Figure 14–3. Relationship of bleeding time to platelet count. The bleeding time relates inversely to circulating platelet count in patients with thrombocytopenia owing to decreased production (closed circles, which also include eight normal subjects) when the count ranges between 100×10^9 per liter and 10×10^9 per liter. Platelet function defects occur in subjects taking aspirin *(open circles)*, and inherited severe von Willebrand's disease *(open triangles)*. Many patients with idiopathic thrombocytopenic purpura have platelets with increased hemostatic competence *(open squares)*. The closed triangles represent patients with uremia-related platelet function defect. (Modified from Thompson, AR and Harker, LA,[87] p 60, with permission.)

est value 3 to 5 days after delivery. However, neonates with a normal platelet count at birth may develop severe thrombocytopenia several days later and require daily platelet counts for approximately 1 week.[110]

Mild ITP (bleeding time normal; platelet count $>50 \times 10^9$ per liter) requires no treatment or small doses of prednisone (up to 20 mg per day). Prednisone may improve the fetal platelet count as well, although much controversy exists about the value of steroids. Mothers with significant hemostatic impairment (bleeding time >20 min; platelet count between 20 and 50×10^9 per liter) require prednisone; 1 mg per kg is the initial dose, which is then tapered to the lowest dose necessary to normalize bleeding time and maintain platelet count above 50×10^9 per liter.

The use of high-dose intravenous immunoglobulin (IVIG) therapy for ITP represents a new short-term treatment, but the indications remain unclear.[111–117] The platelet count rises during the first week of therapy and falls to pretreatment level within approximately 1 month. The mechanism of action remains obscure, but one theory suggests IVIG blocks macrophage Fc receptors and prevents macrophages from mopping up platelets coated with PAIgG. IVIG appears to have a role in the management of patients who are unresponsive to steroids and in the preparation of mothers for cesarean section or splenectomy.

Because corticosteroids and IVIG provide only temporary remission, most adults later need splenectomy to eliminate the primary site of platelet destruction. Improved surgical and anesthesia techniques, corticosteroids, and the availability of platelet transfusions have significantly lowered maternal and perinatal mortality and morbidity for splenectomy in pregnancy. Mothers who fail to respond to steroids may require splenectomy, ideally in the second trimester. In late gestation the operation can be combined with cesarean section.[108]

Platelet transfusions represent temporary measures to control life-threatening hemorrhage or prepare patients for cesarean section or splenectomy. While a single unit of platelet concentrate normally increases platelet count by 7 to 11×10^9 per liter, an increase of approximately 3×10^9 per liter occurs in parturients with ITP, and platelet survival time falls significantly (to 48 to 230 min).[105,118]

Other treatment regimens such as immunosuppressive drugs and plasmapheresis have limited indications in patients who do not respond to other therapy.

Management of the Delivery. The clinician cannot accurately predict whether a parturient will have a thrombocytopenic infant. Territo and colleagues[119] claimed that 80 percent of infants developed thrombocytopenia when mothers had a platelet count below 100×10^9 per liter. In contrast, fetal thrombocytopenia occurred in only 27 percent of cases when the platelets exceeded 100×10^9 per liter. Cines and associates[107] could find no correlation between maternal and neonatal platelet counts, nor did the level of PAIgG in the mothers identify neonates at risk. Kelton and associates[120] compared maternal platelet count and PAIgG with neonatal platelet count in 41 pregnancies and reported that PAIgG predicted the occurrence of neonatal thrombocytopenia but not its severity, while maternal platelet count had no correlation with fetal values. Scott and coworkers[121] also found no consistent relationship between fetal and maternal thrombocytopenia, but they considered fetal scalp platelet count reliable in predicting fetal thrombocytopenia. Other investigators have used this approach to decide the optimal mode of delivery and believe a value below 50×10^9 per liter calls for immediate cesarean section. However, the policy of fetal scalp sampling does not have widespread acceptance and problems have occurred with the procedure.[122] Finally, Laros and Kagan[123] believe decisions on the correct route of delivery cannot be based on maternal platelet count, antiplatelet antibody, or fetal platelet count. They treat mothers with steroids and employ cesarean section only for obstetric indications.

In his careful review of the literature, Colvin,[109] a hematologist, recommends the following approach:

1. Monitor the maternal platelet count.
2. Measure maternal serum antibody levels and, if possible, PAIgG.
3. Give steroids to the mother, if necessary, to maintain her platelet count above 50×10^9 per liter.
4. Use fetal scalp sampling at the beginning of labor, if possible, and make a decision on the route of delivery after assessment of all these factors.

Anesthetic Considerations in ITP. The obstetric anesthesiologist will encounter the full spectrum of ITP, from mothers with mild disease and no thrombocytopenia to those with severe depression of the platelet count and hemorrhagic diathesis. Each requires individualized management, and all benefit from a multidisciplinary approach involving the obstetrician, hematologist, and neonatologist. Mothers with a normal platelet count, whether it is associated with mild disease or the result of previous splenectomy, pose no anesthetic problem if they have a normal bleeding time. However circulating serum antibody persists following splenectomy and has major fetal implications.

If time permits, the therapeutic regimens before labor or cesarean section aim to restore the platelet count to between 50 and 100×10^9 per liter. Steroids or IVIG constitute the principal approaches. After infusion of IVIG, 0.4 mg per kg per day for 5 days, the platelet count rises on or about the fourth infusion day, peaks 5 days later, and gradually subsides over 3 to 4 weeks. All mothers receiving steroids require an augmented dose (intravenous hydrocortisone, 200-mg bolus, then 100 mg every 6 hours for 24 to 48 hours) to cover surgery.

While mothers with an acceptable platelet count and normal bleeding time should present no difficulty, some thrombocytopenic mothers may have a normal bleeding time because of the increased platelet size and competence (see Fig. 14–3). No clear consensus exists among obstetric anesthesiologists regarding anesthesia in this situation. Some insist on a platelet count of 100×10^9 per liter or greater before proceeding to regional anesthesia, while others accept levels down to 70—or even 50— $\times 10^9$ per liter. I believe the decision to employ a regional technique calls for careful assessment of a number of factors, including clinical status (evidence of petechiae, or more extensive bruising), the platelet count, and bleeding time (which provides evidence of platelet behavior). When there is no obvious bleeding and the patient has a normal bleeding time I will undertake regional anesthesia with a platelet count below 100×10^9 per liter, especially if considerations of pain relief or fetal status favor regional techniques. However, an abnormal bleeding time, even with a higher platelet count, would contraindicate regional anesthesia because the impaired hemostatis may lead to persistent oozing from a lacerated epidural vein and compromise spinal cord function. Securing a transient improvement of the bleeding time by platelet transfusion, while it suffices for surgery, does not in my view justify regional anesthesia in mothers with ITP.

Thrombocytopenic mothers with a prolonged bleeding time who need labor analgesia may receive psychoprophylaxis, inhalation analgesia, or intravenous narcotics without added risk. Intramuscular injections or pudendal block in the second stage of labor can cause an unpleasant hematoma, but perineal infiltration supplemented by nitrous oxide or low-dose ketamine provides good delivery conditions for spontaneous or easy forceps deliveries. The need for platelet transfusion to cover vaginal delivery requires consultation with a hematologist, but most will accept a platelet count above 50×10^9 per liter, despite some prolongation of the bleeding time. Because of fetal risk, obstetricians do not favor mid-forceps rotation in ITP, and general anesthesia rarely becomes necessary for vaginal delivery.

An epidural or subarachnoid block can be considered for labor or cesarean section in thrombocytopenic ITP mothers with normal bleeding times. Mothers with impaired hemostasis coming to cesarean section for obstetric or fetal considerations must have general anesthesia and a preoperative platelet transfusion, usually 6 to 8 units of platelet concentrate immediately preoperatively. Despite platelet transfusion, the anaesthesiologist must exercise extreme care with laryngoscopy and tracheal intubation, to avoid an airway hematoma and potential postoperative respiratory obstruction. These mothers need close observation in the recovery room or intensive care unit for 24 hours to guard against upper airway obstruction or bleeding from other sites.

The most feared perinatal complication is intracranial hemorrhage in the thrombocytopenic fetus, from trauma sustained during delivery. The discrepancy between maternal and fetal platelet counts previously discussed, and the unpredictability of fetal/neonatal status, undoubtedly leads to a high cesarean section rate in mothers with ITP. Fetuses most at risk of purpura and severe morbidity are those whose mothers have undergone previous splenectomy, but have considerable circulating levels of IgG antibodies.[108] The neonatologists need to be aware of anticipated fetal status, and must be present for all vaginal or cesarean section deliveries in ITP or thrombocytopenic mothers. The greatest neonatal risk occurs some 4 to 6 days after delivery then gradually resolves over a course of several weeks, since the IgG antibody has a half-life of 23 days.[79]

Drug-Induced Platelet Disorders

Drug administration to a mother may affect her platelets both quantitatively and qualitatively (Table 14–4).[87,90,124,125] Fetal and neonatal platelets show greater susceptibility which may result in adverse fetal effects in the absence of discernible maternal change.[105,126]

Thrombocytopenia. The commonest pathogenetic mechanism involves formation of an immune complex, subsequently recognized and cleared by the reticuloendothelial system in a reaction dependent on FVIIIR : Ag.[127] The antibodies involved, most frequently IgG, can cross the placenta inducing fetal thrombocytopenia. Some 5 to 10 days after therapy commences, petechiae and bleeding appear in the mother's mucous membranes, and once platelets become sensitized thrombocytopenia invariably recurs within 24 hours of commencing an offending drug. The platelet count recovers, usually within 1 to 2 weeks of stopping the drug, and corticosteroids have no proven value in hastening resolution. Other mechanisms of drug-induced thrombocytopenia include general marrow depression (chloramphenicol) and selective marrow effects such as those induced by thiazide diuretics and tolbutamide. In these situations the platelet count declines gradually and demonstrates more prolonged recovery because of megakaryocyte damage.[105] When labor or delivery intervenes in mothers with impaired hemostasis and drug-induced thrombocytopenia, the anesthesia considerations of ITP apply.

Thrombopathia. Many agents inhibit platelet function by a variety of mechanisms.[87,90,124] Aspirin irreversibly acetylates cyclo-oxygenase, a TXA_2 precursor, inhibiting its synthesis. One aspirin tablet (325 mg) daily induces a more than 95 percent inactivation of cyclo-oxygenase. Following a single dose, bleeding time can remain prolonged for 2 to 3 days, until synthesis of new unaffected platelets occurs, since the irreversible inhibition persists for the platelet's lifetime. Sulfinpyrazone, a nonsteroidal anti-inflammatory drug (NSAID) competitively inhibits cyclo-oxygenase reversibly. Bleeding time remains within normal limits, and sulfinpyrazone actually prolongs platelet life in subjects with shortened platelet survival times.[128] Dipyridamole inhibits platelet phosphodiesterase increasing the level of cAMP. Again, dipyridamole normalizes platelet survival in patients with ongoing platelet consumption, and recent interesting evidence suggests a combination of aspirin and dipyridamole may prevent the occurrence of pre-eclampsia.[129]

It is impractical and unnecessary to check the bleeding time of every pregnant woman to exclude the possibility of a drug-induced thrombopathia. Therapy with aspirin and similar drugs only contraindicates regional techniques when patients show evidence of hemostatic impairment (e.g., purpura, ecchymoses, or persistent

Table 14–4. EFFECTS OF DRUGS ON PLATELETS

Drug	Thrombocytopenia	Thrombopathia
Antibacterial agents		
Ampicillin	+	+ rarely
Azlocillin		+
Carbenicillin		+
Cephalothin	+	
Chloramphenicol	+	
Isoniazid	+	
Mithramycin		+
Nafcillin		+
Nitrofurantoin		+
Novobiocin	+	
PAS	+	
Penicillin	+	+ (in high doses)
Piperacillin		+
Rifampicin	+	
Ticarcillin		+
Anticoagulants		
Heparin	+	+
Anticonvulsants		
Barbiturates	+	
Diphenylhydantoin	+	
Antidepressants		
Imidobenzyl derivatives		+
Monoamine oxidase inhibitors		+
Antihistamines		+
Analgesics		
Acetaminophen	+	
Acetylsalicylic acid	+	+
Nonsteroidal anti-inflammatory drugs	+	+
Oxyphenbutazone	+	+
Antihypertensive drugs		
α-Methyldopa	+	
Diazoxide	+	
Hydralazine	+	
Cardiac drugs		
Digitalis	+	
Quinidine	+	
Cytotoxic agents	+	
Diuretics		
Acetazolamide	+	
Furosemide	+	
Thiazides	+	
Oral hypoglycemic agents	+	
Sympatholytic agents		
Propranolol		+
Phentolamine		+
Tranquilizers and psychotropic drugs		
Chlordiazepoxide		+
Diazepam		+
Phenothiazines	+	+
Miscellaneous drugs		
Dextran		+
Ethanol		+

(Modified from Horger, EO and Keane, MW[105] and Romero, R and Duffy, TP,[125] with permission.)

bleeding). However, mothers on long-term antiplatelet treatment should have a bleeding time estimation before proceeding to regional anesthesia.

Thrombotic Thrombocytopenic Purpura (TTP)

This rare disorder has generated considerable interest in the last 5 years.[130] A multisystem disease (or, more precisely, syndrome), TTP has its peak incidence in women of child-bearing age. The original characteristic triad[131]—microangiopathic hemolytic anemia, thrombocytopenic purpura, and neurologic symptoms—now includes renal disease, leading to progressive renal failure, and fever. In the majority of cases, TTP develops without any known causal event, but pregnancy can precipitate the syndrome.[132] Most of the less than 70 pregnancy-associated cases reported up to 1983 have resulted in death of both mother and fetus.[133] A recent review involving patients of both sexes quoted a mortality rate of 54 percent, with a 28-percent stillbirth rate for pregnancy-associated TTP.[132]

The syndrome shares features with hemolytic uremic syndrome (HUS) and pre-eclampsia, a similarity that sheds interesting light on the pathogenesis of TTP. Diffuse microvascular thrombosis of unknown etiology is the hallmark of the disorder. Hyaline thrombi containing varying amounts of fibrin and platelets, occlude capillaries and precapillary arterioles supplying pancreas, adrenals, brain, heart, and kidneys. In association with this thrombus formation, endothelial cells proliferate excessively and partially cover the thrombi. Whether the basic defect results from abnormal damage to vascular endothelium or hyperaggregable circulating platelets remains unclear. Deficient synthesis or release of prostacyclin (PGI_2) plays a role in the syndrome's genesis. Healthy endothelial cells synthesize PGI_2 and release it into the circulation to induce local vasodilation and inhibit platelet aggregation. A stimulatory factor present in plasma (and serum),[134,135] which the plasma from patients with TTP lacks, appears to control this PGI_2 release.[136] Cultured endothelial cells produce less PGI_2 in the presence of TTP plasma, and some TTP plasma induces aggregation of both normal and TTP platelets.[136, 137] Normal plasma contains an IgG that inhibits the TTP platelet aggregating factor, but the IgG purified from TTP plasma lacks this inhibition.[138] Thus, Lian[138] proposes an IgG deficiency with resultant inappropriate and excessive platelet activation. Finally, the two Factor VIII proteins (vWF and FVIII), normally circulate as multimers, which can become quite large. In TTP, unusually large FVIII multimers circulate which appear to bind and agglutinate platelets in vivo, initiating the agglutination that heralds a TTP episode.[139]

TTP must be considered in patients who demonstrate features of the classic pentad, especially fluctuating neurologic abnormalities, progressive renal failure, fever, and thrombotic lesions.[140] Most have a hemolytic anemia, and the peripheral blood film reveals numerous bizarre fragmented RBCs. Thrombocytopenia, usually less than 40×10^9 per liter, marked hyperplasia of marrow megakaryocytes, and shortened platelet survival occur. The lack of coagulation abnormalities distinguishes TTP from DIC, and fibrinogen levels are invariably normal. Biochemical changes, including elevated indirect bilirubin and increased LDH, reflect the intravascular hemolysis. The hemoglobin and hematocrit confirm the severity of the hemolytic anemia, while renal function studies frequently demonstrate elevated BUN and creatinine. The neurologic disturbances may be mild with some confusion, headache, and transient episodes of numbness, or more frank with visual disturbance, hemiplegia, and dysphasia.

Exciting developments in the management of TTP have reduced mortality in recent years. Many reports confirm that infusion of fresh frozen plasma (FFP) produces improvement in 60 to 70 percent of patients.[141–144] A few remit dramatically after infusion of just 2 units, but the majority require significantly more plasma. Long-term maintenance may become necessary during pregnancy, with infusion of 2 units FFP each time the platelet count begins to fall. The important factor in FFP, which is deficient in TTP, inhibits platelet aggregation and the formation of large FVIII multimers. Failure to respond to FFP calls for plasmapheresis and replacement of some 2 to 3 liters of plasma.[109,143] Platelet concentrates accelerate the disease process (cf. the "fuelling" of disseminated intravascular coagulation which follows administration of FFP or fibrinogen). Oral antiplatelet drugs such as aspirin and dipyridamole, while they do not affect the underlying mechanisms of the disorder, supplement plasma exchange.

The similarity between severe pre-eclampsia and TTP emphasizes that PGI_2-TXA_2 imbalance may also underlie severe PET.

Anesthetic Considerations. The bleak picture of TTP presented in the first edition of this book has significantly improved with plasma therapy. The generally prompt response to FFP means that the mother will usually present for labor analgesia or cesarean section in a more controlled nonthrombocytopenic state. Preoperative evaluation must include CBC, hematocrit, platelet count, and bleeding time, together with assessment of serum electrolytes, BUN and creatinine, and liver function. Severe anemia may require blood transfusion, but this will have little effect unless the underlying disease process is controlled by FFP infusions.

Parenteral analgesia often represents the safest approach for labor and vaginal delivery, but the mother with well-controlled TTP may have regional analgesia. Some TTP–controlled mothers present for cesarean section at 34 to 36 weeks, when amniotic fluid PG confirms fetal lung maturity. With an acceptable platelet count and normal bleeding time, TTP does not contraindicate regional techniques. In contrast to disseminated intravascular coagulation of pregnancy TTP may not necessarily resolve following delivery, but the expeditious performance of cesarean section once fetal maturity is assured removes one complicating factor (the fetus) and may improve maternal well-being.

Rarely, the anesthesiologist may be faced with a seriously ill TTP mother who has a bleeding diathesis. FFP must be immediately available, together with packed fresh RBCs to correct anemia. The severity of the mother's condition obviously necessitates general anesthesia, and the choice of intravenous induction agent depends on assessment of her circulation, hypotension favoring intravenous ketamine. As previously noted, hemorrhagic diathesis calls for extreme care with laryngoscopy and tracheal intubation. These seriously ill mothers have an increased likelihood of postpartum renal failure and require intensive care following delivery.

Uncontrolled TTP may lead to fetal demise, however, mothers who respond to FFP infusions usually deliver a healthy infant, though neonatal platelet function may be compromised if the mother has received antiplatelet agents. The neonatology team must attend in the operating room and be fully apprised of the mother's status.

COAGULATION COMPARTMENT DISORDERS

The Nature of Factor VIII

Factor VIII (FVIII)[145] describes that protein deficient or abnormal in hemophilia A (antihemophilic factor [AHF]). FVIII:C refers to its biologic activity as measured by coagulation assays. Von Willebrand factor (vWF) is the deficient or abnormal protein in von Willebrand's disease (vWd). Its function is reflected by measurement of the bleeding time, platelet adhesion, or platelet aggregation in the presence of ristocetin (ristocetin cofactor activity [VIIIR:RCo]). Factor VIII–related antigen (FVIIIR:Ag) describes the antigenic determinants of vWf measured by bioassay. The vWF circulates in plasma in a multimeric complex with FVIII, and the levels of both factors increase during pregnancy. Von Willebrand factor forms the largest proportion of the FVIII–vWF complex, occurring in a ratio as high as 50 to 1 with respect to FVIII. Hemophilia A, an X-linked disease, results from low or undetectable levels of FVIII. Because vWF levels are normal or even increased bleeding time remains normal.

Von Willebrand's Disease

Usually inherited as an autosomal-dominant disorder, vWD affects approximately one in 10,000 persons and is the commonest hereditary coagulation defect during pregnancy.[10,90,146,147] The disease assumes two main forms: Type I, a quantitative deficiency with a normal multimeric profile, but at a reduced level, and Type II, a qualitative defect with abnormal plasma VIIIR:Ag multimeric profiles (further subdivided into Types IIA, IIB, and IIC). The clinical symptoms and laboratory investigation further classify vWd as mild or severe. The mild form, inherited as an autosomal-dominant, is characterized by a bleeding

Table 14–5. FACTOR ASSAY IN VON WILLEBRAND'S DISEASE (vWd)

	Type I (%)	Type II (%)
Mild vWd (autosomal dominant)		
Ivy bleeding time 12–24 min		
FVIII C*	10–40	25–100
FVIII R:Agt	5–40	60–100
Severe vWd (autosomal recessive)		
Ivy bleeding time >30 min		
FVIII C*	2–5	25–50
FVIII R:Agt	<5	60–100

*FVIII C = Factor VIII procoagulant activity
†FVIII R:Ag = Factor VIII related antigen
(Reprinted, with modifications, from Nilsson IM, et al[147] with permission.)

time in the range of 12 to 24 min. Severe vWd, an autosomal-recessive condition, has a bleeding time longer than 30 min (Table 14–5). The relatively low frequency of complications during pregnancy probably reflects the generally benign nature of vWd.

In patients with severe vWd bleeding begins in childhood but often improves with age. Clinical features may include menorrhagia, epistaxis, bleeding from mucous membranes, and excessive bleeding following surgery or accidental trauma. Muscle and joint bleeds, which characterize hemophilia A, occur very rarely in vWd. Patients with mild vWd, in contrast, may have no symptoms, and the diagnosis becomes suspect only after excessive postsurgical bleeding. Coagulation tests may demonstrate prolongation of the aPTT, reflecting the depression of FVIII:C and impairment of the coagulation pathway. Prothrombin time and TCT remain unchanged.

In normal pregnancy FVIII:C and FVIIIR:Ag gradually increase to, approximately, 200 and 375 percent, respectively.[95] In vWd these factor levels similarly increase as pregnancy advances but peak, at term, at about one half the normal nonpregnant level.[148] Along with the increase in factor levels bleeding time can also improve.

Von Willebrand's disease does not increase maternal mortality or fetal loss, but patients have an increased risk of postpartum hemorrhage when FVIII:C and FVIIIR:Ag fall to nonpregnant levels after delivery. Mothers who fail to normalize their bleeding time during pregnancy or have persistently low levels of FVIII:C (<50 percent at term) require supportive transfusion, preferably with cryoprecipitate (or FFP) to bring factor levels above 50 percent.[149] Typically, they respond by producing new FVIII in vivo and improve even if the plasma comes from hemophilia A subjects, since FVIIIR:Ag (vWf) is the missing factor. Mothers having cesarean section need higher FVIII:C levels (approximately 80 percent) and a normal bleeding time. Caldwell and colleagues[89] recommend 15 to 20 units of cryoprecipitate twice daily for patients who fail to correct their bleeding time or increase FVIII:C levels in pregnancy to 50 percent or greater.

Anesthetic Considerations. The risk of spontaneous bleeding in patients with hereditary coagulopathies increases the likelihood of an epidural hematoma, and permanent neurologic damage, following epidural, caudal, or spinal anesthesia. An epidural vein lacerated during the procedure may not bleed excessively in labor (when clotting parameters remain normal), but can bleed significantly when FVIII levels decline postpartum. Therefore, labor analgesia should generally be restricted to narcotic and inhalation techniques, since conduction anesthesia requires complete investigation of the hemostatic deficit and planned cryoprecipitate therapy. (However, I believe mothers with mild or variant [Type II] vWd who have minimal symptoms when not pregnant and a normal bleeding time during pregnancy can have safe conduction anesthesia.) Von Willebrand's disease remains an unpredictable entity, and anesthesiologists would always be wiser to employ narcotic and inhalation techniques in the first instance. While outlet forceps deliveries can be performed under ketamine analgesia (0.25 mg per kg and increments of 10 mg to a maximum of 100 mg), supplemented with nitrous oxide if required, more complex maneuvers, such as Kielland's rotation, require general anesthesia. The proximity of the pudendal vessels makes pudendal nerve block inadvisable, although perineal infiltration of local anesthetic should not cause significant postoperative hematoma.

Because elective cesarean section requires full preoperative hemostatic evaluation, including an assessment of factor levels and planned cryoprecipitate therapy, I consider regional anesthesia feasible, especially in the mother with mild disease. The cryoprecipitate must normalize the bleeding time, aPTT, and factor levels. Subarachnoid block with a 25- or 26-gauge needle is probably the technique of choice, and the one least likely to lacerate a blood vessel. If the anesthesiologist employs epidural anesthesia and the block proves difficult or if significant bleeding occurs during catheter insertion the technique must be abandoned and the patient carefully observed postpartum for neurologic signs of developing cord compression.

Emergency cesarean section mandates general anesthesia, since complete hematologic evaluation may not prove feasible. Cryoprecipitate should be infused immediately before surgery to minimize intraoperative bleeding. As in other hemostatic disorders, extreme care must be taken to avoid airway trauma, and the gentle insertion of a small (6.0- to 6.5-mm), well-lubricated, low-pressure cuffed endotracheal tube will help to minimize airway trauma. Extubation also demands care, and the mother requires observation in an intensive care area during the immediate postpartum period because of the possibility of bleeding and respiratory obstruction.

Hemophilia A and B[89]

Being X-linked recessive disorders, classic hemophilia (FVIII : C deficiency) and Christmas disease (FIX deficiency, hemophilia B) normally produce an asymptomatic carrier female. Approximately 2 percent of hemophilia A carriers have symptoms of bleeding and unusually low factor levels, as a result of inactivation of the normal X chromosome during development. Hemophilia B carriers usually remain asymptomatic.

FVIII : C levels categorize the severity of the disease. Patients with severe hemophilia (FVIII : C <1 percent of the normal mean) have spontaneous, sometimes severe bleeding, and hemarthroses. Those with factor levels in the 1- to 4-percent range rarely bleed spontaneously or suffer hemarthroses but they may experience severe bleeding from minor trauma. Patients who have mild hemophilia (factor levels between 5 and 30 percent) have no spontaneous bleeding and may not recognize that they have a bleeding deficiency until, for example, postsurgical bleeding occurs unexpectedly. The clinical features of hemophilia B are indistinguishable from those of hemophilia A.

Laboratory findings in hemophilia A include prolonged aPTT, normal PT and TCT, reduced FVIII : C, variable levels of VIIIR : Ag, and a normal bleeding time (which distinguishes hemophilia from vWd). In FIX, deficiency factor levels similar to those in hemophilia A help classify the disease as mild or severe. These patients also have a prolonged aPTT, and usually normal PT (although this may be prolonged by 1 or 2 seconds).

FVIII : C and VIIIR : Ag rise steadily during normal pregnancy, and hemophilia A carriers may reach or exceed normal levels by term. Caldwell[89] reviews four cases of women with symptomatic hemophilia A, only one of whom had abnormal bleeding following delivery, presumably because of the post-delivery fall in FVIII : C levels. Delivery normally poses little hemorrhagic risk, even for affected male offspring, but fetal scalp electrodes should be avoided when the fetus is known to be male. Cord blood samples obtained at delivery will reveal a prolonged aPTT and reduced FVIII : C levels in affected males.

In hemophilia B, variable factor changes occur during pregnancy, although the levels of two other vitamin K–dependent factors (II and VII) increase, the former falling toward term. Pregnancies in affected hemophilia-B carriers, similarly, have an unpredictable outcome, and some may require plasma infusion or FIX concentrate (sometimes with concurrent plasmapheresis to avoid circulatory overload) to maintain a satisfactory factor level.[89] Factor IX concentrate carries a significant risk of hepatitis and AIDS (HIV) transmission.

Anesthetic Considerations in Hemophilia A and B. Asymptomatic hemophilia A carriers (factor levels >50 to 60 percent, aPTT normal) rarely experience bleeding problems during pregnancy and delivery and present no anesthetic hazard. In contrast, symptomatic carriers constitute a major anesthetic risk which contraindicates regional techniques. Preoperative assessment, in consultation with the hematologist and obstetrician, mandates a careful study of the patient's factor levels and indications for cryoprecipitate. A single donor product, cryoprecipitate carries less risk of disease transmission. Failure to detect the transmissible agent of non–A, non–B hepatitis means that FVIII concentrates, on the other hand, carry a high hepatitis risk as well as a risk of AIDS in areas where donor blood is not screened for HIV antibody. Cryoprecipitate contains 80 to 100 units per 10- to 15-ml bag, and uncomplicated vaginal delivery requires factor replacement to a 30- to 40-percent level. Cesarean section and extensive bleeding at vaginal delivery need replacement to between 80 and 100 percent. Calculation of the required cryoprecipitate dose involves estimation of the mother's plasma volume and a knowledge of the desired factor level. Plasma volume at term approximates 80 to 100 ml per kg, and a symptomatic 60-kg hemophilia–A carrier with an existing factor level of 5 percent would require 60 (kg) × 80 (estimated plasma volume: ml per kg) × 0.35 (percent factor increase required), or 1680 units (17 cryoprecipitate bags, dissolved and pooled) for vaginal delivery. To maintain an acceptable FVIII: C, the mother needs 50 percent of the initial replacement dose every 8 to 12 hours for 3 to 5 days after uncomplicated vaginal delivery or for 10 to 14 days after cesarean section. The poor prognosis of transfusional liver disease,[150] resistance to replacement therapy in 5 to 10 percent of patients, and the threat of treatment-related AIDS cause hemophiliacs understandable concern. Recent evidence suggests that 1-deamino-8-D-arginine vasopressin (DDAVP), a synthetic analog of antidiuretic hormone, produces a three- to sixfold increase in FVIII: C activity. It may be given intranasally, but intravenous administration in a dose of 0.3 μg per kg produces a more reliable response.[151] In subjects with mild hemophilia A, DDAVP has been employed successfully to treat minor bleeding episodes, to allow tooth extraction, and even for major surgery. Intravenous DDAVP may, in future, assume greater popularity as treatment for those with mild to moderate hemophilia or for symptomatic carriers, although no controlled studies have evaluated its use in pregnancy. (DDAVP may also prove beneficial in Type I von Willebrand's disease.)

FIX deficiency requires more aggressive replacement, because of a distribution volume 2.5 times plasma volume. However, factor levels of 40 to 50 percent suffice for normal delivery or cesarean section. Thus a 60-kg female with a factor level of 5 percent scheduled for vaginal delivery requires 60 × 200 (volume of distribution: ml per kg) × 0.45 FIX units. The hazards of FIX concentrates (hepatitis, AIDS, and inappropriate thrombosis) may call instead for plasma replacement, with concurrent plasmapheresis to avoid overload.

Although factor replacement may normalize factor levels and prevent bleeding, the coagulation defect in symptomatic hemophilia A and -B carriers contraindicates conduction anesthesia. The risk always exists that unexpected depletion of the appropriate factor may occur, with slow and steady bleeding from an epidural vein damaged by catheter insertion. In labor, intravenous narcotics and inhalation analgesia constitute acceptable alternatives to conduction anesthesia. These techniques also suffice for uncomplicated vaginal delivery, but more complicated procedures call for general anesthesia. Mothers who require factor replacement also have a significant risk of postoperative bleeding from damaged mucous membranes, and the anesthesiologist must exercise extreme care, as previously advised, in the performance of laryngoscopy and tracheal intubation. For cesarean section also, these mothers require general anesthesia after appropriate preoperative factor replacement.

Other Hereditary Factor Deficiencies in Pregnancy

Caldwell and associates[89] discuss in detail the extremely rare occurrence of other factor deficiencies in pregnancy. The anesthetic principles that apply to these conditions follow those outlined above.

THROMBOEMBOLIC DISEASE

Pulmonary Embolism

Pulmonary embolism remains a major cause of maternal mortality. In the triennium 1978 to 1981, 28 deaths occurred in England and Wales (9.4 per 1 million pregnancies).[152] This represented a 50-percent reduction from 1976–1978, largely due to reduced mortality from pulmonary embolism following vaginal delivery. Despite this improvement, pulmonary embolism was the second leading cause of maternal mortality. The quoted incidence of nonfatal pulmonary embolism and deep venous thrombosis varies between 2 and 12 per 1000 deliveries, depending on the diagnostic techniques employed. The risk of thromboembolism in pregnancy and postpartum increases fivefold over that in the nonpregnant state, and thrombosis occurs three to six times more frequently postpartum than antepartum. Recent studies found deep-vein thrombosis in 0.7 per thousand pregnancies.[153,154] Risk factors include increased maternal age and parity, obesity, cesarean section, prolonged bed rest during pregnancy, estrogen therapy for lactation suppression, ABO blood group other than O, and antithrombin III (AT III) deficiency.[154,155]

Antithrombin III functions as the major inhibitor of thrombin, FXa, and other proteases, and inhibits coagulation in vivo.[86,89] An autosomal dominant AT III deficiency occurs, with estimated prevalence between 1 in 2000 and 1 in 5000.[156,157] The deficiency assumes two forms: classical AT III deficiency, in which the level of AT III antigen (AT III Ag) is below 50 percent of normal, and variant AT III in which AT III Ag level is normal but functional abnormalities exist in the molecule.[158] Between 70 and 94 percent of women with hereditary AT III deficiency develop thromboembolism in pregnancy or when taking the contraceptive pill. The majority of thrombotic incidents in AT III deficient women occur antepartum, in contrast to other causes of thromboembolism in pregnancy.

Pulmonary thromboembolism classically presents with pleuritic chest pain, sudden dyspnea, and hemoptysis leaving little doubt of the diagnosis. However, the patient may experience only mild pleuritic chest pain, with or without physical signs, and nonspecific or absent chest x-ray changes.

On physical examination the clinician may note tachycardia, atelectatic rales, increased jugular venous pressure, and a fourth heart sound in the left parasternal area. Massive embolization causes a left parasternal heave and fixed splitting of P_2. Nonspecific signs include tachypnea and a pleural friction rub.

Electrocardiography in significant embolization reveals an S wave in lead I, and a Q wave and inverted T in lead III ($S_IQ_3T_3$). T-wave inversion also occurs in leads V_1 to V_3, and a P pulmonale and right bundle branch block may also be evident. The chest x-ray may show diminished vascular markings, diaphragmatic elevation, and pleural effusion. Arterial blood gases may reveal a lowered PaO_2 and $PaCO_2$, but the normal respiratory alkalosis of pregnancy may limit their value. After a large pulmonary embolism, $PaCO_2$ increases abruptly, while end-tidal PCO_2 falls and may prove detectable on capnography.[159] Later, $PaCO_2$ values may be normal or decreased due to tachypnea. CVP and pulmonary artery pressures increase, while PCWP remains normal.[159] A ventilation-perfusion lung scan enables the most accurate diagnosis, and the short-duration isotopes expose the mother to no more radiation than a chest x-ray.[155,160]

Amniotic Fluid Embolism

On rare occasions (estimated incidence 1 in 8000 to 1 in 80,000) amniotic fluid embolism occurs. Differentiation from thrombotic embolism can be difficult, but occurrence in labor or in association with delivery, severe respiratory distress, cardiovascular collapse, and the onset of disseminated intravascular coagulation suggest amniotic fluid embolism. Thrombotic embolism, in contrast, more usually occurs in the puerperium.

Treatment of Pulmonary Embolism

Treatment depends on the severity of embolism and the magnitude of shock. A mother who sustains massive embolism with persistent shock and hypotension, PaO_2 below 60 mmHg, and oliguria may require cardiopulmonary bypass and pulmonary embolectomy. Inferior vena cava (IVC) ligation, or transvenous insertion of an umbrella filter under local anesthesia into the IVC are other possibilities.[161,162] Supportive therapy for these critically ill women, prior to transfer to the operating room for pulmonary embolectomy, includes tracheal intubation and ventilation with 100-percent oxygen; two large-bore intravenous lines; infusion of intravenous fluid to maintain a high venous pressure; augmentation of venous return (in the pregnant mother by left uterine displacement); an arterial line for direct estimation of arterial blood pressure and blood gas monitoring; intravenous sodium bicarbonate to correct acidosis; and infusion of inotropes (dopamine, dobutamine, or isoproterenol) for hypotension.

The majority of mothers with deep venous thrombosis and nonfatal pulmonary embolism receive anticoagulant therapy to avoid serious or fatal sequelae. The drug of choice, heparin, a high-molecular-weight (20,000 daltons) thrombin inhibitor that is highly polar in nature, does not cross the placenta or enter breast milk. Because of its relatively short half-life (1.5 hours) continuous intravenous infusion gives the best control. After a loading dose of 5000 to 10,000 units, infusion continues at a rate of 30,000 to 40,000 units per 24 hours. For life-threatening pulmonary embolism the aPTT (or TCT) should be maintained at least two or three times control, or the ACT at 1.5 to 2.5 times control, by continuous adjustment of the infusion rate. After stopping the intravenous infusion, de Swiet[155] recommends subcutaneous heparin, 10,000 units twice daily. Most patients readily learn to inject themselves and may be treated on an ambulatory basis. If heparin assay indicates a level in excess of 0.4 units per ml the dose must be reduced. Subcutaneous heparin does not increase bleeding if heparin levels remain below 0.4 unit per ml and may be given before and during labor. Alternative regimens employ heparin doses between 5000 and 15,000 units twice daily, or a dose to maintain the aPTT at 1.5 times control 6 hours following injection.

Patients with artificial heart valves generally require warfarin to prevent embolism.[155] This means these mothers must accept the increased risk of abortion and a small risk of teratogenesis. Very strict control of anticoagulation, maintaining the aPTT at 1.5 to 2 times normal, limits fetal loss to 15 percent. At 36 weeks the risk of fetal bleeding mandates stopping warfarin and switching to heparin, initially at 40,000 units per day then adjusted to maintain a level of 1 unit per ml. Two weeks after stopping warfarin, delivery can safely be accomplished, if necessary with the temporary discontinuance of heparin, which the mother recommences 6 to 12 hours following delivery.

Anticoagulant Prophylaxis in High-Risk Parturients

One episode of thromboembolism implies a 12-percent risk of repeat thrombosis during the same pregnancy, and a 5- to 10-percent chance of recurrence in subsequent pregnancies.[155,160] The use of prophylactic anticoagulants in such high-risk patients remains controversial. Former regimens employed warfarin until approximately 36 weeks' gestation followed by subcutaneous heparin in the last few weeks of pregnancy, but warfarin's adverse fetal effects make its general use less desirable. As an alternative, some obstetricians use subcutaneous heparin throughout the pregnancy, while others institute heparin prophylaxis only after the 34th week. Long-term heparin prophylaxis also causes adverse maternal effects, including thrombocytopenia, bone demineralization, alopecia, and possibly an increased risk of premature delivery. In view of heparin's adverse skeletal effects, some authorities use it for shorter periods (e.g., from 34 weeks' gestation onward) or in smaller doses (short-term use of 10,000 units daily appears to carry no increased risk of osteoporosis). Others substitute dextran prophylaxis in labor, and recommence heparin for 6 weeks postpartum. Indications for heparin prophylaxis include, in addition to previous thromboembolism, multiparity, obesity, immobilization during pregnancy, diabetes, hypertension, some cardiac diseases, and severe varicose veins.[163]

Pregnancy contraindicates the prostaglandin inhibitors, such as indomethacin, since they cross the placenta and promote premature closure of the ductus arteriosus.[164]

AT III deficiency, because of the extreme risk of thromboembolism, requires special management. Mothers switch from warfarin, which they take routinely when not pregnant, to subcutaneous heparin, 10,000 units twice daily, aiming for a 10-sec prolongation of aPTT *before* conception. The aPTT monitors heparin therapy at least twice weekly during pregnancy, until delivery. Immediately before delivery, heparin is reduced to 5000 units twice daily, administered concurrently with AT III infusions on alternate days, to achieve AT III levels greater than 80 percent. The reduction of heparin and institution of AT III normalizes aPTT, and the regimen continues until 7 days postpartum, when the mother recommences warfarin. Affected neonates (cord blood AT III 20 to 30 percent of normal activity) also need AT III by infusion, since they have an increased risk of aortic occlusion.[155,158,165]

Anesthetic Considerations for Patients Receiving Anticoagulants. From the anesthesiologist's viewpoint, parturients receiving anticoagulants fall into two groups: (1) Low-dose (prophylactic) regimens, given to reduce the incidence of thromboembolism, and usually not associated with abnormality of any coagulation tests; and (2) High-dose (therapeutic) regimens, administered to treat existing thromboembolism or, less frequently, as prophylaxis in high-risk parturients, and *deliberately* intended to prolong the coagulation tests (aPTT 1.5 to 2.5 times control). Mothers in this second group carry an increased risk of epidural or spinal hematoma with subsequent spinal cord compression, should they undergo epidural or subarachnoid anesthesia.

Epidural, subdural, and subarachnoid bleeding, although rare, have occurred spontaneously, in association with anticoagulant or antiplatelet therapy, and following needle insertion into the epidural or subarachnoid space. Odoom and Sih[166] refer to more than 100 cases of spinal and epidural hematoma (some anesthesia-related), approximately one third of which were associated with anticoagulant therapy. Owens and colleagues,[167] in a case report and comprehensive review of spinal hematoma after lumbar puncture and heparinization, cite 33 cases of spinal hematoma with neurologic dysfunction, following attempted lumbar puncture (n = 27) or spinal anesthesia (n = 6). Thirteen (40 percent) had received anticoagulant therapy, the majority of them *after* the lumbar puncture; another thirteen had coagulation abnormalities, predominantly thrombocytopenia ($<50 \times 10^9$ per liter); in addition, some were receiving antiplatelet therapy while others had pathologic states with an associated coagulopathy. Of the six cases following spinal anesthesia, one exhibited a prolonged bleeding time and two had received antiplatelet therapy. Owens[167] also documents approximately 48 spontaneous spinal hematomas in association with anticoagulants or clotting abnormalities.

Rao and El-Etr[168] reported more than 3000 continuous epidural blocks, and approximately 850 patients receiving continuous subarachnoid anesthesia, all of whom commenced therapeutic heparin (ACT 174 ± 30 sec, approximately twice baseline), about 1 hour after institution of regional anesthesia. None developed signs of subarachnoid or epidural hematoma. A similar report described intrathecal morphine administration to 40 cardiac surgery patients 50 min before heparinization, without neurologic sequelae.[169] Odoom and Sih[166] document their experience of 1000 lumbar epidural blocks in patients undergoing vascular surgery, all of whom received preoperative oral anticoagulants, which prolonged the aPTT. The majority also received intraoperative heparin following establishment of the block, and in many cases the anticoagulants continued into the postoperative period. No patient developed neurologic complications, but 10 percent had poorly localized backache for 3 to 5 days following anesthesia. The authors excluded patients with blood dyscrasias, thrombocytopenia, leukemia, hemophilia, and those who are receiving preoperative intravenous heparin or prolonged aspirin. They consider epidural anesthesia safe, if the ACT remains below 200 sec, and analgesia wears off at intervals to allow assessment of motor and sensory function before each top-up.

Collectively, the above case reports demonstrate that spinal and epidural hematomas can occur spontaneously and in association with anticoagulants, with or without anesthetic intervention. They also demonstrate that some authors successfully employ subarachnoid and epidural techniques in anticoagulated patients, and in those about to receive anticoagulants. I do not consider the use of epidural or subarachnoid anesthesia justifiable in parturients receiving *therapeutic* doses of anticoagulants. The risk of spinal cord compression and resultant paraplegia, I believe, outweighs any advantages of conduction techniques in this situation. However, regional anesthesia for mothers receiving low-dose ("minidose") heparin remains a source of controversy. To date, no case reports or prospective studies document the safety or danger of spinal or epidural techniques in these subjects, and anesthesiologists in many institutions administer epidural or subarachnoid block to those receiving minidose heparin. Low-dose heparin combines with AT III to inhibit FXa, usually without disturbing coagulation, although variable effects occur in different subjects. Cooke and others[170] demonstrated that approximately 50 percent of patients receiving heparin prophylaxis (5000 units twice daily) have therapeutic, rather than prophylactic, heparin blood levels for up to 4 hours following the last dose. Therefore, ACT or aPTT should be checked, and confirmed to be normal, before commencing epidural or subarachnoid anesthesia. However, on the basis of currently available information, Owens and colleagues[167] recommend avoiding subarachnoid anesthesia in patients receiving minidose heparin unless "strong indications" favor this type of technique.

I believe that many conditions — obesity, diabetes, hypertension, severe varicose veins — indicate epidural or subarachnoid block for parturients undergoing cesarean section. Epidural anesthesia causes less postoperative morbidity than general anesthesia and may reduce the incidence of pulmonary embolism and venous thrombosis in lower limb vessels.[171,172] Postoperative fibrinolytic activity also increases following epidural block in healthy premenopausal women who have abdominal hysterectomy.[173] I therefore employ epidural anesthesia for cesarean section in high-risk thromboembolism patients receiving minidose heparin prophylaxis but consider it advisable to take the following precautions:

1. The technique applies only to mothers receiving heparin no more frequently than every 12 hours.
2. Before institution of epidural or subarachnoid block, the ACT or aPTT must be within normal limits.
3. Perform epidural block with the patient in the left lateral position to reduce aortic compression and distension of epidural veins.
4. Use a midline approach to the epidural space, since lateral techniques will more likely lacerate epidural vessels.
5. Abandon the procedure and proceed to alternate anesthesia if a traumatic tap or significant bleeding occurs, suggesting damage to an epidural vein.

In labor, the choice of regional techniques also depends on weighing advantages against potential disadvantages. Parturients at high risk for thromboembolism deserve strong consideration of regional techniques. In the absence of other contraindications (e.g., thrombocytopenia), epidural block can be undertaken, but should be allowed to wear off at intervals to confirm the return of sensory and motor function. Any signs or symptoms suggesting spinal or epidural hematoma call for early surgical assessment, and possible intervention, to minimize the incidence of permanent neurologic sequelae.[167]

Hemolytic Disease of the Newborn

Hemolytic disease of the newborn (HDN) describes a group of conditions that usually result from the transplacental passage of fetal erythrocytes (RBCs), having an antigen foreign to the mother (e.g., Rh – D antigen), into the maternal circulation. After exposure to the antigen, the mother at first produces "saline-reacting" (complete) antibody. This high-molecular-weight IgM antibody (890,000 daltons) does not cross placenta and poses no risk to the fetus, but indicates that maternal isoimmunization has occurred. Soon afterward the mother produces a 7S – IgG antibody (160,000 daltons; blocking or incomplete antibody), which crosses the placenta and coats the fetal D – positive RBCs by attaching to surface receptors.[174] Those fetal RBCs coated with immunoglobulins bind rapidly to splenic macrophages, which readily induce their destruction.[175] The IgG−3 antibody causes a much more severe form of HDN, while infants with IgG−1 coated RBCs undergo hemolysis of variable severity.

Usually, the fetal RBCs enter the maternal circulation during pregnancy or immediately after delivery. Etiologic factors include placental accidents, spontaneous or induced abortions, ectopic pregnancy, and amniocentesis. Significant transplacental hemorrhage follows therapeutic abortion. Maternal sensitization to the Rh−D antigen and to several "irregular" antigens (e.g., Lewis, Kell, Duffy) may follow previous blood transfusion. In one study, 70 percent of Rh−positive women, with non−Rh antibodies, gave a history of previous blood transfusion, in contrast to an incidence of previous transfusion in 5 to 6 percent of healthy women.[176] Since maternal antibodies may induce HDN, such figures emphasize the hazards of unnecessary blood transfusion to women in the reproductive years.

Fetomaternal ABO incompatibility represents the commonest cause of HDN, and "irregular" antibodies (Lewis, Kell, etc.) account for only 2 to 5 percent of incompatibility.[175,177] However, irregular antibodies rarely cause severe HDN, and maternal alloantibody to the fetal Rh−D antigen remains the commonest cause of severe fetal hemolytic anemia and hydrops fetalis.

Erythroblastosis fetalis has been classically associated with an Rh−D positive fetus in an Rh−D negative mother, but the tremendous strides in Rh isoimmunization prophylaxis, by the use of Rh immune globulin (RhIG), have reduced the prevalence of such alloimmunization from, approximately, 10 to 1.5 per 1000 total births.[178] Unfortunately, Rh alloimmunization still occurs, due to failure to administer RhIG, its failure to have an effect, or the spontaneous occurrence of maternal antibodies before 28 weeks' gestation. Without treatment, 45 to 50 percent of isoimmunized infants survive. Twenty-five to 30 percent, although born alive, succumb to their disease in the first few days of life, and the remaining 20 to 25 percent will be stillborn or hydropic before term.[174,179] Although accurate fetal assessment, and intrauterine fetal transfusion, improve the outcome for these fetuses, obstetric anesthesiologists may still encounter mothers who have cesarean section for severely anemic or hydropic infants.

PATHOPHYSIOLOGY OF ERYTHROBLASTOSIS FETALIS

Irrespective of antibody type, all HDN cases demonstrate similar pathogenesis. The maternal alloantibody crosses the placental barrier and attaches to fetal RBCs. The subsequent destruction of these antibody-coated fetal RBCs initiates a fetal hemolytic anemia and a compensatory increase in erythropoietin production in an attempt to counter RBC depletion. Initially, all fetal marrow resources respond to the anemia; then extramedullary sites, especially liver and spleen, and release immature nucleated RBCs (erythroblasts) into the circulation. When hemolysis exceeds compensation, anemia, hyperbilirubinemia, and hepatosplenomegaly develop as the reticuloendothelial (RE) system adopts the dual role of extramedullary hematopoiesis and RBC destruction.

In 20 to 25 percent of fetuses with Rh erythroblastosis, severe hemolysis occurs, and the fetus ultimately develops generalized edema and extreme ascites (hydrops fetalis).[179] Hydrops results not from heart failure but from marked distortion and enlargement of liver parenchyma by erythropoiesis. As a consequence portal and umbilical venous hypertension occur. The fetus also develops hypoalbuminemia because of the liver's impaired synthesizing capacity. This exacerbates the ascites, and edema becomes more severe and generalized, with pleuropericardial effusions (hydrops). In the final stage of hydrops, hydrothorax causes compression hypoplasia of the lungs which, together with pulmonary edema, makes neonatal respiratory exchange virtually impossible. The hydropic fetus looks pale and bloated, with marked edema and jaundice. Petechial hemorrhages often result from thrombocytopenia. Bile discolors the amniotic fluid, and placental edema results from umbilical veinous hypertension. Since hepatic dysfunction, not anemia, causes the hydrops, hydropic fetuses demonstrate variable hemoglobin levels.[180] All such infants require immediate intensive care and exchange transfusion with compatible O Rh D− negative whole blood, crossmatched against the mother. Immediate exchange transfusion usually becomes necessary in mature neonates with cord hemoglobin levels less than 120 g per liter.[76,179]

HDN presents a variable spectrum at birth, from fully developed hydrops fetalis to barely perceptible hemolytic anemia. Less severely affected fetuses transfer bilirubin, as normally in utero, transplacentally to the mother's circulation. Conjugation and excretion take place in maternal liver, accounting for the absence of icterus at delivery. However, following birth, the increased hemolysis elevates the neonate's indirect bilirubin and increases the risk of bilirubin encephalopathy (kernicterus). Indirect bilirubin binds to albumin, but its free fraction crosses the blood-brain barrier. A bilirubin level exceeding 20 mg per dl (345 μmol per liter) represents a significant risk for kernicterus.[175]

ANTENATAL MANAGEMENT OF THE RH-SENSITIZED WOMAN

When maternal antibodies exist at the onset of pregnancy or develop before RhIG prophylaxis the mother's management involves predicting the severity of fetal erythroblastosis and modifying it by early delivery, sometimes combined with intrauterine transfusion.[179] The introduction of amniotic fluid spectrophotometry[181] and further refinements of the technique[182] enable an accurate assessment of fetal status. Factors involved in timing amniocentesis include the antibody titer, duration of any high titer, and previous maternal history. The initial "tap" may be undertaken as early as 20 weeks' gestation or as late as 36 weeks', depending on these criteria. The obstetrician must balance the risks of intrauterine fetal transfusion (IUT) and continued intrauterine life against those of respiratory distress syndrome, immaturity, and extrauterine survival. Because approximately 8 percent of affected fetuses succumb before 32 weeks' gestation IUT is the principal treatment in this group. Improved neonatal care may, in future, advance the delivery date to between 28 and 30 weeks, but most authorities presently recommend IUT up to 30 to 32 weeks' gestation and early delivery after that.[174,179,180]

Some centers now use direct intravascular fetal transfusion (IVT) in second-trimester fetuses.[180,183] The technique accurately defines the severity of Rh hemolytic disease (by measurement of fetal hemoglobin), confirms fetal blood group, and facilitates rapid correction of anemia. The development of hydrops (as reflected by reticulocytosis and circulating erythroblasts) correlates with cord hemoglobin concentrations of 40 g per liter or less. Intravascular transfusion involves puncture of an umbilical cord artery under direct vision at fetoscopy, fetal blood sampling for hematologic and biochemical indices, and infusion of fresh Rh–negative blood (hematocrit 0.6 to 0.8, and compatible with the mother) manually through a 5-ml syringe, at a rate of 1 to 3 ml per minute. Because amniotic fluid spectrophotometry correlates poorly with the degree of fetal anemia in second-trimester pregnancies, fetoscopic IVT will probably become the technique of choice for this group of babies.

Other therapeutic approaches to the management of Rh–isoimmunized pregnancies have included maternal plasmapheresis, prevention of fetal hemolysis by immunosuppression of the fetal phagocytic system, maternal ingestion of Rh D–positive red-cell extracts, and alteration of the fetal blood group by bone marrow transplantation. None of these compares with fetoscopic IVT or, later, IUT.

Anesthetic Considerations in Rh Hemolytic Disease

The exciting advances in the prevention of Rh hemolytic disease have reduced the number of mothers with hydropic fetuses who present for cesarean section. However, the 8-percent failure rate of RhIG and the occurrence of severe isoimmunization to irregular antigens (notably Kell and Duffy), account for some mothers who require cesarean section at 32 to 34 weeks for delivery of a hydropic or severely anemic fetus. Inappropriate anesthesia in this situation increases fetal risk.

Preoperative assessment requires careful consideration of the anticipated fetal status and should exclude significant maternal complications. Fetal problems may include anemia, preterm gestation, a nonreactive nonstress test, and severe acidosis (Fig. 14–4). When compared with spinal anesthesia, epidural block carries less risk of hypotension, and the high-risk fetus tolerates poorly decreases in intervillous perfusion and oxygenation. The asphyxiated and compromised fetus transfers less local anesthetic to the mother, increasing its risk of local anesthetic toxicity.[184] Although some local an-

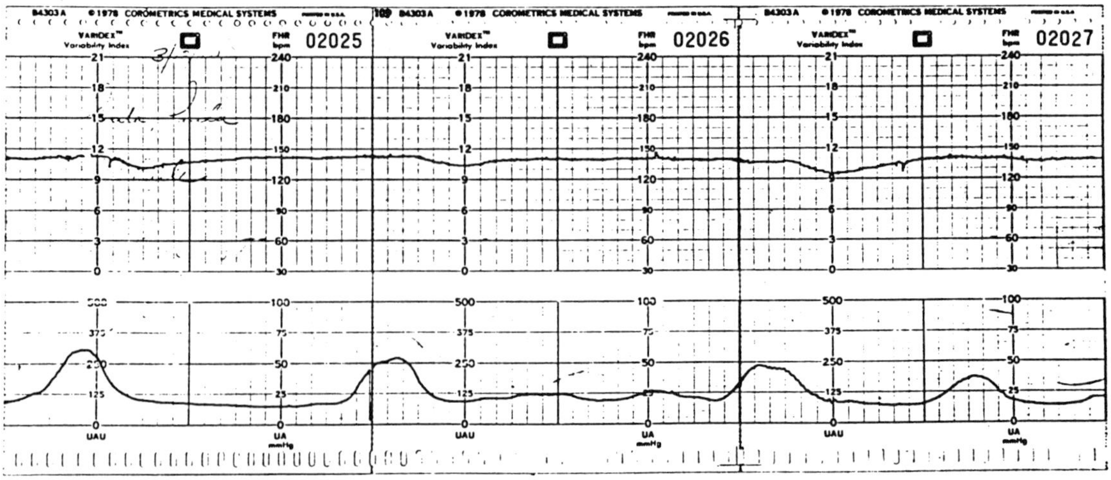

Figure 14–4. Fetal heart tracing of a fetus with severe Rh hemolytic disease recorded shortly before delivery and showing almost no beat-to-beat variability, with late decelerations. Contractions are Braxton-Hicks contractions, and gestational age was 34 weeks. A severely hydropic infant was born, with a hemoglobin of 37 g per liter, and hematocrit of 0.14. Umbilical vein pH was 6.9, and the severely depressed infant needed immediate resuscitation and respiratory care.

esthetics (e.g., lidocaine and mepivacaine; pKa 7.7 and 7.6, respectively), demonstrate ion trapping and higher blood levels in the acidotic fetus,[185] this finding may be more theoretical than practical. No single agent appears to possess obvious advantages for cesarean section in fetal hydrops. The amide compounds cause less hypotension but result in higher fetal blood levels, while 2-chloroprocaine undergoes rapid maternal metabolism (with consequently low fetal levels) but carries an increased risk of hypotension.[186] Whichever drug the anesthesiologist chooses should be administered incrementally, with great care to avoid hypotension and to immediately correct any fall in blood pressure with ephedrine. Maternal prehydration with Ringer's lactate 30 ml per kg, while not affecting the incidence of maternal hypotension, diminishes its severity.[187] The mother should breathe 100-percent oxygen from the commencement of anesthesia to ensure maximum fetal and neonatal $PuvO_2$.[36]

When obstetric urgency contraindicates epidural block, spinal or general anesthesia become necessary, but the former carries a significant risk of hypotension and fetal compromise. General anesthesia, like epidural block, demands a left lateral tilt and careful maternal preoxygenation. The four-deep-breaths technique effectively increases maternal PaO_2.[188] If time permits, I preoxygenate the mother with 100-percent oxygen for 3 to 5 min. The premature hydropic fetus has a significant risk of intracranial hemorrhage in the neonatal period, as a result of intrapartum asphyxia. Pickering[189] and coworkers, in asphyxiated sheep fetuses with increased regional cerebral blood flow (rCBF), identified a potentially deleterious fall in cerebral perfusion when inducing maternal anesthesia with thiopental. Ketamine, in contrast, had no adverse effect in this situation, suggesting that its use may be preferable in the mother with a potentially asphyxiated, preterm, hydropic fetus. The mother should receive 100-percent oxygen until delivery of the infant, to maximize fetal PO_2, with the addition of enflurane 1- to 1.5-percent, or halothane 0.5- to 0.7-percent. These doses of volatile agent have no adverse effect on uterine blood flow.[41] End-tidal carbon dioxide monitoring lessens the possibility of maternal hyperventilation and diminished uteroplacental flow.

The severely distressed condition of the hydropic fetus mandates the presence of a neonatology team, fully equipped to handle the emergency, in the operating room well in advance of delivery. Possible heart failure, neonatal asphyxia, and stiff congested lungs require immediate tracheal intubation and ventilation with 100-percent oxygen. Umbilical cord blood must be obtained immediately for measurement of hemoglobin, hematocrit, bilirubin, blood-gas values, and a Coombs' test. Exchange transfusion may prove necessary in the delivery room in the most severe cases.

Summary

The formed elements of blood circulating in a protein-rich plasma subserve the functions of oxygen transport, defense of the organism by inflammation, cell-mediated and humoral immunity, and hemostasis. Hematologic disorders affect one or more of these functions.

Anemias result from impaired hemoglobin synthesis (e.g., deficiency anemias, thalassemias), or excessive RBC destruction (hemolytic anemias). For labor and vaginal delivery most anemic mothers tolerate narcotic techniques or regional anesthesia well. More severe anemia requires CVP (sometimes PCWP) monitoring, and epidural block must be carefully titrated to the mother's response, to avoid hypotension, reduced intervillous blood flow, and impaired maternal-fetal oxygen delivery. Epidural block offers particular advantages for cesarean section, but the more extensive sympatholysis requires careful attention to blood pressure and oxygen delivery with appropriate monitoring. General anesthesia superimposes risks of maternal hypoxia, and cardiac decompensation in severely hypervolemic parturients. Blood transfusion to correct anemia should generally be avoided in women of child-bearing age. Severe anemia rarely occurs, and maternal compensation, not hemoglobin concentration, defines the maternal status.

Sickling disorders represent a severe hemolytic anemia, due to structurally defective Hb. In response to adverse stimuli like hypoxia and acidosis, RBCs aggregate and occlude the microcirculation. The resultant anemia may seriously affect oxygen transport. These disorders merit exceptional obstetric and anesthesia care to avoid sickling crises. Prenatal care aims to achieve an HbA concentration in excess of 40 percent by prophylactic or therapeutic transfusion. Anesthesia requires careful preanesthetic assessment, close attention to intraoperative hydration and electrolyte balance, and an "obsessive" avoidance of hypotension and hypoxemia. Epidural block gives excellent labor analgesia, but most centers employ balanced general anesthesia for cesarean section. The anesthesiologist should use continuous pulse oximetry to monitor maternal oxygenation.

The anesthetic management of leukemic mothers depends on the degree of maternal anemia and thrombocytopenia. Preanesthetic care should optimize the mother's status, and regional techniques are preferred in patients with a normal platelet count and bleeding time. Chemotherapy increases the risk of fetal loss or malformation.

The coagulation disorders pose a potpourri of problems. Thrombocytopenia (<80 to 100×10^9 per liter) generally contraindicates regional techniques because of the risk of epidural hematoma. In immunologic thrombocytopenic purpura (ITP), an IgG antibody, which crosses placenta, induces maternal, and variable fetal, thrombocytopenia. The mother may have a normal bleeding time because of enhanced platelet competence, allowing epidural or subarachnoid block. In severe ITP, however, platelet transfusion only transiently corrects thrombocytopenia and abnormal hemostasis, and these mothers require intravenous narcotics for labor analgesia and general anesthesia for cesarean section. Intravenous immunoglobin G may generate short-term (3 to 4 weeks) improvement in ITP and make possible the use of regional techniques.

Von Willebrand's disease (vWd) and hemophilia A and B variably affect coagulation. Mild or asymptomatic cases may not contraindicate regional anesthesia, but more severe defects require alternative labor analgesia. Pregnancy generally improves these coagulopathies, and anesthesiologists selecting regional block should recognize that coagulation may deteriorate immediately after delivery, increasing the risk of epidural hematoma. In vWd, preoperative administration of cryoprecipitate gives prolonged correction of hemostasis, enabling regional techniques for parturients having planned cesarean section. However, cryoprecipitate produces only temporary improvement in hemophilia, negating epidural or subarachnoid block. Parturients requiring general anesthesia because of their coagulopathy risk postpartum respiratory obstruction from any airway trauma and severe postpartum hemorrhage. Hemophiliacs may need cryoprecipitate for up to 10 to 14 days; intravenous DDAVP may also improve coagulation in vWd and hemophilia A.

Anticoagulated parturients, at high risk for thromboembolism, remain a source of controversy for anesthesiologists. Therapeutic anticoagulation contraindicates regional block; in contrast, regional techniques deserve serious consideration in high-risk parturients on minidose heparin. Preoperative evaluation should exclude an unexpected prolongation of the ACT or aPTT, and the regional technique demands great care to minimize trauma to epidural veins.

References

1. Longo, LD: Maternal blood volume and cardiac output during pregnancy: A hypothesis of endocrinologic control. Am J Physiol 245:720, 1983.
2. Hytten, F: Blood volume changes in normal pregnancy. Clin Haematol 14:601, 1985.
3. Taylor, DJ and Lind, T: Red cell mass during and after normal pregnancy. Br J Obstet Gynaecol 86:364, 1979.
4. Pitkin, RM and Witte, DL: Platelet and leukocyte counts in pregnancy. JAMA 242:2696, 1979.
5. Fletcher, J and Suter, PE. The transfer of iron by the human placenta. Clin Sci 36:209, 1969.
6. Chanarin, I: Folate and cobalamin. Clin Haematol 14:629, 1985.
7. Harrison, KA: Anaemia, malaria and sickle cell disease. Clin Obstet Gynaecol 9:445, 1982.
8. Mayet, FG: Anaemia of pregnancy. S Afr Med J 67:804, 1985.
9. Bentley, DP: Iron metabolism and anaemia in pregnancy. Clin Haematol 14:613, 1985.
10. Levin, J: Hematologic disorders of pregnancy. In Burrow, GN and Ferris, TF (eds): Medical Complications During Pregnancy, ed 2. WB Saunders, Philadelphia, 1982, p 62.
11. Worwood, M: Ferritin in human tissues and serum. Clin Haematol 11:275, 1982.
12. Taylor, DJ: Prophylaxis and treatment of anaemia during pregnancy. Clin Obstet Gynaecol 8:297, 1981.
13. Letsky, E: Blood volume, haematinics, anaemia. In de Swiet, M (ed): Medical Disorders in Obstetric Practice. Blackwell Scientific, Oxford, 1984, p 35.
14. Knispel, JW, Lynch, VA and Viele, BD: Aplastic anemia in pregnancy: A case report, review of the literature and a re-evaluation of management. Obstet Gynecol Surv 31:523, 1976.
15. Doney, K, et al: Marrow transplantation for treatment of pregnancy-associated aplastic anemia. Exp Hematol 13:1080, 1985.
16. Lehman, G and Alcoff, J: Reversible pure red cell hypoplasia in pregnancy. JAMA 247:1171, 1982.
17. Picot, C, et al: Relapsing pure red-cell aplasia during pregnancy. N Engl J Med 311:196, 1984.
18. Slater, LM, et al: Aplastic anemia occurring as amegakaryocytic thrombocytopenia with and without an inhibitor of granulopoiesis. Am J Hematol 18:251, 1985.
19. Evans, IL: Aplastic anaemia in pregnancy remitting after abortion. Br Med J 3:166, 1968.
20. Crisp, AJ: Remission of pregnancy hypoplastic anaemia and "malignant" pre-eclampsia after delivery: A case report and discussion. Br J Clin Pract 34:304, 1980.
21. Watson-Williams, EJ: Hematologic and hemostatic considerations before surgery. Med Clin North Am 63:1165, 1972.
22. Gillies, ID: Anaemia and anaesthesia. Br J Anaesth 46:589, 1974.
23. Allen, JB and Allen, FB: The minimum acceptable level of hemoglobin. Int Anesthesiol Clin 20:1, 1982.
24. Eltherington, LG: Anesthesia for the patient with hematologic disease. In 35th Annual Refresher Course Lectures. American Society of Anesthesiologists, Park Ridge, IL, 1984, p 101.
25. Sproule, BJ, Mitchell JH and Miller, WF: Cardiopulmonary physiological responses to heavy exercise in patients with anemia. J Clin Invest 39:378, 1960.
26. Varat, MA, Adolph, RJ and Fowler, NO: Cardiovascular effects of anemia. Am Heart J 83:415, 1982.
27. Kelman, GR, et al: The influence of cardiac output on arterial oxygenation: A theoretical study. Br J Anaesth 39:450, 1967.
28. Bevan, DR, et al: Closing volume and pregnancy. Br Med J 1:13, 1974.
29. Russell, IF and Chambers, IF: Closing volume in normal pregnancy. Br J Anaesth 53:1043, 1981.
30. Joynson, DH, et al: Defect of cell mediated immunity in patients with iron deficiency anaemia. Lancet 2:1058, 1972.
31. Srikantia, SG, et al: Anaemia and immune response. Lancet 1:1307, 1976.
32. Kowalyshyn, TJ, Prager, D and Young, J: A review of the present status of preoperative hemoglobin requirements. Anesth Analg 51:75, 1972.
33. Myhre, BA: Fatalities from blood transfusion. JAMA 24:1333, 1980.
34. Bromage PR: Epidural Analgesia. WB Saunders, Philadelphia, 1978.
35. Robinson, JO, et al: Self-administered intravenous and intramuscular pethidine: A controlled trial in labour. Anaesthesia 35:763, 1980.
36. Ramanathan, S, et al: Oxygen transfer from mother to fetus during cesarean section under epidural anaesthesia. Anesth Analg 61:576, 1982.
37. Jouppila, P and Kirkinen, P: Umbilical vein blood flow in the human fetus in cases of maternal and fetal anemia and uterine bleeding. Ultrasound Med Biol 10:365, 1984.
38. Lah, F, Giles, WR and Trudinger, BJ: Epidural anaesthesia for caesarean section and its effect on maternal uterine and foetal umbilical placental arterial blood flow velocity-time waveforms (abstr). Can Anaesth Soc J 32:S76, 1985.
39. Moir, DD: Anaesthesia for cesarean section: An evaluation of a method using low concentrations of halo-

thane and 50 percent of oxygen. Br J Anaesth 42:136, 1970.

40. Abboud, TK, et al: Comparative maternal neonatal effects of halothane and enflurane for cesarean section. Acta Anaesthesiol Scand 29:663, 1985.
41. Shnider, SM, et al: Plasma norepinephrine and uterine blood flow changes during endotracheal intubation and general anaesthesia in the pregnant ewe (abstr). In Abstracts of Scientific Papers, Annual Meeting. American Society of Anesthesiologists, Chicago, 1978, p 115.
42. Hansen, JM and Ueland, K: The influence of caudal analgesia on cardiovascular dynamics during labor and delivery. Acta Anaesthesiol Scand Suppl 23:449, 1966.
43. Bay, J, Nunn, JF and Prys-Roberts, C: Factors influencing arterial PO_2 during recovery from anesthesia. Br J Anaesth 40:398, 1968.
44. Lehmann, H and Hunstman, RG: An introduction to the structure and function of haemoglobin. Clin Haematol 3:217, 1974.
45. Perutz, MF: Hemoglobin structure and respiratory transport. Sci Am 239:92, 1978.
46. Morrison, JC: Hemoglobinopathies and pregnancy. Clin Obstet Gynecol 22:819, 1979.
47. McLaughlin, BN, Martin, RW and Morrison, JC: Clinical management of sickle cell hemoglobinopathies during pregnancy. Clin Perinatol 12:585, 1985.
48. Gibson, JR: Anesthetic implications of sickle cell anemia and other hemoglobinopathies. In 36th Annual Refresher Course Lectures. American Society of Anesthesiologists, Park Ridge, IL, 1985, p 231.
49. McKay, ML, Martin, JN, Jr and Morrison, JC: Disseminated intravascular coagulation, idiopathic thrombocytopenic purpura, and hemoglobinopathies. In Knuppel, RA and Drukker, JE (eds): High Risk Pregnancy. A Team Approach. WB Saunders, Philadelphia, 1986, p 440.
50. Charache, S and Niebyl, JR: Pregnancy in sickle cell disease. Clin Haematol 14:729, 1985.
51. Kaufmann, L and Sumner, E: Anaemia. In Medical Problems and the Anaesthetist. Edward Arnold, London, 1979, p 139.
52. Noguchi, CT and Schechter, AN: The intracellular polymerization of sickle hemoglobin and its relevance to sickle cell disease. Blood 58:1057, 1981.
53. Walsh, TD: Antidepressants in chronic pain. Clin Neuropharmacol 6:271, 1983.
54. Martin, JN and Morrison, JC: Managing the parturient with sickle cell crisis. Clin Obstet Gynecol 27:39, 1984.
55. Morrison, JC, Blake, PG and Reed CD: Therapy for the pregnant patient with sickle hemoglobinopathies: A national focus. Am J Obstet Gynecol 144:268, 1982.
56. Huehns, ER: The structure and function of haemoglobin: Clinical disorders due to abnormal haemoglobin structure. In Hardisty, RM and Weatherall, DJ (eds): Blood and Its Disorders, ed 2. Blackwell Scientific, Oxford, 1982, p 364.
57. Foster, HW, Jr: Maternal death associated with sickle cell trait (correspondence). Am J Obstet Gynecol 153:346, 1985.
58. Cohen, SE, et al: Epidural fentanyl/bupivacaine combinations for labor analgesia: Effect of varying dosages (abstr). Anesthesiology 65:A368, 1986.
59. Hughes, SC: Intraspinal opiates in obstetrics. In Shnider, SM and Levinson, G (eds): Anesthesia for Obstetrics, ed 2. Williams & Wilkins, Baltimore, 1987, p 123.
60. Baraka A, Noueihid, R and Hajj, S: Intrathecal injection of morphine for obstetric analgesia. Anesthesiology 54:136, 1981.
61. Leicht, CH, et al: Epidural morphine sulfate for analgesia after cesarean section: A prospective report of 1000 patients (abstr). Anesthesiology 65:A366, 1986.
62. Rawal N, et al: Influence of naloxone infusion on analgesia and respiratory depression following epidural morphine. Anesthesiology 64:194, 1986.
63. Pastorek, JG and Seiler, B: Maternal death associated with sickle cell trait. Am J Obstet Gynecol 151:295, 1985.
64. Dunn, A, et al: Intraoperative death during cesarean section in a patient with sickle-cell trait. Can Anaesth Soc J 34:67, 1987.
65. Weatherall, DJ: The New Genetics and Clinical Practice. Oxford University Press, Oxford, 1985.
66. Weatherall, DJ: Prenatal diagnosis of inherited blood disorders. Clin Haematol 14:747, 1985.
67. Liang, DT, et al: Homozygous α-thalassaemia: Clinical presentation, diagnosis and management — A review of 46 cases. Br J Obstet Gynaecol 92:680, 1985.
68. Wong, SC, Ali, MA and Benzie, R: The intrauterine diagnosis of hemoglobin disorders. Clin Perinatol 11:283, 1984.
69. Grech, ES, Silva, LJ and Ventura, CS: Homozygous beta thalassaemia and pregnancy. Aust NZ J Obstet Gynaecol 24:45, 1984.
70. Alger, LS, Golbus, MS and Laros, RK: Thalassemia and pregnancy: Results of an ante-natal screening program. Am J Obstet Gynecol 134:662, 1979.
71. Cooley, TB and Lee, P: A series of cases of splenomegaly in children with anemia and peculiar bone changes. Trans Am Pediatr Soc 37:29, 1925.
72. Wolman, IJ: Transfusion therapy in Cooley's anemia: Growth and health as related to long-range hemoglobin levels — A progress report. Ann NY Acad Sci 119:736, 1964.
73. Greenwalt, TJ and Zelensky, KR: Transfusion support for haemoglobinopathies. Clin Haematol 13:151, 1984.
74. Propper, RD, Button, LN and Nathan, DG: New approaches to the transfusion management of thalassemia. Blood 55:55, 1980.
75. Meadows, K: A successful pregnancy outcome in transfusion dependent thalassaemia major. Aust NZ J Obstet Gynaecol 24:43, 1984.
76. Weatherall, DJ: Haemolytic anaemia. Practitioner 221:194, 1978.
77. Roizen, MF: Anesthetic implications of concurrent diseases. In Miller, RD (ed): Anesthesia, ed 2. Churchill Livingstone, New York, 1986, p 255.
78. Lux, SE and Wolfe, LC: Inherited disorders of the

red cell membrane skeleton. Pediatr Clin North Am 27:463, 1980.

79. Willoughby, ML: Haematological disorders. Clin Obstet Gynaecol 4:371, 1977.
80. Kickler, TS: The hemolytic anemias. In Harvey, A McC, et al (eds): The Principles and Practice of Medicine, ed 21. Appleton-Century-Crofts, Norwalk, CT, 1984, p 494.
81. Mitchell, MS and Capizzi, RL: Neoplastic diseases. In Burrow, GN and Ferris, TF (eds): Medical Complications During Pregnancy, ed 2. WB Saunders, Philadelphia, 1982, p 510.
82. MacLain, CR: Leukemia in pregnancy. Clin Obstet Gynecol 17:185, 1984.
83. Ewing, PA and Whittaker, JA: Acute leukemia in pregnancy. Obstet Gynecol 42:245, 1973.
84. Nicholson, HO: Leukaemia and pregnancy. J Obstet Gynaecol Br Commonw 75:517, 1968.
85. Gokal, R, et al: Successful pregnancy in acute monocytic leukaemia. Br J Cancer 34:299, 1976.
86. Brandt, JT: Current concepts of coagulation. Clin Obstet Gynecol 28:3, 1985.
87. Thompson, AR and Harker, LA: Manual of Hemostasis and Thrombosis, ed 3. FA Davis, Philadelphia, 1983.
88. Bennett, JS: Blood coagulation and coagulation tests. Med Clin North Am 68:557, 1984.
89. Caldwell, DC, Williamson, RA and Goldsmith, JC: Hereditary coagulopathies in pregnancy. Clin Obstet Gynecol 28:53, 1985.
90. Lind, SE: Prolonged bleeding time. Am J Med 77:305, 1984.
91. Duke, WW: The relation of blood platelets to hemorrhagic disease: Description of a method for determining the bleeding time and coagulation time and report of three cases of hemorrhagic disease relieved by transfusion. JAMA 55:1185, 1910.
92. Harker, LA and Slichter, SJ: The bleeding time as a screening test for evaluation of platelet function. N Engl J Med 287:155, 1972.
93. Kumar, R, et al: Clinical trial of a new bleeding time device. Am J Clin Pathol 70:642, 1978.
94. Hamblin, TJ: What about the bleeding time? (editorial). Br Med J 291:91, 1985.
95. Stirling, Y, et al: Haemostasis in normal pregnancy. Thromb Haemost 52:176, 1984.
96. Plauche, WC: Henoch-Schonlein (anaphylactoid) nephropathy in pregnancy. Obstet Gynecol 56:515, 1980.
97. McCoy, MJ: Henoch-Schonlein purpura and pregnancy. Am J Obstet Gynecol 141:469, 1981.
98. Ray, M and Posen, GA: Henoch-Schonlein purpura in pregnancy. Can Med Assoc J 132:1385, 1985.
99. Pitkin, RM: Auto-immune diseases in pregnancy. Semin Perinatol 1:161, 1977.
100. de Swiet, M: Systemic lupus erythematosus and other connective tissue diseases. In de Swiet, M (ed): Medical Disorders in Obstetric Practice. Blackwell Scientific, Oxford, 1984, p 260.
101. Tan, EM, et al: The 1982 revised criteria for the classification of systemic lupus erythematosus. Arthritis Rheum 25:1271, 1982.
102. Prentice, CR: Acquired coagulation disorders. Clin Haematol 14:413, 1985.
103. Boey, ML, et al: Thrombosis in systemic lupus erythematosus: Striking association with the presence of circulating lupus anticoagulant. Br Med J 2:1020, 1983.
104. Lubbe, WF, et al: Lupus anticoagulant in pregnancy. Br J Obstet Gynaecol 91:357, 1984.
105. Horger, EO and Keane, MW: Platelet disorders in pregnancy. Clin Obstet Gynecol 22:843, 1979.
106. McMillan, R: Chronic idiopathic thrombocytopenic purpura. N Engl J Med 304:1135, 1981.
107. Cines, DB, et al: Immune thrombocytopenic purpura and pregnancy. N Engl J Med 306:826, 1982.
108. Martin, JN, Jr, Morrison, JC and Files, JC: Autoimmune thrombocytopenic purpura: Current concepts and recommended practices. Am J Obstet Gynecol 150:86, 1984.
109. Colvin, BT: Thrombocytopenia. Clin Haematol 14:661, 1985.
110. Kelton, JG: Management of the pregnant patient with idiopathic thrombocytopenic purpura. Ann Intern Med 99:796, 1983.
111. Morgenstern, GR, Measday, B and Hedge, UM: Autoimmune thrombocytopenia in pregnancy: A new approach to management. Br Med J 287:584, 1983.
112. Hegde, UM: Immune thrombocytopenia in pregnancy and the newborn. Br J Obstet Gynaecol 92:657, 1985.
113. Newland, AC, et al: High dose intravenous IgG in adults with autoimmune thrombocytopenia. Lancet 1:84, 1983.
114. Mizunuma, H, et al: A new approach to idiopathic thrombocytopenic purpura during pregnancy by high-dose immunoglobulin G infusion. Am J Obstet Gynecol 148:218, 1984.
115. Adderley, RJ, et al: High-dose intravenous therapy with immune globulin before delivery for idiopathic thrombocytopenic purpura. Can Med Assoc J 130:894, 1984.
116. Besa, EC, et al: High-dose intravenous IgG in the management of pregnancy in women with idiopathic thrombocytopenic purpura. Am J Hematol 18:373, 1985.
117. Lavery, JP, et al: Immunologic thrombocytopenia in pregnancy: Use of antenatal immunoglobulin therapy: Case report and review. Obstet Gynecol 66:41S, 1985.
118. Anguillo, J, Temple, JT and Corrigan, JJ: Management of cesarean section in a patient with idiopathic thrombocytopenic purpura. Anesthesiology 46:145, 1977.
119. Territo, M, et al: Management of autoimmune thrombocytopenia in pregnancy and in the neonate. Obstet Gynecol 41:579, 1973.
120. Kelton, JG, et al: The prenatal prediction of thrombocytopenia in infants of mothers with clinically diagnosed immune thrombocytopenia. Am J Obstet Gynecol 144:449, 1982.
121. Scott, JR, Rote, NS and Cruikshank, DP: Antiplatelet antibodies and platelet counts in pregnancies

complicated by autoimmune thrombocytopenic purpura. Am J Obstet Gynecol 145:932, 1983.
122. Wahbeh, CJ, et al: Pregnancy and immune thrombocytopenic purpura. Am J Obstet Gynecol 149:238, 1984.
123. Laros, RK and Kagan, R: Route of delivery for patients with immune thrombocytopenic purpura. Am J Obstet Gynecol 148:901, 1984.
124. Barrer, MJ: Platelet function. Anesthesiology 46:202, 1977.
125. Romero, R and Duffy, TP: Platelet disorders in pregnancy. Clin Perinatol 7:327, 1980.
126. Andrews, NP, Pipkin, FB and Heptinstall, S: Blood platelet behaviour in mothers and neonates. Thromb Haemost 53:428, 1985.
127. Pfueller, SL, Hosseinzadeh, PK and Firkin, BG: Quinine- and quinidine-dependent antiplatelet antibodies: Requirement of factor VIII–related antigen for platelet damage and for in vitro transformation of lymphocytes from patients with drug-induced thrombocytopenia. J Clin Invest 67:907, 1981.
128. Steele, P, et al: Effect of sulfinpyrazone on platelet survival time in patients with transient cerebral ischemic attacks. Stroke 8:396, 1977.
129. Beaufils, M, et al: Prevention of pre-eclampsia by early antiplatelet therapy. Lancet 1:840, 1985.
130. Machin, SJ: Thrombotic thrombocytopenic purpura. Br J Haematol 56:191, 1984.
131. Moschowitz, E: An acute febrile pleiochromic anaemia with hyaline thrombosis of the terminal arterioles and capillaries. Arch Intern Med 31:89, 1925.
132. Ridolfi, RL and Bell, WR: Thrombotic thrombocytopenic purpura. Medicine 60:413, 1981.
133. Caggiano, V, et al: Thrombotic thrombocytopenic purpura: Report of fourteen cases — occurrence during pregnancy and response to plasma exchange. J Clin Apheresis 1:71, 1983.
134. Macintyre, DE, Pearson, JD and Gordon, JL: Localisation and stimulation of prostacyclin production in vascular cells. Nature 271:549, 1978.
135. Ritter, JM, et al: Prostacyclin synthesis is stimulated by a serum factor formed during coagulation. Thromb Haemostas 49:58, 1983.
136. Remuzzi, G, et al: Prostacyclin generation by cultured endothelial cells in haemolytic uraemic syndrome. Lancet 1:656, 1980.
137. Lian, EC, et al: Presence of a platelet aggregating factor in the plasma of patients with thrombotic thrombocytopenic purpura (TTP) and its inhibition by normal plasma. Blood 53:333, 1979.
138. Lian, EC, et al: Properties and identification of a plasma factor which inhibits the platelet aggregation induced by TTP plasma (abstr). Thromb Haemost 50:101, 1983.
139. Moake, JL, et al: Unusually large plasma factor VIII: Von Willebrand factor multimers in chronic relapsing thrombotic thrombocytopenic purpura. N Engl J Med 307:1432, 1982.
140. Kennedy, SS, Zacharski, IR and Beck, JR: Thrombotic thrombocytopenic purpura: Analysis of 48 unselected cases. Semin Thromb Haemostas 6:341, 1980.
141. Walker, BK, Ballas, SK and Martinez, J: Plasma infusion for thrombotic thrombocytopenic purpura during pregnancy. Arch Intern Med 140:981, 1980.
142. Byrnes, JJ: Plasma infusion in the treatment of thrombotic thrombocytopenic purpura. Semin Thromb Haemostas 7:9, 1981.
143. Madden, M and Kettle, P: Thrombotic thrombocytopenic purpura. Ir Med J 76:388, 1983.
144. Ambrose, A, Welham, RT and Cefalo, RC: Thrombotic thrombocytopenic purpura in early pregnancy. Obstet Gynecol 66:267, 1985.
145. Peake, IR: The nature of factor VIII. Clin Sci 67:561, 1984.
146. Aronstam, A and Arblaster, PG: The haemorrhagic disorders including haemophilia. Practitioner 221:176, 1978.
147. Nilsson, IM, Bergentz, S-E and Larsson, SA: Surgery in von Willebrand's disease. Ann Surg 190:746, 1979.
148. Hanna, W, et al: Variant von Willebrand's disease and pregnancy. Blood 58:873, 1981.
149. Lipton, RA, Ayromlooi, J and Coller, BS: Severe von Willebrand's disease during labor and delivery. JAMA 248:1355, 1982.
150. Mannucci, PM, Ronchi, G and Rota, L: A clinicopathological study of liver disease in haemophiliacs. J Clin Path 31:779, 1978.
151. Gill, FM: Congenital bleeding disorders: Hemophilia and von Willebrand's disease. Med Clin North Am 68:601, 1984.
152. Department of Health and Social Security: Report on Confidential Enquiries into Maternal Deaths in England and Wales 1979–81. HMSO, London, 1986, p 30.
153. Kierkegaard, A: Incidence and diagnosis of deep vein thrombosis associated with pregnancy. Acta Obstet Gynecol Scand 62:239, 1983.
154. Bergqvist, A, Bergqvist, D and Hallbrook, T: Deep vein thrombosis during pregnancy: A prospective study. Acta Obstet Gynecol Scand 62:443, 1983.
155. de Swiet, M: Thromboembolism. Clin Haematol 14:643, 1985.
156. Rosenberg, RD: Actions and interactions of antithrombin and heparin. N Engl J Med 292:146, 1975.
157. Thaler, E and Lechner, K: Antithrombin III deficiency and thromboembolism. Clin Haematol 10:369, 1981.
158. Samson, D, et al: Management of planned pregnancy in a patient with congenital antithrombin III deficiency. Br J Haematol 56:243, 1984.
159. Mangano, DT: Immediate hemodynamic and pulmonary changes following pulmonary thromboembolism. Anesthesiology 52:173, 1980.
160. Bolan, JC: Thromboembolic complications of pregnancy. Clin Obstet Gynecol 26:913, 1983.
161. Neiderman, MS: Asthma and other severe respiratory diseases during pregnancy. In Berkowitz, RL (ed): Critical Care of the Obstetric Patient. Churchill Livingstone, New York, 1983, p 335.
162. Mobin-Uddin, K, et al: Transvenous caval interrup-

tion with umbrella filter. N Engl J Med 286:55, 1972.
163. Editorial: Thromboembolism in pregnancy. Br Med J 1:1661, 1979.
164. Laros, RK, Jr and Alger, LS: Thromboembolism and pregnancy. Clin Obstet Gynecol 22:871, 1979.
165. Hellgven, M, Tengborn, L and Abildgaard, U: Pregnancy in women with congenital antithrombin III deficiency: Experience of treatment with heparin and antithrombin. Gynecol Obstet Invest 14:127, 1982.
166. Odoom, JA and Sih, IL: Epidural analgesia and anticoagulant therapy: Experience with one thousand cases of continuous epidurals. Anaesthesia 38:254, 1983.
167. Owens, EL, Kasten, GW and Hessel, EA II: Spinal subarachnoid hematoma after lumbar puncture and heparinization: A case report, review of the literature, and discussion of anesthetic implications. Anesth Analg 65:1201, 1986.
168. Rao, TL and El-Etr, AA: Anticoagulation following placement of epidural and subarachnoid catheters: An evaluation of neurologic sequelae. Anesthesiology 55:618, 1981.
169. Matthews, ET and Abrams, LD: Intrathecal morphine in open heart surgery. Lancet 2:543, 1980.
170. Cooke, ED, et al: Monitoring during low-dose heparin prophylaxis. N Engl J Med 294:293, 1976.
171. Morgan, BM, et al: Anaesthetic morbidity following cesarean section under epidural or general anesthesia. Lancet 1:328, 1984.
172. Modig, J, Malmberg, P and Saldeen, T: Comparative effects of epidural and general anesthesia on fibrinolysis function, lower limb rheology and thromboembolism after total hip replacement (abstr). Anesthesiology (Suppl) 53:S34, 1980.
173. Simpson, PJ, et al: The fibrinolytic effects of anaesthesia. Anaesthesia 37:3, 1982.
174. Peddle, LJ: The antenatal management of the Rh sensitized woman. Clin Perinatol 11:251, 1984.
175. Kurtz, EM, Pappas, AA and Cannon, A: Laboratory identification of erythroblastosis fetalis. Ann Clin Lab Sci 12:388, 1982.
176. Hardy, J and Napier, JA: Red cell antibodies detected in antenatal tests on rhesus-positive women in South and Mid Wales, 1948–1978. Br J Obstet Gynaecol 88:91, 1981.
177. Weinstein, L: Irregular antibodies causing hemolytic disease of the newborn: A continuing problem. Clin Obstet Gynecol 25:321, 1982.
178. Baskett, TF, Parsons, ML and Peddle, LJ: The experience and effectiveness of the Nova Scotia Rh program, 1964–84. Can Med Assoc J 134:1259, 1986.
179. Bowman, JM: The management of Rh-isoimmunization. Obstet Gynecol 52:1, 1978.
180. Nicolaides, KH, Rodeck, CH and Mibashan, RS: Obstetric management and diagnosis of haematological disease in the fetus. Clin Haematol 14:775, 1985.
181. Bevis, DC: Blood pigments in haemolytic disease of the newborn. J Obstet Gynaecol Br Commonw 63:68, 1956.
182. Liley, AW: Liquor amnii analysis in the management of the pregnancy complicated by rhesus sensitization. Am J Obstet Gynecol 83:1359, 1961.
183. Rodeck, CH, et al: Direct intravascular fetal blood transfusion by fetoscopy in severe rhesus isoimmunisation. Lancet 1:625, 1981.
184. Moroshima, HO and Covino, BG: Toxicity and distribution of lidocaine in nonasphyxiated and asphyxiated baboon fetuses. Anesthesiology 54:182, 1981.
185. Brown, WU, Jr, Bell, GC and Alper, MH: Acidosis, local anesthetics and the newborn. Obstet Gynecol 48:27, 1976.
186. James, FM III, et al: Chloroprocaine vs. bupivacaine for lumbar epidural analgesia for elective cesarean section. Anesthesiology 52:488, 1980.
187. Gibbs, CP, et al: Prevention of hypotension with hydration (abstr). Anesthesiology 55:A308, 1981.
188. Norris, MC and Dewan, DM: Preoxygenation for cesarean section: A comparison of two techniques. Anesthesiology 62:827, 1985.
189. Pickering, BG, et al: Cerebral vascular responses to ketamine and thiopentone during foetal acidosis. Can Anaesth Soc J 29:463, 1982.

CHAPTER 15

BLEEDING PROBLEMS

MICHAEL H. PLUMER, M.D.

Joyful and natural though childbirth may be, the specter of death attends every birth. Women still bleed to death during childbirth, though modern medical care could save 75 to 90 percent of them. Once the leading cause of maternal mortality,[1] hemorrhage remains an important cause of death in developed countries despite elimination of maternal anemia and availability of blood transfusion.[2,3] Kaunitz and colleagues[4] found hemorrhage to be the third leading cause of reported maternal deaths in the United States between 1974 and 1978, though reports from individual states show wide variation in the rate of hemorrhagic death.[5-8] Hemorrhage remains among the leading causes of death in reports from the Nordic countries,[9] Sweden,[10] England, and Wales,[11] and Canada.[12]

Hogberg[13] estimates that worldwide reproductive mortality may approach a half million women per year, with maternal mortality rates for individual nations ranging from less than 10 to more than 2000 maternal deaths per 100,000 live births. Hemorrhage compounded by anemia represents the major cause of maternal mortality throughout the world.[14-21]

Women older than 35 suffer four times the obstetric mortality of women aged 20 to 34;[9,22] hemorrhage primarily causes death in this older group (14.3 deaths per 100,000 live births).[22] A religious group in the United States which rejects all medical care suffers 100 times the predicted maternal mortality, with 66 percent of the deaths due to hemorrhage.[23]

Pregnancy-related hemorrhage occurs not only with birth but also with ectopic pregnancy and abortion. Deaths from spontaneous abortion explain 5 percent of the United States maternal mortality; hemorrhage accounts for one in five.[24] Hemorrhage is the leading cause of death following legal abortion.[25,26]

Cesarean section introduces more risks, including hemorrhage, than vaginal delivery.[10,27,28] Petitti[29] identifies transfusion as the second most common source of significant morbidity after cesarean section.

Obstetric complications have become an uncommon cause of death in young women. Of North American women aged 15 to 24, 38 will die in motor vehicle accidents for each one who dies of any complication of pregnancy, and 40 more will die of murder, suicide, or nonvehicular accidents.[30] Obstetric bleeding problems pose a public health problem not because of their numbers but because almost all women who bleed to death should not have died. A low death rate makes an individual death no less tragic, especially if prevention could have averted that death.

Physiology

This section briefly reviews placental function, maternal blood volume changes with pregnancy, and the features of normal hemostasis. For details, see Chapters 1 and 2.

FETAL ASPECTS

The parasitic human fetus draws life through the hemochorial placenta, a network of exteriorized fetal vessels implanted in maternal tissue. Maternal blood surrounds the fetal blood vessels of the placental villi, allowing metabolic exchange between fetal and maternal circulations. As much as a liter of maternal blood escapes the spiral arteries each minute to momentarily occupy extravascular areas within the placenta's intervillous space before re-entering maternal uterine veins through venous sinuses. Ironically, the very adaptation that enables fetal life imperils maternal life. Maternal blood may escape its accustomed vascular confinement to become irretrievably lost; amniotic fluid, air, infected debris, or thromboplastic material may invade the mother's once inviolable circulation (Fig. 15–1).

As the placenta separates from the uterine wall, maternal vessels supplying it shear off. Blood that would have perfused the placenta flows into the uterine cavity. The vascular system would empty in minutes if not for the simultaneous uterine contraction that normally compresses spiral arteries to stop blood loss. Not only can blood escape as the placenta separates, but material within the uterus or beneath the placenta can also enter the maternal circulation through venous sinuses. The hemochorial placenta which makes human reproduction possible thus introduces to childbirth the risks of bleeding and embolism.

MATERNAL ASPECTS

Pregnancy induces maternal physiologic adaptations to nourish a growing organism within the mother's body. Those changes essential to our consideration of bleeding problems include blood volume adaptations and alterations in the hemostatic mechanism.

Changes in Blood Volume

Pregnancy prepares patients well for the hemorrhage that inevitably accompanies delivery.

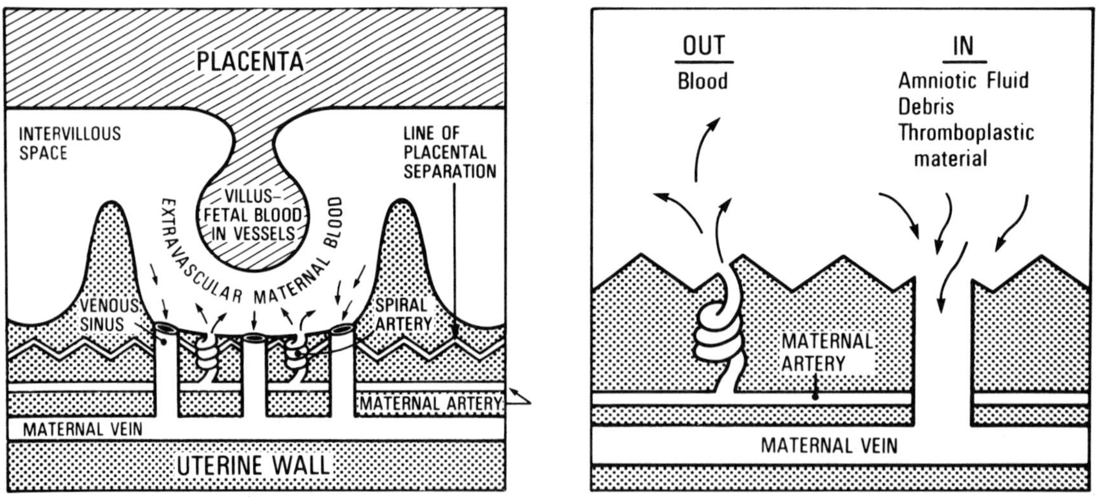

Figure 15–1. Maternal blood momentarily becomes extravascular as it perfuses the hemochorial human placenta *(left)*. After placental separation *(right)*, spiral arteries lose blood which would have perfused the placenta, and venous sinuses remain open to invasion by foreign material. Uterine contraction normally compresses these vessels, sealing the maternal circulation again.

Blood volume increases markedly with pregnancy; total blood volume near term exceeds nonpregnant volume by 35 to 50 percent, an increase of 1000 to 1500 ml.[31,32] Both plasma volume and red cell mass increase, but a greater increase in plasma volume produces the physiologic "anemia" of pregnancy by hemodilution. Pregnant patients withstand hemorrhage well because of their increased blood volume and because the blood-containing space becomes smaller immediately after delivery. The intervillous space disappears with the placenta, and uterine vasculature shrinks with uterine contraction to reduce the maternal vascular space by 300 to 500 ml.

Normal Hemostasis

Blood is a remarkable substance: free-flowing within the intact vascular system, it quickly blocks its own egress following vascular damage. Vascular injury initiates three groups of reactions that contribute to formation of a firm clot at the site of injury. First, a platelet plug forms at the injured site. Second, the coagulation mechanism evolves fibrin to stabilize the fragile platelet plug. Third, a group of limiting reactions restrict the clot to the area of injury.[33]

Platelet Plug. Vascular injury exposes subendothelial collagen, to which platelets adhere, releasing ADP and thromboxanes. Platelets aggregate in the presence of these substances, releasing more ADP and thromboxanes, causing further aggregation and making platelet phospholipids available for coagulation.

Formation of the primary hemostatic plug requires both functional platelets in adequate numbers and constriction of blood vessels in the injured area, since unimpeded blood flow would otherwise wash away any aggregating platelets. Because primary hemostasis is independent of coagulation, coagulation tests *do not* measure the ability to form this primary hemostatic plug; only bleeding time is a reliable test.

Coagulation. Secure hemostasis requires reinforcement of the temporary platelet plug by fibrin gel, a protein polymer composed of the fibrin monomers produced when thrombin digests fibrogen. The central reaction of the coagulation process involves generation of thrombin from prothrombin, with subsequent cleavage of fibrinogen to fibrin. The coagulation process (Fig. 15–2), a series of proteolytic reactions,[34] includes at each step conversion of an inactive precursor to an activated clotting factor, which, in turn, transforms the next factor into its active form.

Thrombin production proceeds through either of two pathways. Vascular injury activates the intrinsic pathway, so named because all of its components are present in circulating blood. The extrinsic pathway requires the presence of tissue factor, a generic term for certain proteins released by injured cells. Subsequent to activation of Factor X by either route (Fig. 15–2), the coagulation sequence follows the same common pathway, regardless of the initiating stimulus. The thrombin produced cleaves fibrinogen to the fibrin monomer. Fibrin monomers rapidly polymerize to form insoluble strands that wind around the platelet aggregates at the site of injury, providing a reinforced fibrin plug.

Limiting Reactions. Thrombin is a potent enzyme that not only cleaves fibrinogen to fibrin but also promotes its own formation, directly aggregates human platelets, activates Factor XIII, and converts plasminogen to plasmin.[35] Although unchecked generation of thrombin could rapidly clot all the blood in the body, a series of limiting reactions usually confine the clot to the injured area.

Several types of limiting reactions act simultaneously. Much of the thrombin generated becomes unavailable for further reaction after it is absorbed onto the surface of the developing fibrin gel. Simultaneously, blood flow to an injured area dilutes activated clotting factors and slows coagulation, while the force of the flow itself disrupts the clot and opposes further propagation. In addition, the liver clears blood of activated clotting factors. Conditions producing poor regional and hepatic blood flow, such as hemorrhagic shock, can unbalance the limiting mechanisms, an important effect in initiating disseminated intravascular coagulation (DIC).

Fibrinolysis is the most important limiting reaction. Plasmin, the major agonist in the fibrinolytic system, may serve as the most important defense against generalized clotting.[36] A potent proteolytic enzyme that digests both fibrin and fibrinogen, plasmin originates from plasminogen by thrombin, by activated Factor XIII, and by plasminogen activators from injured cells. Plasmin generation occurs as a normal part of the coagulation sequence.

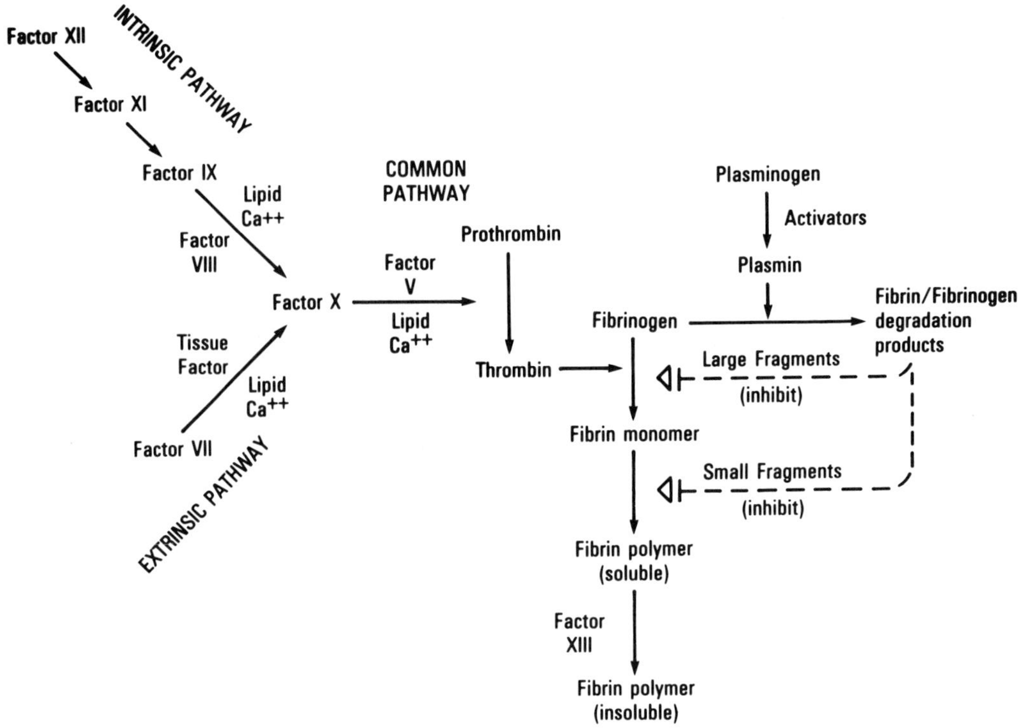

Figure 15–2. Thrombin evolves by one of two pathways, with a final common step to cleave fibrinogen to fibrin monomers, the structural units of the fibrin polymer, which stabilizes the platelet plug. In one of the limiting reactions, plasmin also cleaves fibrinogen to anticoagulant fragments which help confine coagulation to the site of vascular injury.

Plasmin digestion of fibrinogen removes a few small fragments first, leaving large fibrinogen remnants which can still react with thrombin but which clot very slowly (see Fig. 15–2). These large fragments act as potent anticoagulants, tying up thrombin with slowly reactive substrates. Further fibrinogenolysis produces smaller fragments, which no longer react with thrombin but, when incorporated into the developing fibrin gel, slow its rate of formation and weaken the resulting polymer. Therefore, the fibrin-fibrinogen degradation products produced when plasmin digests fibrinogen, interfere with production of further fibrin by thrombin. This point bears emphasis: Thrombin acts on fibrinogen to form fibrin; plasmin acts on fibrinogen to form anticoagulant degradation products. Both processes contribute to normal coagulation, and both normally take place only at the site of injury.

Changes With Pregnancy. Levels of Factors VII, VIII, IX, and X increase during pregnancy, though not significantly.[31] Plasma fibrinogen increases during pregnancy to levels of 400 to 600 mg per dl; severe pre-eclampsia may produce fibrinogen levels as high as 800 to 1000 mg per dl.[37] The platelet count does not change in normal pregnancy, remaining between 150,000 and 300,000 per mm^3. Pregnancy does not alter the results of coagulation tests.

The Anesthesiologist's Role in Obstetric Hemorrhage

An anesthesiologist caring for a hemorrhaging patient functions as resuscitator to prevent death and organ damage, and as anesthetist to facilitate diagnostic examination or operative repair of bleeding sites. In addition, an obstetric anesthesiologist may direct resuscitation of an infant born to a hemorrhaging patient.

Good care requires good communication. Obstetrician and anesthesiologist must clearly define resuscitative needs and plans for therapy. An experienced obstetric anesthesiologist anticipates hemorrhage, understands the differential diagnosis, and participates in planning definitive therapy.

In the face of obstetric bleeding, one may need to summon additional help from within the obstetric suite or from elsewhere in the hospital. Don't hesitate—saving the life of a mother or her child takes priority over almost all other concerns within the hospital. A bleeding patient receives the best care from anesthesiologists who are fully involved in obstetric anesthesia care and who know the patient, the facility, and the members of the patient care team.

RESUSCITATION

Resuscitation during hemorrhage aims to ensure oxygen delivery to the tissues, maintaining good tissue perfusion by fluid with adequate oxygen content. Perfusion depends on both the fluid volume and the pump. Since hemorrhaging obstetric patients generally have sound hearts, the resuscitator can concentrate on fluid volume. Oxygen delivery depends on the oxygen content of the blood, a function of its hemoglobin content and of the quality of respiratory exchange within the lungs. Hemorrhaging obstetric patients usually start with healthy lungs, which allows the resuscitator to concentrate on hemoglobin content.

Effects of Hemorrhage

Volume Loss. Although pregnant patients may tolerate hemorrhage more readily, no study specifically delineates that tolerance. A healthy nonpregnant human can compensate for acute loss of up to 15 percent of the blood volume without change in blood pressure by constricting venous capacitance vessels. Loss of 15 to 30 percent of the blood volume leads to arterial vasoconstriction, tachycardia, and a slight drop in cardiac output. Acute volume loss of 30 to 50 percent produces decreased cardiac output with tachycardia, hypotension, and the α-adrenergic features of clinical shock, with preferential perfusion of heart and brain. Untreated loss of more than 50 percent of the blood volume leads to irreversible shock and death.[38]

Oxygen-Carrying Capacity. Little oxygen is dissolved in the fluid elements of blood compared with the amount carried by hemoglobin (0.30 ml dissolved oxygen per 100 ml of blood versus 20 ml per 100 ml of blood combined with hemoglobin at a PaO_2 of 100). Tissue under resting conditions normally extracts about 5 ml of oxygen from each 100 ml of blood. Dissolved oxygen represents less than 3 percent of that oxygen.[39] Even a patient breathing 100-percent oxygen with an arterial PO_2 over 600 will have only 2 ml of dissolved oxygen per 100 ml of blood—not even enough for half the resting tissue oxygen demand. Up to a point, the body can compensate for the loss of oxygen-carrying hemoglobin by increasing cardiac output and tissue perfusion. Beyond that point, tissue oxygenation will fail, leading to anaerobic metabolism, acidosis, and cellular death.

Hemostatic Ability. Hemorrhage per se has little effect on the blood's ability to remain fluid within blood vessels and to clot at the site of damage. However, a coagulopathy may develop upon depletion of clotting factors at the site of hemorrhage, and limiting reactions become unbalanced from the poor perfusion that accompanies hemorrhagic shock. Treatment of severe hemorrhage with massive fluid replacement often compounds a problem by diluting available clotting factors.

Extracellular Fluid. Hemorrhage initiates a shift of interstitial fluid into blood vessels to restore plasma volume and an apparent shift into cells to produce intracellular edema. The functional deficit of extracellular fluid thus induced may require up to 4 liters of clear fluid replacement beyond the correction of blood volume deficit.[40] Replacement of protein-containing intravascular fluid with noncolloidal fluid reduces colloid osmotic pressure, allowing fluid to shift to the interstitial space. Although colloid fluids should remain intravascular better than crystalloids, colloid resuscitation remains controversial owing to concerns about leakage into the interstitial space across shock-damaged capillaries.

Fluids Available to the Resuscitator

The resuscitator aims to restore intravascular volume and to maintain oxygen-carrying capacity; correction of coagulation defects is initially of secondary importance but may later be essential for successful therapy. Table 15–1 lists major resuscitative fluids and clotting factor concentrates available in North America and indicates whether the fluid provides volume, oxygen-carrying capacity, colloid osmotic (oncotic) pressure, or hemostatic capacity. (Table 15–1 also identifies fluids acceptable to patients who refuse blood products.)

Crystalloid Solutions. Crystalloids, or balanced salt solutions, are mixtures of water and salts that approximate the composition of body fluids. Adding dextrose provides an energy source. Although they are inexpensive, easy to store, sterile, and virtually without risk of infection or immunoreactivity, crystalloids leave the vascular space readily and provide neither oxygen-carrying capacity nor hemostatic ability.

Ringer's lactate, the most ubiquitous crystalloid solution, is widely used in resuscitation. Some clinicians feel that the calcium in Ringer's lactate (3 mEq per liter) may reverse the anticoagulant effect of citrate in banked blood and discourage its use for diluting packed red blood cells (RBCs) prior to infusion. Others avoid Ringer's lactate in the presence of shock,[41] though no evidence links lactate in the solution (28 mEq per liter) to lactic acidosis. Normal saline is an acceptable crystalloid resuscitation solution and may be the fluid of choice for dilution of packed cells or for concurrent administration with blood.

Colloid Solutions. Large molecules in colloid solutions pass poorly through undamaged capillaries and, so, contribute to colloid osmotic pressure. Commercially prepared solutions, though sterile, easy to store, and free of infection risk, are more expensive than crystalloids, especially those protein products derived from blood. Untoward side effects are rare. Colloid solutions provide neither oxygen-carrying capacity nor hemostatic ability.

A 6-percent solution of hydroxyethyl starch (hetastarch, Hespan) expands plasma volume as effectively as albumin[42] but complicates blood typing and antibody screening if blood samples contain more than 30 percent starch.[43] Hetastarch has a lower cost and a longer shelf life than albumin.

Dextran 40 (Rheomacrodex) as "low–molecular weight dextran" (mw 40,000 dal-

Table 15–1. RESUSCITATIVE FLUIDS AND CLOTTING FACTORS

	Volume	Oncotic Pressure	Oxygen Carrying	Hemostasis
Crystalloids				
Ringer's lactate*	+			
Normal saline*	+			
Colloids				
Hetastarch*	+	+		
Dextran*	+	+		
Albumin, 5%	+	+		
Albumin, 25%		+		
Purified protein fraction	+	+		
Hemoglobin Substitutes				
Fluosol†			+	
Blood Products				
Fresh whole blood	+	+	+	+
Banked whole blood	+	+	+	
Packed red blood cells	+		+	
Fresh frozen plasma	+	+		+
Platelets				+
Fibrinogen				+
Cryoprecipitate				+
Factor VIII concentrate				+
Factor IX concentrate				+

*Products acceptable to a patient refusing all blood products. Such fluids (with the exception of Fluosol) possess neither hemostatic ability nor oxygen-carrying capacity.
†Experimental.

tons) reduces blood viscosity. Some have used it to improve microcirculation during low-flow states. Dextran 40 remains in the vascular space longer than crystalloids but not as long as dextran 70.

Dextran 70 (Macrodex), a glucose polysaccharide (mw 70,000 daltons), expands volume effectively but has little clinical use in the bleeding patient because it causes crossmatching problems, induces a bleeding diathesis due to reduced platelet adherence, and produces an occasional severe anaphylactic reaction.[44]

Albumin, 5-percent, in isotonic saline, a pooled plasma derivative, effectively expands volume, carries no risk of infection, and requires no ABO typing. However, it is expensive.

Albumin, 25-percent, in saline expands volume less effectively than the 5-percent solution, since it contains only one fifth the fluid volume of the more dilute solution. Water drawn from the extracellular fluid space by the concentrated solution may aggravate an extracellular volume deficit.

Plasma protein fraction (PPF), a heat-treated pooled plasma product, contains albumin plus alpha- and beta globulins. Though free of infection risk, PPF is expensive and has been associated with transient hypotension attributed to generation of bradykinin by an activator in the globulin fraction.

Hemoglobin Substitutes. Perfluorochemical emulsion (Fluosol-DA), the only resuscitative fluid besides blood that possesses any oxygen-carrying capacity, has limited usefulness, since it carries oxygen only at an arterial PO_2 above 300 mm Hg,[45] is available only to investigators, and has significant adverse effects.[46]

Blood Products. Human blood is the only available substance with both hemostatic properties and oxygen-carrying capacity. Though expensive, difficult to obtain and store, capable of transmitting all blood-borne diseases and of producing immune-mediated disease itself, blood and its components are irreplaceable in the treatment of hemorrhage. The availability of blood-banking services directly accounts for much of the recent decline in hemorrhagic maternal mortality. Fresh whole blood—if it is truly fresh—performs all the functions of a patient's own blood. However, clotting functions and, to a lesser extent, oxygen-carrying capacity decline with storage. Platelets lose their ability to function within 48 hours when stored at 4°C. After 1 week of storage, activity of the labile clotting factors (Factors V and VIII) falls to 50 percent of normal. Intracellular 2,3-DPG increases for the first 10 days of storage, then declines. Blood deficient in 2,3-DPG releases oxygen from hemoglobin less well, making less oxygen available to the tissues though the lower storage pH of blood partly counters this questionably significant clinical effect.[38] Despite the appeal of fresh whole blood, logistic difficulties usually make it unavailable as an emergency resuscitation fluid. Blood risks include not only infectious diseases such as hepatitis and acquired immune deficiency syndrome (AIDS), but also potentially fatal transfusion reactions which require crossmatching blood from donor and recipient before administration.

Platelets and labile clotting factors are deficient in stored whole blood in proportion to the time stored, while pH, 2,3-DPG levels, and perhaps temperature are lower than those of fresh blood. Risks and compatibility requirements parallel those for fresh blood. Stored blood should be warmed before administration and filtered through a standard 170-μ transfusion filter. Micropore filters are not needed. The need for acute replacement of both intravascular volume and oxygen-carrying capacity calls for administering whole blood. Difficulty in obtaining whole blood instead of components from some blood banks has led to its replacement by packed RBCs with supplemental colloid or crystalloid volume.

Removing most of the plasma from a unit of whole blood leaves packed RBCs—all the red cells of a unit of blood but a hematocrit near 70 instead of 40. Risks and compatibility requirements are those of whole blood. Packed cells can be diluted before administration with normal saline but not with Ringer's lactate (contains calcium) or 5-percent dextrose in water (forms aggregations of red cells).

Fresh frozen plasma, prepared from the plasma of a single unit of fresh blood, presents the same risks as a unit of blood, and should be ABO compatible. A unit of fresh frozen plasma contains most of the plasma proteins of a unit of fresh blood, including the labile Factors V and VIII. An NIH Consensus Development Conference in 1984 reported overuse of fresh frozen plasma, citing "little scientific evidence to support the increasing use of fresh frozen plasma in clinical medicine." Participants did agree on its value in replacement of documented isolated factor deficiencies and, rarely, after massive blood transfusion when Factors V and VII decrease to less than 25 percent of normal.[47]

Platelets, prepared from a single unit of fresh blood, present the same infectious risks as the unit of blood and should be ABO compatible. Each pack raises the platelet count by 7,000 to 10,000 platelets per mm^3. Platelet survival decreases significantly if platelets are refrigerated, but if stored at room temperature they remain viable for 5 days. To reduce platelet destruction, platelets should be administered through a filter no smaller than 170 microns, using a needle no smaller than 19-gauge. Platelets are used to treat thrombocytopenia (less than 75,000 platelets per mm^3) associated with clinical bleeding. Dilutional thrombocytopenia is the most common cause of a coagulation defect in a patient who has received multiple units of banked blood.[48]

Fibrinogen, prepared by Cohn fractionation of 500 to 1000 pooled plasma donations, carries a correspondingly high risk of hepatitis. If needed, one may obtain a better supply of fibrinogen from fresh frozen plasma (400 mg per 200 ml) or by cryoprecipitate (50 mg per 15 to 20 ml). Cryoprecipitate, possessing the same infectious risk as the single unit of blood from which it originates, commonly serves as treatment for hemophiliacs (Factor VIII deficiency).[49]

Freeze-dried concentrates of Factor VIII and Factor IX now available undergo heat treatment to reduce the risk of transmitting infection.

Emergency Availability of Blood

Each obstetric suite should have immediate access to a blood bank which can provide type-specific blood within minutes after saline crossmatch to patients who have previously undergone ABO and Rh typing and antibody screen. Such a system may not always be practical, especially in small hospitals or in cities with a single central blood bank, but alternatives can compromise patient safety.

A patient of unknown blood type who needs immediate transfusion can receive O-negative blood. However, this introduces the risk of a transfusion reaction in a patient with an undetected rare antibody to a non–ABO antigen. Further, the anti–A or anti–B antibodies which may be present in O negative plasma may be detrimental to recipients with type A, B, or AB blood (55 percent of the population). Giving only O negative packed cells reduces but does not eliminate this problem. A patient who has received 500 to 600 ml of type O plasma should be tested for anti–A and anti–B antibodies before she receives new units of the proper ABO type.[38]

Even in an emergency, obstetric patients should have type-specific blood available. Rarely is a patient's blood type unknown. In that situation, if the patient urgently needs blood but can be managed temporarily with other fluids; rapid ABO and Rh typing enable the patient to receive type-specific blood. Without antibody screen or crossmatch, an undetected rare antibody could still cause a reaction, but the risk with type-specific blood is less than with O-negative blood.

Performing blood type determination and antibody screening in advance enables the patient to receive type-specific uncrossmatched blood without delay and with minimal risk if the antibody screen was negative. In only a few more minutes, an immediate spin (saline) crossmatch provides a check against ABO incompatibilities and errors in typing. Shortening all incubation times to the minimum allows "stat" crossmatch in 30 to 45 minutes, while a complete crossmatch using optimal incubation times takes an hour.[50] Optimally, all blood administered will undergo full cross-matching. Given sufficient fluid, patients rarely die from lack of blood as they await crossmatch.

All patients at significant risk of hemorrhage (i.e., all patients in labor) should have blood drawn in advance for type and screen. Immediate access to blood banking allows patient typing and screening, which usually suffice for most obstetric situations, including most obstetric procedures. Patients at higher risk for transfusion (e.g., cesarean hysterectomy, cesarean section for low anterior placenta previa after previous cesarean section) should have fully crossmatched blood available. Predeposited autologous blood avoids the risks of homologous blood, but few obstetric and gynecologic patients have used this technique.[51]

Techniques of Infusion

Rapid intravenous fluid infusion initially restores tissue perfusion and oxygenation during hemorrhage. One must establish adequate perfusion before oxygen-carrying capacity becomes meaningful. Patients can tolerate severe hemorrhage if they receive *some* physiologic fluid infusion; obstetric patients die not because they receive the wrong fluid, but because they don't receive enough of any fluid to prevent irreversible shock and organ damage. Rapid fluid infusion initially takes priority over the choice of fluid or selection of hemodynamic monitoring.

Intravenous Equipment. Every parturient is a candidate for hemorrhage, and rapid fluid infusion may be life saving. Every parturient should have a large-bore intravenous cannula in place, inserted as painlessly as possible with local anesthesia. For ambulation a "heparin-locked" cannula can replace the connecting intravenous tubing. Optimistic individuals who resist dealing with the catastrophic potential of obstetrics find this recommendation controversial; it has not entirely gained favor even in the author's institution.

The importance of a large-bore cannula to fluid infusion cannot be overemphasized. A cannula smaller than 16-gauge should not routinely be used in obstetrics (Fig. 15–3). Routine use of plastic intravenous bags compressible by a pressure infuser set allows rapid fluid administration under pressure when necessary; an intravenous set with an in-line blood pump permits rapid pumping of fluid or medication boluses. When standard intravenous equipment seems inadequate, a special high-volume infusion system can infuse fluid through a central vein at rates up to 41 liters per hour.[52]

Fluid Management. Reported fluid management schemes for major hemorrhage and trauma resemble each other in concept but vary considerably in details. All investigators initially replace lost blood with clear fluid (crystalloid,

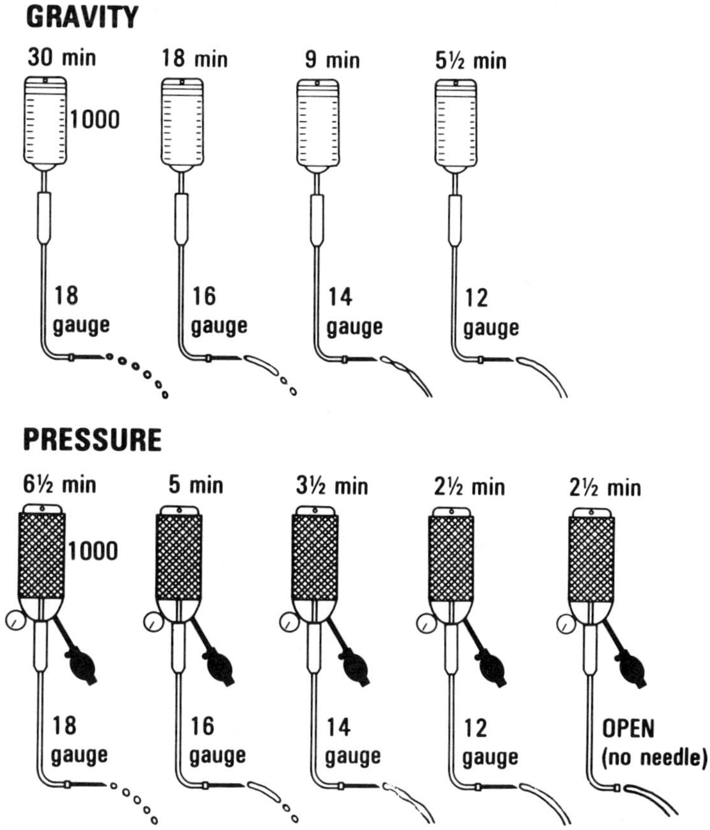

Figure 15–3. Intravenous cannula size affects rate of fluid administration. This figure shows approximate times to infuse 1 liter of fluid through various cannulas. Upper fluids infuse by gravity alone; lower fluids infuse under 300 mmHg constant pressure. Internal diameters of cannulas vary among manufacturers, even for identical gauge; the infusion rate rises with larger diameter and falls with longer length. Cannulas smaller than 16-gauge have no place in obstetrics.

colloid, or a combination) until losses approach 20 to 50 percent of the blood volume, then they administer erythrocytes as packed cells or whole blood.[53-56] For losses exceeding 100 percent of the estimated blood volume, most add platelets from either fresh whole blood[53] or platelet packs.[38,41,54,57] Recommended quantities of platelets range from one pack per six units of blood[41] to two or three packs per unit.[38,57] Most authors also recommend fresh frozen plasma when replacing more than the patient's original blood volume, 1 unit of FFP per 4 or 5 units of blood.[38,41] Prophylactic calcium replacement proves unnecessary,[38] though the physician may administer calcium for inotropic effect when blood replacement exceeds twice the original blood volume.[57]

Monitoring Volume Replacement and Oxygenation. The resuscitator faces the difficult decisions of when to start giving fluid and when to stop. In the nonpregnant patient, traditional signs of tachycardia, hypotension, and sympathetic hyperactivity may not surface until blood loss approaches 50 percent of blood volume. Since a pregnant patient in the lithotomy position can undergo substantial blood loss before manifesting unequivocal changes, vital sign surveillance alone does not adequately signal the onset of significant hemorrhage. An experienced obstetric attendant's observation of "excessive" blood loss probably constitutes the best early warning of hemorrhage.

Rapid infusion of fluids is the most important response to hemorrhage. Since the best approach to shock involves prevention, not treatment, recognition of excessive blood loss dictates infusion of fluids as rapidly as possible, even though vital signs remain unchanged. The infusion continues while the resuscitator assesses the patient, secures additional vascular access, seeks other appropriate fluids, and makes monitoring decisions. Initiating fluid resuscitation takes priority over all other steps.

Blood pressure, heart rate, and mental status guide the first moments of fluid replacement. An automated blood pressure device provides reliable data and frees hands for other tasks. Ideally, the clinical team should monitor shivering or significantly hypotensive patients with an indwelling arterial line after beginning vigorous fluid resuscitation.

Massive or prolonged blood loss justifies other monitoring. An indwelling urinary catheter measures urine output, a reliable indicator of renal perfusion in the absence of diuretics. Pritchard[31] recommends maintaining urine output at 60 ml per hr, 30 ml being the minimum acceptable output. A central venous pressure catheter measures right heart filling pressure, a good indicator of changes in intravascular volume in patients with a normal heart. If insertion of a jugular or subclavian line seems unwise in a patient with a coagulopathy, a long line from an antecubital vein serves the same function. A Swan-Ganz pulmonary artery catheter provides a more sensitive index of volume status in the presence of abnormal myocardial function or pulmonary edema.

Pulse oximetry aids assessment of oxygenation by giving beat-to-beat readings of hemoglobin saturation, though oximetry proves less helpful during shock, since it examines peripheral blood flow. In addition, oximetry may be a poor predictor of tissue oxygenation with very low hemoglobin levels. The best assessment of oxygenation remains periodic arterial blood gas sampling, to measure arterial PO_2, hemoglobin level, and acid-base balance. Metabolic acidosis may reflect inadequate tissue oxygenation with anaerobic metabolism.

Laboratory monitoring during volume replacement includes hemoglobin determination after clear fluid replacement, to evaluate the need for transfusion, as well as periodic assessment of platelet count and coagulation status during massive transfusion (blood replacement greater than original blood volume).

The Patient Who Refuses Blood

Many patients are reluctant to accept blood transfusion because of the medical risks, but few would prefer certain death to the risks of transfusion. Jehovah's Witnesses, however, refuse on religious grounds to accept blood and blood products, including packed cells, plasma, and platelets; most would accept death rather than submit to transfusion. Commercial products prepared from blood are apparently a matter of individual conscience, but serious Witnesses uniformly refuse transfusion.[58]

Jehovah's Witnesses now number more than 650,000 in the United States. Though the denomination was founded in 1884, blood transfusions were not proscribed until July 1, 1945.[59] Biblical references supporting this proscription, such as *Genesis* 9 : 1 – 6, *Leviticus* 7 : 22 – 27 and 17 : 1 – 4, and *Acts* 17 : 22 – 29, prohibit eating blood and describe its sacrificial use.

The bleeding patient who refuses blood leaves few options for maintaining oxygen-carrying capacity. Prior withdrawal of blood for reinfusion at the time of need is useless in an emergency, and is usually unacceptable to Witnesses anyway.[60] Some patients refusing prior withdrawal may accept autotransfusion if the medical team can keep the blood in continuity with the circulation.[61] Acceptable systems for immediate preoperative blood withdrawal and contiguous storage[62,63] do not provide for emergency. Fluosol, though not widely available, has been used successfully in two patients whose hemoglobin values dropped to 3 mg per dl after postpartum hemorrhage.[64]

Patients can often survive hemorrhage without blood replacement, even when transfusion might normally have been given.[65,66] However, a hemorrhagic complication of pregnancy with coagulopathy means almost certain death if the patient refuses blood and blood products.[66,67] The obstetric anesthesiologist in particular often must contend with the painful dilemma created when a bleeding patient needs emergency care but refuses blood. An anesthesiologist on emergency call can neither refuse care nor engage in extensive discussion with the patient before providing care. Acceding to the patient's wishes may require the anesthesiologist to permit the preventable death of a young mother. Disregarding her wishes may expose the anesthesiologist to professional isolation and litigation, and the patient may suffer rejection by her own religious community.[68]

A physician who withholds blood in accord with a competent patient's wishes faces no legal jeopardy. A competent adult has the right to refuse a recommended therapy if fully informed of the consequences of refusal; the physician has no obligation to pursue legal efforts to force treatment. If requested, the court may order a mother to accept treatment intended to preserve the life and health of a fetus.[69] Courts are increasingly less likely to order a parent to accept medical treatment on behalf of minor children when other adult family members could care for the children if the parent dies.

A physician who gives blood despite a patient's refusal may face a law suit for battery and for any negligence in the medical treatment provided, though no one has yet successfully pursued such a suit. A decision to transfuse a Jehovah's Witness may commit an anesthesiologist to continuing care of a very ill patient with little support from physicians who disagree, to dealing with untoward consequences of transfusion in addition to the underlying illness, and to facing the displeasure of the patient and the patient's family.

ANESTHESIA

The bleeding patient's anesthesia needs depend upon the obstetrician's plans for diagnosis and definitive treatment, taking into account the individual patient's physical and emotional status. If the obstetrician can define plans and needs clearly, the anesthesiologist can provide the safest and most appropriate anesthetic.

Anesthesia for Examination

Examination of a patient with postpartum bleeding requires manual exploration of the uterus and inspection of the perineum, vagina, and cervix. A skillful examiner can accomplish this without anesthesia in a tolerant patient, but many patients need help. Examination requires no additional anesthesia in the patient with spinal, lumbar epidural, or caudal anesthesia for delivery. Analgesia without loss of consciousness or airway reflexes may permit brief examination of an unanesthetized patient. Nitrous oxide, 50- to 60-percent in oxygen, administered by an attentive anesthetist using mask or mouthpiece, effectively produces brief but profound analgesia without significant residual depression. Small doses of an intravenous narcotic can supplement inhalational analgesia, though the anesthetist must guard against loss of consciousness. Intravenous ketamine in 10- to 20-mg increments provides analgesia, amnesia, and immobility, and can likewise supplement inhalation analgesia. Though some vocal expression of discomfort may persist, patients tolerate examination and even definitive therapy well and seem to accept the technique readily.

Some patients recall having vivid dreams under low-dose ketamine, but if told in advance that dreams may occur, most do not find them unpleasant.

Conditions requiring general anesthesia call for endotracheal intubation to guard against regurgitation and aspiration of gastric contents. If the anesthetist cannot predict obstetric needs or patient response with confidence, general anesthesia with immediate intubation may be preferable to the risk of inducing anesthesia midway through a procedure when the patient is semiconscious and out of control.

Rapid induction of anesthesia with intravenous thiopental (3 to 5 mg per kg) or ketamine (0.8 to 1 mg per kg) and paralysis with succinylcholine (1 mg per kg) permits rapid tracheal intubation. Cricoid pressure applied by an experienced assistant until the airway is secure reduces the likelihood of regurgitation.[70] Pretreatment with a small dose of a nondepolarizing muscle relaxant (e.g., 3 mg d-tubocurarine) eliminates succinylcholine-induced fasciculations, though the dose of succinylcholine required for complete paralysis is then increased to 1.5 mg per kg.[71] A balanced technique maintains anesthesia: ventilate the lungs with nitrous oxide and oxygen, maintain muscle relaxation as necessary, and give small additional intravenous doses of thiopental, ketamine, or a narcotic. Volatile agents may be used in concentrations less than two-thirds MAC; uterine relaxation requires higher concentrations.

Perineal Anesthesia

Anesthesia of the perineum facilitates vaginal delivery, allows examination of the birth canal and repair of vaginal or perineal lacerations, and simplifies examination and manipulation of the uterus (since the examining hand must pass through the perineum). Local infiltration reduces perineal sensation, but bilateral pudendal block produces better and more widespread anesthesia. Major neuraxis blocks—spinal, lumbar epidural, or caudal—anesthetize the sacral roots of the pudendal nerve (S2–S4) but produce sympathectomy and loss of vasomotor tone in the affected areas, which may impair the normal vasoconstrictor response to hemorrhage. Thus major regional anesthesia is relatively contraindicated in an actively bleeding patient, and absolutely contraindicated in the presence of uncorrected hypovolemia. If regional anesthesia of the perineum is inadequate, contraindicated, or impossible to establish, analgesia for examination can be provided with inhaled nitrous oxide in oxygen or by small intravenous doses of a narcotic or ketamine. Balanced general anesthesia with tracheal intubation is an acceptable last resort.

Uterine Anesthesia

The uterus receives visceral innervation from fibers that enter the spinal cord at the T11 and T12 levels. Fibers from the fundus may pass to the tenth thoracic segment[72] (see Chap. 6). A patient may remain unaware of a punctate stimulus such as a suture needle in an area of visceral innervation, but stretching and distention of the cervix or uterus by cervical traction or intrauterine manipulation produces pain. Analgesia or anesthesia may be required, depending on the procedure, the skill of the operator, and the patient.

Patients with adequate spinal, lumbar epidural, or caudal anesthesia for delivery need no further uterine anesthesia. Initiation of major regional anesthesia after delivery can provide uterine anesthesia, though an actively bleeding or hypovolemic patient is a poor candidate for de novo block.

Inhaled nitrous oxide in oxygen, intravenous narcotics, or ketamine may provide adequate analgesia for brief intrauterine manipulation in selected patients. However, unless the obstetrician can ensure brief manipulation and the anesthetist feels confident that conscious analgesia seems appropriate for the patient, general endotracheal anesthesia from the outset may present the best choice. A volatile anesthetic added to the inhaled mixture can enhance uterine relaxation for rapid removal of retained placental fragments or reduction of an inverted uterus.

Uterine Relaxation

The bleeding patient seldom requires uterine relaxation. Indeed, relaxation (atony) is the commonest cause of postpartum hemorrhage. However, if the uterus contracts well but continues to bleed because remaining placental fragments prevent complete contraction, then momentary uterine relaxation may allow the obstetrician to empty the uterus and facilitate complete contraction. Uterine relaxation may also facilitate reduction of an inverted uterus which has been allowed to contract in the inverted position. However, with prompt recognition and proper management of inversion, uterine relaxation not only proves unnecessary but probably contributes to the problem. Unless the uterus contracts promptly after reduction, reinversion may occur.

Halothane has become the standard anesthetic agent for uterine relaxation, replacing diethyl ether. Halothane concentrations above 2 MAC (1.6 percent) reversibly relax the uterus and block the response to oxytocin infusion,[73] though an equipotent dose of enflurane or isoflurane produces a similar degree of uterine relaxation in vitro[74] and is equally effective. Inhaled anesthetics produce rapid uterine relaxation which abates rapidly when the inhaled agent is withdrawn. The use of inhaled anesthetics as relaxants presents a major disadvantage: Effective concentrations also produce general anesthesia, with the attendant risks and side effects.

Despite the drawbacks of inhaled anesthetics as uterine relaxants, clinical experience with their emergency use is substantially greater than with nonanesthetic uterine relaxants such as tocolytic agents and amyl nitrite. Among tocolytics, selective β_2-adrenergic agonists such as ritodrine and terbutaline produce rapid but persistent uterine relaxation when given as an intravenous bolus; magnesium sulfate acts too slowly and persists too long for emergency use. Amyl nitrite produces rapid smooth muscle relaxation and vasodilation when inhaled from a crushed ampule and appears capable of producing rapid uterine relaxation. It may also produce hypotension in a hypovolemic patient.

Anesthesia for Laparotomy

The bleeding patient may require laparotomy for cesarean section, for ligation of the uterine blood supply, or for removal or repair of a ruptured or atonic uterus. Women who require laparotomy for control of obstetric hemorrhage are among the most desperately ill patients encountered in obstetrics. However, restoring circulatory volume and oxygen carrying capacity as completely as possible before anesthesia induction enables young, previously healthy patients to tolerate anesthesia and operation satisfactorily.

Major Conduction Anesthesia. Major conduction anesthesia (spinal, lumbar epidural, caudal) produces sympathetic block and is generally not appropriate for laparotomy in the actively bleeding patient. However, unexpected bleeding problems during cesarean section under regional anesthesia (e.g., placenta accreta) do not mandate conversion to general anesthesia unless this is required by the patient's emotional state or by the duration or anatomic extent of the procedure. If necessary, a vasopressor such as ephedrine, which affects both resistance and capacitance vessels, counters the pharmacologic sympathectomy of regional anesthesia. A patient facing possible major bleeding (e.g., repeat cesarean section with placenta previa) but currently neither actively bleeding nor hypovolemic should have the same anesthetic options offered to her as any other cesarean section patient. Quality of venous access carries much more significance to such a patient than choice of anesthesia.

Emergency cesarean section in the absence of a capable anesthetist may occasionally call for local infiltration anesthesia by the obstetrician, though obstetricians no longer receive adequate training in this approach and the absence of an anesthetist seems inexcusable except in the most isolated locations. This approach may sacrifice patient comfort but should not compromise patient safety. In the absence of an anesthetist, a physician member of the team should assume the role of resuscitator, monitoring and maintaining vital functions.

General Endotracheal Anesthesia. General endotracheal anesthesia is usually the best choice for laparotomy in a bleeding patient. An adequately resuscitated patient will tolerate rapid-sequence induction with either thiopental or ketamine, followed by succinylcholine-induced paralysis and rapid tracheal intubation with cricoid pressure. When rapid and uncontrollable blood loss prevents adequate fluid replacement prior to surgical control of the bleeding, no anesthetic technique appears ideal. If rapid-sequence induction seems inadvisable, the anesthetist can secure the airway of an unconscious patient by inserting an orotracheal or nasotracheal tube without anesthesia, ventilate with oxygen, then administer a muscle relaxant to provide sufficient immobility to operate. For the conscious patient, small doses of ketamine (0.2 to 0.5 mg per kg) provide amnesia during airway manipulation. However, these approaches present real hazards. Unskilled attempts at intubation in unanesthetized patients can rapidly produce a bloody and compromised airway, perhaps causing hypoxia or provoking vomiting and pulmonary aspiration. Ketamine, which depends on catecholamine release to maintain blood pressure, may depress the cardiovascular system as much as any other anesthetic when given to the hypovolemic patient already experiencing maximal sympathetic activity.[75]

In short, there is no substitute for adequate resuscitation before anesthesia. General anesthesia cannot safely be provided to a hypovolemic patient hovering on the brink of profound shock. Though paralysis and ventilation with oxygen may suffice for surgical control of hemorrhage in a rapidly exsanguinating patient, the presence of an obstetric team prepared for resuscitation should preclude this desperate compromise.

Obstetric Hemorrhage

Obstetric hemorrhage arises either from the placental implantation site or from disrupted blood vessels in the uterus or birth canal. Uterine contraction normally arrests bleeding from the placental site by blood vessel compression, not by coagulation. In contrast, coagulation normally stops bleeding from disrupted blood vessels. Rapid bleeding or disruption of large vessels may require manual compression or surgical intervention to reduce blood flow so clotting can occur; if blood clots poorly, bleeding may persist despite effective control of large vessel bleeding.

This section examines the causes of obstetric hemorrhage. Obstetric considerations for each entity include the nature of the problem, its usual clinical presentation, and the treatment. Anesthesia considerations include brief discussion of both resuscitation and anesthetic management.

ANTEPARTUM HEMORRHAGE

Up to two thirds of antepartum bleeding episodes originate in the placental site, including nearly every instance of life-threatening hemorrhage.[76] Placenta previa and abruptio placentae account for nearly all serious antepartum bleeding; uterine rupture and fetal bleeding, though more grave, occur less frequently.

Placenta Previa

Obstetric Considerations. Placenta previa (literally, the placenta going ahead) implies abnormal implantation of the placenta on the lower uterine segment with some encroachment on the cervical os. A complete placenta previa covers the os entirely; a partial or marginal previa does so incompletely. Placenta previa occurs in 1 in 345 to 1 in 53 deliveries.[77-79] Singh, Rodriques, and Gupta[78] found twice the normal incidence (1 in 26) in patients with a previous cesarean section, peaking in the pregnancy immediately after the section. As noted later, the incidence of morbidly adherent placentas also increases with the number of previous cesarean sections.

Placenta previa causes significant morbidity, but rarely produces maternal death. Although nearly one third of the patients with placenta previa in one series[79] delivered without antepartum hemorrhage, others[80,81] have suggested that 90 percent of patients with placenta previa have at least one hemorrhage, and 10 to 25 percent develop hypovolemic shock. Patients with placenta previa and previous cesarean section run an increased risk for placenta accreta, massive hemorrhage, and hysterectomy to control bleeding.[82] Perinatal mortality, though it greatly exceeds maternal mortality, has improved. As high as 17 to 25 percent a decade ago,[76] perinatal mortality has more recently been reported to be 4.2 to 8.1 percent.[82,83]

Patients with placenta previa most commonly present with painless vaginal bleeding in the third trimester of pregnancy. The first bleeding episode usually ceases spontaneously, and fatalities rarely occur in the absence of rectal or vaginal manipulation. Subsequent episodes may occur at any time, and the bleeding may be severe. Ultrasound examination reliably establishes the diagnosis of placenta previa, largely eliminating the need for the risky double set-up vaginal examination, which requires equipment and personnel in readiness for emergency cesarean section, should a vaginal examination provoke uncontrolled bleeding from the placenta.

Third-trimester bleeding is assumed to be a significant problem until proven otherwise. A bleeding patient should be admitted to the hospital, with immediate attention to vascular access and availability of resuscitative fluid during evaluation. A large-bore intravenous cannula allows immediate infusion of crystalloid fluid to restore intravascular volume; if bleeding has ceased and the obstetrician plans no immediate intervention, a type and screen suffices when the blood bank is located in the hospital. The blood bank director should be consulted with questions and kept aware of the clinical situation.

Management depends on the volume of blood lost, on the presence or absence of further bleeding, and on the gestational age. In all cases, resuscitation takes priority, and should be underway as clinical evaluation and diagnostic examination occur. Occasionally, bleeding from a disrupted placenta may be so heavy that complete fluid resuscitation becomes impossible without control of bleeding; resuscitation and definitive therapy then proceed simultaneously.

Indications for prompt delivery include continued bleeding that threatens the mother, fetal distress, or sufficient fetal maturity to render additional time in utero unnecessary (35 weeks or more). With firm diagnosis and satisfactory resuscitation, delivery proceeds at once, usually by cesarean section.

If mother and fetus remain stable, the obstetrician must weigh the maternal and fetal risks of keeping the fetus in utero against the fetal risks of premature delivery. For severe or repeated hemorrhage before 35 weeks in a stable patient the obstetrician will probably confirm fetal lung maturity by amniocentesis as soon as the fetus reaches 35 to 36 weeks and then proceed to cesarean section. If bleeding has been slight, expectant management may allow the fetus to mature beyond 35 weeks before delivery. Silver and colleagues[83] "aggressive expectant management" consists of multiple transfusions, volume expansion, tocolysis, and periodic determination of fetal lung maturity. Keeping the fetus in utero until 37 weeks' gestational age with mature lung function reduces the morbidity of prematurity and the cost of newborn care.[84] Patients managed expectantly usually remain in the hospital to minimize risks in the event of recurrent hemorrhage.

Cesarean section is almost always the preferred method of delivery with complete placenta previa to reduce maternal hemorrhage; rarely, vaginal delivery may be possible for a multiparous patient with a low-lying placenta. Even a dead fetus dictates delivery by cesarean section, for the mother is still at risk of hemorrhage.

Significant blood loss often accompanies cesarean section for placenta previa. Because the uterine incision may enter an anterior placenta, producing both maternal and fetal hemorrhage, the infant care team should recognize the possibility of fetal hemorrhage in all cases of placenta previa. The obstetrician may favor a vertical uterine incision to reduce placental injury and avoid extending the incision laterally through the poorly developed lower uterine segment into uterine vessels.

Placenta previa increases the risk of postpartum hemorrhage, since the lower uterine segment implantation site contracts less well than the usual fundal site and compresses spiral arteries poorly. Should this occur despite good uterine contraction, the obstetrician can oversew individual bleeding sites or compress the area with the overinflated balloon of a Foley catheter inserted through the cervix.[85,86] Ligation of the hypogastric (internal iliac) arteries may reduce pulsatile flow enough to achieve hemostasis. If not, the patient may require hysterectomy, which entails substantial additional blood loss (see the discussion of uterine atony in the section on postpartum hemorrhage).

Coagulation problems common with abruption rarely occur with placenta previa. Placenta accreta, more common with previous cesarean section, should lead to prompt hysterectomy without attempts to dislodge the placenta piecemeal. (See discussion of placental abnormalities in the section on postpartum hemorrhage.)

Anesthetic Considerations. Resuscitation of the patient bleeding from a placenta previa follows the general principles outlined in the section on resuscitation. The patient with placenta previa and a history of prior cesarean section especially needs additional massive fluid resuscitation. More than half of such patients in one series[87] required hysterectomy for placenta accreta.

A patient with placenta previa requires anesthesia for cesarean section. Normovolemic patients can receive regional anesthesia, but those with uncorrected hypovolemia must not undergo this procedure. An unstable patient with continued bleeding and possible hypovolemia should receive general endotracheal anesthesia (see discussion of anesthesia techniques above).

Abruptio Placentae

Obstetric Considerations. Abruptio placentae (literally, breaking away of the placenta) involves separation of the normally implanted placenta before birth. Abruption occurs in 1 in 500 to 1 in 37 pregnancies.[76,77,88,89] More than half appear before the 36th week of gestation;[76] in a series of patients with premature rupture of the membranes, abruption occurred at two to eight times the normal rate.[90] Hypertension is unexpectedly common among patients with placental abruption;[91] one study found abruption in 23 percent of eclamptic patients, 10 percent of chronic hypertensives, and 2 to 3 percent of patients with pre-eclampsia, in contrast to 1.17 percent in the general population.[88] A history of abruptio placentae with a previous pregnancy is associated with a 10-fold increase in the rate of abruption in the current pregnancy.[89] The practice of medicine is itself associated with an increased risk of abruption; one report found evidence of abruption in 12 percent of pregnancies among female physicians.[92]

Though hemorrhage from abruptio placentae appears less dramatic than hemorrhage from placenta previa, abruption is the more lethal condition. Maternal mortality from abruption ranged in 1976 from 1.8 to 11 percent;[76] more recent reviews report maternal mortality from zero to 5 percent.[77,93] Perinatal mortality rates range from 19 to 67 percent with vaginal delivery and 8 to 22 percent with cesarean section.[77,94,95]

Abruption has been reported in association with up to 66 percent of abdominal trauma during pregnancy,[96] usually within the first 24 to 48 hours.[97] Though maternal death from trauma is the leading cause of traumatic fetal death,[98] when mothers survive their infants[99] abruption is the leading cause of fetal death. Individual reports describe abruption in association with snake bite,[100] cocaine use,[101] and congenital hypofibrinogenemia.[102]

Open venous sinuses beneath the abrupted placenta allow thromboplastic material to enter maternal veins and initiate DIC. Coagulation problems occur in up to 50 percent of patients with abruption,[77,95,103,104] becoming more severe with increasing placental separation. Abruption doubles the risk of postpartum hemorrhage; with DIC the incidence of postpartum hemorrhage quadruples again. The blood-suffused Couvelaire uterus of severe abruption responds normally to oxytocics and uterine massage, posing no additional threat of uterine atony.[105] Abruption severe enough to produce hypovolemic shock and DIC may initiate renal failure[103,105] or Sheehan's syndrome of anterior pituitary insufficiency secondary to posthemorrhagic necrosis.[106]

Although bleeding from placenta previa nearly always becomes visible, placental margins, adherent fetal membranes, or a fetal head that completely fills the lower uterine segment may conceal bleeding from abruptio placentae. Fewer than 80 percent of patients with abruption in one series experienced vaginal bleeding.[95]

A patient with severe abruptio placentae classically presents with vaginal bleeding, a painfully hypertonic uterus, hypovolemia, and absent or inaudible fetal heart tones. The extent and duration of separation determine the severity of presenting symptoms. Abruption presents a grave continuing threat to those fetuses who remain alive in utero. In one series, half of the fetuses alive at the time of hospital admission manifested fetal distress.[95]

A patient with suspected abruptio placentae should be evaluated in the hospital. Preventing hypovolemic shock avoids most maternal problems associated with abruption; fluid resuscitation should begin during evaluation of the patient. A large-bore intravenous needle allows restoration of circulating volume with crystalloid while awaiting blood; improved peripheral perfusion and hepatic blood flow reduce the risk of DIC. Blood bank personnel should be notified that the patient may need volume replacement for hemorrhage and component therapy for DIC.

Once the diagnosis of abruptio placentae has

been confirmed by ultrasound examination, obstetric management usually proceeds with vigorous maternal resuscitation and delivery of the infant. In the absence of fetal distress, the obstetrician may attempt vaginal delivery with careful fetal monitoring. Vaginal delivery is the preferred approach if the fetus is already dead, especially in the presence of coagulation problems, unless deteriorating maternal condition necessitates cesarean section. Pagano, Adey and Butterfield[107] recommend cesarean section for moderate to severe abruption when the fetus is viable, the uterus exhibits generalized tenderness and tenseness, and vaginal delivery is not imminent. For severe abruption with coagulopathy, Sher and Statland[108] recommend vigorous fluid resuscitation and expeditious vaginal delivery, avoiding cesarean section if the baby has died except to reduce worsening maternal complications. They also advocate the use of aprotonin (Trasylol), an antifibrinolytic, antithromboplastic, antikallikrein agent not available in the United States. Aprotonin reportedly produces rapid control of DIC, spontaneous resolution of uterine inertia, and rapid progress toward vaginal delivery. A later section discusses treatment of DIC.

Anesthetic Considerations. Since sudden exsanguinating hemorrhage occurs less frequently with abruption than with placenta previa, surgical intervention in the face of inadequate resuscitation seldom proves necessary. As with other hemorrhagic complications, fluid resuscitation should be the first course of action, not only to ensure oxygenation of maternal and fetal tissues but also to dilute activated clotting factors and restore hepatic blood flow as the first steps in preventing or treating DIC. Abruption severe enough to kill the fetus involves considerable maternal blood loss. Pritchard[31] found 1500 to 5000 ml of concealed hemorrhage in such cases, and Brame and associates[103] reported that patients with severe abruption required an average blood replacement of 2650 ml.

For the patient without hypovolemia or coagulopathy, the usual anesthetic options for labor, delivery, and cesarean section apply. Increased uterine irritability with abruption often produces rapid labor, which may reduce the duration if not the degree of pain relief needed. The compromised fetus requires careful electronic monitoring, since one cannot always predict the effects of an anesthetic on uterine blood flow and fetal oxygenation. As with any compromised fetus, supplemental oxygen administered to the mother may help maintain fetal oxygenation should placental perfusion fall.

Uterine Rupture

Obstetric Considerations. Rupture of the gravid uterus, a significant but often unrecognized cause of maternal and fetal mortality, classically occurs in a multigravid patient in tumultuous labor who experiences sudden severe abdominal pain. The abdominal contour changes, labor stops, and the patient becomes "shocky." Fetal heart tones diminish or disappear. However, this classic picture accurately describes only a portion of cases. Recent literature emphasizes a much wider variety of presentations and associations with uterine rupture.

Schrinsky and Benson's extensive review[109] notes the differences between incomplete rupture, usually due to dehiscence of a uterine scar, and the much more catastrophic true or complete rupture of an unscarred uterus. They describe traumatic rupture from instrumentation, violence, or obstetric causes (both direct application of force and indirect application by myometrial contraction) and spontaneous rupture, with or without a history of uterine surgery.

The incidence of uterine rupture of all types appears to fall between 1 in 1000 and 1 in 1500 deliveries in the United States,[109] with traumatic rupture in the majority. Spontaneous rupture represented only 25 percent of Schrinsky's own series, occurring before labor in 4.3 percent of cases. Uterine rupture happens much more commonly in developing countries. Reported African rates range from 1 in 943 in a South African hospital[100] to 1 in 93 at a rural Nigerian hospital.[111]

Uterine rupture contributes significantly to maternal mortality even in the United States, accounting for half the obstetric deaths from uterine hemorrhage and 5 percent of the total maternal mortality.[109] In Schrinsky and Benson's own series no maternal mortality followed rupture of a uterine scar, but maternal mortality rose to 13.6 percent with rupture of an intact uterus. African reports indicate higher maternal mortality—from 3 percent at a South African hospital to 41 percent at a hospital in Nigeria, where half of the deaths occurred before the patients reached the operating room.[110,112–115] Two reports specifically mention that all maternal deaths were associated with rupture of the unscarred uterus;[113,115] one cites hemorrhage as the cause of eight out of nine maternal deaths.[115]

The fetus is even more likely to die than the mother when the uterus ruptures. Some larger series report fetal mortality over 80 percent after rupture of the intact uterus;[109] even Schrinsky's own series had fetal mortality of 28 percent after rupture of a scarred uterus, rising to 45.5 percent with rupture of the intact uterus.[109]

Uterine rupture most commonly originates from a scar at the site of prior cesarean section[116] or uterine surgery.[117] An unscarred uterus is more likely to rupture in the presence of thinning or increased fibrosis of the myometrium, previous curettage, infection, infarction, adenomyosis, and trophoblastic invasion.[118] The recent literature has firmly documented the relationship to trophoblastic invasion. A review of uterine rupture associated with placenta percreta (placental villi penetrating the myometrium) noted postpartum hemorrhage in 39 percent of patients, 90 percent of whom underwent postpartum hysterectomy.[119] All patients lacked decidua at the site of placental implantation; 30 percent had previously undergone cesarean section. Other reports document uterine rupture before labor due to placenta increta or percreta from 15 weeks to near term,[120–126] or during labor with a breech presentation at 34 weeks.[127] Though uterine rupture is frequent with placenta percreta (7 to 15 percent), the rarity of placenta percreta makes it an uncommon cause of uterine rupture.[121,126]

A number of reports describe uterine rupture when prostaglandins are used to induce labor. Prostaglandin $F_{2\alpha}$ has been associated with uterine rupture when used to induce abortion in the second trimester.[128,129] Uterine rupture has accompanied prostaglandin E_2 therapy for the induction of labor, usually after fetal demise.[122,130–134] In two of these instances a pre-eclamptic patient who suffered a seizure in the immediate postpartum period had a ruptured uterus at laparotomy.[133,134]

Several additional reports describe spontaneous rupture of the uterus in patients without evident predisposing factors at gestational ages ranging from 19 weeks to term,[135–138] emphasizing that uterine rupture may occur outside the intrapartum period.

Clinical presentations of uterine rupture vary; no individual sign is pathognomonic. Bleeding is the most common feature,[110,115] by one report present in two thirds of patients after rupture of the intact uterus and in 40 percent after rupture of a uterine scar.[115] Shock develops in one fourth of patients.[110] Abdominal pain or tenderness occurs more frequently when rupture has been unrecognized or untreated.[111] Fetal distress, uncommon with rupture of a scar, develops commonly with rupture of the intact uterus,[115] and delaying treatment increases its frequency.[111] Lenke[139] describes a single case in which rupture of a scar allowed the umbilical cord to prolapse into the abdomen, producing fetal distress.

Contractions may appear to cease if the uterus ruptures during labor, particularly if the uterine contents are extruded through the rupture into the abdominal cavity. In the presence of posterior rupture, a monitor may continue to show apparently normal contractions[140] or may show a hypertonic contraction pattern similar to that seen in abruption.[137] Significant rupture may remain entirely asymptomatic, only to be discovered as an incidental finding at the time of cesarean section[141,142] or postpartum tubal ligation.[143]

Effective treatment of uterine rupture cannot precede recognition. Even in a large center where uterine rupture occurred frequently, clinicians recognized only 35 percent of ruptures before delivery,[110] finding the remainder either at emergency cesarean section (20 percent) or after vaginal delivery (45 percent). Ultrasound examination can demonstrate scar rupture before it progresses to clinical catastrophe[116] and may help differentiate rupture from severe abruption. However, uterine rupture cannot be found unless it is sought. Gibbs[144] remarks on the tragedy of failing to consider uterine rupture because of its rarity, only to have it appear as a surprising autopsy finding.

Uterine rupture requires operation. Repair may be possible when the rupture has occurred in a scarred area; Fakhoury and coworkers even described fetal survival in utero after repair.[145] However, when an intact uterus ruptures or a scarred uterus tears beyond the scar, hysterectomy almost always becomes necessary. Since hemorrhage is the leading cause of maternal death with uterine rupture, this complication calls for an urgent laparotomy to control bleeding. Prompt maternal resuscitation and immediate operation may also save the baby. Ideally complete maternal resuscitation should take place before operation, but fetal distress or rapid blood loss may necessitate proceeding to operate as resuscitation continues.

Anesthetic Considerations. Prompt restoration of circulatory volume and replacement of blood loss are the most important measures in preparing to treat uterine rupture. Reports of catastrophic rupture describe 2000 to 3500 ml of obvious blood within the abdomen at the time of operation; eventual replacement volume sometimes exceeds 30 units of blood. Since control of bleeding requires surgical hemostasis, anesthesia may need to be induced while resuscitation continues to progress. The section on anesthesia for laparotomy describes anesthesia options.

The anesthesiologist should also consider whether analgesia provided for labor would interfere with recognition and prompt treatment of uterine rupture should it occur. Though some have questioned whether patients allowed to labor after previous cesarean section should receive epidural analgesia for labor,[146] no evidence suggests that epidural analgesia for labor impairs recognition of uterine rupture when it occurs.[147,148] Just as scar separation or significant rupture may be asymptomatic even without analgesia, uterine rupture can be painful even in the presence of epidural blockade.[149,150] Uppington[151] found no reason to withhold epidural block from patients undergoing trial of labor. Fetal distress remained the most common sign of scar separation independent of analgesia, while pain and tenderness were unreliable symptoms of rupture whether or not a patient had received epidural block.

Some have questioned the relationship between epidural block and rupture, noting that uterine rupture in one study occurred more frequently in patients given epidural anesthesia (1 in 596) than in unanesthetized patients (1 in 1362).[115] Since epidural anesthesia was freely available to patients in pain, this observation may simply emphasize the painful nature of yet-unrecognized uterine rupture. Others suggest a causal relationship between uterine rupture and extreme anteflexion in the sitting position for initiation of epidural anesthesia.[115,146] Although some authorities[148] dispute such a relationship, good sense dictates that anesthetists avoid the extremes of pressure that could result when an assistant forcefully flexes the patient by pulling down on the neck and shoulders.

Fetal Bleeding

Obstetric Considerations. Vaginal bleeding before birth almost always comes from the mother: fetal bleeding is unusual and difficult to identify but poses a much more immediate threat to the fetus. The great disparity between maternal and fetal blood volumes may render failure to identify a relatively small quantity of fetal bleeding fatal to the baby. The 80 ml of blood in a fully soaked perineal pad[152] is an insignificant portion of the mother's 5000-ml circulatory volume, but it could represent half the blood volume of a preterm fetus. As with uterine rupture, one must consider fetal bleeding in the differential diagnosis of every antepartum hemorrhage, especially in the presence of fetal distress. Diagnosis of fetal bleeding rests on identification of fetal hemoglobin by laboratory testing.

Iatrogenic fetal hemorrhage may follow disruption of fetal vessels in the placenta or, rarely, in the scalp. Incision through the placenta during cesarean section inevitably allows some fetal bleeding from incised placental villi and larger vessels, though such bleeding lasts only briefly. Fetal scalp blood sampling is rarely complicated by continued fetal bleeding,[153,154] but almost half of the reported cases of bleeding involve mortality.

Spontaneous fetal hemorrhage comes from disrupted placental or umbilical vessels. Acute fetomaternal hemorrhage from placental vessels directly into the intervillous space, invisible and difficult to diagnose before birth, accounts for some cases of intrauterine death or hypovolemia at birth. Rupture of a vasa previa, a fetal umbilical vessel traversing the fetal membranes, produces visible hemorrhage with rapid fetal exsanguination.

Detection of fetomaternal hemorrhage, direct fetal bleeding into the maternal bloodstream, involves testing for fetal hemoglobin in maternal blood. The ratio of fetal cells to maternal cells allows calculation of the volume of fetal blood infused. Fetomaternal bleeding is not rare; for example, Gjode, Rasmussen, and Jorgensen[155] found evidence of some fetomaternal bleeding in 28 percent of mothers after attempted breech version. However, extensive bleeding is uncommon. Fay[156] estimates that macrotransfusion (fetomaternal bleeding in excess of 10 ml) occurs in 1 in 714 to 1 in 200 births; Hoag[157] reports massive transfusion (fetomaternal bleeding $>$150 ml) in 1 in 800 deliveries, accounting for 3 percent of perinatal mortality. In contrast to the high fetal mortality, fetomaternal bleeding carries no recognized threat of maternal mortality and little maternal morbidity unless maternal-fetal incompatibility exists. Unexplained fetal death or neonatal anemia should trigger a search for fetomaternal bleeding by testing for fetal hemoglobin in maternal blood.

Velamentous insertion of the umbilical cord occurs when the cord inserts into the fetal membranes rather than the surface of the placenta, allowing the ramifying fetal vessels to lie unsupported in the membranes. Vasa previa (literally, "vessel going ahead") exists when a vessel traverses the membranes in front of the presenting part. Velamentous insertion of the cord occurs in 1 in 417 to 1 in 56 deliveries,[158] nine times more frequently with twins, and most commonly with triplets.[159]

Vasa previa poses no threat to the mother, but the fetal risk is substantial. Perinatal mortality approaches 50 to 60 percent with intact membranes and increases to 75 to 100 percent when membranes rupture.[159] However, correct diagnosis apparently improves therapy; definitive antepartum or intrapartum diagnosis of vasa previa was associated with perinatal mortality in only 23 percent of cases in an extensive review.[158]

Signs of vasa previa include fetal bradycardia and hemorrhage. Fetal monitoring observations have included bradycardia with a "cord compression" pattern as the presenting part compressed an intact vasa previa,[160] and a sinusoidal pattern with vasa previa in twins.[159] Though vasa previa usually produces painless vaginal bleeding after rupture of the membranes, bleeding may occur in the presence of intact membranes or it may not begin for an hour or more after rupture.[161] Fetal distress appears as hemorrhage progresses; if diagnosis and delivery are not immediate, fetal death soon follows.

The obstetrician most readily diagnoses vasa previa before the vessel ruptures. He or she can sometimes palpate a pulsatile vessel on vaginal examination; amnioscopy allows direct examination of the membranes, and some physicians recommend it as a routine measure before artificial rupture of the membranes.[158,162] If hemorrhage has already begun, testing vaginal blood for fetal hemoglobin establishes the presence of fetal bleeding.[159] The hematocrit of a fetal scalp blood sample will resolve doubt about the significance of fetal bleeding, particularly if the bleeding has occurred slowly.[163]

Ruptured vasa previa represents a true obstetric emergency requiring immediate delivery, almost always by cesarean section. Fetal salvage requires a high index of suspicion, rapid action upon diagnosis, and skillful resuscitation of the baby at birth. Though the infant resuscitator must first establish adequate ventilation, an infant who has bled also needs immediate attention to volume replacement. Some of the baby's own blood drawn from vessels on the placental surface into a heparinized syringe can serve as an initial fluid bolus; however, adequate volume replacement usually requires balanced salt solution and perhaps colloid until type-specific or crossmatched blood arrives from the blood bank.

Anesthesia Considerations. As in many other situations, the anesthesiologist may have to function as the mother's guardian while all others concentrate on the distressed fetus. Upon diagnosis, immediate operation represents the appropriate response if the fetus remains alive. Anesthesia is risky, particularly for patients (e.g., those with airway abnormalities, severe asthma, cardiac defects, or malignant hyperthermia susceptibility). The anesthetist must not become so pressured by concern for the fetus that rescue imperils the mother.

In the absence of known maternal contraindications, general anesthesia may be the speediest anesthetic approach for immediate cesarean section. A skilled anesthesiologist can institute spinal anesthesia rapidly. Added maternal safety makes regional anesthesia the technique of choice for some patients.

POSTPARTUM HEMORRHAGE

Every mother bleeds at birth; few have bleeding problems. The contracting uterus normally arrests its own hemorrhage after expelling the placenta, while the mother's physiologic hypervolemia enables her to withstand normal blood loss even without intravenous fluid replacement. The wonder is not that postpartum hemorrhage occurs but that it so infrequently becomes a problem.

Postpartum hemorrhage has classically been defined as loss of more than 500 ml of blood in the postpartum period,[164] implying that substantially less blood loss usually occurs and that precise measurement of shed blood customarily takes place. Neither implication appears accurate. One recent study of measured blood loss in a small series found that 10 percent of patients lost more than 500 ml;[165] a larger study of weighed and measured loss found an average loss of 308 ml at vaginal delivery without episiotomy, 417 ml with episiotomy, and an association of greater blood loss with larger babies and episiotomy.[166] Older measurements of blood volume changes rather than measured blood loss suggest average blood loss of 600 ml with vaginal delivery, 1000 ml with cesarean section, and 1500 ml with cesarean hysterectomy.[167] Applying the above definition, "postpartum hemorrhage" might accompany more than half of all deliveries instead of the 5 percent now expected. In any event, the definition remains meaningless in practice. Estimates of obstetric blood loss are notoriously inaccurate, and clinicians seldom measure shed blood precisely. The implication of quantitative precision ignores reality.

For purposes of this discussion, postpartum hemorrhage includes any hemorrhage that occurs after the birth of the baby and threatens maternal health or survival. Most bleeding problems occur within the first 24 hours, primarily around the time of placental delivery. Donald's[168] dramatic statement, "The third stage is always a time of anxiety which no obstetrician ever wholly outlives," applies equally to the obstetric anesthetist. The anesthetist responsible for a patient's anesthetic care (e.g., a patient having epidural analgesia for labor) clearly must be available to the patient at birth and during the third stage of labor.

Excess postpartum bleeding usually comes from the placental implantation site, either because the uterus fails to contract (uterine atony) or because it cannot contract effectively (retained placental fragments, lower segment implantation, placenta accreta, or uterine inversion). Traumatically disrupted blood vessels in the uterus and birth canal also allow major bleeding. Only uterine atony surpasses lacerations as a source of postpartum hemorrhage. Uterine rupture can produce life-threatening hemorrhage that may not be recognized until after birth.

Uterine Atony

Obstetric Considerations. The normal uterus contracts as the placenta separates, compressing spiral arteries within the myometrium to stop the flow of blood in minutes. The ability of the uterus to arrest its own hemorrhage by contraction is largely a mechanical phenomenon, independent of blood coagulation. The myometrium fails to contract effectively in 2 to 5 percent of vaginal deliveries,[169] making uterine atony the commonest cause of pastpartum hemorrhage and the most frequent antecedent of maternal hemorrhagic death.[170]

Whenever conditions leading to ineffective myometrial contraction occur, the clinician should anticipate uterine atony. Since smooth muscle fibers do not contract effectively when stretched to their full fiber length, uterine atony may occur with the overdistension of polyhydramnios or multiple gestation. Even a macrosomic singleton fetus causes enough uterine distension to produce a sevenfold increase in postpartum hemorrhage when fetal weight exceeds 4500 grams (10 lb).[171] Metabolic interference with contraction may produce atony during hypoxia or ischemia; atony occurs more commonly with arrested labor or after pitocin has augmented labor.[87] Infection such as chorioamnionitis makes atony more probable and increases the likelihood of hysterectomy for atony.[87]

Pharmacologic agents can impede or entirely abolish uterine contraction (see the section on uterine relaxation). Volatile anesthetics produce dose-related uterine relaxation that interferes with spontaneous uterine activity at about 1 MAC and blocks oxytocin-induced contractions entirely at 2 MAC. Tocolytic agents such as ritodrine, terbutaline, and isoxsuprine reduce uterine contractility and could produce atony if given within several hours of delivery, though Essed and co-workers[166] found no increase in peripartum blood loss in patients who received chronic β-sympathomimetic agents. Magnesium sulfate, a tocolytic agent also used to treat pre-eclampsia, reduces contraction in both smooth and skeletal muscle. Atony has followed use of intravenous dantrolene for malignant hyperthermia prophylaxis.[172] Atony occurs more commonly in the presence of DIC, leading to speculation that fibrin degradation products interfere with uterine contraction. Atony also occurs more often with increasing parity and in patients with a previous history of postpartum hemorrhage.

Uterine atony usually produces painless vaginal bleeding which continues longer than a few minutes after delivery of the placenta; yet bleeding due to atony is not always apparent, since the atonic uterus can hold a large volume of blood before vaginal bleeding begins. The uterine fundus should feel firmly contracted to the examining hand after placenta expulsion, and the fundal height should not change on subsequent examinations. A rising fundus without vaginal bleeding suggests intrauterine bleeding with the cervical os obstructed by blood clots.

Treatment of uterine atony consists of vigorous intravascular volume replacement while attempting to stimulate uterine contraction by uterine manipulation and appropriate pharmacologic maneuvers. Persistent bleeding may necessitate operative or embolic interruption of the uterine blood supply; uncontrollable bleeding may require hysterectomy.

Gentle kneading external massage of the uterus is the first step in stimulating uterine contraction; bimanual massage allows simultaneous exploration of the uterine cavity for placental fragments or disruption.[173] Although packing has not gained universal favor, some obstetricians may elect to pack an atonic uterus with gauze, removing the pack in 12 to 24 hours. Such a patient needs continued careful surveillance since bleeding behind the pack may not be evident.[173]

Pharmacologic agents that interfere with contraction should be withdrawn or discontinued, and pharmacologic stimulation of contraction should be initiated. Many obstetricians routinely administer oxytocin after delivery of the placenta, and this is essential if the uterus contracts poorly. Although intramuscular agents can be given, uterine atony should not be treated without a functioning intravascular line to permit fluid replacement. A patient who refuses an intravenous line for delivery should understand the risks and sign a waiver releasing the hospital and the medical staff from liability for harm caused by her refusal of recommended care.

Rapid intravenous infusion of synthetic oxytocin, 10 to 30 units per 1000 ml of balanced salt solution, can serve to supplement endogenous oxytocin and maintain uterine contraction. An intravenous bolus of more than 5 units rarely produces better contraction than a continuous infusion, and the bolus may be dangerous. Oxytocin causes significant but transient vasodilation;[174] rapid intravenous administration can produce profound hypotension in a hypovolemic patient, though Beeby[175] found no cardiovascular effects of a 10-unit bolus in healthy patients undergoing dilatation and curettage after spontaneous abortion. Oxytocin does have some antidiuretic activity, but brief postpartum administration in balanced salt solution has not been associated with water intoxication.

Calcium chloride is sometimes administered intravenously to treat uterine inertia, particularly that due to magnesium sulfate.

Ergot alkaloids produce rapid and sustained uterine contraction. Though usually administered intramuscularly in doses of 0.2 to 0.3 mg, either ergonovine or methylergonovine may be given cautiously in intravenous doses up to 0.2 mg if more rapid action is essential.[176] Ergot alkaloids can produce hypertension by a complex pharmacologic interaction which appears to include both agonist and antagonist activity at α–adrenergic and tryptaminergic receptors; they should be used cautiously in patients receiving vasopressors, particularly intramuscular pressors. A hypertensive patient should not receive ergot preparations as arteriospasm with catastrophic consequences could result. Ergonovine has been implicated in coronary spasm causing myocardial infarction in a previously asymptomatic 22-year-old patient.[177]

Prostaglandins are local hormones that produce uterine contraction. Prostaglandin $F_{2\alpha}$ as the 15-methyl analog has been the most useful of the prostaglandins in treating postpartum uterine atony. Hayashi, Castillo, and Noah[178] reported that intramuscular or intramyometrial injection of 0.25 to 0.5 mg 15-methyl prostaglandin $F_{2\alpha}$ for intractable postpartum uterine atony successfully stopped hemorrhage in 86 percent of patients. Mild, infrequent side effects included nausea, vomiting or diarrhea, or slight temperature elevation. Among the patients in whom therapy was ineffective, more than half had chorioamnionitis. Buttino and Garite[179] reported similar results. They successfully arrested hemorrhage in 85 percent; half the failures had placenta accreta. The authors conclude that prostaglandins will successfully treat atony except in the presence of placenta accreta, lacerations, or retained products of conception.

Prostaglandin E_2 has served less frequently in the treatment of uterine atony. In one case vaginal prostaglandin E_2 effectively arrested late postpartum hemorrhage after uterine curettage and three doses of methylergonovine were ineffective.[180] In another, intravenous prostaglandin E_2 at 10 μg per min stopped a single case of primary postpartum hemorrhage within 20 min.[181]

When pharmacologic attempts to stimulate contraction fail, the obstetrician must interrupt the blood supply or remove the bleeding uterus. Interrupting the blood supply without surgery involves either direct infusion of a vasoconstrictor such as pitressin into the bleeding vessel or embolization of the bleeding vessel. Magrina and colleagues[182] successfully controlled hemorrhage with pitressin infusion after oxytocin, methylergonovine, prostaglandin $F_{2\alpha}$, subtotal hysterectomy, and hypogastric artery ligation had failed. Embolization of pelvic arteries with Gelfoam effectively controls postpartum hemorrhage,[183] though the 2-hour procedure more effectively controls pelvic bleeding after gynecologic surgery.[184] Complications such as nerve ischemia or tissue loss leading to vesicovaginal fistula occur more frequently in older patients who have received radiotherapy for malignancy.[185,186]

Ligation of the uterine blood supply can effectively reduce uterine hemorrhage. Blood comes to the uterus from uterine arteries and from anastomoses with ovarian arteries. The uterine artery branches from the hypogastric (internal iliac) artery, one of two branches of the common iliac artery. The posterior division of the hypogastric artery supplies the fascia, viscera, and muscles of the pelvis as well as the perineal, gluteal, and anorectal regions; the anterior division gives rise to internal pudendal, uterine, vaginal, and superior vesical arteries. When possible, Cruikshank and Stoelk[187] recommend ligation of the anterior division of the hypogastric arteries as well as the ovarian arteries.

Hypogastric artery ligation does not render the uterus avascular but reduces pulsatile flow and allows clotting to occur. Unilateral ligation reduces distal ipsilateral flow by only 48 percent but reduces pulse pressure by 77 percent (85 percent following ligation of both arteries).[188] Control of hemorrhage still requires an intact clotting mechanism. The rich collateral blood flow makes pregnancy possible even after uterine artery ligation. O'Leary[189] reported 12 pregnancies after uterine artery ligation; interestingly, 3 of the 12 women had a repeat postcesarean hemorrhage requiring a second hypogastric artery ligation.

Hypogastric artery ligation is drastic therapy requiring surgery in a seriously ill patient; it is neither uniformly effective nor innocuous. In one series of 19 patients treated with hypogastric artery ligation for bleeding, the procedure was effective in 42 percent; the remaining 58 percent went on to hysterectomy.[190] Another series of 18 patients achieved similar results,[191] though two serious complications occurred in this series. One patient developed not only ischemic lower motor neuron damage but also ischemic breakdown of the central pelvic area; the other developed obstruction of the right common iliac artery and required femoral-femoral bypass grafting.

When all else fails, hysterectomy is the therapy of choice for uterine bleeding. Peripartum hysterectomy is a major operation. Maternal mortality approaches 1 percent in major centers,[146,192] a 10-fold increase over the mortality for cesarean section alone.[193] Reported blood loss before and during the procedure ranges from 500 to 10,000 ml,[194] with replacement of up to 35 units.[192,194] Indications for emergency peripartum hysterectomy include not only uterine atony unresponsive to other measures but also placenta accreta, uterine rupture, extension of a uterine incision laterally into vessels, abruption with DIC, chorioamnionitis, and leiomyomata. Unfortunately, only one-fourth of the patients who will require hysterectomy can be identified in advance.[87]

If hysterectomy fails to control bleeding, few options remain. Selective pitressin infusion and arterial embolization have been mentioned above. Jackson, Liebermann, and Smith[195] describe a single case in which deliberate hypotension induced by sodium nitroprusside slowed bleeding after hypogastric artery ligation in a patient who became hypertensive. Cassels, Greenberg, and Otterson[196] describe use of a mushroom pack for pelvic tamponade after hysterectomy for postpartum bleeding.

Anesthetic Considerations. Uterine atony may be treated simply by uterine massage, or it may require escalating therapy in a progressively more compromised patient, culminating in laparotomy and massive transfusion. The fundamental principal of resuscitative management with uterine atony is to maintain intravascular volume as attempts to treat atony proceed. Prompt and vigorous volume resuscitation should begin at once when the uterus fails to contract and should continue until hemostasis is established. Patients should not have to become hypotensive or exhibit signs of shock to command attention on an obstetric floor; any hint of excess bleeding should prompt vigorous volume replacement while diagnosis and therapy proceed.

Anesthesia depends on obstetric needs. Examination, uterine massage, fluid resuscitation, and oxytocics may require little anesthesia. Laparotomy for control of hemorrhage calls for balanced general endotracheal anesthesia in an adequately and continuously resuscitated patient. (See the section on anesthetic options above.)

Lacerations

Obstetric Considerations. Lacerations of the cervix, vagina, and perineum are the second most common cause of excessive maternal blood loss at delivery. Serious cervical or vaginal lacerations occur more frequently with operative delivery (e.g., use of forceps), particularly when the infant is high in the birth canal, the operator is relatively inexperienced, or the patient is poorly anesthetized and highly mobile. Vaginal rupture is a rare condition that may occur spontaneously or may follow traumatic delivery.[197]

Lacerations should be suspected when vaginal bleeding continues despite good uterine contractions. Diagnosis rests on direct visualization during examination. Vaginal rupture may allow the examiner to see intestinal loops with fatty epiploic appendages during vaginal exam, a presentation which could also be seen with ruptured uterus. Treatment of lacerations consists of maintaining intravascular volume, conducting a thorough examination of the uterus and birth canal, and repairing lacerations surgically. Vaginal rupture may require laparotomy;[197] other lacerations can be repaired vaginally. The obstetrician requires good lighting and assistance with retraction; the patient requires good anesthesia.

Anesthetic Considerations. Resuscitation should be as extensive as necessary for the amount of bleeding; lacerations do not usually produce major hemorrhage unless large vessels are involved. Anesthesia requirements depend on the affected areas. Perineal lacerations frequently involve only the area innervated by the pudendal nerve; when local infiltration does not suffice, careful bilateral pudendal nerve block with supplemental intravenous or inhalation analgesia often proves satisfactory even for extensive repairs. However, major conduction anesthesia (spinal, lumbar epidural, or caudal) produces more widespread and dependable block, allowing not only comfortable perineal repair but also uterine and cervical examination and repair. Repair of extensive lacerations may require general endotracheal anesthesia with appropriate precautions to prevent aspiration of gastric contents. General anesthesia or major conduction anesthesia are equally appropriate for laparotomy in the well-resuscitated patient with vaginal rupture.

Retained Placenta

Obstetric Considerations. When all or part of the placenta stays within the uterine cavity after separation from the implantation site, the uterus cannot contract completely, and hemorrhage continues. Retention of the placenta or placental fragments is the third most frequent cause of postpartum hemorrhage. The diagnosis is suspected when bleeding continues from the cervical os in spite of apparently firm uterine contraction. Though therapeutic examination and curettage usually confirm the diagnosis, one group has reported detecting placental fragments and clots in the postpartum uterus on ultrasound examination, saving some patients the necessity of examination and curettage should the uterus prove empty.[198] Therapy for retained placenta may be as simple as brief manual examination with placental extraction or as complex as immediate hysterectomy for placenta accreta.

Anesthetic Considerations. Adequate resuscitation must take place before anesthetic intervention. The parturient seldom hemorrhages so rapidly from a retained placenta that resuscitation cannot be accomplished before induction.

Obstetric plans dictate anesthetic management. Good perineal and uterine anesthesia expedite manual removal of the placenta or uterine curettage. Analgesia using nitrous oxide, small doses of narcotics, or ketamine may permit expeditious removal if the placenta has already separated; if not, or if the obstetrician plans curettage or removal of small fragments, more adequate anesthesia is best instituted before beginning. Lumbar epidural, caudal, or spinal block suffice for all placental manipulations; if the patient was not anesthetized for delivery, the anesthesiologist can institute major regional anesthesia de novo for removal of placental fragments, particularly in the absence of hypovolemia and if the obstetrician anticipates extensive examination or curettage. The patient who needs more than brief analgesia but does not qualify for regional anesthesia can receive general endotracheal anesthesia. Inhalation of volatile anesthetics or amyl nitrite can provide uterine relaxation, when required.

Placenta Accreta, Increta, Percreta

Obstetric Considerations. Placenta accreta, an abnormality of placentation in which placental villi attach directly to the myometrium without intervening decidua basalis, makes separation of the intact placenta from the uterus virtually impossible. Placental villi invade or penetrate the myometrium in placenta increta and placenta percreta, respectively. Placenta increta and -percreta have been discussed earlier in relation to antepartum uterine rupture, with which they are strongly associated. Incidence of placenta accreta in recent reviews ranges from 1 in 2562 to 1 in 4348 pregnancies.[199,200] Read, Cotton, and Miller[199] estimate maternal mortality of 3.1 percent from placenta accreta in the period from 1970 to 1980, a decline from previous reports of 37 percent before 1934 and 10 percent between 1945 and 1969.

Placenta accreta shows a strong association with placenta previa and with previous uterine surgery. Not only does the incidence of placenta previa increase after cesarean section, but the incidence of placenta accreta among the previae increases markedly. Singh, Rodrigues, and Gupta[78] found placenta accreta in 15 percent of patients with placenta previa and prior cesarean section, but only 1 percent of patients with placenta previa and an unscarred uterus. Other studies confirm the relationship between placenta accreta, placenta previa, and previous cesarean section.[87,199,201] Clark, Koonings, and Phelan reported that the risk of placenta accreta with placenta previa and an unscarred uterus was 5 percent; with placenta previa and one prior cesarean section, the incidence rose to 26 percent and continued to rise until the risk of placenta accreta reached 67 percent with placenta previa and four or more previous sections.

Recognition of placenta accreta before the placenta is damaged by unsuccessful attempts at manual removal simplifies management, since a completely adherent placenta provokes no maternal bleeding. If untreated, a morbidly adherent placenta undergoes slow postpartum involution over almost 2 months, with continued risk of infection or hemorrhage; methotrexate has successfully hastened involution,[203] with no ultrasound evidence of the placenta 13 days after delivery. However, this would seldom be the treatment of choice in a major North American medical center.

Placenta accreta usually calls for immediate peripartum hysterectomy.[87,119,199] Recognition of placenta accreta before placental disruption reduces blood loss, but morbid adherence may not be obvious until attempts at removal are unsuccessful. Partial or focal placenta accreta may be treated conservatively without hysterectomy,[199] though placenta accreta in these cases remains a clinical diagnosis without pathologic confirmation.

Anesthetic Considerations. Resuscitation is the first priority, but a partially destroyed placenta accreta may bleed so copiously that complete resuscitation is difficult without simultaneous surgical control of bleeding. In Clark and associates[87] series of emergency hysterectomies for hemorrhage, average blood loss with placenta accreta reached 3506 ml—less bloody than uterine atony (4013 ml) or extension of the uterine incision into the great vessels (4780 ml).

In most cases of placenta accreta, patients will need anesthesia for laparotomy. When placenta accreta becomes evident during cesarean section under regional anesthesia, continued regional anesthesia is appropriate if the patient tolerates additional time and surgical manipulation without difficulty. If enough supplemental sedation to cause loss of airway reflexes becomes necessary, establish general endotracheal anesthesia. Most anesthesiologists employ general endotracheal anesthesia when anesthesia is required de novo for hysterectomy in the presence of placenta accreta, particularly in the unstable or bleeding patient.

Lower Segment Placental Implantation

Postpartum hemorrhage often follows placental implantation in an area of the uterus that contracts poorly, since constriction of the placental bed may be ineffective. Postpartum hemorrhage may occur with placenta previa, with any implantation in the lower uterine segment, or with implantation at the site of an old uterine scar.

When massage and uterotonic agents cannot control the bleeding, surgical control may be necessary. In the patient already undergoing cesarean section, hemostatic suturing of discrete bleeding sites may control bleeding. If this proves ineffective, or control of bleeding requires laparotomy, ligation of uterine blood supply is usually the procedure of choice. Hysterectomy may be necessary as a last resort.

Uterine Rupture

The obstetric and anesthetic considerations with uterine rupture have been discussed in the section on antepartum hemorrhage. Uterine rupture deserves mention in a discussion of postpartum hemorrhage because the diagnosis may not become apparent until the postpartum period, even though rupture is usually an antepartum event. For example, 29 of 129 patients with uterine rupture in one series presented with postpartum bleeding; diagnosis took place in the postpartum period in 45 percent of all uterine ruptures.[110] We emphasize that differential diagnosis of postpartum hemorrhage must include uterine rupture to ensure proper diagnosis and appropriate treatment—in this case, hysterectomy or repair of the uterine defect.

Uterine Inversion

Obstetric Considerations. The inverted uterus actually everts, turning inside out so that the placental surface appears on the outside. Inversion may be partial, with the fundus inverted inside the lower uterine segment, or complete, with the inside-out uterus actually protruding from the vagina. Reported incidence ranges upward from 1 in 1700 deliveries,[204] though unreported institutional rates may be higher. Inversion can be fatal, yet mortality rates are not available from the literature.

Inversion produces profuse and continued postpartum bleeding. Hemorrhage occurred in 94 percent of such cases in one series;[204] 39 percent of these patients were in shock, but the shock related proportionally to blood loss. The uterus inverts more frequently when atonic or when the obstetrician has applied inappropriate traction to the umbilical cord to hasten delivery of the placenta.[205,206]

Treatment of uterine inversion consists of immediate reduction of the inversion while restoring intravascular volume. Continued firm pressure against the fundus from inside the uterus is necessary for reduction, which can be performed with relative ease without uterine relaxation if undertaken at once. However, if inversion is not recognized or reduction is delayed until after a cervical contraction ring has formed, uterine relaxation may be required.[204,205] This is particularly likely in the hands of an inexperienced attendant; oxytocics and massage fail to stop the bleeding, but contract the inverted uterus so firmly on itself that reduction without relaxation is impossible. Even after reduction, a uterus which has been inverted may remain atonic, and recurrent inversion may occur. Heyl[206] describes successful management of such a patient with 15-methyl prostaglandin $F_{2\alpha}$ and uterine packing. Additional steps to control hemorrhage may be necessary, including laparotomy for control of uterine blood supply or for hysterectomy. (See the section on uterine atony for further discussion.)

Anesthetic Considerations. Resuscitation is the first priority. Though hypotension out of proportion to apparent blood loss was once considered characteristic of uterine inversion, this arose from our inability to estimate obstetric blood loss rather than from any special characteristic of obstetric shock. Postpartum hematocrits usually reflect blood losses much greater than initial estimates. A patient with uterine inversion needs vigorous replacement of current and continuing losses until the uterus is positioned and satisfactory uterine tone is restored.

Reduction of an inverted uterus that has begun to contract on itself can be painful. The process is easily accomplished in patients who have satisfactory regional anesthesia (spinal, caudal, or lumbar epidural) for delivery. Reduction can otherwise be accomplished under balanced general endotracheal anesthesia, usually without uterine relaxation unless the uterus has become tightly contracted on itself. Uterine relaxation, if needed, can be provided by adding a volatile agent to the inhaled anesthetic mixture. However, a patient who has been bleeding from an inverted uterus may be so hypovolemic despite vigorous resuscitation that high concentrations of a volatile agent are unwise. In our experience, uterine reduction has usually occurred by the time the patient is able to tolerate volatile agents.

Cesarean Section

Blood loss at cesarean section ranges from 500 to 1500 ml. Some of the loss comes from the placental site, just as in a vaginal delivery; the remainder comes from vessels disrupted by incisions in the abdominal wall and in the uterus. In spite of the relatively large blood losses, few patients require replacement of RBCs or even colloid. Crystalloid replacement of three to four times the estimated blood loss usually is satisfactory.

However, blood loss at routine cesarean section may approach 20 percent of a parturient's blood volume. Unanticipated bleeding—as from an atonic uterus, an adherent placenta, or a lateral extension of the uterine incision—could rapidly compromise intravascular volume and tissue oxygenation. For this reason, all patients undergoing cesarean section should have a large-bore intravenous cannula in place and should have blood available. When the blood bank is in the hospital, advance blood typing and antibody screen suffice. Except in cases where unusual blood loss is anticipated, patients having cesarean section do not need typed and cross-matched blood set up in advance.

COAGULATION DEFECTS

Congenital defects of the coagulation process, such as hereditary factor deficiencies, have been discussed in Chapter 14. Normal coagulation is reviewed in the physiology section at the beginning of this chapter. This section discusses acquired problems of hemostasis, which may be induced by drugs or by pathologic processes. The section on resuscitation covers dilution of coagulation factors during massive transfusion.

Drug-Induced Coagulation Defects

Heparin, oral anticoagulants such as warfarin, and drugs such as aspirin that alter platelet function can affect the coagulation process. Heparin acts through a plasma cofactor, antithrombin III, to inactive thrombin and neutralize several activated clotting factors (XII, XI, X, IX, and VII).[207] Though heparin is used infrequently in pregnancy, patients with a history of deep venous thrombosis have received it in low doses. In the extremely rare event of bleeding due to anticoagulation with heparin, intravenous protamine (1 mg for every 100 units of heparin remaining in the patient) provides rapid reversal.

A pregnant patient rarely takes warfarin, except in the event of accidental ingestion. Warfarin inhibits production of vitamin K–dependent clotting factors (prothrombin, VII, IX, X) in the liver. Intravenous administration of up to 50 mg of vitamin K_1 serves as treatment for severe warfarin-induced hemorrhage;[207] continued intravascular volume support will be needed, however, as the drug requires several hours to produce effects. In a bleeding crisis the anesthesiologist may consider administration of the deficient clotting factors themselves.

Pregnant patients often have used aspirin because they regard it as a benign drug and because it may have some therapeutic role. For example, some have suggested that aspirin prevents maternal symptoms of pre-eclampsia,[208] although Goodlin[209] contends that only the mother benefits from such therapy. Aspirin interferes with platelet function by inhibiting release of ADP and inhibiting synthesis of the prostaglandins and thromboxane which stimulate aggregation. The effects on platelets are irreversible, lasting the life of the platelet. Prolonged bleeding times may persist for several days after aspirin therapy ceases.[207] Stuart and colleagues[210] found hematologic abnormalities in 60 percent of mothers and 90 percent of newborns when mothers took aspirin within 5 days of delivery.

Acquired Coagulation Defects

Blood's ability to clot helps stop bleeding; however, defective clotting does not by itself cause bleeding. Bleeding follows disruption of blood vessels; coagulation problems only make such bleeding more difficult to stop. The most common hemostatic defect is inadequate surgical hemostasis;[55] discovery of a coagulation problem should not divert attention from mechanical hemostasis. Surgical hemostasis must be even more meticulous when blood clots poorly.

Acquired coagulation defects with pregnancy include disseminated intravascular coagulation (DIC), coagulopathy with pre-eclampsia, and the dilutional changes with massive transfusion. The last has been discussed earlier in the chapter.

Disseminated Intravascular Coagulation. Generalized activation of the clotting system can occur when a disease causes widespread vascular damage or when thromboplastic materials enter the circulation.[33] Obstetric patients are particularly at risk for the latter because of the open venous sinuses beneath the placental site. Abruptio placentae is the commonest obstetric cause of DIC; significant coagulation abnormalities occur in 10 percent of abruptions overall but in up to 30 percent of severe abruptions.[211] Twenty percent of those with coagulopathy develop uterine inertia that is refractory to oxytocin.[212] The catastrophic cardiovascular collapse thought to accompany amniotic fluid embolism is accompanied by significant DIC so frequently that the presence of DIC helps establish the diagnosis. Additionally, DIC can also occur in the patient who carries a retained dead fetus in utero, as products of fetal or placental degeneration enter her circulation. The incidence of coagulation abnormalities exceeds 25 percent if the fetus has been dead for more than 4 weeks.[211]

Whatever the initiating event, DIC results from generalized activation of a usually local process. Thrombin and plasmin generation leads to the evolution not only of fibrin but also of fibrin-fibrinogen degradation products, which behave as anticoagulants. Though some patients remain asymptomatic, most patients will display signs of either excessive bleeding or of intravascular thrombosis, depending on the balance between the evolution of thrombin and the limiting reactions. Shock will worsen the problem by reducing peripheral blood flow and hepatic perfusion, thereby reducing dilution and clearance of activated clotting factors while producing further cell damage.

Diagnosis. No single laboratory test establishes the presence of disseminated intravascular coagulation, nor is any specific constellation of signs and symptoms unique. Clinical suspicion prompts laboratory testing. Suspicion may be based on increased likelihood of DIC — the patient with abruption, amniotic fluid embolus, or retained dead fetus — or on a clinical presentation that unmistakably suggests a clotting problem, with bleeding from the gums, from venipuncture sites, from surgical wounds, and into the urine. The diagnosis rests on laboratory evidence that clotting factors are being consumed, with activation of both coagulation and fibrinolysis.

Laboratory findings consistent with DIC include decreased fibrinogen level, decreased platelet count, prolonged thrombin time, abnormal levels of fibrin-fibrinogen degradation products, and a peripheral smear showing red-cell fragmentation.

Plasma fibrinogen levels normally range from 400 to 600 mg per dl in pregnancy, with levels as high as 800 to 1000 mg per dl in severe pre-eclampsia. A "normal" level of 150 to 250 mg per dl may represent marked depletion in a pregnant patient. Comparison with a baseline value is helpful; serial tests establish a decline.

The platelet count remains normal in pregnancy. Laboratory levels that would otherwise be abnormally low are likewise low in pregnancy.

Fibrin-fibrinogen degradation products can be demonstrated by a variety of tests which fall into three groups: immunologic tests (Fi test, tanned red-cell agglutination), staphylococcal clumping, or paracoagulation (protamine sulfate precipitation, ethanol gelation). Though the effect of pregnancy on FDPs is not resolved, it appears that they should not normally be present, even in pregnancy.[37] Individual laboratories can best interpret the significance of the tests which they use.

The thrombin time, measured by adding dilute thrombin to plasma and recording the time necessary to form a clot, tests the reactivity of the fibrinogen in plasma. This reactivity remains normal in pregnancy but is reduced in DIC.

Treatment of DIC. Treating obstetric DIC consists primarily of maintaining circulatory volume while removing the stimulus that triggered DIC. Blood volume replacement and circulatory support are the resuscitator's first priorities. Replacement of specific clotting factors is usually unnecessary and may be dangerous. Treatment with heparin or with inhibitors of fibrinolysis appears to have little place in obstetrics.

Volume replacement follows the guidelines outlined earlier in the section on resuscitation. Restoring the circulation improves regional circulation and hepatic blood flow, both important as thrombin-limiting forces. If massive blood replacement is necessary, the deficiencies of stored blood (Factor V, Factor VIII, platelets) may become more of an issue. Fresh frozen plasma and platelets can be administered as needed in the presence of severe clotting factor deficiency. However, in the absence of frank bleeding from open vessels, replacement of clotting factors is usually unnecessary. Deficient factors will be repleted after the initiating stimulus has been corrected — in most obstetric cases, after the uterus has been emptied. If the stimulus persists, infusion of additional clotting factors may stimulate further consumption, perhaps tilting the balance in favor of clotting rather than lysis.

Fibrinogen replacement, once emphasized in treating obstetric DIC, now seems unsupportable. Bleeding in DIC results more from anticoagulant breakdown products of fibrinogen than from depletion of clotting factors; adding fibrinogen may worsen the process. The high risk of hepatitis with commercial pooled-plasma fibrinogen reduces its appeal even further.

Antifibrinolytic agents such as ε-aminocaproic acid have no role in treatment of obstetric DIC; such agents remove the important thrombin-limiting action of plasmin and may result in generalized thrombosis. Sher[93] has championed the use of aprotonin (Trasylol), an antifibrinolytic, antithromboplastic, antikallikrein agent currently unavailable in the United States, claiming improvement in consumption coagulopathy and in uterine activity with its use.

Although some suggest that antithrombin action of heparin should make it useful for treatment of DIC, nothing recommends its use. It has not been shown effective, may be frankly dangerous in the presence of open blood vessels, and is not necessary because most obstetric DIC clears by itself with adequate resuscitation and removal of the initiating stimulus.

Obstetric DIC has no specific treatment beyond applying sound principles of resuscitation to support the patient while removing the initiating stimulus and recovery begins. Obstetric need, the patient's intravascular volume status, and the bleeding which follows all vascular injury dictate anesthetic considerations.

Coagulation Defects With Pre-eclampsia. Pre-eclamptic patients may exhibit coagulopathy manifested primarily by thrombocytopenia, with normal levels of fibrinogen, normal prothrombin time and partial thromboplastin time, and no evidence of fibrin degradation products.[211] Platelet counts may drop to 20,000,[213] often associated with a corresponding derangement of liver function.[214] Weinstein[215] has coined the acronym HELLP for the syndrome of *H*emolysis, *E*levated *L*iver enzymes, and *L*ow *P*latelets which appears as a variant of severe pre-eclampsia. Available evidence suggests that the thrombocytopenia of pre-eclampsia results not from a change in platelets themselves nor from increased thrombin activity but rather from an apparent increase in platelet turnover as platelets adhere to damaged vascular endothelium.[216–221] Weenink and associates[222] report that platelet counts and antithrombin III levels correlate inversely with the degree of placental infarction in pre-eclampsia and suggests that increased consumption in the maternal vasculature also depresses antithrombin III levels.

Treatment consists of supportive therapy, including platelet transfusions for counts under 20,000, while expediting delivery. If severe thrombocytopenia and significantly prolonged bleeding time exist, major neuraxis block (spinal, epidural, caudal) may present an unacceptable risk of bleeding into the subarachnoid or epidural space.

Other Acquired Problems. Two recent reports[223,224] describe patients with acquired Factor VIII inhibitors who experienced late postpartum bleeding (10 days after vaginal delivery or cesarean section). Patients were treated successfully with Autoplex, an anti-inhibitor coagulant complex, when other treatment had failed.

Nonobstetric Hemorrhage in the Obstetric Patient

In addition to the bleeding that follows trauma and accidents, obstetric patients face a greater risk of hepatic bleeding and intracranial hemorrhage. Pregnancy may complicate treatment of other nonobstetric hemorrhage.

HEPATIC BLEEDING

Intrahepatic bleeding, subcapsular hematoma, and rupture of the liver are rare complications of pregnancy associated with pre-eclampsia. The incidence is difficult to determine; maternal mortality ranges from 40 to 75 percent when the liver ruptures.[225,226] Liver enzyme elevation, coagulopathy, and right upper quadrant pain accompany hepatic bleeding. Ultrasonography or CAT scan can identify intraparenchymal or subcapsular bleeding before liver rupture.[227] Rupture may occur suddenly, usually in the right lobe, with rapid deterioration due to intra-abdominal bleeding.

Once the liver ruptures, prompt recognition of the problem facilitates resuscitation of the patient and surgical control of bleeding.[228] Control of hemorrhage almost always requires laparotomy, though Loevinger[225] reports a single case in which transcatheter embolotherapy using Gelfoam pledgets successfully treated bleeding from hepatic rupture.

Anesthesia considerations are those of other massive hemorrhage. Resuscitation is the first priority, but it may not be accomplished until bleeding is surgically controlled. Laparotomy calls for general endotracheal anesthesia. The patient, usually severely pre-eclamptic (see Chap. 21), will remain quite ill even if she survives the operation and merits attention to hemodynamic and ventilatory monitoring which should continue postoperatively.

INTRACRANIAL AND OTHER BLEEDING

Intracranial hemorrhage is a rare event, occurring in fewer than 1 : 10,000 pregnancies; however, the mortality exceeds 80 percent.[229] The risk of intracranial hemorrhage increases with pregnancy-induced hypertension. Treatment depends on the lesion and on the stage of pregnancy. Although a viable fetus might be removed by cesarean section at the time of craniotomy for bleeding, Reece and colleagues[229] report craniotomy for intracerebral hematoma at 24 weeks' gestation, after which the fetus was left in utero until vaginal delivery at 33 weeks.

Howard[230] reports recurrent epistaxis in a normotensive pregnant patient that was so severe that the patient underwent simultaneous cesarean section and external carotid artery ligation at 36 weeks' gestation. The patient recovered uneventfully after an episode of aspiration pneumonia secondary to inhalation of blood.

Summary

Birth is bloody, but bleeding at birth should seldom be fatal. Rapid and adequate fluid resuscitation is the most important response to obstetric hemorrhage, followed by immediate measures to stop the bleeding. The anesthetist must ensure resuscitation, assist in diagnosis, and facilitate repair.

References

1. Hogberg, U and Brostrom, G: The demography of maternal mortality: Seven Swedish parishes in the 19th century. Int J Gynaecol Obstet 23:489, 1985.
2. Hogberg, U and Joelsson, I: The decline in maternal mortality in Sweden, 1931–1980. Acta Obstet Gynecol Scand 64:583, 1985.
3. Varner, MW, et al: Maternal mortality in a major referral hospital, 1926 to 1980. Am J Obstet Gynecol 143:325, 1982.
4. Kaunitz, AM, et al: Causes of maternal mortality in the United States. Obstet Gynecol 65:605, 1985.
5. Wiener, WB: Maternal mortality in Mississippi: 1977–1978. J Miss St Med Assoc 22:208, 1981.
6. Benedetti, TJ, Starzyk, P and Frost, F: Maternal deaths in Washington state. Obstet Gynecol 66:99, 1985.
7. Sachs, BP, et al: Maternal mortality in Massachusetts: Trends and prevention. N Engl J Med 316:667, 1987.
8. Thompson, JP: Maternal deaths in New Jersey: 1979. J Med Soc NJ 78:825, 1981.
9. Augensen, K and Bergsjo, P: Maternal mortality in the Nordic countries 1970–1979. Acta Obstet Gynecol Scand 63:115, 1984.
10. Hogberg, U: Maternal deaths in Sweden: 1971–1980. Acta Obstet Gynecol Scand 65:161, 1986.
11. Boulton, FE and Letsky, E: Obstetric hemorrhage: Causes and management. Clin Haematol 14:683, 1985.
12. Steinberg, WM and Farine, D: Maternal mortality in Ontario from 1970 to 1980. Obstet Gynecol 66:510, 1985.
13. Hogberg, U: Maternal mortality: A worldwide problem. Int J Gynaecol Obstet 23:463, 1985.
14. Chattopadhyay, SK, et al: Maternal mortality in Riyadh, Saudi Arabia. Br J Obstet Gynaecol 90:809, 1983.
15. Mashini, I, Mroueh, A and Hadi, H: Maternal mortality in the American University of Beirut Medical Center: 1971–1982. Int J Gynaecol Obstet 22:275, 1984.
16. Chi, IC, et al: In-hospital maternal mortality risk by cesarean and vaginal deliveries in two less developed countries: A descriptive study. Int J Gynaecol Obstet 24:121, 1986.
17. Crowther, CA: Maternal deaths at Harare Maternity Hospital during 1893. S Afr Med J 69:180, 1986.
18. De Groot, HAV: Maternal mortality in Cape Town: 1978–1983. S Afr Med J 69:797, 1986.
19. Walker, GJA, et al: Maternal mortality in Jamaica. Lancet i(8479):486, 1986.
20. Melrose, EB: Maternal deaths at King Edward VIII Hospital, Durban. S Afr Med J 65:161, 1984.
21. Hartfield, VJ and Woodland, M: Prevention of maternal death in a Nigerian Village. Int J Gynaecol Obstet 18:150, 1980.
22. Buehler, JW, et al: Maternal mortality in women aged 35 years or older: United States. JAMA 255:53, 1986.
23. Kaunitz, AM, et al: Perinatal and maternal mortality in a religious group avoiding obstetric care. Am J Obstet Gynecol 150:826, 1984.
24. Berman, SM, et al: Deaths from spontaneous abortion in the United States. JAMA 253:3119, 1985.
25. Grimes, DA, et al: Fatal hemorrhage from legal abortion in the United States. Surg Gynecol Obstet 157:461, 1983.
26. Atrash, HK, et al: Legal abortion mortality in the United States: 1972 to 1982. Am J Obstet Gynecol 156:605, 1987.
27. Petitti, DB, et al: In-hospital maternal mortality in the United States: Time trends and relation to method of delivery. Obstet Gynecol 59:6, 1982.
28. Moldin, P, Hokegard, K-H and Nielsen, TF: Cesarean section and maternal mortality in Sweden: 1973–1979. Acta Obstet Gynecol Scand 63:7, 1984.
29. Petitti, DB: Maternal mortality and morbidity in cesarean section. Clin Obstet Gynecol 28:763, 1985.
30. U.S. Department of Health, Education, and Welfare (Public Health Service): Vital statistics of the United States 1974, vol II, Mortality: Part A. Hyattsville, MD, 1978.
31. Pritchard, JA: Haematological problems associated with delivery, placental abruption, retained dead fetus and amniotic fluid embolism. Clin Haematol 2:563, 1973.
32. Ueland, K: Maternal cardiovascular dynamics VII: Intrapartum blood volume changes. Am J Obstet Gynecol 126:671, 1976.
33. Deykin, D: Hemostasis. In Reich, RR: Hematology: Physiopathologic Basis for Clinical Practice. Little, Brown & Co, Boston, 1978.
34. Brandt, JT: Current concepts of coagulation. Clin Obstet Gynecol 28:3, 1985.
35. Wintrobe, MM, et al: Clinical Hematology. Lea & Febiger, Philadelphia, 1974.
36. Deykin, D: The clinical challenge of disseminated intravascular coagulation. N Engl J Med 283:636, 1970.

37. Bonnar, J: Coagulation disorders. J Clin Pathol (Suppl)10:35, 1976.
38. Moore, SB: Management of transfusion in the massively bleeding patient. Hum Pathol 14:267, 1983.
39. Guyton, AC: Textbook of Medical Physiology. WB Saunders, Philadelphia, 1980.
40. Giesecke, AH, Jr and Egbert, LD: Perioperative fluid therapy: Crystalloids. In Miller, RD (ed): Anesthesia, ed 2. Churchill Livingstone, New York, 1986.
41. Marsden, DE and Cavanagh, D: Hemorrhagic shock in the gynecologic patient. Clin Obstet Gynecol 28:381, 1985.
42. Puri, V, Paidipty, B and White, L: Hydroxyethyl starch for resuscitation of patients with hypovolemia and shock. Crit Care Med 9:833, 1981.
43. Daniels, MJ, Strauss, RG and Smith-Floss, AM: Effects of hydroxyethyl starch on erythrocyte typing and crossmatching. Transfusion 22:226, 1981.
44. Ljungstrom, KG, et al: Adverse reactions to dextran in Sweden: 1970 – 1979. Acta Chir Scand 149:253, 1983.
45. Tremper, KK, et al: The preoperative treatment of severely anemic patients with perfluorochemical oxygen-transport fluid, Fluosol-DA. N Engl J Med 307:277, 1982.
46. Waxman, K, et al: Perfluorocarbon infusion of bleeding patients refusing blood transfusions. Arch Surg 119:721, 1984.
47. National Institutes of Health: Fresh Frozen Plasma: Indications and Risks Consensus Development Conference Statement. NIH, Bethesda, 1984.
48. Miller, RD, et al: Coagulation defects associated with massive blood transfusions. Ann Surg 174:794, 1971.
49. Entwhistle, CC: Clotting factor concentrates. Int Anesth Clin 23:49, 1985.
50. Milam, JD: The emergency transfusion. Tex Med 80:52, 1984.
51. Toy, PTCY, et al: Predeposited autologous blood for elective surgery: A national multicenter study. N Engl J Med 316:517, 1987.
52. Iserson, KW and Reeter, AK: Rapid fluid replacement for severe hypovolemia: Human subject trials. West J Med 146:313, 1987.
53. Lundsgaard-Hansen, P and Pappova, E: Component therapy of surgical hemorrhage: Red cells, plasma substitutes and albumin. Ann Clin Res (Suppl)13:26, 1981.
54. Wiklund, L and Thoren, L: Intraoperative blood component and fluid therapy. Acta Anaesthesiol Scand 29:1, 1985.
55. Blajchman, MA, Herst, R and Perrault, RA: Blood component therapy in anaesthetic practice. Can Anaesth Soc J 30:382, 1983.
56. Orlin, JB: Current trends in whole blood and red cell therapy. Postgrad Med 72:63, 1982.
57. Zauder, HL: Massive transfusion. Int Anesth Clin 20:157, 1982.
58. Findley, LJ and Redstone, PM: Blood transfusion in adult Jehovah's Witnesses: A case study of one congregation. Arch Intern Med 142:606, 1982.
59. Sacks, DA and Koppes, RH: Blood transfusion in Jehovah's Witnesses: Medical and legal issues in obstetrics and gynecology. Am J Obstet Gynecol 154:483, 1986.
60. Oneson, R, Douglas, DK and Mintz, PD: Letter to the editor. Transfusion 25:179, 1985.
61. Popovsky, MA and Moore SB: Letter to the editor. Transfusion 25:444, 1985.
62. Lichtiger, B, Dupuis, JF and Seski, J: Hemotherapy during surgery for Jehovah's Witnesses: A new method. Anesth Analg 61:618, 1982.
63. Kaplan, RF, et al: Letter to the editor. Anesth Analg 62:122, 1983.
64. Karn, KE, et al: Use of a whole blood substitute, Fluosol-DA 20%, after massive postpartum hemorrhage. Obstet Gynecol 65:127, 1985.
65. Reid, MF, Nohr, K and Birks, RJS: Letter to the editor. Anaesthesia 41:324, 1986.
66. Bonakdar, MI, et al: Major gynecologic and obstetric surgery in Jehovah's Witnesses. Obstet Gynecol 60:587, 1982.
67. Jewett, JF: Report from the Committee on Maternal Welfare: Total exsanguination. N Engl J Med 305:1216, 1981.
68. Anderson, GR: Medicine versus religion: The case of the Jehovah's Witnesses. Health Soc Work 8:31, 1983.
69. Drake, K: What to do when a patient refuses treatment. Leg Aspects Med Pract 7:22, 1979.
70. Sellick, BA: Cricoid pressure to control regurgitation of stomach contents during induction in anesthesia. Lancet 2:404, 1961.
71. Cullen, DJ: The effect of pretreatment with nondepolarizing muscle relaxants on the neuromuscular blocking action of succinylcholine. Anesthesiology 35:572, 1971.
72. Bonica, JJ: The nature of pain of parturition. Clin Obstet Gynecol 2:511, 1975.
73. Naftalin, NJ, et al: The effects of halothane on pregnant and non-pregnant human myometrium. Anesthesiology 46:11, 1977.
74. Munson, ES and Embro, WJ: Enflurane, isoflurane, and halothane and isolated human uterine muscle. Anesthesiology 46:11, 1977.
75. Zsigmond, EK, Kelsch, RC and Kothary, SP: Rise in plasma free norepinephrine during anesthetic induction with ketamine. Behav Neuropsych 6:81, 1975.
76. Abdul-Karim, RW and Chevli, RN: Antepartum hemorrhage and shock. Clin Obstet Gynecol 19:533, 1976.
77. Green-Thompson, RW: Antepartum haemorrhage. Clin Obstet Gynaecol 9:479, 1982.
78. Singh, PM, Rodrigues, C and Gupta, AN: Placenta previa and previous cesarean section. Acta Obstet Gynecol Scand 60:367, 1981.
79. Hill, DJ and Beischer, NA: Placenta praevia without antepartum haemorrhage. Aust NZ J Obstet Gynaecol 20:21, 1980.
80. Crenshaw, C, Jr, Jones, DED and Parker, RT: Placenta previa: A survey of twenty years' experience with improved perinatal survival by expectant therapy and cesarean delivery. Obstet Gynecol Surv 28:461, 1973.
81. Hibbard, LT: Placenta previa. Am J Obstet Gynecol 104:172, 1969.

82. McShane, PM, Heyl, PS and Epstein, MF: Maternal and perinatal morbidity resulting from placenta previa. Obstet Gynecol 65:176, 1985.
83. Silver, RD, et al: Placenta previa: Aggressive expectant management. Am J Obstet Gynecol 150:15, 1984.
84. Tomich, PG: Prolonged use of tocolytic agents in the expectant management of placenta previa. J Reprod Med 30:745, 1985.
85. Bowen, LW and Beeson, JH: Use of a large Foley catheter balloon to control postpartum hemorrhage resulting from a low cervical implantation. J Reprod Med 30:623, 1985.
86. Reginald, PW, Reid, JE and Paintin, DB: Control of bleeding in cervical pregnancy: Two case reports. Br J Obstet Gynaecol 92:1199, 1985.
87. Clark, SL, et al: Emergency hysterectomy for obstetric hemorrhage. Obstet Gynecol 64:376, 1984.
88. Abdella, TN, et al: Relationship of hypertensive disease to abruptio placentae. Obstet Gynecol 63:365, 1984.
89. Karegard, M and Gennser G: Incidence and recurrence rate of abruptio placentae in Sweden. Obstet Gynecol 67:523, 1986.
90. Nelson, DM, Stempel, LE and Zuspan, FP: Association of prolonged, preterm rupture of the membranes and abruptio placentae. J Reprod Med 31:249, 1986.
91. Pritchard, JA, et al: Genesis of severe placental abruption. Am J Obstet Gynecol 108:22, 1970.
92. Schwartz, RW: Pregnancy in physicians: Characteristics and complications. Obstet Gynecol 66:672, 1985.
93. Sher, G: Trasylol in the management of abruptio placentae with consumption coagulopathy and uterine inertia. J Reprod Med 25:113, 1980.
94. Okonofua, FE and Olatunbosun, OA: Cesarean versus vaginal delivery in abruptio placentae associated with live fetuses. Int J Gynaecol Obstet 23:471, 1985.
95. Hurd, WW, et al: Selective management of abruptio placentae: A prospective study. Obstet Gynecol 61:467, 1983.
96. Higgins, SD and Garite, TJ: Late abruptio placentae in trauma patients: Implications for monitoring. Obstet Gynecol 63:10S, 1984.
97. Kuhn, W, Ulbrich, R and Rath, W: Changes of the clinical presentation of abruptio placentae. Eur J Obstet Gynaecol Reprod Biol 17:131, 1984.
98. Crosby, WM: Traumatic injuries during pregnancy. Clin Obstet Gynecol 26:902, 1983.
99. Lavin, JP and Polsky, SS: Abdominal trauma during pregnancy. Clin Perinatol 10:423, 1983.
100. Zugaib, M, et al: Abruptio placentae following snake bite. Am J Obstet Gynecol 151:754, 1985.
101. Acker, D, et al: Abruptio placentae associated with cocaine use. Am J Obstet Gynecol 146:220, 1983.
102. Ness, PM, et al: Congenital hypofibrinogenemia and recurrent placental abruption. Obstet Gynecol 61:519, 1983.
103. Brame, RG, et al: Maternal risk in abruption. Obstet Gynecol 31:224, 1968.
104. Gilabert, J, et al: Abruptio placentae and disseminated intravascular coagulation. Acta Obstet Gynecol Scand 64:35, 1985.
105. Pritchard, JA and MacDonald, PC: Williams' Obstetrics, ed 15. Appleton-Century-Crofts, New York, 1976.
106. Sheehan, HL and Stanfield, JP: Spasm of the anterior pituitary arteries as a cause of postpartum necrosis of the pituitary. Acta Endocrinol 37:479, 1961.
107. Pagano, R, Adey, FD and Butterfield, LJH: The management of antepartum haemorrhage (excluding placenta praevia). Aust NZ J Obstet Gynaecol 23:20, 1983.
108. Sher, G and Statland, BE: Abruptio placentae with coagulopathy: A rational basis for management. Clin Obstet Gynecol 28:15, 1985.
109. Schrinsky, DC and Benson, RC: Rupture of the pregnant uterus: A review. Obstet Gynecol Surv 33:217, 1978.
110. Lachman, E, et al: Rupture of the gravid uterus. S Afr Med J 67:333, 1985.
111. Elkins, T, et al: Uterine rupture in Nigeria. J Reprod Med 30:195, 1985.
112. Megafu, U: Factors influencing maternal survival in ruptured uterus. Int J Gynaecol Obstet 23:475, 1985.
113. Rahman, J, Al-Sibai, MH and Rahman, MS: Rupture of the uterus in labor: A review of 96 cases. Acta Obstet Gynecol Scand 64:311, 1985.
114. Heij, HA, TeVelde, ER and Cairns, JM: The treatment of rupture of the pregnant uterus: Analysis of 93 cases treated in a rural hospital in Zambia. Int J Gynaecol Obstet 22:415, 1984.
115. Golan, A, Sandbank, O and Rubin, A: Rupture of the pregnant uterus. Obstet Gynecol 56:549, 1980.
116. Suonio, S, et al: Intrapartum rupture of uterus diagnosed by ultrasound. Int J Gynaecol Obstet 22:411, 1984.
117. Shortle, B and Jewelewicz, R: Uterine rupture following tubal reimplantation: Review of the literature and report of three additional cases. Obstet Gynecol Surv 39:407, 1984.
118. Felmus, LB, Pedowitz, P and Nassberg, S: Spontaneous rupture of the apparently normal uterus during pregnancy: A review. Obstet Gynecol Surv 8:155, 1953.
119. Breen, JL, et al: Placenta accreta, increta, and percreta: A survey of 40 cases. Obstet Gynecol 49:43, 1977.
120. Camlibel, FT: Spontaneous rupture of uterus caused by placenta percreta. NY St J Med 81:1373, 1981.
121. Innes, G and Rosen, P: An unusual cause of abdominal pain and shock in pregnancy: Case report and review of the literature. J Emerg Med 2:261, 1985.
122. Bromham, DR and Anderson, RS: Letter to the editor. Lancet 2:485, 1980.
123. Gribble, RK and FitzSimmons, JM: Placenta previa percreta with fetal survival. Am J Obstet Gynecol 153:314, 1985.
124. Bezdek, J: Placenta percreta causing uterine rupture: Case report. Br J Obstet Gynaecol 92:853, 1985.
125. Cario, GM, Adler, AD and Morris, N: Placenta percreta presenting as intra-abdominal antepartum hem-

orrhage: Case report. Br J Obstet Gynaec 90:491, 1983.
126. Moldin, P and Nielsen, TF: Spontaneous uterine rupture in late pregnancy caused by placenta percreta. Acta Obstet Gynecol Scand 62:87, 1983.
127. Arkutu, AA: Spontaneous uterine rupture with placenta percreta: A case report. Int J Gynaecol Obstet 17:485, 1980.
128. Vergote, I, et al: Letter to the editor. Lancet 2(8312):1402, 1982.
129. Malmstrom, H and Hemmingsson, E: Uterine rupture as a complication of second-trimester abortion when using prostaglandin F-2 alpha together with other oxytocic agents. Acta Obstet Gynecol Scand 63:271, 1984.
130. Larsen, JV, Brits, CIJ and Whittal, D: Uterine hyperstimulation and rupture after induction of labour with prostaglandin E2: Case reports. S Afr Med J 65:615, 1984.
131. Valenzuela, G, et al: Uterine rupture at term with vaginal prostaglandin E_2. Am J Obstet Gynecol 138:1223, 1980.
132. Sawyer, MM, et al: Third-trimester uterine rupture associated with vaginal prostaglandin E2. Am J Obstet Gynecol 140:710, 1981.
133. Keller, F and Joyce, TH III: Uterine rupture associated with the use of vaginal prostaglandin E2 suppositories. Can Anaesth Soc J 31:80, 1984.
134. Claman, P, Carpenter, RJ and Reiter, A: Uterine rupture with the use of vaginal prostaglandin E2 for induction of labor. Am J Obstet Gynecol 150:889, 1984.
135. DeWane, JC and McCubbin, JH: Spontaneous rupture of an unscarred uterus at 19 weeks' gestation. Am J Obstet Gynecol 141:222, 1981.
136. Dainer, MJ: Spontaneous uterine rupture. J Reprod Med 26:35, 1981.
137. Nel, JT: An unusual case of uterine rupture: A case report. S Afr Med J 65:60, 1984.
138. Wiswedel, K: Rupture of the uterus in a primigravida: A case report. S Afr Med J 65:182, 1984.
139. Lenke, R and Osterkamp, T: A prolapsed umbilical cord into the abdominal cavity in a woman with a previous cesarean section. Am J Obstet Gynecol 138:1224, 1980.
140. Zuidema, LJ, Goldkrand, JW and Work, BA: Uterine contractility after rupture of the gravid uterus: A case report. Am J Obstet Gynecol 150:783, 1984.
141. Olobo-Lalobo, JH: A hole in a primigravid uterus: An unusual finding at elective cesarean section. Postgrad Med J 60:559, 1984.
142. Cotton, DB: Infant survival with prolonged uterine rupture. Am J Obstet Gynecol 142:1059, 1982.
143. Alper, MM and Dudley, DK: Asymptomatic rupture of the uterus: A case report. Can Med Assoc J 130:153, 1984.
144. Gibbs, CE and Locke WE: Maternal deaths in Texas, 1969–1973: A report of 501 consecutive maternal deaths from the Texas Medical Association's Committee on Maternal Health. Am J Obstet Gynecol 126:687, 1976.
145. Fakhoury, GW and Eddie, DAS: Continuation of pregnancy and vaginal delivery following incomplete uterine tear during pregnancy. Br J Obstet Gynaecol 91:299, 1984.
146. Plauche, WC, Von Almen, W and Muller, R: Catastrophic uterine rupture. Obstet Gynecol 64:792, 1984.
147. Meier, PR and Porreco, RP: Letter to the editor. Obstet Gynecol 66:296, 1985.
148. Chestnut, DH: Letter to the editor. Obstet Gynecol 66:295, 1985.
149. Eckstein, K-L, Oberlander, SG and Marx, GF: Uterine rupture during extradural blockade. Can Anaesth Soc J 20:566, 1973.
150. Carlsson, C, Nybell-Lindahl, G and Ingemarsson, I: Extradural block in patients who have previously undergone caesarean section. Br J Anaesth 52:827, 1980.
151. Uppington, J: Epidural analgesia and previous cesarean section. Anaesthesia 38:336, 1983.
152. Higgins, PG: Measuring nurses' accuracy of estimating blood loss. J Adv Nurs 7:157, 1982.
153. Reti, LL, Adey, FD and Brown, MF: Excessive bleeding from fetal scalp blood sampling. Aust NZ J Obstet Gynaec 20:55, 1980.
154. Chawla, R, et al: Hemorrhage after fetal scalp sampling. Am J Obstet Gynecol 149:92, 1984.
155. Gjode, P, Rasmussen, TB and Jorgensen, J: Fetomaternal bleeding during attempts at external version. Br J Obstet Gynaecol 87:571, 1980.
156. Fay, RA: Feto-maternal haemorrhage as a cause of fetal morbidity and mortality. Br J Obstet Gynaecol 90:443, 1983.
157. Hoag, RW: Fetomaternal hemorrhage associated with umbilical vein thrombosis: Case report. Am J Obstet Gynecol 154:1271, 1986.
158. Kouyoumdjian, A: Velamentous insertion of the umbilical cord. Obstet Gynecol 56:737, 1980.
159. Antoine, C, et al: Sinusoidal fetal heart rate pattern with vasa previa in twin pregnancy. J Reprod Med 27:295, 1982.
160. Pallewela, CS: Antepartum diagnosis of vasa previa: Report of a case causing sudden foetal death. Postgrad Med J 50:723, 1974.
161. Hanretty, KP: Ruptured vasa previa. Scott Med J 30:115, 1985.
162. Carp, HJA, Mashiach, S and Serr, DM: Vasa previa: A major complication and its management. Obstet Gynecol 53:273, 1979.
163. Silva, PD, et al: Use of fetal scalp hematocrit in the diagnosis of severe hemorrhage from vasa previa. Am J Obstet Gynecol 153:307, 1985.
164. Hughes, EC (ed): Obstetric-Gynecologic Terminology. FA Davis Company, Philadelphia, 1972.
165. Haswell, JN: Measured blood loss at delivery. J Indiana St Med Assoc 74:34, 1981.
166. Essed, GGM, et al: The influence of long term betamimetic drug administration during pregnancy on blood loss postpartum. Eur J Obstet Gynecol Reprod Biol 13:159, 1982.
167. Pritchard, JA, et al: Blood volume changes in pregnancy and the puerperium: II. Red blood cell loss and changes in apparent blood volume during and follow-

ing vaginal delivery, cesarean section, and cesarean section plus total hysterectomy. Am J Obstet Gynecol 84:1271, 1962.
168. Donald, I: Practical Obstetric Problems, ed 4. JB Lippincott, Philadelphia, 1969.
169. Newton, M: Postpartum hemorrhage. Am J Obstet Gynecol 54:51, 1967.
170. Cruikshank, SH: Management of postpartum and pelvic hemorrhage. Clin Obstet Gynecol 29:213, 1986.
171. Lazer, S, et al: Complications associated with the macrosomic fetus. J Reprod Med 31:501, 1986.
172. Weingarten, AE, et al: Postpartum uterine atony after intravenous dantrolene. Anesth Analg 66:269, 1987.
173. Herbert, WNP and Cefalo, RC: Management of postpartum hemorrhage. Clin Obstet Gynecol 27:139, 1984.
174. Weis, FR, et al: Cardiovascular effects of oxytocin. Obstet Gynecol 46:211, 1975.
175. Beeby, D and Hughes, JOM: Oxytocic drugs and anaesthesia. Anaesthesia 39:764, 1984.
176. Rall, TW and Schleifer, LS: Oxytocin, prostaglandins, ergot alkaloids, and other drugs; tocolytic agents. In Gilman, AG, et al (eds): The Pharmacological Basis of Therapeutics, ed 7. Macmillan, New York, 1985.
177. Taylor, GJ and Cohen, B: Ergonovine-induced coronary artery spasm and myocardial infarction after normal delivery. Obstet Gynecol 66:821, 1985.
178. Hayashi, RH, Castillo, MS and Noah, ML: Management of severe postpartum hemorrhage with a prostaglandin F2 alpha analogue. Obstet Gynecol 63:806, 1984.
179. Buttino, L, Jr and Garite, TJ: The use of 15-methyl F2-alpha prostaglandin (Prostin 15M) for the control of postpartum hemorrhage. Am J Perinatol 3:241, 1986.
180. Goldstein, AI, Kent, DR and David, A: Prostaglandin E2 vaginal suppositories in the treatment of intractable late-onset postpartum hemorrhage: A case report. J Reprod Med 28:425, 1983.
181. Henson, G, Gough, JD and Gillmer, MDG: Control of persistent primary postpartum haemorrhage due to uterine atony with intravenous prostaglandin E2: Case report. Br J Obstet Gynaecol 90:280, 1983.
182. Magrina, JF, et al: Selective arterial infusion of pitressin for the control of puerperal hemorrhage after hypogastric artery ligation. Obstet Gynecol 58:646, 1981.
183. Pais, SO, et al: Embolization of pelvic arteries for control of postpartum hemorrhage. Obstet Gynecol 55:754, 1980.
184. Rosenthal, DM and Colapinto, R: Angiographic arterial embolization in the management of postoperative vaginal hemorrhage. Am J Obstet Gynecol 151:227, 1985.
185. Benham, K and Jarmolowski, CR: Vesicovaginal fistula following hypogastric embolization for control of intractable pelvic hemorrhage. J Reprod Med 27:304, 1982.
186. Hare, WSC and Holland, CJ: Paresis following internal iliac artery embolization. Radiology 146:47, 1983.
187. Cruikshank, SH and Stoelk, EM: Surgical control of pelvic hemorrhage: Bilateral hypogastric artery ligation and method of ovarian artery ligation. South Med J 78:539, 1985.
188. Burchell, RC: Internal iliac artery ligation: Hemodynamics. Obstet Gynecol 24:737, 1964.
189. O'Leary, JA: Pregnancy following uterine artery ligation. Obstet Gynecol 55:112, 1980.
190. Clark, SL, et al: Hypogastric artery ligation for obstetric hemorrhage. Obstet Gynecol 66:353, 1985.
191. Evans, S and McShane, P: The efficacy of internal iliac artery ligation in obstetric hemorrhage. Surg Gynecol Obstet 160:250, 1985.
192. Plauche, WC: Cesarean hysterectomy: Indications, technique, and complications. Clin Obstet Gynecol 29:318, 1986.
193. Park, RC and Duff, WP: Role of cesarean hysterectomy in modern obstetric practice. Clin Obstet Gynecol 23:601, 1980.
194. Chestnut, DH, et al: Peripartum hysterectomy: A review of cesarean and postpartum hysterectomy. Obstet Gynecol 65:365, 1985.
195. Jackson, SH, Liebermann, MC and Smith, DE: Sodium nitroprusside-induced hypotension as a supplemental therapeutic modality in postpartum hemorrhage. Obstet Gynecol 58:649, 1981.
196. Cassels, JW, Jr, Greenberg, H and Otterson, WN: Pelvic tamponade in puerperal hemorrhage: A case report. J Reprod Med 30:689, 1985.
197. Herbert, WNP: Complications of the immediate puerperium. Clin Obstet Gynecol 25:219, 1982.
198. Lee, CY, Madrazo, B and Drukker, BH: Ultrasonic evaluation of the postpartum uterus in the management of postpartum bleeding. Obstet Gynecol 58:227, 1981.
199. Read, JA, Cotton, DB and Miller, FC: Placenta accreta: Changing clinical aspects and outcome. Obstet Gynecol 56:31, 1980.
200. Sturdee, DW and Rushton, DI: Caesarean and postpartum hysterectomy 1968–1983. Br J Obstet Gynaecol 93:270, 1986.
201. Hutton, L, Yang, SS and Bernstein, J: Placenta accreta: A 26-year clinicopathologic review (1956–1981). NY St J Med 83:857, 1983.
202. Clark, SL, Koonings, PP and Phelan, JP: Placenta previa/accreta and prior cesarean section. Obstet Gynecol 66:89, 1985.
203. Arulkumaran, S, et al: Medical treatment of placenta accreta with methotrexate. Acta Obstet Gynecol Scand 65:285, 1986.
204. Watson, P, Besch, N and Bowes, WA, Jr: Management of acute and subacute puerperal inversion of the uterus. Obstet Gynecol 55:12, 1980.
205. Harris, BA, Jr: Acute puerperal inversion of the uterus. Clin Obstet Gynecol 27:134, 1984.
206. Heyl, PS, Stubblefield, PG and Phillippe, M: Recurrent inversion of the puerperal uterus managed with 15(s)-15-methyl prostaglandin F2-alpha and uterine packing. Obstet Gynecol 63:263, 1984.
207. O'Reilly, RA: Anticoagulant, antithrombotic,

and thrombolytic drugs. In Gilman, AG, et al (eds): The Pharmacological Basis of Therapeutics. Macmillan, New York, 1985.

208. Wallenburg, HCS, et al: Low-dose aspirin prevents pregnancy-induced hypertension and pre-eclampsia in angiotensin-sensitive primigravidae. Lancet 1:1, 1986.

209. Goodlin, RC: Correction of pregnancy related thrombocytopenia with aspirin without improvement in fetal outcome. Am J Obstet Gynecol 146:862, 1983.

210. Stuart, MJ, et al: Effects of acetylsalicylic-acid ingestion on maternal and neonatal hemostasis. N Engl J Med 307:909, 1982.

211. Naumann, RO and Weinstein, L: Disseminated intravascular coagulation: The clinician's dilemma. Obstet Gynecol Surv 40:487, 1985.

212. Sher, G: Pathogenesis and management of uterine inertia complicating abruptio placentae with consumption coagulopathy. Am J Obstet Gynecol 129:164, 1977.

213. Schwartz, ML and Brenner, WE: Pregnancy-induced hypertension presenting with life-threatening thrombocytopenia. Am J Obstet Gynecol 146:756, 1983.

214. Thiagarajah, S, et al: Thrombocytopenia in preeclampsia: Associated abnormalities and management principles. Am J Obstet Gynecol 150:1, 1984.

215. Weinstein, L: Preeclampsia/eclampsia with hemolysis, elevated liver enzymes, and thrombocytopenia. Obstet Gynecol 66:5, 1985.

216. Socol, ML, et al: Platelet activation in preeclampsia. Am J Obstet Gynecol 151:494, 1985.

217. Oian, P, et al: Enhanced platelet release reaction related to arterial plasma adrenaline and blood pressure in preeclampsia. Br J Obstet Gynaecol 93:548, 1986.

218. Bern, MM, Driscoll, SG and Leavitt, T, Jr: Thrombocytopenia complicating preeclampsia: Data to support a new model. Obstet Gynecol 57:28 S, 1981.

219. Kelton, JG, Hunter, DJS and Neame, PB: A platelet function defect in preeclampsia. Obstet Gynecol 65:107, 1985.

220. Gibson, B, et al: Thrombocytopenia in preeclampsia and eclampsia. Semin Thromb Hemost 8:234, 1982.

221. Inglis, TCM, et al: Haemostatic and rheological changes in normal pregnancy and pre-eclampsia. Br J Haematol 50:461, 1982.

222. Weenink, GH, et al: Antithrombin III levels in preeclampsia correlate with maternal and fetal morbidity. Am J Obstet Gynecol 148:1092, 1984.

223. Files, JC, Morrison, FS and Halbrook, J: Letter to the editor. N Engl J Med 305:1650, 1981.

224. Reece, EA, Fox, HE and Rapoport F: Factor VIII inhibitor: A cause of severe postpartum hemorrhage. Am J Obstet Gynecol 144:985, 1982.

225. Loevinger, EH, et al: Hepatic rupture associated with pregnancy: Treatment with transcatheter embolotherapy. Obstet Gynecol 65:281, 1985.

226. Statler, KD and Sterling, WA, Jr: Hepatic subcapsular hemorrhage associated with pregnancy. Surgery 98:112, 1985.

227. Winer-Muram, HT, et al: Hepatic rupture in preeclampsia: The role of diagnostic imaging. J Can Assoc Radiol 36:34, 1985.

228. Gonzalez, GD, et al: Spontaneous hepatic rupture in pregnancy: Management with hepatic artery ligation. South Med J 77:242, 1984.

229. Reece, EA, et al: The perinatal management of pregnancy complicated by massive intracerebral hemorrhage. Am J Perinatol 1:266, 1984.

230. Howard, DJ: Life-threatening epistaxis in pregnancy. J Laryngol Otol 99:95, 1985.

PART 4

FETAL PROBLEMS

CHAPTER 16

FETAL SURGERY

FRED J. SPIELMAN, MD

Pioneering work in fetal surgery began in 1884 when Cohnstein and Zuntz performed surgery on the exteriorized fetuses of sheep.[1] Liley's[2] use in 1963 of the peritoneal cavity of the fetus for administration of blood in the treatment of infants suffering from erythroblastosis fetalis represents the first successful application on humans. Using fluoroscopy, he introduced the blood via a needle placed in the abdominal wall of the mother.

Liley's success motivated others to treat fetal deficiencies, either by administration of medications to the mother or by direct injection into the amniotic cavity. Massive maternal doses of vitamin B_{12} or biotin served to treat fetuses with vitamin B_{12}-responsive methylmalonic acidemia and biotin-dependent multiple carboxylase deficiency respectively.[3,4] Other fetuses received hormones and amino acids to remedy fetal goiter and intrauterine growth retardation.[5,6] These interventions often represented futile attempts to salvage severely affected fetuses. Frequently, the diagnosis became evident only after irreversible damage had taken place. The use of the mother as a conduit for fetal treatment often proved inefficient and placed the parturient at considerable risk. However, as currently practiced, fetal surgery has the potential for significantly reducing the morbidity and mortality of affected fetuses without greatly endangering the health of the mother. Advances in ultrasound imaging, surgical techniques, biotechnology, and the development of safe and effective drugs for tocolysis and anesthesia primarily account for the recent growth and success of fetal medicine.

Fetal surgery has become a well-defined and organized division of perinatal medicine as evidenced by the formation of the Society of Fetal Medicine in 1983. The society established a set of general and specific criteria for fetal treatment in order to maximize the likelihood of successful outcomes of therapy and created a voluntary international registry of fetal surgery. As of 1986, 21 centers from seven countries have reported on their experience.[7] In 1983 the Council on Scientific Affairs of the American Medical Association passed a resolution which called for a study of surgical procedures in utero.[8]

Fetal surgery strives to reverse or arrest a destructive process before irreversible damage occurs. For example, urinary tract obstruction produces hydronephrosis and renal damage. Without adequate urine production, amniotic fluid volume decreases, resulting in fetal growth retardation and pulmonary insufficiency. Prenatal intervention may arrest progressive organ damage while allowing continued intrapartum fetal growth and development. Definitive correction of the problem can then be attempted in the neonatal period.[9]

The fetus has unique anatomic and physiologic characteristics that may provide for an excellent outcome following surgery. The underdeveloped fetal immune system infrequently rejects foreign materials such as catheters. During embryogenesis, limb buds retain regenerative capabilities. Rapid postoperative healing characteristically occurs in utero as the environment receives maternal immune factors transplacentally.[8,10]

Institutions that perform fetal surgery must meet certain standards. They must have a high-risk obstetric unit and an intensive care nursery. Each pair of patients, mother and fetus, must undergo extensive diagnostic evaluations to determine whether the fetus might benefit from treatment. Psychologists, social workers, and bioethical support personnel should be available.[11] In order to deliver optimal care for the parturient and fetus a multidisciplinary team effort must be organized, consisting of an obstetrician, a pediatric surgeon, a neonatologist, and an anesthesiologist. The team must understand the physiologic and anatomic changes of pregnancy and the factors that will affect fetal morbidity and mortality, such as intrauterine hypoxia and premature labor. Finally, the team must know and consider the legal and ethical aspects and psychological needs of each patient and of surgical intervention.[12]

Diagnosis

The advent and availability of high-resolution ultrasound have made early antenatal diagnosis of fetal anomalies possible and have allowed perinatologists to delineate and monitor the natural history and progression of congenital defects early in gestation. This process makes the successful treatment of fetuses more realistic. Real-time ultrasound has produced successful and safe placement of needles and catheters directly into the amniotic sac and drainage of fluid from hydrocephalic heads, distended bladders, and thoracic cavities. Fiberoptics makes fetoscopy possible and enables physicians to perform fetal skin and liver biopsies and to sample blood.

Appropriate selection of candidates for fetal surgery is an important, difficult, and challenging goal in perinatal management. Careful assessment of fetal anatomy and organ function excludes fetuses with abnormalities serious enough to prevent salvage and those so mildly affected that they will do well without antenatal treatment.[13] Accurate diagnosis is essential and often includes ultrasonographic studies, amniocentesis, maternal and fetal blood sampling, chorionic villus biopsy, and fetoscopy.

ULTRASOUND

Ultrasound imaging effectively fosters the diagnosis of fetal anomalies. Unexplained collections of fluid or marked changes in the anatomic configuration of the fetus often characterize congenital defects. Sonography readily detects problems involving the central nervous system, heart, visceral organs, and skeletal system. This form of evaluation proves most effective at 16 weeks' gestation, when fetal structures have completed development. Real-time sonographic evaluation may yield important information on fetal breathing movements and other vital functions.[14] Many perinatologists place so much importance on the results of ultrasound that they require confirmation by an independent observer and permanent documentation on either hard copy or videotape.[15]

AMNIOCENTESIS

By about 16 weeks' gestation sufficient amniotic fluid has formed to simplify the technical aspects of amniocentesis, and the concurrent use of ultrasound increases its safety. Amniocentesis directly causes an incidence of fetal loss of less than 0.06 percent, and less than 10 percent of the patients require more than one tap.[15] Cells obtained by amniocentesis help determine chromosomal defects, detect inherited metabolic abnormalities, evaluate pulmonary maturity, and quantify fetal hemolysis.[14] Measurement of serum α fetoprotein, an established method for identification of patients at risk for having children with central nervous system defects, may also facilitate screening for congenital nephrosis, esophageal and duodenal atresia, Turner's syndrome, and fetal death. It is most accurate when performed at 16 to 20 weeks' gestation.

CHORIONIC VILLUS BIOPSY

Chorionic villus biopsy, a new diagnostic tool, can help determine fetal sex, cytogenic disorders, and DNA sequence. With the aid of ultrasound for identification of the biopsy site, this test is safe for mother and fetus and is easily performed as early as 8 to 10 weeks' gestation.[15]

FETOSCOPY AND BLOOD SAMPLING

Fetoscopy and fetal blood sampling are invaluable diagnostic techniques in the evaluation of congenital abnormalities. These invasive procedures have the same anesthetic requirements, complications, and need for multidisciplinary cooperation as fetal surgery.

Although obstetricians first attempted fetoscopy through a dilated cervix, it evolved from an experimental procedure to a major diagnostic tool of proven safety and efficacy after the perfection of fiberoptics and real-time ultrasound. Direct fetal visualization offers the potential for a precise and expanded approach to antenatal evaluation. The perinatologist uses fetoscopy primarily to detect small external anatomic abnormalities that cannot be appreciated by ultrasound. For example, fetoscopy helps assess abnormalities of the face, digits, and genitalia which may be markers for serious syndromes.[16] It is also used for obtaining samples of fetal tissues, most notably skin and liver. Using light and electron microscopy, skin biopsies can be performed to help diagnose Ehlers-Danlos syndrome, epidermolysis bullosa, and albinism, among other problems. The fetoscope can be introduced so as to achieve access to the ventral surface of the liver and therefore to obtain specimens for biochemical and histologic analysis in order to diagnose enzyme deficiencies and tumors.

Fetal blood can be used for the prenatal diagnosis of hemoglobinopathies and bleeding, chromosomal, and metabolic disorders as well as infections and anemia. The perinatologist may obtain blood by direct visualization of umbilical and placental vessels through the fetoscope or percutaneous sampling of the cord with a needle under sonographic guidance.[17] Fetoscopy is best performed at 15 to 18 weeks' gestation, when the fetus is large enough for transabdominal entry but still small enough for efficient visualization. Fifteen to 20 weeks' gestation is the optimal time for blood sampling. Small blood vessels and the relatively large fetal blood loss in proportion to the total blood volume render blood sampling less satisfactory before this time.[18]

Trauma and safety qualify as important considerations, for the operator must avoid injuring the fetus and placenta. Placental trauma causing bleeding will make visualization difficult, while uterine trauma can precipitate contractions. Use of the smallest possible trocar and cannula reduces the risks involved, however a fetoscope of small diameter provides poor lighting, limits magnification, and offers a small field of vision. Maternal risks are negligible, while the incidence of fetal loss prior to 28 weeks' gestation is approximately 2 percent.[16]

Surgery in Utero

EXCHANGE TRANSFUSION

The incidence of Rhesus isoimmunization has greatly diminished due to the widespread use of immunoprophylaxis, but some fetuses continue to become severly anemic while still too immature to deliver. In 1963 Liley[2] first reported the intrapartum treatment of affected fetuses. Using radiography, he introduced a catheter through the maternal and fetal abdomens and transfused Rh-negative erythrocytes into the fetal peritoneal cavity. The success of treatment depends upon absorption of transfused blood through fetal subdiaphragmatic lymphatic vessels. However, erratic and nonuniform absorption often occurs in the hydropic fetus.[19] In addition, intraperitoneal transfusion does not allow the sampling of fetal blood for hematocrit determination. In an attempt to transfuse fetuses in a more efficient and therapeutically beneficial manner, Rodeck[20] introduced fetoscopically directed intravascular transfusion in 1981. Direct access to the fetal circulation via the umbilical vessels makes hematocrit estimation possible. The posttransfusion hematocrit can verify that the optimal amount of blood has been administered. Recently, with the aid of ultrasound, percutaneous umbilical vessel cannulation has become popular. The percutaneous approach uses a 22-gauge needle versus a 2.2-mm endoscope and therefore avoids the inherent risks of employing a large-bore instrument, especially in the second trimester.[19] Any evidence of cardiac irregularities or bradycardia as detected by ultrasound monitoring of the fetal heart rate throughout the procedure calls for termination of the treatment.

TREATMENT OF HYDROCEPHALUS

The treatment of fetal hydrocephalus attempts to minimize gross disfigurement caused by hydrocephalus and maximize potential brain growth and development. Most children born with severe obstructive hydrocephalus die or are left severely retarded. Early diagnosis and prompt treatment offer the best opportunity for normal brain development, since decompressing the ventricles may reverse the adverse effects of high-pressure obstruction.[14,21] Hydrocephalus, rarely an isolated anomaly, most often associates with other malformations, most notably meningomyelocele, or it may follow intrauterine infections. The detection of hydrocephalus calls for a thorough search for additional pathology, with particular attention to the evaluation of the spinal column, relative size of the head and abdomen, motion of the lower extremities, and symmetry of the cerebral anatomy.[22] After fully evaluating the fetus the perinatologist must decide whether in utero treatment is required, or even possible. Alternatives for treatment depend on the gestational age and the extent and severity of additional anomalies. In those instances, such as anecephaly, in which gross abnormalities of the central nervous system render neonatal survival unlikely, induction of labor or even abortion may be the best plan. Cases in which hydrocephalus occurs independently of other fetal anomalies and the fetus demonstrates pulmonary maturity indicate early delivery. The fetus with a progressive obstruction without major dysmorphic brain development, as occurs in stenosis of the aqueduct of Sylvius, and too premature to survive delivery qualifies as an ideal candidate for intrauterine surgery.[22]

Intermittent ventricular aspiration or percutanously placed ventriculoamniotic shunt catheters can decompress hydrocephalus. Intermittent aspiration provides only transient relief of elevated intracranial pressure because of prompt reaccumulation of fluid, while shunt displacement and malfunction are common and frustrating problems associated with this approach to ventricular drainage.

The International Fetal Surgery Registry has compiled data on 44 fetuses who underwent drainage procedures for obstructive hydrocephalus. Although 34 of 44 fetuses (83 percent) survived, the procedure-related death rate was 10 percent; 18 of the 34 survivors (53 percent) had serious neurologic handicaps; four (12 percent) had less severe handicaps; and only 12 (35 percent) displayed normal development. Aqueductal stenosis of unknown etiology was the most common cause of the hydrocephalus, and all normal survivors had this disorder.[7] The natural history of hydrocephalus must be better defined to allow selection of only those cases where in utero treatment is both necessary and beneficial.

TREATMENT OF URINARY TRACT OBSTRUCTION

Urinary tract anomalies are one of the congenital abnormalities most frequently detected by ultrasound. This happens because sonography easily detects the fluid-filled masses and because decreased fetal urine excretion results in oligohydramnios, a common indication for ultrasound. In a review of 73 fetuses with urinary obstruction, the mean gestational age at the time of diagnosis was 23 $\pm$ 5 weeks (range, 16 to 34 weeks), and the mean age at the time of in utero therapy was 24 $\pm$ 5 weeks (range, 17 to 36 weeks). The posterior urethral valve syndrome (29 percent) was the most common diagnosis. Unknown causes for obstructive uropathy occurred in 45 percent of the cases. Forty-eight percent of fetuses survived the in utero surgery. Perinatal survival related strongly to the type of obstruction; 77 percent of fetuses with posterior urethral valves survived.[7]

Urinary obstruction can produce widespread sequelae and demands decompression of severe obstruction. Urinary obstruction causes hydronephrosis and progressive renal damage. Decreased fetal urine output produces oligohydramnios, which in turn causes fetal growth retardation, pulmonary hypoplasia, abnormal foot and hand development, and abdominal wall and facial deformities. Pulmonary hypoplasia, the primary cause of neonatal mortality, relates to both the severity of the oligohydramnios and the degree of intra-abdominal distention caused by the massively dilated urinary tract organs. Since nephrogenesis occurs primarily between 20 and 36 weeks, successful fetal surgery at this period can restore normal amniotic fluid dynamics and thus prevent or reduce pulmonary and renal damage.[23] Many of the fetuses with obstruction may also have other malformations as well as chromosomal and metabolic disorders, so that serial sonographic observations, fetal karyotyping, and examination of the fetus for additional anomalies will aid in the identification of those fetuses who will benefit from in utero surgery.

The wide spectrum of fetal urinary tract anomalies requires different perinatal management plans. Some fetuses with non–life-threatening problems do not require intervention and will do well with appropriate treatment after birth; a fetus with unilateral hydronephrosis with a normally functioning contralateral kidney is one example.[24] Other fetuses such as one with bilateral renal agenesis or ureteral obstruction with severe oligohydramnios already present before 20 weeks' gestation have a poor prognosis, and no currently available treatment can help them. For them selective abortion may be the most reasonable management decision.[25] Finally, appropriate prenatal therapy exists for some fetal malformations that cause mild but progressive bilateral renal disease.

The goal of surgery is to decompress the obstructed fetal urinary tract. Similar to the treatment of hydrocephalus, intermittent drainage of the accumulated fluid, although technically easy, offers only temporary relief, especially since the fetus makes a large amount of urine (5 ml per kg per hr) and will rapidly refill the bladder.[26] The risks of infection and trauma increase with repeated procedures. Although catheters can effectively relieve the obstruction, dislodgement and blocking of catheters frequently complicate this drainage technique.

Obstetric Considerations

LEGAL AND ETHICAL CONCERNS OF FETAL SURGERY

Until recently, the diagnosis of fetal malformations presented the mother with the choice of either doing nothing or having an abortion. The ability to successfully treat some fetal disorders has raised complex legal and ethical questions.[27] Uniquely, in utero therapy involves two patients, the fetus and the mother. For the fetus, the risks of the procedure are balanced by the possibility of correcting the malformation or minimizing the damage it may produce. The risks and benefits for the mother are more complicated as most fetal malformations do not directly threaten the mother's health, yet she bears some risk from the procedure.[14]

The National Commission for the Protection of Human Subjects of Biomedical and Behavioral Research has made fetal intervention a high priority. Confusion, nevertheless, persists concerning the definition of and legislation for in utero intervention. The federal government states that fetal therapy experimentation must meet the health needs of the fetus and should place the fetus at risk only to the minimum extent necessary to meet such need. Some states, however, have legislated that in utero research is a criminal activity, and others have restricted fetal research more stringently than the federal government.[28]

What if the mother refuses surgery which her physicians think is necessary for the well-being of the fetus? The mother has no legal responsibility to have a procedure performed that is considered experimental. An operation that has a reasonable chance of saving the fetus's life or of increasing the quality of life after birth constitutes the strongest claim for court-ordered fetal surgery. When fetal surgery moves from experimental to established therapy, the refusal by the parents to have it performed would place them at risk for prosecution for feticide or child abuse if the viable fetus died in utero or was born handicapped.[29]

Prior to signing the consent for surgery, the

parents need to comprehend the alternative treatments available, the expected prognosis with each plan, the maternal and fetal risks of surgery, as well as the limited evidence of benefit that the procedure may produce. The mother and father must understand that irreversible fetal damage may have already occurred.

TIMING AND MODE OF DELIVERY

Fetal abnormalities can influence the timing and mode of delivery. Early delivery may be indicated for those fetuses with anomalies most effectively treated after birth and with lungs mature enough to sustain them after delivery —for example, fetuses with hydrops fetalis, gastroschisis, or obstructive hydrocephalus or hydronephrosis. With this treatment plan, the risk of premature delivery must be weighed against the risk of continued gestation. Steroid administration prior to delivery and advances in neonatal medicine have greatly improved the outcome for premature infants with respiratory distress syndrome.[14] Some malformations, such as large hydrocephalus, ruptured meningomyelocele, omphalocele, cystic hygroma, cause dystocia and call for elective cesarean rather than vaginal delivery. Failure to progress during labor or fetal distress may necessitate cesarean section instead of a planned preterm vaginal delivery.[14]

PREMATURE LABOR

Induction of labor and/or premature delivery represents a great risk of fetal intervention. All of the factors responsible for premature rupture of membranes or preterm labor have not been elucidated; no specific anesthetic agent or technique increases the incidence of premature labor. Only placement of a large trocar through the mother's abdomen, uterus, and amniotic membranes provides fetal access. The uterus of primates is highly sensitive to stimulation and is prone to generalized contractions.[30]

Monitoring uterine activity continuously with an external tocodynamometer in the immediate postoperative period minimizes the risk of premature labor. Prophylactic tocolytic drugs are not universally employed, for no convincing evidence of their efficacy exists in these circumstances. Beta-adrenergic agents can cause significant maternal complications such as hypotension, dysrhythmias, pulmonary edema, and metabolic abnormalities. Some perinatologists routinely use prophylactic medications, infusing intravenous terbutaline intraoperatively and continuing oral terbutaline until the 36th week of gestation.[31] Others administer preoperative indomethacin to block prostaglandin synthesis.[27] Premature labor that begins after surgery should not be stopped if the gestational age exceeds 34 to 36 weeks, a time when neonatal survival can be expected.

Risk of respiratory distress syndrome accompanies premature delivery, hence some fetal surgeons given betamethasone to all patients between 26 and 34 weeks' gestation to encourage accelerated pulmonary development.[32]

Anesthetic Considerations

PHYSIOLOGIC CHANGES OF PREGNANCY

As with any type of surgery, proper anesthesia can greatly enhance the overall outcome of the procedure. The same anesthetic considerations hold for fetal surgery as for nonobstetric surgery during pregnancy, including maternal safety, avoidance of teratogenic drugs, fetal asphyxia, and premature delivery.[33] The physiologic changes of pregnancy influence the maternal considerations for fetal surgery. Hormones and the effects of the enlarging uterus cause these changes and often occur during the first and second trimesters. The parturient possesses less cardiovascular and pulmonary reserve than the nonpregnant patient. Use of lateral uterine displacement may reduce the risks of hypotension and diminished uterine blood flow from aortocaval compression during the final two trimesters. The fetus depends on adequate uteroplacental blood flow to maintain homeostasis; if uteroplacental perfusion diminishes due to aortocaval compression, α-adrenergic drugs, endogenous catecholamines, or maternal hypotension, the fetus will suffer. The best anesthetic is directed at anticipating potential problems. Increased oxygen consumption and carbon dioxide production place the parturient at significant risk for hypoxia and hypercarbia. Therefore, all patients should receive supplemental oxygen. Elevated gastric volumes and lower pH make regurgitation and aspiration a leading cause of maternal mortality and morbidity. The risk of this complication may be reduced by giving nothing by mouth for at least 8 hours prior to surgery, administering sodium citrate shortly before surgery, and closely monitoring mental status and airway patency during local and regional anesthesia. All patients who have entered the second trimester must be intubated for general anesthesia after preoxygenation, rapid-sequence induction, and cricoid pressure.

PREOPERATIVE VISIT

A thorough and thoughtful preoperative discussion with the mother is essential. She is often very anxious about the outcome of the surgery for herself and her child. A detailed explanation of what to expect during intraoperative monitoring, the anesthetic and the recovery process can reduce her apprehensions. Questions should be encouraged.

ANESTHESIA TECHNIQUE

No anesthetic agent or adjunctive medication qualifies as totally free of side effects. However, children of women who receive general, regional, or local anesthesia do not exhibit an increased incidence of congenital anomalies.[34,35]

General, regional, and local infiltration have facilitated fetal surgery.[24,32,33] Local infiltration with intravenous supplementation is the most common and safest anesthetic technique. The surgeon establishes local analgesia while the anesthesiologist administers small incremental amounts of intravenous narcotics and sedatives as warranted for the mother's comfort. Avoiding general anesthesia has several advantages: it reduces the risk of aspiration, and it diminishes wide swings in blood pressure and heart rate that accompany tracheal intubation and extubation. Endogenous catecholamine release is associated with light general anesthesia and intubation. These vasopressors have α-adrenergic activity, which decreases uterine blood flow. In addition mother and fetus should receive only small amounts of cardiovascular and respiratory depressing drugs. Many parturients really want to be awake for the operation, and many couples wish to have the husband in the operating room for emotional support. The successful use of local infiltration and intravenous sedation requires several factors. The surgeon must be sensitive to the patient's awake status and must operate with a soft touch. Adequate premedication well in advance of surgery is required. The anesthesiologist must establish rapport with the patient during the preoperative visit, communicate effectively during surgery, and display compassion. Numerous drugs or combinations of drugs have served to supplement local analgesia. Unanimity concerning the best drug does not exist; however, the short action of fentanyl makes it ideal for outpatient fetal surgical procedures that require early discharge. Midazolam (Versed) produces superior sedation, can cause amnesia when employed for cesarean section, and hence may deprive patients of their memory of fetal surgery.[36]

Local analgesia is insufficient for more extensive fetal surgery that requires hysterotomy, such as repair of diaphragmatic hernia or spina bifida. These operations have been reported only in animal models but if their human application becomes reality, they will require regional or general anesthesia. Regional or general anesthesia may also be necessary when the parturient refuses local analgesia or the obstetrician proposes lengthy or technically difficult surgery requiring multiple needle placements.[11] Regional anesthesia would be expected to be superior to general anesthesia in the pregnant patient, since it exposes the fetus to fewer drugs and reduces the risk of aspiration. Studies, however, have failed to demonstrate the superiority of either form of anesthesia as long as anesthesia personnel meticulously maintain maternal blood pressure, oxygenation, airway control, and acid-base balance.[37] Maternal oxygenation directly affects fetal oxygenation, but only up to a point. As maternal PO_2 increases beyond 100 mmHg, fetal PO_2 rises to about 40 to 46 mmHg.[38] The inspired oxygen concentration administered to the mother must be sufficient to fully saturate her hemoglobin; 40 percent inspired oxygen concentration is usually adequate.

FETAL ANALGESIA

In the absence of proof that preterm infants remember pain many anesthesiologists assume that the fetus cannot feel noxious stimuli. Functioning neurologic structures necessary for pain sensation, skin nociceptors, and electrical activity in the spinal cord and thalamus have developed by the end of the first trimester. Fetuses move and demonstrate increased heart rate, autonomic activity, and hormone secretion in response to noxious stimuli.[11,32,33] Both practical and moral concerns mandate fetal anesthesia in the event of surgery.

Maternal administration of parenteral or inhalation anesthesia supplies fetal pain relief, but regional anesthesia does not. The degree of fetal movement and increase in heart rate in response to surgical stimulation indicate the adequacy of anesthesia. Since all parenteral analgesics are nonionized, lipid soluble, and have a low molecular weight, they traverse the placenta with ease and accumulate in the fetus. The concentration of these drugs in the fetus depends on fetal pH, amount of drug passing through the portal circulation, plasma protein and tissue binding, and metabolism. The equilibration between mother and fetus of intravenous drugs and nitrous oxide occurs more quickly than that of potent inhalation agents, such as halothane and isoflurane, which take much longer for fetal concentrations to approach maternal levels. Small to moderate doses of inhalation agents (one MAC) do not depress the fetal cardiovascular system; however, anesthesia with 1.5 percent halothane or 2 percent isoflurane causes significant decreases in fetal blood pressure, heart rate, and oxygen saturation with a progressive fetal acidosis.[39]

FETAL MOVEMENT

Control of intraoperative fetal movement is a primary anesthetic goal. Fetal movement during invasive procedures may cause trauma, displace needles and catheters, and interrupt surgery. Placental passage of narcotics and sedatives can reduce fetal response to surgical stimulation, but this does not always succeed, and the operation may need to be abandoned. The use of excessive amounts of narcotics and tranquilizers places the parturient at substantial risk for regurgitation and aspiration. The injection of pancuronium (0.5 mg) into the gluteal area of the fetus with a 22-gauge spinal needle helps by temporarily eliminating fetal movement during the invasive procedure without heavy maternal sedation. Fetal movement returns within 2 hours. No maternal or fetal side effects have been observed using this technique.[40]

The Future of Fetal Surgery

Fetal intervention has opened up a new area of perinatology, and a more complete understanding of normal and abnormal fetal development has been achieved. As more experience is gained in fetal pathophysiology, uterine physiology, and medical technology, continued success in this science will follow.

The possibilities for in utero endocrine therapy include prevention of fetal masculinization in the adrenogenital syndrome and the treatment of fetal hypothyroidism. Allogenic bone transplantations have been successfully performed in the Rhesus monkey and may offer potential help for the repair of skeletal anomalies in utero, such as the closure of neural tube defects.[10,28] Congenital diaphragmatic hernia, which occurs in 1 in 2000 to 1 in 5000 births, is another malformation that may be corrected prior to birth. In the fetal lamb decompression of the lungs permits them to develop sufficiently to allow for survival after birth.

Although hope and enthusiasm for fetal intervention abound, we must not generate false hopes for fetal surgery, and must understand that experience with fetal surgery in the laboratory animal does not necessarily transfer to the human.[10] Fetal sheep survive more readily after surgery than human fetuses for preterm labor is difficult to control in humans. The need for hysterotomy automatically increases the maternal risk. The mother may die from the operation or its complications, including postoperative bleeding or infection, or reoperation and hysterectomy may be required. Fetal surgery requires hysterotomy location in the upper segment of the uterus and therefore necessitates cesarean section for all future deliveries. Attempts to repair fetal malformations in the human should not be undertaken until sufficient experience and success have been achieved in a primate model.[14] Because a procedure can be done does not mean that it should be done. We must proceed with caution.[41]

References

1. Adamsons, RK, Jr: Current concepts: Fetal surgery. N Engl J Med 275:204, 1966.
2. Liley, AW: Intrauterine transfusion of foetus in haemolytic disease. Br Med J 2:1107, 1963.
3. Ampola, MG, et al: Prenatal therapy of a patient with vitamin B_{12}–responsive methylmalonic acidemia. N Engl J Med 293:313, 1974.
4. Golbus, MS, et al: In utero treatment of urinary tract obstruction. Am J Obstet Gynecol 142:383, 1982.
5. Weiner, S, et al: Antenatal diagnosis and treatment of a fetal goiter. J Reprod Med 24:39, 1980.
6. Renaud, R, et al: Injections intra-amniotiques d'acides amines dans les cas de malnutrition foetale. J Gynecol Obstet Biol Reprod 1:231, 1972.
7. Manning, FA, Harrison, MR and Rodeck, C: Catheter shunts for fetal hydronephrosis and hydrocephalus. N Engl J Med 315:336, 1986.
8. Beljian, TR, et al: In utero fetal surgery. JAMA 250:1443, 1983.
9. Berkowitz, RL, et al: Fetal urinary tract obstruction: What is the role of surgical intervention in utero? Obstet Gynecol 144:367, 1982.
10. Hodgen, GD: Antenatal diagnosis and treatment of fetal skeletal malformations. JAMA 246:1079, 1981.
11. Michejia, M: Antenatal treatment of neural tube defects. In Kurjak, A (ed): The Fetus as a Patient. Elsevier Science Publishers, Amsterdam, 1984, p 131.
12. Fainstat, T and Bhat, N: Surgical resolution of non-obstetric abdominal crises complicating pregnancy. In Baden, JM and Brodsky, JB (eds): The Pregnant Surgical Patient. Futura Publishing Company, Mt. Kisco, NY, 1985, p 149.
13. Dudenhausen, JW: Risks and benefits of fetal therapy. In Kurjak, A (ed): The Fetus as a Patient. Elsevier Science Publishers, Amsterdam, p 279, 1985.
14. Harrison, MR, Golbus, MS and Filly, RA: Management of the fetus with a correctable congenital defect. JAMA 246:774, 1981.
15. Lange, IR: Congenital anomalies: Detection and strategies for management. Semin Perinatol 9:151, 1985.
16. Rodeck, CH and Nicolaides, KH: Fetoscopy. Br Med J 42:296, 1986.
17. Chervenak, FA, Isaacson, G and Mahoney, MJ: Current concepts: Advances in the diagnosis of fetal defects. N Engl J Med 315:305, 1986.
18. Grannum, PA, et al: In utero exchange transfusion by direct intravascular injection in severe erythroblastosis fetalis. N Engl J Med 314:1431, 1986.
19. Bowman, JM and Manning, FA: Intrauterine fetal transfusions: Winnipeg, 1982. Obstet Gynecol 61:203, 1983.
20. Rodeck, CH, et al: Direct intravascular fetal blood transfusion by fetoscopy in severe Rhesus isoimmunisation. Lancet 1:625, 1981.
21. Harrison, MR, Golbus, MS and Filly RA: Congenital hydrocephalus. In Harrison, MR, Golbus, MS and Filly, RA (eds): The Unborn Patient. Grune and Stratton, Orlando, 1984, p 349.
22. Redwine, F and Petres, RE: Fetal surgery: Past, present, and future. Clin Perinatol 10:399, 1983.
23. Harrison, MR, et al: Correction of congenital hydronephrosis in utero. II: Decompression reverses the effects of obstruction on the fetal lung and urinary tract. J Pediatr Surg 17:965, 1982.
24. Harrison, MR, et al: Management of the fetus with congenital hydronephrosis. J Pediatr Surg 17:728, 1982.
25. D'Addario, V: Ultrasound prenatal diagnosis and perinatal management of fetal urinary tract anomalies. In Kurjak A (ed): The Fetus as a Patient. Elsevier Science Publishers, Amsterdam, 1985, p 198.
26. Harrison, MR, et al: Management of the fetus with a urinary tract malformation. JAMA 246:635, 1981.
27. Harrison, MR, et al: Fetal surgery for congenital hydronephrosis. N Engl J Med 306:591, 1982.
28. Elias, S and Annas, GJ: Perspectives on fetal surgery. Am J Obstet Gynecol 145:807, 1983.
29. Robertson, JA: Legal considerations: The duties of mothers and physicians in fetal treatment. In Harrison, MR, Golbus, MS and Filly, RA (eds): The Unborn Patient. Grune and Stratton, Orlando, 1984, p 171.
30. Brodsky, JB: Anesthesia and surgery for the pregnant patient and fetal outcome. In Baden, JM and Brodsky, JB (eds): The Pregnant Surgical Patient. Futura Publishing Company, Mt. Kisco, NY, 1985, p 247.
31. Gustavii, B, et al: Fetoscopy. Acta Obstet Gynecol Scand 58:409, 1979.
32. Spielman, FJ, Seeds, JW and Corke, B: Anaesthesia for foetal surgery. Anaesthesia 39:756, 1984.
33. Rosen, MA: Anesthesia for fetal surgery. In Shnider, SM and Levinson G (eds): Anesthesia for Obstetrics. Williams & Wilkins, Baltimore, 1987, p 206.
34. Duncan, PG: Fetal risk of anesthesia and surgery during pregnancy. Anesthesiology 64:790, 1986.
35. Brodsky, JB, et al: Surgery during pregnancy and fetal outcome. Am J Obstet Gynecol 138:1165, 1980.
36. Camann, W, Cohen, MB and Ostheimer, GW: Is midazolam desirable for sedation in parturients? Anesthesiology 65:441, 1986.
37. Coe, VL: Physiologic effects of regional anesthesia during pregnancy. In Baden, JM and Brodsky, JB (eds): The Pregnant Surgical Patient. Futura Publishing Company, Mt. Kisco, NY, 1985, p 133.
38. Wood, C: Use of fetal blood sampling and fetal heart rate monitoring. In Adamsons, K (ed): Diagnosis and treatment of fetal disorders. Springer-Verlag, New York, 1968, p 169.
39. Palahniuk, RJ and Shnider, SM: Maternal and fetal cardiovascular and acid-base changes during halothane and isoflurane anesthesia in the pregnant ewe. Anesthesiology 41:462, 1974.
40. Seeds, JW, Corke, BC and Spielman, FJ: Prevention of fetal movement during invasive procedures with pancuronium bromide. Am J Obstet Gynecol 155:818, 1986.
41. Harrison, MR, Golbus, MS and Filly, RA: Medical considerations. In Harrison, MR, Golbus, MS and Filly, RA (eds): The Unborn Patient. Grune and Stratton, Orlando, 1984, p 145.

CHAPTER 17

PRETERM DELIVERY

RICHARD J. PALAHNIUK, M.D., F.R.C.P.C.

Preterm delivery, by definition, occurs prior to week 37 of gestation, whereas abortion indicates delivery of the fetus earlier than 20 weeks. Unfortunately, birth weight does not necessarily correlate with gestational age. For instance, full-term infants with severe intrauterine growth retardation may weigh less than 1500 g.[1] In this chapter, I shall make every effort to restrict discussion to preterm deliveries, although some information may relate to low-birth-weight infants as well.

General Considerations

MATERNAL FACTORS

Creasy and coworkers[2] graded maternal risk factors contributing to preterm delivery (Table 17–1). Correlation between risk factors and preterm delivery has been inconsistent, leading to significant numbers of false-negatives and false-positives.[3,4]

Even when high-risk patients can be identified early during pregnancy, there appears to be little that can be done to prevent the onset of labor.[4] A thorough patient education program, including frequent visits to the obstetrician, will help in the early recognition of premature labor and the prompt institution of systemic tocolytic therapy.

Improved antenatal fetal assessment techniques have reduced the number of unintentional deliveries of premature infants resulting from misdiagnosed gestational age. Our incidence of preterm delivery at elective cesarean section decreased from approximately 5 percent to nearly zero over the past 10 years. Table 17–2[5] lists factors that can help minimize the risk of inadvertent preterm elective section.

Despite the current awareness of the problem and attempts to identify the population at risk, a significant number of preterm deliveries occur in otherwise healthy patients for no apparent reason.[6]

INCIDENCE

Preterm births, accounting for 3 to 19 percent of all deliveries,[7] remain the major cause of neonatal morbidity and mortality,[8] contributing to as many as 80 percent of early neonatal deaths (excluding congenital anomalies).[9] The

Table 17–1. MATERNAL RISK FACTORS FOR PRETERM DELIVERY

Major Risk Factors
Previous premature delivery
Previous second-trimester abortion
Polyhydramnios
Multiple gestation
Moderate Risk Factors
Low socioeconomic status
Uterine anomaly
Small weight gain during pregnancy
Low maternal prepregnant weight
Mother's age over 40 or under 18
Minor Risk Factors
Mother smokes
Mother has hypertension
Poor attitude toward pregnancy

incidence varies widely from one obstetric unit to another, depending on the referral patterns in the area and the type of population served. Of the estimated 14 percent preterm deliveries occurring at our institution, 82 percent of premature babies arrive at 34 to 37 weeks' gestation, 12 percent at 30 to 33 weeks', and 6 percent at less than 30 weeks.

THE PRETERM FETUS

More babies previously considered previable now reach the intensive care nursery because of improved care for tiny infants.[10] Despite the improved long-term outlook for premature babies, however, the preterm fetus remains vulnerable because of several factors that differ from the full-term fetus[11] (Table 17–3). The anesthesiologist often is involved in preterm labors owing to the frequency of operative deliveries (cesarean or forceps). By becoming familiar with the risk factors in the preterm fetus, he or she can effectively minimize asphyxia and drug-related depression in premature newborns.

Table 17–2. MINIMIZING THE RISK OF PRETERM ELECTIVE CESAREAN SECTION

Clinical Assessment
Impeccable menstrual history
Bimanual uterine size estimates correspond to menstrual history throughout pregnancy
First trimester pregnancy test
Ultrasound Assessment in First Trimester
Amniocentesis (mature L/S ratio prior to section)
X-ray Confirmation of Maturity (presence of distal femoral and proximal tibial epiphyses), used only when other assessments are unavailable

Table 17–3. RISK FACTORS IN THE PRETERM FETUS

Low hemoglobin levels
Decreased glycogen stores
Decreased fat stores
Predisposition to subependymal venous bleeding
Relative deficiency of clotting factors
Hypoxia developing during uterine contractions
Increased risk of intrauterine infection
Deficiency of surfactant
Tendency to deliver as a breech

Inhibition of Preterm Labor

Once preterm labor has been diagnosed, the obstetrician has several possible courses of action. He or she may allow labor to progress normally if gestation exceeds 34 weeks and if the fetal size seems appropriate for gestational age, since the survival rate for such infants approaches 100 percent. When gestation is less than 34 weeks, the obstetrician may try to delay delivery for 48 to 72 hours in order to assess the fetal status and attempts to enhance pulmonary maturity by maternal steroid administration. Finally, attempts to pharmacologically delay labor for a prolonged period will allow greater fetal maturation, especially for gestations of less than 30 to 33 weeks. Table 17–4 lists drugs that can inhibit labor.

The pharmacologic inhibition of labor for gestations under 34 weeks has achieved success rates as high as 90 percent.[12] Systemic tocolysis costs less than intensive care of the premature neonate at gestations under 34 weeks.[13] Nevertheless, some obstetric units do not subscribe to the use of tocolytic drugs.[14]

BETA-SYMPATHOMIMETIC AGENTS

When stimulated, β_2 receptors residing in uterine muscle, vascular smooth muscle, bronchioles, and diaphragm elicit smooth muscle relaxation. In the myocardium, β_1 receptors increase heart rate and contractility. Only the β_2

Table 17–4. DRUGS USED TO INHIBIT LABOR

Beta-sympathomimetic agents
Epinephrine
Fenoterol
Isoprenaline
Isoxsuprine
Orciprenaline
Ritodrine
Salbutamol
Terbutaline
Calcium channel blockers
Nifedepine
Verapamil
Diazoxide
Ethanol
Magnesium sulfate
Prostaglandin inhibitors
Aspirin
Indomethacin
Phenylbutazone
17-α-hydroxyprogesterone
Theophylline

agonists ritodrine and terbutaline are suitable for delaying labor, since combined β_1 and β_2 agonists (isoprenaline, orciprenaline, and isoxsuprine) accelerate heart rate. Although ritodrine and terbutaline may cause tachycardia, it is usually minimal. They are, however, associated with an impressive list of minor and major side effects (Table 17–5). Pulmonary edema, possibly resulting from fluid overload, occurs in up to 5 percent of treated patients.[15] This complication occurs more frequently in patients with twin pregnancies or chorioamnionitis. Although increased capillary permeability rather than cardiac failure has been suggested as the cause of this complication,[16] recent evidence suggests this may not be the problem.[17]

Table 17–5. SIDE EFFECTS OF BETA-SYMPATHOMIMETIC THERAPY

Major
Pulmonary edema
Myocardial ischemia
Arrhythmias
Cerebral vasospasm
Hypotension
Ketoacidosis
Minor
Hyperglycemia
Lactic acidosis
Hypokalemia
Anemia
Headache

Beta-sympathomimetic therapy may be associated with myocardial ischemia.[18] If a patient on ritodrine or terbutaline therapy develops chest pain, she should receive supplemental oxygen, have the β-mimetic drug discontinued, and have an immediate ECG. Persistent chest pain may call for nitrate or β-blocker therapy.

Other major complications that might necessitate discontinuation of a beta agonist include cardiac arrhythmias (ventricular, nodal, or atrial), cerebral vasospasm, hypotension, and ketoacidosis. Terbutaline in combination with anesthesia reportedly contributes to pulmonary edema, ventricular dysrhythmias, and severe tachycardia.[19] Although both agents appear equally effective,[20,21] terbutaline seems slightly more toxic than ritodrine.[12] Anesthetizing a patient who is receiving this type of therapy can provoke numerous complications.[22] Aside from the major problems listed above, hypokalemia, anemia, and hyperglycemia may occur.[23] Preanesthetic laboratory investigations should include hemoglobin, blood sugar, serum electrolytes, and an ECG. Perioperative management requires close patient monitoring, limited fluid administration, and avoidance of halothane because of its potential to cause arrhythmias and myocardial depression.

Another interesting and potentially serious side effect of ritodrine involves its ability to inhibit hypoxic pulmonary vasoconstriction.[24] If this occurs in patients with underlying pulmonary disease (or pulmonary edema), ventilation-perfusion abnormalities could worsen with resultant arterial hypoxemia. For a more thorough review of the complications of β-mimetic tocolytic agents, consult the review by Benedetti.[16]

ETHANOL

Because of the effectiveness of other forms of tocolytic therapy and because of its frequent side effects, the obstetric use of ethanol should rarely occur. The excellent review by Caritis and associates[7] provides more information about ethanol.

MAGNESIUM SULFATE

Clinicians have long recognized the inhibitory effect on labor when magnesium sulfate was used to treat pre-eclampsia.[25] More recent evidence points to its efficacy as a primary tocolytic agent,[26] proving as effective as the β-mimetic agents but with fewer side effects.[12] Noted side effects include nausea, flushing, drowsiness, and headache, as well as a few cases of pulmonary edema[27] and myocardial ischemia reportedly related to its use. Ritodrine in combination with magnesium sulfate appears to interfere with myocardial function.[28]

Magnesium sulfate's weak muscle relaxant effect[29] should concern the anesthesiologist, since it can potentiate the effects of other muscle relaxants and perhaps interfere with neuromuscular function in the neonate.[30] In addition, its action as a central nervous system (CNS) depressant introduces the threat of augmented anesthetic depression and/or depression of the neonate.

Calcium preparations antagonize some of the adverse effects of magnesium on neuromuscular and CNS activity in cases of magnesium overdose.

17-α-HYDROXYPROGESTERONE CAPROATE

This substance may provide prophylaxis against preterm labor in high-risk patients.[31,32] Weekly intramuscular injection avoids expensive hospitalization, and there have been no reported major or minor complications to date.

The potential to produce birth defects or delayed carcinogenic effects causes concern, and widespread use is unlikely until much further work is done on its efficacy and toxicity. The anesthesiologist must also realize that progesterone depresses the CNS and may reduce the requirement for other anesthetics.[33]

OTHER AGENTS

Although calcium-channel blockers, diazoxide, prostaglandin inhibitors, and theophylline have all shown an ability to inhibit uterine activity, their use for this purpose seems unlikely in the near future.

Other Maternal Therapy

STEROIDS

Since the publication of Liggins' study[34] in 1972, there have been varying degrees of enthusiasm for the use of corticosteroids in preterm patients.[35] A short course of maternal steroid therapy prior to delivery may increase the fetal production of surfactant and lessen the severity of the neonatal respiratory distress syndrome.[36] Steroids should not affect the anesthetic management of the mother or adversely affect the neonate.[37]

ANTIBIOTICS

Antibiotic therapy in the preterm laboring patient may reduce the risk of intrauterine infection associated with prolonged rupture of the membranes. The anesthesiologist should remember that some antibiotics can interact with muscle relaxants and anesthetic agents.

AMINOPHYLLINE

Although aminophylline reportedly reduces the incidence of neonatal respiratory distress syndrome in preterm deliveries,[38] its clinical use remains investigative.

AMNIOINFUSION

Saline amnioinfusion in preterm patients reduces the incidence of fetal distress when premature rupture of the membranes occurs.[39] No serious maternal complications have resulted, and subsequent anesthetic management does not appear to be affected.

The Premature Infant

The neonatal complications of prematurity (Table 17–6) pose two primary concerns for the anesthesiologist: 1) to avoid using drugs and techniques that might complicate the neonatal course of the premature baby, and 2) to partici-

Table 17–6. NEONATAL COMPLICATIONS OF PREMATURITY

Respiratory distress syndrome
Ischemic cerebral damage
Intracranial hemorrhage
Prolonged effects of depressant medications
Hypoglycemia
Hypocalcemia
Hyperbilirubinemia

pate fully in the resuscitation of these high-risk neonates.

INFANT RESPIRATORY DISTRESS SYNDROME (IRDS)

With improved antepartum evaluation of pulmonary maturity, active management of premature labor, and improvements in neonatal intensive care, IRDS is no longer the major cause of death in the premature infant. Intrapartum asphyxia and maternal stress during labor may increase the incidence and severity of IRDS in premature newborns by interfering with the production of surfactant.[36] The anesthesiologist can facilitate the prevention of IRDS by administering effective analgesia and avoiding factors that contribute to fetal hypoxia.

CEREBRAL ISCHEMIA

The premature infant shows greater susceptibility to developing ischemic cerebral lesions secondary to intrapartum asphyxia, hypotension, and bradycardias than the term infant.[40] Ischemic areas develop in the periventricular region and may produce mental retardation, seizure disorders, or cerebral palsy. The anesthesiologist should avoid complications and drugs that can lead to fetal cerebral ischemia, namely fetal asphyxia, fetal bradycardia, and fetal hypotension. Readily available and rapid anesthesia to facilitate delivery of the distressed premature newborn undoubtedly contributes to the prevention of this disorder.

INTRACRANIAL HEMORRHAGE

Intracranial bleeding resulting from a multitude of determinants occurs more frequently in the premature newborn, but there are two main preventable causes: bleeding related to birth trauma and bleeding related to loss of cerebral autoregulation and hypertension. The anesthesiologist contributes to the prevention of traumatic cerebral hemorrhage by providing those conditions necessary for controlled delivery of the neonatal head. Regional or general anesthetic techniques can prevent precipitous delivery, reduce extreme degrees of maternal effort, relax the perineum, and provide analgesia for a generous episiotomy and early application of forceps, all of which will prevent sudden wide swings in intracranial pressure that could lead to hemorrhage.

Intracranial bleeding related to neonatal hypertension represents a more recently recognized phenomenon,[41] occurring subsequent to a period of asphyxia (either intrapartum or postpartum), which abolishes normal cerebral autoregulation and subjects the capillary system to the direct effects of arterial hypertension. In addition to trying to avoid conditions that predispose to this complication,[42,43] the anesthesiologist may actively contribute to the pharmacologic prevention of hypertensive episodes in the premature neonate.

PROLONGED EFFECT OF DEPRESSANT MEDICATIONS

Immature enzyme and renal systems complicate the metabolism and excretion of drugs and their metabolites in the premature neonate. In addition, the premature newborn binds less drug to serum proteins and has a poorly developed blood-brain barrier.[44] Consequently, narcotics, phenothiazines, barbiturates, and other sedatives, hypnotics, and anesthetics that may be used without hesitation for birth at term may profoundly affect the premature infant.[45] The anesthesiologist faces the challenge of choosing the safest and most appropriate analgesic and anesthetic techniques in these patients.

HYPOGLYCEMIA AND HYPOCALCEMIA

These two metabolic disorders occur more frequently in preterm newborns, and perinatal asphyxia increases the incidence.

HYPERBILIRUBINEMIA

The neurotoxic effects of unconjugated bilirubin affect the premature newborn more frequently; kernicterus is a potential complication even at low serum bilirubin levels. Since kernicterus produces permanent neurologic damage, drugs that displace bilirubin from the protein-binding sites (e.g., sodium benzoate, a buffer in diazepam) could prove harmful.

Obstetric Considerations

Much controversy exists regarding the use of cesarean section for preterm deliveries, since breech presentation is twice as common in these infants as in full-term infants. Some reports claim markedly improved outcomes with cesarean section,[46,47] while others recommend cesarean only for the footling breech.[48] In some series, cesarean section improved outcome for all tiny fetuses,[49] irrespective of presentation, while in others this was not true.[50] An overall trend reflects an increasing tendency toward operative intervention in the delivery of preterm babies. Many obstetricians prefer the more controlled conditions provided by low forceps for vaginal delivery of premature infants. Outlet forceps permit gentle delivery of the fetal head, thus preventing the wide fluctuations in intracranial pressure that can accompany a precipitous, uncontrolled, spontaneous delivery. The increased use of forceps in preterm deliveries has led to more frequent requests for anesthesia for operative vaginal delivery.

The vaginal breech delivery deserves special consideration. Because of the relatively small body and large head of the preterm fetus, the after-coming head may become trapped by the lower birth canal. This can result in cerebral hypoxia and damage unless rapid delivery and resuscitation ensue. If the patient has not received an epidural anesthetic, the anesthesiologist must anticipate these complications by preparing to give a rapid general anesthetic and uterine relaxants.

Anesthetic Considerations

The relationship between obstetric anesthesia and fetal prematurity has generated little direct investigation, either basic or clinical. Many clinical considerations have originated by extrapolation from studies involving full-term patients or animals, with allowance for the increased risk of drug effects and alterations in placental perfusion in the premature fetus. Although maternal considerations usually differ little from those in full-term patients, the anesthesiologist must carefully evaluate the maternal safety of any technique or drug that is considered. Also, the concurrent use of tocolytic and anesthetic substances demands caution. The β-sympathomimetic agents in particular exert additive effects when combined with anesthetic agents. Regional anesthetics or potent cardiovascular depressants aggravate β-agonist–induced hypotension. The possibility exists that tachycardia could develop after atropine or pancuronium administration in the presence of β-mimetic agents. Since the half-life of these drugs is measured in hours, discontinuing β-mimetic therapy at least 12 hours prior to anesthesia would seem preferable.

For the patient receiving magnesium sulfate as a tocolytic drug, the anesthesiologist must remember the neuromusuclar blocking properties of this drug and the potential interaction with other muscle relaxants.[51] In addition, central depression might prove additive to that of the anesthetic agents.

Notwithstanding maternal safety, fetal and neonatal well-being usually receive prime consideration during anesthetic administration for preterm delivery.

SYSTEMIC MEDICATION

For the reasons stated above, most obstetrics and anesthesia textbooks advise avoiding depressant systemic medication in preterm patients, if possible. Narcotics, barbiturates, phenothiazines, benzodiazepines, and other sedative-hypnotic agents can cause greater than expected CNS depression in the premature neonate. Most authors recommend using regional anesthesia techniques for analgesia.

PARACERVICAL BLOCK

The fetal bradycardia and neonatal depression frequently seen following paracervical block make this technique inadvisable for preterm patients.[52]

SPINAL ANESTHESIA

Spinal anesthesia offers the advantage of producing major conduction blockade with a very small dose of local anesthetic, thereby avoiding potential fetal and neonatal local anesthetic toxicity. Spinal anesthesia provides optimal conditions for cesarean or forceps deliveries, but not for labor analgesia. Maternal hypotension can occur quickly and with severity, thus contributing to fetal asphyxia.

EPIDURAL ANALGESIA

Many obstetric anesthesiologists prefer continuous lumbar epidural analgesia because of the superior control of anesthetic level and maternal blood pressure. This technique has become the preferred method of producing safe, maximally effective analgesia in most obstetric situations. For the preterm patient, epidural analgesia seems especially appropriate for first-stage analgesia, operative vaginal delivery, and cesarean section.[48,53,54] Prevention or rapid treatment of maternal hypotension proves essential. Minimal doses of local anesthetics can achieve effective analgesia while avoiding local anesthetic toxicity in the neonate. Agents with limited placental transfer least affect the preterm fetus. Thus, bupivacaine, with its high degree of maternal protein binding, appears to be ideal.[52] Two-chloroprocaine, an ester-linked local anesthetic that is rapidly hydrolyzed by maternal plasma cholinesterase, presents another reasonable choice, as it reaches the fetus in minimal amounts.[55] (See Chapter 2 for a more comprehensive discussion of local anesthetic agents.)

Disadvantages of lidocaine theoretically include higher maternal free plasma levels, greater placental transfer to the fetal circulation, and ion trapping in the acidotic fetus.[56] Teramo and associates[57] demonstrated that preterm sheep fetuses exhibit less sensitivity to lidocaine than animals near term. This holds true for CNS effects and for cardiovascular responses to toxic doses of lidocaine. The late gestational development of cardiac sympathetic innervation may, in part, account for the decreased cardiovascular reactivity in the preterm fetus.[58] The little clinical data available from preterm studies seem to indicate the superiority of regional anesthesia over general anesthesia or systemic medication.

The actual technique of performing the epidural puncture lies beyond the scope of this chapter, but the following general principles should be followed:

1. Improve maternal FiO_2 by continuous oxygen administration (4 liters per min by nasal prongs or 6 to 8 liters per min by loosely fitting mask).
2. Prehydrate the mother using an appropriate intravenous solution (500 to 1000 ml lactated Ringer's or 0.9-percent NaCl).
3. Maintain the lateral position or lateral tilt using a wedge under one maternal buttock.
4. Monitor vital signs frequently (every minute for the first 5 to 7 min following each injection; every 2 min up to 15 min; and every 5 min thereafter).
5. Carefully titrate each dose of local anesthetic to use the least amount necessary to obtain the desired block. We currently use bupivacaine without adrenaline (0.125- or 0.25-percent) for labor and delivery and lidocaine (2.0-percent with adrenaline 1:400,000) for cesarean section.

GENERAL ANESTHESIA

Regional anesthesia generally proves safer for both mother and baby during operative vaginal delivery or cesarean section, while both intravenous and inhalation anesthetics possess a definite potential to depress the neonate. This depression may become severe and complicate the management of the premature newborn. When conditions necessitate general anesthesia, no one technique qualifies as preferable, although certain general principles bear observing:

1. Either ketamine, 1 mg per kg, or thiopental, 3 to 4 mg per kg, can safely induce anesthesia.
2. To reduce the incidence of anesthetic depression of the newborn, the anesthesiologist should keep the induction-to-delivery period as short as possible.
3. Avoid light anesthetic techniques since convincing evidence shows that during such procedures maternal catecholamine output decreases placental perfusion.[59]
4. The maternal inspired oxygen concentration should remain at no less than 50 percent. Marx[60] presented evidence that maximal fetal oxygenation results when the maternal PaO_2 exceeds 300 mmHg.
5. Halothane (<0.5 percent), enflurane (<1 percent), or isoflurane (<0.75 percent) can safely serve as supplements to inhalational anesthetics.

I recommend the following general anesthetic technique:

1. Maintain left uterine displacement with a wedge under the mother's right buttock.
2. Preoxygenate the patient for 3 min while prepping and draping the abdomen.
3. Prior to induction, administer 3 mg d-tubocurarine or 1 mg pancuronium.
4. Apply cricoid pressure.
5. Use a rapid-sequence induction consisting of 3 mg per kg thiopental and 1.5 mg per kg succinylcholine.
6. Intubate the trachea with a cuffed endotracheal tube.
7. Maintain anesthesia with 50 percent oxygen, 50 percent nitrous oxide, and up to 0.75 percent isoflurane.
8. Maintain paralysis with pancuronium, atracurium, or vecuronium.
9. Control ventilation to maintain $PaCO_2$ near preanesthetic values (10 ml per kg tidal volume, rate 10 per min).

INHALATION ANALGESIA

When epidural analgesia is unsuitable or becomes unavailable, subanesthetic doses of nitrous oxide, or possibly enflurane, can provide safe and effective alternatives during labor and delivery.

AVOIDING ANALGESIA

Maternal catecholamine output associated with the pain and anxiety of labor may reduce uterine blood flow and contribute to fetal asphyxia.[61] Even mild reductions in uterine perfusion may endanger the preterm fetus. Evidence suggests that the potential benefits of providing the preterm parturient with good analgesia (lumbar epidural) far outweigh the potential danger of maternal hypotension. Few reasons can justify allowing these patients to suffer through a painful labor given the availability and usefulness of epidural analgesia.[61]

Mother-Child Interaction

The premature birth of a child can provoke extreme anxiety in the mother. For the premature infant, more likely to experience a prolonged stay in an intensive or intermediate care nursery, the current trend toward early maternal-child interaction has even greater meaning.[62] The anesthesiologist can facilitate maternal-newborn interaction by ensuring an awake, alert mother and an infant free of drug depression.

Summary

Despite advances in recognizing the causes of preterm delivery and increasingly aggressive attempts to delay early labor, more than 10 percent of babies still deliver prematurely and account for more than 80 percent of early neonatal morbidity and mortality. Beta-sympathomimetic amines and magnesium sulphate currently are the most widely used drug therapy for early preterm labor. An impressive list of serious complications accompanies the use of these drugs, however, and the anesthesiologist presented with patients receiving these agents faces a significant challenge.

The preterm fetus and premature newborn tolerate asphyxial episodes much more poorly than mature babies, so the obstetrician more readily intervenes with operative delivery. Also, these immature babies cannot withstand depressant analgesic and sedative drugs resulting in severe depression with many of the usual obstetric anesthetic regimens. Unfortunately, they also respond poorly to maternal pain and anxiety, thus challenging the anesthesiologist to provide effective maternal analgesia and anesthesia with the least depressant effect on the fetus and newborn.

Currently, lumbar epidural analgesia for labor and lumbar epidural or spinal anesthesia for cesarean section best meet the requirements for maximal maternal safety and efficacy with minimal fetal and neonatal depression.

References

1. Goldenberg, RL, et al: Low birth weight, intrauterine growth retardation, and preterm delivery. Am J Obstet Gynecol 152:980, 1985.
2. Creasy, RK, Gummer, BA and Liggins, GH: System for predicting spontaneous preterm birth. Obstet Gynecol 55:692, 1980.
3. Berkowitz, GS: An epidemiological study of preterm deliveries. Am J Epidemiol 113:81, 1981.

4. Main, DM, et al: Can preterm deliveries be prevented? Am J Obstet Gynecol 151:892, 1985.
5. Manitoba College of Physicans and Surgeons: Guidelines to Confirm Fetal Maturity Prior to Elective Caesarean Section or Elective Induction of Labour. Winnepeg, 1985.
6. Fedrick, J and Anderson, ABM: Factors associated with spontaneous preterm birth. Br J Obstet Gynaecol 83:342, 1976.
7. Caritis, SN, Edestone, DI and Mueller-Huebach, E: Pharmacologic inhibition of preterm labor. Am J Obstet Gynecol 133:557, 1979.
8. Brans, YW, et al: Perinatal mortality in a large perinatal center: Five-year review of 31,000 births. Am J Obstet Gynecol 148:284, 1984.
9. Rush, RW, Davey, DA and Segall, ML: The effect of preterm delivery on perinatal mortality. Br J Obstet Gynaecol 85:806, 1978.
10. Goldenberg, RL, et al: Neonatal mortality in infants born weighing 501 to 1000 grams. Am J Obstet Gynecol 151:608, 1985.
11. Bowes, WA: Delivery of the very low birth weight infant. Clin Perinatol 8:183, 1981.
12. Beall, MH, et al: A comparison of ritodrine, terbutaline, and magnesium sulfate for the suppression of preterm labor. Am J Obstet Gynecol 153:854, 1985.
13. Korenbrot, CC, Aalto, LH and Laros, RK: The cost effectiveness of stopping preterm labor with beta-adrenergic treatment. N Engl J Med 310:691, 1984.
14. Boylan, P and O'Driscoll, K: Improvement in perinatal mortality rate attributed to spontaneous preterm labor without the use of tocolytic agents. Am J Obstet Gynecol 145:781, 1983.
15. Wagner, JM, et al: Terbutaline and maternal cardiac function. JAMA 246:2697, 1981.
16. Benedetti, TJ: Maternal complications of parenteral beta-sympathomimetic therapy for premature labor. Am J Obstet Gynecol 145:1, 1983.
17. MacLennan, FM: Fatal pulmonary oedema associated with the use of ritodrine in pregnancy: Case Report. Br J Obstet Gynaecol 92:703, 1985.
18. Tye, KH, Desser, KB and Benchimol, A: Angina pectoris associated with terbutaline for premature labor. JAMA 244:692, 1980.
19. Ravindran, R, Padilla, LM and LaBlonde, P: Anesthetic considerations in pregnant patients receiving terbutaline therapy. Anesth Analg 59:391, 1980.
20. Ingemarsson, I and Bengtsson, B: A five-year experience with terbutaline for preterm labor: Low rate of severe side effects. Obstet Gynecol 66:176, 1985.
21. Beniarz, J, Motew, M and Scommegna, A: Uterine and cardiovascular effects of ritodrine in premature labor. Obstet Gynecol 40:65, 1972.
22. Knight, RJ: Labour retarded with beta-agonist drugs. Anaesthesia 32:639, 1977.
23. Main, DM, et al: The effect of oral ritodrine therapy on glucose tolerance in pregnancy. Am J Obstet Gynecol 152:1031, 1985.
24. Conover, WB, Benumof, JL and Key, TC: Ritodrine inhibition of hypoxic pulmonary vasoconstriction. Am J Obstet Gynecol 146:652, 1983.
25. Hall, DG, et al: The effects of magnesium therapy on the duration of labor. Am J Obstet Gynecol 18:27, 1959.
26. Steer, CM and Petrie, RH: A comparison of magnesium sulfate and alcohol for the prevention of premature labor. Am J Obstet Gynecol 129:1, 1977.
27. Elliott, JP: Magnesium sulfate as a tocolytic agent. Am J Obstet Gynecol 147:277, 1983.
28. Ferguson, JE, Hensleigh, PA and Kredenster, D: Adjunctive use of magnesium sulfate with ritodrine for preterm labor tocolysis. Am J Obstet Gynecol 148:166, 1984.
29. Morris, R and Giesecke, AH: Potentiation of muscle relaxants by magnesium sulfate therapy in toxemia of pregnancy. South Med J 61:25, 1968.
30. Lipsitz, PJ: The clinical and biochemical effects of excess magnesium in the newborn. Pediatrics 47:3, 1971.
31. Johnson, JWC, et al: High-risk prematurity: Progestin treatment and steroid studies. Obstet Gynecol 54:412, 1979.
32. Yemini, M, et al: Prevention of premature labor by 17-alpha-hydroxyprogesterone caproate. Am J Obstet Gynecol 151:574, 1985.
33. Selye, H: Studies concerning the anesthetic action of steroid hormones. J Pharmacol Exp Ther 73:127, 1941.
34. Liggins, GC and Howie, RN: A controlled trial of antepartum glucocorticoid treatment for prevention of respiratory distress syndrome in premature infants. Pediatrics 50:515, 1972.
35. Simpson, GF and Harbert, GM: Use of beta-methasone in management of preterm gestation with premature rupture of membranes. Obstet Gynecol 66:168, 1985.
36. Quirk, JG, et al: The role of glucocorticoids, unstressful labor, and atraumatic delivery in the prevention of respiratory distress syndrome. Am J Obstet Gynecol 134:768, 1979.
37. Taeuch, HW: Glucocorticoid prophylaxis for respiratory distress syndrome: A review of potential toxicity. J Pediatr 87:617, 1975.
38. Hadjigeorgiou, E, et al: Antepartum aminophylline treatment for prevention of the respiratory distress syndrome in premature infants. Am J Obstet Gynecol 135:257, 1985.
39. Nageotte, MP, et al: Prophylactic intrapartum amnioinfusion in patients with preterm premature rupture of membranes. Am J Obstet Gynecol 153:557, 1985.
40. Pape, KE and Wigglesworth, JS: Ischaemic lesions of the preterm and term brain. Clin Dev Med 69:100, 1979.
41. Fujimura, M, et al: Clinical events relating to intraventricular hemorrhage in the newborn. Arch Dis Child 54:409, 1979.
42. Lou, HC, et al: Pressure-passive cerebral blood flow and breakdown of the blood-brain barrier in experimental fetal asphyxia. Acta Pediatr Scand 68:57, 1979.
43. Ong, BY, et al: Acidemia impairs autoregulation of cerebral blood flow in newborn lambs. Can Anaesth Soc J 33:5, 1986.
44. Van Petten, GR: Principles of fetal pharmacology. In Goodwin, JW, Godden, JO and Chance, GW (eds):

Perinatal Medicine: The Basic Science Underlying Clinical Practice. Williams & Wilkins, Baltimore, 1976, p. 286.

45. Dubowitz, V: Neurologic fragility in the newborn: Influence of medication in labour. Br J Anaesth 47:1005, 1975.
46. Goldenberg, RL and Nelson, KG: The premature breech. Am J Obstet Gynecol 127:240, 1977.
47. Smith, ML, Spencer, SA and Hull, D: Mode of delivery and survival in babies weighing less than 2,000 g at birth. Br Med J 281:1118, 1980.
48. Karp, LE, et al: The premature breech: Trial of labor or cesarean section? Obstet Gynecol 53:88, 1979.
49. Haesslein, HC and Goodlin, RC: Delivery of the tiny newborn. Am J Obstet Gynecol 134:192, 1979.
50. Kitchen, W, et al: Cesarean section or vaginal delivery at 24 to 28 weeks' gestation: Comparison of survival and neonatal and two-year morbidity. Obstet Gynecol 66:149, 1985.
51. DeVore, JS and Asram, R: Magnesium sulfate prevents succinylcholine-induced fasciculations in toxemic parturients. Anesthesiology 52:76, 1980.
52. Ralston, DH and Shnider, SM: The fetal and neonatal effects of regional anesthesia in obstetrics. Anesthesiology 48:34, 1978.
53. Second Report of Perinatal Mortality Study in Ten University Hospitals. Ontario Department of Health, Toronto, 1967.
54. Finucane, BT and Bramwell, RSB: Regional anesthesia is preferable for the premature fetus (letter to the editor). Anesthesiology 54:435, 1981.
55. O'Brian, JE, et al: Metabolism and measurement of 2-chloroprocaine, an ester-type local anesthetic. J Pharm Sci 66:75, 1979.
56. Biehl, D, et al: Placental transfer of lidocaine: Effects of fetal acidosis. Anesthesiology 48:409, 1978.
57. Teramo, K, et al: Gestational differences in lidocaine toxicity in the fetal lamb. Anesthesiology 44:133, 1976.
58. Lebowitz, EA, Novick, JS and Rudolph, AM: Development of myocardial sympathetic innervation in the fetal lamb. Pediatr Res: 6:887, 1972.
59. Palahniuk, RJ and Cumming, M: Foetal deterioration following thiopental-nitrous oxide anaesthesia in the pregnant ewe. Can Anaesth Soc J 24:361, 1977.
60. Marx, GF and Mateo, CV: Effects of different oxygen concentrations during general anaesthesia for elective cesarean section. Can Anaesth Soc J 18:587, 1971.
61. Myers, RE and Myers SE: Use of sedative, analgesic, and anesthetic drugs during labor and delivery: Bane or boon? Am J Obstet Gynecol 133:83, 1979.
62. Gorski, PA, Davison, MF and Brazelton, TB: Stages of behavioural organization in the high risk neonate: Theoretical and clinical considerations. Semin Perinatol 3:61, 1979.

CHAPTER 18

BREECH PRESENTATION AND MULTIPLE GESTATION

A. SCOTT WHEELER, M.D.

Few situations in obstetrics generate more interest and controversy than the breech presentation and multiple gestation. Prematurity, congenital anomalies, peripartal hypoxia, and birth trauma occur in both events,[1] often necessitating difficult management decisions by members of the perinatal care team. Thoughtfully chosen and skillfully administered anesthesia can contribute to the successful outcome of these pregnancies. However, differences of opinion commonly exist regarding the best method of management. Despite individual preferences, the obstetrician and anesthesiologist should appreciate that no single anesthetic can produce perfect results in all cases. Rather, the preferred approach for each delivery depends upon the experience and expertise of attending physicians and nurses, clinical status of mother and fetus, quality of facilities and equipment, and patient preference. Appropriate management of pain relief serves to improve fetal and maternal outcome,[1] whereas poorly conducted analgesia may complicate patient care.

This chapter presents the fetal and maternal problems occurring in breech and twin deliveries and attempts to inform health care professionals about pertinent obstetric and anesthetic considerations. The reader will gain more knowledge in how to deliver safe and effective anesthesia and analgesia, particularly suited for each patient.

Breech Presentation

GENERAL PERSPECTIVES

Breech position occurs in 3 to 4 percent of term fetuses. Some of the etiologic factors might be anatomic, yet Luterkort and coworkers[2] attribute the breech position to anatomic problems of the fetus, uterus, placenta, or pelvis in 15 percent of cases and cannot discern a single cause in the remaining 85 percent. Ultrasonography and palpation detect most breech fetuses by 32 weeks' gestation.[3] During the third trimester nearly 60 percent of breech babies undergo spontaneous version (from breech to vertex position).[3] Spontaneous version occurs more frequently in multigravidas near term and less commonly in primigravidas and in women who have had a previous breech presentation.

Centuries ago "breech presentation was considered advantageous, because midwives could pull the legs and quickly extract the fetus when life-threatening bleeding was noticed."[4] While avoiding the maternal hazards of cesarean section, rapid breech extraction frequently traumatized the fetus, leading to more gentle delivery of the after-coming head by means of the Mauriceau and Bracht maneuvers or by the use of Piper forceps.[5] Vaginal delivery remained commonplace until after the 1950s.

Over the past three decades, retrospective studies[6-12] examining perinatal outcome demonstrated significantly higher morbidity and mortality rates for breech fetuses compared with vertex singletons delivered vaginally. Accurate figures for fetal morbidity and mortality could not be established, owing to variations in composition of series (patient selection), methods of management, and data analysis.[10] Rovinsky, Miller, and Kaplan[13] emphasized the influence of imprecise obstetric terminology on the misinterpretation of data in some studies (Table 18–1). They found corrected perinatal morbidity and mortality rates to be 12 and 3 times higher, respectively, in vaginally delivered breech infants than in vertex infants at term. Other authors reported similar findings.[11,14] Higher corrected perinatal death rates (23 percent) followed vaginal delivery of the premature breech.[15]

Based upon the results of these retrospective analyses, obstetricians advocated more liberal or even routine use of cesarean section to improve outcome of breech presentation.[6,15,16] Yet, cesarean delivery has not eliminated unfavorable outcomes.[17-20] Possible mechanisms include hypoxia and trauma resulting from difficult delivery of the after-coming head through an inadequate abdominal or uterine incision, and the complications of prematurity in the neonate. In addition, obstetricians select cesarean section more frequently for the management of already compromised babies.

Westgren, Songster, and Paul[21] discuss the limited value of such nonrandomized retrospective studies for evaluating obstetric procedures for the breech. They conclude that the retrospective design of their study, as in most published studies on the subject, confounds the results and makes conclusions precarious. Although clouded by methodologic difficulties, the results of these retrospective assessments support the following conclusions: (1) as a group, breech fetuses are at increased risk for significant morbidity and mortality; (2) deleterious factors often associated with the breech position may influence perinatal outcome more than the breech presentation itself; and (3) the true neonatal benefit of cesarean section depends upon the circumstances involved in each individual case and does not relate to all breech pregnancies.

Table 18–1. DEFINITION OF OBSTETRIC TERMS FOR THE BREECH

Breech presentation: A longitudinal fetal lie in which the fetal pelvis is the leading pole.
Frank breech: A breech presentation in which the fetal lower extremities are flexed at the hips and extended at the knees.
Complete breech: The lower extremities are flexed at both hips and knees.
Footling breech: One or both lower extremities are extended at the hip and one or both feet are presenting.
Spontaneous breech delivery: Delivery is produced by natural maternal forces with no assistance other than the support of the baby as it is being born.
Assisted breech delivery: Natural forces propel the fetus to the umbilicus; the obstetrician extracts the remainder. This includes application of forceps, usually Pipers, to the after-coming head.
Partial breech extraction: Similar to assisted delivery except that the fetus is not delivered spontaneously to the umbilicus; assistance is initiated when a small part of the fetus, such as the buttocks, protrudes below the pelvic floor.
Complete breech extraction: No portion of fetus extends below the pelvic floor; the obstetrician extracts the entire body (includes digital traction in groins to deliver buttocks of frank breech or traction on lower extremity of a footling breech).
Breech decomposition: The intrauterine conversion of a frank into a footling breech by flexing the fetus' knees and extending the hips followed by complete extraction.

PROBLEMS OF BREECH PRESENTATION

Breech presentation poses many problems, including intracranial hemorrhage, trauma, hypoxia, umbilical cord prolapse, fetopelvic disproportion, prematurity, congenital anomalies, uterine abnormalities, placenta previa, and abruptio placentae.[1] Prematurity, congenital malformations, trauma, and asphyxia are the major causes of death.[10,12,22]

Prematurity

Statistics demonstrate the significance of prematurity. Forty percent of infants delivering prior to 28 weeks' gestation present as breech, in contrast to 17 percent at 28 to 38 weeks and 3 to 4 percent at term.[2,23] Fetuses previously diagnosed as breech deliver significantly earlier in pregnancy than vertex infants, yet the reason for prematurity remains unexplained.[3,12] Perinatal mortality rates exceed 60 percent in breech fetuses weighing less than 1000 g, regardless of the method of delivery.[24,25] Infants weighing from 1000 to 1500 g display a mortality rate of 25 to 45 percent, while mortality falls to less than 5 percent in neonates exceeding 1500 g (32 weeks).[18,24–26] These data clearly demonstrate that, within the entire breech population, very-low-birth-weight babies (<1500 g) presently account for most deaths as well as most sustained neurologic sequelae.[19,20,25] Much of this pathology relates directly to prematurity (e.g., from respiratory distress, necrotizing enterocolitis, kernicterus, or sepsis). However, peripartum and intrapartum hypoxia, prolapsed umbilical cord, and head entrapment occur more frequently and are gravely dangerous events in the low-birth-weight breech.[27,28] Main, Main, and Maurer[24] note an alarmingly high incidence of intraventricular hemorrhage (30 to 60 percent of cases) in prematures weighing less than 1500 g (whether delivered vaginally or abdominally). Their findings demonstrate the increased susceptibility of the premature neonate to perinatal trauma and asphyxia. Whether the method of delivery improves outcome for the premature breech is controversial.[19,24,25,27,29,30] On the basis of present evidence, one can conclude that the inherent immature physiology of the 500- to 1000-g infant limits its prognosis. However, most authors agree that abdominal delivery enhances outcome of infants in the 1000- to 1500-g range.[11,21]

Congenital Anomalies

The association between breech position and congenital anomalies also raises concern. Brenner, Bruce, and Hendricks[12] reported a higher incidence of fetal anomalies in breech (6.3 percent) than in vertex infants (2.4 percent). Malformations occurred most commonly in the breech beyond 35 weeks. However, a later study[31] of premature breech deliveries noted the presence of anomalies in 18 percent of neonates weighing less than 2500 g. Less discussion about anomalies exists in recent investigations on perinatal outcome, since most authors exclude malformed infants from data analyses. However, the current incidence of major or more lethal congenital anomalies approximates 2 to 5 percent in both term and preterm breech infants.[24,26–28] Minor anomalies occur most frequently in the musculoskeletal system. Major defects most commonly involve the central nervous, urogenital, musculoskeletal, cardiovascular, and gastrointestinal systems.[32] In a survey on the preterm breech, Van Eyk and Huisjes[27] designated congenital anomalies and respiratory distress syndrome as the most frequent causes of neonatal death. Recent reviews[18,26] identify congenital anomalies as the leading cause of death in breech babies at term. Therefore, diagnosis of breech position should be followed by ultrasonographic assessment, and perhaps chromosome studies, which assist the obstetrician in planning the time and method of delivery should malformations be discovered.[32]

Fetal Distress

During labor, fetal distress develops three to eight times more frequently in breech than in cephalic presentations.[12,13,18] Umbilical cord accidents (prolapse, compression, etc.) produce most episodes of fetal distress, although increased incidences of low placental weight, abruptio placentae, and placenta previa account for some cases of peripartum hypoxia in the breech.[13]

Umbilical Cord Prolapse. This phenomenon constitutes a leading cause of severe asphyxia and occurs in approximately 5 percent of breech presentations.[10,12] Most prolapsed cords (72 percent) accompany the footling breech,[10] but the frequency also increases in prematures, multiparas, and when rupture of membranes precedes labor. Immediate cesarean section improves infant outcome when this catastrophe occurs in the second stage.[12]

Hypoxic Heart Rate Changes. Recent studies,[33,34] monitoring fetal heart rate (FHR) electronically throughout labor observed the development of abnormal FHR tracings in approximately 60 to 70 percent of breech pregnancies. Ominous patterns include severe variable decelerations and variable declerations with a late component, both of which occur frequently and correlate with low Apgar scores, fetal acidosis, and increased mortality, especially when associated with persistent tachycardia or a flat baseline.[33,34] Labor often necessitates continuous FHR monitoring and fetal capillary pH measurements, since breech fetuses appear to deteriorate more rapidly than vertex babies during periods of hypoxia.[35]

Head Entrapment. Head entrapment during delivery also produces severe asphyxia, because some degree of umbilical cord compression invariably takes place between delivery of the trunk and head. Collea and associates[22] infrequently note low Apgar scores with umbilicus-to-head delivery intervals of less than 3.5 min.

Trauma

Trauma occurs in 6 to 12 percent of breech vaginal deliveries and usually results from difficult delivery of the after-coming head, breech extraction, or breech decomposition.[10,13,14] The most common injuries include intracranial hemorrhage; cervical spine and cord damage; fractures of the clavicle, arms, and femur; and brachial plexus palsy.[11,14,23,36] During difficult extraction maneuvers, excessive manipulation (hyperextension and traction) traumatizes the after-coming head and neck, but abdominal organs (liver, spleen, adrenals) can be damaged as well. Arm injuries and brachial plexus palsy commonly occur in infants presenting with nuchal arms.[22] Approximately 6 percent of breech fetuses have a hyperextended head in utero, which prevents an easy vaginal delivery and calls for cesarean section.[37,38] A most precarious situation develops when the mother prematurely pushes the fetal trunk through an incompletely dilated cervix, producing entrapment of the after-coming head. Safe means do not exist for immediate resolution of this catastrophe; severe hypoxia, trauma, or death usually occurs. Therefore, to avoid fetal trauma during labor and delivery, the mother should not push prematurely, the body should be handled gently, and delivery of the head should be managed appropriately.[17] Many obstetricians prefer spontaneous vaginal delivery with gentle assistance and place forceps, when necessary, to facilitate delivery of the head. Spontaneous or assisted delivery necessitates controlled and effective expulsive efforts by a cooperative mother.

OBSTETRICAL CONSIDERATIONS

Method of Delivery

In the 1970s several authorities[10,11,14] recommended cesarean delivery in 25 to 45 percent of breech pregnancies. The use of cesarean section increased from 4 to 10 percent in the 1950s, to exceed 80 to 90 percent in the early 1980s.[4] Near routine cesarean section obviates many of the fetal risks previously associated with vaginal delivery; difficult management decisions are simplified. However, Collea and coworkers[22] and Lyons and Papsin[39] question such routine usage for the term *frank* breech, noting the development of significant maternal complications, primarily infection and excessive hemorrhage, in approximately 30 percent of abdominal deliveries. Also, cesarean section increases the duration of hospitalization. Several authors[14,22] suggest a trial of labor for the *term* frank breech. Karp and others[31] propose a trial of labor for the *premature* frank or complete breech, since most episodes of asphyxia and trauma occur in footling presentations. These initial reports[22,31,39] triggered considerable debate regarding the propriety of vaginal delivery versus cesarean section.[4,18–21,25,26,28,29,35,40–42] Currently, some advocate near-routine use of cesarean section, while others believe that a trial of labor and delivery deserves consideration in selected cases. The controversy will likely continue, but one can conclude that neither method produces a substantially different risk of sustained asphyxia, irreversible trauma, long-term neurologic sequelae, or death, *provided vaginal delivery follows careful selection and appropriate intrapartum management* (Table 18–2). As a result, the pendulum is swinging back to more liberal use of vaginal delivery.

Vaginal Delivery

In a thoughtful review of the breech dilemma, Confino and colleagues[4] discuss the difficulties involved in selecting patients for vaginal delivery. The risk of vaginal delivery is mainly determined by evaluating pelvic adequacy or attempting to rule out cephalopelvic disproportion (CPD). Yet the clinical and laboratory indices used to exclude CPD in vertex presentations are not always reliable prognosticators for an easy vaginal delivery in the breech, although ultrasonography and x-ray pelvimetry do offer useful data for the obstetrician. Newer methods, Ball pelvimetry[43] and computed tomography scanning,[44] may prove to be more useful, while exposing the fetus to similar or lower radiation, respectively. Meanwhile, the obstetrician understands clearly that safe delivery of the head is unpredictable and cannot always be guaranteed. The point of no return is reached once the trunk is delivered, since no easy cure exists for a trapped after-coming head. Therefore, normal fetopelvic dimensions, assessed by clinical and laboratory methods, are utilized only to allow a trial of labor. Once initiated, labor must be thoroughly and continuously reappraised. Vaginal delivery can be employed when labor progresses normally. However, inadequate dilatation and descent in the presence of good uterine contractions imply the presence of CPD, indicating the use of cesarean section. Abdominal delivery becomes necessary in approximately 20 to 40 percent of planned labor trials.[28,35] Sound judgment by an experienced obstetrician helps to prevent and resolve many of the problems posed by the breech in labor and likely influences outcome more than any other factor involved.[4]

Cesarean Section

When considering the various indications for cesarean section (Table 18–3) one can assume that obstetricians will continue to employ abdominal delivery in a relatively high percentage of cases. This is especially so since the routine use of cesarean section may have produced a

Table 18–2. PROTOCOL FOR BREECH TRIAL OF LABOR AND VAGINAL DELIVERY*

Selection	Mangement
Frank or complete breech	Prerequisites:
Fetal weight 2000–3600 g	Immediate cesarean section capability
Gestational age >34 wk	Anesthesia support
Normal x-ray pelvimetry	Pediatric support
Flexed fetal head	Obstetrician skilled in vaginal breech delivery
Possible sonar evaluation	Labor
Fetal dimensions and weight	Spontaneous, Friedman curve
Congenital malformations	Continuous electronic fetal monitoring
Neuromuscular function	Oxytocin for dysfunctional labor, if necessary, after careful evaluation
No other maternal or fetal indications for cesarean section	Delivery
	Generous episiotomy
	Spontaneous delivery to umbilicus; assisted breech extraction
	Piper forceps to after-coming fetal head, with any delay in delivery
	Cesarean section for fetal distress or failure to progress in labor with adequate contractions

*Method used at University of Alabama at Birmingham.
(From Tatum et al,[26] with permission.)

Table 18–3. INDICATIONS FOR CESAREAN SECTION IN THE BREECH PRESENTATION

Prolapse of umbilical cord
Fetal distress
Rupture of membranes before labor
Cephalopelvic disproportion (CPD)
Very premature fetus (1000–1500 g)
Footling presentation
Hyperextension of fetal head
Nuchal arms
Low-lying placenta
Abruptio placentae
Dysfunctional labor
Failure to progress
Complicated obstetric history (e.g., diabetes, pre-eclampsia, etc.)
Available anesthesia personnel
Inexperienced obstetrician (in breech vaginal delivery)

generation of obstetricians with insubstantial experience in the management of breech labor and delivery.[4] Renewed interest in external cephalic version with tocolysis in the third trimester may eventually decrease the incidence of breech presentation, thus diminishing fetal risks at vaginal delivery and maternal sequelae from cesarean section.[45–48]

ANESTHETIC CONSIDERATIONS

To provide optimal services for breech deliveries, the anesthesiologist must understand the obstetrician's plan for management soon after admission. This gives the anesthesia team sufficient time to obtain the preanesthetic history, procure necessary drugs and equipment, and discuss the choice of anesthesia with obstetrician and patient. Members of the obstetric and anesthetic teams must communicate. Only by doing so can the best possible conditions exist for each parturient and her fetus.

Labor and Vaginal Delivery

Regardless of the anesthetic method initially chosen, the anesthesia team should be readily available since portentous changes in maternal and fetal status may necessitate changes in the original obstetric and anesthesia plans. Irrespective of the type of anesthesia, the anesthesia team should administer pure oxygen with a tightly fitted face mask throughout delivery. Maternal oxygen inhalation lessens fetal hypoxia during a difficult delivery[1] and denitrogenates the mother in case general anesthesia becomes necessary for a trapped after-coming head. Positive verbal and emotional support and encouragement by anesthesia team members help to allay the mother's anxiety, so that she can more effectively participate in the delivery. The increased possibility of neonatal depression following breech vaginal delivery also warrants the presence of anesthesia personnel who can help to resuscitate the newborn. Since emergency general anesthesia may be required, the obstetrician and anesthesiologist should consider the use of antacids and histamine-2 antagonists throughout labor to decrease the risk of acid aspiration. An effective regimen consists of Bicitra, 30 ml orally every 1 to 2 hours, or ranitidine (Zantac), 50 mg intravenously every 6 to 8 hours.[49,50] For maximum efficacy, Bicitra is given immediately prior to delivery.

The optimal method of analgesia/anesthesia for labor and vaginal delivery remains controversal,[4] yet few of the obstetric reports on the breech have correlated anesthesia with perinatal outcome. One study[12] noted that regional blocks, when compared with local or general anesthesia, produced lower mortality and higher Apgar scores. However, conduction analgesia was used more frequently in pregnancies beyond 31 weeks. Another report[10] utilized general anesthesia with cyclopropane in 94 percent of cases for the purpose of maintaining quiescent patients during vaginal breech deliveries. General anesthesia requires breech extraction and introduces substantial maternal risks. Thus, it should be employed only when indicated and not routinely.[10,13,17] Several negative attributes arise in the use of any method, when reflecting on the following anesthetic prerequisites for the breech:

1. Provision of sufficient analgesia to prevent undue maternal stress, catecholamine release, and uterine hypoperfusion, especially in long, poorly tolerated labors
2. Avoidance of fetal drug depression, particularly in prematures or distressed fetuses
3. Minimal effect on uterine contractility and progress of labor, especially when the obstetrician desires to avoid oxytocin

4. Maintenance of adequate but controlled maternal pushing efforts in stage II
5. Production of good perineal analgesia and relaxation, creating adequate conditions for spontaneous expulsion or an assisted delivery with forceps
6. Rapid initiation of uterine relaxation, when necessary, to promote delivery of a trapped head

Anesthetic requirements often vary from patient to patient and from one period to the next in the same laboring mother. Therefore, no technique can be universally ideal; selection and maintenance of anesthesia should be individualized for each patient and fetus, while optimizing conditions for the obstetrician.

Prepared Childbirth. James[1] calls attention to the many advantages offered by prepared childbirth techniques to parturients with breech presentations: "An informed, motivated patient well in control of her emotions cooperates nicely with the obstetric team and requests little analgesia. This decreases the risk of drug depression in the newborn and permits the woman to have full use of her accessory abdominal muscles to facilitate spontaneous vaginal delivery." However, analgesia should not be withheld or avoided when the prepared mother becomes stressed during a long labor or begins pushing prematurely (prior to complete cervical dilatation). This author believes that childbirth education also enables the mother to cooperate advantageously with the anesthesia team during selection and placement of regional blocks.

Intravenous Analgesia. For shorter, less painful labors, carefully titrated doses of intravenous analgesia with meperidine, butorphanol, etc., often suffice to provide adequate analgesia (see Chap. 6). Excessive parenteral analgesia may impair the mother's ability to cooperate fully with controlled pushing efforts in stage II. Significant narcotic levels also carry the possibility of neonatal depression after delivery.

Paracervical and Lumbar Sympathetic Block. Paracervical and lumbar sympathetic blocks effectively suppress pain from uterine contractions. The association of paracervical block with the uterine vasoconstriction[51] and fetal bradycardia and acidosis[52] limits its use in the breech presentation. Lumbar sympathetic block requires caution as well, since the technique can increase uterine activity.[53,54] Without coexisting sacral blockade, this could prompt uncontrolled pushing efforts before complete cervical dilatation.

Inhalation Analgesia. Inhalation of methoxyflurane produces adequate analgesia for labor but is rarely used. Some mothers object to the smell while others become excessively sedated. For maximal effectiveness and safety, the method also requires the continuous presence of anesthesia personnel.

Pudendal Block. The methods described above require a second anesthetic technique for delivery. Bilateral pudendal blockade, either alone or combined with local perineal infiltration of local anesthetic, often produces sufficient analgesia for episiotomy and application of Piper forceps. The technique preserves maternal bearing-down efforts and minimally affects the neonate. However, a hastily administered pudendal, given immediately prior to delivery, frequently fails to provide satisfactory perineal analgesia either because of inadequate time or technical problems. The mother who experiences both uterine and perineal pain may become uncooperative and resist the efforts of the obstetrician to deliver the after-coming head, especially during forceps application. In that event, the anesthesia team can supplement pudendal-local analgesia with nitrous oxide, 25 to 40 percent, methoxyflurane, 0.25 to 0.50 percent, or enflurane, 0.2 to 0.8 percent, by means of a snuggly fitted face mask. This technique provides a high FIO_2 and enhances fetal oxygenation.

General Anesthesia. Should the approach above prove unsatisfactory, general endotracheal anesthesia with thiopental, nitrous oxide, a halogenated agent, and muscle relaxant becomes necessary. General anesthesia facilitates delivery of a retained head primarily by producing perineal muscle relaxation. Halothane (1 to 2 percent), enflurane (2 to 3 percent), or isoflurane (2 to 3 percent) relaxes the lower uterine segment but does not dilate the cervix. Thiopental and succinylcholine are given in rapid sequence, cricoid pressure is applied, and, following tracheal intubation, halothane, enflurane, or isoflurane is combined with nitrous oxide (30 to 50 percent) and oxygen. Immediately after delivery, one discontinues the halogenated agent and rapidly infuses oxytocin to overcome uterine relaxation and postpartum hemorrhage.[55]

Spinal Anesthesia. For mothers near to delivery and particularly for the small, premature fetus, spinal anesthesia warrants consideration[1,17] and is quite helpful during a rapidly progressing second stage in parturients with poor pain tolerance. The technique offers ease of administration, rapid onset of profound analgesia, good perineal relaxation, and negligible fetal drug exposure (see Chap. 6). By preventing a precipitous or poorly controlled delivery, subarachnoid block lessens the possibility of intracranial trauma in the premature breech. Disadvantages include the need for late and often hasty administration in the delivery room and unpredictable degrees of motor blockade, possibly resulting in diminished bearing down efforts. The anesthesiologist circumvents the latter concern by injecting 1.5 percent lidocaine (1.5 to 2.0 ml) in D7.5W, which preserves motor function while providing good analgesia (i.e., establishes a differential block).[1]

Lumbar Epidural Block. Continuous lumbar epidural blockade furnishes good analgesia for both labor and delivery (see Chap. 6).[56–60] Recently, several authors[1,4,17] referred to it as the method of choice for labor and vaginal delivery of the breech. When compared to other techniques, the procedure best satisfies the anesthetic requirements previously outlined in this section. Epidural analgesia particularly suits premature labors because it lessens maternal stress and neonatal drug depression and provides a controlled delivery through a relaxed perineum. The method warrants consideration in any parturient not coping with the pain of labor, especially when uncontrolled pushing efforts precede complete cervical dilatation. Individuals manifesting such responses to pain and pressure are expected to fare poorly and have marginal ability to cooperate adequately in the delivery room. Satisfactory epidural analgesia will provide better conditions for all involved. An indwelling epidural catheter also avoids the hazards of general anesthesia when fetal distress indicates emergency abdominal delivery.[61,62]

However, several concerns exist about lumbar epidural analgesia in the breech. First, the possible depressant effect on uterine contractions can perplex the obstetrician, who usually relies on the progress of labor to determine the ease of delivery. Epidural analgesia may introduce another variable into this assessment process. Second, extention of a segmental epidural block to involve sacral nerve roots reduces the *urge* to push in stage 2. Profound epidural block may additionally decrease the mother's *ability* to push, promoting fears about the necessity of breech extraction. In response to the first concern, several authors[63,64] demonstrate a minimal effect on duration of stage 1 of labor when a segmental epidural block is given using local anesthetics without epinephrine in the active phase. Also, intravenous oxytocin can safely reinstitute effective labor when used in conjunction with intrauterine pressure monitoring.[4,26,35,58,63] Bowen-Simpkins and Fergusson[57] and Confino and coworkers[65] report comparable durations of stage 1 in patient groups managed with either segmental epidural analgesia or parenteral analgesia. The frequency of oxytocin augmentation is similar in the epidural group (53 percent) and the nonepidural group (36 percent).[65] Epidural blockade moderately prolongs the second stage, which still remains within clinically acceptable time limits.[56,57,59] Most importantly, the frequency of breech extraction does not increase[65] and may actually decrease, since epidural blockade produces better perineal analgesia and more controlled pushing efforts.[56] Parturients with epidural blockade *can* push adequately if the level of motor blockade remains below T10 and the mother receives proper coaching.[66] This is especially so with epidural administration of dilute bupivacaine (0.125 to 0.25 percent) which avoids significant motor blockade.

Prospective studies[56,57,59] reveal similar Apgar scores in breech infants delivered by parenteral-local analgesia or lumbar epidural block. Crawford[56] implies that lumbar epidural analgesia decreases the frequency of prolonged, severe neonatal depression, regardless of birth weight. Another study of primigravidas finds significantly higher 5-minute Apgar scores in babies whose mothers receive epidural analgesia when compared with those managed with meperidine for labor and nitrous oxide–local anesthesia for delivery.[59] These findings presumably result from controlled maternal pushing efforts, preserved uteroplacental perfusion, and less head entrapment during epidural analgesia. Measurements of fetal pH during stage 2, fetal heart rate, and umbilical cord blood pH verify that lumbar epidural analgesia does not compromise—and may benefit—the breech fetus. Therefore, the method provides many advantages for both mother and newborn, and proves especially beneficial for the premature fetus and the mother with poor pain tolerance.

Cesarean Section

In comparison to vaginal delivery, the choice of anesthesia for cesarean section is relatively straightforward; lumbar epidural, spinal, or general anesthesia can be used (see Chap. 6). Selection of method should not be based upon the breech presentation per se but rather upon other obstetric and medical factors. For example, the prolapsed cord usually demands expeditious delivery, indicating general anesthesia, which is the fastest method. However, the anesthesia team should remain cognizant of the possibility of failed intubation and acid aspiration.[67,58] The increased vulnerability of premature infants to drug depression bears consideration in planning anesthesia techniques.[1] Epidural, and especially spinal, anesthesia reduce the possibility of neonatal depression while maintaining better uteroplacental perfusion than general anesthesia.[69] Women in premature labor often receive tocolytic agents (β_2 mimetics, magnesium sulfate, and occasionally ethanol) which may alter the response to anesthesia (Chap. 17). The anesthesia team must keep possible effects of these agents in mind and make necessary adjustments.

Regardless of anesthesia method used for cesarean section, a high fraction of inspired oxygen should be employed, since neonatal depression is more likely. Parturients delivering with regional blocks should inhale 100-percent oxygen through an anesthesia mask until delivery of the head. Nitrous oxide (20 to 40 percent) or methoxyflurane (0.2 to 0.5 percent) can be used for supplementary analgesia. Following induction of general anesthesia, the anesthesia team should provide maintenance with nitrous oxide (30 to 50 percent), oxygen (50 to 70 percent), and a low concentration of halogenated agent, thus facilitating fetal oxygenation and preventing maternal awareness.[70] When necessary, higher inspired concentrations of halothane, enflurane, or isoflurane relax the uterus, promoting delivery of a retained aftercoming head. Inadequate relaxation of abdominal muscles also complicates delivery of the head. During general anesthesia, the use of a peripheral nerve stimulator for determination of sufficient doses of muscle relaxant avoids this complication. With regional blocks, a sensory level above T6 provides adequate muscle relaxation and suitable conditions for abdominal delivery. I believe that spinal anesthesia with tetracaine, bupivacaine, or lidocaine (5-percent) or epidural blockade with 2-chloroprocaine (3-percent) or lidocaine (2-percent) provides excellent relaxation of abdominal muscles. Regional techniques do not provide uterine relaxation. General anesthesia must be considered when a regional block fails to function well prior to incision.

Multiple Gestation

GENERAL PERSPECTIVES

Twinning occurs in approximately 1 in 90 pregnancies and has considerable importance because of frequent maternal and fetal hazards. Ovulation-inducing agents increase the rate of multiple pregnancies with more than two fetuses.[1] Maternal risk factors include higher rates of pregnancy-induced hypertension, abruptio placentae, premature rupture of membranes with amnionitis, anemia, uterine atony, postpartum hemorrhage, and obstetric trauma.[71–78] In comparison to singleton pregnancies, greater increases in blood volume, cardiac index, and total peripheral resistance place more stress on the cardiovascular system in women with twins.[79] Greater combined fetal weight and hydramnios potentiate the development of aortocaval compression and the supine hypotensive syndrome. The enlarged uterus increases gastric distortion, escalating the risk of aspiration pneumonitis. Hypoxia develops more rapidly when mothers assume the supine position, due to upward displacement of the diaphragm.[1]

In regards to the fetus and neonate, perinatal morbidity and death ensue more often, the latter occurring in 5 to 15 percent of twins (3 to 6 times that in singletons)![71–74,77,80–84] Keith and coworkers[84] report the highest rate of twin wastage in mothers under 20 years of age and low parity who deliver prematurely. Their survey reveals that nearly one third of twins remain unsuspected until ater the onset of labor. This finding has significant importance, since approximately 40 percent of fetal deaths occur in the antepartum period (Table 18–4).[81,83,85] Most missed diagnoses of twins result from prematurity and growth retardation, both of which occur quite frequently in multiple gestations[71] and account for a majority of neonatal deaths (see Table 18–4).[81,82,84,86] At present fetal electrocardiography, roentgenography, and ultrasonography reliably detect twins. Ultrasound has become the method of choice, allowing diagnosis by 8 to 12 weeks while avoiding fetal radiation exposure. Its reliability for twin detection exceeds 90 percent after 20 weeks' gestation,[85,87] and fetal gestational age, viability, anomalies, placentation, and growth can also be determined.[87–94] Although screening with ultrasonography has not yet become routine, the technique successfully delineates high-risk factors such as growth retardation, prematurity, anomalies, and monoamniotic twins, promulgating the referral of these pregnancies to perinatal centers for continuing evaluation of fetal status in the antenatal period and provision of critical care for mother and fetuses in the peripartum period.[77,81]

Table 18–4. CAUSES OF PERINATAL DEATH OCCURRING MORE FREQUENTLY IN TWINS

Antepartum death
Twin transfusion syndrome
Abruptio placentae
Placental infarcts
Prolapsed cord
Premature rupture of membranes
Amnionitis
Vasa previa
Hypoxia of unknown cause
Hydramnios
Fetus papyraceus
Pre-eclampsia
Congenital anomalies
Intrapartum and postpartum death
Prematurity
Hyaline membrane disease
Necrotizing enterocolitis
Intracranial hemorrhage
Sepsis
Hyperbilirubinemia
Growth retardation
Second twin retained, breech, or transverse
Asphyxia
Trauma
Twin transfusion syndrome
Abruptio placentae, placental separation
Placenta previa
Other hemorrhage, maternal
Premature rupture of membranes—amnionitis
Pneumonitis
Meningitis
Congenital anomalies
Intrapartum asphyxia
Uteroplacental insufficiency
Cord compression
Prolapsed cord
Vasa previa
Interlocked twins

PROBLEMS OF TWINS

Antepartum Problems

Antepartum fetal demise occurs three times more often in twins than in singletons.[95] Many intrauterine deaths are unexplained, yet antepartum hemorrhage, cord accidents, and placental dysfunction from pre-eclampsia, abruptio placentae, or infarction are commonly responsible.[81,83,84,86] Velamentous insertion of the cord combined with vasa previa occurs in 7 percent of twin pregnancies, compared to 1 percent in singletons.[73] Possible tearing of umbilical vessels during spontaneous rupture of membranes makes this condition particularly dangerous. Abnormalities of the umbilical-placental vasculature develop commonly in monozygotic (identical) twins, which usually have monochorial placentas (one placental disc, one chorion, and one or two amnions). Arteriovenous connections between the two fetal circulations occur frequently and can produce the twin-to-twin transfusion syndrome. The donor twin becomes malnourished, growth retarded, and anemic, while the recipient develops congestive heart failure, polycythemia, and hydramnios.[96,97] The syndrome is associated with a perinatal death rate of 70 percent, partly accounting for a three times higher mortality rate in monozygotic than in dizygotic (nonidentical) twins.[74,98] Monochorionic, monoamniotic twinning occurs infrequently (1 percent of cases), but assumes importance, since fetal mortality rates approximate 40 to 50 percent.[93,94] In the antenatal period, ultrasound and nonstress fetal heart rate testing most reliably assess fetal status; serial estriol determinations are not dependable for detection of compromised twins.[95]

Congenital Anomalies

Congenital anomalies[83,84,86] develop three times more often in twins (10 percent) than in singletons (three percent) and contribute to antepartum and neonatal death. According to Hendricks,[71] less than 10 percent of malformed twins expire, indicating that anomalies do not represent a major source of mortality. Duncan and others[85] disagree: anomalies rank as the third leading cause of mortality and account for 18 percent of twin deaths. The significance of hydramnios, which occurs in approximately 12 percent of twin gestations, is controversial. Hydramnios develops most commonly in malformed, monozygotic, and very premature infants[73,74,99] and is associated with a perinatal death rate of 41 percent. It remains unknown whether hydramnios actually endangers the fetuses or, rather, develops as a by-product of fetal or placental pathology. Naeye and coworkers[74] suggest that increased uterine distention from hydramnios contributes to the higher frequency of amnionitis and premature labor.

Prematurity

As in the breech presentation, prematurity accounts for many neonatal problems (Table 18–4), especially when coupled with growth retardation. For example, a majority of twin neonates with traumatic morbidity, low 5-minute Apgar scores, and prolonged neurologic sequelae deliver before 34 weeks' gestation and weigh less than 2000 grams.[83,84,86,90,100] The following magnifies the significance of the problem: 40 to 50 percent of twins deliver preterm (before 37 weeks) and nearly 25 percent weigh less than 1500 grams at birth.[71,72,81,101,102] Twin growth resembles that of the singleton in the initial 20 weeks of gestation[103] but declines after 32 weeks, so that the average term twin weighs 600 grams less than the average term singleton.[71,72,98] Twenty-three percent of twin offspring fall below the tenth percentile in weight for gestation.[81]

The predominant influence of prematurity and growth retardation on morbidity and mortality raises an important question: "What can be done to prevent premature labor and poor growth from occurring when ultrasound provides early diagnosis of twins?" At present, no generally accepted answer exists, primarily because the etiology of these problems remains unclear. Premature labor likely has a multifactorial basis, making analysis of the event difficult at best. In regards to growth retardation, various causes—fetal crowding, placental dysfunction, decreased placental perfusion, marginally inserted cords, and twin transfusion syndrome—have been proposed[72,81,98,104] without substantiation. Attempts to prevent premature labor (i.e., bed rest, circlage, and tocolysis) have produced equivocal results while increasing risk and expense.[72,100,105,106] Therefore, the following approach presently provides the best chance for decreasing perinatal death and long-term morbidity: (1) early diagnosis, (2) referral of mother and twins to a high-risk perinatal center prior to delivery, and (3) appropriate intrapartum and postpartum management of mother and infants, with immediate admission of premature and low-birth-weight infants to the neonatal ICU. In such centers, most obstetricians attempt to inhibit premature labor with β_2-mimetic compounds but obtain poor results once labor is well established.[100]

METHOD OF DELIVERY

At any stage of gestation, vaginal delivery often produces a poorer outcome for the second twin as compared to the first.[81,82,107] In the past, morbidity and mortality rates for the second twin correlated positively with the time interval between delivery of twin A and twin B. The frequency of asphyxia and death increased for twin B when this interval exceeded 15 to 30 minutes.[108] This relationship was attributed to obstetric complications (placental separation, uterine atony, hemorrhage, prolapsed cord), prolonged aortocaval compression in supine-lithotomy position, lengthy exposure to general anesthesia, and difficult version or extraction maneuvers for a malpresenting second twin. As a result, many obstetricians delivered the second twin by cesarean section when the delivery interval exceeded 30 minutes, status of twin B deteriorated intrapartally, or concern existed about the use of cephalic version or breech extraction. However, recent reports[100,109–111] find no relationship between the delivery interval and the fate of twin B, provided the mother is maintained in left lateral tilt position, general anesthesia is avoided, electronic fetal heart rate monitoring continues until delivery, and twin B receives immediate resuscitation. These studies link most episodes of asphyxia and trauma to low birth weight (<1500 g) and to fetal malposition. Twin A presents by the breech 15 to 20 percent of the time; twin B is nonvertex in approximately 40 percent of cases.[81,110] Thus, most considerations given to method of delivery should be similar to those for the breech singleton; cesarean section seems advised when either twin is breech and weighs less than 1500 g.[86,110,112]

OBSTETRIC CONSIDERATIONS

Following diagnosis of a multiple gestation, the obstetrician must determine whether he or she has the support services and facilities available for provision of necessary maternal and fetal care. The coexistence of maternal or fetal pathophysiology influences the obstetrician's assessment. Ultrasound or roentgenograms should facilitate confirmation of fetal position soon after admission. Pre-existing fetal problems (Table 18–4), malpresentation, or maternal risk factors such as severe pre-eclampsia frequently necessitate cesarean section. The obstetrician may decide to inhibit premature labor with β_2-mimetic agents or alcohol, which have potentially harmful side effects (See Chap. 17). Soon after admission, patients in labor should receive clear antacids intermittently; intravenous ranitidine, 50 mg every 8 hours, also decreases the risk of acid aspiration when emergency general anesthesia is required.

During labor, intensive obstetrical care with thorough maternal and fetal surveillance is necessary. If labor progresses unremarkably, the obstetrician usually employs vaginal delivery when twin A is vertex. He or she may utilize outlet forceps to protect the head of a premature fetus. After delivery of twin A, electronic monitoring of twin B continues while the laterally tilted mother inhales an enriched oxygen mixture. Uterine atony may develop, prompting the obstetrician to initiate an oxytocin infusion.[109,112] In addition, good maternal pushing efforts serve to promote a spontaneous or assisted delivery, especially in case of a breech second twin. The obstetrician may attempt external cephalic version of the breech, provided the estimated fetal weight exceeds 2000 g and the amniotic sac of twin B remains intact.[110] This maneuver requires a cooperative mother and a quiescent uterus; ongoing oxytocin infusions are discontinued. During this period, the perinatal team should remain cognizant of the possible need for rapid abdominal delivery since cord prolapse or placental separation may occur, threatening the status of twin B. Cesarean section may also be required for failure of cephalic version, retention of the second twin, or the obstetrician's preference to avoid breech extraction-decomposition procedures.

ANESTHESIA CONSIDERATIONS

Successful intrapartum management of a multiple pregnancy requires expert anesthetic care, which cannot be provided unless the anesthesia team evaluates maternal and fetal status, has equipment prepared, and remains readily available to the obstetric suite. Due to the high incidence of maternal and fetal complications in twin pregnancies, anesthesia must be individualized for each case. For example, the coexistence of severe pre-eclampsia decreases the safety margin for most anesthetics, making the selection and maintenance of anesthesia more difficult. Increased abdominal girth with marked lumbar lordosis and edema of the back may hamper placement of spinal column blocks. Consequently, the mother's back should be examined before deciding on anesthetic technique; a paramedian approach to spinal and epidural blocks or the use of continuous caudal analgesia may be preferred.[113] James and coworkers[114] caution against the use of larger local anesthetic doses necessary for caudal analgesia because this may contribute to depression of the second twin. Regardless of the method used for vaginal delivery or cesarean section, the anesthesia team must anticipate the effects of the enlarged uterus on cardiopulmonary and gastrointestinal function. Adjustments may be necessary in patients receiving β_2-mimetics (Chap. 17).

Labor and Vaginal Delivery

Many of the anesthetic considerations pertaining to the breech apply as well to management of a multiple gestation. Infants are often premature and are more susceptible to depression with narcotics and sedatives which, when coupled with asphyxia, may decrease their chances for survival. However, lengthy labors often require profound analgesia, to obviate the effects of stress on an already burdened maternal cardiovascular system and to avoid the effects of catecholamines on the uterine vasculature. In addition, a controlled delivery with forceps, cephalic version, and/or assisted breech extraction of the second twin frequently demands good analgesia and perineal relaxation. The ideal anesthetic provides such conditions while minimally affecting uterine contractions and maternal pushing efforts in stage 2. Regardless of method, all mothers should inspire a gas mixture containing high oxygen concentrations until after delivery of the second twin. The anesthesia team must be prepared to provide anesthesia for emergency cesarean section and uterine relaxation for intrauterine manipulations.

Lumbar Epidural Analgesia. For the reasons above, continuous segmental lumbar epidural analgesia with bupivacaine (0.125 to 0.25 percent) is a good approach for labor and delivery of twins, especially prematures.[1,17] The technique produces satisfactory pain relief for both stages of labor, obviating maternal increases in cardiopulmonary workload, preventing neonatal drug depression, and allowing good conditions for a difficult vaginal delivery. Additionally, extension of the block provides anesthesia for cesarean section, when necessary, for a retained second twin. Gullestad and Sagen[115] note that epidural analgesia decreases the need for general anesthesia.

Yet, concern has existed about the effect of epidural blocks on the duration of labor and on the twin A to twin B delivery interval.[116] Most reservations pertain to supression of maternal bearing down efforts and the failure of epidural analgesia to provide uterine relaxation for version-extraction maneuvers.[117] These sentiments surfaced at a time when caudal blocks were primarily employed to achieve epidural analgesia.[116,117] Segmental lumbar epidural blockade with bupivacaine affects the mother's urge and ability to push less than the caudal approach. In comparison to parenteral methods, lumbar epidural analgesia prolongs stage 1 of labor by approximately 2 hours,[115] but the second stage is not significantly altered.[118] Most important, the technique does not significantly increase the twin-to-twin delivery interval,[118] nor does it produce a higher incidence of operative interventions for delivery of twin B.[119] Recent studies fail to associate lumbar epidural analgesia with increased morbidity or mortaility rates in twin infants.[114,115,118–120] In a retrospective analysis of neonatal outcome, Berger and others[100] find no consistent relationship between anesthesia method and the outcome for either twin; low Apgar scores and death relate mainly to prematurity and fetal malposition. Daniels and Hehre[121] and James and coworkers[114] prospectively assessed neonatal status following use of lumbar epidural analgesia and reported similar findings.

Parenteral and Pudendal Analgesia. Even though segmental lumbar epidural analgesia offers many advantages, some obstetricians prefer using low-dose narcotics for labor and pudendal blockade combined with perineal infiltration of local anesthetic for delivery. Prepared childbirth techniques greatly assist women managed with this approach, which has minimal effect on labor and preserves the urge to push. However, the method may not suffice for cephalic version, breech extraction, or difficult forceps deliveries. In such cases, the anesthesia team can provide supplemental analgesia with nitrous oxide (25 to 40 percent), methoxyflurane (0.2 to 0.5 percent), or enflurane (0.3 to 0.8 percent) delivered by face mask. In cases managed with a narcotic-pudendal approach, general endotracheal anesthesia becomes necessary approximately 50 percent of the time,[115] primarily when the mother poorly tolerates a difficult, painful delivery or when a distressed or retained second twin dictates delivery by cesarean section.

Spinal Anesthesia. Spinal anesthesia is considered for delivery of twins when the patient care team anticipates the need for profound analgesia and the mother has not received an epidural block. Following injection of tetracaine or 5 percent lidocaine, unpredictable levels of motor blockade may impair the mother's ability to bear down effectively. However, 1.5-percent lidocaine (25 mg in D7.5W) produces excellent pain relief while preserving the auxiliary forces of labor.[1]

None of the techniques above produces uterine relaxation. Whenever the obstetrician decides to perform an intrauterine manipulation and requires a relaxed uterus, halothane (1 to 2 percent), enflurane (2 to 3 percent), or isoflurane (2 to 3 percent) should be administered following an intravenous induction and tracheal intubation during cricoid pressure. Careful monitoring helps to avoid combined effects of the halogenated agent and vena caval compression on the mother's cardiovascular system. To minimize postpartum uterine atony and hemorrhage, the anesthesia team discontinues these agents immediately after delivery of twin B.

Cesarean Section

No studies prospectively compare maternal and neonatal outcome with the use of regional or general anesthesia for abdominal delivery of twins. Therefore, the anesthesia team must use experience and exercise good judgment to make appropriate decisions. The occurrence of maternal and fetal pathophysiology rather than the presence of a multiple gestation will often determine the choice of anesthesia. However, several points should be emphasized. First, multiple gestation accentuates the development of hypotension during regional blocks; thus, thorough prehydration with crystalloid intravenous fluids, maintenance of left lateral tilt position, provision of close cardiovascular monitoring, and use of ephedrine, if necessary, are important. In pregnancies near term, the enlarged uterus presents some difficulties during placement of the mother in the tilt position. Manual support by an assistant helps to prevent the distended uterus from falling excessively to the side. Second, patients scheduled for general anesthesia deserve thorough preoxygenation prior to induction, since hypoxia develops rapidly during periods of apnea. This results from substantial reductions in functional residual capacity. In addition, every effort is made to avoid the increased likelihood of acid aspiration during general anesthesia. Third, premature twins are prediposed to the depressant effects of hypnotics, narcotics, and sedatives. For this reason, regional blocks seem advantageous for abdominal delivery of prematures, although no studies presently exist to substantiate this viewpoint. On the other hand, severe maternal or fetal compromise from abruptio placentae, cord proplase, and so on may require rapid delivery, indicating general endotracheal anesthesia, which takes less time than regional techniques. Regardless of the method used, regional or general, clear antacids and histamine-2 antagonists are administered preoperatively; the mother inhales a high inspired oxygen mixture throughout cesarean delivery, and one member of the anesthesia team remains ready to assist in the resuscitation of two neonates.

Summary

Breech presentation and multiple gestation present special problems to mothers and their neonates. In both settings, prematurity, congenital anomalies, hypoxia, and birth trauma most frequently are responsible for neonatal morbidity and mortality. Although numerous reports address the issue of neonatal outcome and different methods of management, the retrospective nature of most studies makes it difficult to form definite conclusions. Thus, the obstetric and anesthetic care of breech presentation and of twins remains controversial, especially regarding the conduct of labor and vaginal delivery. Obviously, no single anesthetic provides best results for all situations. More importantly, optimal outcome depends upon the presence of practitioners with substantial experience, sound judgment, and the ability to communicate freely and effectively. Soon after admission, the anesthesia team must be aware of the obstetrician's concerns and plans for the delivery. Sufficient time must be allowed for thorough patient evaluation and preparation of equipment, and the anesthesia team must be readily available. In the absence of contraindications, continuous segmental lumbar epidural analgesia provides better conditions than other methods for vaginal delivery of breech and twin pregnancies.

References

1. James, FM: Anesthetic considerations for breech or twin delivery. Clin Perinatol 9:77, 1982.
2. Luterkort, M, Persson, P and Weldner, B: Maternal and fetal factors in breech presentation. Obstet Gynecol 64:55, 1984.
3. Westgren, M, et al: Spontaneous cephalic version of breech presentation in the last trimester. Br J Obstet Gynaecol 92:19, 1985.
4. Confino, E, et al: The breech dilemma: A review. Obstet Gynecol Surv 40:330, 1985.

5. Pritchard, JA and MacDonald, PC: Williams' Obstetrics. Appleton-Century-Crofts, New York, 1980, p 1064.
6. Hall, JE and Kohl, SG: Breech presentation. Am J Obstet Gynecol 72:977, 1956.
7. Morgan, HS and Kane, SH: An analysis of 16,327 breech births. JAMA 187:108, 1964.
8. Hall, JE, et al: Breech presentation and perinatal mortality. Am J Obstet Gynecol 91:665, 1965.
9. Fischer-Rasmussen, W and Trolle, D: Abdominal versus vaginal delivery in breech presentation. Acta Obstet Gynecol Scand 46:69, 1967.
10. Johnson, CE: Breech presentation at term. Am J Obstet Gynecol 106:865, 1970.
11. Neilson, DR: Management of the large breech infant. Am J Obstet Gynecol 107:345, 1970.
12. Brenner, WE, Bruce, RD and Hendricks, CH: The characteristics and perils of breech presentation. Ann J Obstet Gynecol 118:700, 1974.
13. Rovinsky, JJ, Miller, JA and Kaplan, S: Management of breech presentation at term. Am J Obstet Gynecol 115:497, 1973.
14. Wolter, DE: Patterns of management with breech presentation. Am J Obstet Gynaecol 125:733, 1976.
15. Benson, WL, Boyce, DC and Vaughn, DL: Breech delivery in the primigravida. Obstet Gynecol 40:417, 1972.
16. Wright, RC: Reduction of perinatal mortality and morbidity in breech delivery through routine use of cesarean section. Obstet Gynecol 14:758, 1959.
17. Crawford, JS and Weaver, JB: Anaesthetic management of twin and breech deliveries. Clin Obstet Gynecol 9:291, 1982.
18. Green, JE, et al: Has the increased cesarean section rate for term breech delivery reduced the incidence of birth asphyxia, trauma, and death? Am J Obstet Gynecol 142:643, 1982.
19. Cox, C, Kendall, AC and Hommers, M: Changed prognosis of breech-presenting low birth weight infants. Br J Obstet Gynaecol 89:881, 1982.
20. Faber-Nijholt, R, et al: Neurologic follow-up of 281 children born in breech presentation: A controlled study. Br Med J 286:9, 1983.
21. Westgren, IMR, Songster, G and Paul RH: Preterm breech delivery: Another retrospective study. Obstet Gynecol 66:481, 1985.
22. Collea, JV, et al: The randomized management of term frank breech presentation: Vaginal delivery vs cesarean section. Am J Obstet Gynecol 131:186, 1978.
23. Bilodeau, R and Marier, R: Breech presentation at term. Am J Obstet Gynecol 130:555, 1978.
24. Main, DM, Main, EK and Maurer, MM: Cesarean section versus vaginal delivery for the breech fetus weighing less than 1500 grams. Am J Obstet Gynecol 146:580, 1983.
25. Rosen, MG and Chik, L: The effect of delivery route on outcome in breech presentation. Am J Obstet Gynecol 148:909, 1984.
26. Tatum, RK, et al: Vaginal breech delivery of selected infants weighing more than 2000 grams. Am J Obstet Gynecol 152:145, 1985.
27. Van Eyk, EA and Huisjes, HJ: Neonatal mortality and morbidity associated with preterm breech presentation. Am J Obstet Gynecol 148:909, 1984.
28. Confino, E, et al: Vaginal delivery versus cesarean section oriented approaches in the management of breech delivery. Int J Gynaecol Obstet 23:1, 1985.
29. Ingemarsson, I, Westgren, M and Svenningson, NW: Long-term follow-up of preterm infants in breech presentation delivered by cesarean section. Lancet 2:172, 1978.
30. Yu, VYH, et al: Effect of mode of delivery on outcome of very-low-birth-weight infants. Br J Obstet Gynaecol 91:633, 1984.
31. Karp, LE, et al: The premature breech: Trial of labor or cesarean section? Obstet Gynecol 53:88, 1979.
32. Mazor, M, et al: Fetal malformations associated with breech delivery: Implications for obstetric management. J Reprod Med 30:884, 1984.
33. White, PC and Cibils, LA: Clinical significance of fetal heart rate patterns during labor: VIII. Breech presentations. J Reprod Med 29:45, 1984.
34. Eilen, B, et al: Fetal acidosis and the abnormal fetal heart rate tracing: The term breech fetus. Obstet Gynecol 63:233, 1984.
35. Watson, W and Benson, WL: Vaginal delivery for the selected frank breech infant at term. Obstet Gynecol 64:638, 1984.
36. Tank, ES, Davis, R and Holt, JF: Mechanisms of trauma during breech delivery. Obstet Gynecol 38:761, 1971.
37. Ballas, S and Toaff, R: Hyperextension of the fetal head in breech presentation: Radiologic evaluation and significance. Br J Obstet Gynaecol 83:201, 1976.
38. Phelan, JP, et al: Use of ultrasonography in the breech presentation with hypertension of the fetal head. J Ultrasound Med 2:373, 1983.
39. Lyons, ER and Papsin, FR: Cesarean section in the management of breech presentation. Am J Obstet Gynecol 130:558, 1978.
40. Svenningson, NW, Westgreen, M and Ingemarsson, I: Modern strategy for the term breech delivery: A study with a 4-year follow-up of the infants. J Perinat Med 13:117, 1985.
41. Anderman, S, et al: Is term breech presentation in primigravida an absolute indication for cesarean section? Eur J Obstet Gynecol Reprod Biol 18:11, 1984.
42. Granati, B, et al: The premature breech presentation: Outcome of newborn infants born by vaginal or abdominal delivery. Am J Perinatol 1:145, 1985.
43. Capeless, EL and Mann, LI: A vaginal deivery protocol for the term breech infant utilizing Ball pelvimetry. J Reprod Med 30:545, 1985.
44. Gimovsky, ML, et al: X-ray pelvimetry in a breech protocol: A comparison of digital radiography and conventional methods. Am J Obstet Gynecol 153:887, 1985.
45. Wallace, RL, et al: External cephalic version with tocolysis. J Reprod Med 29:745, 1984.
46. Phelan, JP, et al: Observations of fetal heart rate characteristics related to external cephalic version and tocolysis. Am J Obstet Gynecol 149:658, 1984.

47. Stine, LE, et al: Update on external cephallic version performed at term. Obstet Gynecol 64:642, 1985.
48. Dyson, DC, Ferguson, JE II and Hensleigh, P: Antepartum external cephalic version under tocolysis. Obstet Gynecol 67:63, 1986.
49. Gibbs, CP and Banner, TC: Effectiveness of Bicitra as a preoperative antacid. Anesthesiology 61:97, 1984.
50. Gillett, GB, Watson, JD and Langford, RM: Ranitidine and single-dose antacid therapy as prophylaxis against acid aspiration syndrome in obstetric practice. Anaesthesia 39:638, 1984.
51. Greiss, FC, Still, JG and Anderson, SG: Effects of local anesthetic agents on the uterine vasculature and myometrium. Am J Obstet Gynecol 120:791, 1976.
52. Asling, JH, et al: Paracervical block anesthesia in obstetrics: II. Etiology of fetal bradycardia following paracervical block. Am J Obstet Gynecol 107:626, 1970.
53. Meguiar, RV and Wheeler, AS: Lumbar sympathetic block with bupivacaine: Analgesia for labor. Anesth Analg 57:486, 1978.
54. Hunter, CA: Uterine motility studies during labor: Observations on bilateral sympathetic nerve block in the normal and abnormal first stage of labor. Am J Obstet Gynecol 85:681, 1963.
55. Munson, ES and Embro, WJ: Enflurane, isoflurane, and halothane and isolated human uterine muscle. Anesthesiology 46:11, 1977.
56. Crawford, J: An appraisal of lumbar epidural blockade in patients with a singleton fetus presenting by the breech. J Obstet Gynaecol Br Commonw 81:867, 1974.
57. Bowen-Simpkins, P and Fergusson, ILC: Lumbar epidural block and the breech presentation. Br J Anaesth 46:42, 1974.
58. Donnai, P and Nicholas, ADG: Epidural analgesia, fetal monitoring, and condition of the baby at birth with breech presentation. Br J Obstet Gynaecol 82:360, 1975.
59. Darby, S and Hunter, DJ: Extradural analgesia in labour when the breech presents. Br J Obstet Gynaecol 83:35, 1976.
60. Breeson, AJ, et al: Extradural analgesia: The preferred method of analgesia for vaginal breech delivery. Br J Anaesth 50:1227, 1978.
61. Marx, GF, Luykx, WM and Cohen, S: Fetal-neonatal status following cesarean section for fetal distress. Br J Anaesth 56:1009, 1984.
62. Gale, R, Zalkinder-Luboshitz, I and Slater, PE: Increased neonatal risk from use of general anesthesia in emergency cesarean section. J Reprod Med 27:715, 1982.
63. Phillips, JC, et al: Epidural analgesia and its effects on the normal progress of labor. Am J Obstet Gynecol 129:316, 1977.
64. Jouppila, R, et al: Segmental epidural analgesia in labour: Related to the progress of labour, fetal malposition and instrumental delivery. Acta Obstet Gynecol Scand 58:135, 1979.
65. Confino, E, et al: Extradural analgesia in the management of singleton breech delivery. Br J Anaesth 57:892, 1985.
66. Johnson, WL, et al: Effect of pudendal, spinal and peridural block anesthesia in the second stage of labor. Am J Obstet Gynecol 113:166, 1972.
67. Morgan, BM: Maternal death: A review of maternal deaths at one hospital from 1958 to 1978. Anaesthesia 35:334, 1980.
68. Gibbs, CP, Rolbin, SH and Norman, P: Cause and prevention of aspiration. Anesthesiology 61:111, 1984.
69. Jouppila, R, et al: Effect of the anesthetic method, epidural and general anesthesia on intervillous blood flow. Region Anesth 2:2, 1977.
70. Warren, TM, et al: Comparison of the maternal and neonatal effects of halothane, enflurane, and isoflurane for cesarean delivery. Anesth Analg 62:516, 1983.
71. Hendricks, CH: Twinning in relation to birth weight, mortality, and congenital anomalies. Obstet Gynecol 27:47, 1966.
72. Powers, WF: Twin pregnancy: Complications and treatment. Obstet Gynecol 42:795, 1973.
73. Benirshke, L and Kim, CH: Multiple pregnancy. N Engl J Med 288:1276, 1973.
74. Naeye, RL, et al: Twins: Causes of perinatal death in 12 United States cities and one African city. Am J Obstet Gynecol 131:267, 1978.
75. Foster, HW: Twin pregnancy: A three-year report. J Natl Med Assoc 69:139, 1970.
76. Starder, RW: Abnormalities of the placenta, membranes, and fetus. In Danforth, DN (ed): Obstetrics and Gynecology, ed. 2. Harper & Row, New York, 1977, p 347.
77. Medearies, AL, et al: Perinatal deaths in twin pregnancies. Am J Obstet Gynecol 134:413, 1979.
78. Kauppila, M, et al: Twin pregnancy: A clinical study of 355 cases. Acta Obstet Gynecol Scand (Suppl) 44:5, 1975.
79. Rovinsky, JJ and Jaffin, H: Cardiovascular hemodynamics in pregnancy: III. Cardiac rate, stroke volume, total peripheral resistance, and central blood volume in multiple pregnancy: Synthesis of results. Am J Obstet Gynecol 95:787, 1966.
80. Farooqui, P, Groosmam, KJ and Shannon, RA: A review of twin pregnancy and perinatal mortality. Obstet Gynecol Surv 28:144, 1973.
81. Ho, SK and WU, PYK: Perinatal factors and neonatal morbidity in twin pregnancy. Am J Obstet Gynecol 122:979, 1973.
82. Johnson, DR: Twin pregnancy: A review of 214 cases. J Arkansas Med Soc 75:453, 1979.
83. Sehgal, NN: Perinatal mortality in twin pregnancies: Implications for clinical management. Postgrad Med 68:231, 1980.
84. Keith, L, et al: The Northwestern University multihospital twin study: I. A description of 588 twin pregnancies and associated pregnancy loss, 1971 to 1975. Am J Obstet Gynecol 138:781, 1980.
85. Duncan, SB, Ginz, B and Wahab, H: Use of ultrasound and hormonal assays in the diagnosis, management, and outcome of twin pregnancy. Obstet Gynecol 53:367, 1979.

86. MacGillivray, I and Campbell, DM: The outcome of twin pregnancies in Aberdeen. Prog Clin Biol 69A:203, 1981.
87. Kurjak, A and Latin, V: Ultrasound diagnosis of fetal abnormalities in multiple pregnancy. Acta Obstet Gynecol Scand 58:153, 1979.
88. Haney, AF, Crenshaw, MC and Dempsey, PJ: Significance of biparietal diameter difference between twins. Obstet Dynecol 51:609, 1978.
89. Levine, SC and Filly, RA: Rapid B-scan (real-time) ultrasonography in the identification and evaluation of twin pregnancies. Obstet Gynecol 51:170, 1978.
90. Secher, NJ, Kaern, J and Hansen, PK: Intrauterine growth in twin pregnancies: Prediction of fetal growth retardation. Obstet Gynecol 66:63, 1985.
91. Divens, WA and Hensell, DL: The use of ultrasound in multiple gestations. Obstet Gynecol 53:500, 1979.
92. Bessis, R and Papiernik, E: Echographic imagery of amniotic membranes in twin pregnancies. Prog Clin Biol Res 69A:183, 1981.
93. Mantoni, M and Pedersen, JF: Monoamniotic twins diagnosed by ultrasound in the first trimester. Acta Obstet Gynecol Scand 59:551, 1980.
94. Brzezinski, A, Mor-Yosef, S and Granat, M: Antepartum diagnosis of monoamniotic twin pregnancy. Int J Gynaecol Obstet 23:335, 1985.
95. Blake, GD, et al: Evaluation of nonstress fetal heart rate testing in multiple gestations. Obstet Gynecol 63:528, 1984.
96. Rausen, AR, Saki, M and Strauss, L: Twin transfusion syndrome: A review of 19 cases studied at one institution. J Pediatr 66:613, 1965.
97. Naeye, RL: Human intrauterine parabiotic syndrome and its complications. N Engl J Med 268:804, 1963.
98. Bleker, OP, Breur, W and Huidekoper, BL: A study of birth weight, placental weight, and mortaility of twins as compared to singletons. Br J Obstet Gynecol 86:111, 1979.
99. Farrell, AGW: Twin pregnancy: A study of 1000 cases. S Afr J Obstet Gynecol 2:35, 1964.
100. Berger, GS, et al: The Northwestern University multihospital twin study: III. Obstetric characteristics and outcome. Prog Clin Biol Res 69A:207, 1981.
101. Dunn, PM: Some perinatal observations on twins. Dev Med Child Neurol 7:121, 1975.
102. Persson, P, et al: On improved outcome of twin pregnancies. Acta Obstet Gynecol Scand 58:3, 1979.
103. Iffy, L, et al: The rate of early intrauterine growth in twin gestation. Am J Obstet Gynecol 146:970, 1983.
104. Bjoro, K and Bjoro, K: Disturbed intrauterine growth in twins: Etiological aspects. Acta Genet Med Gemellol (Rome) 34:73, 1985.
105. Beisher, NA and O'Sullivan, EF: The effect of rest and intravenous infusion of hypertonic dextrose on subnormal estriol excretion in pregnancy. Am J Obstet Gynecol 113:771, 1972.
106. Hartikainen-Sorri, A and Jouppila, P: Is routine hospitalization needed in antenatal care of twin pregnancy? J Perinat Med 12:31, 1984.
107. Ware, HH: The second twin. Am J Obstet Gynecol 110:865, 1971.
108. Adeleye, JA: Retained second twin in Ibadan: Its fate and management. Am J Obstet Gynecol 114:204, 1972.
109. Rayburn, WF, et al: Multiple gestation: Time interval between delivery of the first and second twin. Obstet Gynecol 63:502, 1984.
110. Chervenak, FA, et al: Intrapartum management of twin gestation. Obstet Gynecol 65:119, 1985.
111. Eskes, TAB, et al: The second twin. Eur J Obstet Gynecol Reprod Biol 19:159, 1984.
112. Kelsick, F and Minkoff, H: Management of the breech second twin. Am J Obstet Gynecol 144:783, 1982.
113. Abouleish, E: Caudal analgesia for quadruplet delivery. Anesth Analg 55:61, 1976.
114. James, FM III, et al: Lumbar analgesia for labor and delivery twins. Am J Obstet Gynecol 127:176, 1976.
115. Gullestad, S and Sagen, N: Epidural block in twin labour and delivery. Acta Anaesth Scand 21:504, 1977.
116. Little, WA and Friedman, EA: Anesthesia for the twin delivery. Anesthesiology 19:515, 1958.
117. Hingson, RA and Hellman, LM: Anesthesia for Obstetrics. FA Davis, Philadelphia, 1957.
118. Crawford, JS: An appraisal of lumbar epidural blockade in labour in patients with multiple pregnancy. Br J Obstet Gynaecol 82:929, 1975.
119. Weeks, ARL, Cheridjian, VE and Mvenje, DK: Lumbar epidural analgesia in labour in twin pregnancy. Br Med J 2:730, 1977.
120. Jaschevatzsky, OE, et al: Epidural analgesia during labour in twin pregnancy. Br J Obstet Gynecol 84:327, 1977.
121. Daniels, JC and Hehre, FW: Anesthetic considerations for complicated obstetrics. I. A retrospective study of 527 twin deliveries. Anesth Analg 46:527, 1967.

CHAPTER 19

FETAL DISTRESS

DAVID H. CHESTNUT, M.D.

Prior to 1970, the major advances in obstetrics focused on reducing maternal morbidity and mortality. Improved fetal/neonatal outcome largely resulted from improved maternal care. Subsequently, techniques of fetal assessment have fostered the concept of the fetus as a patient. As more women choose to delay and/or limit child bearing and as medical and medicolegal costs escalate, each pregnancy should be regarded as a premium pregnancy. Thus physicians are challenged to deliver a healthy baby to every parturient. The anesthesiologist is often asked to provide anesthesia in the presence of fetal stress or distress. The anesthesiologist must be prepared to provide anesthesia in an expeditious manner consistent with maternal safety without further compromising fetal well-being.

Pathophysiology

ETIOLOGY

The diagnosis of fetal stress/distress can be made before or during labor. Detection of fetal stress before the development of frank distress, as reflected by fetal acidosis, is one goal of fetal assessment.

Chronic Fetal Stress

Each of the following conditions may be accompanied by evidence of intrauterine fetal stress.

Fetal Anomaly. The anomaly can result from a chromosomal abnormality, exposure to a teratogen, or an unknown factor. Regardless, the anesthesiologist should realize that anomalous fetuses have an increased incidence of heart rate abnormalities.[1,2] The anesthesiologist may need to provide reassurance and comfort to the awake patient who has just delivered (expectedly or unexpectedly) an anomalous infant.

Inadequate Maternal Oxygenation and/or Nutrition. The asthmatic patient may have chronic and/or acute hypoxemia; it is often preferable to avoid instrumentation of the airway in such a patient. Poor nutrition is commonly seen in parturients addicted to alcohol, narcotics, or other drugs. Difficult intravenous access and the potential for drug withdrawal may complicate anesthetic management.

Inadequate Delivery of Oxygen to the Placenta. Maternal heart disease or anemia can compromise delivery of oxygen to the uterine circulation. Hypertension and diabetes (Chaps. 21 and 20, respectively), as well as nicotine abuse, may cause chronic compromise of uteroplacental blood flow. Further, the chronic airway irritability associated with smoking can be troublesome during general or regional anesthesia.

Inadequate Transfer of Oxygen Across the Placenta. Placenta previa and partial placental abruption can decrease the transfer capabilities of the placenta. Patients with placenta previa have an increased risk of placenta accreta, especially if there is a history of a previous cesarean section.[3] Even in the absence of preoperative bleeding, significant intraoperative hemorrhage may occur, necessitating hysterectomy.[4]

Inadequate Fetal Circulation of Hemoglobin and Oxygen. Fetal tachyarrhythmia can compromise fetal cardiac output. Hemolytic disease (e.g., Rh sensitization) can cause fetal anemia and high-output heart failure.

Acute Fetal Distress

Acute fetal distress has three primary etiologies.

Uteroplacental Dysfunction. The usual decrease in uteroplacental blood flow associated with uterine contractions, when superimposed on chronic uteroplacental insufficiency (e.g., diabetes, postdatism), may result in acute fetal distress. In contrast, maternal hypotension (e.g., after induction of spinal or epidural anesthesia) can cause acute fetal distress despite the presence of a normal uteroplacental unit.

Cord Compression. Frank prolapse of the umbilical cord commonly occurs with abnormal fetal presentations (e.g., footling breech, transverse lie). However, intermittent cord compression often appears during labor in otherwise normal pregnancies and can occur before labor in patients with oligohydramnios. Mann[5] recently suggested that undetected antenatal umbilical cord compression may be a possible cause of "unexplained brain damage." Finally, Marx and associates[6] suggested that maternal catecholamines cross the placenta during labor and cause umbilical vasoconstriction; they demonstrated that epidural analgesia decreases umbilical artery vascular resistance.

Uterine Tachysystole or Tetany. While uterine hypertonus may be associated with placental abruption, more often it signifies dehydration or hyperstimulation by parenteral oxytocin.

DIAGNOSIS

Biophysical methods of assessment of fetal well-being (e.g., ultrasound, fetal heart rate [FHR] testing) have supplanted biochemical methods of assessment (e.g, measurements of estriol or human placental lactogen). The anesthesiologist should understand the three types of periodic changes in FHR that can be detected with FHR monitoring.[7] Early decelerations (Fig. 19–1A) have a uniform pattern. The onset, nadir, and recovery of the FHR coincide with the onset, peak, and end of the uterine contraction, respectively. Head compression probably causes these generally benign decelerations. In my experience, early declerations are often discussed but infrequently seen. Late decelerations (Fig. 19–1B) also have a uniform pattern. However, the deceleration begins well after the onset of the uterine contraction, the nadir of the FHR occurs after the time of maximal contraction intensity, and the FHR does not recover until after completion of the uterine contraction. Late decelerations indicate fetal hypoxia, usually due to uteroplacental insufficiency. Variable decelerations (Fig. 19–1C), the most common of the periodic FHR changes, appear nonuniform in both pattern and timing. They denote umbilical cord compression. The occurrence of variable decelerations before labor may signal the presence of oligohydramnios and/or a vulnerable umbilical cord.

Antepartum Assessment

Fetal Movement Counting. A simple method of antepartum fetal surveillance involves asking the mother to record the frequency of fetal movement twice a day, at the same time at home. However, variations in the fetal sleep-wake cycle produce a nonuniform distribution of fetal movements during a 24-hour period. Further, ultrasound imaging re-

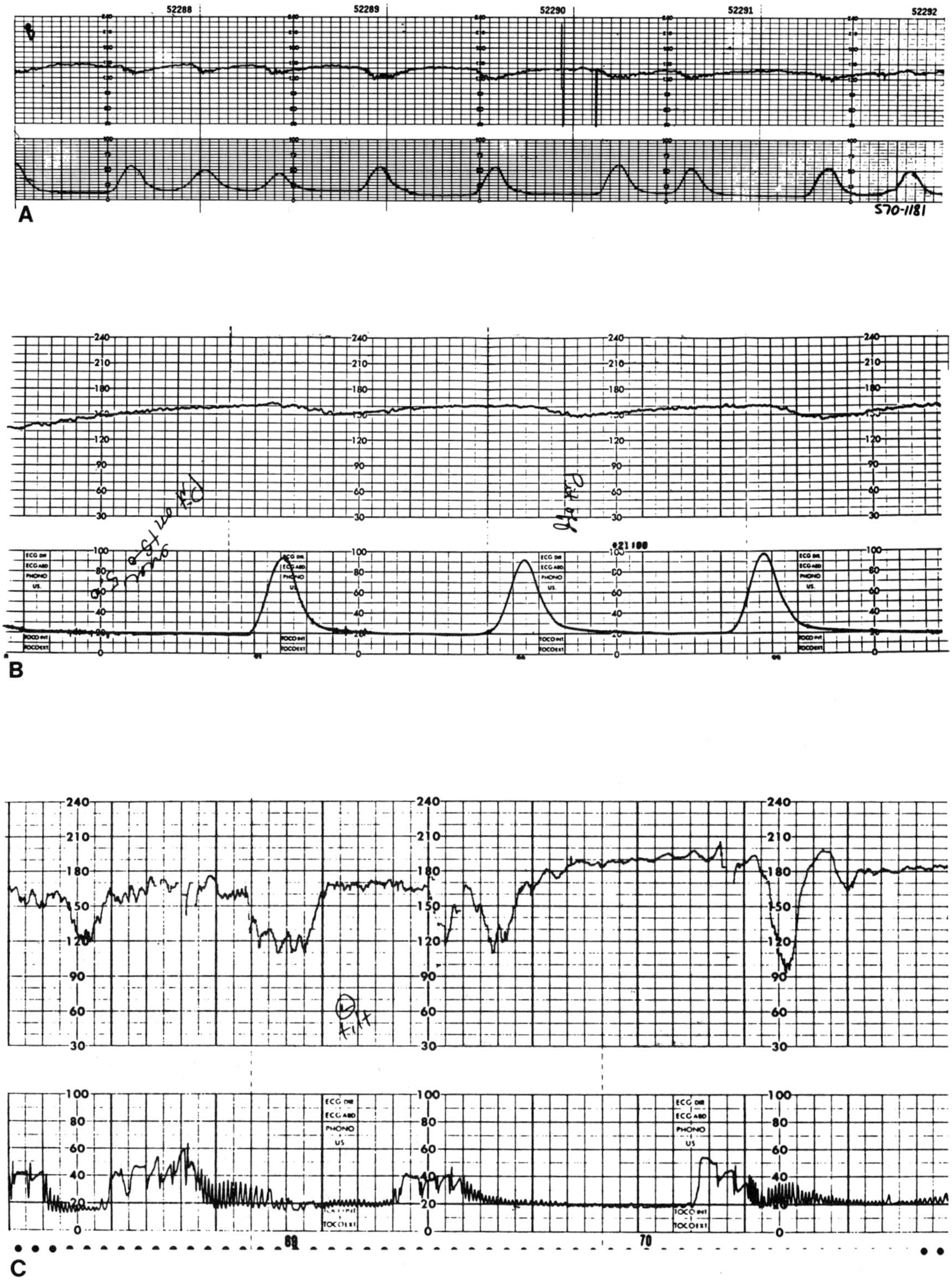

Figure 19–1. Examples of periodic changes of fetal heart rate: *(A)* early decelerations, *(B)* late decelerations, *(c)* variable decelerations.

veals that mothers fail to detect all fetal movements. No consensus exists regarding the minimum number of fetal movements that should be felt within 1 hour. The obstetrician may instruct a patient to call if she has not noted five or ten fetal movements within one of two 1-hour periods. Fetal movement counting is inexpensive and noninvasive, and it allows the mother to actively participate in antepartum fetal surveillance. While low in specificity, it may alert the obstetrician to unsuspected fetal compromise. Further, it encourages the patient to rest periodically, since the fetal movements should be counted while the mother lies on her side.

Ultrasound. Ultrasound can serve to evaluate fetal growth, in an effort to detect the small- or large-for-gestational-age fetus. The term *small for gestational age* (SGA) is preferable to *intrauterine growth retardation,* as parents often focus on the word *retardation*. The obstetrician may elect to deliver the SGA infant (either vaginally or by cesarean) from a hostile intrauterine environment. Similarly, he or she may deliver the severely macrosomic infant (e.g., >4500 g) by elective cesarean section in order to decrease the risk of fetal trauma at delivery.

Fetal Heart Rate (FHR) Testing. The contraction stress test (CST), also known as the oxytocin challenge test (OCT), evaluates changes in the FHR in response to spontaneous or induced contractions. (Either parenteral oxytocin or nipple stimulation will induce contractions.) Uterine contractions decrease uteroplacental blood flow and thus can expose uteroplacental insufficiency. Repetitive late decelerations (i.e., occurring after at least 50 percent of the uterine contractions) constitute a positive result. Three contractions lasting at least 40 sec, occurring in a 10-min period, and not associated with late decelerations constitute a negative test. A negative test indicates a low risk (i.e., 2 in 1000) of intrauterine death from uteroplacental insufficiency within the next 7 days.[8] Disadvantages of the CST include 1) a frequent need for intravenous access; 2) 60 to 90 min to complete the test; and 3) a high false-positive rate. Up to 50 percent of patients with a positive test will labor without further evidence of fetal or neonatal distress.

The nonstress test (NST) takes advantage of the phenomenon that the FHR of a healthy fetus accelerates with movement. The criteria for a reactive test vary, but most require two or three accelerations of at least 15 beats per min, of at least 15-sec duration, within a 20-min period. Zlatnik[9] has stated, "one should be able to read the accelerations with dirty glasses from across the room." This noninvasive procedure typically can be performed in half the time of the CST. However, the NST may not detect uteroplacental insufficiency as early as the CST. Late decelerations with uterine contractions indicate uteroplacental insufficiency earlier than does a loss of FHR accelerations in response to fetal movement. Thus, the sensitivity of the CST may exceed that of the NST.

Fetal Biophysical Profile (FBP). In an effort to improve the sensitivity of the NST, Manning and coworkers[10,11] integrated the NST and real-time ultrasound into the FBP. The obstetrician awards two points for each of the following: 1) a reactive NST; 2) occurrence of at least one 30-sec episode of fetal breathing movements in a 30-min period; 3) occurrence of at least three axial trunk rotations in a 30-min period; 4) presence of fetal tone (at least one episode of active extension, with return to flexion, of a fetal limb); and 5) adequate amniotic fluid volume (at least one pocket of amniotic fluid measuring ≥1 cm in two perpendicular planes). A score of 8 or 10 suggests the presence of a normal fetus at low risk for chronic asphyxia. A score of 6 or less warrants repeat testing or delivery, depending upon the gestational age.[10,11] The advantages of the FBP are its noninvasive character, its ability to diagnose fetal anomalies by employing ultrasound in conjunction with the NST, and its capacity to estimate both amniotic fluid volume and fetal weight. However, the FBP requires the presence of a physician and an ultrasound machine in the antepartum testing center. If the fetus is normal, the ultrasound typically can be completed within 10 min, although the full 30 min will be required in some patients. It remains uncertain whether the FBP is a more sensitive indicator of fetal stress/distress than the CST.

Newer Methods of Assessment. These include: 1) percutaneous umbilical cord blood sampling; 2) echocardiography; and 3) umbilical artery flow velocity waveform analysis. Advances in ultrasound imaging now permit sonographically guided percutaneous umbilical cord blood sampling (also known as cordocentesis) during the second and third trimesters of pregnancy. This procedure allows direct access to the fetal circulation for diagnostic and/or therapeutic purposes. Daffos' group[12] and Hobbins and associates[13] have described its utility in the antenatal assessment of fetuses at risk for isoimmunization, hemophilia, idiopathic thrombocytopenic purpura, hypoxia, and chromosomal disorders. M-mode and two-dimensional echocardiography serve to evaluate the cardiac structure, function, and rhythm of fetuses with arrhythmia and/or nonimmune hydrops.[14] Finally, umbilical artery velocimetry, performed with continuous-wave Doppler ultrasound, can identify a normal umbilical circulation versus one with increased vascular resistance. Fleischer and coworkers[15] have suggested that this technique may prove useful for identification and management of the SGA fetus. Bracero and associates[16] recently reported a positive correlation between umbilical artery velocity waveforms and the risk of adverse outcome in diabetic pregnant women.

Intrapartum Assessment

Meconium. The presence of meconium-stained amniotic fluid has long been associated with an increased likelihood of fetal stress/distress. Nevertheless, most fetuses with meconium-stained amniotic fluid have no other evidence of distress during labor and are in good condition at birth. Meis and coworkers[17] prospectively evaluated 2933 pregnancies during labor; the incidence of meconium passage was 22 percent. Light meconium staining present from the start of labor was not associated with any increase in fetal/neonatal morbidity or death. Meconium staining appearing during the second stage when the fluid had been initially clear, and heavy staining at any time, were associated with increased fetal/neonatal morbidity. Regardless of whether an infant delivered through meconium-stained amniotic fluid is acidotic at birth, that infant may have a low 1-min Apgar score because of the performance of laryngoscopy, intubation, and tracheal suctioning. This obligatory sequence, which should be preceded by DeLee catheter suctioning by the obstetrician, reduces the likelihood of neonatal meconium aspiration syndrome and takes precedence over a high 1-min Apgar score.

Electronic FHR Monitoring. Electronic FHR monitoring (supplemented by fetal scalp blood pH determination) remains the mainstay of intrapartum assessment. Periodic changes of the FHR are discussed earlier in this chapter. Additionally, the physician should observe the baseline FHR. Traditionally an FHR of 120 to 160 beats per min (bpm) is considered normal. These norms were derived prior to umbilical cord blood gas analysis. At our hospital an FHR greater than 150 bpm concerns us. Tachycardia may be the consequence of maternal fever or thyrotoxicosis, but it may also be a response to hypoxia. Mild bradycardia (100 to 120 bpm) does not necessarily represent fetal distress, especially in a fetus of advanced gestational age with normal FHR variability and no periodic changes.

Assessment of FHR variability may be the most important aspect of intrapartum FHR monitoring. A normal well-oxygenated fetus should have both long-term and short-term (beat-to-beat) variability. The presence of normal variability implies normal central nervous system (CNS) regulation of FHR, although some uncertainty remains as to the relative contributions of the sympathetic and parasympathetic nervous systems to FHR variability.[18] A scalp ECG electrode allows the physician to accurately assess beat-to-beat variability. In contrast, external monitors of FHR do not reliably indicate the presence of beat-to-beat variability. However, if variability is *absent* on an external FHR tracing, normal variability will not be detected with a fetal scalp electrode.

Historically, fetal scalp capillary blood sampling for pH determination has been the "gold standard" of intrapartum fetal assessment. The conventional view held that a scalp blood pH greater than 7.25 was normal and regarded a pH under 7.20 as representing acidosis, which should prompt delivery, pending the result of a repeat sample. Some obstetricians believe that these criteria are too strict; they contend that in most instances FHR monitoring equals or surpasses scalp blood pH determination in the prediction of fetal/neonatal outcome.[19] At our hospital and at a major European university hospital,[20] 7.14 represents the lower tenth percentile for umbilical artery blood pH at birth. Clark and associates[21,22] have suggested the scalp stimulation test as an alternative to scalp blood sampling. They reported that an FHR acceleration of 15 bpm for 15 sec in response to fetal scalp stimulation assures the physician of a nonacidotic fetus, even in the presence of an FHR tracing suggesting acidosis. However, when doubt persists regarding fetal well-being or distress, fetal scalp blood pH determination remains useful.

Obstetric Management

CHRONIC FETAL STRESS

Detection of fetal stress *before* the development of frank distress and acidosis qualifies as an important goal of antepartum assessment. Once the diagnosis of chronic fetal stress is made, the obstetrician must decide whether to effect delivery. The obstetrician will opt for delivery if the parturient is at or near term, but prematurity complicates the decision. The obstetrician must decide whether the intrauterine condition of the fetus can be improved. For example, continuous bed rest in the lateral decubitus position may enhance uteroplacental blood flow in the patient with chronic hypertension and/or mild preeclampsia. An antiarrhythmic drug may be given to the mother whose fetus has a tachyarrhythmia; transplacental passage of the drug may result in conversion of the tachyarrhythmia to sinus rhythm. The Rh-sensitized fetus can undergo blood transfusion, either intraperitoneally or via the umbilical vein. Finally, delivery may be delayed for 24 to 48 hours for glucocorticoid administration to accelerate fetal lung maturity. Two doses of glucocorticoid (e.g., betamethasone, dexamethasone) given 12 or 24 hours apart will not render the parturient or her fetus steroid dependent.

Deferral of delivery necessitates frequent reassessments of fetal condition. However, when electing to effect delivery, the obstetrician must decide whether to attempt vaginal delivery or to perform a cesarean section. As stated earlier, a positive CST does not preclude an uneventful labor. Factors that may lead the obstetrician to favor cesarean section over induction of labor and attempted vaginal delivery include: 1) prematurity; 2) abnormal presentation; and 3) an unfavorable cervix.

ACUTE FETAL DISTRESS

In Utero Resuscitation

When possible, in utero resuscitation is preferable to delivery of an acidotic infant.

Maternal Positioning. Unfortunately, a significant number of obstetricians and nurses continue to allow parturients to remain supine during labor. Uteroplacental blood flow and fetal condition often improve once aortocaval compression is relieved by asking the parturient to assume the lateral decubitus position. Cord compression may be relieved by having the patient move into any of a variety of positions (e.g., Trendelenburg, knee-chest).

Oxygenation. Supplemental oxygen administration is mandatory at the first sign of fetal distress. Contrary to earlier reports, supplemental oxygen does not cause uterine vasoconstriction and fetal acidosis. Willcourt and coworkers[23] concluded that administration of oxygen elevates fetal transcutaneous Po_2 in both healthy and high-risk parturients during labor. Edelstone and associates[24] and Caine and coworkers[25] demonstrated in pregnant sheep that administration of supplemental oxygen increases oxygen delivery to the fetus during times of reduced umbilical and uterine perfusion and "provides an oxygen reserve with which the fetus can maintain oxidative metabolism."

Maintenance of Maternal Circulation. Hypotension, if present, should be corrected. Again, aortocaval compression should be avoided. The patient may be placed in the Trendelenburg position, provided that uterine displacement is maintained. Dextrose-containing solutions may cause maternal and fetal hyperglycemia and hyperinsulinemia, which can later lead to neonatal hypoglycemia; thus, dextrose-free balanced salt solutions (e.g., Ringer's lactate) are preferred.[26,27] Finally, ephedrine, a mixed alpha and beta agonist, more favorably influences uterine blood flow in gravid ewes than do other vasopressors.[28,29] Conventional wisdom has been that the increase in cardiac output secondary to beta-receptor stimulation compensates for alpha receptor–mediated uterine vasoconstriction. Recently Ramanathan and associates[30] and Chestnut and coworkers[31] reported data that suggest that ephedrine more effectively increases cardiac preload than afterload in pregnant women and pregnant guinea pigs. Lawson and Wallfisch[32] concluded that ephedrine "produces venoconstriction to a greater degree than arterial constriction . . . [and] causes a redistribution of blood centrally, improves venous return . . . , increases cardiac output, and restores uterine perfusion."

Tocolysis. As stated earlier, injudicious administration of parenteral oxytocin represents one cause of uterine tachysystole or tetany. Parenteral oxytocin should be discontinued in the presence of fetal distress, whether or not uterine hypertonus is present. Further, some obstetricians have suggested the administration of a uterine relaxant to allow restoration of uteroplacental perfusion. Ingemarsson and coworkers[33,34] administered an intravenous bolus of 250 μg of terbutaline to 33 parturients with prolonged fetal bradycardia. The FHR improved after injection of terbutaline in 30 cases, and 23 patients subsequently delivered vigorous infants per vagina. They also confirmed the report of Freeman and colleagues[35] that fetal acidosis occurs more often if the fetal bradycardia continues for 10 min or more. While a single bolus injection of terbutaline may facilitate in utero fetal resuscitation and spare some women emergency operative delivery, the investigators emphasized, "in cases with an ominous fetal heart rate pattern preceding the bradycardia and in abruptio placentae immediate operative intervention without delay is probably better. . . . Preparation for emergency delivery should be made while a recovery is awaited."[33] The anesthesiologist should realize that the cardiovascular effects of β-mimetic tocolytic agents may persist for 10 to 30 min, or longer, following their administration.[36,37]

Saline Amnioinfusion. Gabbe and associates[38] induced variable decelerations in rhesus monkeys by removing amniotic fluid; replacing the amniotic fluid with normal saline resulted in resolution of the decelerations. Subsequently, Miyazaki and Taylor [39] observed that saline amnioinfusion relieved repetitive variable decelerations in 19 of 20 laboring women and relieved prolonged decelerations in 12 of 14 cases. Recently Miyazaki and Nevarez[40] obtained similar results in a prospective randomized study of 96 patients. Similarly, Nageotte and coworkers[41] reported that prophylactic saline amnioinfusion decreases the incidence and severity of variable decelerations in patients with preterm premature rupture of membranes. The procedure involves infusion of approximately 500 ml (range: 200 to 1500 ml) of normal saline into the uterine cavity through the intrauterine pressure catheter. This can be accomplished while transferring the patient to the operating room and preparing for cesarean section, should the amnioinfusion fail. At the University of Iowa Hospitals, we believe that this simple procedure can help reduce the incidence of cesarean section for fetal distress. Additional controlled studies involving large numbers of patients are needed.

Delivery

When in utero fetal resuscitation fails, delivery must be effected. Full cervical dilatation warrants consideration of vaginal delivery. Although most obstetricians will not hestiate to perform a low pelvis instrumental (forceps or vacuum) delivery, many are now reluctant to attempt mid-pelvis delivery in the presence of fetal distress. In such circumstances, or when acute fetal distress occurs and persists prior to complete cervical dilatation, delivery must be accomplished by cesarean section.

Anesthetic Management

LABORATORY INVESTIGATION

Several recent studies have examined the effects of anesthetic agents on asphyxiated fetal lambs. Palahniuk and colleagues[42] incrementally inflated an umbilical cord occlusion loop to effect fetal respiratory and metabolic acidosis (mean arterial pH, 7.05). Following induction of maternal anesthesia with 4 percent halothane in oxygen, anesthesia was maintained with 1 percent halothane in oxygen for 15 min. Maternal administration of halothane reduced fetal arterial pH (mean, 6.85), blood pressure, cerebral blood flow (CBF), and cerebral oxygen delivery. Yarnell and coworkers[43] also used an umbilical cord occlusion loop to induce asphyxia in fetal lambs. Maternal administration of 1.5-percent halothane for 15 min abolished the fetal hypertensive response to asphyxia, but no significant change in fetal arterial pH (means, 7.14 and 7.09 before and after 15 min of halothane, respectively), cardiac output, or CBF resulted. They concluded that low levels of halothane anesthesia "do not cause further deterioration in the asphyxiated foetus if the duration of anaesthesia is less than 15 minutes."

Subsequently, Swartz and associates[44] performed a similar study with three groups of animals: Group A, the controls; Group B, which received intravenous sodium thiopental, 3 mg per kg, followed by 50 percent nitrous oxide and 0.5 percent halothane in oxygen for 15 min; and Group C, which received intravenous sodium thiopental, 3 mg per kg, followed by 1 percent halothane in oxygen for 15 min. The administration of general anesthesia in both Groups B and C abolished the fetal hypertension and bradycardia produced by asphyxia but did not produce a significant fall in fetal cerebral or myocardial blood flow. During administration of anesthesia (or oxygen alone in Group A), fetal pH progressively decreased in each group, but no significant difference developed between the three groups. Two fetuses in the nitrous oxide group died after 10 min of anesthesia, although the cause of the demise was unclear. Swartz's group[44] concluded that general anesthesia does not improve fetal oxygenation or acid-base status, and that "rapid delivery is essential."

The results of these three studies do not necessarily contradict each other. In the first study,[42] the fetal lambs were more acidotic before induction of anesthesia, and the ewes initially received 4 percent halothane in oxygen. Yarnell and coworkers[43] speculated that this longer and greater exposure to halothane may have produced higher halothane concentrations in the fetuses.

Cheek and coworkers[45] described a model of fetal lamb asphyxia using adjustable *uterine* artery occlusion. After sequential induction of fetal asphyxia and general anesthesia, each pregnant ewe received 1 percent halothane in oxygen for 15 min. Mean fetal arterial pH before and after 15 min of halothane exposure was 7.13 and 7.00, respectively. Again, halothane abolished the fetal hypertension and bradycardia produced by asphyxia, but it did not significantly reduce fetal CBF. Subsequently Baker and coworkers[46] used the same model to study the effects of 1 percent isoflurane in oxygen. Administration of isoflurane decreased fetal cardiac output, renal blood flow, and mean arterial pH (7.16 and 6.99 before and after isoflurane, respectively), and blunted the compensatory increase in fetal CBF. In both of these studies, induction of anesthesia was accomplished with inhalation of a halogenated agent (e.g., 5 percent halothane[45]), rather than with a rapidly acting intravenous agent, as would occur clinically.

Pickering and colleagues[47] used the model of umbilical cord occlusion to evaluate the effects of sodium thiopental and ketamine on asphyxiated fetal lambs (mean fetal arterial pH, 7.10). Each ewe received either high-dose sodium thiopental (10 mg per kg), low-dose sodium thiopental (6 mg per kg), high-dose ketamine (4 mg per kg), or low-dose ketamine (2 mg per kg). High-dose sodium thiopental and ketamine resulted in marked reductions in fetal blood pressure, CBF, and cerebral oxygen delivery. Fetal blood pressure and CBF were better preserved after administration of low-dose sodium thiopental or ketamine, and low-dose ketamine appeared to cause the least reduction of CBF. Leicht and colleagues[48] used the model of uterine artery occlusion to compare the administration of sodium thiopental and ketamine in the presence of fetal lamb asphyxia. They induced anesthesia with either sodium thiopental (4 mg per kg) or ketamine (3 mg per kg). Subsequently they administered either drug intravenously "in doses sufficient to keep the animals anesthetized" for 15 min. Induction of anesthesia with either agent caused no significant change in fetal blood pressure, CBF, or cerebral metabolic oxygen consumption. Their preliminary results suggested no clear difference between sodium thiopental and ketamine for induction of anesthesia in the presence of fetal asphyxia. Parenthetically, the aforementioned studies did not address the contention that maternally administered anesthetics (e.g., barbiturates) might protect the fetal brain from hypoxic damage during asphyxia.[49,50]

Friesen and associates[51] used the model of partial umbilical cord occlusion to evaluate maternal lidocaine infusion in the presence of fetal lamb asphyxia. Fetal arterial blood lidocaine concentrations of 1.4 to 1.5 μg per ml produced an increase in fetal heart rate and CBF when compared with control acidotic fetuses. No significant change in fetal blood pressure or acid-base status occurred. The authors speculated that a direct vasodilating effect of lidocaine on cerebral vessels may have accounted for the increased CBF. The failure of lidocaine to reduce fetal blood pressure, as occurred with administration of halothane in earlier studies,[42-44] caused the authors to suggest that in situations of fetal distress regional anesthesia might promote better neonatal outcome.[51]

During the 30 min of lidocaine infusion, fetal concentrations of lidocaine did not increase,[51] as might be expected from the "ion-trapping" phenomenon previously demonstrated in the fetal lamb.[52] Morishima and coworkers[53] also administered intravenous lidocaine to pregnant ewes in which umbilical cord occlusion had caused asphyxia (mean arterial pH, 7.23). Although plasma concentrations of lidocaine did not differ between nonasphyxiated and asphyxiated fetuses, markedly higher tissue uptake of lidocaine took place in the asphyxiated fetuses. Fetal plasma lidocaine concentrations of 1.0 to 1.5 μg per ml generated no significant alterations in fetal hemodynamic or acid-base status in these mature fetal lambs. However, in a subsequent study, Morishima's group[54] observed that similar fetal concentrations of lidocaine reduced pH, cardiac output, and blood pressure in preterm fetal lambs.

These studies of asphyxiated fetal lambs do not perfectly mimic clinical practice. First, if fetal distress occurs following increased uterine activity, halogenated anesthetic agents may decrease uterine activity and thus improve uteroplacental blood flow. Even cord compression may be relieved by uterine relaxation. In the aforementioned animal studies, umbilical cord and uterine artery occlusion remained constant during administration of anesthesia. Second, in situations of dire fetal distress the duration of fetal anesthetic exposure may be significantly less than 15 to 30 min. A skilled obstetrician typically can deliver the infant within 1 or 2 min of making a midline skin incision. Such limited exposure to the halogenated anesthetic agents will not likely influence neonatal outcome significantly. Third, intravenous infusion of lidocaine should not be equated with the induction of epidural or spinal anesthesia, which may produce hemodynamic changes unrelated to the maternal and fetal arterial blood concentrations of lidocaine. Finally, one should be circumspect in extrapolating animal data to clinical practice. I conclude that at present no laboratory data clearly favor one intravenous anesthetic agent over another or one potent halogenated agent over another.

PREANESTHETIC EVALUATION

Each paturient admitted to the labor and delivery suite is a potential candidate for an emergency anesthetic for either vaginal or abdominal delivery. Ideally, each patient will undergo preanesthetic evaluation at the time of admission. Unfortunately this may not be possible in all hospitals providing obstetric care. However, the obstetrician should notify the anesthesiologist of any potential need for anesthesia care as soon as he or she suspects that need. In the event that anesthesia is required for acute fetal distress in a patient who has not had a preanesthetic evaluation, the anesthesiologist may need to perform that evaluation even as he or she makes other preparations for anesthesia (e.g., establishment of intravenous access, placement of blood pressure cuff and ECG electrodes, and so on). While the presence of fetal distress should not lead the anesthesiologist to proceed in a manner that will compromise maternal safety, he or she should limit the history and physical examination to those areas essential for safe anesthetic administration. For example, while the anesthesiologist should inquire of previous anesthetic complications or medical illnesses in every patient, one may forgo a thorough reading of each page of the patient's chart in the presence of acute fetal distress. Further, the anesthesiologist should evaluate the airway and potential difficulty of intubation in every patient presenting for anesthesia. On the other hand, the anesthesiologist might forego preanesthetic auscultation of the heart and lungs in every patient with acute fetal distress.

Even as the degree of urgency may vary, so will the duration and extent of the preanesthetic evaluation. The obstetrician and anesthesiologist should communicate honestly regarding the urgency of delivery. Specifically, chronic fetal stress, or even acute fetal distress that was resolved, should not be confused with ongoing fetal distress.

PREANESTHETIC PREPARATION

The following standards apply to both vaginal and abdominal deliveries, regardless of choice of anesthetic technique. First, avoid aortocaval compression. In my experience, elevation of the right buttock is more effective than lateral tilting of the entire operating table. Second, administer a clear antacid (e.g., 30 ml of 0.3 M sodium citrate) in anticipation of the need, or potential need, for general anesthesia. Third, administer supplemental oxygen before and during induction of either general or regional anesthesia.[55] However, do not delay induction of general anesthesia while awaiting 3 to 5 min of preoxygenation. Norris and Dewan[56] demonstrated that four maximally deep inspirations of 100 percent oxygen provide as much benefit as 3 min of oxygen breathing before rapid sequence induction of general anesthesia for cesarean section. Fourth, avoid hypotension and treat it promptly if it occurs. Fifth, continue electronic FHR monitoring until delivery. A further deterioration of the FHR may prompt a more expeditious delivery; conversely, an improved FHR pattern may allow a more "leisurely" approach to delivery. In the latter circumstance, the obstetrician may be more willing to await establishment of adequate regional anesthesia and/or may elect to perform a more cosmetically pleasing transverse (rather than vertical) skin incision. Not infrequently an improved FHR pattern will allow deferral of cesarean section with subsequent vaginal delivery of a vigorous infant. Finally, be sensitive to the emotional needs of the mother and father. Often the anesthesiologist qualifies as the best person to reassure and comfort distressed parents. The anesthesiologist and other members of the obstetric team should remember that chaos need not accompany urgency.

CHOICE OF ANESTHETIC TECHNIQUE

Few specialists in obstetric anesthesia would dispute the contention that either regional or general anesthesia may be safely administered in the presence of chronic fetal stress. However, some physicians contend that the speed, reliability, and hemodynamic stability associated with general anesthesia mandate its use in all cases of cesarean section for acute fetal distress. Clearly, general anesthesia qualifies as the best choice when either dire distress (e.g., placental abruption, prolapsed cord, unremitting fetal bradycardia) or a contraindication to regional anesthesia (e.g., coagulopathy, hypovolemia) exists. Many cases of less severe distress fall between chronic fetal stress and dire distress. Decisions regarding anesthetic technique for these cases prove more difficult, and may cause misunderstanding and disagreement between the anesthesiologist and the obstetrician. Clearly a need exists for honest communication and mutual understanding among members of the obstetric team.

Marx and associates[57] reported on the anesthetic management of 126 emergency cesarean sections of fetal distress. Fetal scalp capillary blood pH was determined preoperatively in each case, and the mother selected the anesthetic technique. Seventy-one women received general anesthesia, and 55 chose regional anesthesia (spinal, 33; extension of epidural block, 22). All operations commenced within 20 min of the last scalp blood pH determination, and no patient experienced hypotension. At delivery umbilical artery blood pH values were higher than the last scalp blood pH in 63 percent and 80 percent of the general and regional anesthesia cases, respectively. In five cases umbilical artery blood pH fell significantly below the last scalp blood pH, but the authors did not identify the anesthetic technique for those five cases. Umbilical vein and artery blood-gas and pH values and 5-min Apgar scores were similar in the two anesthesia groups, but regional anesthesia was associated with significantly better 1-min Apgar scores. The authors did not randomly select either general or regional anesthesia, and one must wonder whether the general anesthesia group included a higher percentage of patients whose FHR tracings demonstrated further deterioration between the last scalp blood pH determination and induction of anesthesia. Further, one may question whether fetal distress existed in each case, as the mean (±S.D.) scalp blood pH determinations for the two groups were 7.20 ± 0.05 and 7.20 ± 0.04, respectively. Nevertheless, this study represents the most exemplary report to date of the use of regional anesthesia in cases of fetal distress.

If an epidural catheter is in place and a partial level of anesthesia already exists, extension of the epidural anesthetic for cesarean section is appropriate. Epidural anesthesia adequate for performance of cesarean section does not significantly decrease placental perfusion, provided the anesthesiologist avoids aortocaval compression and hypotension.[58–60] Epidural anesthesia may even improve intervillous blood flow in women with pre-eclampsia, provided no decrease in blood pressure accompanies the induction of anesthesia.[61,62] I give an intravenous bolus of Ringer's lactate and inject 15 to 20 ml of 3-percent 2-chloroprocaine in 5-ml increments epidurally while preparations are being made for surgery (e.g., insertion of urethral catheter, preparation and draping of the abdomen). Often adequate anesthesia develops by the time the obstetrician is ready to make the skin incision. If not, the decision as to whether to delay surgery should be based on the ongoing FHR pattern. This illustrates the importance of continuing FHR monitoring until delivery in all cases of fetal distress. Clearly there must be no delay in the presence of ongoing distress. When partial but inadequate epidural anesthesia results, one should consider supplemental local infiltration, especially if there is a contraindication to rapid sequence induction of general anesthesia. Otherwise, the combination of inadequate anesthesia and ongoing fetal distress mandate: 1) application of cricoid pressure; 2) rapid sequence induction of general anesthesia; and 3) placement of a cuffed endotracheal tube.

In Marx and coworkers'[57] study of anesthesia for emergency abdominal delivery, 33 of 55 women in the regional anesthesia group received spinal anesthesia. Spinal hypotension occurs less often in laboring patients than in women undergoing elective cesarean section,[63] but the incidence of hypotension in such circumstances remains significant. Ongoing fetal distress precludes the opportunity for infusing a large volume of intravenous crystalloid before performance of the spinal block, since the urgency of the situation limits the time available for that purpose. The potential for rapid onset of sympathetic block, with resultant hypotension and decreased uteroplacental perfusion, prompts my reluctance to institute spinal or epidural anesthesia de novo in the presence of ongoing acute fetal distress. However, the administration of a low spinal (saddle) block to facilitate emergent instrumental vaginal delivery represents a valid indication for conduction anesthesia.

After transfer of the parturient to the delivery room, the FHR abnormality may resolve. For example, the administration of oxytocin may have caused late decelerations or bradycardia. Even though the FHR abnormality may disappear after discontinuing oxytocin, the obstetrician may conclude that the fetus is unlikely to tolerate further labor. In this or a similar circumstance, epidural, spinal, or general anesthesia can be administered, depending upon the wishes of the mother and the presence or absence of other medical considerations. Remember that the mother and fetus have shown evidence of marginal uteroplacental reserve; therefore FHR monitoring should be established before induction of anesthesia and continued until delivery. Regardless of indication for cesarean or choice of anesthetic technique, the uterine incision-to-delivery interval should be less than 3 min.[64,65]

CHOICE OF ANESTHETIC AGENTS

General Anesthesia

No laboratory or clinical data clearly favor either sodium thiopental (4 mg per kg) or ketamine (1 mg per kg) for induction of anesthesia. Administration of 1 mg per kg of ketamine should not significantly increase uterine tone. Marx and coworkers[57] administered a combination of ketamine (0.75 mg per kg) and sodium thiopental (1.0 to 1.5 mg per kg) to 54 of 71 women receiving general anesthesia. Subsequently Marx[66] has advocated giving approximately 0.5 mg per kg ketamine, followed by 1.0 to 1.5 mg per kg sodium thiopental. The choice of sodium thiopental or ketamine appears of little consequence provided the dose employed remains low.

For intubation, succinylcholine (1.0 to 1.5 mg per kg) is the muscle relaxant of choice in the absence of contraindications to its use.

The mother should receive an inspired oxygen concentration of at least 50 to 70 percent until delivery.[55,64,67] A low concentration (<1 MAC) of a potent halogenated agent will reduce the incidence of maternal awareness. For most patients I prefer 0.5-percent halothane.

After delivery, the anesthetic considerations do not differ from those for any other cesarean section. Fetal considerations no longer present an immediate issue. However, I prefer to avoid giving agents (e.g., diazepam, droperidol) that can result in prolonged postoperative sedation and interference with early maternal-infant bonding and breast feeding.

Regional Anesthesia

For elective cesarean section for chronic fetal stress, 0.5 percent bupivacaine offers the advantage of a slow onset, which may reduce the risk of a sudden decrease in blood pressure and uteroplacental blood flow.[68] When extending a pre-existing epidural block in the presence of acute fetal distress, 3 percent 2-chloroprocaine offers two advantages: 1) rapid onset of action, and 2) limited placental transfer. In the presence of fetal acidosis, amide local anesthetic agents (e.g., lidocaine, bupivacaine) may become "trapped" in their ionized forms on the fetal side of the placenta, resulting in increased fetal levels of drug.[52,53] Philipson and associates[69] demonstrated that even in the presence of fetal acidosis, placental transfer of 2-chloroprocaine does not increase, probably because of its rapid metabolism.

For spinal anesthesia, hyperbaric lidocaine may have a faster onset than either tetracaine or bupivacaine, and is my choice for vaginal or cesarean delivery when speed is of the essence. The faster onset may produce a somewhat greater potential for hypotension.

As stated earlier, two situations call for local infiltration: 1) supplementation of a "patchy" or inadequate epidural block; and 2) acute fetal distress combined with a contraindication to rapid sequence induction of general anesthesia (e.g., unavailability of a skilled anesthesia care provider or anticipated difficulty with intubation). In either situation a dilute solution of local anesthetic (e.g., 1 percent 2-chloroprocaine or 0.5 percent lidocaine) should be administered. A dilute solution should be used because, in the first circumstance, a significant dose of local anesthetic has probably already been given epidurally. In the second circumstance, a large volume (e.g., 60 to 80 ml) of local anesthetic solution will be needed to achieve some semblance of satisfactory anesthesia.[70]

Summary

1. Complete the preanesthetic assessment of all parturients as soon as possible after admission to the labor and delivery suite. During acute fetal distress limit the assessment to the most pertinent areas.
2. Avoid aortocaval compression.
3. Administer a clear antacid (e.g., 30 ml of 0.3-M sodium citrate).
4. Administer a high concentration of supplemental oxygen before, during, and after induction of either general or regional anesthesia. Prior to induction of general anesthesia, administer at least four deep breaths of 100-percent oxygen.
5. Avoid hypotension; administer a balanced salt solution containing no dextrose (e.g., Ringer's lactate).
6. Continue electronic FHR monitoring until delivery.
7. Provide emotional support for the mother and her family.
8. Extend epidural anesthesia (previously established for labor) if time and hemodynamic stability permit; however, do not delay surgery in the presence of ongoing distress. Consider supplementation of inadequate epidural anesthesia with infiltration of local anesthetic by the obstetrician. Otherwise, apply cricoid pressure, perform rapid sequence induction of general anesthesia, and insert a cuffed endotracheal tube.
9. In the absence of pre-existing epidural analgesia, consider administration of low spinal anesthesia to facilitate emergent instrumental *vaginal* delivery.

The presence of fetal distress results in emotional stress for the mother and father as well as for all members of the obstetric team. Few clinical situations demand better judgment and greater skill. Each anesthesiologist who cares for obstetric patients should be: 1) *alert* to the potential for fetal distress; 2) *aware* of maternal-fetal physiology and pharmacology; 3) physically *available* should fetal distress mandate rapid delivery; and 4) *adaptable*—one anesthetic technique is not equally appropriate for all parturients.

References

1. Phillips, WDP and Towell, ME: Abnormal fetal heart rate associated with congenital abnormalities. Br J Obstet Gynaecol 87:270, 1980.
2. Navot, D, et al: Antepartum fetal heart rate pattern associated with major congenital malformations. Obstet Gynecol 63:414, 1984.
3. Clark, SL, Koonings, PP and Phelan, JP: Placenta previa/accreta and prior cesarean section. Obstet Gynecol 66:89, 1985.
4. Clark, SL, et al: Emergency hysterectomy for obstetric hemorrhage. Obstet Gynecol 64:376, 1984.
5. Mann, LI: Pregnancy events and brain damage. Am J Obstet Gynecol 155:6, 1986.
6. Marx, GF, et al: Umbilical blood flow velocity waveforms in different maternal positions and with epidural analgesia. Obstet Gynecol 68:61, 1986.
7. Pritchard, JA, MacDonald, PC and Gant, NF: Williams' Obstetrics, ed 17. Appleton-Century-Crofts, Norwalk, 1985, p 267.
8. Huddleston, JF and Freeman, RK: Assessment of fetal well-being by antepartum fetal heart rate testing. In Bolognese RJ, Schwarz RH and Schneider J (eds): Perinatal Medicine: Management of the High-Risk Fetus and Neonate, ed 2. Williams & Wilkins, Baltimore, 1982, p 129.
9. Zlatnik, F: Antepartum fetal surveillance. Iowa Perinatal Letter 5:5, 1984.
10. Manning, FA, et al: Fetal biophysical profile scoring: A prospective study in 1,184 high-risk patients. Am J Obstet Gynecol 140:289, 1981.
11. Manning, FA, et al: Fetal assessment based on fetal biophysical profile scoring: Experience in 12,620 referred high-risk pregnancies. I. Perinatal mortality by frequency and etiology. Am J Obstet Gynecol 151:343, 1985.
12. Daffos, F, Capella-Pavlovsky, M and Forestier, F: Fetal blood sampling via the umbilical cord using a needle guided by ultrasound. Prenat Diagn 3:271, 1983.
13. Hobbins, JC, et al: Percutaneous umbilical blood sampling. Am J Obstet Gynecol 152:1, 1985.
14. Kleinman, CS, et al: Fetal echocardiography for evaluation of in utero congestive heart failure. N Engl J Med 306:568, 1982.
15. Fleischer, A, et al: Umbilical artery velocity waveforms and intrauterine growth retardation. Am J Obstet Gynecol 151:502, 1985.
16. Bracero, L, et al: Umbilical artery velocimetry in diabetes and pregnancy. Obstet Gynecol 68:654, 1986.
17. Meis, PJ, et al: Meconium passage: A new classification for risk assessment during labor. Am J Obstet Gynecol 131:509, 1978.
18. Dalton, KJ, Dawes, GS and Patrick, JE: The autonomic nervous system and fetal heart rate variability. Am J Obstet Gynecol 146:456, 1983.
19. Clark, SL and Paul, RH: Intrapartum fetal surveillance: The role of fetal scalp blood sampling. Am J Obstet Gynecol 153:717, 1985.
20. Eskes, TKAB, Jongsma, HW and Houx, PCW: Percentiles for gas values in human umbilical cord blood. Eur J Obstet Gynecol Reprod Biol 14:341, 1983.
21. Clark, SL, Gimovsky, ML and Miller, FC: Fetal heart rate response to scalp blood sampling. Am J Obstet Gynecol 144:706, 1982.
22. Clark, SL, Gimovsky, ML and Miller, FC: The scalp stimulation test: A clinical alternative to fetal scalp blood sampling. Am J Obstet Gynecol 148:274, 1984.
23. Willcourt, RJ, King, JC and Queenan, JT: Maternal oxygenation administration and the fetal transcutaneous PO_2. Am J Obstet Gynecol 146:714, 1983.
24. Edelstone, DI, Peticca, BB and Goldblum, LJ: Effects of maternal oxygen administration on fetal oxygenation during reductions in umbilical blood flow in fetal lambs. Am J Obstet Gynecol 152:351, 1985.
25. Caine, ME, Hebrank, G and Edelstone, DI: Effects of maternal O_2 administration on fetal oxygenation during reductions in uterine blood flow (abstr). Proceedings of the 1986 Meeting of the Society for Gynecologic Investigation, Toronto, CA, p 107.
26. Kenepp, NB, et al: Fetal and neonatal hazards of maternal hydration with 5% dextrose before caesarean section. Lancet 1:1150, 1982.
27. Grylack, LJ, Chu, SS and Scanlon, JW: Use of intravenous fluids before cesarean section: Effects on perinatal glucose, insulin, and sodium homeostasis. Obstet Gynecol 63:654, 1984.
28. James, FM, Greiss, FC and Kemp, RA: An evaluation of vasopressor therapy for maternal hypotension during spinal anesthesia. Anesthesiology 33:25, 1970.
29. Ralston, DH, Shnider, SM and deLorimier, AA: Effects of equipotent ephedrine, metaraminol, mephentermine, and methoxamine on uterine blood flow in the pregnant ewe. Anesthesiology 40:354, 1974.
30. Ramanathan, S, Grant, G and Turndorf, H: Cardiac preload changes with ephedrine therapy for hypotension in obstetrical patients (abstr). Anesth Analg 65:S125, 1986.
31. Chestnut, DH, et al: The effect of ephedrine upon uterine artery blood flow velocity in the pregnant guinea pig subjected to terbutaline infusion and acute hemorrhage (abstr). Anesthesiology 65:A386, 1986.
32. Lawson, NW and Wallfisch, HK: Cardiovascular pharmacology: A new look at the "pressors." In Stoelting, RK, Barash, PG and Gallagher, TJ (eds): Advances in Anesthesia. Year Book Medical Publishers, Chicago, 1986, p 195.
33. Ingemarsson, I, Arulkumaran, S and Ratnam, SS: Single injection of terbutaline in term labor: I. Effect on fetal pH in cases with prolonged bradycardia. Am J Obstet Gynecol 153:859, 1985.
34. Ingemarsson, I, Arulkumaran, S and Ratnam, SS: Single injection of terbutaline in term labor: II. Effect on uterine activity. Am J Obstet Gynecol 153:865, 1985.
35. Freeman, RK, et al: Fetal cardiac response to paracervical block anesthesia: Part I. Am J Obstet Gynecol 113:583, 1972.
36. Ravindran, R, et al: Anesthetic considerations in pregnant patients receiving terbutaline therapy. Anesth Analg 59:391, 1980.
37. Shin, YK and Kim, YD: Anesthetic considerations in

patients receiving ritodrine therapy for preterm labor (abstr). Anesth Analg 65:S140, 1986.

38. Gabbe, SG, et al: Umbilical cord compression associated with amniotomy: Laboratory observations. Am J Obstet Gynecol 126:353, 1976.
39. Miyazaki, FS and Taylor, NA: Saline amnioinfusion for relief of variable or prolonged decelerations. Am J Obstet Gynecol 146:670, 1983.
40. Miyazaki, FS and Nevarez, F: Saline amnioinfusion for relief of repetitive variable declerations: A prospective randomized study. Am J Obstet Gynecol 153:301, 1985.
41. Nageotte, MP, et al: Prophylactic intrapartum amnioinfusion in patients with preterm premature rupture of membranes. Am J Obstet Gynecol 153:557, 1985.
42. Palahniuk, RJ, et al: Maternal halothane anesthesia reduces cerebral blood flow in the acidotic sheep fetus. Anesth Analg 59:35, 1980.
43. Yarnell, R, et al: The effect of halothane anaesthesia on the asphyxiated foetal lamb in utero. Can Anaesth Soc J 30:474, 1983.
44. Swartz, J, et al: The effects of general anaesthesia on the asphyxiated foetal lamb in utero. Can Anaesth Soc J 32:577, 1985.
45. Cheek, DBC, et al: The effect of halothane anesthesia on the asphyxiated fetal lamb (abstr). Anesthesiology 63:A356, 1985.
46. Baker, BW, et al: Effects of isoflurane on the asphyxiated fetal lamb (abstr). Anesthesiology 65:A394, 1986.
47. Pickering, BG, et al: Cerebral vascular responses to ketamine and thiopentone during foetal acidosis. Can Anaesth Soc J 29:463, 1982.
48. Leicht, CH, et al: The effect of ketamine or sodium thiopental rapid sequence induction on the asphyxiated fetal lamb (abstr). Anesthesiology 65:A387, 1986.
49. Myers, RE and Myers, SE: Use of sedative, analgesic, and anesthetic drugs during labor and delivery. Bane or boon? Am J Obstet Gynecol 133:83, 1979.
50. Rurak, DW and Taylor, SM: Oxygen consumption in fetal lambs after maternal administration of sodium pentobarbital. Am J Obstet Gynecol 154:674, 1986.
51. Friesen, C, et al: The effect of lidocaine on regional blood flows and cardiac output in the non-stressed and the stressed foetal lamb. Can Anaesth Soc J 33:130, 1986.
52. Biehl, D, et al: Placental transfer of lidocaine: Effects of fetal acidosis. Anestheisology 48:409, 1978.
53. Morishima, HO, et al: Effects of asphyxia on the pharmacodynamics of lidocaine in the mature fetal lamb (abstr). Anesthesiology 63:A443, 1985.
54. Morishima, HO, et al: Pharmacodynamics of lidocaine in the asphyxiated preterm fetal lamb (abstr). Anesthesiology 65:A372, 1986.
55. Ramanathan, S, et al: Oxygen transfer from mother to fetus during cesarean section under epidural anesthesia. Anesth Analg 61:576, 1982.
56. Norris, MC and Dewan, DM: Preoxygenation for cesarean section: A comparison of two techniques. Anesthesiology 62:827, 1985.
57. Marx, GF, Luykx, WM and Cohen, S: Fetal-neonatal status following caesarean section for fetal distress. Br J Anaesth 56:1009, 1984.
58. Wallis, KL, et al: Epidural anesthesia in the normotensive pregnant ewe: Effects on uterine blood flow and fetal acid-base status. Anesthesiology 44:481, 1976.
59. Jouppila, R, et al: Placental blood flow during caesarean section under lumbar extradural analgesia. Br J Anaesth 50:275, 1978.
60. Huovinen, K, et al: Changes in placental intervillous blood flow measured by the ^{133}Xenon method during lumbar epidural block for elective caesarean section. Acta Anaesth Scand 23:529, 1979.
61. Jouppila, R, et al: Epidural analgesia and placental blood flow during labour in pregnancies complicated by hypertension. Br J Obstet Gynaecol 86:969, 1979.
62. Jouppila, P, et al: Lumbar epidural analgesia to improve intervillous blood flow during labor in severe preeclampsia. Obstet Gynecol 59:158, 1982.
63. Clark, RB, Thompson, DS and Thompson, CH: Prevention of spinal hypotension associated with cesarean section. Anesthesiology 45:670, 1976.
64. Crawford, JS, et al: A further study of general anaesthesia for caesarean section. Br J Anaesth 48:661, 1976.
65. Datta, S, et al: Neonatal effect of prolonged anesthetic induction for cesarean section. Obstet Gynecol 58:331, 1981.
66. Marx, GF: Editor's note. Obstet Anesth Digest 5:113, 1985.
67. Marx, GF and Mateo, CV: Effects of different oxygen concentrations during general anesthesia for elective cesarean section. Can Anaesth Soc J 18:587, 1971.
68. James, FM, et al: Chloroprocaine vs. bupivacaine for lumbar epidural analgesia for elective cesarean section. Anesthesiology 52:488, 1980.
69. Philipson, EH, Kuhnert, BR and Syracuse, CD: Fetal acidosis, 2-chloroprocaine, and epidural anesthesia for cesarean section. Am J Obstet Gynecol 151:322, 1985.
70. Ranney, B and Stanage, WF: Advantages of local anesthesia for cesarean section. Obstet Gynecol 45:163, 1975.

PART 5

SPECIAL PROBLEMS

CHAPTER 20

THE DIABETIC PARTURIENT

SANJAY DATTA, M.B., F.F.A.R.C.S. (Eng)

Diabetes mellitus, the third most common metabolic disorder (after obesity and thyroid disease), has two interrelated components: metabolism and vascularity. The former refers to a relative or absolute lack of insulin, leading to abnormal elevation of blood glucose and alterations in lipid and protein metabolism. The latter complication, evidenced by accelerated nonspecific atherosclerosis and a more specific microangiopathy, mainly affects the eyes and kidneys.

Diabetes is a common medical problem during pregnancy, occurring in 1 in 700 to 1 in 1000 gestations. With the advent and application of better medical skills, the probability of a viable birth for the diabetic parturient has increased significantly in recent years. Advances in diagnosis and obstetric management, anesthetic medication and technique, and in the neonatal management of diabetic parturients have dramatically reduced overall perinatal mortality for insulin-dependent diabetic parturients. In some centers perinatal mortality for the offspring of diabetic mothers is approximately the same as that in the general population (1.6 to 2 percent).[1] The anesthetic management either for vaginal delivery or cesarean section should be based on an understanding of the pathophysiology of pregnant diabetics and of the advantages and disadvantages of different anesthetic techniques and medications.

Metabolic Changes in Normal Pregnancy

Pregnancy generates substantial changes in body fuel metabolism and consequently causes hyperplasia of the beta cells of maternal islets of Langerhans. Animal experiments provide evidence of increased insulin secretion from the islets during pregnancy as well as greater sensitivity to a lower dose of glucose. Gestational hormones such as estrogen, progesterone, and human placental lactogen bring about these morphologic and secretory changes.[2] Human placental lactogen, progesterone, and cortisol have also been described as anti-insulin factors,[3] but the mechanism of insulin interference is still incompletely understood. Recent evidence suggests that the site of action may be the postreceptor level.[4] Plasma concentrations of glucose in the postabsorptive state decline as pregnancy advances, owing to increasing placental uptake of glucose and a probable limitation of hepatic output of glucose.

The metabolic changes of pregnancy peak in the latter half of gestation during which the basal plasma concentration of immunoreactive insulin increases compared with nonpregnant controls. Diabetic parturients respond to a glucose load by increasing insulin levels more quickly and to a higher peak plasma concentration. Even with the associated hyperinsulinism, the metabolism of glucose is inhibited, producing higher maternal blood glucose levels. Effects on fat metabolism also exist; for example, fat deposition increases during early pregnancy. However, in the later part of pregnancy lipolysis increases, with associated enhanced production of glycerol and free fatty acids. The lipolytic action of human placental lactogen overrides the antilipolytic effects of insulin. Ketogenesis increases in the postabsorptive state.

Diabetic Ketoacidosis

Insulin deficiency in type I insulin-dependent pregnant patients increases postprandial blood glucose concentrations. The liver can produce more glucose by glycogen breakdown due to lower insulin levels. Insulin-sensitive branched-chain amino acids such as leucine, isoleucine, and valine also increase in diabetic subjects with fasting hyperglycemia (fasting glucose >105 mg per dl).[5] Gluconeogenesis takes place with the mobilization of amino acids and glycerol from muscle and fat stores. Free fatty acids can ultimately be converted in the liver to triglycerides, cholesterol, and phospholipids.[6] Thus, lack of insulin in diabetic parturients can contribute to increasing amounts of free fatty acids available for conversion to ketone bodies, acetoacetate, and β-hydroxybutyric acid.

Diabetic ketoacidosis is the major factor in the increased incidence of perinatal morbidity and mortality. Evidence exists that ketone can readily cross the placenta. When women in early pregnancy fast for 84 hours prior to elective abortion, the β-hydroxybutyrate and acetoacetic acid levels in amniotic fluid increase by 30- and 10-fold, respectively.[7] These levels correlate well with maternal blood concentration. Ketones also increase in the amniotic fluid of poorly controlled diabetic parturients.[8] Measurement of ketone concentrations in cord blood reveals a ratio of 1 in 2 in relation to maternal blood.[9] Thus, simple diffusion probably occurs across a concentration gradient. The placenta contains enzymes that can convert acetylcoenzyme A to β-hydroxybutyric acid and thus can contribute to the supply of ketones that reaches the fetus.[9] The placenta may also utilize ketones as a source of fuel and does so preferentially over glucose in vitro in the presence of increased maternal ketones. The placenta can contribute to the fetal supply of free fatty acids as well. Although free fatty acids provide the major source of energy-yielding fuel for extracerebral tissues in the adult, the fetus principally uses glucose. Glucose consumption at term occurs at a rate of approximately 6 mg per kg per min, a pace two to three times greater than that in the normal adult.[10] Normally, energy derived from ketone bodies amounts to only about 6 percent of that derived from glucose. The fetus can also use lactate, free fatty acids, and amino acids in limited amounts. The clinical effects on neonates of ketosis during pregnancy remain unclear. However, recent studies in pregnant sheep suggest that hyperketonemia, alone or associated with hyperglycemia, can cause a significant decrease in fetal PaO_2, together with increases in fetal lactate levels and fetal heart rate.[11,12] The authors suggest that these observations may partially explain the increased perinatal mortality with uncontrolled diabetes.

Patients with diabetic ketoacidosis usually present with vomiting, thirst, polyuria, weakness, altered sensorium, and air hunger, and they may complain of abdominal pain. Clinical signs include poor turgor, soft or sunken eyeballs, hypotension, tachycardia, and hypothermia. Hyperventilation (deep sighing Küssmaul respiration) indicates acidosis. The face may appear flushed. The characteristic fruity odor on the patient's breath comes from the large amounts (up to 12 mmol per liter) of acetone in the blood, formed by spontaneous decarboxylation of acetoacetic acid. Biochemical findings include: plasma glucose >300 mg per dl, plasma HCO_3 <15 mEq per liter, arterial pH <7.30, and serum acetone positive at 1:2 dilution. The treatment of diabetic ketoacidosis should provide enough insulin to correct the acidosis and to carefully balance fluid and electrolyte levels. Continuous fetal heart rate (FHR) monitoring should be instituted for fetal surveillance.

Insulin treatment should include administration of an intravenous loading dose of regular insulin (0.4 units per kg) to reduce ketones in the first 2 hours of therapy. The loading dose should be repeated in 1 hour if the plasma glucose has not declined by 10 percent. Correction of maternal acidosis represents the goal of treatment. Five to 10 units per hour of insulin should be used as an intravenous infusion. Potassium administration will be necessary, for patients with ketoacidosis have a marked deficit of body potassium, which correction of acidosis and treatment with insulin further aggravates. Phosphate should also be given with the potassium. Use of bicarbonate for the treatment of diabetic ketoacidosis remains controversial. Prompt correction of the acidosis could reduce morbidity and mortality and avoid potentially harmful effects on myocardial function. However, the problems with bicarbonate treatment include the possibility of a transient paradoxical intracerebral acidosis and reduced oxygen unloading to tissues due to increased affinity. Most clinicians use bicarbonate for patients with severe acidosis (pH <7). A suggested regimen includes the addition of 89.2 mEq sodium bicarbonate to each liter of half-normal or normal saline. Bicarbonate infusion should be stopped when pH reaches 7.20.

Effects on Fetus and Causes of Fetal Morbidity and Mortality

All metabolic products, both normal and abnormal, reach the fetus from the mother. In poorly controlled diabetic parturients, the fetus receives increased energy fuels including glucose, ketones, certain amino acids, and free fatty acids and consequently, responds by releasing insulin. The combination of hyperinsulinemia and excessive substrate for fat synthesis will cause deposition of fetal fat and glycogen. It was originally thought that maternal hyperglycemia alone accounted for fetal macrosomia.[13] However, this hypothesis does not explain the poor correlation between maternal blood glucose and fetal weight.[14] Thus, other metabolites might be responsible for inducing lipogenesis in utero.

Main causes of fetal morbidity and mortality in diabetic parturients include maternal ketoacidosis, major congenital anomalies, intrauterine fetal distress, prematurity, respiratory distress syndrome, macrosomia, birth trauma, and neonatal hypoglycemia. Polyhydramnios and pre-eclampsia constitute the major causes of prematurity in pregnant diabetics. If diabetics receive synthetic corticosteroids to induce fetal lung maturation of β-mimetic drugs for tocolysis, one must remember that these drugs can initiate hyperglycemia and ketoacidosis. The chances of hypoglycemia, hyperbilirubinemia, and hypoglycemia are much greater for infants of diabetic parturients.

Obstetric Management

In the patient with a history of diabetes, a fasting blood glucose value of 120 mg per dl or more makes the diagnosis. In asymptomatic patients, one should incorporate the glucose screening into routine blood testing at around 28 weeks' gestation. The glucose tolerance test still represents the standard for identifying gestational diabetes. Any of the following symptoms place the parturient at risk for gestational diabetes:[15] (1) abnormal glucose screen, (2) history of adult-onset diabetes in parents, siblings, or grandparents, (3) previous delivery of an infant with birth weight of more than 4000 g, and (4) obstetric history complicated by toxemia, glucosemia, excessive weight gain, premature delivery, previous stillbirth, neonatal death, polyhydramnios, or congenital anomaly.

DIET AND INSULIN

Diabetic parturients should follow a diet of 30 to 35 kcal per kg ideal body weight. Carbohydrates usually provide 40 to 50 percent of the total calories, with the remaining calories divided equally between fat and protein. A high-protein diet has been suggested for the maintenance of a more constant glucose level.

The ultimate goal of insulin therapy during pregnancy should include an avoidance of both fasting and postprandial hyperglycemia and hypoglycemic reactions. Hemoglobin A_{1C} (Hb A_{1C}) correlates well with mean daily capillary blood glucose over a few weeks during pregnancy. A sequential measurement of Hb A_{1C} (range 5 to 10 percent) will provide the physician with another indicator of long-term control. However, since insulin dosage must be adjusted frequently during the metabolically dynamic state of pregnancy, urine- or capillary blood glucose must be measured several times each day to assist in insulin management. Self-monitoring of capillary blood glucose at home with glucose oxidase strips and portable reflectance colorimeter has proved reliable in the hands of almost all patients and provides an excellent end-point of therapy. In Brigham and Women's Hospital, the obstetrician strives for an average fasting capillary blood glucose of 100 mg per dl or less and average 2-hour postprandial values below 140 mg per dl. Most insulin-dependent parturients require at least two injections of a 1 to 2 mixture of regular and intermediate insulin daily in order to prevent fasting and postprandial hyperglycemia. Usually, two thirds of the insulin is given before breakfast and one third before supper. Occasionally, administration of regular insulin three or four times each day, continued with intermediate insulin at one or two injections, becomes necessary to manage unstable cases. A few perinatal centers employ small portable pumps for continuous infusion of regular insulin.

MONITORING OF THE FETUS

In the past, the incidence of sudden intrauterine death in the third trimester ranged as high as 5 to 10 percent, mainly because of poor diabetic control with ketoacidosis, pre-eclampsia, and diabetic nephropathy. Other factors included a combination of relative fetal hypoxia and hyperglycemia with ketoacidosis, severe hypoglycemia, or fetal myocardial dysfunction. Advances in technology have developed more sophisticated methods to detect fetal distress and prevent stillbirth. Quantitative studies of fetal activity pattern employ ultrasound more often. Measurement of maternal urinary and serum estriol levels serves to evaluate functioning of the fetal placental unit; the placenta produces estriol from aromatization of dehydroepiandrosterone sulfate, which the fetal adrenals produce and the fetal liver hydroxylates further. Low maternal levels (<95 percent confidence limits for stage of gestation) or a rapid fall below 40 percent from the mean estriol level of the previous 3 days may indicate fetal distress. Estriol assays should be performed daily to be of value in preventing stillbirths in high-risk pregnancies. Fetal heart rate should also be monitored regularly. Nonstress tests showing good long-term variability of the fetal heart rate and accelerations greater than 15 beats per min with fetal movements predict fetal well-being. A nonstress test nonreactive even with stimulation calls for a full oxytocin challenge test. Deceleration of fetal heart rate following uterine contractions after oxytocin infusion signifies transient fetal hypoxia and abnormal uteroplacental function. Poor control of diabetes, significant hypertension, or suspicion of fetal jeopardy demands early hospitalization. Brigham and Women's Hospital experience shows that diabetic gravidas with superb control of capillary blood glucose in the third trimester are at very low risk for antepartum fetal distress. However, from 36 weeks on they visit the clinic biweekly to assess results of home blood glucose monitoring and nonstress tests.

TIMING AND ROUTE OF DELIVERY

The incidence of stillbirths in diabetic pregnancy increases as gestation extends beyond 36 weeks. On the other hand, the benefits of premature delivery must be weighed against the risks of respiratory distress syndrome. The obstetrician usually faces the problem of identifying the infant at risk of dying before delivery and the infant too immature to survive in an extrauterine environment. At present, most obstetricians individualize the timing of delivery based on various assessments of fetoplacental function as well as fetal lung maturity.

Termination of pregnancy in normal circumstances is considered at 38 weeks or after, in order to reduce neonatal morbidity from preterm deliveries. Before delivery, lecithin-sphingomyelin (L-S) ratio is obtained by amniocentesis. According to our experience, the incidence of severe RDS with an L-S ratio of 3.5 is minimal. Other amniotic fluid assays such as saturated phosphatidylcholine, phosphatidylglycerol, or the so-called "foam test" are being evaluated for greater diagnostic specificity. Route of delivery depends on the usual obstetric indications. A large fetus (4300 g, 9.5 lb) dictates delivery by cesarean section because of the possibility of shoulder dystocia. On the other hand, if the cervix and pelvis seem favorable, the induction of labor can be planned for vaginal delivery. The insertion of lamineria the night before anticipated delivery can serve to ripen a cervix that is unfavorable for induction. Continuous fetal heart rate monitoring with an internal electrode and scalp pH back-up is used routinely during labor. A high incidence of intrapartum fetal distress occurs in diabetic pregnancies. If progress of cervical effacement and dilation is minimal on the first day, a "stage induction" is performed. Beta-mimetic drugs used to arrest premature labor have a potential hyperglycemic effect in diabetic subjects. Severely uncontrolled diabetes can develop within a few hours of starting treatment, leading to a substantial increase in insulin requirement. The continuous intravenous administration of low doses of regular insulin can effectively prevent the problem of hyperglycemia.

GLUCOSE AND INSULIN THERAPY DURING LABOR OR PRIOR TO CESAREAN SECTION

The intrapartum period requires rigid control of diabetes, for maternal hypoglycemia may interfere with the progress of labor while hyperglycemia might increase the chances of fetal distress. Well-planned insulin management for labor and delivery consists of administering only one third to one half the prepregnancy dose in the morning because sensitivity to insulin increases after delivery, and insulin shock may develop if delivery occurs earlier than anticipated. West and Lowry described an infusion of low-dose intravenous insulin and glucose during labor.[16] In their study, patients received a normal dose of insulin on the day before delivery and began fasting after 10 PM. The next morning patients were given 1 liter of 5-percent dextrose every 6 hours together with actrapid insulin, usually 1 to 2 units per hour. The insulin infusion was adjusted to maintain blood glucose concentrations between 90 and 125 mg per dl. None of the neonates developed hypoglycemia. Soler and Malins also achieved good metabolic control of both mothers and babies by the use of a standard dose of intermediate-acting insulin (24 units in patients who had required more than 60 units per day in the third trimester and 16 units for women needing less than 60 units per day).[17] During labor, they infused 200 ml of 5-percent dextrose (10 g glucose) hourly. This regimen proved very successful when the fasting blood glucose level was less than 100 mg per dl on the day of induction. They recommended an intravenous infusion of insulin during labor for management of higher fasting blood glucose levels. Jovanovich and coworkers studied glucose and insulin requirements during induction of labor in 10 previously well-controlled insulin-dependent women.[18] These investigators maintained the blood glucose concentration in the range of 70 to 90 mg per dl by placing an external monitor connected to the biostator on all patients and infusing glucose (5-percent dextrose with Ringer's lactate) at a rate of 150 ml per hour. Normoglycemia persisted during the administration of 7.5 g per hour of dextrose, and no patient required intrapartum insulin. Our protocol for administration of insulin during labor varies according to the fasting blood glucose. If fasting blood glucose levels are less than 120 mg per dl, we administer one third the pregnancy daily dose as intermediate insulin, and measure capillary blood glucose every 1 to 2 hours during labor. If capillary blood glucose levels subsequently exceed 120 mg per dl during labor, the patient receives an intravenous infusion of 0.5 to 2.0 units of regular insulin per hour. If the original fasting blood glucose levels exceed 120 mg per dl, we infuse insulin intravenously from the very beginning. We withhold insulin until after surgery for patients having cesarean sections early in the morning but follow the protocol for labor for those planned later in the day.

Anesthetic Management

Ideal anesthetic management of diabetic parturients requires an understanding of the important pathophysiologic changes associated with diabetic pregnancy.

MATERNAL FACTORS

Placental abnormalities occur even in association with mild, well-controlled gestational diabetes. Nylund and associates compared uteroplacental blood flow index in the last trimester of pregnancy in 26 women with diabetes mellitus to that of 41 healthy parturients.[19] They recorded radiation over the placentas of diabetic parturients with a computer-linked gamma camera after injecting intravenous indium-113m. and noted a decrease of 35 to 45 percent in uteroplacental blood flow index. Interestingly, blood flow index tended to be further impaired in those diabetic women who had higher blood glucose values. However, the reduction in the blood flow index in gestational diabetes did not differ statistically from that in severe diabetes. Bjork and Persson observed that enlarged villi increase the density of the diabetic placenta and can compromise uteroplacental blood flow by reducing the intervillous space.[20] These changes in placental perfusion render the infants of diabetic parturients more vulnerable to decrease in placental blood flow.

Hemoglobin A_{1C} measures two to three times higher in insulin-treated diabetics than in control subjects.[21] Glucose enters the internal cavity of Hb A_{1C} as it binds covalently to the two beta chains, preventing the approximation of the H-helices to each other. This movement represents a normal allosteric response of the hemoglobin molecule for oxygen loading. In contrast to hemoglobin A, the in vitro addition of 2,3-diphosphoglycerate (2,3-DPG) minimally affects the oxygen affinity of Hb A_{1C}, for the presence of a hexose on the N-terminal residues of Hb A_{1C} impairs the binding of 2,3-DPG to hemoglobin. Madsen and Ditzel observed that insulin-dependent patients demonstrate impaired red blood cell oxygen transport, saturation, and oxygen tension.[22] Those with higher concentrations of Hb A_{1C} and lower levels of 2,3-DPG may release oxygen at the tissue level even less efficiently.

FETAL FACTORS

In 1981, Brouillard and coworkers observed an interesting phenomenon which suggests that the infants of diabetic mothers have decreased buffering capacity, causing them to respond differently to an increased acid load.[23] Hemoglobin of infants of diabetic mothers has an increased affinity for oxygen. The P50 (mmHg) values were significantly less in infants of diabetic mothers when compared to control infants (17.9 vs. 22.6 mmHg). Normally, as blood levels of carbon dioxide and fixed acid increase, oxyhemoglobin affinity decreases, oxygen leaves the hemoglobin complex, and the amount of reduced hemoglobin increases and becomes available for buffering. The principle is called the "Bohr effect." When blood levels of carbon dioxide or fixed acid decrease, oxyhemoglobin affinity increases, thus, more hemoglobin becomes available for binding with oxygen because of the hydrogen release. This mechanism is the "Haldane effect." The higher intracellular pH values noted in the infants of diabetic mothers correlate with the higher oxyhemoglobin affinity which also occurs in the neonate. These multiple phenomena render the infants of diabetic mothers more vulnerable to hypoxia and mandate careful anesthesia management.

LABOR AND DELIVERY

During labor and vaginal delivery, small doses of narcotics provide moderate pain relief early in the first stage of labor. The principal risks of larger doses of systemic medication include maternal and neonatal respiratory depression. Prolonged labor and decreased placental perfusion, caused by altered maternal hemodynamics following intravenous narcotics administration, may result in fetal acidosis. The development of fetal acidosis can significantly affect placental transfer of the drugs, interfere with perinatal homeostasis, and ultimately potentiate the depressant effects of these drugs. Natural childbirth may also interfere with placental perfusion, causing fetal acidosis if pain and anxiety significantly elevate maternal catecholamine levels. Paracervical block can cause fetal hypoxia due to umbilical and uterine arterial vasoconstriction. Reduced placental perfusion affects infants of diabetic mothers more adversely since they display greater vulnerability to hypoxia. Lumbar epidural block offers excellent pain relief both for labor and delivery. Pearson noted that fetuses commenced the second stage in a less acidotic state when their mothers received epidural anesthesia as compared to those whose mothers did not receive major nerve conduction anesthesia.[24] The acidosis, metabolic in origin, related to high lactate concentrations. In 1980, Shnider and associates observed that epidural anesthesia reduces maternal endogenous catecholamines during labor; this might enhance placental perfusion, an important advantage in this special group of patients.[25] Patients who have not received an epidural and who require a forceps delivery can benefit from spinal anesthesia, which nicely relaxes the perineum and, so, reduces the likelihood of birth trauma. This is especially important for delivery of a large baby. One must remember to use a separate intravenous line for the rapid infusion of a nondextrose solution to prevent, and when needed to treat, hypotension, as the infants of diabetic mothers are highly susceptible to hypoxia during maternal hypotension.

CESAREAN SECTION

Anesthesia for abdominal delivery requires special attention for diabetic parturients. Cardiovascular depression with associated hypotension occurs more often during regional anesthesia than during vaginal delivery because of the higher sympathetic blockade produced. Compression of the inferior vena cava and aorta by the gravid uterus accentuates the problem of hypotension by decreasing venous return and lowering uterine blood flow. In 1977, Datta and Brown compared spinal and general anesthesia for cesarean section in healthy mothers and diabetic parturients.[26] Infants of diabetic mothers who received spinal anesthesia demonstrated more acidosis than infants of diabetic mothers who received spinal anesthesia. The acidosis appeared to be related to both maternal diabetes and maternal hypotension. Subsequently, we examined maternal and neonatal acid-base values after administering epidural anesthesia to this special group of parturients[27] and noted a 60-percent incidence of neonatal acidosis (umbilical artery pH, ≤ 7.20). The fetal acidosis related to both the severity of maternal diabetes and the presence of maternal hypotension. The umbilical artery pH was exceeded 7.20 in the absence of maternal hypotension. We used 5-percent dextrose with lactated Ringer's solution for acute volume expansion in both studies.

The factors responsible for fetal acidosis in diabetic parturients remain unclear; however, several mechanisms might be involved. The human placenta in vitro produces lactate, especially under conditions of hypoxia in the presence of increased glycogen deposition, as occurs in maternal diabetes.[28] The glycogen-rich placenta of a diabetic parturient might contribute lactate to fetal blood under conditions of relative hypoxia, such as decreased uterine blood flow, which may happen during hypotension.

In human pregnancies, associations have been reported between elevated fetal blood glucose levels and acidosis at birth. Swanstrom and Bratteby observed a significant correlation between blood glucose concentration and base deficit in infants with low 1-minute Apgar scores.[29] In a randomized controlled study of maternal intravenous fluid administration with or without dextrose in healthy patients who have cesarean section, Kenepp and coworkers found significantly lower umbilical artery pH values in glucose-loaded infants. Hypoxia following maternal hypotension might cause fetal lactic acidemia in the presence of hyperglycemia after acute volume loading with dextrose-containing solutions.[30] To test this possibility Kitzmiller and coworkers observed the effect of acute hyperglycemia on monkey fetuses subjected to acute maternal hypoxia.[31] Hyperglycemic fetuses exhibited: greater reduction in arterial oxygen tension and content than normoglycemic controls, despite similar maternal arterial oxygen partial pressure in each group, and severe metabolic acidosis (compared with a modest reduction of arterial pH in normoglycemic fetuses). Carson and associates observed that chronic infusion of insulin directly into the sheep fetus increased fetal glucose uptake and oxidative utilization of glucose and, surprisingly, reduced arterial oxygen content.[32] The authors hypothesized that hyperinsulinemia can increase oxygen consumption and that fetal hyperglycemia and hyperinsulinemia might result in reduced fetal oxygenation in pregnancies complicated by uncontrolled diabetes. Datta and colleagues recently re-evaluated acid-base status in 10 rigidly controlled insulin-dependent diabetic mothers and in 10 healthy nondiabetic control women, all having spinal anesthesia for cesarean section.[33] We employed dextrose-free intravenous solutions for volume expansion before induction of anesthesia, and prevented hypotension in all cases by prompt treatment with ephedrine. No significant differences evolved in acid-base values between the diabetic and nondiabetic mothers, or between infants of diabetic and control subjects (Table 20–1). We concluded that: (1) if maternal diabetes is well controlled, dextrose-containing solutions for maternal volume expansion are avoided, and (2) if maternal hypotension is prevented, spinal anesthesia can be used safely for diabetic mothers having cesarean section. Neonatal hypoglycemia signifies an additional risk of maternal and fetal hyperglycemia accompanying acute volume expansion with dextrose-containing solutions before cesarean section in diabetic parturients. Soler and Malins reported an incidence of over 40 percent in their studies when the mean maternal blood glucose at delivery exceeded 130 mg per dl.[34] Although theoretical, an advantage of epidural anesthesia for cesarean section may be related to the better regulation of glucose homeostasis.[35] This might be due to less increase in the plasma catecholamine and serum cortisol concentrations during epidural anesthesia when compared to general anesthesia. Finally, anesthesiologists should remember that the "stiff-joint syndrome"—a rare condition consisting of juvenile-onset diabetes, nonfamiliar short stature, and joint contractures—increases the risk of difficult tracheal intubation.

In summary, properly administered regional or general anesthesia should provide good maternal and fetal outcome. After delivery, insulin management must be carefully regulated. Lev-Ran noted a drop of insulin requirement to zero for 1 to 2 days in 11 of 12 patients undergoing cesarean section. Hypoglycemia appeared in three of these eleven.[37] A steep rise in blood glucose levels followed this temporary drop in insulin requirement.

Newborn Resuscitation

A neonatologist should attend both vaginal and abdominal deliveries of infants of diabetic parturients, and birth should take place in a hospital with access to facilities for neonatal intensive care. Infants of diabetic mothers have an increased risk of respiratory distress syndrome (RDS). However in recent years the incidence of RDS has declined throughout the country. Serious RDS has to be differentiated from milder and more transient (48 hours) tachypnea of the newborn (TTN), which may be due to retained fetal lung fluid. The diagnosis of RDS is made mainly by: (1) clinical signs including grunting, retractions, and a respiratory rate of more than 60 per minute, (2) a roentgen finding of diffuse reticulogranular patterns, and (3) an increased oxygen requirement to maintain PaO_2 at 50 to 70 mmHg for more than 48 hours with no other causes of respiratory problems. With the advent of modern ventilatory support, including high-frequency ventilation, the survival rate of RDS infants has increased dramatically.

Table 20–1. ACID-BASE AND BLOOD GAS DATA

	Diabetic* (N = 10)	Control* (N = 10)
Maternal artery		
pH	7.40 ± 0.006	7.42 ± 0.01
PO_2 (mmHg)	205 ± 8	200 ± 9
PCO_2 (mmHg)	33 ± 1	33 ± 2
Base deficit (mEq/liter)	2.7 ± 0.5	1.3 ± 0.6
Umbilical artery		
pH	7.27 ± 0.01	7.30 ± 0.01
PO_2 (mmHg)	20 ± 2	22 ± 2
PCO_2 (mmHg)	56 ± 2	50 ± 2.5
Base deficit (mEq/liter)	4 ± 1	3 ± 0.7
Transplacental base deficit difference†	1.4 ± 1	1.7 ± 0.3

*Values are means ±SE

†Transplacental base deficit difference = umbilical arterial base deficit − maternal arterial base deficit

High hematocrit poses another problem for the infant of a diabetic mother. If extreme, this condition can produce thrombosis, especially in the renal veins. Hyperbilirubinemia and hypocalcemia can also develop more frequently in these infants. The high incidence of complex congenital anomalies remains a major problem because these defects require a multitude of therapies.

Summary

Metabolic changes which take place during pregnancy can affect the well-being of the diabetic parturient and her baby. Uncontrolled diabetes with unstable blood glucose concentrations can increase the incidence of ketoacidosis. Material ketoacidosis, major congenital anomalies, prematurity, the respiratory distress syndrome, macrosomia, birth trauma, and neonatal hypoglycemia all contribute to fetal morbidity and mortality. A strict control of maternal blood glucose is mandatory throughout gestation as well as during labor and delivery. For the anesthesiologists the preservation of uteroplacental blood flow remains the most important task. Epidural anesthesia offers several major advantages for the management of labor and delivery and is also associated with good neonatal outcome. For cesarean section a properly managed general or regional anesthesia should be associated with optimal maternal and neonatal conditions. A neonatologist should be in the delivery room during both vaginal and abdominal deliveries to take care of these high-risk neonates.

References

1. Adashi, EY, Pinto, H and Tyson, JE: Impact of maternal euglycemia on fetal outcome in diabetic pregnancy. Am J Obstet Gynecol 74:133, 1979.
2. Kitzmiller, JL: The endocrine pancreas and maternal metabolism. In Tulchinsky, DT and Ryan, KJ (eds): Maternal-Fetal Endocrinology. WB Saunders, Philadelphia, 1980, p 56.
3. Tyson, JE and Felig, P: Medical aspects of diabetes in pregnancy and the diabetogenic effects of oral contraceptives. Med Clin North Am 55:947, 1971.
4. Puavilai G, et al: Insulin receptors and insulin resistance in human pregnancy: Evidence for a postreceptor defect in insulin action. J Clin Endocrinol Metab 21:507, 1972.
5. Knopp, RH, et al: Metabolic adjustments in normal and diabetic pregnancy. Clin Obstet Gynecol 24:21, 1981.
6. Rudolf, MC and Sherwin, RS: Maternal ketosis and its effects on the fetus. Clin Endocrinol Metals 12:417, 1981.
7. Kim, YJ and Felig P: Maternal and amniotic fluid substrate levels during calorie deprivation in human pregnancy. Metabolism 21:507, 1972.
8. Seeds AE, et al: Changes in amniotic fluid glucose, β-hydroxybutarate, glycerol and lactate concentration in diabetic pregnancy. Am J Obstet Gynecol 135:887, 1979.
9. Patterson, P, et al: Maternal and fetal ketone concentrations in plasma and urine. Lancet 1:862, 1967.
10. Felig, P: Pregnancy and diabetes: The endocrine pancreas: diabetes mellitus. In Felig, P, Baxter, JD, Broadus, AE and Frohman, LA (eds): Endocrinology and Metabolism. McGraw-Hill, New York, 1980, pp 853–859.
11. Miodovnik, M, et al: Effects of maternal ketoacidemia on the pregnant ewe and her fetus. Am J Obstet Gynecol 144:585, 1982.
12. Miodovnik, M, et al: Effect of maternal hyperketonemia in hyperglycemic pregnant ewes and their fetuses. Am J Obstet Gynecol 154:394, 1986.
13. Pedersen, J and Osler, M: Hyperglycemia as the cause of characteristic features of the fetus and newborn of diabetic mothers. Dan Med Bull 8:78, 1961.
14. Karlsson, K and Kjellmer, I: The outcome of diabetic pregnancies in relation to the mother's blood sugar level. Am J Obstet Gynecol 112:213, 1972.
15. O'Sullivan, JB, Mahan, CM and Charles D: Screening criteria for high risk gestational diabetic patients. Am J Obstet Gynecol 116:895, 1973.
16. West, TET and Lowy C: Control of blood glucose during labor in diabetic women with combined glucose and low dose insulin infusion. Br Med J 1:1252, 1977.
17. Soler, NG and Malins, JM: Diabetic pregnancy: Management of diabetes on the day of delivery. Diabetologia 15:441, 1978.
18. Jovanovic, L and Peterson, CM: Insulin and glucose requirements during the first stage of labor in insulin-dependent diabetic women. Am J Med 75:607, 1983.
19. Nylund, L, Lunnel, NO and Lew, AR: Utero placental blood flow in diabetic pregnancy: Measurements with indium-113 m and a computer linked gamma camera. Am J Obstet Gynecol 144:298, 1982.
20. Bjork, O and Persson, B: Placental changes in relation to the degree of metabolic control in diabetes mellitus. Placenta 3:367, 1982.
21. Trivelli, LA, Ranney, HM and Lai, HT: Hemoglobin components in patients with diabetes mellitus. N Engl J Med 284:353, 1971.
22. Madsen, H and Ditzel, J: Changes in red blood cell oxygen transport in diabetic pregnancy. Am J Obstet Gynecol 143:421, 1982.
23. Broulliard, RG, Kitzmiller, JL and Datta S: Buffering capacity and oxyhemoglobin affinity in infants of diabetic mothers. Anesthesiology 55:A318, 1981.
24. Pearson, JF: The effects of continuous lumbar epidural block on maternal and fetal acid-base balance during labor and delivery. In Proceedings of the Sym-

posium on Epidural Analgesia in Obstetrics. HK Lewis, London, 1968, p 26.
25. Shnider, SM, et al: Maternal endogenous catecholamine decrease during labor after epidural anesthesia. Am J Obstet Gynecol 147:13, 1983.
26. Datta, S and Brown, WV: Acid-base status in diabetic mothers and their infants following general or spinal anesthesia for cesarean section. Anesthesiology 47:272, 1977.
27. Datta, S, et al: Epidural anesthesia for cesarean section in diabetic parturients: Maternal and neonatal acid-base status and bupivacaine concentration. Anesth Analg 60:574, 1981.
28. Gabbe, SG, Deiner, DLM and Greep, RO: The effects of hypoxia on placental glycogen metabolism. Am J Obstet Gynecol 114:540, 1972.
29. Swanstrom, S and Bratteby, LE: Metabolic effects of obstetric regional analgesia and of asphyxia in the newborn infant during the first two hours after birth. Acta Paediatr Scand 70:791, 1981.
30. Kenepp, NB, et al: Effects on newborn of hydration with glucose in patients undergoing cesarean section with regional anesthesia. Lancet 1:1150, 1980.
31. Kitzmiller, JL, et al: Hyperglycemia hypoxia and fetal acidosis in rhesus monkey. Abstracts of the Proceeding of the Society of Gynecological Investigation. BR 1981, p 45.
32. Carson, BS, et al: Effects of a sustained insulin infusion upon glucose uptake and oxygenation of the ovine fetus. Pediatr Res 14:147, 1980.
33. Datta, S, et al: Acid-base status of diabetic mothers and their infants following spinal anesthesia for cesarean section. Anesth Analg 61:662, 1982.
34. Soler, NG and Malins, JM: Diabetic pregnancy: Management of diabetes on the day of delivery. Diabetologia 15:441, 1978.
35. Lund, L, et al: Effects of extradural analgesia on glucose metabolism and gluconeogenesis, studies in association with upper abdominal surgery. Br J Anaesth 58:851, 1986.
36. Salzarulo, HH and Taylor LA: Diabetic "stiff joint syndrome" as a cause of difficult endotracheal intubation. Anesthesiology 3:366, 1986.
37. Lev-Ran A: Sharp temporary drop in insulin requirement after cesarean section in diabetic patients. Am J Obstet Gynecol 120:905, 1974.

CHAPTER 21

PREGNANCY-INDUCED HYPERTENSION

FRANCIS M. JAMES III, M.D.

Pregnancy-induced hypertension (PIH) develops in 5 to 10 percent of pregnancies[1] and progresses to eclampsia in 0.05 to 0.2 percent of all deliveries.[2] The American College of Obstetricians and Gynecologists recognizes four categories of hypertension associated with pregnancy: pre-eclampsia and eclampsia (PIH), chronic hypertension, chronic hypertension with superimposed pre-eclampsia, and late or transient hypertension.[1] Clinicians have difficulty distinguishing between pre-eclampsia, essential or secondary hypertension, renal disease, and combinations of these entities. Renal biopsies have proved the clinical impression of pre-eclampsia wrong in about 15 percent of nulliparas and 50 percent of multiparas and detected unsuspected renal disease in 10 to 20 percent of cases.[1] Pre-eclampsia falls into two categories: (1) gestational hypertension limited to blood pressure levels of either ≥140/90 mmHg noted on two occasions at least 6 hours apart or an increase of 30 mmHg systolic or 15 mmHg diastolic above nonpregnant levels and (2) pre-eclampsia consisting of at least two of three possible conditions—hypertension, proteinuria, and edema. Any of the following criteria qualifies pre-eclampsia as severe: systolic blood pressure ≥160 mmHg or diastolic pressure ≥110 mmHg on at least two occasions more than 6 hours apart; poteinuria of ≥5 g per 24 hours; oliguria (≤400 ml per 24 hours); cerebral or visual disturbances, or cyanosis. Pre-eclampsia progresses to eclampsia when seizures occur. Pre-eclampsia occurs after the 20th week of gestation but can develop earlier with trophoblastic disease.[3]

PIH, hemorrhage, and infection are the leading causes of maternal mortality[3] with pre-eclampsia and eclampsia possibly accounting for 40 percent of obstetric-related maternal deaths.[4] Table 21–1 depicts the leading causes of maternal death. Perinatal mortality in pre-eclampsia more than doubles that of normotensive gestation and increases with the severity of maternal hypertension.[3] Placental infarcts, growth retardation, and abruption provoke most fetal deaths.

Etiology

Science has not unraveled the etiology of PIH. Wormlike organisms observed in peripheral

Table 21-1. ETIOLOGY OF MATERNAL DEATH IN PIH

Cause of Death	% of Deaths
Cerebral hemorrhage	30–40
Pulmonary edema/congestive heart failure	33–38
Cerebral edema	19
Hepatic coma	15
Renal failure	10
Intravascular coagulation	9
Airway obstruction	6

(From Wright, JP,[3] with permission.)

blood and the placental surface of women with PIH[5] represented a possible explanation until a subsequent study identified them as artifacts.[6] Hereditary and acquired immune factors may play a role.[7,8] One intriguing theory involving angiotensin II (A II) and prostaglandin E_2 (PGE_2) hypothesizes that, in normal pregnancy, the fetus governs placental blood flow by local and distal effects on the maternal vascular tree.[9] In the placental bed, the local release of A II, the most potent vasoconstrictor peptide known, promotes uteroplacental blood flow by stimulating the release of PGE_2, a vasodilator, while the release of A II into the maternal circulation raises systemic blood pressure, thus enhancing placental perfusion. Decreased PGE_2 production or excessive A II levels would constrict the uteroplacental circulation, causing maternal blood pressure to rise, thereby provoking the "cascade of events which only the termination of pregnancy breaks."[10] The sequence of causative events would continue, with reduced uteroplacental circulation associated with vasoconstriction, which damages the placenta, and release of placental trophoblasts into the circulation, which precipitates disseminated intravascular coagulation (DIC), fibrin deposition, glomerular endothelial lesions, reduced glomerular filtration rate (GFR), sodium retention, and intracellular sodium shifts with reduced plasma volume and further compromised placental perfusion. Fibrin deposition probably follows both increased fibrin production and impaired removal of fibrin by decreased fibrinolytic activity, while an array of potential vasoactive peptides might account for the humoral induction of vasospasm.[9] The response to A II decreases markedly in normal pregnancy, but increases in PIH by the 18th week of gestation,[11] before hypertension develops. Angiotensin-converting enzyme (ACE), responsible for converting angiotensin I to A II, appears to increase in PIH at about the same time the clinical disease manifests itself.[12] The local vasodilator activity of PGE_2 may negate the vasoconstrictive effect of A II in normal pregnancies.

During normal pregnancy, rising maternal and fetal blood levels of prostaglandin I_2 (PGI_2, prostacyclin)[13] produce vasodilation, decreased platelet adhesiveness, and prevention of fibrin deposition.[12] Reduced PGI_2 in PIH creates a relative imbalance with increased thromboxane A_2 (TxA_2). TxA_2 released from platelets exerts opposing effects to PGI_2, causing vasoconstriction, platelet adhesiveness, and fibrin deposition.[12] A deficiency of PGI_2 in maternal and/or fetal vasculature may relate to the occurrence of PIH; evidence suggests that umbilical PGI_2 deficiency is a specific feature of PIH.[14]

Pathophysiology

MATERNAL

Blood Volume and Hemodynamics

The pathophysiology of PIH involves numerous maternal organ systems plus the uteroplacental-fetal unit. Hypovolemia often coexists with increased total body water. Chesley[15] concluded that the mean blood volume decrease of 9 percent occurring in pre-eclampsia still represented a blood volume greatly exceeding that of nonpregnant women. In severe PIH, blood volume may contract by 30 to 40 percent.[3] Arteriolar vasoconstriction diminishes the intravascular space. The low central venous pressure accompanying pre-eclampsia varies inversely with the severity of hypertension.[16] Increased vascular permeability fosters the loss of fluid and protein from the intravascular space, thereby contributing to hypovolemia and hypoproteinemia. Fluid shifts from intravascular to extravascular spaces may disguise a decreased circulating red cell mass by generating a deceptively normal or elevated hematocrit. The interstitial accumulation of water and sodium exceeds that of normal pregnancy. An increased capacity for tubular reabsorption together with the impaired ability to excrete sodium probably causes that ion's retention. PGE_2 possesses both vasodilator and natriuretic effects. The lower renal PGE_2 and/or PGI_2 levels noted in PIH could explain the triad of decreased renal blood flow (RBF), GFR, and sodium excretion.[13]

The contracted plasma volume accompanied by sodium retention in pre-eclampsia provokes a major controversy about management involving two conflicting beliefs.[1] One theory holds that decreased intravascular volume represents a primary event and produces the rise in blood pressure. Placental hypoperfusion causing the release of a uterine pressor substance or relative hypovolemia stimulating excess secretion of catecholamines represent two mechanisms by which hypovolemia might elevate blood pressure. Physicians who adhere to this first theory employ intravascular expansion as a method of treatment and avoid diuretics. The second theory postulates that vasoconstriction precedes hypovolemia, and its advocates recommend the use of diuretics in conjunction with vasodilating drugs, warning that volume expansion may aggravate hypertension or produce pulmonary edema.[1] The literature supports the first theory, for hypovolemia appears to precede the occurrence of hypertension.[1] Whatever the cause, generalized arteriolar spasm characterizes PIH.[17] Increased sodium in vascular walls heightens vascular reactivity, inducing vasospasm with underlying degrees of tissue hypoxia.[10] Isolated human omental vessels in pre-eclamptics have an increased ratio of media thickness-to-lumen diameter and demonstrate an exaggerated response to A II together with a decreased rate of relaxation. These functional responses suggest the absence of a change in vascular function which normally occurs during pregnancy.[18] Increased systemic vascular resistance (SVR) in the presence of PIH places greater demands on the heart than in normal pregnancy. SVR may reach an average of 1709 dynes per sec per cm^{-5}.[19]

One cannot classify all patients with severe PIH under one diagnostic "umbrella," for hemodynamic manifestations vary.[20] The differences probably relate to the degree of hypertension. With early hypertension in nonpregnant patients, cardiac output (CO) increases while SVR remains unchanged or falls. As hypertension progresses, CO declines in response to increasing SVR. Total blood volume decreases in conjunction with these changes. The pattern in PIH appears similar. The cardiovascular hemodynamics represent a spectrum from high CO and low SVR to low CO and high SVR.[20] Studies[20–23] show that most patients with severe PIH have hyperdynamic cardiac function (Fig. 21 – 1). Using echocardiography to calculate CO, Kuzniar and coworkers[24] compared the hemodynamic profiles of 20 women with gestational hypertension with those of 47 normal pregnant women matched for gestational age. The hypertensive group exhibited an increase of heart rate, stroke volume, and CO; this pattern resembles that noted in early forms of essential hypertension. These findings support the theory that gestational hypertension may represent latent essential hypertension, for women with gestational hypertension more frequently develop hypertension 3 to 6 years after pregnancy than women with normal pregnancies or with pre-eclampsia/eclampsia.[24] The increase in CO which usually takes place early in the puerperium does not occur in patients with severe pre-eclampsia. The contracted blood volume combined with the excessive blood loss at delivery in pre-eclamptics may account for this phenomenon.[21] An average loss of 1000 ml can occur with vaginal delivery.[25]

Pulmonary Artery Measurements

Neither Benedetti and coworkers[21] nor Clark[26] noted pulmonary artery pressures significantly different from those observed in normal pregnancy (mean about 10 mmHg) or in nonpregnant women. Therefore, the primary vasospastic process of severe PIH spares the pulmonary vasculature.[22] Pulmonary artery catheterization fails to detect any difference in systemic or pulmonary vascular resistance, cardiac index (CI), left ventricular stroke work index (LVSWI), or any other hemodynamic parameter between eclamptics and pre-eclamptics.[27] In 25 percent of pre-eclamptics, marked discrepancies exist between right and left ventricular preload as assessed by simultaneous measurements of central venous pressure (CVP) and pulmonary capillary wedge pressure (PCWP). Hence, pulmonary artery catheters prove useful in managing patients with low urinary output or cardiac failure. Following delivery, women with severe

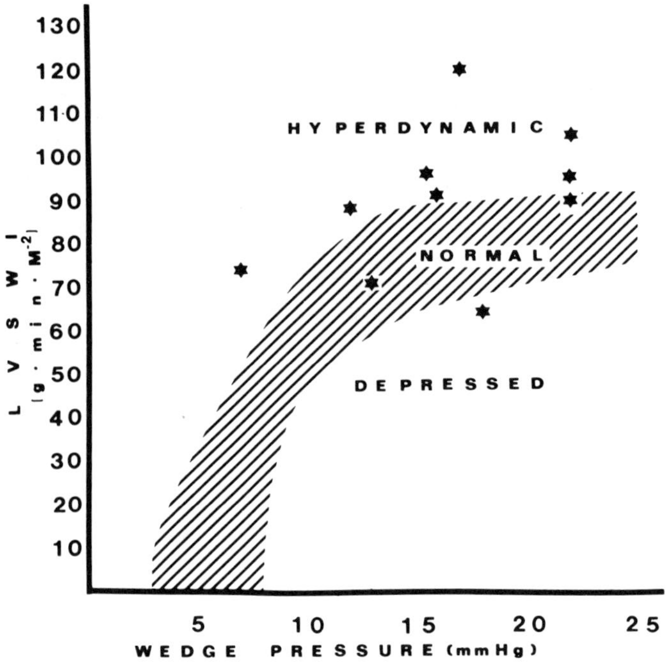

Figure 21–1. Ventricular function measurement (left ventricular stroke work index [LVSWI] versus wedge pressure) in 10 patients with severe pre-eclampsia. (From Phelan, JP and Yurth, DA: Severe pre-eclampsia. I: Peripartum hemodynamic observations. Am J Obstet Gynecol 144:17, 1982, with permission.)

pre-eclampsia may experience an increase in PCWP, which reflects an increase in circulating blood volume rather than left ventricular failure.[22] Cardiomyopathy can occur but does not usually contribute to the postpartum increase in PCWP.[22]

Renal Changes

Both effective renal blood flow (ERBF) and glomerular filtration rate (GFR) decrease in PIH. Specific renal lesions include swelling of glomerular endothelial cells to the extent of greatly compromising capillary lumina. Morris[28] detected fibrinoid material deposited between the swollen endothelial cells along the basement membrane. The severity of PIH relates to the extent of the glomerular lesion and proteinuria.[29] Electron microscopy and renal biopsy unveil a distinct pattern of intracapillary vacuolization and cell swelling. The extent of glomerular capillary endotheliosis correlates with the amount of proteinuria and not with the degree of hypertension.[30] The selectivity of the glomerulus to the passage of protein macromolecules measures the degree of capillary damage. A disproportionate loss of large proteins signifies poor selectivity, while highly selective proteinuria primarily consists of small and intermediate-sized molecules. High glomerular selectivity occurs with mild PIH while increasingly poor selectivity typifies moderate to severe disease.[29] Additional renal changes include juxtaglomerular cell hyperplasia, localized degeneration of tubular epithelium of the loop of Henle, and afferent arteriolar spasm. These lesions account for the decrease in glomerular filtration and renal plasma flow. Urea clearance falls to 50 to 70 percent that of normal gravidas. Urinary protein loss may increase from 300 to 400 mg per 24 hours in normal pregnancy to more than 5 g daily in severe pre-eclampsia.

Altered sodium and uric acid excretion often characterize PIH.[31] Both decreased GFR and increased tubular reabsorption account for the compromised ability to excrete sodium.[32] Serum uric acid provides an excellent guide to the severity of PIH.[33,34] The increased renal clearance of uric acid in pregnancy lowers uric acid levels to 3.0 to 3.5 mg per dl, a range below that of normal nonpregnant women. In mild PIH, uric acid values average 4 mg per dl, climbing to 7.5 mg per dl in severe PIH and eclampsia.

As the severity of PIH increases, renal function falters and daily urine output declines, sometimes progressing to anuria. Rarely do women with PIH develop acute renal failure (ARF), one of the most serious complications of pregnancy. ARF occurs in 1 in 1400 to 1 in 5000 pregnancies.[35] Smith and coworkers[35] noted that 62 percent of 29 patients who developed ARF in late pregnancy were hypertensive. The number of these patients with hypertension prior to pregnancy was not known. Those patients with severe PIH experienced renal failure following either eclamptic seizures or successful induction of labor for severe PIH. Renal ischemia associated with hemorrhagic hypotension represents the most common single factor leading to ARF. PIH increases the likelihood of major hemorrhage and also produces tissue ischemia and even infarction unassociated with hemorrhagic hypotension.[35] Histologic changes in the kidney during ARF vary from almost undetectable alterations to gross bilateral cortical necrosis (Chap. 11).[32,36]

Pulmonary Effects

Templeton and Kelman[37] measured pulmonary function in 31 women with proteinuric pre-eclampsia. In 22 patients with moderate proteinuria (0.25 to 2.0 g per liter), arterial blood gas values, physiologic dead space, or venous admixture (physiologic shunt) were not different from measurements in normal pregnant women. Nine patients with severe pre-eclampsia (proteinuria >2 g per liter) displayed a significant increase in the alveolar-arterial oxygen gradient (A-a PO_2) and physiologic shunt, indicating some ventilation/perfusion mismatch. Leakage of fluid from pulmonary capillaries into the interstitium could account for the shunting.[38] However, none of the nine women with severe pre-eclampsia developed hypoxia, and PaO_2, dead space (V_D), and V_D/V_T were similar in pre-eclamptic and in normal individuals. Littler and coworkers[39] observed a decrease in pulmonary blood flow during PIH. This could explain the increase in A-a PO_2 in the presence of normal whole body oxygen consumption. In severe pre-eclampsia and eclampsia, left ventricular failure or marked hypoalbuminemia or both may produce pulmonary edema. Colloid osmotic pressure (COP) decreases to 18 mmHg and 14 mmHg in the antepartum and postpartum periods, respectively, in women with PIH.[40,41] These values range significantly lower than in normal pregnancy (antepartum 22.0 mmHg, postpartum 17.2 mmHg).[41] Further pulmonary compromise occurs when aspiration of gastric contents complicates eclamptic seizures. Severe PIH may also involve the larynx. Jouppila and others[42] reported two patients with severe PIH and marked generalized edema who had severe laryngeal edema which complicated tracheal intubation.

Coagulation Abnormalities

Debate persists regarding the incidence and significance of coagulation abnormalities. Low platelet count and prolonged thrombin time represent the two most common observations.[3] Increased platelet consumption due to slow disseminated intravascular coagulation (DIC) or adherence to sites of disrupted vascular epithelium explain thrombocytopenia,[3] which develops chronically in pre-eclampsia.[31] In a study of 67 eclamptics, Sibai[43] found no evidence of DIC and no significant difference in platelet count, serum fibrinogen, or bilirubin values in comparison to control subjects. Only one of 67 patients had a platelet count below 100,000 per mm^3; however, 42 percent exhibited increased activated partial thromboplastin times. Other investigators[44] have found a usually mild but at times severe consumptive thrombocytopenia in approximately 20 percent of pre-eclamptics. The platelet count usually ranges from 100,000 to 150,000 per mm^3, denoting a small hemostatic risk. However, abnormal platelet function can occur, since a significant number of pre-eclamptic patients have in vivo and in vitro platelet function defects evidenced by prolonged bleeding times.[44] This acquired platelet dysfunction frequently develops in severe pre-eclampsia and increases the potential for bleeding.

Hepatic Involvement

Physicians rarely appreciate the degree of liver compromise that can take place at both cellular and enzymatic levels. Subcapsular hepatic hemorrhage, swelling, pain, and jaundice may occur. Immunofluorescent techniques reveal fibrinoid deposits in hepatic venous sinusoids.[45] Abnormal liver enzyme levels develop inconstantly in pre-eclampsia and have no established prognostic value.[32] In severe PIH, the presence of ascitic fluid with colloid osmotic pressures of 3 to 12 mmHg hints at possible leakage from the liver and other abdominal viscera.[39] Hepatic hemorrhage rarely occurs, but the inception of computerized axial tomography (CT) has increased the diagnosis of this complication. Symptoms include the abrupt onset of constant acute epigastric and right upper-quadrant pain. Liver function tests show nonspecific changes coinciding with the development of pain, while platelet counts fall in conjunction with a mean decrease in hematocrit of 10.8 percent within several hours of the onset of pain.[46] When hepatic rupture ensues, maternal mortality ranges from 56 to 75 percent and triples in conservatively managed patients as opposed to those undergoing surgery.[46] Surgery may be avoided if the capsule has not torn and the patient receives blood product replacement and careful monitoring. Weinstein[47] reported on the development of a syndrome of hemolysis, elevated liver enzymes, and low platelet count (HELLP) in 57 patients (Table 21–2). Severe hypertension does not always accompany the other changes. MacEnna and coworkers[48] maintain that the syndrome does not represent an entity but rather a cluster of signs seen in some patients with PIH, not necessarily requiring aggressive management and prompt delivery unless associated with rapid maternal or fetal deterioration.

Table 21–2. HELLP ADMISSION FINDINGS

Finding	% of Patients
SGOT ↑	100
SGPT ↑	100
Proteinuria ≥2+	96
Right upper quadrant tenderness on palpation	86
Epigastric pain	86
Nausea with or without vomiting	84
Demonstrable edema	67
Hyperbilirubinemia	62
Creatinine ↑	53
BUN ↑	53

(From Weinstein, L,[47] with permission.)

Central Nervous System

The central nervous system (CNS) is generally edematous, hyperirritable, and more sensitive to all depressant drugs. Convulsions may appear without warning in seemingly stable patients with only minimal hypertension, although most often definite premonitory symptoms and signs do appear.[1] Twenty seven percent of 179 eclamptics observed by Sibai and coworkers[49] experienced their first seizure postpartum. Nearly one half of these had the onset of convulsions more than 48 hours postpartum.

Cerebral blood flow and oxygen consumption remain normal in PIH, indicating that cerebral vascular resistance must increase to maintain normal cerebral blood flow.[32] Intracranial pressure increases in some cases, but cerebral edema is uncommon and probably represents a postmortem change.[32] Cerebral edema may result from anoxia associated with eclamptic seizures, loss of cerebral autoregulation associated with severe hypertension,[38] or low plasma colloid osmotic pressures. Clinical findings include disorientation, headache, amaurosis, and, rarely, papilledema.[50] CT confirmed the presence of occipital lobe edema in a patient who became blind at 36 weeks' gestation prior to convulsing. Vision returned 24 hours postcesarean section and CT confirmed the resolution of cerebral edema.[50] Loss of cerebral autoregulation secondary to hypertension (mean arterial pressure $>$140 mmHg) can also disrupt cerebral capillary integrity.[37] In a study of 533 fatal cases of PIH, cerebral dysfunction accounted for 180 deaths, with gross evidence of intracranial hemorrhage occurring in 17 percent of deaths.[51]

Uterine and Placental Effects

Uterine and placental blood flow decrease in the presence of PIH. Lunell and associates[52] studied intervillous blood flow with an indium. (^{133}In) technique and noted levels 50 percent below those of normal pregnancy in pre-eclampsia with a decrease of up to 70 percent in severe cases. Reasons for decreased uterine blood flow (UBF) include increased vascular resistance, greater vascular activity, decreased plasma volume, and intimal changes which narrow the lumina of placental arteries. A 30-percent increase in blood viscosity may occur by 32 weeks' gestation in pre-eclamptics.[53] Elevation of the fetal hematocrit causes a 13-percent increase in fetal blood viscosity.[53] Vasoconstriction and blood hyperviscosity impair blood flow to all vital organs in pre-eclamptic women.[52] The decreased ability of red blood cells to alter their morphology also compromises both maternal and fetal peripheral blood flow. Premature placental aging may compromise its function, even in gestational hypertension. Placental infarcts develop with underlying occlusion of the uterine spiral arteries by fat-laden cells and fibrin.[54] Uterine hypertonicity and hypercontractility often cause premature labor and precipitous delivery, and aggravate uteroplacental insufficiency. In severe PIH, uterine sensitivity to oxytocin increases.[32] Abruptio placentae seems to occur more frequently in these patients. Pritchard and Bretten[55] noted a 48-percent incidence of hypertension in women with abruptio placentae, an incidence five times greater than that occurring in their pregnant population in general. One half of the hypertensive women had chronic hypertension; the other half had PIH.[55] The link between severe abruption and hypertension appears closer than for lesser degrees of abruption and hypertension.[35] Paterson[56] failed to find a higher incidence of hypertension in patients with abruptio placentae than in the general pregnant population.

PERINATAL

Svenningsen and others[57] looked at a large population of pre-eclamptic women and recorded a 23-percent incidence of intrauterine fetal death in pregnancies complicated by hypertension. In addition, they noted a significantly higher cesarean section rate and lower 1-minute Apgar scores in the pre-eclamptic group. At 2 years of age, the rate of neurodevelopmental handicaps was similar in the study population and in the children of normotensive controls.

The fetus encounters special problems associated with pre-eclampsia—prematurity, placental insufficiency, and placental abruption. Severe intrauterine growth retardation (IUGR; $<$2.5th percentile), hypoglycemia (blood glucose $<$ 30 mg per dl), asphyxia neonatorum, respiratory distress syndrome (RDS), and hyperbilirubinemia ($>$15 mg per dl) occur, in decreasing order of frequency.[58] Intrauterine growth retardation presented in 56.6 percent and hypoglycemia in 24.5 percent of Martin's[58] series of newborns delivered after less than 36 weeks' gestation of mothers with severe PIH. Uteroplacental insufficiency abets IUGR which, in turn, is associated with the high incidence of hypoglycemia.[58] The respiratory distress syndrome, when present, usually appears mild. Chronic stress may stimulate fetal cortisol levels and pulmonary surfactant formation. Accelerated clinical neurologic maturation occurs in association with accelerated fetal lung maturation in some chronically stressed fetuses. The chronicity of the hypertension may prove more important than its severity in accelerated fetal cerebral maturation. Many infants born of mothers with PIH are depressed at the time of birth. The delivery room must have available appropriate personnel and equipment for resuscitation.

Obstetric Management

Obstetric management depends on numerous factors, especially the maternal condition, the ability of the fetus to cope with the intrauterine environment, and the degree of fetal pulmonary maturity. Therapy strives to control maternal hypertension by keeping diastolic pressure below 110 mmHg to decrease central nervous system irritability, to improve renal function, and to assure fetal viability. Termination of pregnancy represents the only definitive remedy. Severe hypertension which persists beyond 24 to 48 hours of therapy calls for delivery of the fetus regardless of gestational age, for further delay rarely saves the fetus and the mother remains at risk.[1] When severe PIH continues, most infants weighing more than 1500 g have a better chance for survival in a neonatal intensive care unit than in utero.[1] Clotting or liver abnormalities, decreasing renal function, and signs of imminent convulsions (epigastric pain, headache, hyperreflexia) are additional indications for termination of pregnancy.[1] If the fetus can benefit by remaining in utero without jeopardizing maternal outcome, the obstetric staff usually allows the pregnancy to continue while working to improve maternal status. An intrauterine environment that threatens fetal viability necessitates delivery.

Mild PIH calls for bed rest, light sedation with

drugs such as diazepam or phenobarbital, and occasionally antihypertensive medication (hydralazine or methyldopa). This condition calls for careful observation of blood pressure, fluid balance, weight change, and CNS irritability.

Patients with more severe PIH usually receive aggressive therapy consisting of anticonvulsants, sedatives, antihypertensive agents, intravascular volume adjustment, and rigorous monitoring.

MAGNESIUM THERAPY

Magnesium sulfate decreases central nervous system irritability and may prevent seizures from occurring. Therapeutic anticonvulsant levels of magnesium range from 4 to 8 mEq per liter.[3,59] Higher blood levels can cause disappearance of deep tendon reflexes (10 mEq per liter), skeletal muscle relaxation (12 mEq per liter), respiratory arrest (15 mEq per liter), and cardiac arrest (30 mEq per liter)[3,32] In addition, magnesium sulfate produces mild sedation and vasodilation and decreases uterine tone and contractility. The anticonvulsant effect does not relate to its neuromuscular activity and probably acts specifically on the cerebral cortex. When given intravenously to monkeys, magnesium suppresses seizure foci experimentally induced by penicillin. Seizure suppression occurs at blood levels below those that cause paralysis and corresponds proportionately to the serum magnesium concentration.[3] Seizures can occur despite magnesium therapy. Up to one third of patients who experience seizures may do so in spite of obstetric care that meets or exceeds all current standards.[60]

Magnesium affects the neuromuscular junction by 1) decreasing the amount of acetylcholine released by the motor nerve terminals, 2) decreasing the depolarizing action of acetylcholine at the motor end-plate, and 3) decreasing the excitability of the muscle fiber membrane. In vitro, it increases the neuromuscular blockade of d-tubocurarine and succinylcholine in both duration and intensity by factors of 4.1 and 1.9, respectively.[3] It also potentiates pancuronium and vecuronium.[59] Fasciculation frequently fails to follow succinylcholine administration in patients receiving magnesium.[61]

When given as an intravenous bolus, magnesium can transiently lower mean arterial blood pressure, primarily by causing peripheral arterial vasodilation. Hypovolemia enhances this response. Intravenous infusion at a rate of 1.0 to 1.5 g per hour rarely lowers the blood pressure.[62] Magnesium may produce vasodilation by decreasing angiotensin converting enzyme (ACE) levels in the arteriolar endothelium.[63] By reducing uterine hypercontractility, magnesium sulfate theoretically improves placental perfusion, permitting better fetal nutrition and oxygenation. In a study of pregnant ewes, Krames and others[64] noted that magnesium sulfate decreased uterine vascular resistance but did not increase uterine blood flow (UBF) because of a concomitant fall in arterial pressure. Magnesium readily crosses the placenta and may cause neonatal hypotonia and respiratory depression.

ANTIHYPERTENSIVE THERAPY

Various physicians dispute the degree of blood pressure reduction needed in PIH, but Lindheimer and associates[1] recommend diastolic levels between 90 and 105 mmHg. Magnesium proves relatively inadequate for blood pressure control, often necessitating oral or parenteral antihypertensive therapy. The α_2-adrenergic agonists, α-methyldopa and clonidine, prove equally effective and safe in counteracting PIH.[65] Alpha-methyldopa may also act through a false transmitter effect. Problems associated with its use include hepatitis, hemolytic anemia, postural hypotension, and sedation.[66] Clonidine slows the heart rate by stimulating the vagal nuclei.[65] Prazosin, a selective α_1 antagonist, reduces both arterial and venous resistance, thus encouraging the pooling of blood in peripheral organs and causing postural hypotension.

Hydralazine

Obstetricians frequently use hydralazine, an arterio-selective dilator causing postural hypotension, to counteract hypertension. Peak effects occur 10 to 20 min after intravenous administration, and significant activity persists for several hours. Smooth muscle relaxation may cause vascular headaches, facial flushing, nausea, and vomiting.[66] Following monitored blood volume expansion, a 10-mg bolus of hydralazine produces a significant increase in heart rate and CI and a decrease in mean arterial pressure

(MAP) and SVR in women with severe PIH. The compensatory tachycardia caused by hydralazine may limit its effectiveness, and sustained, profound hypotension and decreased placental perfusion may occur if hypovolemia has not been corrected.[67] In a study of pregnant ewes,[68] hydralazine increased UBF by decreasing uterine vascular resistance. Following the administration of hydralazine to women with PIH, nondepressed newborns displayed abnormally low blood pressures, a response that could interfere with the conversion to an adult circulatory pattern.[69] Neonatal thrombocytopenia has followed maternal hydralazine therapy as well.[1]

Diazoxide

Obstetricians occasionally employ diazoxide for patients with refractory hypertension. A lower margin of safety and a significant incidence of side effects reduce the usefulness of this potent vasodilator, which may cause profound maternal hypotension. Chesley[32] cautions against its use, citing decreased uterine blood flow and primate studies that reveal fetal tachycardia, acidosis, and prolonged hypotension. Diazoxide may also inhibit labor and cause both maternal and neonatal hyperglycemia.[66] A high incidence of fetal mortality in animal studies has discouraged the use of captopril, an ACE inhibitor, during pregnancy.[66]

Calcium Entry Blockers

These drugs exert an antihypertensive effect by relaxing vascular smooth muscle and thereby decreasing SVR. They may also inhibit uterine contractions. Nifedipine and verapamil prove equally effective in countering norepinephrine-induced hypertension in gravid ewes without adversely affecting UBF or fetal hemodynamics during short-term therapy.[70] Verapamil may prove preferable since it does not cause maternal tachycardia.

Beta-Adrenergic Blockers

These antagonists form a first line of therapy for hypertension and are becoming more important in PIH treatment as well. Increased uterine tone and fetal bradycardia, theoretical problems with β-blocker therapy, have not followed treatment with small doses of propranolol. Cardioselective (β_1) blockers such as metoprolol seem less liable to affect uterine activity, glucose homestasis, and respiration than propranolol, yet they decrease heart rate just as effectively.[66] Reduced heart rate represents an advantage, since tachycardia frequently occurs in PIH. Metoprolol works primarily by altering cardiac dynamics while pindolol, another β-adrenoreceptor blocker, exhibits pronounced intrinsic sympathomimetic activity which stimulates β_2 receptors, promoting vasodilation and decreasing peripheral vascular resistance.[71] Pindolol significantly reduces maternal mean arterial pressure (MAP) without compromising the uteroplacental blood flow index, an effect it shares with metoprolol.[71] Michael, in Australia, has employed the combined alpha/beta-adrenoreceptor blocker labetalol for treatment of PIH.[72] Labetalol may work by inhibiting thromboxane A_2 (TxA_2) or stimulating the vasodilatory action of prostacyclin (PGI_2), but Jouppila and coworkers debate this mechanism.[73] Labetalol, 1 mg per kg, infused intravenously over 10 to 15 min in pre-eclamptic women at 30 to 39 weeks' gestation, reduced maternal blood pressure without compromising placental or fetal blood flow.[73] Van Assche and coworkers[74] first reported the use of a specific TxA_2 blocker, dazoxiben, in PIH in 1984.

Serotonin facilitates platelet aggregation, constricts peripheral vessels, and enhances the vasoconstrictive effect of other neurohumoral mediators. Ketanserin, a highly selective competitive antagonist of serotonin, significantly reduced blood pressures in 20 postpartum women with PIH while causing minimal side effects.[75] No published information exists which describes its antepartum use.

Diuretics

Diuretics, once important drugs in PIH therapy, have become less widely used since they can aggravate hypovolemia, compromise placental perfusion, and produce electrolyte imbalance. During pregnancy, thiazides and loop diuretics now serve primarily for cases of heart failure and fluid overload, in certain cases of hypervolemic hypertension, and occasionally in non-prerenal oliguria. Despite the condemnation of their use, a review of randomized trials of diuretics in PIH uncovered a 33-percent reduction in the incidence of stillbirth.[76] The ability of diuretics to decrease venous tone and to increase venous capacitance may account for this finding.

Other Drugs

Ganglionic blockers, reserpine, and guanethidine have not achieved popularity for long-term treatment of PIH. Trimethaphan reduces both CO and cerebral blood flow (CBF).[77] These effects make it unsuitable for controlling blood pressure in PIH. Reserpine increases tracheal/bronchial secretions in the newborn.[66]

MONITORING

Monitoring requirements depend upon the severity of PIH. Noninvasive blood pressure monitoring and a Foley catheter for urine output determination suffice in mild to moderate PIH. Severe PIH requires an arterial cannula for continuous blood pressure measurement and a central venous catheter for central venous pressure (CVP) monitoring. The problems of assessing central volume status, the prospect of pulmonary edema, and the presence of compromised renal function necessitate Swan-Ganz catheterization in patients with severe PIH. Twenty-five percent of women with severe pre-eclampsia exhibit a marked discrepancy between right and left ventricular preload measurements as assessed by CVP and PCWP.[78] Using pulmonary artery catheters, Henderson and coworkers[79] recorded hemodynamic data showing a broad range of measurements for various parameters. Patients with severe PIH are not a homogeneous population, and volume management requires individualization. Depending on the phase of severe pre-eclampsia, fluid management should focus on volume expansion, fluid restriction, a reduction in afterload, or combination therapy only after monitoring identifies the problems involved.[20] Joyce and coworkers[16] recommended using CVP measurements to guide fluid therapy, after finding that the degree of diastolic hypertension relates inversely to CVP values and directly to the volume of intravenous fluid needed to restore CVP to a normal level (6 to 8 cm H_2O). The most severe pre-eclamptics (diastolic pressure >110 mmHg) had initial CVP measurements of -1 to -4 cm H_2O and required >750 ml plasmanate plus 2 liters of lactated Ringer's solution to restore CVP to 6 cm H_2O, while mild pre-eclamptics needed only 1 liter of lactated Ringer's to achieve the same CVP. In another study, Joyce and Loon[80] infused 25-percent albumin to raise the CVP to 6 to 8 cm H_2O while limiting intravenous crystalloids to ≤ 75 ml per hour. Subjects with severe PIH required 75 to 100 g of albumin (300 to 400 ml of 25-percent solution) to achieve a normal CVP, while those with mild hypertension needed only 25 g. While helpful, CVP measurement may also be dangerously misleading in severe PIH, where right and left ventricular function can differ significantly. In the presence of a low or normal CVP, intravenous fluid therapy may produce pulmonary edema. Infusion of crystalloids alone decreases oncotic pressure and can lead to pulmonary and cerebral edema.[1] Severe PIH calls for serial measurements of plasma oncotic pressure.

Oliguria usually responds to a fluid challenge (300 to 400 ml crystalloid) and to delivery of the fetus,[81] since the hemodynamic state in most pre-eclamptics consists of moderately elevated systemic vascular resistance, hyperdynamic ventricular function, and a low PCWP. Benedetti and Quilligan[38] reported on three patients who developed cerebral edema without pulmonary edema following vigorous crystalloid therapy for oliguria. They suggested that the brain, contained within fixed cranial boundaries, might be more vulnerable to interstitial edema than the lungs and recommended restricting crystalloids to no more than 125 ml per hour despite a decreased urine output. Several mechanisms may produce oliguria, and each requires different therapy. Relative intravascular volume depletion accompanied by systemic arteriospasm responds to volume infusion with hemodynamic improvement and decreased SVR. Selective renal arteriospasm requires both preload expansion and afterload reduction, while decreased renal perfusion due to profound vasospasm and reduced cardiac output benefits from fluid restriction and afterload reduction.[81]

Recommendations for management of the HELLP syndrome vary. An established diagnosis dictates prompt delivery of the fetus.[82] Evidence of a coagulation defect mandates use of fresh frozen plasma, and continuing hemolysis often necessitates transfusion of fresh whole blood or packed cells. Some workers advise against giving platelets, for they may trigger DIC with platelet consumption following soon after administration. However, Weinstein[47] recommends giving platelets before or after delivery if excessive bleeding occurs or if the platelet count falls below 20,000 per mm^3. Plasmapheresis, a plasma-exchange transfusion, can return coagulation parameters to normal when HELLP develops postpartum.[47]

METHOD OF DELIVERY

Once the obstetrician decides to deliver the fetus, several options become available. In the parturient with spontaneous labor, vaginal delivery usually ensues as long as fetal status remains acceptable. The onset of fetal distress often necessitates an abdominal delivery. If labor has not begun, the obstetrician may induce labor carefully by periodic uterine stimulation with oxytocin over several days. Should this approach fail, or if deterioration of maternal or fetal status occurs, the obstetrician usually proceeds with cesarean section. The method of delivery greatly influences the anesthetic options for the parturient.

Anesthetic Management

Keeping the above problems in mind, the difficulty of anesthetic management for these patients becomes obvious. Well-managed anesthesia will help mother and child by facilitating obstetric management, whereas poor analgesia or anesthesia will compound the problems of PIH. For the best results, obstetric and anesthesia personnel must communicate freely, with the obstetrician capitalizing on the anesthesiologist's expertise in managing cardiovascular, respiratory, acid-base, and electrolyte problems. Factors that influence anesthesia and analgesia include fetal condition, maternal condition, personnel available, previous drug administration, monitoring capability, and time and type of delivery.

In severe pre-eclampsia, oxygen consumption rises with increased maternal metabolism. Both mother and fetus may benefit from oxygen given during labor and delivery. Maternal oxygen administration, 5 to 10 liters per min by mask, will elevate mean maternal PaO_2 from 88 to 380 mmHg and fetal PaO_2 from a normal mean value of 19 to 24 mmHg without changing maternal or fetal acid-base balance.[17] If a seizure should occur, the increased maternal and fetal PaO_2 may help to protect against hypoxia. Table 21−3 lists a number of basic principles of anesthetic management. Strictly following the principles proves difficult.

LABOR

Parenteral Sedation and Analgesia

Heavy sedation with parenteral morphine and phenobarbital provides one approach for managing labor during PIH. Advantages include the analgesic properties of morphine and the anticonvulsant and sedative effects of phenobarbital. These attributes help to control maternal blood pressure and to prevent seizures. However, these drugs have a number of disadvantages. Both morphine and phenobarbital can depress the fetus and the newborn. The premature newborn has difficulty metabolizing narcotics.[64] Although phenobarbital reputedly protects the fetal central nervous system from hypoxia, it yields little benefit in combating asphyxia and produces feeding problems in sedated infants.[83] Both morphine and phenobarbital depress maternal respiration and can cause respiratory acidosis and decreased maternal and, subsequently, fetal oxygenation. Narcotics increase maternal CSF pressure when given in doses that cause respiratory depression. Finally, narcotics have antidiuretic properties, hardly an attribute for parturients with compromised renal function. Meperidine and morphine cause

Table 21−3. BASIC PRINCIPLES OF ANESTHESIA MANAGEMENT

Avoid stressing organs with compromised function: central nervous system, heart, kidneys, liver, lungs.
Avoid hypoxia and hypercarbia.
Avoid further elevation of blood pressure or severe hypotension.
Avoid further increases in cardiac output.
Avoid exciting the parturient.
Avoid agents depressing the fetus or newborn.
Avoid drugs excreted unchanged by kidney or that may accentuate liver dysfunction.

a significant decrease in GFR and effective renal plasma flow (ERPF) with diminished urine flow and higher urinary concentrations of sodium, potassium, and chloride and a fall in total electrolyte excretion.[84] Small doses of tranquilizers such as promethazine and hydroxyzine can help to relax the mother and reduce the amount of narcotics she requires.

Lumbar Sympathetic Block

The uterus is already hyperirritable in PIH. Lumbar sympathetic block frequently increases uterine activity.[85] The injection of local anesthetic solution proximal to the lumbar sympathetic chain quite likely produces rapid profound sympathetic denervation of the uterus, perhaps explaining why labor accelerates more often following lumbar sympathetic block than during lumbar epidural analgesia. Therefore, the anesthesiologist should avoid lumbar sympathetic block in PIH since further increases in uterine activity might lead to tumultuous labor or uterine tetany with reduced placental perfusion and subsequent fetal hypoxia. This could have disastrous results for the already compromised fetus.

Paracervical Block

Paracervical blocks correlate with a 5- to 20-percent incidence of fetal bradycardia.[86] Occasional local anesthetic constriction of uterine arteries could explain the etiology of fetal bradycardia.[87] The resultant reduction of uterine blood flow superimposed on the uteroplacental hypoperfusion of PIH would be detrimental to the fetus, contraindicating the use of paracervical block analgesia.

Natural Childbirth

Although permissible, natural childbirth techniques ineffectively control blood pressure and fail to diminish the threat of convulsions. The active participation of the parturient during labor and the associated mental stimulation provided by her husband and/or natural childbirth coach probably aggravate the condition. Active pushing, especially if prolonged during the second stage, can result in marked variations in blood pressure and pulse rate. Such fluctuations especially threaten patients with low myocardial reserve. A prepared childbirth patient unable to cope with her labor may have additional problems. Fear and pain increase endogenous catecholamine levels, which in turn lead to additional vasoconstriction and compromise of uteroplacental circulation.[88]

Lumbar Epidural Analgesia

"Epidural block should be avoided, since in pre-eclampsia it is associated with sudden marked falls of blood pressure and on occasion with vascular collapse."[1] This statement typifies the archaic thinking that persists in the minds of physicians who remain unaware of the progress obstetric anesthesiologists have made during the past decade in improving the management of labor and delivery of women with PIH. Continuous lumbar epidural analgesia (LEA) qualifies as the best overall technique for helping these women through this perilous period. Numerous workers have documented the safety of LEA when administered to parturients with PIH.[89–98] This method provides excellent pain relief, facilitates control of hypertension, can improve uteroplacental perfusion, preserves renal function, supports and may improve the fetal condition, and does not depress ventilation. Additionally, LEA may abolish maternal bearing-down impulses, thereby avoiding increases in CSF pressure, which can climb above 50 mmHg with expulsive efforts.[99] Several mechanisms control maternal blood pressure. Sympathetic block to T8 to T10 produces vasomotor blockade with resultant vasodilation and reduced peripheral vascular resistance. Effective analgesia helps to prevent hypertension resulting from pain and the anxiety it provokes. Pre-eclamptic patients have higher plasma levels of catecholamines than normal parturients. LEA administration to the pre-eclamptic during labor promotes significant reductions in these levels without adverse effects on maternal blood pressure, uterine activity, fetal heart rate or the neonate.[94] Epidural analgesia permits the use of outlet forceps, which avoids prolonged maternal pushing and the marked fluctuations in cardiovascular function associated with the Valsalva maneuver.

Because women with PIH are often hypovolemic, justified concern exists regarding the potential problem of hypotension during LEA. Pritchard[100] warns that major conduction analgesia may cause peripheral pooling of blood and decrease cardiac output, thereby compromising placental blood flow, fetal well-being or both. To the contrary, Ueland and Hansen[101,102] failed to find changes in cardiac output with caudal analgesia for vaginal delivery or with LEA for cesarean section in normal parturients. A study of 10 women with severe PIH documents that LEA for labor and delivery fails to decrease and may even slightly increase cardiac output.[93] Proper management will prevent hypotension. Placement of a central venous pressure line monitors changes in right ventricular function and helps assess the response to intravascular volume expansion with colloid or crystalloid solutions. With severe PIH, the CVP should register at least 4 to 6 cm H_2O prior to initiation of LEA. Pulmonary artery and pulmonary capillary wedge pressure monitoring with a Swan-Ganz catheter prove helpful in severe pre-eclampsia, since right and left ventricular function may show unequal compromise. Initiation of LEA necessitates avoiding the supine position to prevent aortocaval compression. If blood pressure decreases more than 25 percent, rapid intravenous infusion of a balanced salt solution and placement of the patient in the left lateral position usually rapidly correct the problem. Intravenous infusions of ephedrine or mephentermine may begin if needed. These patients respond more readily to vasopressors; accordingly, ephedrine should be given in 5-mg increments. Vasopressors with alpha predominance should be avoided.[103]

In a series of 150 pre-eclamptic women with proteinuria and blood pressures of at least 160/100 mmHg, hypotension rarely accompanied LEA.[89] A 20-percent average decrease in systolic pressure occurred (from 167 to 133 mmHg), with systolic levels dropping below 100 mmHg in only five of 150 patients (3 percent). My experience with LEA in parturients with gestational hypertension revealed even more moderate decreases, with mean arterial pressure never dropping more than 10 percent.[90] Over a 9-year period, approximately 2000 patients with PIH received LEA for labor and vaginal delivery at the Birmingham (England) Maternity Hospital. That large series involved an average of four to five injections per patient, with only 6 percent of injections leading to a decline in systolic levels of more than 20 mmHg.[91] In a large series of pre-eclamptic women delivering vaginally, Moore and coworkers[96] noted no difference at any time during the course of labor in the incidence of hypotension in women receiving LEA versus those receiving no anesthesia (6 and 7 percent, respectively). Newsome[97] adjusted intravenous fluid administration to maintain PCWP between 8 and 12 mmHg in a series of severe pre-eclamptics receiving $MgSO_4$ and noted no significant changes in CI, SVR, and pulmonary vascular resistance (PVR) accompanying LEA during labor, at delivery, or 2 hours postpartum. Mean maternal arterial pressure fell from 120 mmHg to 97 mmHg.

In the past, proponents of LEA championed the possibility of improved renal function. James and coworkers[90] could not demonstrate sustained or significant changes in renal function (glomerular function and urine output) in parturients with gestational hypertension who received LEA. However, LEA may facilitate renal function through avoiding narcotics, since these drugs possess antidiuretic activity.[104]

Pre-eclampsia prolongs the total body clearance and elimination half-life of lidocaine. Changes accompanying pre-eclampsia, such as decreased plasma volume, increased interstitial fluid volume, decreased plasma proteins, and compromised hepatorenal function, can alter maternal responses to drug therapy and disposition.[105]

During pregnancy-induced hypertension, LEA prevents further increases in CSF pressure. However, rapid injection of 10 to 20 ml of local anesthetic into the epidural space over 20 to 30 sec markedly elevated intracranial pressure in two nonpregnant patients with reduced intracranial compliance.[106] The magnitude and duration of increased intracranial pressure was less with 5 ml increments.

Even with sensory block to the upper midthoracic region, LEA fails to compromise ventilation. LEA can relieve pulmonary edema, if present, by producing decreased left ventricular work, increased peripheral venous pooling, and reduced peripheral vascular resistance.

Debate continues regarding the advantages and disadvantages of adding epinephrine to local anesthetics to produce LEA. Albright and others[107] observed that the inclusion of epinephrine had no significant effect on placental blood flow in normotensive parturients. Heller[108] used 2 percent lidocaine with 1 in 200,000 epinephrine in four women with pre-eclampsia without producing maternal or fetal compromise. Epinephrine injection through the epidural space may prove safe, but intravascular administration of small amounts of epinephrine may markedly decrease UBF. In sheep, 5-, 10-, and 20-μg intravenous boluses compromised UBF for up to 3 min.[109] The UBF decline of 55 to 65 percent of control with the larger doses[109] could endanger a fetus already experiencing the problems of compromised placental function associated with PIH. Chestnut and coworkers[110] noted nearly identical compromise of UBF with similar intravenous doses of epinephrine in guinea pigs. My advice would be to avoid the potential risks of epinephrine in pre-eclamptics, for they outweigh any possible benefit it might provide.

Fetal outcome with LEA has been good. Moir[89] reported a perinatal mortality of 3.9 percent in his series of 150 severe pre-eclamptics managed with LEA. Prematurity and placental insufficiency accounted for the fetal deaths (three stillbirths, three neonatal deaths). Lumbar epidural analgesia makes controlled delivery over a relaxed perineum possible, thereby diminishing fetal trauma. The decreased need for maternal narcotics, sedatives, and tranquilizers results in less newborn drug depression. Effective LEA reduces the time-dependent increase in maternal metabolic acidosis and placental transport of hydrogen by decreasing maternal motor activity and stress.[111] In a study comparing parturients with gestational hypertension to normotensive controls, LEA resulted in normal acid-base status in mothers and newborns of both groups.[92] Epidural analgesia also suppresses the increase in free fatty acid levels observed in women receiving narcotic analgesia.[112] The prevention of maternal metabolic acidosis and free fatty acid production helps to avoid an incremental contribution to fetal acidosis during labor and delivery.

Some physicians worry that LEA interferes with uteroplacental exchange, causing fetal compromise. In normal pregnancy, uteroplacental vessels are widely dilated; therefore, UBF is pressure dependent and a decrease in perfusion pressure compromises UBF. Since most of the work on UBF and conduction analgesia derives from normotensive animals, one cannot conclude that any reduction in blood pressure will inevitably diminish UBF in the hypertensive patient. Uteroplacental vessels probably remain constricted in parturients with PIH. Thus, a decrease in perfusion pressure during LEA may be accompanied by a reduction in uterine vascular resistance, possibly resulting in unchanged or increased UBF. Lumbar epidural analgesia quite likely produces an effect similar to that observed with hydralazine hydrochloride, which improves uterine blood flow while decreasing maternal blood pressure in hypertensive pregnant ewes.[68] Using a ^{133}Xe clearance technique before and after segmental epidural analgesia during the first stage of labor in pregnancies complicated by essential hypertension or severe pre-eclampsia, Jouppila and coworkers[92] noted that placental blood flow increased slightly, although insignificantly, in most patients with PIH and in half of those with essential hypertension. Subsequently, these same investigators[113] noted that LEA improved UBF more in pre-eclamptics than in women with normal pregnancies and that the response was better with a larger volume of a dilute bupivacaine solution (10 ml of 0.25-percent) than with a smaller volume of a more concentrated solution (4 ml of 0.5 percent; Fig. 21–2). They demonstrated the safety of LEA in hypertensive pregnancies in the absence of any substantial change in systemic blood pressure.

The anesthesiologist should 1) avoid LEA in parturients with DIC, since penetration of epidural vessels by needle or catheter occurs in about 10 percent of parturients and an epidural hematoma could result, producing serious sequelae, and 2) carefully assess coagulation capability prior to attempting LEA. Platelet count and/or function may decrease in PIH. Bassell[114] insists on an Ivy bleeding time of ≤ 10 min as a prerequisite for regional block when the platelet count falls below 100,000 per ml^3.

In patients with severe PIH, epidural analgesia requires management by anesthesiologists well versed in LEA and the peculiarities of obstetric anesthesia. LEA must proceed carefully and well or not at all.

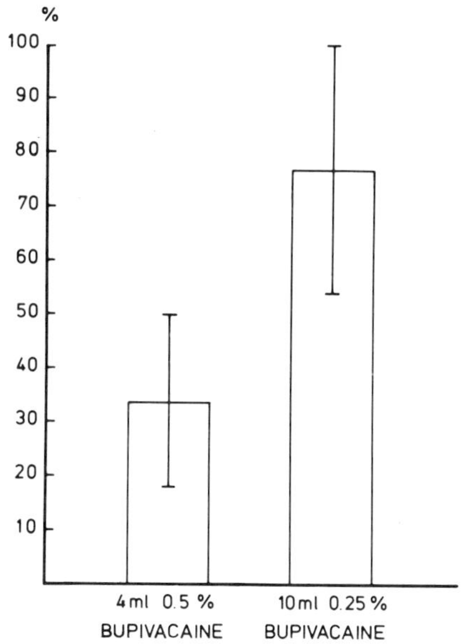

Figure 21–2. Mean (± SEM) percentage changes in intervillous blood flow after epidural analgesia with 4 ml 0.5-percent bupivacaine and 10 ml 0.25-percent bupivacaine. (Reprinted with permission from the American College of Obstetricians and Gynecologists. Obstet Gynecol 59:158, 1982.)

Subarachnoid Morphine

One mg subarachnoid morphine without preservative offers a good alternative to LEA. Good analgesia develops in approximately 45 min without motor or sympathetic blockade, thereby preserving cardiovascular stability. Analgesia persists for several hours.

VAGINAL DELIVERY

Lumbar Epidural Analgesia

Analgesia and anesthesia for vaginal delivery can be managed in several ways. LEA, beneficial in labor for the previously mentioned reasons, provides excellent analgesia for delivery as well. It permits a controlled delivery without last-minute urgency and facilitates the application of forceps to prevent additional maternal cardiovascular stress.

Spinal Analgesia

If LEA has not been used for labor, low spinal or saddle block analgesia offers an attractive alternative for delivery. The incidence of hypotension during spinal analgesia for vaginal delivery of parturients with PIH is no greater than during general anesthesia.[115] As with LEA, spinal analgesia avoids maternal pushing by facilitating the use of outlet forceps, permitting a controlled delivery over a relaxed perineum. Prophylactic intravenous fluid preloading is advisable and equipment for ventilatory support must be present prior to initiating spinal analgesia. If subarachnoid morphine has provided labor analgesia, a pudendal block will be necessary for perineal analgesia for episiotomy or forceps delivery.

Pudendal Block

Pudendal block with or without nitrous oxide analgesia offers a third alternative for vaginal delivery. The pudendal artery travels in close proximity to the pudendal nerve, necessitating extra care to avoid intravascular injection, since the increased CNS irritability of patients with PIH might intensify their susceptibility to seizures from the toxic effects of local anesthetics. Pudendal block can provide satisfactory analgesia for low forceps delivery. We frequently administer nitrous oxide (25 to 40 percent) to supplement the perineal and vaginal analgesia of the pudendal block and to furnish additional pain relief for uterine contractions. Though helpful, this technique offers considerably less effective analgesia than LEA or spinal.

General Anesthesia

At times, general anesthesia, which poses many hazards (Chap. 6), becomes necessary for vaginal delivery. Pharyngolaryngeal edema, possibly accompanying facial and neck edema in women with pre-eclampsia, can create respiratory embarrassment and difficulty in endotracheal intubation. In five of seven reported cases of laryngeal edema, the patient also displayed facial edema.[116] Therefore, the anesthesiologist should anticipate intubation problems in the presence of nuchal or facial edema and employ gentle direct laryngoscopy to determine the appropriateness of an awake intubation versus one carried out after the induction of general anesthesia. A variety of endotracheal tubes 7.0

mm and smaller must be available since edema may markedly decrease the size of the tube that will pass into the trachea.

Preventing the aspiration of gastric contents mandates tracheal intubation. This maneuver, however, often evokes a marked hypertensive response which may prove disastrous.[117] Plasma concentrations of epinephrine and norepinephrine can increase by 300 percent after tracheal intubation, together with a rise in mean arterial blood pressure of 30 percent.[118] Severe postintubation hypertension may exceed the upper limit of cerebral autoregulation, approximately 130 mmHg mean arterial pressure in normotensive people. Although chronic hypertensives exhibit a higher autoregulatory limit, women with PIH may not have had time to adapt. Forced dilation of brain arterioles at multifocal points disrupts the blood-brain barrier, allowing plasma proteins to penetrate into the brain, thereby producing cerebral edema and possibly hypertensive encephalopathy. Systolic pressures exceeding 180 mmHg may rupture intracranial aneurysms which exist in 0.4 to 2.0 percent of the population,[119,120] making intracranial hemorrhage a real concern in severe PIH. Pulmonary edema may also result from the hypertensive response to intubation or extubation. It is essential to avoid a difficult induction accompanied by respiratory obstruction, hypoventilation, hypoxia, and hypercarbia.

The technique of general anesthesia should consist of intravenous thiopental, 3 to 4 mg per kg, followed by intravenous succinylcholine, 100 mg, and tracheal intubation during cricoid pressure to prevent aspiration. Recommended precautions to prevent the hypertensive response to tracheal intubation will be discussed under the general anesthesia for cesarean section. Nitrous oxide, oxygen, and a succinylcholine drip should be used for maintenance. Intravenous narcotics given after delivery can facilitate analgesia and augment blood pressure control. Hepatic involvement in these patients may contraindicate the use of halogenated agents; enflurane and isoflurane as well as halothane have the potential to produce hepatic damage.[121–123] However, the advantage of improved fetal oxygenation offered by the increased FIO_2 made possible by employing low doses of halogenated agents (isoflurane 0.5 to 1.0 percent; enflurane 0.75 to 1.5 percent) outweighs this potential problem. The lesser degree of metabolism of the former two agents recommends them over halothane for patients with PIH.

The potential renal toxicity of several volatile anesthetics warrants discussion. Extensive documentation of high-output renal failure accompanied by increased serum fluoride levels in the presence of methoxyflurane anesthesia renders this agent undesirable.[124,125] Methoxyflurane analgesia during labor can produce serum inorganic fluoride levels as high as 56 to 62 μmol per liter.[126] Enflurane undergoes considerably less metabolism than methoxyflurane, but questions regarding its safety for patients with renal compromise have arisen since renal failure following enflurane anesthesia has been reported,[127,128] and significant serum fluoride levels and decreased creatine clearance may follow use of enflurane in normal subjects.[129] The possibility of enflurane defluorination increases in animals that receive phenobarbital for prolonged periods.[130] The effect of phenobarbital on enflurane metabolism in humans[131] remains controversial and varies among individuals.[132] However, Crowhurst and Rosen[133] believe that even severe PIH does not contraindicate the use of enflurane—and probably not halothane—as volatile supplements during general anesthesia. They found no evidence of nephrotoxicity following use of enflurane (mean 0.24 MAC hours) or halothane (mean 0.23 MAC hours) and 50-percent nitrous oxide and 50-percent oxygen for general anesthesia in severe pre-eclamptics and normotensive controls. The metabolism of enflurane produced plasma inorganic fluoride levels well below toxic values. The peak level recorded, 15 μmol per liter, occurred in only one patient. Postoperative liver function tests also failed to differ significantly from preoperative levels. Seizure type activity, found in association with both enflurane and ketamine use, makes these agents less appealing in PIH, since increased CNS irritability already exists. Ketamine's ability to aggravate hypertension should preclude its use for this reason.

Isoflurane represents the volatile agent of choice for general anesthesia in patients with PIH. It lowers systemic arterial pressure in a dose-related manner, but causes less cardiac depression than other volatile anesthetics.[134] Humans and other animals metabolize isoflurane less than other anesthetics.[135-138] Serum fluoride levels increase after isoflurane anesthesia but reach only about one tenth the amount detected with enflurane.[139] Animal studies fail to indicate significant hepatic effects associated with isoflurane anesthesia, and only one report of human hepatic dysfunction exists.[123] The lack of renal compromise and minimal evidence for hepatic danger with isoflurane make this an appealing agent for use in patients with PIH where compromise of these organs may already exist.

CESAREAN SECTION

Anesthesia for cesarean section presents multiple problems. The advantages and limitations of the various techniques parallel those for labor and vaginal delivery. The perfect approach does not exist, and anesthesia personnel must employ only those techniques with which they have significant experience.

Major Conduction Analgesia

Lumbar epidural analgesia is safe in these patients. Intravascular volume expansion should accompany this procedure, with careful monitoring to prevent a fluid overload. Patients should receive an intravenous preload of ≥ 1000 ml of a balanced salt solution. A central venous pressure increase of 4 to 5 cm of water or a pulmonary capillary wedge pressure exceeding 15 mmHg calls for curtailment of the saline infusion. Some authorities[140] use plasma products to expand the vascular space in preference to balanced salt solutions. The vasodilation produced by LEA and the blood loss associated with the operation should protect against cerebral edema resulting from intravascular volume expansion with crystalloid solutions. Left uterine displacement avoids the complications of aortocaval compression, namely decreased maternal blood pressure and/or UBF and the possible extension of pre-existing placental abruption due to increased venous pressure at the placental site. Once initiated, epidural analgesia should continue with the patient breathing oxygen by mask to raise fetal PO_2. After delivery, if necessary, intravenous narcotics and tranquilizers may supplement epidural analgesia. Magnesium sulfate administration should cease prior to initiation of LEA, for magnesium may increase the likelihood of hypotension through its vasodilating properties. Accidental rapid intravenous administration of solutions containing magnesium sulfate would oppose compensatory vasoconstriction occurring above the level of sympathetic block during conduction analgesia. Elevated serum magnesium levels will persist after infusion of the medication stops, since compromised renal function limits the rate of magnesium excretion. Check blood pressure at least every 2 min until delivery of the infant, and do not permit a fall of more than 25 percent in systolic levels. In normal term gravid ewes, the fetus tolerates decreases in UBF to 50 percent of normal, but a fetus already coping with diminished uteroplacental function, as in PIH, could suffer further compromise by such a drop in UBF. If additional intravenous fluid administration and positioning in a slight Trendelenburg position do not correct hypotension, give intravenous ephedrine, 4 to 10 mg. The presence of CVP or pulmonary artery catheters facilitates intravenous fluid management in women with severe PIH.

The relatively slow onset of sympathetic block with LEA permits time for both mother and anesthesiologist to compensate for sympathetic blockade. I recommend using bupivacaine in preference to chloroprocaine, since the latter disturbs maternal blood pressure and pulse rate more in normotensive parturients receiving LEA for elective cesarean section.[141] A faster onset of sympathetic block by chloroprocaine probably explains the more impressive cardiovascular changes with this local anesthetic. A continuous catheter technique, allowing the gradual establishment of analgesia with 5- to 10-ml increments of local anesthetic until the desired level is achieved, thus avoids unnecessarily high levels of analgesia more readily than with spinal analgesia.

A higher incidence of hypotension makes spinal anesthesia less preferable than LEA. However, spinal analgesia provides a reasonable second choice. As with LEA, intravenous fluid preloading, left uterine displacement, and maternal oxygen administration by mask are important. The potential problem of hypotension represents the greatest drawback. Contraindications to major conduction analgesia include maternal coagulopathies, acute fetal distress, and a parturient emotionally unsuitable for major surgery while awake.

Local Infiltration and Field Block

Local infiltration and field block for cesarean section offer an alternative for an obstetrician adept in this technique. It bypasses both the dangers of hypotension secondary to major conduction techniques and the disadvantages of general anesthesia. Supplementation with 25 to 40 percent nitrous oxide by mask can significantly potentiate local anesthetic analgesia. The surgeon must handle the patient's tissues gently to avoid pain with resulting exacerbations of hypertension and possible seizures. The possibility of increased CNS sensitivity to the toxic effects of local anesthetic demands limitation of the amount infiltrated into maternal tissues. Obstetricians unfamiliar with this technique should not use it in women with PIH. The resultant prolonged, painful experience could prove disastrous for such parturients by exacerbating their hypertension and perhaps causing seizures.

General Anesthesia

This procedure should include uterine displacement, achieved by tilting the patient at least 15 degrees to the left, since this position produces less birth asphyxia and better Apgar scores than the supine position.[142] For the reasons mentioned in discussing vaginal delivery, general anesthesia should include the thiopental-succinylcholine, isoflurane, oxygen, nitrous oxide technique. Jouppila and others[143] noted a fall in intervillous blood flow of 20 to 50 percent in normotensive humans given thiopental, 4 mg per kg, and succinylcholine, 1 mg per kg, prior to tracheal intubation. This obviously could threaten a fetus already experiencing problems from compromised UBF. However, the maternal risks associated with ketamine outweigh the potential fetal problems related to thiopental. Maternal denitrogenation with 100-percent oxygen may help to blunt the fetal effects of reduced intervillous blood flow by raising fetal oxygen levels. Four breaths of 100-percent oxygen increase maternal and umbilical levels of oxygen as effectively as 3 min of continuous oxygen inhalation.[144] Limit nitrous oxide concentrations to 33 percent until delivery, for maternal PaO_2 plateaus at an FIO_2 of 66 percent.[145] After delivery, inspired nitrous oxide levels may be increased to 50 percent. Until delivery, use inspired isoflurane concentrations of 1 percent or less, as this level usually does not decrease UBF. After delivery of the placenta, intravenous oxytocin will overcome the uterine relaxant effects of less than 1 MAC isoflurane. Narcotic administration at this point will allow the parturient to tolerate lower levels of isoflurane.

Cardiovascular response to tracheal intubation. Maternal hypertension secondary to laryngoscopy and tracheal intubation represents the greatest drawback of general anesthesia.[117] Direct laryngoscopy and tracheal intubation not only raise blood pressure but can also compromise uterine blood flow and cause marked increases in plasma norepinephrine levels.[146] Hodgkinson and others[147] noted impressive elevations of pulmonary artery pressure, systemic arterial pressure, and pulmonary artery wedge pressure together with a decreased cardiac index in PIH patients during endotracheal intubation and at the time of extubation (Fig. 21–3). Pulmonary artery pressures and pulmonary wedge pressures climbed to 75/40 mmHg and 55 mmHg, respectively. Frank pulmonary edema may follow intubation or extubation.

Several approaches to diminish the cardiovascular response to laryngoscopy and intubation exist, but none qualifies as ideal. Each of the following drugs has either been used clinically or proposed for trial: esmolol, calcium entry blockers, trimethaphan, hydralazine, sodium nitroprusside (SNP), lidocaine, nitroglycerin (NTG), and fentanyl.

Esmolol. Esmolol, a cardioselective β-adrenergic blocking agent, has a brief duration of action because of its rapid metabolism by blood esterase.[148] Beta blockade ends rapidly once esmolol infusion ceases. The ability to modify tachycardia is esmolol's main effect in attenuating the cardiovascular response to tracheal intubation.[148] This quality might improve the ability of vasodilators like SNP to modify the cardiovascular response to tracheal intubation. Although theoretically attractive, clinical studies must determine esmolol's effect on uterine blood flow and the fetus.

Calcium Entry Blockers. Nifedipine, used

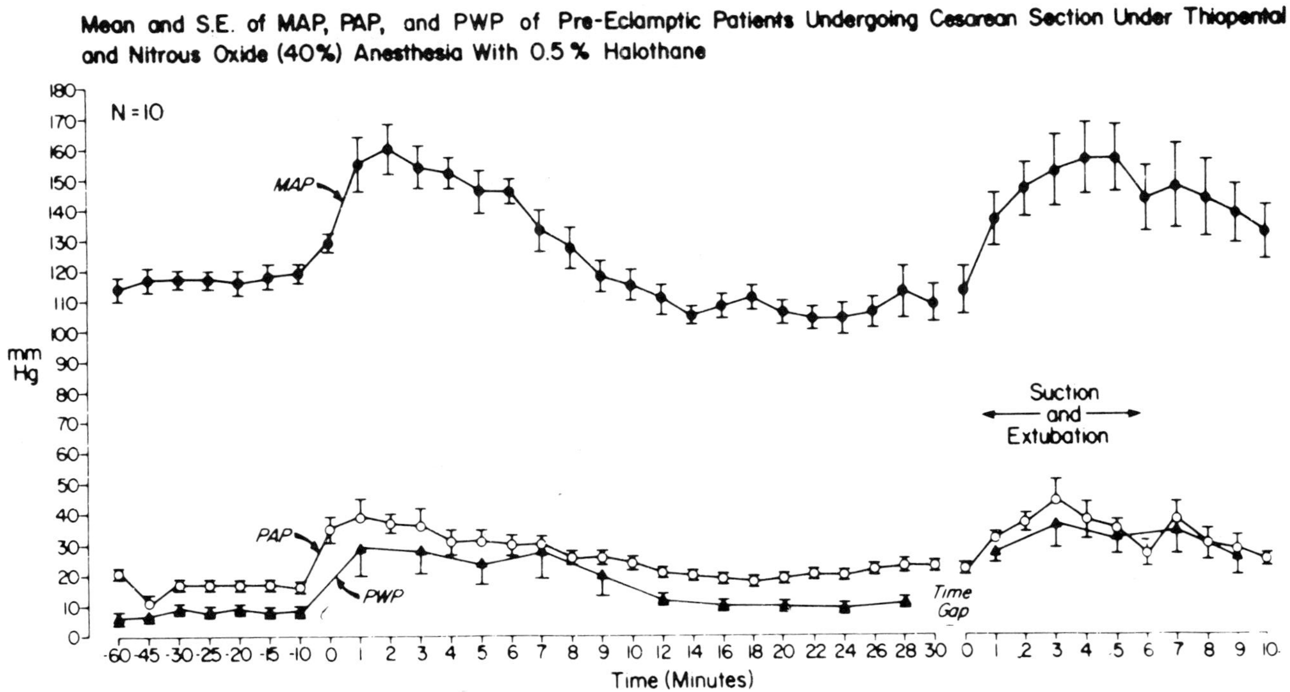

Figure 21–3. The left and right zero points on the time scale represent the initiation of laryngoscopy and intubation and suction plus extubation, respectively. (From Hodgkinson, R, et al,[147] with permission.)

for long-term treatment of severe pre-eclampsia,[149] has an onset of action within 5 min of sublingual administration, with significant increases in heart rate and cardiac output occurring as MAP decreases.[150,151] Nifedipine does not appear to compromise UBF in normotensive pregnant ewes.[152] Verapamil decreases UBF in normotensive gravid ewes by 10 to 25 percent, an effect probably related to an 11-percent fall in MAP and reduced uterine perfusion pressure.[153] The negative chronotropic and inotropic effects of verapamil together with its vasodilating properties make it theoretically more attractive than nifedipine, which causes tachycardia. Furthermore, no preparation of nifedipine suitable for intravenous administration is currently available in the United States. Norris and coworkers[70] noted that both drugs rapidly reversed the hypertensive effect of norepinephrine infusion in pregnant ewes without further compromising UBF. Although verapamil readily crosses the placenta,[154] they failed to note any effect of either drug on fetal blood pressure, heart rate, or acid-base status. Calcium movement through cell membranes governs uterine contractility,[155] and both nifedipine[156] and verapamil[157] inhibit spontaneous uterine activity. Hence, increased blood loss could accompany their use during cesarean section. When nifedipine administration takes place immediately postpartum, no increase in uterine size or bleeding occurs.[156] Calcium entry blockers deserve additional clinical investigation based on these preliminary studies.

Trimethaphan. The ganglionic blocker trimethaphan can effectively modify cardiovascular responses to tracheal intubation but has a number of shortcomings. It has a slower onset of action than SNP or NTG, produces widespread autonomic effects, and large doses can prolong the action of succinylcholine.[158] Animal studies suggest that trimethaphan may be the "worst" of the potent antihypertensive agents, in terms of cerebral, coronary, and renal blood flow.[159–161]

Hydralazine. The relatively slow onset and long duration of action prevent intravenous hydralazine from being an ideal agent to prevent the exacerbation of hypertension by laryngoscopy and endotracheal intubation. Its long-lasting effect could cause problems with hypotension following the magnitude of blood loss frequently occurring with abdominal delivery.

Sodium Nitroprusside. Strauss and coworkers[162] reported success with SNP used to control hypertension during cesarean section in a woman with PIH. Fetal problems did not develop during SNP infusion and a healthy newborn was delivered. Three reports describe the successful use of SNP in pregnant women undergoing intracranial aneurysm surgery.[163–165] In theory, SNP seems preferable to nitroglycerin for controlling maternal hypertension since it primarily decreases afterload while nitroglycerin exerts a greater effect on preload. Concern regarding fetal cyanide toxicity followed a study of normotensive ewes showing resistance to the hypotensive effect of SNP.[166] The fetus possesses less thiosulphate substrate for rhodanase detoxification of cyanide than the adult[167] and may therefore be especially prone to develop cyanide toxicity from SNP infusion. Using a mean dose of 2.3 μg per kg per min, we[168] promptly decreased MAP to control levels during norepinephrine-induced hypertension in gravid ewes and observed no signs of maternal or fetal compromise during 50 minutes of SNP therapy. Maternal and fetal plasma cyanide levels were below 50 μg per liter, ruling out cyanide toxicity. When infused with norepinephrine, SNP caused a progressive increase in UBF which became significant at 40 min of therapy (Fig. 21–4). Fetal heart rate, blood pressure, arterial blood gas levels, and acid-base status remained stable throughout SNP infusion, and all fetuses survived. Both clinical use and our animal data indicate that SNP, when used for only 5 to 10 min to modify the cardiovascular response to tracheal intubation, seems effective and safe for mother and fetus. This vasodilator, like the calcium entry blockers, merits further clinical investigation for this purpose.

Nitroglycerin. Intravenous NTG offers many advantages over SNP for inducing hypotension in adults.[169] It usually produces a smooth and gradual reduction in blood pressure with a lesser chance of producing severe hypotension. In addition, it avoids cyanide toxicity, and tachyphylaxis does not occur. In gravid ewes, both SNP and NTG effectively counteract maternal hypertension and antagonize the uterine

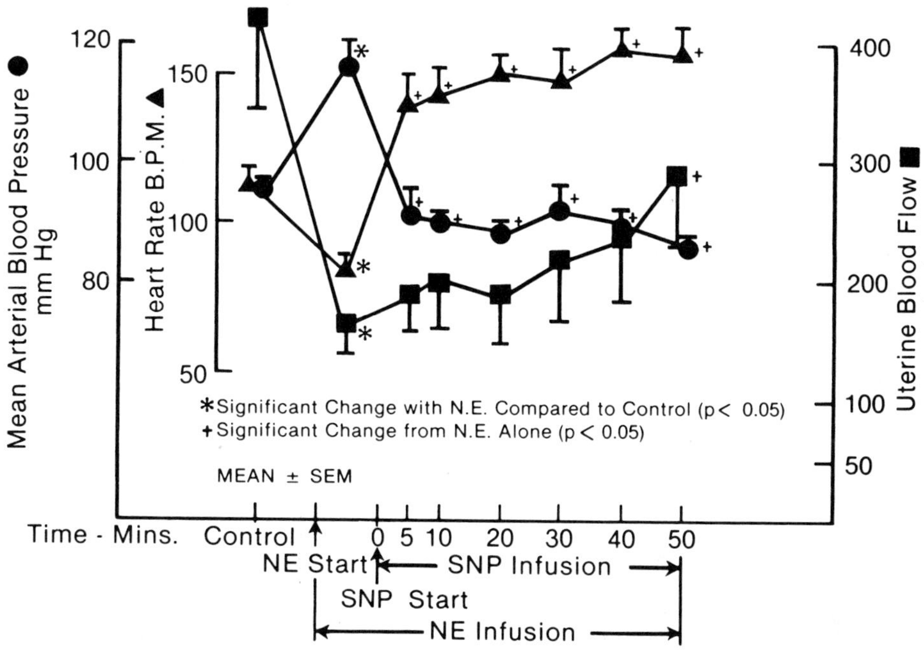

Figure 21–4. Sodium nitroprusside infusion successfully reverses the detrimental effects of norepinephrine on maternal blood pressure, heart rate, and uterine blood flow in the gravid ewe. (From Ellis, SC, Wheeler, AS and James, FM III: Fetal and maternal effects of sodium nitroprusside used to counteract hypertension in gravid ewes. Am J Obstet Gynecol 143:776, 1982, with permission.)

vasoconstriction induced by α-adrenergic stimulation with norepinephrine without shunting or stealing blood flow away from the uterine vasculature.[170] Hood and coworkers[171] used NTG to reduce MAP from 127 ± 12 mmHg to 103 ± 18 mmHg during the preoxygenation of severely pre-eclamptic women and compared findings with a control group not receiving NTG. Following induction with thiopental, laryngoscopy, and tracheal intubation, MAP increased significantly to 155 ± 14 mmHg in controls and to 119 ± 21 mmHg in the NTG group. Maternal heart rates remained similar in both groups. A dose of 0.5 to 1.5 μg per kg per min usually proves effective in lowering maternal blood pressure by 20 to 25 percent so that, as the pressure increases with laryngoscopy and intubation, it will usually not exceed pretreatment levels. Nitroglycerin, un-ionized and having a molecular weight of 227, crosses the placenta readily but causes no significant changes in newborn blood pressure, heart rate, umbilical vessel gases and pH, or Apgar scores.[171] Contrary to our findings, Cotton and others[172] noted that severely pre-eclamptic patients receiving blood volume expansion proved markedly resistant to the hypotensive effect of NTG, whereas NTG readily reduced the blood pressure of patients not undergoing volume expansion. Our patients may have responded more effectively to NTG either because of less effective restoration of blood volume or due to more aggressive treatment with antihypertensive therapy by the obstetric staff. The parturient's baseline intravascular volume status may govern the efficacy of NTG in reducing blood pressure. The same group of workers[173] used NTG to successfully reverse pulmonary edema in three antepartum patients with severe PIH. They reduced mean systemic arterial pressure from 148 to 125 mmHg and PCWP fell from 27 to 14 mmHg, thereby improving the mean colloid osmotic pressure-to-PCWP gradient from 10 to 2. Heart rate did not change. NTG may potentiate pancuronium-induced neuromuscular blockade,[174] necessitating carefully titrated doses and use of a peripheral nerve stimulator. Since NTG may produce a dose-related increase in intracranial pressure (ICP) and a decrease in intracranial compliance,[175] some clinicians caution against its use in severe pre-eclampsia, when cerebral edema may already be present. However, hydralazine,[176] nifedipine,[177] trimethaphan,[178] and SNP[179] each can increase ICP as well.

Lidocaine. Proponents of intravenous lidocaine recommend its use for decreasing the cardiovascular response to intubation in surgical patients. However, Terrasi and coworkers[180] failed to confirm its effectiveness for this purpose in pregnant women. In addition, intravenously administered local anesthetics decrease UBF and increase uterine tone and could further jeopardize the fetus in pre-eclampsia.[181]

Fentanyl. Large doses of fentanyl (>5 μg per kg) can modify the cardiovascular response to laryngoscopy and intubation, but could produce respiratory depression of the newborn. Uteroplacental dysfunction renders the compromised fetus more susceptible to the depressant effects of narcotics.

Recommendations for Cardiovascular Response Control. The ability to easily titrate drug administration to blood pressure control qualifies SNP and NTG as the best agents currently available to blunt the cardiovascular effects of laryngoscopy and intubation. SNP needs further study to provide additional confirmation of fetal safety but seems unlikely to cause cyanide toxicity when given for only a few minutes prior to delivery. In the future, esmolol and verapamil may prove useful, either alone or in combination with SNP or NTG. Labetalol also warrants investigation.

Summary

Although the perfect anesthetic technique for analgesia and anesthesia for vaginal delivery or for cesarean section for patients with PIH still eludes anesthesiologists, they can increase the safety of mother and child by becoming familiar with the pathophysiology involved and how it relates to the various anesthetic options.

PIH involves the mother's cardiovascular and central nervous systems, renal and hepatic function, and coagulation mechanism. Hypovolemia, low colloid osmotic pressure, and increased cardiac afterload due to increased peripheral vascular resistance all present maternal problems. The pre-eclamptic woman may be receiving many potent drugs, including hydralazine, α-methyldopa, and magnesium sulfate. The fetus must cope with compromised uteroplacental function, vulnerability to cardiorespiratory depression from medications, hypoxia and acidosis, and prematurity.

The anesthesiologist's goals include prevention of wide swings in maternal blood pressure, reduction of maternal cardiac stress, appropriate pain relief, protection of central nervous system function, and support of uteroplacental circulation with the aim of preserving fetal well being. Maternal blood volume, coagulation parameters, and airway status deserve special attention. Monitoring must appropriately match the severity of the illness. Severe PIH calls for direct arterial pressure measurement and pulmonary artery catheterization. Central venous pressure measurement, sufficing in women with moderate pre-eclampsia, proves unnecessary in mild PIH. A PCWP of 12 mmHg or CVP levels of 6 to 8 cm H_2O represent measurements consistent with adequate volume restoration. A confirmed platelet count of at least 100,000 per mm^3 must precede initiation of LEA. If the platelet count falls below this level, the Ivy bleeding time must be 10 min or less before attempting LEA.

LEA represents the method of choice for labor and vaginal delivery. The anesthesiologist must assess and, if necessary, restore intravascular volume before initiating LEA, which should be established gradually to allow slow onset of sympathetic nervous system blockade. Limit local anesthetic injections to 5-ml increments given over at least 60 sec to prevent transient increases in ICP, and repeat this dose until achieving the desired level of analgesia. Subarachnoid morphine, 1 mg, represents a reasonable alternative to LEA for labor and can be followed by pudendal nerve blockade for delivery analgesia. When conduction analgesia is contraindicated, small doses of parenteral narcotics and tranquilizers offer a reasonable alternative for labor management combined with pudendal block and inhalation analgesia with 25 to 40 percent nitrous oxide for delivery.

For cesarean section, LEA provides the best

alternative. Follow the same principles for abdominal delivery as when employing this technique for labor and vaginal delivery. When acute fetal distress, coagulopathy, maternal emotional state, or other factors contraindicate LEA or spinal anesthesia, general anesthesia must follow, paying careful attention to preserving fetal oxygenation and preventing marked maternal cardiovascular response to laryngoscopy and endotracheal intubation. Nitroglycerin or SNP therapy should proceed slowly by controlled intravenous administration during the 5 to 10 min before induction to lower maternal blood pressure by 20 to 25 percent. Generally, the vasodilator infusion can be discontinued shortly after intubation but may need reinitiation prior to extubation. I recommend a technique using thiopental (3 mg per kg) plus succinylcholine (1 mg per kg) for induction, followed by nitrous oxide (33-percent), isoflurane (0.5 to 1.0 percent inspired), and oxygen (66-percent) until delivery, at which point inhalation of nitrous oxide can be increased to 50 percent and narcotics may be given intravenously.

The increased likelihood of newborn depression demands careful preparation of appropriate personnel and equipment for carrying out resuscitation.

References

1. Lindheimer, MD and Katz, AI: Hypertension in pregnancy. N Engl J Med 313:675, 1985.
2. Sibai, BM, McCubbin, JH and Anderson, GD: Eclampsia. I: Observations from 67 recent cases. Obstet Gynecol 58:609, 1981.
3. Wright, JP: Anesthetic considerations in preeclampsia-eclampsia. Anesth Analg 62:590, 1983.
4. Gibbs, CE and Locke, WE: Maternal deaths in Texas 1969 to 1973: A report of 501 consecutive deaths from the Texas Medical Association's Committee on Maternal Health. Am J Obstet Gynecol 126:687, 1976.
5. Lueck, J, et al: Observation of an organism found in patients with gestational trophoblastic disease and in patients with toxemia of pregnancy. Am J Obstet Gynecol 145:15, 1983.
6. Ayala, AR, et al: Evidence that a toxemic related organism (Hydratoxilualba) is an artifact. Obstet Gynecol 67:47, 1986.
7. Birkeland, SA and Kristofferson, K: Preeclampsia: A state of mother-fetus immune balance. Lancet 2:720, 1979.
8. Beer, AE: Possible immunologic basis of preeclampsia/eclampsia. Semin Perinatol 2:39, 1978.
9. Symonds, EM: Aetiology of preeclampsia: A review. J R Soc Med 73:871, 1980.
10. Page, EW: On the pathogenesis of preeclampsia and eclampsia. J Obstet Gynaecol Br Commonw 79:883, 1972.
11. Gant, NF, et al: The nature of pressor responsiveness to angiotensin II in human pregnancy. Obstet Gynecol 43:854, 1974.
12. Goldkrand, JW and Fuentes, AM: The relation of angiotensin-converting enzyme to the pregnancy-induced hypertension-preeclampsia syndrome. Am J Obstet Gynecol 154:792, 1986.
13. Pedersen, EB, et al: Preeclampsia: A state of prostaglandin deficiency? Hypertension 5:105, 1983.
14. Makila, U-M, Viinkka, L and Ylikorkala, O: Evidence that prostacyclin deficiency is a specific feature in preeclampsia. Am J Obstet Gynecol 148:772, 1984.
15. Chesley, LC: Disorders of the kidney: Fluids and electrolytes. In Assali, NS (ed): Pathophysiology of Gestation. Academic Press, New York, 1972.
16. Joyce, TH, Debrath, KS and Baker, EA: Preeclampsia-relationship of CVP and epidural analgesia. Anesthesiology (Suppl)51:297, 1979.
17. Lerner, SM: Anesthetic considerations for complicated obstetrics. II: Preeclampsia and hypertensive vascular disease. Anesth Analg 48:771, 1969.
18. Aalkjaer, C, et al: Abnormal vascular function and morphology in preeclampsia: A study of isolated resistance vessels. Clin Sci 69:477, 1985.
19. Clark, SL, Divon, MY and Phelan, JP: Preeclampsia/eclampsia: Hemodynamic and neurologic correlations. Obstet Gynecol 66:337, 1985.
20. Phelan, JP and Yurth, DA: Severe preeclampsia. I: Peripartum hemodynamic observations. Am J Obstet Gynecol 144:17, 1982.
21. Benedetti, TJ, et al: Hemodynamic observations in severe preeclampsia with a flow directed pulmonary artery catheter. Am J Obstet Gynecol 136:465, 1980.
22. Rafferty, TD and Berkowitz, RL: Hemodynamics in patients with severe toxemia during labor and delivery. Am J Obstet Gynecol 138:263, 1980.
23. Hankins, GDV, et al: Longitudinal evaluation of hemodynamic changes in eclampsia. Am J Obstet Gynecol 150:506, 1984.
24. Kuzniar, J, et al: Hemodynamics of gestational hypertension: Pathophysiological and clinical considerations. Clin Exp Hypertens (B)B5(1):79, 1986.
25. Pritchard, JA and Stone, SR: Clinical and laboratory observations on eclampsia. Am J Obstet Gynecol 99:754, 1967.
26. Clark, SL and Phelan, JP: Ob uses for the pulmonary artery catheter. Contemp OB/Gyn 24:172, 1984.
27. Clark, SL, Divon, MY and Phelan, JP: Preeclampsia/eclampsia: Hemodynamic and neurologic correlations. Obstet Gynecol 66:337, 1985.
28. Morris, RH, et al: Immunofluorescent studies of renal biopsies in the diagnosis of toxemia of pregnancy. Obstet Gynecol 24:32, 1964.
29. Eden, RD, Williams, AY and Gall, MA: Pregnancy-induced hypertension and postpartum maternal morbidity. Obstet Gynecol 68:86, 1986.
30. Fisher, KA, et al: Hypertension in pregnancy: Clini-

cal pathological correlations and remote prognosis. Medicine 60:267, 1981.
31. Dieckmann, WJ, Pottinger, RE and Rynkiewicz, LM: Etiology of preeclampsia-eclampsia: IV sodium chloride test for the diagnosis of preeclampsia. Am J Obstet Gynecol 63:783, 1952.
32. Chesley, LC: Hypertensive Disorders in Pregnancy. Appleton-Century-Crofts, New York, 1978.
33. Handler, JS: The role of lactic acid in the reduced excretion of uric acid in toxemia of pregnancy. J Clin Invest 39:1526, 1960.
34. Hayashi, T: Uric acid and endogenous creatinine clearance studies in normal pregnancy and toxemia of pregnancy. Am J Obstet Gynecol 71:859, 1956.
35. Smith, K, et al: Acute renal failure of obstetric origin. Lancet 2:351, 1965.
36. Pritchard, JA and MacDonald, PE: Williams Obstetrics. Appleton-Century-Crofts, New York, 1980.
37. Templeton, AA and Kelman, GR: Arterial blood gases in preeclampsia. Br J Obstet Gynaecol 84:290, 1977.
38. Benedetti, TJ and Quilligan, EJ: Cerebral edema in severe pregnancy induced hypertension. Am J Obstet Gynecol 137:860, 1980.
39. Littler, WA, et al: Reduced pulmonary arterial compliance in hypertensive pregnancy. Lancet 1:1274, 1973.
40. Benedetti, TJ, Kates, R and Williams, V: Hemodynamic observations in severe preeclampsia complicated by pulmonary edema. Am J Obstet Gynecol 152:330, 1985.
41. Benedetti, TJ and Carlson, RW: Studies of colloidal osmotic pressure in pregnancy induced hypertension. Am J Obstet Gynecol 135:308, 1979.
42. Jouppila, R, Jouppila, P and Hollmen, A: Laryngeal edema as an obstetric anesthesia complication: Case reports. Acta Anaesthesiol Scand 24:97, 1980.
43. Sibai, BM, Anderson, GD and McCubbin, JH: Eclampsia. II: Clinical significance of laboratory findings. Obstet Gynecol 59:153, 1982.
44. Kelton, JG, Hunter, DJS and Neame, P: A platelet function defect in preeclampsia. Obstet Gynecol 65:107, 1985.
45. Arias, F and Mancilla-Jimenez, R: Hepatic fibrinogen deposits in preeclampsia. N Engl J Med 295:578, 1978.
46. Manas, KJ, et al: Hepatic hemorrhage without rupture in preeclampsia. N Engl J Med 312:424, 1985.
47. Weinstein, L: Preeclampsia/eclampsia with hemolysis, elevated liver enzymes and thrombocytopenia. Obstet Gynecol 66:657, 1985.
48. MacEnna, J, Dover, NL and Brame, RG: Preeclampsia associated with hemolysis, elevated liver enzymes, and low platelets: An obstetric emergency? Obstet Gynecol 62:751, 1983.
49. Sibai, BM, et al: Eclampsia. V: The incidence of nonpreventable eclampsia. Am J Obstet Gynecol 154:581, 1986.
50. Beeson, JH and Duda, EE: Computed axial tomography scan demonstration of cerebral edema in eclampsia preceded by blindness. Obstet Gynecol 60:529, 1982.
51. Donnelly, JF and Lock, FR: Causes of death in 533 fatal cases of toxemia of pregnancy. Am J Obstet Gynecol 68:184, 1954.
52. Lunell, NO, et al: Uteroplacental blood flow in preeclampsia measurements with indium-133m and a computer linked gamma camera. Clin Exp Hypertens B1:105, 1982.
53. Buchan, PC: Preeclampsia: A hyperviscosity syndrome. Am J Obstet Gynecol 42:111, 1982.
54. Dixon, HG and Robertson, W: A study of the vessels of the placental bed in normotensive and hypertensive women. J Obstet Gynaecol Br Commonw 65:803, 1958.
55. Pritchard, JA and Bretten, AL: Clinical and laboratory studies in severe abruptio placentae. Am J Obstet Gynecol 97:681, 1967.
56. Paterson, MEL: The aetiology and outcome of abruptio placentae. Acta Obstet Gynecol Scand 58:31, 1979.
57. Svenningsen, NW, Liedholm, H and Aberg, A: Hypertension in pregnancy and the infant. Acta Obstet Gynecol Scand (Suppl)118:103, 1984.
58. Martin, TR and Tupper, WRC: The management of severe toxemia in patients of less than 36 weeks gestation. Obstet Gynecol 54:602, 1979.
59. Sinatra, RS, et al: Prolonged neuromuscular blockade with vecuronium in a patient treated with magnesium sulfate. Anesth Analg 64:1220, 1985.
60. Sibai, BM, et al: Eclampsia. V: The incidence of nonpreventable eclampsia. Am J Obstet Gynecol 154:581, 1986.
61. DeVore, JS and Asrani, R: Magnesium sulfate prevents succinylcholine-induced fasciculations in toxemic parturients. Anesthesiology 52:76, 1980.
62. Cotton, DB, Gonik, B and Dorman, KF: Cardiovascular alterations in severe pregnancy induced hypertension: Acute effects of intravenous magnesium sulfate. Am J Obstet Gynecol 148:162, 1984.
63. Goldkrand, JW and Fuentes, AM: The relation of angiotensin-converting enzyme to the pregnancy-induced hypertension-preeclampsia syndrome. Am J Obstet Gynecol 154:792, 1986.
64. Krames, E, et al: The effect of magnesium sulfate on uterine blood flow and fetal well-being in the pregnant ewe. (abstr). Annual Meeting of American Society of Anesthesiologists, 287, 1975.
65. Horvath, JS, et al: Clonidine hydrochloride: A safe and effective antihypertensive agent in pregnancy. Obstet Gynecol 66:634, 1985.
66. Liedholm, H and Melander, A: Drug selection in treatment of pregnancy hypertension. Acta Obstet Gynecol Scand (Suppl)118:49, 1984.
67. Cotton, DB, Gonik, B and Dorman, KF: Cardiovascular alterations in severe pregnancy induced hypertension seen with an intravenously given hydralazine bolus. Surg Gynecol Obstet 161:240, 1985.
68. Ring, G, et al: Comparison of nitroprusside and hydralazine in hypertensive pregnant ewes. Obstet Gynecol 50:598, 1977.
69. Marx, GF, et al: Neonatal blood pressures. Anaesthetist 25:318, 1976.
70. Norris, MC, Rose, JE and Dewan, DM: Nifedipine or verapamil counteracts hypertension in gravid ewes. Anesthesiology 65:254, 1986.

71. Lunell, NO, et al: Uteroplacental blood flow in pregnancy hypertension after the administration of a beta-adrenoreceptor blocker, pindolol. Gynecol Obstet Invest 18:269, 1984.
72. Michael, CA: Use of labetalol in the treatment of severe hypertension during pregnancy. Br J Clin Pharmacol (Suppl)8:211, 1979.
73. Jouppila, P, et al: Labetalol does not alter the placental and fetal blood flow or maternal prostanoids in preeclampsia. Br J Obstet Gynaecol 93:543, 1986.
74. Van Assche, FA, et al: Preliminary observations on treatment of pregnancy-induced thromboxane hypertension with a synthetase inhibitor. Am J Obstet Gynecol 148:216, 1984.
75. Weiner, CP, Socol, ML and Vaisrub, N: Control of preeclamptic hypertension by ketanserin, a new serotonin receptor antagonist. Am J Obstet Gynecol 149:496, 1984.
76. Goodlin, RL: Expanded toxemia syndrome or gastosis. Am J Obstet Gynecol 154:1227, 1986.
77. Stoyka, WW and Schultz, H: The cerebral response to sodium nitroprusside and trimethaphan controlled hypotension. Can Anaesth Soc J 22:275, 1975.
78. Clark, SL and Phelan, JP: Ob uses for the pulmonary artery catheter. Contemp OB/Gyn 24:172, 1984.
79. Henderson, DW, et al: The role of Swan-Ganz catheterization in severe pregnancy-induced hypertension. Am J Obstet Gynecol 148:570, 1984.
80. Joyce, TH and Loon, M: Preeclampsia: Effect of albumin 25 percent infusion (abstr). Anesthesiology 55:313, 1981.
81. Clark, SL, et al: Severe preeclampsia with persistent oliguria: management of hemodynamic subsets. Am J Obstet Gynecol 154:490, 1986.
82. Oian, P, Maltau, JM and Abyholm, T: HELLP syndrome: A serious complication of hypertension in pregnancy. Acta Obstet Gynecol Scand 63:727, 1984.
83. Goodlin, RC: Fetal medication in high risk pregnancies. Obstet Gynecol 34:109, 1969.
84. Loughridge, L: Kidneys and anaesthesia. In Scurr C and Feldman S (eds): Scientific Foundation of Anaesthesia. William Heinemann Medical Books, London, 1974, p 319.
85. Hunter, CA: Uterine motility studies during labor. Am J Obstet Gynecol 85:681, 1963.
86. Shnider, SM and Gildea, J: Paracervical block anesthesia in obstetrics. III: Choice of drug: Fetal bradycardia following administration of lidocaine, mepivacaine, and prilocaine. Am J Obstet Gynecol 116:320, 1973.
87. Gibbs, CP and Noel, SC: Human uterine artery responses to lidocaine. Am J Obstet Gynecol 126:313, 1976.
88. Shnider, SM, et al: Uterine blood flow and plasma norepinephrine changes during maternal stress in the pregnant ewe. Anesthesiology 50:524, 1979.
89. Moir, DD, et al: Epidural analgesia during labor in patients with preeclampsia. J Obstet Gynaecol Br Commonw 79:465, 1972.
90. James, FM III and Davies, P: Maternal and fetal effects of lumbar epidural for labor and delivery in patients with gestational hypertension. Am J Obstet Gynecol 126:195, 1976.
91. Crawford, JS: Epidural analgesia in pregnancy hypertension. Clin Obstet Gynaecol 4:735, 1977.
92. Jouppila, R, et al: Epidural analgesia and placental blood flow during labour in pregnancies complicated by hypertension. Br J Obstet Gynaecol 86:969, 1979.
93. Graham, C and Goldstein, A: Epidural analgesia and cardiac output in severe preeclamptics. Anaesthesia 35:709, 1980.
94. Abboud, T, et al: Sympathoadrenal activity, maternal, fetal, and neonatal responses after epidural anesthesia in the preeclamptic patient. Am J Obstet Gynecol 144:915, 1982.
95. Jouppila, P, et al: Lumbar epidural analgesia to improve intervillous blood flow during labor in severe preeclampsia. Obstet Gynecol 59:158, 1982.
96. Moore, TR, et al: Evaluation of the use of continuous lumbar epidural anesthesia for hypertensive pregnant women in labor. Am J Obstet Gynecol 152:404, 1985.
97. Newsome, LR, Bramwell, RS and Curling, PE: Severe preeclampsia: Hemodynamic effects of lumbar epidural anesthesia. Anesth Analg 65:31, 1986.
98. Neri, A, et al: Lumbar epidural analgesia in hypertensive patients during labour. Eur J Obstet Gynecol Reprod Biol 22:1, 1986.
99. Donaldson, JO: Neurology of Pregnancy. WB Saunders, Philadelphia, 1978.
100. Pritchard, JA and Pritchard, SA: Standardized treatment of 154 consecutive cases of eclampsia. Am J Obstet Gynecol 123:543, 1975.
101. Ueland, K and Hansen, JM: Maternal cardiovascular dynamics. III: Labor and delivery under local and caudal analgesia. Am J Obstet Gynecol 103:8, 1969.
102. Hansen, JM and Ueland, K: Maternal cardiovascular dynamics during pregnancy and parturition. In Marx, GF: Clinical Anesthesia: Parturition and Perinatology. FA Davis, Philadelphia, 1973.
103. James, FM III, Greiss, FC and Kemp, RA: An evaluation of vasopressor therapy for maternal hypotension during spinal anesthesia. Anesthesiology 33:25, 1970.
104. Jaffe, JH and Martin, WR: Narcotic analgesics and antagonists. In Goodman LS and Gilman A (eds): The Pharmacological Basis of Therapeutics. Macmillan, New York, 1975.
105. Ramanthan, J, Bottorff, M and Jeter, JN: The pharmokinetics and maternal and neonatal effects of epidural lidocaine in preeclampsia. Anesth Analg 65:120, 1986.
106. Hilt, H, Gramm, H-J and Link, J: Changes in intracranial pressure associated with extradural anesthesia. Br J Anaesth 58:676, 1986.
107. Albright, G, et al: Epinephrine does not alter human intervillous blood flow during epidural anesthesia. Anesthesiology 54:131, 1981.
108. Heller, PJ and Goodman, C: Use of local anesthetics with epinephrine for epidural anesthesia in preeclampsia. Anesthesiology 65:224, 1986.
109. Hood, DD, Dewan, DM and James, FM III: Maternal

and fetal effects of epinephrine in gravid ewes. Anesthesiology 64:610, 1986.
110. Chestnut, DH, et al: Effect of intravenous epinephrine on uterine artery blood flow in the pregnant guinea pig. Anesthesiology 65:633, 1986.
111. Pearson, JF and Davies, P: The effect of continuous lumbar epidural analgesia upon fetal acid base status during the first stage of labor. J Obstet Gynaecol Br Commonw 81:971, 1974.
112. Malthau, JM, et al: Obstetrical analgesia assessed by free fatty acid mobilization. Acta Anaesth Scand 19:245, 1975.
113. Jouppila, P, et al: Lumbar epidural analgesia to improve intervillous blood flow during labor in severe preeclampsia. Obstet Gynecol 59:158, 1982.
114. Bassell, GM: Editorial Comments. Obstet Anesth Digest, 1984.
115. Smith, BE, Cavanagh, D and Moya, F: Anesthesia for vaginal delivery of the patient with toxemia of pregnancy. Anesth Analg 45:853, 1966.
116. Heller, PJ, Scheider, E and Marx, GF: Pharyngolaryngeal edema as a presenting symptom in preeclampsia. Obstet Gynecol 62:523, 1983.
117. Fox, EJ, et al: Complications related to the pressor response of endotracheal intubation. Anesthesiology 47:524, 1977.
118. Fell, D, et al: Measurement of plasma catecholamine concentrations: An assessment of anxiety. Br J Anaesth 57:770, 1985.
119. Toole, JF and Patel, AN: Cerebrovascular Disorders. McGraw-Hill, New York, 1974.
120. Adams, RD: The nervous system. In Harrison TR (ed): Principles of Internal Medicine, ed. 3. McGraw-Hill, New York, 1958.
121. Denlinger, JK, Lecky, JH and Nahn, HL: Hepatocellular dysfunction without jaundice after enflurane anesthesia. Anesthesiology 41:86, 1974.
122. Sadove, MS and Kim, SI: Hepatitis after use of two different fluorinated anesthetic agents. Anesth Analg 53:336, 1974.
123. Gregoire, S and Smiley, RK: Acute hepatitis in a patient with mild factor IX deficiency after anesthesia with isoflurane. Canadian Medical Association Journal 135:645, 1986.
124. Taves, DR, et al: Toxicity following methoxyflurane anesthesia. II: Fluoride concentrations in nephrotoxicity. JAMA 214:91, 1970.
125. Mazze, RI, Trudell, JR and Cousins, MJ: Methoxyflurane metabolism and renal dysfunction: Clinical correlation in man. Anesthesiology 35:247, 1971.
126. Creasser, CW, et al: Methoxyflurane metabolism and renal dysfunction after methoxyflurane analgesia during labor and delivery. Anesthesiology 41:62, 1974.
127. Eichhorn, JH, et al: Renal failure following enflurane anesthesia. Anesthesiology 45:557, 1976.
128. Hartnett, MN, Lane, W and Bennett, WM: Nonoliguric renal failure and enflurane. Ann Intern Med 81:560, 1964.
129. Mazze, RI, Calverly, RK and Smith, NT: Inorganic fluoride nephrotoxicity. Anesthesiology 46:265, 1977.
130. Norgate, CE, Sharp, JH and Cousins, MH: Metabolism of enflurane in man following a second exposure. Anaesth Intensive Care 4:186, 1976.
131. Dooley, JR, et al: Is enflurane defluorination inducible in man? Anesthesiology 50:213, 1979.
132. Corall, IM, Knights, KM and Strunin, L: Enflurane (Ethrane) anesthesia in man. Br J Anaesth 49:881, 1977.
133. Crowhurst, JA and Rosen, M: General anesthesia for caesarean section in severe preeclampsia: Comparison of the renal and hepatic effects of enflurane and halothane. Br J Anaesth 56:587, 1984.
134. Stevens, WC, et al: The cardiovascular effects of a new inhalation anesthetic, forane, in human volunteers at constant arterial carbon dioxide tension. Anesthesiology 35:8, 1971.
135. Holaday, D, et al: Resistance of isoflurane to biotransformation in man. Anesthesiology 43:313, 1975.
136. Rehder, K, et al: Halothane biotransformation in man: A quantitative study. Anesthesiology 28:711, 1967.
137. Holaday, DA, Rudofsky, S and Treuhaft, PS: Metabolic degradation of methoxyflurane in man. Anesthesiology 33:579, 1970.
138. Chase, RE, et al: The biotransformation of ethrane in man. Anesthesiology 35:262, 1971.
139. Eger, EI: Pharmacology of isoflurane compared to other general anesthetics. Annual Refresher Course Lectures of the American Society of Anesthesiologists, St. Louis, October, 1980.
140. Cloeren, SE, Lippert, TH and Hinselmann, M: Hypovolemia in toxemia of pregnancy: Plasma expansion therapy with surveillance of central venous pressure. Arch Gynaecol 215:123, 1973.
141. James, FM III et al: Chloroprocaine vs. bupivacaine for lumbar epidural analgesia for elective cesarean section. Anesthesiology 52:488, 1980.
142. Crawford, JS, Burton, M and Davies, P: Time and lateral tilt at cesarean section. Br J Anaesth 44:447, 1972.
143. Jouppila, P, et al: Effect of induction of general anesthesia for cesarean section on intervillous blood flow. Acta Obstet Gynecol Scand 58:249, 1979.
144. Norris, MC and Dewan, DM: Preoxygenation for cesarean section: A comparison of two techniques. Anesthesiology 62:827, 1985.
145. Marx, GF and Mateo, CV: Effects of different oxygen concentrations during general anesthesia for elective caesarean section. Canad Anaesth Soc J 18:587, 1971.
146. Shnider, SM, et al: Plasma norepinephrine and uterine blood flow changes during endotracheal intubation and general anesthesia in the pregnant ewe (abstr). Abstracts of the Annual Meeting of the American Society of Anesthesiologists, October 23, 1978, Chicago.
147. Hodgkinson, R, Husain, FJ and Hayashi, RH: Systemic and pulmonary pressure during cesarean section in parturients with gestational hypertension. Can Anaesth Soc J 27:389, 1980.
148. Liu, PL, et al: Esmolol for control of increases in heart rate and blood pressure during tracheal intuba-

tion after thiopentone and succinylcholine. Can Anaesth Soc J 33:556, 1986.
149. Walters, BNJ and Redman, CWG: Treatment of severe pregnancy-associated hypertension with the calcium antagonist nifedipine. Br J Obstet Gynaecol 91:330, 1984.
150. Singh, BN, et al: Electrophysiologic and hemodynamic effects of slow channel blocking drugs. Prog Cardiovasc Dis 25:103, 1982.
151. Guazzi, M, et al: Nifedipine, a new antihypertensive with rapid action. Clin Pharmacol Ther 22:528, 1977.
152. Norris, MC, Rose, JC and Dewan, DM: Maternal and fetal effects of nifedipine in the gravid ewe (abstr). Anesthesiology 63:430, 1985.
153. Murad, SHN, et al: Effects of verapamil on uterine blood flow and maternal cardiovascular function in the awake pregnant ewe. Anesth Analg 64:7, 1985.
154. Murad, SHN, et al: Verapamil: Placental transfer and effects on maternal and fetal hemodynamics and atrioventricular conduction in the pregnant ewe. Anesthesiology 62:49, 1985.
155. Haszar, G: Biology and biochemistry of myometrial contractility and cervical maturation. Semin Perinatol 5:216, 1981.
156. Forman, A, et al: Effects of nifedipine on spontaneous and methylergometrine-induced activity post-partum. Am J Obstet Gynecol 144:442, 1982.
157. Hahn, DW, et al: Evaluation of drugs for arrest of premature labor in a new animal model. Am J Obstet Gynecol 148:775, 1984.
158. Poulton, TJ, James, FM III and Lockridge, O: Prolonged apnea following trimethaphan and succinylcholine. Anesthesiology 50:54, 1979.
159. Michenfelder, JD and Theye, RA: Canine systemic and cerebral effects of hypotension induced by hemorrhage, trimethaphan, halothane, and nitroprusside. Anesthesiology 46:188, 1977.
160. Artu, A, Wright, K and Colley, PS: Cerebral effects of hypocapnia plus nitroglycerin-induced hypotension in dogs. J Neurosurg 64:924, 1986.
161. Fyman, PN, et al: Vasodilator therapy in the perioperative period. Canad Anaesth Soc J 33:629, 1986.
162. Strauss, RG, et al: Hemodynamic monitoring of cardiogenic pulmonary edema complicating toxemia of pregnancy. Obstet Gynecol 55:170, 1980.
163. Donchin, Y, Amirav, B and Yarkoni, S: Sodium nitroprusside for aneurysm surgery in pregnancy. Br J Anaesth 50:849, 1978.
164. Rigg, D and McDonagh, A: Use of sodium nitroprusside for deliberate hypotension during pregnancy. Br J Anaesth 53:985, 1981.
165. Willoughby, JS: Sodium nitroprusside, pregnancy and multiple intracranial aneurysms. Anaesth Intensive Care 12:358, 1984.
166. Lewis, PE, et al: Placental transfer and fetal toxicity of sodium nitroprusside. Gynecol Invest 8:46, 1977.
167. Naulty, J, Cefalo, RC and Lewis, PE: Fetal toxicity of nitroprusside in the pregnant ewe. Am J Obstet Gynecol 139:708, 1981.
168. Ellis, SC, Wheeler, AS and James, FM III: Fetal and maternal effects of sodium nitroprusside used to counteract hypertension in gravid ewes. Am J Obstet Gynecol 143:776, 1982.
169. Yaster, M, et al: A comparison of nitroglycerin and nitroprusside for inducing hypotension in children: A double blind study. Anesthesiology 65:175, 1986.
170. Wheeler, AS, et al: Effects of nitroglycerin and nitroprusside on the uterine vasculature in gravid ewes. Anesthesiology 52:390, 1980.
171. Hood, DD, et al: The use of nitroglycerin in preventing the hypertensive response to tracheal intubation in severe preeclamptics. Anesthesiology 63:329, 1985.
172. Cotton, DB, et al: Cardiovascular alterations in severe pregnancy-induced hypertension: Effects of intravenous nitroglycerin coupled with blood volume expansion. Am J Obstet Gynecol 154:1053, 1986.
173. Cotton, DB, et al: Role of intravenous nitroglycerin in treatment of severe pregnancy-induced hypertension complicated by pulmonary edema. Am J Obstet Gynecol 154:91, 1986.
174. Glisson, SN, El-Etr, AA and Lim, R: Prolongation of pancuronium-induced neuromuscular blockade by intravenous infusion of nitroglycerin. Anesthesiology 51:47, 1979.
175. Ghani, GA, et al: Effects of intravenous nitroglycerin on the intracranial pressure and volume-pressure response. J Neurosurg 58:562, 1983.
176. Overgaard, J and Skinhoj, E: A paradoxical cerebral hemodynamic effect of hydralazine. Stroke 6:402, 1975.
177. Giffin, JP, et al: Intracranial pressure during nifedipine-induced hypotension. Anesth Analg 62:1078, 1983.
178. Stullken, EH and Sokoll, MD: Intracranial pressure during hypotension and subsequent vasopressor therapy in anesthetized cats. Anesthesiology 42:425, 1975.
179. Turner, JM, et al: Intracranial pressure changes in neurosurgical patients during hypotension induced with sodium nitroprusside or trimethaphan. Br J Anaesth 49:419, 1977.
180. Terrasi, J, et al: IV lidocaine in obstetrics: Placental transfer and cardiovascular response to intubation (abstr). Abstracts of 18th Annual Meeting of Society for Obstetric Anesthesia and Perinatology, 1986.
181. Greiss, FC, Jr., Still, JG and Anderson, SG: Effects of local anesthetic agents on uterine vasculatures and myometrium. Am J Obstet Gynecol 124:889, 1976.

CHAPTER 22

THE FEBRILE PARTURIENT

FRANK R. STORNIOLO, M.D.
THEODORE G. CHEEK, M.D.
W. CLYDE SHELLEY, M.D.
BRETT B. GUTSCHE, M.D.

The presence of fever or infectious disease in the parturient is an important issue confronting the obstetric anesthetist. This chapter covers current information on the issues of anesthetizing the febrile parturient and includes discussions of herpes genitalis and acquired immune deficiency syndrome, diseases that have gained greater importance since the first edition of this book.

Pathophysiology of Fever

The human, as a homoiothermic animal, attempts to maintain body temperature within a range of 36.1° to 37.4°C (97° to 99.3°F).[1] Fever is considered a hallmark of disease; temperature readings above this range indicate the presence of disease or cellular metabolic disorder. In health, chemical reactions[2] and muscle activity, which alone account for about one third of daily metabolic heat production, generate body heat. Body temperature varies in a rhythmic pattern with changes from morning to evening being greater in women than in men.[3] Ranging widely among individuals, temperature rhythm tends to be consistent in any single person, being an inherent biorhythm that returns after a febrile episode abates.[3]

The body regulates its temperature by means of the thermoregulatory center located in preoptic hypothalamic nuclei near the floor of both third ventricles.[3,4] When blood at an elevated temperature perfuses this region, an associated increase in autonomic outflow initiates sweating and increased blood flow to the periphery. This, in turn, facilitates heat dissipation through conduction, convection, radiation, and evaporation.

In contrast the mechanism responsible for heat conservation is disputed. One concept postulates the existence of deep and surface thermal receptors, which initiate signals promoting vasoconstriction (decreased heat loss) and shivering (increased heat production). Various disease states may alter normal autoregulatory functions thereby augmenting heat production, blocking heat dissipation, or both, resulting in fever. Studies in some febrile patients indicate that the central set-point around which the body temperature is usually maintained is elevated during the onset of fever.[2–5] When the body temperature has risen to the new point, heat loss and gain are again finely balanced at this higher level. This alteration in set-point usually occurs in the presence of pyrogens. For example, febrile response can be prevented in animals given endotoxin when the hypothalamus is heated during the latent period preceding the onset of fever.[4]

Pyrogens, both endogenous and exogenous, can initiate fever.[1,3-5] Exogenous pyrogens, including infectious agents or their products, do not produce a direct effect upon the thermoregulatory center.[3] Rather, they activate the leukocytes to produce endogenous pyrogens. Following a latent period of approximately 90 min after injection of exogenous pyrogen, heat-labile endogenous pyrogens begin to appear in the circulation. Concomitant increases in oxygen consumption occur in response to augmented metabolic activity, yet peripheral vasoconstriction yields the sensation of feeling cold. Shivering may begin at this time. Owing to the central pooling of blood, less heat dissipates peripherally, resulting in increased core temperature and fever.

Endogenous pyrogens apparently initiate this process by induction of prostaglandin synthesis.[3] Prostaglandins may function as central neurotransmitters for stimulating febrile responses. Prostaglandins E_1 and E_3 produce fever when injected intravenously or into the CNS. Conversely, the well-known ability of aspirin and similar antipyretics to reduce fever relates to their ability to block prostaglandin synthesis. Increased levels of prostaglandin present during fever decrease with the use of antipyretics or with spontaneous abolishment of fever.

Prostaglandins increase the levels of cyclic AMP, a substance important in the production of fever. Cerebrospinal fluid levels of cyclic AMP double during fevers produced by endogenous pyrogens.[3] Cyclic AMP apparently functions as a neuromediator in the scheme of fever production. Other neuromediators, serotonin and norepinephrine, function as hypothalamic regulators of normal body temperature. These monoamines raise levels of cyclic AMP and prostaglandins in the central nervous system. Therefore, a possible mechanism for hyperthermia (Fig. 22–1) would be the production of endogenous pyrogens by bacteria, antigen, lysosome damage, and so forth, followed by initiation of prostaglandin synthesis. Prostaglandins then increase cyclic AMP, which mediates the hypothalamic signals responsible for vasoconstriction (heat conservation) and increased metabolic activity (heat production). Perhaps temperature increases can be initiated at any

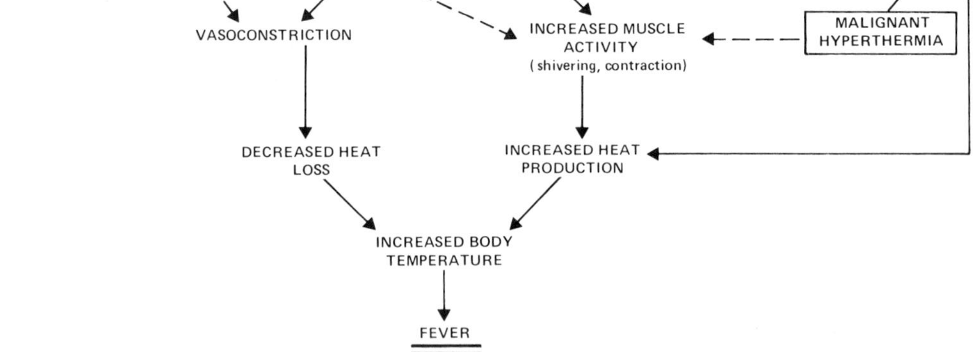

Figure 22–1. Various pathways of fever production. Boxes represent inciting or triggering factors.

point in this scheme (Fig. 22–1). Any disease state associated with increased levels of catecholamines or catecholamine sensitivity may manifest an increased body temperature. Since monoamines increase prostaglandins and cyclic AMP, they may initiate fever higher up on the pathway. Additionally, they directly produce peripheral vasoconstriction, thereby inhibiting an important mechanism of heat dissipation.

Changes in body temperature, whether a result of environmental variations, infections, or metabolic or toxic insults, produce profound effects on the biologic systems within the body.[1,5–9] The presence of high temperatures decreases the ability of body systems to withstand additional stress, as indicated by decreased ability of animals to survive shock from any cause.[2] Fever significantly increases heart rate, cardiac output, oxygen consumption, basal metabolic rate, and the incidence of arrhythmias (Table 22–1). When seen in combination with the normal physiologic changes of pregnancy, these pathologic alterations cause significant maternal and fetal morbidity during prolonged high fevers. For example, Cefalo[10] noted maternal cardiovascular collapse when temperature increased by only 2°C in the pregnant ewe.

Fever During Pregnancy

Fever and pregnancy also affect the respiratory system. Increased ventilation during pregnancy does not produce notable changes in arterial pH, due to increased renal excretion of bicarbonate.[11] However, the additional rise in alveolar ventilation caused by fever yields a significantly increased pH, especially during the pain of labor. Alkalemia shifts the oxyhemoglobin dissociation curve to the left, decreasing oxygen transport; lactic acidosis may occur in mother and fetus.[10]

Maternal fever has a deleterious effect upon the fetus and intrauterine environment, much of which may be attributed to increased uterine activity. Kullander[12] notes premature labor in 50 percent of rabbits with pyrogen-induced fever. Ahlgren[13] reports that elevated maternal temperature increases the motility of human gravid uterine muscle fibers in vitro. Intravenous injection of pyrogen into women at term gestation produces a two- to threefold increase in uterine activity. Increased myometrial activity during fever may be due, in part, to activation of the neurohypophyseal axis, resulting in secretion of oxytocin. Certainly, premature labor and delivery threaten the possibility of a successful pregnancy.

Although increased uterine tonicity may endanger fetal status by means of reduced uterine blood flow, Kullander's[12] data suggest that other factors partly account for fetal mortality during hyperthermia. Maternal stress of any type may adversely affect the fetus. Kim[7] detected increased plasma norepinephrine levels during hyperthermia. Endogenous and exogenous catecholamines constrict the uterine vascular bed and decrease uterine blood flow, resulting in fetal asphyxia. Since hyperthermia also increases catecholamine production, it may prove deleterious in the same manner. In pregnant ewes, Cefalo[10] found insignificant changes in uterine blood flow during mild increases of maternal temperature (0.5° to 1.0°C), while elevations of 1.0° to 2.5°C above normal decreased uterine blood flow to less than 50 percent of control (Table 22–2).

Fetal-maternal temperature difference, which correlates with uterine blood flow, has been used experimentally as an indicator of fetal well-being.[10] In sheep, the fetus' temperature is 0.61°C higher than the mother's. With maternal hyperthermia, a biphasic effect occurs in this difference. Initially, with a 1°C increase in

Table 22–1. CARDIOVASCULAR EFFECTS OF HYPERTHERMIA IN GRAVIDAS AND NONGRAVIDAS

Parameter	Nongravidas	Gravidas
Heart rate	↑10 bpm/°F[2]	↑15 bpm over nonpregnant
Cardiac output	↑50–75% at 39.2°C[9]	↑30–50%[209]
Oxygen consumption	↑60% at 41°C[195]	↑21%[192]
BMR	↑13%/°C[194]	↑14%[192]
Incidence of arrhythmias	↑	↑

Table 22–2. EFFECTS OF INCREASING MATERNAL TEMPERATURE ON UTERINE BLOOD FLOW AND FETAL TEMPERATURE IN THE EWE

	Control	+1.0°C	+2.5°C
Uterine blood flow (ml/kg/min)	111.38	122	53
Fetal-maternal temperature difference	0.61°C	0.19°C	1.27°C

(From Cefalo, RC[10] with permission.)

maternal temperature, the fetal-maternal temperature difference decreases. As the maternal temperature increases further (Table 22–2), the fetal-maternal temperature difference begins to increase. The increased temperature difference between the fetus and mother has been associated with both distressed fetuses and neonates.[10]

An increased fetal heart rate accompanies increasing maternal temperature.[10,14] Fetal heart rate irregularities may develop and persist even after the maternal fever subsides.[8] Fetal scalp pH values progressively fall, depending upon the duration, etiology, absolute elevation in temperature, and fetal cardiovascular reserve to the fever. At delivery, the neonate of the febrile septic mother often requires resuscitation from the effects of its previous environment. Some circumstances call for emergency cesarean section to remove the fetus from the unfavorable uterine environment of the febrile mother.

Mechanisms of Fever

The parturient may become febrile by several mechanisms. The following sections discuss the more common etiologies and their ramifications on parturient and anesthetic management.

CHORIOAMNIONITIS

Infection represents the major cause of fever in the parturient. A temperature in excess of 100.2°F (37.8°C) qualifies as a sign of infection until proven otherwise. Pregnancy tends to alter host defense mechanisms, as demonstrated by decreased circulating immunoglobulin levels, specifically IgG. Alterations in cellular function also occur, with lymphocytes diminishing in numbers and decreasing in immunologic reactivity.[15] These changes may explain the less favorable outcome in gravidas than in nonpregnant women with serious systemic infection.

Chorioamnionitis, one of the most frequently encountered infectious processes during parturition, produces maternal sepsis, antepartum and intrapartum fetal infection, and congenital pneumonia.[16] Neonatal problems resulting from premature delivery are common.[17] The mechanism of this infective process is somewhat complex. With intact membranes, evidence indicates direct placental transport of maternal blood-borne infectious agents to the fetus and amniotic fluid.[15] Bacteria may also gain access to the fetus by ascending through ruptured membranes into the intrauterine cavity. Yet premature rupture of membranes may be a result of maternal infectious processes.[18] The common organisms responsible for chorioamnionitis include both aerobes and anaerobes found in the lower genital tract.[15,17] Infections may be mixed, but the predominant bacteria isolated from the neonate usually include group B streptococci and *E. coli.*[17]

Amniotic fluid has specific antibacterial activity which protects against infection,[15,18] accounting for a low incidence of chorioamnionitis in the absence of operative intervention or rupture of membranes. The capacity of amniotic fluid to inhibit bacterial growth increases with duration of pregnancy; marked inhibition occurs after 20 weeks' gestation.[18] These antibacterial substances are lysozymes, immunoglobulins, and a zinc-protein complex.[15] Wide individual variations in the levels of these substances help explain the differences in susceptibility to chorioamnionitis following premature rupture of membranes.

As the length of time from rupture of membranes until delivery increases, the incidences of intrauterine infection and perinatal morbidity and mortality also increase.[15] For example, the fetal mortality rate increases from about 3 percent at 24 hours to 10 percent at 48 hours after rupture of membranes.

Rupture of the amniotic membranes sets the stage for infection. Usually, membranes rupture during labor, and termination of pregnancy occurs before infection. However, after premature rupture of membranes or during prolonged labor, the incubation period may be sufficient for infection to occur.

Following rupture of membranes, labor, manual examinations, and monitoring devices have all been implicated in increasing the bacterial inoculum within the uterus.[15,16,19] Larsen[19] found that prolonged internal fetal monitoring was associated with an increased rate of intrauterine infections when the interval since rupture of the membranes exceeded 8 hours. In contrast, Ledger[15] found no correlation between the incidence of infections and the length of time of internal monitoring. Evacuation of uterine contents represents the only definitive cure for amnionitis. When evaluating the time between diagnosis of chorioamnionitis and delivery, Gibbs[17] could not identify a critical interval beyond which maternal complications, neonatal infection, or low Apgar scores increased. However, nearly all of his patients delivered within 8 to 12 hours after the diagnosis of chorioamnionitis was established.

The use of antibiotic therapy remains controversial and depends upon the philosophy of the individual obstetrician and the existing condition of the mother. Some prefer delaying maternal antibiotics until after delivery to prevent antibacterial drugs from altering culture results of the newborn.[17] Prophylactic antibiotics given to the mother have proven ineffective in preventing perinatal infection.[15] Yet, other clinicians recommend initiation of antibiotic therapy soon after diagnosis of amnionitis and procurement of appropriate cultures.[17] Various antibiotic regimens have been recommended, but most obstetricians prefer single coverage with ampicillin or cephalosporin or a combination of penicillin and an aminoglycoside.[17] Bacteria commonly associated with amnionitis usually prove sensitive to these antibiotics.

RESPIRATORY INFECTION

Maternal respiratory tract infections occur in approximately 1 percent of deliveries,[12] are usually viral in origin, and pose no specific threat to the healthy parturient. Unfortunately, the "common cold" predisposes the patient to other more serious respiratory problems and greatly alters her anesthetic care. Possible secondary bacterial infections include sinusitis, otitis media, bronchitis, and pneumonia. An upper respiratory tract infection precedes half of all cases of pneumonia in pregnant women.[20] The physiologic alterations in pregnancy may be the predisposing, or at least aggravating, factors in these infections. Hyperemia, hypersecretion, and edema characterize the respiratory mucosa as pregnancy progresses.[12,20] A concomitant viral infection intensifies this obstructive situation, producing a confined, poorly-drained space which creates a perfect environment for secondary bacterial infection. Furthermore, the altered host defense mechanisms can transform a simple upper respiratory infection into a much more serious condition.

Pneumonia occurs in 0.10 to 0.84 percent of all deliveries, accounting for 3.5 to 24 percent of nonobstetric deaths.[12,15] Leontic states that influenza and pneumonia combined are the second leading cause of maternal morbidity and mortality.[20] In addition, 71 percent of patients who have pneumonia during the 25th through 36th weeks of gestation deliver prematurely.[12] After finding high maternal and fetal death rates in deliveries complicated by acute pneumonia, Hopwood[21] advised against inducing labor unless indicated until improvement of the pneumonic process. Treatment should include appropriate antibacterial therapy based on culture and sensitivity results, antipyretics, increased inspired oxygen, hydration, and pulmonary toilet. Such therapy has significantly reduced maternal mortality, from 20 to 3.5 percent.[21] Since the era preceding antibiotics, mortality in term babies has decreased from 19 percent to a negligible number.[21]

UROLOGIC INFECTIONS

The common occurrence of urinary tract infections during pregnancy and parturition makes them a leading cause of maternal fever. Dilation of the calyces, renal pelvis, and ureters following the third month of pregnancy predispose the gravida to urinary tract infections. In addition, increased progesterone levels during pregnancy produce hypotonia of smooth muscle in the collecting system, resulting in decreased ureteral peristalsis with stasis of urine. These changes mimic the permanent abnormalities found in patients with chronic, recurrent urinary tract infections.[22] While it remains unknown whether pregnancy predisposes to bladder infection, a 2- to 7-percent incidence of asymptomatic bacteriuria occurs during gestation.[22-24] Unless treated, this bacteriuria results in a 20- to 40-percent incidence of pyelonephritis, most likely due to ascension of bacteria in the static ureteral urine.[22,24,25]

THYROID DISEASE

Thyrotoxicosis occurs in 0.04 to 0.2 percent of pregnancies, as compared with 0.4 to 0.5 percent in the general nonpregnant population.[26] It is not known whether pregnancy ameliorates thyrotoxicosis or masks its symptomatology. Thyrotoxicosis does decrease the likelihood of successful conception.[26] Should thyrotoxicosis occur during pregnancy, diagnosis and control become mandatory to prevent maternal and fetal morbidity and mortality. For detailed information on the parturient with thyroid disease the reader should refer to Chapter 13. We have included a discussion of thyrotoxicosis for completeness, since it can cause fever. Severe hypermetabolism and fever invariably occur during thyroid storm and form the sine qua non for diagnosis.[27,28] Some workers[27] have recorded temperatures exceeding 106°F.[27] The thyroid hormones play an important role in the control of body temperature and heat production. This heat production, the source of homoiothermic control of body temperature, ultimately arises from the mitochondria. About 60 percent of the energy liberated by mitochondrial oxidative phosphorylation normally becomes incorporated into ATP, while the other 40 percent escapes as heat.[29] During storm, the oxidative phosphorylative system uncouples completely, releasing energy in the form of heat rather than through ATP formation. Control of hyperthyroidism in the parturient not only prevents early gestational fetal wastage but also guards against the occurrence of thyroid storm. Thyroid storm usually develops in undiagnosed, poorly treated, or uncooperative patients.[26,30] Nonthyroidal conditions that sometimes precipitate it include infection, labor, ketoacidosis, trauma, surgery, or pregnancy-induced hypertension.[26,27,30]

Genital Herpes Simplex

Since 1970 the incidence of genital herpes simplex virus (HSV) has risen sharply, the majority of those infected coming from middle and upper socioeconomic groups.[31-33] Over the same period, the incidence of neonatal herpes has risen to a reported frequency of one case in 3500 to 7500 live births.[34] Obstetricians increasingly perform cesarean section to avoid the devastating effects of this neonatal disease. According to some reports, more than 50 percent of women with recurrent herpes genitalis in pregnancy receive cesarean section.[35] This means that this disease accounts for more than 25,600 cesarean sections a year in the United States.[36] Despite efforts to avoid neonatal HSV, the incidence of neonatal infection with the virus continues to rise.[37] Anesthesiologists caring for pregnant women must be aware of these perinatal issues as well as the anesthetic implications to the mother and fetus with intercurrent HSV genitalis. This section reviews the natural history of HSV genitalis, the obstetric management of this disease, and considerations for obstetric anesthesia care in the presence of active disease.

NATURAL HISTORY OF GENITAL HSV

The understanding of genital HSV, particularly during pregnancy, continually evolves, as considerable variation exists in the manifestation of the disease. Initial infection, usually more severe than recurrent infections, involves adenopathy and ulceration which lasts 10 to 16 days in women. Occasionally the host fails to notice genital HSV.[38] Indeed, recurrence of genital HSV disease may range from unnoticeable to severe symptoms in the same patient. This implies that history and physical exam may not always indicate the presence of HSV infection or viral shedding in the pregnant patient. Unfortunately prohibitive laboratory costs prevent routine screening of all parturients for the disease. Physical signs and symptoms of HSV genitalis include painful lesions of genital skin and mucous membranes in most patients, while 40 to 50 percent have fever, malaise, myalgia, photophobia, headache, and tender inguinal lymphadenopathy. In the initial infections, 4 to 10 percent manifest viral meningitis with nuchal rigidity, photophobia, fever, emesis, and prostration.

HSV usually resolves without sequelae; encephalitis is extremely rare.[39] In 1 to 3 percent of subjects, lower motor neuron dysfunction occurs transiently resulting in lower extremity numbness, weakness, urinary retention, and impotence in men. Viral shedding from labia, urethra, and cervix lasts from 3 to 14 days. Table 22–3 summarizes the major findings of this disease in pregnancy. Although the incidence of HSV varies, a recent study[43] found that in 215 pregnant women, a positive history placed 25 at risk for HSV, of whom 15 had positive HSV cultures and eight had active shedding of the virus.

OBSTETRIC MANAGEMENT OF GENITAL HSV

In 1980, the American Academy of Pediatrics published its recommendations for management of pregnant women with a history of HSV.[44] These include weekly examinations beginning at the 34th week of gestation and vaginal delivery only if virologic, cytologic, and clinical findings show no evidence of HSV 1 week before delivery. The report considered the following risks: probability of neonatal HSV infection, status of fetal membranes, gestational age, and maternal complications following cesarean section.[14] Patients who need prospective monitoring during pregnancy are: (1) those with documented or probable HSV infection occurring 12 to 18 months prior to established gestation; (2) those who develop herpetic vulvovaginitis during gestation; (3) those with frequent episodes of labial herpes; or (4) any woman whose sexual consort has experienced genital or oral herpes infections. Additionally, all active lesions of the thighs and buttocks require virologic and cytologic assessment.[45] To permit vaginal delivery in women with gestational HSV, most obstetricians require the absence of symptoms for 15 days and at least one, preferably two, negative cultures prior to labor.[37] Some obstetricians criticize this practice, as it may lead to an unnecessarily high cesarean section rate. Brown[37] recently modified these suggestions to include a careful history and tactile examination at the onset of labor. If a patient or partner has lesions or symptoms of HSV at the time of labor, cesarean section should proceed. Patients with a history of HSV can deliver vaginally when physical examination rules out the presence of lesions and when viral cultures are available. Positive cultures mandate close following of the infant and initiation of therapy prior to the onset of symptoms. This approach carries a small risk of neonatal exposure to the virus. In review, few disagree that the presence of active genital herpes at the onset of labor precludes vaginal delivery. The indications for cesarean section in an asymptomatic parturient with a history of recurrent HSV remain controversial and require the clinician's judgment.

Table 22–3. PRIMARY AND RECURRENT GENITAL HERPES IN WOMEN

	Study	Primary (days)	Recurrence (days)
Incubation		3–6	7–10
Viremia		Yes	Rare
Number of lesions		6	4
Mean duration of pain (days)	Adams[40]	13.0	8.6
	Nilsen[41]	9.6	
Mean duration of lesion (days)	Adams[40]	16.6	10.5
	Nilsen[41]	9.6	7
	Bryson[42]	13.7	
Mean duration of viral shedding (days)	Adams[40]	8.0	4.5
	Nilsen[41]	12.6	3
	Bryson[42]	13.9	
Virus in cervical secretions		87%	4 %

NEONATAL CONSIDERATIONS IN THE PRESENCE OF GESTATIONAL HSV

Maternal HSV infection introduces little maternal risk as sequelae rarely develop. In contrast, neonatal effects of this disease can be devastating, causing permanent sequelae or death even with proper treatment. For this reason, clinicians must make every effort to avoid transmission of HSV from mother to fetus and to promptly diagnose and treat the disease in the neonate.

The incidence of neonatal HSV continues to rise. Sullivan-Bolyai and associates[46] recently reported the highest incidence, 1 in 1500 births, in a survey in Washington state. Parturients experiencing their first HSV infection during pregnancy present the fetus with the greatest risk of infection since in primary maternal infection as many as one third to one half of women transmit HSV to the fetus. In contrast, about 3 percent of women with recurrent disease transmit HSV to the newborn.[47]

Neonatal HSV presents in two forms, localized and disseminated. Localized HSV is confined to the skin, eyes, and mucous membranes (SEM), in which vesicles and keratoconjunctivitis develop. Neonatal HSV can also localize in the CNS, producing symptoms of encephalitis. Of those infants who survive HSV encephalitis, almost all experience permanent neurologic sequelae.[48] Pneumonitis, rash, hepatitis, and disseminated intravascular coagulopathy, with or without encephalitis or SEM involvement, characterize disseminated neonatal HSV. Twenty percent of neonates with diagnosed HSV develop dissemination and of these more than half die.

Infants born to mothers with confirmed or suspected HSV infection must be observed and tested carefully for at least 2 weeks for possible neonatal infection. Cultures must be taken from the eyes, nose, mouth, throat, rectum, and any skin lesion. Urine, buffy white blood cell coat, and CSF are also cultured for the virus. Therapy includes the use of the antiviral drug vidarabine in addition to supportive measures. Recent studies[49] report that acyclovir, a parenteral antiviral drug, is more effective and is tolerated well by the neonate. Mothers are confined to isolated rooms but allowed to care for their babies. Breast feeding is discouraged until complete resolution of active maternal disease.

ANESTHETIC CONSIDERATIONS

A search of a 15-year period of the literature elicited little information on the subject of anesthetic management of the pregnant patient with herpes. An absence of complications following the use of either regional or general anesthesia in patients afflicted with this disease, or an incidence of complications too rare to be reported may explain the paucity of data. The primary issue revolves around these questions: Does a chance of seeding the epidural or subarachnoid space with HSV in active disease exist and does herpes ever contraindicate regional anesthesia? Definitive answers have not evolved, but examination of current anesthesia practice in the presence of similar types of infection proves useful.

Regional Block

Anesthesiologists commonly perform regional block in the presence of infections such as chorioamnionitis, urinary tract infection, viral infection, or rectal-perineal abscess in the absence of severe systemic dissemination. Indeed, lumbar sympathetic or epidural injection of local anesthetics and steroids for prevention of postherpetic neuralgia represents one accepted therapy for acute herpes zoster.[50] Herpes genitalis generally remains in the perineal region, while epidural and spinal blocks take place in the midlumbar region. Ravindran and coworkers,[51] evaluating 30 parturients with active HSV type 2 who received continuous lumbar epidural, reported good outcomes with no complications. Though HSV rarely produces meningitis, no evidence exists that regional anesthesia disseminates HSV genitalis or that the presence of this disease contraindicates regional anesthesia. Joyce and Marx[52] recently surveyed 123 anesthesiologists and 20 obstetricians who actively practice obstetric anesthesia in the United States, to gain insight into the standard of care regarding the presence of this disease and the frequency of complications. The respondents collectively saw approximately 3000 patients per year with herpes, diagnosed either by active lesions or by history. The majority of respondents had not seen a complication which one could associate with regional anesthesia in the presence of HSV, and none defined a known complication in their own practice. In the presence of an active vulvar, vaginal, or cervical lesion, 52 of 143 respondents would not use regional anesthesia. Of the remaining 87 who would use regional anesthesia, 10 percent would defer regional anesthesia when a primary lesion existed. Most respondents (136 of 143) would use spinal or epidural anesthesia in a patient with a history of HSV. If the sexual consort had an active lesion, 107 would administer regional anesthesia and 13 would not; 23 had no opinion. If the obstetrician decided on cesarean section to prevent fetal HSV exposure, 107 respondents would use regional anesthesia and 36 would employ general anesthesia. Conclusions drawn from this survey include the following:

1. Of some 3000 pregnant patients per year with either active primary or recurrent herpes genitalis, at least 65 percent (more than 2000 per year for several years) have received regional anesthesia without complications.
2. Clinicians surveyed almost universally agree that a history of HSV alone, without active lesions, does not contraindicate regional anesthesia.
3. Seventy percent of clinicians surveyed routinely use regional anesthesia for cesarean sections performed to prevent neonatal HSV and find no maternal complications.
4. The presence of active lesions on buttocks or back may be a reason to avoid regional techniques.
5. A history of a previous positive culture, active lesion in the male partner, or recurrent disease does not deter the majority from using regional anesthesia in the obstetric patient.
6. Some respondents have medical and medicolegal concerns regarding the use of regional techniques in the presence of active herpetic lesions, which may not be justified.

We routinely use regional anesthesia in most parturients with active herpes lesions when the obstetrician chooses cesarean section to avoid HSV in neonates. However, if HSV lesions exist near or over the site of the planned needle puncture, we prefer general anesthesia. Labor floor personnel with active HSV infection on the face or hands should have limited patient contact and observe infection control procedures (hand washing, gloves, and mask).

The use of epidural narcotics for postcesarean analgesia may be associated with reactivation of oral herpes in the postpartum period. Crone and coworkers[53] retrospectively surveyed 291 parturients who received epidural analgesia. Thirteen of 134 women given epidural morphine developed recurrent oral herpes, compared with one of 157 women who did not receive epidural morphine. Douglas and others[54] studied the incidence of recurrent oral herpes in 556 women who delivered by cesarean section, finding that 20 patients (3.59 percent) developed recrudescent HSV-1 lesions. Of this number, 18 had received epidural morphine. In comparison, 5 of 255 vaginal delivery patients (1.96 percent) developed recrudescent lesions, none of whom received epidural morphine. Because of confounding variables and lack of strict controls, careful prospective studies have yet to establish a cause and effect relationship between epidural morphine and recurrent oral herpes. However, epidural morphine and the HSV-1 share the trigeminal ganglion as a site of activity, and itching over the trigeminal distribution of the face due to epidural morphine may reactivate a lesion. In view of these preliminary findings and the possibility of maternal-newborn transmission of this disease, the anesthesiologist must inquire during the preanesthetic visit whether the patient has a history of HSV infection and must weigh potential risks against the advantages of epidural morphine following cesarean section.

Acquired Immunodeficiency Syndrome

Fever commonly occurs in individuals with acquired immunodeficiency syndrome (AIDS). Although AIDS predominantly affects men, 7 percent of AIDS cases occur in women.[55] As of 1986, 1075 cases in women had been reported to the Centers for Disease Control (CDC) in Atlanta, of which 81 percent occurred during child-bearing years.[56]

DEFINITION AND ETIOLOGY

Since the first clinical report of AIDS in 1981, between 5 and 15 million people worldwide, and more than 1 million in the United States, have become infected with the virus. Eventually causing death, AIDS is characterized by alterations in cell-mediated immunity that ultimately render previously healthy men and women vulnerable to unusual opportunistic infections and certain malignancies. The pathogen responsible for the reduction in cell-mediated immunity is a retrovirus, isolated in 1983[57] called human T-cell lymphotrophic virus, type III (HTLV-III). Recently, workers[58] have proposed the designation human immunodeficiency virus (HIV). This virus interacts with and penetrates T cells, particularly helper-inducer T cells (T_4), a subset of lymphocytes responsible for a number of immune system functions, including stimulation of B cells to produce antibody, induction of T_8 suppressor cells to kill infected cells, and stimulation of T_8 cells to suppress the cytotoxic response during resolution of infection. Once in the target cell's cytoplasm, the virus transcribes its genetic information from RNA into a proviral DNA by way of an enzyme called reverse transcriptase. The proviral DNA is then integrated into the host's DNA. The invaded T cell now contains the genetic information needed to produce and assemble HIV, once triggered. What factors stimulate infected T_4 cells to clone HIV remains unclear. With subsequent destruction of T_4 cells, the T_4/T_8 ratio, usually >1, decreases to <0.5, a laboratory finding helpful in making the diagnosis of AIDS. An antibody response does appear; yet the time to develop seroconversion varies extremely. Paradoxically, this antibody response does not confer immunity or viral eradication but instead indicates active infection.

Limited reports indicate that seroconversion takes place anywhere from 19 days[59] to as long as 4 months[60] after viral exposure. The virus can be cultured in 68 to 100 percent of seropositive individuals.[61] Four to 20 percent of antibody-positive individuals develop the complete syndrome of AIDS,[62,63] with symptoms appearing from 9 months to 5 years after becoming seropositive.[64,65] One study[66] reports that, on the average, AIDS patients die 12 months after being diagnosed.

RISK GROUPS

In the United States, an overwhelming majority of adults with AIDS are men, ages 20 to 49, with homosexual experiences or a history of using intravenous drugs (Table 22–4).[67] Recent studies in Haiti,[68] Rwanda,[69] and Zaire[70] reveal an increasing proportion of female cases, resulting from heterosexual transmission. Of the nearly 2000 cases involving American women in 1986, 51 percent resulted from intravenous drug use, 27 percent from sexual contact with high-risk men, 10 percent by transfusions, and 12 percent from unknown means.[67] Recent evidence indicates that the vaginal canal, like the rectum, can introduce or harvest the AIDS virus. Several investigators[71,72] have isolated HIV from cervical secretions in a significant percentage of seropositive women. In a recent study,[73] 34 percent of men with AIDS and no identifiable risk factors gave a history of sexual contact with female prostitutes. Equally important, semen is a likely vector of sexual transmission, since transmission of HIV by artificial insemination has been confirmed.[74] Undoubtedly, HIV can be transmitted by either sex. This mechanism will gradually increase the incidence of infection in women in the United States in years to come.

Table 22–4. DISTRIBUTION OF ADULT AIDS PATIENTS THROUGH DECEMBER, 1986

Patient Group	% of Total Cases Reported
Homosexual and bisexual men only	66
IV drug users only	17
Both homosexuals and IV drug users	8
Hemophilia patients and transfusion recipients	4
Heterosexual contacts	4
Persons with no identified risks	3

(From Morbidity and Mortality Weekly Report 35:49, 1986)

MODES OF TRANSMISSION

Male-to-male transmission through anal intercourse has been the principal route of spread in the United States and in Europe.[62] Horizontal transmission occurs through administration of contaminated blood products (i.e., packed red blood cells, platelets, plasma, whole blood, clotting factor concentrates, and cryoprecipitate), the sharing of contaminated needles by IV drug abusers, and from maternal-fetal contamination. Nearly 1 percent of hemophiliacs are infected;[75] a higher risk follows the use of pooled products such as Factor VIII concentrates. Heat treatment of some of these blood products dramatically reduces transmission, but in some cases it may also decrease their efficacy.[76] One study[77] suggests that IV drug users and hemophiliacs are four to five times more likely to get AIDS than are homosexuals. A smaller yet significant number of cases has been traced to the administration of contaminated blood or plasma.[78] The American Red Cross now screens all donated blood for HIV antibody to minimize this risk.

Reports suggest that maternal-fetal transmission occurs during pregnancy, parturition,[79,80] or ingestion of infected breast milk.[81] About two thirds of pregnancies in HIV infected mothers lead to neonatal infection.[65] AIDS does not appear to spread by casual contact,[82] saliva, tears, or by means of sneezing or coughing.[83] Likewise, no evidence exists that the hepatitis B vaccine transmits AIDS.[84]

CLINICAL MANIFESTATIONS

Although only 28,098 cases of AIDS were reported in the United States by December 1986, estimates place the number of infected persons at approximately 1 million.[67] The disease has a wide spectrum of clinical manifestations, ranging from asymptomatic carrier states to lymphadenopathy-associated syndromes (otherwise known as AIDS-related complex, ARC), to fulminant AIDS with devastating opportunistic infections, malignancies, and ultimately death. The symptoms of ARC, often referred to as persistent generalized lymphadenopathy, consist of swollen lymph glands in the neck, axillae, and inguinal areas lasting for weeks or months, fever of unknown origin, diarrhea, weight loss, and night sweats. The disease may progress to a more sinister state, predisposing the infected individual to protozoal, helminthic, fungal, bacterial, or viral infection, i.e., diseases considered predictive of underlying cellular immunodeficiency (Table 22–5). As a result, patients present with profound alterations in multiple organ systems (Table 22–6). Additionally, several neoplastic diseases occur with much higher frequency among the AIDS population, namely Kaposi's sarcoma, Burkitt's lymphoma, non-Hodgkin's lymphoma, and chronic lymphocytic leukemia.

OBSTETRIC MANAGEMENT

Since women constitute an increasing fraction of infected individuals, obstetricians are becoming more aware of AIDS in the parturient. Given the alterations in immunity known to occur with pregnancy,[85] the mother may have decreased resistance to infectious and neoplastic agents, hence placing her at greater risk of acquiring AIDS.[86] Pregnancy may also suppress an immune system already compromised by HIV, which could promote progression from an asymptomatic infection to ARC or AIDS. For example, Scott and coworkers[87] report on the fate of 16 asymptomatic mothers (carriers) who delivered 22 infants with AIDS. Although the women were well at delivery, five developed fulminant AIDS and seven had ARC within an average postpartum time of 30 months. Welti and others[90] recount the case of a 27-year-old Haitian woman who was initially admitted at 32

Table 22–5. OPPORTUNISTIC INFECTIONS IN AIDS

Protozoal and helminthic infections
Cryptosporidiosis
Pneumocystis carinii
Strongyloidosis
Toxoplasmosis
Fungal infections
Aspergillosis
Candidiasis
Cryptococcosis
Histoplasmosis
Bacterial infections
Atypical mycobacteriosis
Viral infections
Cytomegalovirus
Herpes simplex virus
Progressive multifocal leukoencephalopathy (papovavirus)

Table 22–6. SYSTEMIC MANIFESTATIONS OF AIDS

CNS
Encephalopathies, meningitis, mass lesions, and cerebral vasculitis resulting in dementia paraparesis, ataxia, and seizures terminating in coma and death; 30 percent develop neurologic complications[88]
Respiratory
Pneumonias (in 63% *Pneumocystis carinii* pneumonia[89]), aspergillosis, herpetic lesions, oral and pharyngeal candidiasis, mycobacterium (typical and atypical), coccidioidomycosis resulting in severe respiratory compromise
GI
Cytomegalovirus colitis-proctitis resulting in diarrhea, vomiting, decrease in appetite and subsequent malabsorption, dehydration, negative nitrogen balance, and electrolyte abnormalities
Hematologic
Anemia, leukopenia, and idiopathic thrombocytopenia

weeks' gestation with a fever, sore neck, and slight cough of 1 week's duration. She subsequently developed *Listeria monocytogenes* bacteremia and died of cardiac arrest 3½ hours after giving birth to a premature infant. The presumed underlying cause was AIDS.

The management of the AIDS-infected parturient poses many difficult questions. Although a few reports do trace newborn AIDS to blood transfusions in the neonate,[91] mounting evidence indicates that mothers serve as the likely source of infection in pediatric cases of AIDS or ARC.[92–94] The routes of HIV transmission include (1) uteroplacental,[79–80] (2) perinatal, via contact with maternal blood or cervical secretions during delivery, and (3) postnatal, via breast feeding.[81]

In 1985, the CDC made the following recommendations for preventing perinatal transmission of HIV.[60] In addition to counseling, blood screening should be offered to the following pregnant women: (1) those with clinical evidence of HIV infection, (2) intravenous drug abusers, (3) individuals from countries where heterosexual transmission plays a major role in the epidemiology of the virus, (4) women with multiple sexual encounters or those engaged in prostitution, and (5) women who are or have been sexual partners of high-risk individuals, i.e., bisexual men, hemophiliacs, infected men, or men born in high-risk countries. When screening detects infection, the woman should be strongly advised to avoid pregnancy, and if pregnant, to terminate the pregnancy.[65] This eliminates the risk of neonatal AIDS and the likelihood of acquisition or progression of disease in the parturient. Additionally, infected or high-risk mothers should avoid breast feeding. Last, public education must be instituted to enable those at high risk to identify themselves. Obstetric management of the parturient with AIDS poses many legal and ethical issues. Despite remarkable advances in our understanding of AIDS, much remains to be learned about this tragic disease.

ANESTHETIC CONSIDERATIONS

The parturient with AIDS is at risk of developing perioperative complications due to the presence of multisystem disease (see Table 22–6). We will discuss those conditions most likely to influence anesthetic management and make suggestions concerning management of analgesia for labor and anesthesia for operative obstetrics.

Respiratory System

Oral thrush, common in AIDS patients, increases tissue friability and edema, making airway management difficult. The high incidence of *Pneumocystis carinii* pneumonia and other opportunistic pulmonary infections significantly impairs oxygenation and predisposes to hypoxemia and respiratory failure intraoperatively and postoperatively.

Central Nervous System

As many as 30 percent of AIDS patients manifest central nervous system disease, including disorders that can produce secondary vacuolar degeneration of the spinal cord,[88] dementia, and nonspecific loss of higher brain function from progressive encephalopathy. When considering spinal or epidural anesthesia, careful evaluation and documentation of neurologic deficits are prudent.

Cardiovascular System

Dehydration secondary to profuse diarrhea, fever, and poor oral intake and electrolyte abnormalities requires thorough evaluation and adequate correction prior to induction to anesthesia. The need for intraoperative invasive monitoring depends on the severity of the ongoing deficit and the degree of hemodynamic compromise. Common hematologic alterations include anemia, thrombocytopenia, and leukopenia. Thus, coagulation studies should be obtained in AIDS patients before proceeding with regional anesthesia.

Anesthetic Management

The patient with a fatal and communicable systemic infection such as AIDS poses a dilemma for the anesthesiologist. During labor, the path of least resistance leaves analgesia to the obstetrician, who will generally choose a systemic drug for labor and local or pudendal block for delivery. These techniques may provide adequate but not optimal conditions for many deliveries. One can safely provide more effective analgesia for delivery by adding enflurane (0.5- to 1-percent), or ketamine 0.25 mg per kg to 30 to 40 percent nitrous oxide in oxygen. The use of inhalation analgesia and/or low-dose ketamine does not require endotracheal intubation, provided the mother does not lose consciousness. Unconsciousness warrants rapid tracheal intubation with cricoid pressure and succinylcholine. Neither systemic nor inhalation techniques provide consistently adequate analgesia; many patients require more profound pain relief. Therefore, minimizing the involvement of an anesthesiologist predisposes the pregnant AIDS population to a significant number of unnecessary emergency general anesthetics. Additional airway problems and hemodynamic instability stemming from AIDS-related disease will accompany the usual risks of general anesthesia. The foregoing provides a strong argument for the use of epidural analgesia for labor and delivery in the AIDS patient. Unfortunately, the presence of AIDS-related neuropathy, coagulation disorders, and the possibility of spreading an infectious process to the neuraxis discourage many anesthesiologists from using this technique. We believe that the parturient with AIDS can receive regional anesthesia on a selected basis. In the absence of coagulopathy, severe systemic sepsis, or uncorrected hypovolemia, no evidence presently contraindicates the use of regional analgesia in the parturient with AIDS. If the need for emergency cesarean section emerges during labor, the anesthesiologist can easily extend a functioning epidural block for adequate operating conditions, without further impairing maternal consciousness, protective airway mechanisms, or hemodynamic stability.

In the absence of severe systemic manifestations, coagulopathy, and neuropathy, the type of anesthesia for elective cesarean section depends on the mother's preference in consultation with her anesthesiologist. Epidural analgesia offers a variety of well-known advantages, which include preservation of maternal consciousness, avoidance of airway manipulation, less effect on hemodynamics, the opportunity of extended postoperative analgesia with epidural narcotics, earlier ambulation, and improved patient mood and satisfaction. Given the complex nature of this disease, the obstetrician must consult the anesthesia staff early in the course of labor or prior to admission so that thorough evaluation, necessary therapy, and anesthetic plans can be fully discussed and initiated.

RISKS TO HEALTH PROFESSIONALS

Occupational hazards to those caring for AIDS victims continue to foster intense debate. Of greatest concern are the insidious nature of AIDS and its ultimately fatal outcome. While anesthesia, surgical, and obstetrical personnel directly exposed to body fluids of AIDS patients theoretically have a greater risk of becoming infected than other medical personnel, the overall transmission of HIV risk to health care providers remains low.[95–97] Aggregate data from five separate studies, reviewing 666 workers with either direct parenteral or mucosal exposure to AIDS or HIV infection revealed 26 seropositive individuals. All but three of the persons belonged to groups recognized to be at increased risk for AIDS.[60] The CDC registry of documented exposures reveals that 68 percent of infections occurred by needle stick; 13 percent, by mucosal exposure; 10 percent, by cuts with sharp instruments; and 9 percent, from contaminated open skin lesions. Although blood, semen, saliva, urine, CSF, tears, and breast milk harbor HIV, the CDC report cites blood or semen as the fluid involved in 88 percent of all those with AIDS.[82] Table 22–7 outlines guidelines recommended to reduce contamination with the AIDS virus.

CONCLUSION

Acquired immunodeficiency syndrome is increasing in epidemic proportions. It no longer is a disease of male homosexuals and, in fact, statistics show that an increasing proportion of AIDS victims are women, many of whom are of child-bearing age. AIDS is an insidious but ultimately devastating disease with a variable latency period. Clinically, it unfavorably alters various body systems owing to a breakdown in cell-mediated immunity. Definitive obstetric management of the parturient with AIDS remains undetermined, yet recommendations have been made. Anesthesiologists have an obligation to relieve suffering in parturients with an illness that produces physiologic impairment ranging from mild to morbid, and yet must protect themselves from acquiring the disease. Unfortunately, no cure for AIDS exists; therefore, preventive measures remain critical in containing this disease.

Malignant Hyperthermia (MH)

This discussion of fever would be incomplete without considering malignant hyperthermia

Table 22–7. SAFETY PRECAUTIONS FOR TREATING AIDS PATIENTS

Use disposable supplies; masks, laryngoscopes, CO_2 absorbers, resuscitative equipment.
Discard contaminated objects with as little handling as possible; do not recap or bend needles before disposing into puncture resistant containers.
Avoid body fluids from infected persons, particularly blood.
Wear protective clothing—gloves, gowns, masks, and goggles—when necessary.
Avoid the need for mouth-to-mouth resuscitation by being adequately prepared.
Sterilize and disinfect reusable equipment.
Clearly label potentially infected waste for safe disposal.
Pregnant or immunosuppressed persons should avoid contact with AIDS patients.

(MH), previously considered a rare autosomal-dominant inherited myopathy[98] but now thought to be inherited via two or three genes or alleles as opposed to solely dominant or recessive factors.[99] Estimates of genetic malignant hyperthermia susceptibility (MHS) approximate 1 in 20,000.[100] The highest incidence of MH reactions occurs in children and young adults. Ording,[101] studying the disorder in Danish patients, demonstrated a fulminant MH reaction in 1 in 220,000 general anesthesias and an incidence of milder "abortive" cases in 1 in 16,000 general anesthesias. Ellis and Halsal[102] reported an incidence of MH of 1 in 200,000 anesthesias in the United Kingdom, while Britt and Kalow[103] estimated an incidence of MH in 1 in 14,000 anesthesias in Canada. The few cases of MH reported in the parturient to date have all been treated successfully.[104–108] Several parturients with demonstrated malignant hyperthermia susceptibility (MHS) have undergone both regional and general anesthesia without developing MH, either with[107] or without dantrolene prophylaxis.[109–113] However in an MHS Poland China sow, Lucke[114] observed the development of MH followed by death after induction of anesthesia for cesarean section with halothane. Crawford has postulated that pregnancy may protect against the development of MH in some unknown manner.[100]

Before the introduction of dantrolene therapy, patients who developed MH during general anesthesia had a mortality rate of 53 to 70 percent.[115–117] Dantrolene therapy has decreased the MH mortality occurring under general anesthesia to 28 percent.[118] With early diagnosis and dantrolene therapy mortality should be less than 7 to 10 percent.[118,119] Recognition of MHS individuals proves essential to avoid their exposure to triggering drugs and thereby minimize mortality. Susceptible patients often exhibit increased muscle bulk, localized muscle weakness, frequent muscle cramps or spasms, joint hypermobility, ptosis and squint, kyphoscoliosis, and/or club foot.[120] Patients with muscular dystrophies or those with the King-Denborough[121] syndrome (short stature, musculoskeletal abnormalities, and mental retardation) have a higher incidence of MHS. Infants and neonates of an MHS parent may have an increased incidence of sudden infant death syndrome.[122,123] The history of a relative dying during or shortly after general anesthesia, particularly with high fever, muscle spasm, or from causes unrelated to surgery, should alert the anesthesia team to the possibility of MHS. A previous uncomplicated general anesthetic, even utilizing triggering drugs, does not rule out the risk of MH crisis[115] since nearly 50 percent of MHS patients develop MH during a subsequent anesthetic.[116] Unfortunately, no completely reliable diagnostic procedure currently exists to confirm or to rule out MHS. In approximately 70 percent of MHS patients, the serum creatine phosphokinase (CPK) value will become elevated, perhaps indicating susceptibility. However, a negative test does not rule out MHS as repeated normal CPK results commonly occur in MHS individuals[99,124–126] with as many as one third of them having normal serum CPK values.[120] The most reliable test for MHS involves exposing a sample of the person's muscle to the triggering drugs caffeine and/or halothane. Such exposure causes muscle contraction if MHS is present, with a reliability of 90 percent.[127] While false-negative results do not occur, occasionally false-positive results are obtained.[128] Patients undergoing this muscle contraction test must not receive dantrolene, which may block the muscle contraction.[129] Unfortunately, anesthesia personnel frequently first see the obstetric patient when she is in labor, at the time she requires anesthesia, perhaps the first anesthetic of her life.

FACTORS INITIATING MALIGNANT HYPERTHERMIA

Precipitation of an MH crisis depends on three factors: (1) susceptibility, (2) exposure to a triggering drug or other triggering factor (e.g., extreme muscle activity, emotional stress, infection, high environmental temperature, or muscle injury), and (3) absence of triggering inhibitory factors. Drugs capable of triggering an MH crisis consist of *all* potent inhalation agents (halothane, enflurane, forane, methoxyflurane, ether, cyclopropane, etc.) and the depolarizing muscle relaxants. Other drugs to be avoided include caffeine and related drugs, sympathomimetics (including β_2 agonists used for tocolysis), calcium salts, cardiac glycosides, tricyclic antidepressants, MAO inhibitors, and quinidine. In the past, amide local anesthetics reportedly represented possible triggering drugs; indeed some still caution against their use.[119–130] However, there are no reports of an amide local anesthetic alone[131] or the infusion of amide local anesthetics into an MHS swine[132] causing an MH reaction. Berkowitz and Rosenberg[133] utilized mepivacaine for femoral nerve block, often in combination with lidocaine local infiltration, for obtaining muscle biopsies in 103 patients of whom 52 proved positive for MHS. None of these 52 patients displayed any evidence of MH during or following the procedure. While the amide local anesthetics appear innocuous, the para-aminobenzoic acid esters are known to be safe and may even inhibit an MH reaction.[117] Other anesthetic drugs identified as safe in the MHS individual include narcotics, barbiturates, depressant tranquilizers (phenothiazines, butyrophenones, benzodiazepines), nitrous oxide, and the nondepolarizing relaxants (pancuronium, atracurium, vecuronium).[119] These drugs likewise may actually inhibit MH.[134] MHS does not contraindicate the reversal of nondepolarizing muscle relaxants with an anticholinergic agent (glycopyrrolate) and an anticholinesterase (neostigmine).[135,136]

ANESTHETIC CONSIDERATIONS

The basic approach to MHS patients consists of avoidance of triggering agents, careful monitoring, and prompt aggressive treatment of an MH reaction, should it occur. We advocate regional analgesia, particularly the use of continuous epidural analgesia, as the technique of choice in the MHS parturient because it (1) avoids the use of triggering agents, (2) provides excellent conditions alone for either labor and delivery or cesarean section, (3) may be used with either local anesthetics or epidural narcotics for postpartum pain relief, (4) decreases the stress reaction to parturiation whether it be by the vaginal[137] or abdominal route,[138] (5) allows the patient to remain awake and hence may provide earlier evidence of an MH reaction, and (6) in the event of an MH reaction, facilitates surface cooling by its sympathetic block, which causes peripheral vasodilatation.

While Bromage[139] acknowledges the impracticality of epidural analgesia as a form of treatment, he suggests that its effective interruption of neuraxial activity does appear to prevent the syndrome and may serve as a prophylactic measure during appropriate operations. Douglas and McMorland[140] reported 12 MHS parturients undergoing vaginal delivery (5) or cesarean section (7) with epidural utilizing 2-chloroprocaine without incident, while Wallatts[110] and Rose[141] managed two parturients successfully with bupivacaine epidurals. If a high-risk MH patient undergoes a trial of labor with cesarean section as a possibility, the epidural should begin early in labor and a solid T8 sensory level should be maintained until delivery. This will allow immediate abdominal delivery without the need for general anesthesia if emergency cesarean section is indicated. Douglas and McMorland[140] give an excellent discussion of the overall management of the MHS parturient, particularly as it relates to the use of epidural block.

Should an MHS mother require general anesthesia one must employ a technique that avoids all triggering agents. Induce anesthesia with thiopental and use 0.15 μg per kg pancuronium, 0.1 mg per kg vecuronium, or 0.6 mg per kg atracurium to facilitate rapid intubation. A priming dose of 10 percent of the total calculated dose of vecuronium or atracurium given 3 minutes before induction usually provides adequate relaxation for intubation within a minute following the main dose of the relaxant. Maintain anesthesia with 60 to 70 percent nitrous oxide in oxygen with a small amount of narcotic until delivery. Following delivery, addition of more narcotics, tranquilizers, and thiopental to the nitrous oxide insures that the mother will be unconscious. At the conclusion of surgery, reverse residual paralysis with appropriate doses of an anticholinergic (glycopyrrolate) and an anticholinesterase (neostigmine). When employing general anesthesia, use a fresh disposable carbon dioxide canister not previously exposed to potent inhalation drugs. Ideally use an anesthesia machine without vaporizers for potent inhalation drugs. In the absence of such a machine, empty the vaporizers and the machine for several hours, or, in an emergency, as long as possible before induction, as even trace amounts of the potent agent may trigger an MH reaction.

Monitoring During Anesthesia

Careful patient monitoring is essential to the immediate detection of signs of a developing MH reaction. Table 22–8 summarizes the signs and laboratory findings of MH. Early diagnosis and immediate therapy of MH reaction greatly improve the prognosis. The elevation of temperature usually comes late in an MH crisis. A marked elevation in end-tidal carbon dioxide tension ($P_{et}CO_2$), which returns to normal with successful therapy[142] provides one of the earliest warnings of MH and is easily detected by monitoring $P_{et}CO_2$ with a capnograph[143] or the mass spectrometer.[142] Both esophageal and axillary temperatures should be monitored during general anesthesia in the MHS patient. An automatic patient temperature–triggered heating and cooling blanket should be on the operating table to allow surface cooling, should MH occur. Observe the patient constantly for any of the following signs that can indicate MH: tachycardia, muscle spasm or stiffness, especially follow-

Table 22–8. SIGNS AND LABORATORY FINDINGS IN MALIGNANT HYPERPYREXIA

Signs	Laboratory Findings
Tachycardia	Central venous desaturation
Tachypnea	Central venous and arterial hypercarbia (early)
Cardiac arrhythmias	Marked elevation of $P_{et}CO_2$ (early)
Dark blood in surgical field	Metabolic acidosis
Cyanotic mottling of skin	Hyperkalemia
Unstable blood pressure	Respiratory acidosis
Profuse sweating	Myoglobinemia (late)
Fever	Elevated CPK (late)
Rapid rise (1°F/15 min)	
Sustained rise (to as high as 108°F)	
Rigidity (trismus is an early sign, particularly following the use of succinylcholine)	Myoglobinuria (late)

ing the use of succinylcholine, tachypnea, respiratory and/or metabolic acidosis, cardiac arrhythmias, unstable or rising blood pressure, and cyanosis or skin mottling.

THERAPY FOR MALIGNANT HYPERTHERMIA

As soon as MH is suspected discontinue all potential triggering agents and take steps to prevent further exposure to trace amounts of the agents by changing: (1) all rubber goods in the breathing circuit; (2) the soda lime or placing the patient on a non-rebreathing system, and (3) to a machine without potent inhalation agents or vaporizers. Next initiate specific therapy with dantrolene, a direct-acting skeletal muscle relaxant which itself has no effect on the neuromuscular junction or the electrically excitable surface membrane. Dantrolene inhibits the release of calcium ions from the sarcoplasmic reticulum of skeletal muscle with little effect on cardiac or smooth muscle.[144] Its efficacy in the treatment of an MH crisis in both MHS humans[145] and swine[146] has been documented. Administer dantrolene intravenously at a rate of 1 mg per kg per min to a maximum of 10 mg per kg (mean effective dose, 2.5 mg per kg) until the heart rate slows, the cardiac rhythm becomes more regular, and muscle tone and body temperature decrease. Repeat further infusions every 15 min as necessary if signs of the MH reaction reappear.

Initiate intravenous dantrolene therapy immediately after making the diagnosis of MH. Delay in such therapy causes a greatly increased mortality as shown in Table 22–9. Dantrolene is packaged in ampules containing 20 mg dantrolene and 3 g mannitol, which, when reconstituted with 60 ml water (without a bacteriostatic agent), gives a solution of pH 9.5 from added sodium hydroxide. Initial therapy can require as many as 35 ampules of drug and 2100 ml of sterile water to reconstitute it. Hence, therapy requires not only an adequate supply of drug but also sufficient manpower to reconstitute and to administer it.

Other supportive therapy includes active cooling by a variety of routes, hyperventilation with high flows of 100-percent oxygen to assure adequate oxygenation and removal of excess carbon dioxide, treatment of metabolic acidosis with sodium bicarbonate, and promotion of adequate diuresis. Table 22–10 outlines the therapeutic regimen recommended by the Malignant Hyperthermia Association of the United States (MHAUS).[147] This organization has physicians available 24 hours a day* for emergency consultation; for nonemergency advice or patient referral calls, the association may be contacted in Darien, Connecticut.†

Dantrolene Prophylaxis

While some have recommended dantrolene prophylaxis for MHS patients undergoing general anesthesia, considerable controversy exists as to its necessity, since triggering drugs will be avoided.[148] The need for prophylaxis becomes even more questionable when employing major conduction analgesia, particularly if amide local

*Medic Alert Foundation Information. Ask for index zero. Phone (209) 634-4917.

†MHAUS, PO Box 3231, Darien, Conn. 06821. Phone (203) 655-3007.

Table 22–9. TIME FROM INDUCTION OF ANESTHESIA TO INITIATION OF DANTROLENE THERAPY AS RELATED TO MORTALITY IN PATIENTS HAVING A MALIGNANT HYPERTHERMIA REACTION

Time After Anesthesia Induction (min)	No. Patients Survived	Died	% Survival
0–29	9	0	100
30–59	7	0	100
60–119	12	0	100
120–179	4	2	67
≥180	7	8	47

(From BA Britt,[144] with permission.)

Table 22–10. SUGGESTED THERAPY FOR MALIGNANT HYPERTHERMIA EMERGENCY[147]

1. Discontinue all inhalation anesthetics and begin hyperventilation with 100-percent oxygen.
2. In the absence of blood gas analysis, administer bicarbonate, 1 to 2 mEq/kg.
3. Obtain dantrolene sodium, mix it with sterile distilled water, and administer 2.5 mg/kg intravenously. At present, dantrolene comes packaged as a lyophilized preparation that contains 20 mg of dantrolene and 3 g mannitol per vial.
4. Simultaneously initiate cooling by all routes: surface, nasogastric lavage, intravenous cold solutions, wound, and rectally.
5. Change anesthesia tubing, and if possible, soda lime.
6. Arrhythmias will usually respond to treatment of acidosis and hyperkalemia. If they persist or threaten survival, administer 200 mg procainamide in repeated doses as needed.
7. Administer further doses of dantrolene as necessary, titrated to the heart rate, muscle rigidity, and temperature. Response to dantrolene should begin in minutes; if not, administer more drug. Although the average successful dose of dantrolene approaches 2.5 mg/kg, much higher doses may be needed (10 mg/kg and more). Fortunately, dantrolene does not produce significant myocardial depression in these doses.
8. Determine and closely monitor urine output, serum potassium, calcium, arterial blood gases, and clotting studies. Hyperkalemia commonly occurs in the acute phase of MH and requires treatment with intravenous glucose and insulin.
9. Observe the patient in an ICU setting for at least 24 hours since recrudescence of MH may occur, particularly following a case that was difficult to treat.
10. Follow CPK, calcium, and potassium until such time as they return to normal.
11. Also obtain an ECG and follow postoperatively.
12. Monitor body temperature closely since overvigorous treatment of MH may lead to hypothermia. Temperature instability may persist for several days after the acute episode. Body temperatures of 41°C to 42°C are compatible with survival and normal brain function if treated promptly.
13. Ensure urine output of greater than 1 ml/kg/hour. Consider CVP (and PA) monitoring because of fluid shifts that may occur.
14. When the patient's condition has stabilized, convert from intravenous to oral dantrolene. Although data are not available regarding optimal doses and duration of treatment with dantrolene after an episode, the patient should probably receive a total dose of 4 mg per kg per day in divided doses for 48 hours postoperatively.

CAUTION: This protocol may not apply to every patient and must of necessity be altered according to specific patient needs.

anesthetics with epinephrine are avoided. Britt[144] recommends prophylaxis when any of the following conditions exist:

1. A severely apprehensive patient
2. A prolonged operation
3. An operation associated with skeletal muscle injury
4. If anesthesia or surgery may produce a fall in blood pressure, a period of hypoxia, hypercarbia, or lactic acidosis
5. If the operating room or gas machine is not absolutely free of potent inhalation drugs
6. If the patient is to have awake dental or obstetric procedures with local or conductive anesthesia using amide local anesthetics. (Many would question this indication for dantrolene prophylaxis.)

Dantrolene prophylaxis can proceed by oral administration – 4 mg per kg per 24 hours given in three equal doses per day for 3 days before surgery. Unfortunately, it often causes generalized muscle weakness necessitating placing the patient at bed rest. The intravenous administration of 2.4 mg per kg over 10 to 15 min before induction of anesthesia is as effective as oral administration and represents a more practical means of prophylaxis, particularly for emergency anesthesia.[149,150] Like oral dantrolene, intravenous dantrolene administration produces muscle weakness not reversed by anticholinesterase drugs and lasts as long as 48 hours.[149] Dantrolene does cross the placenta, the fetal-maternal ratio being about 0.4.[151,152] Fortunately, maternal administration of dantrolene has not been associated with neonatal muscle weakness or other ill effects.[151] In the chronically instrumented gravid ewe, intravenous dantrolene injections of 1.2 mg per kg or 2.4 mg per kg caused no negative effects.[153] The maternal blood pressure and cardiac output increased slightly without significant changes of maternal heart rate, central venous pressure, or uterine blood flow. Despite a 25-percent decrease in fetal heart rate lasting 3 min no adverse changes occurred in maternal or fetal acid-base balance.[153] Dantrolene, which is metabolized by the cytochrome oxidase system of the liver, may prolong the metabolism and clearance of the amide local anesthetics.[154]

A recent case report described postpartum uterine atony requiring emergency hysterectomy in an MHS parturient following prophylactic intravenous dantrolene (220 mg) during cesarean section under spinal anesthesia.[155] Though no clear-cut cause-and-effect relationship exists between the drug and the atony, animal studies do demonstrate dantrolene-induced myometrial depression,[156] and a sequence of events similar to those in the case report suggest that dantrolene in therapeutic doses may generate postpartum uterine atony. The need for prophylactic dantrolene during cesarean delivery must be weighed against its potential for causing life-threatening uterine atony. If indeed dantrolene causes significant depression of uterine activity, we believe that prophylaxis in the MHS parturient is unwarranted since one can administer a safe anesthetic by avoiding MH-triggering agents and monitoring carefully.

Antipyretics

Antipyretics often constitute part of the therapy for fever. The undesirable sequelae sometimes produced by these drugs make an understanding of their pharmacodynamic properties important. The most frequently used antipyretics are acetylsalicylic acid (aspirin) and acetaminophen (Tylenol). These compounds alter the set-point mechanisms of the hypothalamus in response to pyrogens. They also suppress prostaglandin synthesis and stabilize white blood cells, thus preventing pyrogen release.[157] Steele and coworkers[158] found a faster onset of action and a greater decrease in temperature with acetaminophen than with equipotent doses of aspirin, but aspirin seemed to produce a longer duration of activity. Another study failed to show a significant difference in the antipyretic effects of the two drugs.[157] Both drugs produced an initial temperature reduction 30 to 60 min after ingestion with the maximal decrease of 1.5° to 3°F occurring 3 hours after ingestion. Increased temperatures reappeared shortly thereafter.

The decision to use antipyretics during pregnancy must, in each case, weigh the clinical indications versus the likelihood of harmful maternal and fetal side effects. The advantages of treatment include increased patient comfort and a reduced stress of fever to both mother and fetus. However, these drugs may obscure the signs of impending problems, possibly resulting in delayed treatment. For example, the use of aspirin or acetaminophen for analgesic purposes may mask febrile symptoms of chorioamnionitis or urinary tract infection. The pharmacologic risks of hypersensitivity and allergic reactions are minimal, but still a possibility. The other dangers of antipyretics relate to the specific compounds.

EFFECT ON HEMOSTASIS

The primary disadvantage of aspirin is its negative effect on hemostasis. By decreasing release of platelet adenosine diphosphate (ADP),[124,159–161] aspirin impairs platelet aggregation, which causes prolonged bleeding times.[162] Weiss and coworkers[162] found that in a single oral dose of 1.8 g, aspirin inhibited platelet aggregation for 4 to 7 days. At that time, they could no longer detect aspirin in the blood, implying that an irreversible effect on platelets occurs during their formation. Lower doses of aspirin[159] can alter hemostasis, as demonstrated by doubled bleeding times seen 2 hours after a standard dose of 650 mg orally.[161] Low-dose aspirin therapy has little clinical significance. Even though mean postaspirin bleeding time is twice the mean control value, most bleeding times remain within the normal range.[161] Thirty-five percent of patients have unaltered values after a 650-mg dose. Conversely, Davies[163] reported excessive surgical blood loss in patients who took small doses 3 to 7 days preoperatively. In parturients ingesting aspirin from twice weekly to 12 times daily throughout pregnancy, Corby[164] noted increased antepartum and postpartum hemorrhage, which necessitated more frequent transfusion.

Unlike aspirin, acetaminophen does not affect hemostasis.[165] The coagulation parameters and the incidence of postoperative bleeding do not differ between acetaminophen-treated patients and control patients. The coagulation profile changes only with overdosage of acetaminophen, which causes hepatic damage.

In light of the hemostatic alterations during aspirin therapy, the risk of regional anesthesia, particularly continuous epidural block, warrants consideration. Greensite[166] reported a case in which an epidural hematoma developed 36 hours after continuous spinal anesthesia. The etiology was ascribed to ingestion of 1850 mg aspirin over the 36-hour period. Locke[167] related the occurrence of a spontaneous epidural hematoma to the ingestion of 1500 mg of aspirin. When the patient has a history of aspirin use within a week preoperatively, a bleeding time should be obtained prior to institution of conduction analgesia.

FETAL CONSIDERATIONS

Long-term aspirin therapy may have teratogenic effects. An increased incidence of neonatal cleft palate correlates with aspirin therapy during the first trimester. At term gestation, patients (e.g., rheumatoid arthritics) taking large doses of antipyretic agents may have alterations in labor with resulting fetal effects. Prostaglandins account partly for initiation of uterine contractions. Since aspirin inhibits prostaglandin synthesis, aspirin therapy may delay the onset of labor. Patients using large doses have significant increases in: length of gestation, frequency of postmaturity, and complicated deliveries.[164] Aspirin rapidly crosses the placenta. In vitro studies have shown that neonatal platelets have greater sensitivity to aspirin than those of the mother. Corby[164] reported minor bleeding tendencies in the neonate. Arcilla[168] documented a case of possible closure of the ductus arteriosus in utero in a fetus whose mother had received aspirin for 2 weeks prior to delivery.

Although it has not been studied as thoroughly as aspirin, acetaminophen has not been associated with complications during pregnancy. Other than in gravidas with hepatitis or liver failure, acetaminophen appears the drug of choice for fever control in the gravid patient.

Anesthesia for the Febrile Parturient

REGIONAL ANESTHESIA

Anesthesiologists continue to debate the use of regional anesthesia in the presence of fever and infection. Despite little or no data directly implicating regional block with abscess formation in the febrile parturient, concern persists that a needle-borne nidus of infection could result in a neuraxial abscess. Phillips[169] reported on 11,802 spinal anesthesias without resulting infectious morbidity. Noble[170] reviewed 78,746 spinal anesthesias in Canadian teaching hospitals over a 10-year period and found no evidence of septic meningitis or epidural abscess. While reports of epidural abscess and meningitis following regional anesthesia[39,170–173] exist, close inspection of these reports fails to establish a direct cause-effect relationship with regional block. Most of the cases occurred in subjects at risk of neuraxial complications in the absence of regional block. In our experience, and following an extensive review of the literature, we are unaware of any reports of epidural abscess or meningitis following regional block in the febrile parturient.

Epidural Abscess

Epidural abscess rarely occurs in clinical practice. In a retrospective survey over a 26-year period, Baker[171] found 39 cases of epidural abscess, an overall incidence of 0.2 to 1.2 per 1000 admissions. Only one of the involved patients had received epidural analgesia. Collecting clinical data from 270 cases appearing between 1920 and 1958, Korbin[174] reported a mortality from epidural abscess of approximately 20 percent. Reviewing 202 cases Heusner[175] found 92-percent mortality in cases before 1927, 60-percent mortality before 1937, and 31-percent mortality after 1937, and 22-percent mortality in a series of cases between 1930 and 1948. The use of antibiotics accounts for this reduction in mortality. The clinical course of epidural abscess includes back and spine pain requiring large doses of narcotics. Headache, fever, and nerve root pain may also develop followed by gradual onset of muscle weakness, bladder dysfunction, and paraplegia. The average interval from onset of back pain to paraplegia is 4.5 days,[171] with a range of 1 to 23 days.[176] The mechanisms for paraplegia include spinal cord compression by the purulent mass,[171] impairment of cord perfusion (anterior spinal artery syndrome),[176] or both. Unfortunately, diagnosis usually follows discovery of the cord dysfunction.[173] Hancock[176] states that 60 percent of patients experience irreversible paraplegia.

Meningitis

The incidence of acute bacterial meningitis varies, depending upon age, sex, time of year, and patient debilitation. Swartz[177] found 207 cases from various series in Massachusetts General Hospital over a 6.5-year period. The mortality of meningitis at present approaches 20 percent.[171] The symptoms include headache, lethargy, confusion, vomiting, irritability, and fever; nuchal rigidity appears in 80 percent of patients.[177] These signs and symptoms may progress over a period of 24 hours to several days. When the patient survives, permanent neurologic deficits, hydrocephalus, seizure disorders, or decreased intellect commonly follow. The inoculum that produces meningitis may originate from one of several sources: (1) a break in sterile technique, (2) contaminated solutions or instruments used in establishing the block, (3) infection in the tract of injection, or (4) hematogenous spread.

Mechanism of Infection

Hematogenous spread appears to be the source of epidural abscess or meningitis in the febrile patient. Of the 39 cases of epidural abscess reported by Baker,[171] 26 to 41 percent apparently resulted from hematogenous spread. Grant[178] estimated a much higher incidence (72 percent) of these infections as being blood borne. Although these studies implicate sepsis as a major source of infection in the epidural or subarachnoid space, it remains unclear why these sites become targets for metastasized bacteria. In epidural abscess, trauma to the area has been advocated as a predisposing factor,[171,176] since it causes localized bleeding which then serves as a source for infection.[179] Bleeding can and often does occur in small amounts during placement of epidural or subarachnoid blocks. Bacteria may then invade this locus during a concomitant or subsequent bacteremia. Epidural abscess could then occur, or infection could traverse the dural hole in the case of spinal anesthesia.[180] However, there are no conclusive data to demonstrate that spinal or epidural blocks increase the incidence of infection at the vertebral column over that seen with bacteremia alone. Therefore, the true impact of vertebral column blocks on the incidence of infection remains unknown. The case reports on epidural abscess and meningitis occurring after regional block are few. However, until controlled data clarify the risk of infection following epidural or lumbar puncture during bacteremia, we feel it prudent to avoid elective epidural or subarachnoid block if bacteremia is suspected.

Healthy individuals without evidence of infection and not being instrumented, have an incidence of transient bacteremia, as documented by blood culture, of less than 1 percent.[181] Once the patient has any type of infection or instrumentation, the incidence of bacteremia may reach 90 percent. Parturition alone produces positive blood cultures in up to 5 percent of deliveries.[181] Urinary bladder catheterization, a common procedure in the parturient, can produce transient bacteremia in nearly 57 percent of patients, even though the urine is sterile.[181] The duration of this bacteremia[182] or whether there is a crucial time interval between it and regional anesthesia remains unknown. Furthermore, host defenses must play an important role in determining whether epidural abscess or meningitis occurs following bacteremia and regional block.

Recommendations

The clinical indication for the procedure and the absence of signs of systemic fulminant sepsis justify the decision to perform regional block in the febrile parturient. In the event of suspected bacteremia clinically manifested by high fever, chills, myalgia, and laboratory data showing newly elevated white blood cell count, we avoid epidural or spinal block. Antibiotic therapy, though present, may induce a false sense of security as serum bacterial inhibitory levels may be inadequate or the organism may be resistant. Andersen[183] found that 22 percent of 237 patients had break-through bacteremia due to subinhibitory levels of antibiotics. Blood cultures, though ordered, are usually unavailable to assess antibiotic efficacy. Conversely, endogenous pyrogens may maintain fever despite antibiotic eradication of bacteremia. To date, no documented cases of meningitis or epidural abscess have followed regional block in febrile parturients without bacteremia. Indeed, physicians commonly perform diagnostic lumbar puncture in febrile patients to rule out bacterial meningitis. The authors recommend that, in the presence of obstetric indications, regional block should not be withheld from the febrile parturient who has a nonsystemic infection.

General Anesthesia

While uncomplicated vaginal delivery rarely requires general anesthesia, it frequently becomes the technique of choice when maternal or fetal complications or inadequate time contraindicate regional anesthesia for cesarean section or complicated vaginal deliveries. Acute fetal distress, maternal hypovolemia, and maternal refusal of major conduction anesthesia require general anesthesia, as does sepsis, septic shock, or the development of fetal distress secondary to amnionitis. The febrile parturient falls prey to the same dangers that confront the uncomplicated gravida undergoing general anesthesia. These include: (1) pulmonary aspiration of gastric contents,[184,185] necessitating a rapid-sequence induction and intubation utilizing cricoid pressure;[186] (2) the need to minimize both the induction-to-delivery interval and the depth of anesthesia to avoid unnecessary newborn depression; (3) the requirement of left uterine displacement to prevent aortocaval compression;[187–191] and (4) the prevention of controlled hyperventilation with maternal $PaCO_2$ values below 25 mmHg, which may decrease uterine blood flow and increase fetal hypoxia and acidosis. In addition, the febrile patient has an increased likelihood of developing hypoxia and an abnormal response to skeletal muscle relaxants.

At term, the gravid patient more rapidly develops hypoxia during apneic episodes, such as laryngoscopy and tracheal intubation, for several reasons: (1) a decreased functional residual capacity, (2) a 14 percent increase in basal metabolic rate, (3) a 21 percent increase in oxygen consumption,[192] and (4) a 30 to 50 percent increase in cardiac output. Archer[193] demonstrated a 139 mmHg decrease in PaO_2 in healthy gravidas compared with a fall of only 58 mmHg in nonpregnant women exposed to 60 sec of apnea. Increased body temperature will raise the basal metabolic rate (oxygen demand) by 13 percent per degree centigrade.[194] Thus, the febrile state may elevate total oxygen consumption as much as 60 percent[195] and raise cardiac output by 50 to 70 percent.[9] These alterations place not only the parturient, but especially the febrile parturient and her fetus, at high risk for severe hypoxia during the induction of general anesthesia and possibly on emergence from anesthesia. These considerations mandate preoxygenation with high flows of pure oxygen for at least 3 min or four deep breaths[196] before induction of general anesthesia. A longer period of preoxygenation is preferable since fetal/maternal blood levels of oxygen require 6 min to equilibrate. During maintenance of general anesthesia, the fraction of inspired oxygen should remain above 0.5 until the birth of the newborn because a high FIO_2 fosters more vigorous newborns with better acid-base values.[197,198] Such a technique demands supplementation of nitrous oxide by a potent inhalation agent (halothane, enflurane, or methoxyflurane) to prevent maternal awareness and unpleasant dreams. In inspired concentrations of less than 1.0 MAC these agents provide additional maternal analgesia without increasing newborn depression or maternal blood loss secondary to decreased uterine contractility.[199–202] On emergence from anesthesia, the febrile parturient becomes particularly likely to experience hypoxia because of (1) the marked increase in oxygen consumption, (2) increased upper airway edema making obstruction more likely, and (3) the decreased functional residual capacity found in pregnancy. Remember not to discontinue respiratory assistance or to extubate the patient prematurely. In the postpartum period, observe the patient's respiratory status closely, give supplemental oxygen, and measure arterial blood gas values to assess adequacy of arterial oxygenation and acid-base status.

The febrile patient often receives antibiotics. Some of these agents, especially the aminoglycosides, can accentuate and prolong the effect of muscle relaxants (Table 22−11).[203,204] Therefore, monitoring with a peripheral nerve stimulator becomes important when using muscle relaxants in the presence of these antibiotics. The induction dose of succinylcholine should not be decreased in mothers receiving these antibiotics because a lower dose may not produce adequate relaxation for rapid intubation, thereby predisposing the mother to a greater chance of pulmonary aspiration of gastric contents. The use of 0.5 to 1.0 MAC concentrations of the potent inhalation drugs with 50 to 60 percent nitrous oxide will decrease relaxant requirements by producing a deeper level of anesthesia.

The development of hyperkalemia following the use of succinylcholine presents another problem in the febrile patient. In patients with severe infection of over 1 week's duration, Kohlshutter[205] found a predisposition to hyperkalemia and cardiac arrest after succinylcholine, emphasizing the need for electrocardiographic monitoring. Pretreatment with a nondepolarizing relaxant may attenuate but not completely prevent the change. Elevated T waves suggesting hyperkalemia often call for administering intravenous calcium chloride and sodium bicarbonate.

Table 22−11. ANTIBIOTICS THAT POTENTIATE NEUROMUSCULAR BLOCKING DRUGS

Streptomycin
Dihydrostreptomycin
Kanamycin
Neomycin
Gentamicin
Polymyxin B
Colistin sulfate
Oxytetracycline
Tetracycline
Lincomycin
Clindamycin HCl
Amikacin

INHALATION ANALGESIA

Inhalation analgesia can provide significant pain relief for the late first and second stage of labor.[206] In the febrile patient delivering vaginally, the technique avoids the possibility of morbidity associated with regional anesthesia. However, it produces inadequate analgesia for episiotomy incision and repair, necessitating supplemental use of perineal infiltration of local anesthetics or pudendal nerve blocks. Although minimal neonatal effects[207] and easy maternal adaptability are features of the technique, it has some disadvantages. During labor, the febrile patient should receive increased inspired oxygen, but self-administered vaporizers do not prove readily adaptable for this purpose. Mouthpiece-type vaporizers only allow intermittent oxygen administration, while mask-type vaporizers used with nasal oxygen limit the FIO_2 to less than 0.3. At delivery, the administration of the agents nitrous oxide (20 to 40 percent) or methoxyflurane (0.25 to 0.5 percent) through a snugly-fitted face mask and a semiclosed circle absorber system provides higher FIO_2's. This approach may not suffice for difficult forceps deliveries, and general endotracheal anesthesia may be necessary.

Although inhalation analgesia has limitations, a reasonable degree of patient acceptance and analgesia can follow proper instruction by the anesthetist. The potential for overdose (loss of consciousness) exists during continuous inhalation analgesia because of: (1) the 25 to 40 percent decrease in MAC of potent agents during pregnancy,[208] (2) the reduced functional residual capacity at term, and (3) the marked increases in minute ventilation during labor and delivery, especially in the febrile patient. Therefore, the anesthesiologist must repeatedly assess maternal responsiveness to avoid pitfalls of general anesthesia in the mother and fetus.

Summary

Fever increases the risks of parturition for both the mother and newborn. Their physiologic parameters may be stressed to a point exceeding adequate reserves, possibly resulting in increased morbidity and mortality. Awareness of the pathophysiologic changes associated with fever, possible side effects of treatment modalities, and possible alteration of response to anesthesia can most effectively prevent these untoward events. The type of anesthesia or analgesia employed must be determined on an individual basis, and the expertise of the anesthetist, the reasons for the fever, and the patient's requests dictate this choice. Once the choice has been made, anesthesia should be preceded by adequate hydration, oxygenation, and attempts to lower body temperature. Additionally, obstetric, anesthesia, and pediatric personnel must work in harmony to decrease the potential morbidity and mortality of both the mother and her newborn.

References

1. Pickering, G: Regulation of body temperature in health and disease. Lancet 1:1, 1958.
2. Wakin, KG: Bodily reactions to high temperature. Anesthesiology 25:532, 1964.
3. Dinarello, CA and Wolff, SM: Pathogenesis of fever in man. N Engl J Med 298:607, 1978.
4. Atkins, E and Bodel, P: Fever. N Engl J Med 286:27, 1972.
5. Pickering, G: Regulation of body temperature in health and disease. Lancet i:59, 1958.
6. Harris, WH, et al: Cardiovascular effects of fever in the ewe and fetal lamb. Am J Obstet Gynecol 128:262, 1977.
7. Kim, YD, et al: Hyperthermic alteration of sympathetic activity. Anesthesiology 51:S127, 1979.
8. Knight, RT: Elevation of body temperature during anesthesia and its control. Anesth Analg 31:117, 1942.
9. Rowell, LB, Brengelmann, GL and Murray, JA: Cardiovascular responses to sustained high skin temperatures in resting man. J Applied Physiol 27:673, 1969.
10. Cefalo, RC and Hellegers, AE: The effects of maternal hyperthermia and fetal cardiovascular and respiratory function. Am J Obstet Gynecol 131:687, 1978.
11. Fishburne, JI: Physiology and disease of the respiratory system in pregnancy: A review. J Reprod Med 22:177, 1979.
12. Kullander, S: Fever and parturition: An experimental study in rabbits. Acta Obstet Gynecol Scand. 66:77, 1977.
13. Ahlgren, M and Kullander, S: The influence of temperature on the motility of the human uterus in vitro. Acta Obstet Gynecol Scand 38:243, 1959.
14. Lucke, JN: Malignant hyperthermia in a parturient Poland China sow. Br J Anaesth 49:1070, 1977.
15. Ledger, WJ: Bacterial infections complicating pregnancy. Clin Obstet Gynecol 21:455, 1978.
16. Driscoll, SG: Significance of acute chorioamnionitis. Clin Obstet Gynecol 22:327, 1979.
17. Gibbs, RS: How to manage acute chorioamnionitis. Contemp Obstet Gynecol 14:68, 1979.
18. Ledger, WJ: Premature rupture of membranes and maternal-fetal infection. Clin Obstet Gynecol 22:239, 1979.
19. Larsen, JW, et al: Intrauterine infection in an obstetric service. Obstet Gynecol 43:838, 1974.
20. Leontic, EA: Respiratory disease in pregnancy. Med Clin North Am 61:111, 1977.
21. Hopwood, HG: Pneumonia in pregnancy. Obstet Gynecol 25:875, 1965.
22. Zacur, HA and Mitchiw, E: Renal disease pregnancy. Med Clin North Am 61:89, 1977.
23. Harris, RE, Thomas, VL and Shelokov, A: Asymptomatic bacturia in pregnancy: Antibody-coated bacteria, renal function and intrauterine growth retardation. Am J Obstet Gynecol 126:20, 1976.
24. Little, PJ: The incidence of urinary infection in 5006 pregnant women. Lancet 2:925, 1966.
25. Fairley, KF, Bond, AC and Adey, ED: The site of infection in pregnancy bacturia. Lancet 1:939, 1966.
26. Innerfield, R and Hallander, CS: Thyroidal complications of pregnancy. Med Clin North Am 61:67, 1977.
27. Ingbar, SH: Management of emergencies: Thyrotoxic storm. N Engl J Med 274:1252, 1968.
28. Mazzaferri, EL and Skillman, TG: Thyroid storm. Arch Intern Med 124:684, 1969.
29. Hoch, FL: Biochemistry of hyperthyroidism and hypothyroidism. Postgrad Med J 44:347, 1968.
30. Komins, JI, Snyder, PJ and Schwarz, RH: Hyperthyroidism in pregnancy. Obstet Gynecol Surv 30:527, 1975.
31. Gardiner, HL and Kaufman, RH: Herpes genitalis: Clinical features. Clin Obstet Gynecol 15:896, 1972.
32. Brown, ZA, et al: Clinical and virologic course of herpes simplex genitalis. West J Med 130:41, 1979.
33. Guinan, ME, et al: Epidemiology of genital herpes simplex virus infection. Epidemiol Rev 7:127, 1985.
34. Nahmias, AJ and Scwahn, MG: Neonatal herpes simplex: A worldwide disease which is potentially preventable and treatable. Prog Clin Biol Res 163b:355, 1985.
35. Daling, JR and Wolf, ME: The role of decision and cost analyses in the treatment of pregnant women with recurrent genital herpes. JAMA 251:2828, 1984.
36. Binkin, NJ, Koplan, JP and Cates, W: Preventing neonatal herpes: The value of weekly viral cultures in pregnant women with recurrent genital herpes. JAMA 251:2816, 1984.
37. Brown, ZA, Berry, S and Vontver, LA: Genital herpes simplex virus infections complicating pregnancy. Natural history and peripartum management. J Reprod Med 31:S420, 1986.
38. Harger, JH, Pazin, GJ and Breinig, MC: Current understanding of the natural history of genital herpes simplex infections. J Reprod Med 31:365, 1986.
39. Corey, L: The diagnosis and treatment of genital herpes. JAMA 248:1041, 1982.
40. Adams, HG, et al: Genital herpetic infection in men and women: Clinical course and effect of topical ap-

plication of adenine arabinoside. J Infect Dis (suppl.) 133:151, 1976.
41. Nilsen, AE, et al: Efficacy of oral acyclovir in the treatment of initial and recurrent genital herpes. Lancet ii:571, 1982.
42. Bryson, YL, et al: Treatment of first episodes of genital herpes simplex virus infection with acyclovir. N Engl J Med 308:916, 1983.
43. Jacob, AJ, et al: Genital herpes infection in pregnant women near term. Obstet Gynecol 63:480, 1984.
44. American Academy of Pediatrics Committee on Fetus and Newborn and Committee on Infectious Disease: Perinatal herpes simplex infections. Pediatrics 66:147, 1980.
45. Monif, GRG and Hardt, NS: Management of herpetic vulvovaginitis in pregnancy. Semin Perinatol 7:16, 1983.
46. Sullivan-Bolyai, J, et al: Neonatal herpes simplex virus infections in King County Washington. JAMA 250:3059, 1983.
47. Nahmias, AJ, Keyserling, HL and Kerrick, GM: Herpes simplex. In Remington, JS and Klein, JO (eds): Infectious Disease of the Fetus and Newborn Infant. WB Saunders, Philadelphia, 1983, p 636.
48. Whitley, RJ: Neonatal herpes simplex virus infections. Presentation and management. J Reprod Med 31:426, 1986.
49. Jeffries, DJ: Management of herpes simplex infection during pregnancy and in the neonate. J Hosp Inf 4:217, 1983.
50. Perkin, HM and Hanlon, PR: Epidural infection of local anesthetic and steroids for relief of pain secondary to herpes zoster. Ann Surg 113:253, 1978.
51. Ravindran, RS, Gupta, CD and Stoops, CA: Epidural analgesia in the presence of herpes simplex virus (type 2) infection. Anesth Analg 61:714, 1982.
52. Joyce, TH and Marx, GF: Regional anesthesia and herpes. Soc Obst Anesth Perinatology Newsletter 14:1, 1983.
53. Crone, L, et al: Relation between oral herpes simplex and the use of epidural morphine in obstetric patients. Society for Obstetric Anesthesia and Perinatology. Scientific abstract. Salt Lake City, May, 1986, p 124.
54. Douglas, MJ, et al: Epidemiology of HSV-1 infection in the puerperal population: Does epidural morphine cause recrudescence? Society for Obstetric Anesthesia and Perinatology. Scientific abstract. Salt Lake City, May, 1986, p 125.
55. Centers for Disease Control: Update on acquired immunodeficiency syndrome (AIDS): United States. MMWR 32:688, 1984.
56. Rogers, MF, et al: Virologic studies of HTLV-III/LAV in pregnancy: Case report of a woman with AIDS. Obst Gynecol 68:2S, 1986.
57. Barre-Sinoussi, F, et al: Isolation of a T-lymphotropic retrovirus from a patient at risk for acquired immune deficiency syndrome (AIDS). Science 220:868, 1983.
58. Coffin, J, et al: Human immunodeficiency viruses (letter). Science 232:697, 1986.
59. Cooper, DA, et al: Acute AIDS retrovirus infection. Lancet 1:537, 1985.
60. Centers for Disease Control: Recommendations for assisting in the prevention of perinatal transmission of human T-lymphotropic virus type III/lymphadenopathy-associated virus and acquired immunodeficiency syndrome. MMWR 34:721, 1985.
61. Safai, B, et al: Seroepidemiological studies of human T-lymphotropic retrovirus type III in acquired immunodeficiency syndrome. Lancet i:1438, 1984.
62. Curran, JW: The epidemiology and preventions of the acquired immunodeficiency syndrome. Ann Intern Med 103:657, 1985.
63. Lee, KG and Soni, N: AIDS and anaesthesia. Anaesthesia 41:1011, 1986.
64. Darrow, WW, et al: AIDS in a cohort of homosexual men. 24th Intensive Conference on Antimicrobial Agents and Chemotherapy. Washington, DC, 1984.
65. Pinching, AJ and Jeffires, DJ: AIDS and HTLV-III/LAV infection: Consequences for obstetrics and perinatal medicine. Br J Obstet Gynaecol 92:1211, 1985.
66. Morgan, MW and Curran, JW: Acquired immunodeficiency syndrome: Current and future trends. Public Health Reports 101:459, 1986.
67. Centers for Disease Control: Update: Acquired immunodeficiency syndrome—United States. MMWR 35:17, 1986.
68. Scullon, DI: Anesthetic implications of the acquired immunodeficiency syndrome (AIDS), Part 1. J Am Assoc Nurse Anesthetists 54:400, 1986.
69. Van De Perre, P, et al: Acquired immunodeficiency syndrome in Rwanda. Lancet 2:62, 1984.
70. Piot, P, et al: Acquired immunodeficiency syndrome in a heterosexual population in Zaire. Lancet 2:62, 1984.
71. Wolfsy, CB, et al: Isolation of AIDS associated retrovirus from genital secretions of women with antibodies to the virus. Lancet i:527, 1986.
72. Vogt, MW, et al: Isolation of HTLV-III/LAV from cervical secretions of women at risk for AIDS. Lancet 1:525, 1986.
73. Center for Disease Control: Heterosexual transmission of human T-lymphotropic virus type III/lymphadenopathy associated virus. MMWR 35:561, 1985.
74. Stewart, GJ, et al: Transmission of human T-cell lymphotropic virus type III (HTLV-III) by artificial insemination by donor. Lancet ii:581, 1985.
75. Curran, JW: AIDS: Two years later. N Engl J Med 309:609, 1983.
76. Petricciani, JC, et al: Case for concluding that heat-treated licensed anti-haemophilic factor is free from HTLV-III. Lancet 2:890, 1985.
77. Fuch, D, et al: Are homosexuals less at risk of AIDS than intravenous drug abusers and haemophiliacs? Lancet 2:1130, 1985.
78. HTLV-III and blood donors. Lancet 1:856, 1985.
79. Lapointe, N, et al: Transplacental transmission of HTLV-III virus (letter). N Engl J Med 312:1325, 1985.
80. Cowan, MJ, et al: Maternal transmission of acquired immune deficiency syndrome. Pediatrics 73:1325, 1985.
81. Thirty, L, et al: Isolation of AIDS virus from cell-free

breast milk of three healthy virus carriers. Lancet 2:382, 1984.
82. Centers for Disease Control: Recommendations for preventing transmission of infection with human T-lymphotropic virus type III/lymphadenopathy-associated virus in the workplace. MMWR 34:682, 1985.
83. Marwick, C: AIDS-associated virus yields data to intensifying scientific study. JAMA 254:2865, 1985.
84. Sevens, CE: No increased incidence of AIDS in recipients of hepatitis B vaccine. N Engl J Med 308:1163, 1983.
85. Weinberg, ED: Pregnancy-associated depression of cell-mediated immunity. Rev Infect Dis 6:814, 1984.
86. Weber, DJ, et al: Acquired immunodeficiency syndrome: Epidemiology and significance for the obstetrician and gynecologist. Am J Obstet Gynecol 155:235, 1986.
87. Scott, BG, et al: Mothers of infants with the acquired immunodeficiency syndrome. JAMA 253:363, 1985.
88. Levy, RM, et al: Neurological manifestations of the acquired immunodeficiency syndrome (AIDS): Experience at UCSF and review of the literature. J Neurosurg 62:475, 1985.
89. Food and Drug Administration: Progress on AIDS. FDA Drug Bull 15:27, 1985.
90. Welti, CV, et al: Listeriosis as a cause of maternal death: An obstetric complication of the acquired immunodeficiency syndrome (AIDS). Am J Obstet Gynecol 147:7, 1983.
91. Thomas, PA, et al: Unexplained immunodeficiency in children. JAMA 252:639, 1984.
92. Oleske, J, et al: Immunodeficiency syndrome in children. JAMA 249:2345, 1983.
93. Rubinstein, A, et al: Acquired immunodeficiency with reversed T4-T8 ratios in infants born to promiscuous and drug addicted mothers. JAMA 249:2350, 1983.
94. Scot, G, et al: Acquired immunodeficiency syndrome in infants. N Engl J Med 310:76, 1984.
95. AIDS in the health professions. Br Med J 290:583, 1985.
96. Hirsch, MS, et al: Risk of nosocomial infection with Human T-cell Lymphotropic Virus III (HTLV-III). N Engl J Med 312:1, 1985.
97. Jones, P and Hamilton, P: HTLV-III antibodies in haematology staff. Lancet 1:217, 1985.
98. Gordon, RA, Britt, BA and Kalow, W: International Symposium on Malignant Hyperthermia. Charles C Thomas, Springfield, IL, 1973.
99. Gronert, GA: Malignant hyperthermia. In Miller, RD (ed): Anesthesia, ed 2. Churchill Livingstone, New York, 1986, p 1971.
100. Crawford, JS: Hyperpyrexia during pregnancy. Lancet 1:1244, 1972.
101. Ording, H: Incidence of malignant hyperthermia in Denmark. Anaesth Analg 64:700, 1985.
102. Ellis, FR and Halsall, PJ: Malignant hyperexia. Br J Hosp Med 24:318, 1980.
103. Britt, BA and Kalow, W: Malignant hyperthermia: A statistical review. Canad Anaesth Soc J 12:293, 1970.
104. Tettambel, M: Malignant hyperthermia in an obstetric patient. J Am Osteopath Assoc 79:773, 1980.
105. Lips, FJ, Newland, M and Dutton, G: Malignant hyperthermia triggered by cyclopropane during cesarean section. Anesthesiology 56:144, 1982.
106. Kiwitt, A and Pingel, E: Ein Fall von maligner Hyperthermia in der operativen Geburtshilfe. Gynakol 107:966, 1985.
107. Cupryn, JP, Kennedy, A and Byric, RJ: Malignant hyperthermia in pregnancy. Am J Obstet Gynecol 150:327, 1984.
108. Augustyniak, B and Uszynski, M: Opis przypadku niewyjasnionej goraczk, W okresie pooperacyingm-zespol hipertermii ztosliwej? Ginekol Pol 50:969, 1972.
109. Wadha, RK: Obstetric anesthesia for a patient with malignant hyperthermia susceptibility. Anesthesiology 46:63, 1977.
110. Wallatts, SM: Malignant hyperthermia susceptibility management during pregnancy and labour. Anaesthesia 34:41, 1979.
111. Katz, JD and Krich, LB: Acute febrile reaction complicating spinal anaesthesia in a survivor of malignant hyperthermia. Can Anaesth Soc J 23:285, 1976.
112. Youngberg, JA: Anesthetic management of a pregnant patient with malignant hyperpyrexia susceptibility. J Med Assoc Georgia 68:1046, 1979.
113. Khalil, SN, Williams, JP, and Bourke, DL: Management of malignant hyperthermal susceptible patient in labor with 2-chloroprocaine epidural anesthesia. Anesth Analg 62:119, 1983.
114. Lucke, JN: Malignant hyperthermia in a parturient Poland China sow. Br J Anaesth 49:1070, 1977.
115. Martin, JT: Fulminant hyperthermia. JAMA 204:729, 1968.
116. Halsall, PJ, Cain, PA, and Ellis, FR: Retrospective analysis of anesthetics received by patients before susceptibility to malignant hyperpyrexia was recognized. Br J Anaesth 51:949, 1979.
117. Britt, BA: Malignant hyperthermia. Tenth Annual Anesthesiology Symposium, 1979.
118. Gronert, GA: Malignant hyperthermia. Semin Anesth 2:197, 1983.
119. Britt, BA: Malignant hyperthermia. Can Anaesth Soc J 32:666, 1985.
120. Ryan, JF: Malignant hyperthermia. In: Refresher Courses in Anesthesiology. 1976, p 87.
121. McPherson, EW and Taylor, CA, Jr: The King syndrome: Malignant hyperthermia, myopathy and multiple anomalies. Am J Med Genet 8:159, 1981.
122. Denborough, MA, Galloway, GJ and Hopkinson, KC: Malignant hyperpyrexia and sudden infant death. Lancet ii:1068, 1982.
123. Peterson, DR and Davis, N: Malignant hyperthermia diathesis and sudden infant death syndrome (letter). Anesth Analg 65:209, 1986.
124. Caseby, NG: Anaesthesia during raised creatine phosphokinase activity (letter). Br Med J 4:520, 1974.
125. Ellis, FR and Zwana, SCV: A study of body temperatures of anesthetized man in the tropics. Br J Anaesth 49:1123, 1977.

126. Austin, KL and Denborough, MA: Drug treatment of malignant hyperpyrexia. Anaesth Intens Care 5:207, 1977.
127. Ellis, FR, et al: Screening for malignant hyperpyrexia. Br Med J 3:559, 1972.
128. Gronert, GA: Controversies in malignant hyperthermia (editorial). Anesthesiology 59:273, 1983.
129. Lambert, W: Dantrolene and caffeine contracture test (letter). Can Anesth Soc J 27:304, 1980.
130. Moore, DC: Ester or amide local anesthetics in malignant hyperthermia, who knows? Anesthesiology 64:294, 1986.
131. Paasuke, RT and Brownell, AKW: Amide local anesthetics and malignant hyperthermia. Can Anaesth Soc J 33:126, 1986.
132. Harrison, GG and Morrell, DF: Response of malignant hyperthermia susceptible swine to intravenous infusion of lignocaine and bupivacaine. Br J Anaesth 52:385, 1980.
133. Berkowitz, A and Rosenberg, H: Femoral block with mepivacaine for muscle biopsy in MH patients. Anesthesiology 62:651, 1985.
134. Gronert, GA and Milde, JH: Variation in onset of porcine malignant hyperthermia. Anesth Analg 60:499, 1981.
135. Ilriby, ME and Rushton, SC: Malignant hyperpyrexia? Anaesthesia 37:862, 1982.
136. Williams, AC: Malignant hyperpyrexia. Anaesthesia 37:95, 1982.
137. Gutsche, BB: Obstetric anesthesia, why? Clin Perinatol 9:215, 1982.
138. Loughran, PG, Moore, J, and Dundee, J: Maternal stress response associated with caesarean section delivery under general and epidural anaesthesia. Br J Obstet Gynecol 93:943, 1986.
139. Bromage, PR: Epidural Analgesia. WB Saunders, Philadelphia, 1978, p 396.
140. Douglas, MJ and McMorland, GH: The anaesthetic management of the malignant hyperthermia susceptible parturient. Can Anaesth Soc J 33:371, 1986.
141. Rose, DJA: Malignant hyperpyrexia susceptibility and childbirth. (letter). Anaesthesia 41:668, 1986.
142. Neubauer, KR and Kaufman, RD: Another use for mass spectrometry detection and monitoring for malignant hyperthermia. Anesth Analg 64:837, 1985.
143. Baudendistal, L, et al: End-tidal CO_2 monitoring: Its use in diagnosis and management of malignant hyperthermia. Anaesth 39:1000, 1984.
144. Britt, BA: Dantrolene. Can Anaesth Soc J 31:61, 1984.
145. Kolb, ME, Horne, ML, and Martz, R: Dantrolene in human malignant hyperthermia: A multicenter study. Anesthesiology 56:254, 1975.
146. Harrison, GC: Control of malignant hyperpyrexia syndrome in malignant hyperthermia susceptible swine by dantrolene sodium. Br J Anaesth 47:62, 1975.
147. Recommendations of the Malignant Hyperthermia Association of the United States. P.O. Box 3231, Darien, CT 06820.
148. Hall, GM: Editorial: Dantrolene and treatment of malignant hyperthermia. Br J Anaesth 52:847, 1980.
149. Flewellen, EH, et al: Dantrolene dose response in awake man: Implications for management of malignant hyperthermia. Anesthesiology 59:275, 1983.
150. Flewellen, EH and Nelson, TE: Prophylactic and therapeutic doses of dantrolene for malignant hyperthermia (letter). Anesthesiology 61:477, 1984.
151. Morison, DH: Placental transfer of dantrolene. Anesthesiology 59:265, 1983.
152. Glassenberg, R and Cohen, H: Intravenous dantrolene in a pregnant malignant hyperthermia susceptible (MHS) patient. Anesthesiology 61:A209, 1984.
153. Cosmi, EV and Shnider, SM: Obstetric anesthesia and uterine blood flow. In Shnider, SM and Levinson, G (eds): Anesthesia for Obstetrics, ed 2. Williams & Wilkins, Baltimore, 1987, p 35.
154. Rosenblatt, R, et al: Dantrolene potentiates the toxicity of bupivacaine. Anesthesiology 61:A209, 1984.
155. Weingarten, AE, et al: Postpartum uterine atony after intravenous dantrolene. Anesth Analg 66:269, 1987.
156. Conte-Camerino, D, et al: Dantrolene sodium: Stimulatory and depressant effects on the contractility of guinea pig uterus in vitro. Eur J Pharmacol 92:291, 1983.
157. Lovejoy, FH: Aspirin and acetaminophen: A comparative view of their antipyretic and analgesic activity. Pediatrics 62:904, 1978.
158. Steele, RW, et al: Oral antipyretic therapy. Am J Dis Child 123:204, 1972.
159. Barrer, MJ and Ellison, N: Platelet function. Anesthesiology 46:202, 1977.
160. Rossi, EC and Green, D: Disorders of platelet function. Med Clin North Am 56:35, 1972.
161. Bick, RL, Adams, T, and Schamlhorst, WR: Bleeding times, platelet adhesion, and aspirin. Am J Clin Pathol 65:69, 1976.
162. Weiss, HJ, Aledort, LM and Kochwa, S: The effects of salicylates on the hemostatic properties of platelets in man. J Clin Invest 47:2169, 1968.
163. Davies, DW and Steward, DJ: Unexpected excessive bleeding during operation: Role of acetylsalicylic acid. Can Anesth Soc 24:452, 1977.
164. Corby, DG: Aspirin in pregnancy: Maternal and fetal effects. Pediatrics 62:930, 1978.
165. Pearson, HA: Comparative effects of aspirin and acetaminophen on hemostasis. Pediatrics 62:926, 1978.
166. Greensite, FS and Katz, J: Spinal subdural hematoma associated with attempted epidural anesthesia and subsequent continuous spinal anesthesia. Anesth Analg 59:72, 1980.
167. Locke, GE, et al: Acute spinal epidural hematoma secondary to aspirin-induced prolonged bleeding. Surg Neurol 5:293, 1976.
168. Arcilla, RA, Thilenius, OG and Ranninger, K: Congestive heart failure from suspected ductal closure in utero. J Pediatr 75:74, 1969.
169. Phillips, OC, et al: Neurologic complications following spinal anesthesia with lidocaine: A prospective review of 10,440 cases. Anesthesiology 30:284, 1969.
170. Noble, AB and Murray, JG: A review of the compli-

cations of spinal anesthesia with experience in Canadian teaching hospitals from 1959 to 1969. Can Anaesth Soc J 18:5, 1971.
171. Baker, AS, et al: Spinal epidural abscess. N Engl J Med 293:463, 1975.
172. Loarie, DJ and Fairley, HB: Epidural abscess following spinal anesthesia. Anesth Analg 57:351, 1978.
173. Saddy, A: Epidural abscess complicating thoracic epidural analgesia. Anesthesiology 44:244, 1976.
174. Korbin, WM: Spinal epidural abscess: Review of the literature and report of a case. Bull Los Angeles Neurol Soc 23:21, 1958.
175. Heusner, AP: Non-tuberculous spinal epidural infections. N Engl J Med 239:845, 1948.
176. Hancock, DO: A study of 49 patients with acute spinal extradural abscess. Paraplegia 10:285, 1973.
177. Swartz, MN and Dodge, PR: Bacterial meningitis: A review of selected aspects. N Engl J Med 272:725, 1965.
178. Grant, FC: Epidural spinal abscess. JAMA 128:509, 1945.
179. Schmalz, A: Uber akute pachymeningitis spinalis externa: Virchow's Arch (Pathol Anat) 257:521, 1925.
180. Berman, RS, and Eisele, JH: Bacteremia, spinal anesthesia and development of meningitis. Anesthesiology 48:376, 1978.
181. Everett, ED and Hirschmann, JV: Transient bacteremia and endocarditis prophylaxis: A review. Medicine 56:61, 1977.
182. McHenry, MC, et al: Gram-negative bacteremia: Variable clinical courses and useful prognostic factors. Clev Clin Quart 42:15, 1975.
183. Andersen, ET, Young, LS, and Hewitt, WL: Simultaneous antibiotic levels in "breakthrough" gram-negative bacteremia. Am J Med 61:493, 1976.
184. Robert, RB and Shirley, MA: Reducing the risk of acid aspiration during cesarean section. Anesth Analg 53:859, 1974.
185. Roberts, RB: Aspiration and its prevention in obstetrical patients. Int Anesth Clin 15:49, 1977.
186. Sellick, BA: Cricoid pressure to control regurgitation of stomach contents during induction of anesthesia. Lancet 2:404, 1961.
187. Ansari, I, Wallace, G, and Clemtson, C: Tilt caesarean section. J Obstet Gynaecol Br Commonw 77:713, 1970.
188. Colon-Morales, MA: A self-supporting device for continuous left uterine displacement during cesarean section. Anesth Analg 49:223, 1970.
189. Downing, JW, et al: Lateral table tilt for caesarean section. Anaesth 29:696, 1974.
190. Eckstein, KC and Marx, GF: Aortocaval compression and uterine displacement. Anesthesiology 40:92, 1974.
191. Kennedy, RL: An instrument to relieve inferior vena cava occlusion. Am J Obstet Gynecol 107:331, 1970.
192. Prowse, CM and Gaensler, EA: Respiratory and acid base changes during pregnancy. Anesthesiology 26:381, 1965.
193. Archer, CW and Marx, GF: Arterial oxygen tension during apnea in parturient women. Br J Anaesth 46:358, 1974.
194. Keusch, GT: The consequences of fever. Am J Clin Nutr 30:1211, 1977.
195. Lees, DE, Kim, YD and Macnamara, MB: Pulmonary shunting with hyperthermia under anesthesia. Anesthesiology 51:S385, 1979.
196. Norris, MC and Dewan, DM: Preoxygenation for cesarean section: A comparison of two techniques. Anesthesiology 62:827, 1985.
197. Crawford, JS, et al: A further study of general anaesthesia for cesarean section. Br J Anaesth 48:661, 1976.
198. Marx, GF and Mateo, CV: Effects of different oxygen concentrations during general anaesthesia for elective caesarean section. Can Anaesth Soc J 18:587, 1971.
199. Coleman, AJ and Downing, JW: Enflurane anesthesia for cesarean section. Anesthesiology 43:354, 1975.
200. Crawford, JS, Burton, M and Davies, PC: Anaesthesia for C-section: Further refinements of a technique. Br J Anaesth 43:726, 1973.
201. Marx, GF, Kim, YI and Lin, CC: Postpartum uterine pressures under halothane or enflurane anesthesia (abstr). Abstracts of Scientific Papers, Am Soc of Anesthesiologists Annual Meeting. Chicago, IL, 1975, p 101.
202. Moir, DD: Anaesthesia for cesarean section: An evaluation of a method using low concentrations of halothane and 50% of oxygen. Br J Anaesth 42:136, 1970.
203. Burkett, L, et al: Mutual potentiation of the neuromuscular effects of antibiotics and relaxants. Anesth Analg 58:107, 1979.
204. Singh, VN, Harvey, AL and Marshall, FG: Antibiotic-induced paralysis of the mouse phrenic nerve: Hemidiaphragm preparations and reversibility by calcium and neostigmine. Anesthesiology 48:418, 1978.
205. Kohlschutter, B, Baur, H and Roth, F: Suxamethonium induced hyperkalemia in patients with severe intra-abdominal infections. Br J Anaesth 48:557, 1976.
206. Cohen, SE: Inhalation analgesia and anesthesia for vaginal delivery. In Shnider, S and Levinson, G (eds): Anesthesia for Obstetrics. Williams & Wilkins, Baltimore, 1979.
207. Shnider, SM, Steffensen, JL and Margolis, A: Methoxyflurane analgesia in obstetrics. Obstet Gynecol 33:594, 1969.
208. Palahniuk, RJ, Shnider, SM and Egers, EI: Pregnancy decreases the requirement for inhaled anesthetic agents. Anesthesiology 41:82, 1974.
209. Metcalfe, J and Ueland, K: Maternal cardiovascular adjustments to pregnancy. Prog Cardiovasc Dis 16:363, 1974.

CHAPTER 23

THE OBESE PARTURIENT

DAVID M. DEWAN, M.D.

"Obesity enables chronic illness to begin prematurely, move faster, and threaten life more frequently."[1] Obesity bears a strong, positive curvilinear relationship with medical complications,[2] increasing the incidence of hypertension, coronary artery disease, cerebrovascular disease, diabetes mellitus, gallbladder disease, and liver disease. Consequently, the obese patient has an increased mortality rate when compared with the nonobese individual. A 20-percent weight gain increases the risk of death from heart disease by 40 percent and from cardiovascular disease by 50 percent.[3] In nonpregnant patients, a 20-percent weight gain may increase mortality as much as a 50 percent,[4] and weight gain after the age of 25 increases the incidence of sudden death.[5] Pregnancy provides neither immunity from obesity nor protection from its complications. Obesity qualifies the parturient as a high-risk patient for the obstetrician and the anesthesiologist, requiring special understanding and care to avert potentially catastrophic events.

Most anesthetists categorize patients as obese or nonobese by observation or perhaps solely on the basis of weight. However, numerous systems have been devised to better characterize obesity (Table 23–1). The failure of previous studies to consistently define obesity causes much of the difficulty in interpreting anesthetic and obstetric outcomes during pregnancy in obese parturients. Furthermore, there are no weight standards for parturients. The use of arbitrary weight limits without regard to height flaws most obstetric and anesthesia investigations. Theoretically, the Body Mass Index (BMI) should correlate better than the ponderal index with obesity. However, gross or morbid obesity is unmistakable and regardless of the definition presents major problems for those involved in patient care.

Pathophysiology

RESPIRATORY SYSTEM

Obese patients have a normal basal metabolic rate. Because of their increased body mass, total body metabolism increases markedly and linearly with weight and surface area. Obese patients consume more oxygen and obligatorily produce more carbon dioxide because of the

Table 23–1. INDICES OF OBESITY AND THEIR PARAMETERS

Index	Definition	Values
Overweight	20% >Ideal	
Obesity	>20% Over ideal	
Morbid obesity	Ideal weight × 2	
Broca index	Ideal female weight	Ht (cm) − 105
Body mass (Quetelet) index	$\frac{\text{wt (kg)}}{(\text{ht(m)})^2}$	Normal 25 Obese >30
Ponderal index	$\frac{\text{ht (in)}}{\sqrt[3]{\text{wt (lbs)}}}$	Obese <11.6

energy expended supporting excess weight. Oxygen consumption approximately doubles as weight doubles.[6]

Greater oxygen consumption and carbon dioxide production increase ventilatory requirements and, in the absence of carbon dioxide retention, minute alveolar ventilation increases to meet demands. Respiratory rate usually increases proportionately more than tidal volume, which most often remains normal in the obese non-Pickwickian patient. This ventilatory pattern requires less energy expenditure than breathing larger tidal volumes less frequently. Increased minute ventilation requires energy expenditure and further increases oxygen consumption and carbon dioxide production. The work of breathing, oxygen consumption, and carbon dioxide production rises in a nonlinear fashion, and the muscles of respiration may function less efficiently in extreme obesity.[2] The oxygen cost of breathing (ml per liter per minute) increases as much as 300 percent in the obese patient.[7]

Increased minute ventilation, decreased muscle efficiency, and decreased total lung compliance all contribute to the obese individual's increased work of breathing. Although alveolar collapse can occur in obese patients and would increase the work of breathing, pulmonary compliance usually remains normal. Chest wall compliance decreases markedly because of the increased chest wall weight. Additionally, the weight of the abdominal contents restricts diaphragmatic movement, especially when the patient assumes a recumbent position. Both chest wall weight and diaphragmatic restriction decrease total lung compliance and thereby decrease maximum voluntary ventilatory capacity.

Obesity decreases functional residual capacity (FRC), inspiratory reserve volume, expiratory reserve volume, and total lung capacity. Closing volume increases and, in severe obesity, may fall within the range of normal tidal ventilation, especially when the patient is supine. Obese patients may become markedly hypoxemic when supine because of their decreased FRC and increased closing volume. Surprisingly, massive weight loss (>20 BMI or 100-percent change in weight) in the obese patient does not necessarily improve forced vital capacity or maximum mid-expiratory flow rate.[8] FEV_1 increases in clinically insignificant amounts following weight loss while expiratory reserve volume increases significantly and oxygenation improves following weight loss when correlated with body mass index.[8]

Pregnancy as well as obesity alter pulmonary function. Both obesity and pregnancy increase lumbar lordosis, and obesity increases thoracic kyphosis. During pregnancy, the chest wall flares outward and the abdominal contents force the diaphragm cephalad. In obesity, and especially in the obese parturient, the inspiratory position of the chest wall promotes diaphragmatic breathing. Pregnancy, like obesity, increases oxygen consumption, carbon dioxide production, and minute ventilation. In contrast to an obese person, a nonobese gravida's tidal volume usually increases proportionately more than her respiratory rate. Functional residual capacity, expiratory reserve volume, and residual volume all decline approximately 20 percent during pregnancy in the nonobese pregnant patient.

Eng[9] measured lung volumes during the third trimester in parturients weighing 50 to 140 percent above normal and compared pregnant values with values obtained in the same patients 2 months postpartum. Functional residual capacity did not decrease as much during pregnancy in obese parturients as it usually does in nonobese patients. Otherwise the respiratory changes of pregnancy in obese patients resembled those observed in nonobese patients.

Chest wall weight and the pressure of the protuberant abdomen on the diaphragm compress alveoli in the dependent portion of the lungs. Small alveoli are less compliant than larger alveoli. Compliance decreases in the compressed alveolar units. Ventilation preferentially goes to the nondependent, uncompressed, more compliant portions of the lungs. The relatively decreased tidal volume can cause an exaggerated shift of ventilation from the dependent portions of the lungs. In contrast, blood flow continues its preferential course to the dependent portion of the lungs as it does in the nonobese patient. This flow pattern produces ventilation-perfusion mismatch and hypoxemia, especially in the supine position.[10] The obese individual's increased cardiac output further minimizes the effects of gravity on the distribution of pulmonary blood flow by attenuating hypoxic pulmonary vasoconstriction. Arterial PaO_2, however, does not decrease linearly with increasing weight, and the progesterone-related hyperventilation of pregnancy may protect against mismatch or hypoxemia. Eng[9] and Blass[11] both reported maternal PaO_2s of approximately 85 to 86 mmHg in morbidly obese pregnant patients which contrasts with the normal or increased PaO_2 usually accompanying pregnancy. However, these values exceed those of morbidly obese nonpregnant patients presenting for gastric bypass.[4] Burwell[12] reported increased PaO_2, oxygen saturation, lowered $PaCO_2$, and tripled maximum breathing capacity following a 17.8-kg weight loss in obese patients.

CARDIOVASCULAR SYSTEM

Both pregnancy and obesity increase blood volume and cardiac output. Pregnancy increases blood volume and cardiac output by approximately 35 to 45 percent, while blood volume increases in obese patients proportionate to the total body mass. Blood volume may double in nonpregnant patients weighing over 200 lb. Each 13.5 kg of fat contains approximately 25 miles of blood vessels,[13] and the large vascular bed increases cardiac work and cardiac output concomitantly. One hundred kilograms of excess weight increases cardiac output 200 percent, with increased stroke volume accounting for most of the increase. Systemic blood pressure usually decreases during pregnancy. In contrast, obesity usually increases the incidence of hypertension, and the obese parturient is more likely than her nonobese counterpart to be hypertensive. Pulmonary artery pressure usually remains normal during pregnancy and in most obese patients. Left ventricular end-diastolic pressure reaches the upper limits of normal in obese patients. Hypoxia and physical compression of the pulmonary vessels by the elevated diaphragm and heavy chest wall may eventually produce pulmonary hypertension. Circulatory changes depend markedly on position, and changing from the sitting to the supine position elevates oxygen consumption by 11 percent and wedge pressure by as much as 30 percent.[14] Airway obstruction may account for some of the increased pressure. Teeple[15] reported a marked decrease in pulmonary wedge pressure from 38 to 5 mm Hg following endotracheal intubation and relief of airway obstruction in an obese patient. Tseuda[16] reported two cases of cardiac arrest upon placing morbidly obese patients supine for surgical procedures. Sudden gross circulatory changes may account for the phenomenon of sudden death.

GASTROINTESTINAL SYSTEM

Obese patients, like pregnant patients, have larger gastric volumes and lower gastric pH than nonobese patients. Eighty-eight percent of obese patients have a pH of less than 2.5, and 86 percent have gastric volumes exceeding 25 ml.[17] These factors along with a reduced rate of gastric emptying increase the threat of aspiration. Some conflict exists regarding the incidence of hiatal hernia in extreme obesity. Although obese patients are reputed to have a greater incidence of hiatal hernia,[18] O'Brien,[19] examining sphincter functions in 25 massively obese patients, found normal mean lower esophageal sphincter pressure in 22 patients and reflux in only four. Nevertheless, the combination of reflux, increased gastric volume, and decreased gastric pH is a major concern, especially when superimposed upon the changes in gastrointestinal function that accompany pregnancy. Finally, liver and gallbladder disease occur more frequently in obese patients than in nonobese controls.

Obstetric Consideration

Six to ten percent of pregnant patients are obese.[20] One of every 26 to 30 parturients weighs more than 200 pounds,[21] and up to 1.7 percent weigh more than 250 pounds.[22] Obese patients are usually older and more parous as well. Obesity confronts the obstetrician with many problems including the technical problems of estimating gestational dates, performing amniocentesis, and operative difficulty during both vaginal and abdominal delivery.

EFFECTS ON PREGNANCY

The effects of obesity on pregnancy are controversial. Most previous studies have been retrospective and did not consistently define obesity or even define obesity in terms of prepregnant or pregnant weights. Actual body weight, weight-to-height ratios, and arbitrary weight limits (such as 200 pounds) have all served as indices of obesity. Despite these varied definitions, reports have consistently noted that the obese parturient has an increased incidence of gestational diabetes and chronic hypertension.[22] Gross[23] identified gestational diabetes in 6.5 percent of obese patients (>90 kg) and 0.8 percent of nonobese patients, and insulin-dependent diabetes in 2.5 and 0.4 percent, respectively. Tracy and Miller[24] noted a 10-fold increase in diabetes mellitus in obese parturients. Kliegman[20] reported a 7-percent incidence of chronic hypertension in obese patients versus 1.5 percent in nonobese patients, while Peckham[25] noted an even more remarkable increase in chronic hypertension, 14.2 percent and 2.3 percent in obese and nonobese patients, respectively. Hypertension occurs more commonly in obese patients, but whether pregnancy-induced hypertension develops more frequently in obese parturients remains unclear. Edwards[26] noted more "mild" pregnancy-induced hypertension, whereas Tracy and Miller[24] observed a sevenfold increase in "toxemia." Johnson[22] reported a borderline increase in preeclampsia in nulliparous obese patients.

Obesity increases the risk of death in pregnant[27,28,29] and nonpregnant patients.[30] Eighteen percent of maternal deaths in Minnesota occurred in women who weighed more than 175 pounds, and women who weighed more than 200 pounds accounted for 12 percent of maternal deaths despite the fact that only 4.5 percent of parturients exceeded 175 pounds and only 2 percent weighed more than 200 pounds.[8] Obesity doubled the risk of death from pulmonary emboli, which were the most common primary cause of death. Obesity obviously increases maternal risk.

EFFECT ON OBSTETRIC COURSE

The effect of obesity on the obstetric course is also controversial. Most obstetricians and anesthesiologists intuitively believe that the obese parturient suffers more frequent and more severe sequelae than her nonobese counterpart. Historically, older studies reported increased cesarean section rates, increased requirements for oxytocin augmentation, more frequent abnormal presentations, and more frequent forceps deliveries among obese patients.[27,29] For example, Freedman[27] noted that when maternal weight exceeded 300 percent of ideal pregnant or nonpregnant weight for height, cephalopelvic disproportion (CPD), malposition, and malpresentation (breech) occurred more frequently. More recent controlled studies identify less clear-cut findings. In 1980 Gross[23] examined the outcomes of 279 parturients who weighed more than 90 kg. He noted more hypertension, diabetes, and weight gain when compared with 2,467 nonobese control patients. Although obese patients experienced more cesarean sections, these were attributable to a larger repeat cesarean section rate. No difference appeared in the incidence of oxytocin augmentation, although obese patients had an increased incidence of oxytocin *induction* for medical complications. Gross[23] did *not* note more intrapartum complications. Dysfunctional labor, oxytocin augmentation, and abnormal presentation, when controlled for medical complications, occurred with equal frequency in obese and nonobese parturients. Similarly, Freedman[27] did not detect increased forceps delivery or cesarean section rates until the patient weight exceeded 300 percent of the ideal nonpregnant weight, emphasizing that obesity is not an all-or-none phenomenon. Edwards[26] examined the outcome of 208 parturients weighing at least 50 percent more than their ideal nonpregnant weight and matched these patients with nonobese controls. Mild pregnancy-induced hypertension, decreased maternal weight gain during pregnancy, and gestational diabetes occurred more frequently in obese patients. Frank diabetes, abnormal presentation, forceps delivery, cesarean section, and pitocin augmentation occurred with equal frequencies in both patient groups. Peckham[25] actually noted more spontaneous vaginal deliveries in obese patients. Johnson[22] noted prolongation of the second stage of labor, greater oxytocin requirements, but no increase in mid-forceps deliveries.

Despite these conflicting reports, most institutions report more cesarean sections in obese patients. Garbaciak[31] explains some of the discrepancies between studies in his excellent review on obesity and outcome. He reviewed the charts of 9,667 patients and subdivided the patients into four weight groups, which in turn were subdivided into patients with and without *antenatal* medical complications. His findings indicate that obese patients experience more antenatal medical complications. Obesity increased the incidence of antenatal hypertension from 1.9 to 17.2 percent, pregnancy-induced hypertension from 4.4 to 6.9 percent, and diabetes from 1.4 to 10.4 percent. Antenatal complications increased perinatal mortality and the primary cesarean section rate in obese and nonobese patients. Medical complications raised the cesarean section rates in obese patients from 19.6 percent to 22.6 percent and in the nonobese from 10.4 percent to 17.9 percent. Despite undergoing more cesarean sections than nonobese patients obese women without antenatal complications did not have increased perinatal mortality. Antenatal complications probably account for the worse perinatal mortality rate. Obesity increases the likelihood of intrapartum complications even in the absence of antenatal complications. Obese parturients with and without medical complications delivered larger infants than nonobese pregnant women. Cord accidents occurred in four percent of nonobese and 6.7 percent of obese patients. Shoulder dystocia occurred in 0.81 percent and 1.78 percent of nonobese and obese patients, respectively. Similarly, obesity increased the incidence of meconium (18 to 23.5 percent) and late decelerations (3.83 to 7.55 percent). Despite late decelerations, umbilical cord pH's were similar. Intrapartum complications account for the increased primary cesarean section rate, but without antepartum medical complications the intrapartum complications do not cause perinatal death. Hence, the obese parturient is more likely than her nonobese counterpart to have a cesarean section, and the probability of an emergent or "stat" cesarean section increases. This holds particularly true in obese patients with antenatal complications. Obese parturients who undergo cesarean section are more likely to experience blood loss of more than 1000 ml.[22]

PERINATAL OUTCOME

Obesity apparently does not alter perinatal outcome. According to Edwards,[26] despite more complicating maternal disease, 5-minute APGAR scores and perinatal mortality rates of offspring of obese patients resemble those of nonobese mothers. This is surprising since Gross[23] documented in 1985 that obesity increased the risk of neonatal asphyxia. The obese parturient is half as likely as her nonobese counterpart to deliver prematurely. This affords a likely explanation for the lack of effect of obesity on perinatal mortality.[23] In fact, the obese parturient is three and one half times more likely than a nonobese parturient to deliver post-date.

Fifteen percent of obese mothers deliver macrosomic infants, increasing the incidence of shoulder dystocia.[22] However, extreme obesity does not reliably predict newborn weight, and only 15 percent of macrosomic infants have obese mothers.[21] Twenty pounds and 16 pounds, respectively, represent optimal weight gain for nonobese and obese parturients.[22] Whenever maternal weight gain exceeds 32 pounds, perinatal mortality increases.[22] Kliegman[20] noted an increased incidence of macrosomia and intrauterine growth retardation in obese patients as well as an increased incidence of newborn asphyxia.

Anesthetic Considerations

Many problems face the anesthesiologist confronted with an obese parturient. For example, Catenacci[32] reported three cardiac arrests among 225 spinal anesthetics administered to patients who weighed more than 200 pounds and were less than 5 feet 6 inches tall. Not least among the problems challenging the obstetric team are the physical problems surrounding the management of the overweight individual. Transporting the patient from one site to another, especially an immobile patient with a functioning epidural anesthetic, presents considerable problems. In these instances, it may be worth considering injecting the local anesthetic to produce epidural analgesia on the operating table rather than prior to transport. Finding an appropriate size labor bed and/or operating table may also pose difficulty. Rarely, two operating room tables may be necessary, although this has not been our experience at Wake Forest. Left uterine displacement can also prove exceedingly difficult. The protuberant abdomen may make leftward tilting of the table difficult, if not impossible, and the weight of the tilted abdomen may place the patient in peril of falling from the table. Hodgkinson[33] reported severe hypotension following cephalic retraction of a large panniculus despite left uterine displacement. Finally, as mentioned before, Tseuda[17] reported acute cardiovascular collapse of supine obese patients.

EQUIPMENT NEEDS

Obese patients may require different equipment. The American Heart Association recommends that the width of a sphygmomanometer cuff should exceed the circumference of the arm by 20 percent, and Schwartz[34] has noted that otherwise systolic and diastolic blood pressures may read 20 mmHg above the true value. Arterial monitoring may be necessary for accuracy. Obtaining appropriate venous access can be particularly difficult in the obese parturient. Pregnancy assists somewhat because progesterone increases vessel size. When the obese parturient needs central monitoring, the neck presents a significant challenge. Establishing vascular access prior to the onset of active labor may save the anesthesiologist and the obstetrician valuable time and stress. Similarly, regional blocks may require needles of significantly greater length than the standard needles included in spinal and epidural trays. Buckley[35] reported that 10 percent of thoracic epidurals required extra-long epidural needles. Blass[11] performed 25 spinal anesthetics in morbidly obese patients because the epidural needles available to him were too short to reach the epidural space. We have not experienced this problem even though our epidural tray includes a needle whose usable length measures approximately three quarters of a centimeter shorter than standard epidural needles (8.75 cm versus 8 cm). Only rarely have we required long needles in a series of patients weighing over 300 pounds.

AIRWAY MANAGEMENT

Irrespective of the anesthetic chosen, the anesthesiologist must first secure an airway. Adequate preoperative assessment of the airway is the first step in this process. Mask ventilation, often required during difficult intubations, may be particularly difficult in the obese patient, force air into the stomach, increase gastric pressure, and increase the likelihood of regurgitation and aspiration. Furthermore, Safar[36] noted that extension of the neck in extreme obesity worsens respiratory obstruction. The anesthesiologist should anticipate problems with intubation in patients with thick necks, fat shoulders, large chests, and pendulous breasts, for pregnancy exaggerates these factors. The proximity of the chin and the chest wall often leaves little room for the laryngoscope handle and mandates the use of a short-handled laryngoscope. The fat pads on the back of the shoulders can restrict head extension and, to make matters worse, it may be exceedingly difficult to identify the cricoid ring for application of cricoid pressure during rapid-sequence inductions. This not only increases the likelihood of regurgitation, but incorrectly applied pressure may obscure landmarks during intubation and prevent passage of the endotracheal tube beyond the area of misapplied pressure. Buckley[35] reported nine difficult intubations among 68 (13 percent) morbidly obese patients. However, four additional patients received elective awake intubations and may have also been difficult to intubate. Lee[37] described difficult intubation in 284 gastric bypass procedures. When weight was 1.5 to 1.75 times ideal, 2.4 percent of intubations were difficult. When weight was 1.75 to 2.0 times ideal, 7.3 percent were difficult, and when the weight was 2.75 times ideal weight, 50 percent of patients received awake intubations. Furthermore, 70 percent of patients whose weight exceeded 2.5 times the ideal required postoperative ventilation. Ancillary personnel must be available not only to lend a pair of hands but also to back up the primary anesthetist who rapidly becomes fatigued during intubation attempts. Venous engorgement of the airway, the inability to administer significant quantities of sedatives prior to awake intubation, and the potential detrimental effects of endogenous catacholamine release during maternal stress on uterine blood flow all relatively contraindicate routine awake intubation in the parturient. Sedatives present special hazards in this population because of probable placental transport, detrimental fetal effects, and because sedated patients may obstruct their airway. Anesthesia personnel may have more difficulty in establishing an airway in a semiconscious patient than in an unconscious patient. Despite problems associated with awake intubation during pregnancy, this approach represents an option because the induction of general anesthesia stakes the parturient's life as well as her infant's on establishing an airway. Fiberoptics may lessen the parturient's discomfort, stress, and trauma and make awake intubation a more viable alternative.

ASPIRATION OF GASTRIC CONTENTS

Delayed gastric emptying, increased gastric volume, and decreased gastric pH increase the risk of aspiration of gastric contents. All parturients should receive "anti-acid" therapy. At Wake Forest we administer 30 ml of 0.3-molar sodium citrate by mouth to all "high-risk" parturients approximately 15 minutes before they enter the delivery room. H_2 blockers prove equally effective if given sufficient time to work. Metoclopramide, which speeds gastric emptying, offers theoretical advantages, especially when combined with another "anti-acid," but it has not been studied in this patient population. All general anesthetics mandate endotracheal intubation. If awake intubation has not been accomplished, the patient should be denitrogenated and anesthesia induced in a rapid sequence while applying cricoid pressure. An assortment of laryngoscope blades and endotracheal tubes of various sizes should be readily available along with other equipment that may prove helpful during difficult intubations. Once in place, the endotracheal tube should remain in situ until the patient awakens fully following termination of the surgical procedure.

RESPONSE TO ANESTHETIC DRUGS

Obesity alters the response to anesthetic drugs. Intravenous thiopental has a longer elimination half-life in obese patients primarily because of their increased volume of distribution.[38] The answer remains unclear as to the "appropriate" dose of thiopental in the obese parturient. We rarely, if ever, exceed 500 mg in patients weighing as much as 170 kg, even though 4 mg per kg is our usual anesthetizing dose of thiopental for cesarean section. The hazards of administering less than 4 mg per kg include potential maternal awareness and stress-related reductions in uterine blood flow.

The choice of intravenous induction agent may be relatively unimportant in the absence of complicating disease. Kumar[39] noted no difference in time to opening eyes following methohexital and althesin administration in obese patients, but did not study ketamine and thiopental.

Succinylcholine requirements are more predictable. Bentley[40] reported increased pseudocholinesterase activity in obese patients when compared with nonobese patients. When injected doses were calculated on a milligram-per-kilogram basis, despite large doses, the duration of action remained normal. Succinylcholine requirements are not based on lean weight, and surface area does not accurately predict succinylcholine requirements. A dose of two times the "normal" dose of succinylcholine in obese patients produces paralysis of normal duration. Since optimal intubating conditions are the primary concern during rapid-sequence inductions *and* since large doses do not increase the duration of paralysis, larger doses of succinylcholine based on body weight seem appropriate. We frequently use as much as 200 mg of intravenous succinylcholine for this purpose.

The parturient responds normally to nondepolarizing muscle relaxants. However, no muscle relaxant relaxes fat, and the weight of the abdominal wall presents significant surgical difficulties for the obstetrician, who may misinterpret this as inadequate relaxation and request additional drug. Blockade monitors are essential to assure the administration of appropriate amounts of muscle relaxants. Nevertheless, the anesthetic must not handicap the obstetrician and should provide the best operating conditions possible, even if this mandates postoperative ventilation.

Reduced FRC in obesity and pregnancy hasten the equilibration between inspired and brain concentrations of inhalation agents. The obese parturient becomes unconscious faster during inhalation inductions than her nonobese counterpart. Obesity decreases blood gas partition coefficients for ethrane (1.73 versus 2.03).[41] The reverse phenomenon occurs with halothane. The increased body fat acts as a tremendous reservoir for inhalation and intravenous agents although the usual short operating time in obstetrics makes this mostly a theoretical problem. The total body metabolism of methoxyflurane, enflurane, and halothane markedly increases because of increased body stores. Flouride ion production and its concomitant potential toxicity increase following methoxyflurane and enflurane administration. Sedative blood levels of bromine could theoretically follow prolonged halothane administration to obese patients.[42] According to Cork,[43] 67 morbidly obese patients receiving nitrous oxide–fentanyl anesthetics opened their eyes in less time following anesthesia than did inhalation patients receiving halothane or enflurane. However, the time to discharge from recovery room and the time to extubation were similar for the two groups. Long induction-to-delivery times increase the potential for mother-to-fetus drug transfer, fetal drug depression, and maternal awareness. Nevertheless, the anesthesiologist must provide adequate operating conditions without jeopardizing maternal and fetal safety.

OXYGENATION

Adequate intraoperative oxygenation is critical. Pregnancy increases oxygen consumption and reduces FRC. Normal parturients rapidly become hypoxemic during apnea, and the obese parturient will almost certainly desaturate more quickly than her nonobese counterpart. Although four deep breaths within 30 seconds effectively denitrogenate nonobese parturients,[44] total oxygen stores may be less utilizing this technique.[45] Three to five minutes of denitrogenation is a better choice for the obese parturient. Even this does not guarantee adequate oxygenation during attempted intubation, and pulse oximetry aids decision-making during the induction of anesthesia. General anesthesia further decreases FRC and shifts closing volumes to the tidal range. Blass[11] notes that FRC decreases as the patient changes from upright to sitting to supine. These positional changes increase the possibility of severe hypoxemia. Vaughn[46] documented that 40-percent oxygen does not uniformly produce adequate oxygenation intraoperatively in moderately obese patients. Seventy-seven percent of obese patients had a PO_2 of less than 80 mmHg while breathing 40-percent oxygen. Oxygenation may improve markedly following elevation of the panniculus from the abdomen.[47] Anesthesiologists dispute whether large tidal volumes or positive end-expiratory pressure (PEEP) best prevents intraoperative hypoxemia. Salem[48] noted improved arterial oxygenation following discontinuation of intraoperative PEEP when combined with large tidal volumes. If PEEP decreases cardiac output, oxygen delivery may not increase despite increased maternal oxygenation.[49] Ericksen[50] compared the effectiveness of PEEP versus a 35 percent increase in tidal volume in providing adequate oxygenation. Both methods increased maternal arterial PO_2, but neither increased oxygen delivery. PEEP is probably not warranted, except when oxygenation remains poor despite high inspired oxygen concentrations. Finally, airway obstruction can markedly raise wedge pressure. Airway maintenance throughout induction avoids hypoxemia and may prevent sudden cardiovascular decompensation. Nevertheless, Hodgkinson[33] reported pulmonary edema following endotracheal intubation in a morbidly obese patient, probably secondary to acute increases in systemic and pulmonary blood pressure.

PULMONARY COMPLICATIONS

Preoperative risk determines the likelihood of postoperative pulmonary complications. Thirty-eight percent of patients with preoperative risk factors develop postoperative pulmonary complications, whereas only 12 percent of those without preoperative risk factors develop postoperative respiratory complications.[35] General anesthesia is more likely to be associated with pulmonary complications.

REGIONAL ANESTHESIA

Spinal Anesthesia

Regional anesthesia is possible in grossly obese parturients. Despite most anesthesia personnels' clinical impression, Greene[51] reports that obesity does not alter the drug requirement for spinal anesthesia. He attributes the exaggerated spinal spread which most believe occurs in obese patients to altered patient position caused by greatly enlarged buttocks. Many supine obese patients assume an "auto-Trendelenburg" position despite a horizontal operating table. In contrast, McCulloch[52] reported that the height of the block during spinal anesthesia with isobaric bupivacaine correlated with weight divided by height, or weight divided by height squared, but not with height above. Similarly, Pitkanin[53] found little correlation between BMI and the height of the block with hyperbaric or isobaric bupivacaine. Catenacci[32] reported 225 spinal anesthetics, which included three cardiac arrests and a 30 percent incidence of hypotension, but he recommended using larger than usual doses of local anesthetics in the subarachnoid space of obese patients because of the anticipated longer duration of surgery.

Despite these differences of opinion, spinal anesthesia has achieved varying success in extremely obese patients. Jacobs[54] reported successful continuous spinal anesthesia in a patient weighing over 500 pounds. Similarly, others[4,55] have also documented successful spinal anesthesia in obese parturients. Blass[11] commented that height, not weight, determines the height of block in obese parturients and that spinal anesthesia does not affect oxygenation in obese parturients. Blass[11] sampled arterial blood gases before and after subarachnoid anesthesia in 27 parturients weighing between 250 and 500 pounds and compared these values with those obtained in nonpregnant obese females. Maternal arterial PO_2 decreased slightly following subarachnoid block in obese parturients, but remained higher than in unanesthetized nonpregnant obese patients. Blass suggests that progesterone has a protective effect on oxygenation. When considering spinal anesthesia in the obese patient, the anesthesiologist should anticipate longer operating times and select local anesthetic agents that provide both the quality and the required duration of anesthesia. Approximately 55 percent of a series of parturients weighing more than 250 pounds had operative times exceeding 2 hours.[22] One should palpate the interspace prior to selecting regional anesthesia and possibly use a probe to locate the spinous processes prior to inserting the spinal needle. One should also document the patient's ability to sit and flex for needle placement as well as her ability to lie supine. The motor block accompanying spinal anesthesia may impair ventilation, especially in the supine position.

Epidural Anesthesia

Like subarachnoid anesthesia, epidural anesthesia may prove exceedingly difficult in obese patients but can be successfully achieved. Maitra[56] administered 20 ml of 3 percent chloroprocaine epidurally to a 182-kg patient, and Neuman[57] successfully performed an epidural in a 430-kg Pickwickian male. Buckley[35] reported 11 failed epidurals in 53 attempts in obese parturients. One developed an inadequate block and he failed to locate the epidural space in the remaining 10 patients. This emphasizes the possible requirement of a probe for identification of midline structures prior to administering the epidural anesthetic. Major advantages of epidural anesthesia over spinal anesthesia include possible easier placement, the ability to titrate drug, less hypotension, and the use of segmental anesthesia, which retains motor power in the lower extremities. Less motor block accompanies high sensory levels during epidural analgesia, which impairs ventilation less than spinal analgesia. Finally, the epidural catheter may be used to administer postoperative narcotics.

Obesity alters the response to epidurally administered local anesthetic. Hodgkinson[58] administered 20 ml of 0.75 percent bupivacaine to a series of obese parturients. He administered the drug at the L_{3-4} interspace over a period of 40 seconds, and patients remained horizontal for 40 minutes following drug injection. No patient with a BMI exceeding 28 required supplemental local anesthesia for cesarean section. Although dermatomal levels occasionally reached C5, no patient required ventilation, and hypotension (defined as systolic blood pressure <100 mmHg) occurred in only 12 percent of patients, while 3 percent required ephedrine. Analysis revealed that the height of the block was proportional to BMI and weight, but not to height. The decreased drug requirement probably relates to the distended epidural veins during pregnancy and obesity. Patient position influences the distribution of block in obese patients. Hodgkinson and Husain[59] administered 20 ml of 0.75-percent bupivacaine to 250 parturients at the L_{3-4} interspace, and patients remained sitting for 5 minutes following injection. According to Hodgkinson, when the body BMI exceeds 30, the sitting position decreases the height of the block following epidural drug administration. This contrasts to lean patients, in whom the sitting position does not influence the height of anesthesia.

At Wake Forest, we have found epidural anesthesia feasible in obese parturients. In a series of 80 obese patients weighing more than 300 pounds, over 90 percent of approximately 30 epidurals administered for elective cesarean section proved successful. In contrast, for vaginal delivery, the epidural rate stands at approximately 50 percent, with a significantly higher failure rate. Faculty and fellows administer most "elective" cesarean section epidural blocks, whereas less experienced residents usually establish labor epidurals. This practice pattern *may* explain the higher failure rate with labor blocks. In addition, anesthesia personnel must institute labor epidurals under less favorable conditions and have less time for placement and correction of failed blocks.

POSTPARTUM PAIN MANAGEMENT

Management of postoperative pain is imperative. Preoperative risk factors most reliably predict postoperative outcome in obese patients. Postoperative thoracic levels of epidural anesthesia decrease oxygen consumption and left ventricular stroke work.[60] Gelman[60] noted decreased arterial venous oxygen difference, oxygen consumption, and left ventricular stroke work in extremely obese patients following thoracic epidurals. Rawal[61] compared intramuscular and thoracic epidural morphine in 30 obese gastroplasty patients. Patients receiving epidural narcotic required seven times less morphine, ambulated earlier, suffered fewer pulmonary complications, and had shorter hospitalizations and no evidence of respiratory depression. These findings underscore the necessity of effectively managing postoperative pain. No information exists in the literature concerning the effects of epidural narcotics on parturients with the Pickwickian syndrome. Epidural anesthesia has been used successfully in one patient with this syndrome.[57] However, respiratory arrest followed epidural narcotic administration in a patient with the sleep apnea syndrome.[62] In contrast, epidural narcotics have been successfully used in obese patients with obstructive sleep apnea.[63] According to Doblar,[64] epidural narcotics depress the ventilatory response to carbon dioxide less than parenteral narcotics. Lumbar epidural narcotics effectively provide postoperative analgesia following cesarean section, but their use mandates intensive care monitoring of the obese patient. Certainly one must weigh the benefits of epidural narcotics against their potential sequelae. Respiratory depression poses a greater hazard in the obese patient than in the lean parturient. Establishing an airway during apnea, hypoxia, and unconsciousness may prove impossible in the obese patient. Naloxone, although effective, can evoke nausea and vomiting, thereby creating its own hazard. Perhaps ambulation and maintaining the patient in the head-up position when possible are the best solution.[65] In addition, the head-up position impedes the ascent of epidural morphine in the spinal fluid.

ANESTHESIA FOR VAGINAL DELIVERY

Although some obese parturients deliver without analgesia, our experience indicates that the majority require some analgesia. Intramuscular and intravenous narcotics can provide sedation and reduce pain, but they have disadvantages. Intramuscular injections in obese parturients may be unintentionally injected subcutaneously and have variable absorption and effectiveness. Intravenous narcotics provide analgesia but increase the risk of maternal and neonatal respiratory depression. Even when effective, the parturient still often requires either infiltration of local anesthesia or a pudendal block at delivery. Local infiltration is more reliable since pudendal blocks present technical difficulties in the morbidly obese patient.

During delivery general analgesia with nitrous oxide can provide analgesia. However, general analgesia may be ineffective in some patients and fails to provide profound pain relief in nearly all patients. Furthermore, the patient may be unintentionally anesthetized, lose her airway, become uncooperative, aspirate, or become severly hypoxemic.

Although saddle block (low spinal) anesthesia qualifies as theoretically safe in this patient population, spinal anesthesia presents technical difficulties in most obese patients, except under the most unhurried circumstances.

Epidural anesthesia offers the most advantages for these parturients. Labor increases oxygen consumption and cardiac output, especially during the second stage. The obese parturient has less cardiac reserve and may be unable to meet the ventilatory requirements of increased oxygen consumption and carbon dioxide elimination demanded by labor and delivery. Epidural anesthesia reduces oxygen consumption during labor and attenuates the wide changes in cardiac output which occur during the first and second stage of labor. Epidural anesthesia obviates the need for intrapartum narcotics and lessens the risk of maternal and newborn respiratory depression.

Segmental epidural provides excellent labor analgesia while sparing perineal anesthesia and lower extremity motor block. This provides a calm, cooperative patient who can assist with her nursing care during labor and delivery. Finally, and perhaps most importantly, epidural analgesia can be extended and provide anesthesia for difficult vaginal procedures and cesarean section.

CESAREAN SECTION ANESTHESIA

Spinal anesthesia may be used for cesarean section. However, it may be technically difficult, cause severe hypotension, and fail to provide a sufficient duration of anesthesia. For these reasons we rarely use it for grossly obese patients.

General anesthesia avoids the problems of spinal anesthesia but substitutes the perils of aspiration, failed intubation, and difficult airway management. Intraoperative and postoperative oxygenation are unpredictable and require monitoring with pulse oximetry or arterial blood gas analysis.

Epidural analgesia is the best anesthetic for the obese parturient. Epidural anesthesia preserves airway reflexes, provides intraoperative analgesia, offers the capability of administering 100 percent oxygen to the mother, and avoids the respiratory depression effects of inhalation anesthetic agents and narcotics. Gradual establishment of the block, with fractionated doses of local anesthetic and following adequate preload and left uterine displacement, produces a low incidence of hypotension. Despite high sensory levels, the corresponding lower levels of motor blockade do not impair ventilation. If necessary, a slight degree of head-up position reassures the patient without obscuring the surgical field. In one of our parturients who was unable to lie supine (when unanesthetized), we established epidural anesthesia and performed the surgery in a 15- to 20-degree head-up (flexed) position. Postoperatively the epidural catheter can be used for postoperative analgesia either with dilute concentrations of local anesthetic or, provided adequate monitoring is available, with epidural narcotics. Although lidocaine and chloroprocaine are excellent local anesthetics, we usually test our epidural catheters with chloroprocaine and subsequently establish the block with 0.5 percent bupivacaine. We believe bupivacaine's slower onset of block and lesser motor block offer advantages in this patient population and reduce the risk of hypotension, ventilatory embarrassment, and intraoperative block failure.

Summary

I recommend the following guidelines for the management of the obese parturient:

Evaluate the patient carefully and, if possible, arrange with the obstetrician to see her well in advance of surgery and/or labor. Take a thorough history, for this predicts outcome. Preoperative anterial blood gases may indicate the severity of respiratory embarrassment when the history is equivocal. Question the patient concerning previous anesthetic history, especially previous cesarean sections. Question the patient concerning the presence of heartburn or fainting and carefully evaluate the airway. Talk to the patients candidly concerning their problems. They need support, but do not "sugar coat" your preoperative interview and minimize risk. Warn the patient about failed block and potential technical difficulties of administering regional anesthesia as well as the hazards of general anesthesia.

Plan ahead. Talk to the obstetrician, and when regional anesthesia is selected, place and "test" the block prior to the onset of active labor. Do not wait until the patient gets "out of control." Have experienced people available for assistance. Regional anesthesia *is* feasible. Our experience suggests that obese parturients do not require unusually long epidural needles. Generously infiltrate the epidural site with local anesthetic. Establish trust and maintain rapport with these patients. Painful insertions of epidurals may result in refusal of further attempts at placement and confront you with a difficult dilemma. Secure epidural catheters well. We usually advance epidural catheters no more than 2 to 3 cm into the epidural space in order to avoid asymmetric blocks. However, in obese patients, we thread them at least 5 cm and generously apply tape, and, when necessary, benzoin to secure the catheter well.

Consider anesthetizing patients on the operating room table if possible. We usually test with chloroprocaine for catheter placement and then switch to bupivacaine. Dose slowly. Give the drugs in increments and, most importantly, don't settle for anything less than a *perfect* block. The intraoperative conversion to general anesthesia can prove catastrophic, and is usually more difficult than the preoperative institution of general anesthesia. Obese patients do tolerate surprisingly high levels of sensory anesthesia. We have never had a problem with spontaneous ventilation despite high sensory levels of anesthesia combined with morbid obesity. If necessary, the head-up position does not greatly impair operating conditions.

Whatever type of anesthesia is chosen, all parturients should receive an "anti-acid" treatment prior to induction. Equipment for resuscitation and intubation of the parturient should be immediately available, along with additional experienced personnel.

For general anesthesia, denitrogenate for 5 minutes with 100 percent oxygen and monitor with a pulse oximeter and capnograph. During the induction of general anesthesia administer a "normal" dose of succinylcholine (not based on lean weight).

Finally, ambulate all patients as soon as possible postoperatively. Administer epidural narcotics only if the patient can be monitored in an intensive care unit with immediate availability of experienced personnel for airway management.

References

1. Vaughn, RW: Definitions and risks of obesity. In Brown, BR, Jr (ed): Anesthesia in the Obese Patient. FA Davis, Philadelphia, 1982, p 107.
2. Bray, G: Complications of obesity. Ann Intern Med 103:1052, 1985.
3. Fisher, A, Waterhouse, TD and Adams, AP: Obesity: Its relation to anesthesia. Anesthesia 30:633, 1975.
4. Katz, J, Benumof, J and Kadis, L: Anesthesia and Uncommon Diseases: Pathophysiologic and Clinical Correlations, ed 2. W.B. Saunders Company, Philadelphia, 1981.
5. Kannel, WB, et al: Relation of body weight to the development of coronary heart disease: The Framingham study. Circulation 35:734, 1967.
6. Dempsey, JA, et al: Alveolar-arterial gas exchange during muscular work in obesity. J Appl Physiol 21:1807, 1966.
7. Sharpe, JT, et al: Total respiratory inertance and its gas and tissue components in normal and obese men. J Clin Invest 43:503, 1964.
8. Vaughn, R, Cork, R and Hollander, D: The effects of massive weight loss on arterial oxygenation and pulmonary function tests. Anesthesiology 54:325, 1981.
9. Eng, M, Butler, J and Bonica, J: Respiratory function in pregnant obese women. Am J Obstet Gynecol 123:241, 1975.

10. Tucker, DH and Sieker, HO: The effects of change in body position on lung volumes and intrapulmonary gas mixing in patients with obesity, heart failure and emphysema. J Clin Invest 39:787, 1960.
11. Blass, NH: Regional anesthesia in the morbidly obese. Reg Anaesth 4:20, 1979.
12. Burwell, C, et al: Extreme obesity associated with alveolar hypoventilation. Am J Med 21:811, 1956.
13. Smart, GA: Diseases of metabolism: Obesity. In Hunter, D (ed): Price's Textbook of the Practice of Medicine, ed 9. Oxford Medical Publications, London, 1956, p 450.
14. Paul, D, Hoyt, J and Boutros, A: Cardiovascular respiratory changes in response to changes of posture in the very obese. Anesthesiology 45:73, 1976.
15. Teeple, E and Ghia, J: An elevated pulmonary wedge pressure resulting from an upper respiratory obstruction in an obese patient. Anesthesiology 59:66, 1983.
16. Tseuda, K, et al: Obesity supine death syndrome: Reports of two morbidly obese patients. Anesth Analg 58:345, 1979.
17. Vaughn, RW, Bauer, S and Wise, L: Volume and pH of gastric juice in obese patients. Anesthesiology 43:686, 1975.
18. Vaughan, R: Anesthetic management of the morbidly obese patient. 1987 Review Course Lecture, International Anesthesia Research Society Annual Meeting, Lake Buena Vista, Florida; March 14, 1987.
19. O'Brien, TF: Lower esophageal sphincter pressure (LESP) and esophageal function in obese humans. J Clin Gastroenterol 2:145, 1980.
20. Kliegman, R and Gross, T: Perinatal problems of the obese mother and her infant. Obstet Gynecol 66:299, 1985.
21. Gould, S and Makowski, E: Obesity and pregnancy. Perinatol Neonatol May-June, 49, 1981.
22. Johnson, S, et al: Maternal obesity and pregnancy. Surg Gynecol Obstet 164:431, 1987.
23. Gross, T, Sokol, R and King, K: Obesity and pregnancy: Risks and outcome. Obstet Gynecol 56:446, 1980.
24. Tracy, T and Miller, G: Obstetric problems of the massively obese. Obstet Gynecol 33:204, 1969.
25. Peckham, CH and Christianson, RE: The relationship between prepregnancy weight and certain obstetric factors. Am J Obstet Gynecol 111:1, 1971.
26. Edwards, L, et al: Pregnancy in the massively obese: Course, outcome, and obesity prognosis of the infant. Am J Obstet Gynecol 131:479, 1978.
27. Freedman, M, Wilds, P and George, W: Grotesque obesity: A serious complication of labor and delivery. South Med J 65:72, 1972.
28. Maeder, E, Barno, A and Mecklenburg, F: Obesity: A maternal high risk factor. Obstet Gynecol 45:669, 1975.
29. Roopnarinesingh, S and Pathak, U: Obesity in the Jamaican parturient. Br J Obstet Gynaecol 77:895, 1970.
30. Postlewait, RW and Johnston, WD: Complications following surgery for duodenal ulcer in obese patients. Arch Surg 104:438, 1972.
31. Garbaciak, J, et al: Maternal weight and pregnancy complications. Am J Obstet Gynecol 152:238, 1985.
32. Catenacci, A, Anderson, J and Boersma, D: Anesthetic hazards of obesity. JAMA 175:111, 1961.
33. Hodgkinson, R and Husain, F: Cesarean section associated with gross obesity. Br J Anaesth 52:919, 1980.
34. Schwartz, H: Problems of obesity in anesthesia. New York State J M 55:3277, 1955.
35. Buckley, FP, et al: Anaesthesia in the morbidly obese: A comparison of anesthetic and analgesic regimens for upper abdominal surgery. Anaesthesia 38:840, 1983.
36. Safar, P, Escarraga, LA and Chang, F: Upper airway obstruction in the unconscious patient. J Appl Physiol 14:760, 1959.
37. Lee, J, et al: Airway maintenance in the morbidly obese. Anesth Rev 7:33, 1980.
38. Jung, D, et al: Thiopental disposition in lean and obese patients undergoing surgery. Anesthesiology 56:269, 1982.
39. Kumar, V, Harvey, J and Cooper, G: Does obesity effect recovery? A study using intravenous methohexitone and althesin for short procedures. Anaesthesia 38:968, 1983.
40. Bentley, J, et al: Weight, pseudocholinesterase activity, and succinylcholine requirement. Anesthesiology 57:48, 1982.
41. Borel, J, et al: Enflurane blood-gas solubility: Influence of weight and hemoglobin. Anesth Analg 61:1006, 1982.
42. Bentley, J, et al: Halothane biotransformation in obese and nonobese patients. Anesthesiology 57:94, 1982.
43. Cork, R, Vaughan, R and Bentley, J: General anesthesia for morbidly obese patients: An examination of postoperative outcomes. Anesthesiology 54:310, 1981.
44. Norris, M and Dewan, D: Preoxygenation for cesarean section: A comparison of two techniques. Anesthesiology 62:827, 1985.
45. Gambee, A, Hertzka, R and Fisher, D: Preoxygenation techniques: Comparison of three minutes and four breaths. Anesth Analg 66:468, 1987.
46. Vaughan, RW and Wise, L: Intraoperative arterial oxygenation in obese patients. Ann Surg 84:35, 1976.
47. Wyner, J, Brodsky, J and Merrell, R: Massive obesity and arterial oxygenation. Anesth Analg 60:691, 1981.
48. Salem, M, et al: Does PEEP improve intraoperative arterial oxygenation in grossly obese patients. Anesthesiology 48:280, 1978.
49. Santesson, J: Oxygen transport and venous addmixture in the extremely obese: Influence of anesthesia and artificial ventilation with and without positive end-expiratory pressure. Acta Anaesth Scand 20:387, 1976.
50. Eriksen, J, et al: Effects of ventilation with large tidal volumes or positive end-expiratory pressure on cardiorespiratory function in anesthetized obese patients. Acta Anaesth Scand 22:241, 1978.
51. Greene, N: Physiology of Spinal Anesthesia, ed 3. Williams & Wilkins, Baltimore, 1981.
52. McCulloch, W and Littlewood, D: Influence of obesity on spinal analgesia with isobaric 0.5-percent bupivacaine. Br J Anaesth 58:610, 1986.
53. Pitkanen, M: Body mass and spread of spinal anesthesia with bupivacaine. Anesth Analg 66:127, 1987.

54. Jacobs, L, Berger, H and Fierro, F: Obesity and continuous spinal anesthesia: A case report. Anesth Analg 42:547, 1963.
55. Sicuranza, B and Tisdall, L: Cesarean section in the massively obese. J Reprod Med 14:10, 1975.
56. Maitra, A, et al: Continuous epidural analgesia for cesarean section in a patient with morbid obesity. Anesth Analg 58:348, 1979.
57. Neuman, G, et al: Perioperative management of a 430-kilogram (946-pound) patient with Pickwickian syndrome. Anesth Analg 65:985, 1986.
58. Hodgkinson, R and Husain, F: Obesity and the cephalad spread of analgesia following epidural administration of bupivacaine for cesarean section. Anesth Analg 1980;59:89. Obesity supine death syndrome: Reports of two morbidly obese patients. Anesth Analg 58:345, 1979.
59. Hodgkinson, R and Husain, F: Obesity, gravity, and spread of epidural anesthesia. Anesth Analg 60:421, 1981.
60. Gelman, S, et al: Thoracic epidural versus balanced anesthesia in morbid obesity: An intraoperative and postoperative hemodynamic study. Anesth Analg 59:902, 1980.
61. Rawal, N, et al: Comparison of intramuscular and epidural morphine for postoperative and analgesia in the grossly obese: Influence on postoperative ambulation and pulmonary function. Anesth Analg 84:583, 1962.
62. Lamarche, Y, et al: The sleep apnoea syndrome and epidural morphine. Can Anaesth Soc J 33:231, 1986.
63. Pellecchia, D, Bretz, A and Barnette, R: Postoperative pain controlled by means of epidural narcotics in a patient with obstructive sleep apnea. Anesth Analg 66:280, 1987.
64. Doblar, D, et al: Epidural morphine following epidural local anesthesia: Effect on ventilatory and airway occlusion pressure responses to CO_2. Anesthesiology 55:423, 1981.
65. Vaughn, RW and Wise, L: Postoperative arterial blood gas measurement: Effect of position on gas exchange. Ann Surg 82:705, 1975.

CHAPTER 24

THE EXTREMES OF AGE: THE TEENAGER AND THE ELDERLY PARTURIENT

MONICA M. JONES, M.D.

Age is not just a "state of mind" when it involves a pregnancy. Parturients at the extremes of their reproductive years represent a unique patient population, which may pose special problems for obstetric and anesthesia team members as well as for the mother and her fetus. An awareness of these problems and their influence on the parturient's anesthetic management should improve the care provided to the mother as well as the outcome of the fetus.

The Pregnant Teenager

Approximately 10 percent of teenagers in the United States will become pregnant with 6 percent giving birth each year. Approximately 30,000 girls 15 years old or younger become pregnant annually, with the majority of conceptions occurring out of wedlock.[1] Since 1960, the number of teenage births has declined progressively, largely due to decreasing birth rates in older teenagers. However, recent experience indicates that even the youngest teens are now reducing their birth rates.[2] Factors involved in this decline include increased availability of birth control, improved sex education, and legalized abortion (adolescents account for one third of the legal abortions performed each year in the United States).

Although the fertility rate may be decreasing, accumulating data strongly suggest that teenage motherhood has adverse and long-term implications for both mother and child. Adolescent mothers generally achieve a lower educational level and become less successful vocationally. Approximately 70 percent of women giving birth to children before age 17 do not finish high school.[3] Also, a woman bearing a child during teenage years more likely has an increased number of children and births more closely spaced than her older counterpart. The young father likewise stands at an educational and economic disadvantage if he assumes his parental responsibilities. Those who marry experience a high rate of separation and divorce, frequently leaving the teenage mother at home as the only adult in the household. This combination of social and economic factors often results in a family with a minimal support system requiring public assistance to provide the basic necessities of life.

The infant may also be adversely affected. For example, six percent of all first babies and 10 percent of second babies born to girls under 15 years of age die in the first year of life—a mortality rate two to four times higher than for babies born to women in their twenties.[1] Additionally, infants with a low birth weight are two to six times as prevalent among teenagers than older women.[1,4] Children born to adolescent mothers are likely to be smaller and receive poorer grades by the time they reach school age and may be more likely to suffer neglect and abuse.[4] Therefore, the teenage pregnancy has far-reaching ramifications for the infant as well as the mother.

OBSTETRIC CONSIDERATIONS

Discussions concerning the pregnant teenager should divide these parturients into two age brackets: 1) adolescents less than 16 years old and 2) those 16 years of age or older. Most studies indicate that the 16- to 19-year-old group generally exhibits no difference or a minimal increase in maternal health risk during pregnancy, assuming good prenatal care is obtained. In fact, the mother at 16 to 19 years may be at her peak reproductive age, biologically.

Nutrition

Girls usually begin their growth spurt at age 10½ and reach their peak by age 14. During this time, surveys[3] indicate that iron, vitamin A, and calcium represent the most commonly deficient nutrients in the normal adolescent diet. Factors contributing to this include 1) frequent intake of "junk foods," 2) participation in fad diets, and 3) concerns about the adolescent's "figure." These factors continue to play a role in her prenatal nutrition unless she learns the importance of an adequate balanced diet. In the young pregnant teenager, the requirements of the developing fetus compound the nutritional needs of the growing adolescent body. These common nutritional deficiencies subsequently result in 1) iron-deficiency anemia due to insufficient iron intake at a time when the blood volume increases due to pregnancy and/or 2) fetal malnutrition and abnormal growth. Therefore, prenatal nutrition counseling becomes imperative to optimize maternal and fetal growth and development.

Pregnancy-Induced Hypertension (PIH)

Usually a disease of primigravidas, PIH is especially prevalent among socioeconomically depressed teenage parturients, particularly those less than 16 years of age. In this young population, various surveys[5–8] report the incidence of PIH to be as high as 34 percent. However, some studies[9] indicate that teenagers with adequate prenatal care do not develop the disease with increased frequency. Adequate prenatal care in itself constitutes a problem, since 50 percent of adolescents receive no health care during the first trimester and 16 percent fail to be seen by a health care practitioner in the second trimester.[10] James discusses the implications of PIH in Chapter 21.

Cephalopelvic Disproportion

Duenhoelter and coworkers[7] used pelvimetry to document pelvic inlet contraction in parturients less than 15 years of age, finding a slightly increased incidence compared with a control group aged 19 to 25 years. Their findings suggest that the bony pelvis has not reached its maximum size by the time of childbirth in the adolescent age group. However, most studies[6–8,11,12] fail to substantiate any statistically significant increase in the teenage cesarean section rate, and cephalopelvic disproportion does not appear to be a major factor in the management of teenage mothers.

Premature Labor

Several reports[3,8,11] confirm a high incidence of prematurity in infants born to girls under 16 years of age. Factors that correlate with premature labor in adolescents include: (1) low prepregnancy weight, (2) ethnic origin, i.e., nonwhite teenagers have a higher incidence than whites, (3) adverse social conditions, (4) unmarried status, (5) smoking, (6) narcotic use, (7) anemia, (8) primigravid mother, and (9) inadequate prenatal care. Additionally, low-birthweight infants have a higher incidence of congenital anomalies. Overall, the adolescent experiences a slightly greater rate of fetal anomalies when compared with 20- to 30-year-old parturients but a lower incidence than for children born to women over 30 years old. Anencephaly, spina bifida, meningomyelocele, and cardiac abnormalities are the specific defects exhibiting an increased rate of occurrence in adolescent gestations.

Prenatal Preparation

Pregnancy is often psychologically traumatic and, in some cases, emotionally disastrous to the teenager who has not fully matured. Special education classes oriented toward the new mother can provide information on appropriate parenting while allowing the parturient to continue her education. Childbirth education classes aid in teaching the teenager about her pregnancy as well as the labor and delivery period while helping her to cope with these changes. A support person with whom the patient feels comfortable should also participate in the psychological preparation for the labor and delivery period. To minimize fear and anxiety, the patient care team should encourage the teenage mother and her support person to tour the labor and delivery area, where they can view the monitors, rooms, and nursing staff prior to the onset of labor. This visit should also include an interview with a member of the anesthesia team, so that anesthetic options can be discussed during a calm, nonstressful time.

ANESTHETIC CONSIDERATIONS

Prior to medical treatment or an anesthetic procedure, informed patient consent must be obtained whenever possible. The parturient should possess a cognitive understanding of the procedure before giving her consent. The basic elements of informed consent for anesthesia include (1) a fair and reasonable explanation of the various available anesthetic procedures; (2) a description of the benefits of different anesthetic options as well as associated discomforts and risks possibly occurring with each; (3) a disclosure of any alternative techniques which might be useful although not the best in the provider's hands; (4) disclosure of other persons to be involved in the patient's care; (5) opportunity for the patient to ask questions, and (6) instruction that the parturient may withdraw consent at any time without future prejudice to the patient's care and treatment.[13]

This description of informed consent seems relatively clear, although several court rulings question the extent to which complications must be explained. For example, a recent court case[14] summarizes that "the obligation to give adequate information does not require the disclosure of all risks of a proposed therapy. . . . The remotely possible risks of a proposed treatment may be almost without limit . . . and we now hold that a physician is not required to inform a patient of remote risks." When a teenager is involved though, questions arise concerning her ability to understand as well as who may legally sign consent forms. The age for legal consent varies among states. In the state of Texas, the law considers the pregnant minor an adult who can consent to medical treatment. In some states, however, the young parturient's parents or legal guardians must agree to treatment and sign the consent. A prudent route is to have both the minor and her parent or legal guardian sign the consent form after the procedures, benefits, and risks have been discussed with both present. Rare situations may arise where the parturient is comatose or sufficiently sedated so that informed consent cannot be obtained. If the family is unavailable to consent for medical treatment, a procedure may be done without a written consent if emminently necessary to provide optimal care and the surrounding situation is documented. If unusual difficulties arise, however, the hospital legal counsel should provide consultation.

Anesthesia for Labor and Delivery

The teenage parturient's response to pain and her subsequent need for analgesia and anesthesia vary greatly. The individual pain threshold and the parturient's psychological preparation, including childbirth preparation classes, strongly influence the adolescent's behavior. The presence of a familiar and effective support person during labor as well as delivery may help to decrease the analgesic requirements and will undoubtedly serve to diminish anxiety.

The most common form of analgesia entails the use of intravenous narcotics or agonist-antagonist drugs (i.e., butorphanol). These drugs relieve pain and anxiety while also providing sedation. Placental transport occurs in various degrees (Chap. 2), potentially producing a depressant effect on the fetus. The extent of neonatal depression depends on the dose, time and route of administration in relation to delivery, as well as existing obstetric complications. For the teenager, this form of analgesia works well during the early stages of labor when contractions cause relatively mild pain. It may well not suffice in late labor when attending physicians prefer to minimize additional fetal drug exposure.

As labor progresses, the teenage parturient typically becomes more anxious and fearful, often experiencing pain of an intensity never before known. The increasing catecholamine levels associated with pain theoretically produce uterine artery vasoconstriction and a subsequent decrease in placental perfusion. Anesthetic techniques that specifically block the pain pathways of labor and delivery will provide more profound pain relief for the adolescent and possibly decrease the catecholamine release associated with the first stage of labor.

A lumbar sympathetic block will provide good first-stage analgesia. However, it requires bilateral needle insertion (which the adolescent may not readily tolerate) and does not provide sacral plexus analgesia for the second stage of labor and delivery.

A paracervical block anesthetizes pain fibers as they leave the uterus, providing good analgesia for Stage I. This form of pain relief has fallen into disfavor owing to a relatively high incidence of fetal bradycardia and, occasionally, fetal death. As with a lumbar sympathetic block, this technique provides no analgesia for the second stage of labor and delivery.

A lumbar epidural provides excellent analgesia for labor as well as delivery although placement may be difficult in the anxious teen. Appropriate fluid management and maintenance of left uterine displacement minimize the risk of hypotension. The anemic teenager, most likely exhibiting poor nutritional intake during her pregnancy, will benefit from the administration of supplemental oxygen during the labor and delivery period. Epidural administration of a dilute local anesthetic solution (i.e., bupivacaine 0.125 percent by continuous infusion) minimizes the degree of motor blockade, an aspect that may be disconcerting for the uninformed teenager. By maintaining a segmental level (T10–L2), the parturient should still feel sacral pressure and the subsequent urge to push during the second stage. This is especially important in the young, minimally motivated adolescent who has never experienced this sensation before. Following completion of pushing, a perineal dose administered with the patient in a sitting position provides sacral analgesia for the delivery period. Lumbar epidural analgesia minimizes exposure of the fetus to various drugs. This is of particular importance in the premature fetus, whose drug metabolism may be impaired (see Chap. 17).

The epidural dosage requirements of the pregnant teenager have yet to be clinically evaluated. Bromage and associates[15] documented that epidural dose requirements are linearly related to age in children, with the maximum dose requirement reached by 18½ years of age. They derived a regression equation which demonstrated that the dose of lidocaine 2 percent (ml) $= 0.1063 +$ age in years $\times\ 0.07531$ ml per spinal segment blocked. Furthermore, epidural dose requirements increase by 0.0799 ml per year of age per segment blocked in children and nonpregnant teenagers. When the changes in local anesthetic requirements in pregnancy are considered, this dose should be decreased by approximately one third. Therefore, smaller volumes of local anesthetic should be sufficient to obtain a specified level of block in the young teenager when compared with adult dosages. The very young parturient frequently has a lower body weight than her adult counterpart, which must be considered when maximum doses of local anesthetics are calculated, to avoid systemic toxicity.

Anesthesia for Cesarean Section

Should cesarean section become necessary, the anesthetic choice depends largely on the parturient's psychological state. If the patient has a well-functioning epidural in place and displays minimal anxiety, lumbar epidural blockade can be extended to provide satisfactory anesthesia for abdominal delivery. The preoperative administration of small doses of sedatives (i.e., benadryl) and intraoperative supplementation with a mixture of 30 percent nitrous oxide and oxygen prior to delivery will facilitate the management of apprehension. After delivery, the use of a short-acting intravenous benzodiazepine (i.e., midazolam) may further increase the patient's acceptance of a regional technique. The continued presence of the support person in the operating room proves invaluable with a regional anesthetic.

If the young parturient is extremely anxious, however, a general anesthetic usually becomes necessary (Chap. 6). When based on the patient's weight, the pentothal dose (3 to 4 mg per kg) needed for anesthetic induction will usually be less than the "standard" 250-mg adult dosage. A small cuffed endotracheal tube (5.0 and 6.0 mm) should be available for the potentially smaller airway, especially in the parturient with pregnancy-induced hypertension who may exhibit laryngeal edema. Whether a regional or general anesthetic is used, appropriate explanations and continual patient reassurance will help to psychologically support the adolescent parturient while awake.

Postpartum, early interaction and bonding should be encouraged between the infant and mother. Special instruction by interested social workers is recommended to assess adequate knowledge of infant care skills. Early involvement of social service agencies may assist the mother in obtaining child care and, hopefully, continuing her education.

The Elderly Gravida

The term "elderly" generates interest when used to refer to a female in her reproductive years, since it is classically defined as "somewhat old; between middle and old age; pertaining to persons in later life."[16] In obstetrics, however, it is frequently used in the context of the "elderly primigravida," referring to the woman who is aged 35 or more at the time of her first delivery. Kirtz and others[17] recommend the use of the term "mature gravida" as a more appropriate representation of this group of parturients, since "mature" is defined as "complete in natural growth or development, fully developed in body or mind."[16]

Whatever term is ultimately used to refer to this category of parturients (age 35 years or older), their number is increasing due to several factors.[18] The total number of women aged 35 to 40 years is projected to increase by 42 percent due to the postwar baby boom of the 1950s. Additionally, the number of births in this age group is expected to increase by 37 percent. Numerous other factors play a role including women's career priorities, advanced education, control over fertility, late and second marriages, and financial concerns.

OBSTETRIC CONSIDERATIONS

Fetal Anomalies

The increased risk of fetal anomalies presents a major concern for the elderly parturient as well as the obstetrician. This problem has resulted in the finding[19] that advanced maternal age is now the most common indication for antenatal cytogenetic studies (amniocentesis). One hypothesis of increased fetal anomalies theorizes that the older parturient has decreased maternal selection against chromosomally abnormal conceptuses. Approximately 7 percent of conceptuses, but only 0.5 percent of liveborns, are chromosomally abnormal, which demonstrates natural selection against further development of defective conceptions. It is therefore reasonable to suggest that decreased maternal selection could result in an increased number of neonates with chromosomal abnormalities. Another hypothesis attributes aneuploidy to intrinsic aging factors, possibly mediated by a decrease in chiasmata or premature desynapsis in aging oocytes. Third, environmental toxins must be considered as a cause of some cases. A fourth hypothesis suggests that genetic factors may cause some cases of trisomy (i.e., a recessive gene causing nondisjunction).

Regardless of etiology, the incidence of trisomy 21 (Down's syndrome) increases with maternal age.[19] At age 20, the risk of trisomy 21 is one in 1667; this likelihood increases to one in 385 by age 35, one in 137 at age 39, and one in 30 by age 45. Trisomy 13, trisomy 18, and chromosomal patterns 47XXX and 47XXY also show an increasing incidence with advancing maternal age. Considering these risks, most obstetricians recommend amniocentesis for parturients 35 years and older. If an abnormality is found, the mature parturient must then face the decision of whether to continue the pregnancy or terminate it, a difficult decision when this may be her last possible pregnancy.

Maternal Problems

Booth and Williams[20] documented uncomplicated pregnancy in seven of every ten elderly gravidas, a rate that appears similar to that in younger women. However, obstetricians have historically considered elderly gravidas to be at an increased risk for maternal and fetal problems. Numerous studies[21-29] report a higher incidence of pre-eclampsia (toxemia) and/or essential hypertension, diabetes, and thyroid disease. Additionally, as more parturients approach their later reproductive years, an increase in cardiac disease is anticipated.[30,31] Many of these complications result from the aging process itself, upon which the physiologic demands of pregnancy are superimposed. Events occurring during labor may provoke further maternal and fetal complications.

Due to the increased frequency of pregnancy complications, labor is more likely to be pharmacologically induced in the mature parturient.[22] Once initiated, labor is more frequently prolonged when compared with parturition in younger women. An increasing development of uterine myomas (fibroids) in this age group is one contributing factor for dysfunctional labor. Other common intrapartum problems include fever, fetal distress, malpresentation (breech and transverse lie), abruptio placentae, and placenta previa.[21,23,24,26,29,32]

The older gravida delivers spontaneously less often than her younger counterparts; most reviews[29,30,32] report a higher rate of forceps. In addition, the use of forceps often entails application at a higher pelvic level than in younger obstetric cases. This may reflect, in part, the obstetrician's heightened concern for this age group of parturients and their neonates. Following vaginal delivery, elderly gravidas experience a greater blood loss in response to injuries to the vagina and perineum, possibly owing to loss of tissue elasticity.[29] The aggressive use of oxytocic drugs minimizes blood loss from the uterus postdelivery.

Most studies[22-30, 32-35] substantiate the greatly increased frequency of cesarean section in older primiparous and multiparous patients. In primiparas, the most common indications include fetal distress, abnormal fetal presentation or size, and "failure to progress." In multiparous women, a high percentage of cesarean sections are scheduled electively due to a prior cesarean delivery. Overall, most surveys reflect that obstetricians liberally employ cesarean section in this age group due to the heightened concerns for fetal survival in a parturient in whom (1) this may be her last pregnancy, (2) maternal complications are diagnosed, and/or (3) medical-legal concerns are present. The last may become more apparent in the present atmosphere of parents expecting (and demanding) a "perfect baby".

Neonatal Outcome

Historically, most perinatal physicians and nurses have considered the neonate at increased risk due to the effects of advanced maternal age. Kajonoja and Widholm[28] site higher rates of stillbirth and prematurity as responsible factors for the increased perinatal death rate. However, when parturients with pre-existing hypertension are excluded, Grimes and Gross[34] noted no increased perinatal mortality in infants of healthy, older black mothers. In fact, Jacobson[29] reports a decreasing perinatal mortality in the neonates of parturients over 35 years old. His study, as well as others, attributes improved neonatal outcome to the liberal use of the cesarean section in older gravidas. Prolonged labor ($>$20 hours), post-term gestations, and the presence of meconium have been associated with increased neonatal morbidity. Therefore, the presence of maternal complications (especially hypertension) should alert the health care team of potential neonatal problems and the subsequent need for close antenatal fetal monitoring during the pregnancy as well as the labor and delivery period (see Chap. 3).

ANESTHETIC CONSIDERATIONS

Labor and Delivery

With more women postponing childbirth until their late 30s, this pregnancy may be her only pregnancy—"a premium pregnancy." To some patients, it may represent the end result of a long period of infertility. Whether she has voluntarily or involuntarily postponed pregnancy, the older parturient frequently participates in childbirth education classes and often completes extensive reading on the various aspects of her pregnancy and delivery. Many misconceptions may come about concerning the available anesthetic techniques. The anesthesia team should ascertain the parturient's understanding of anesthesia and address specific concerns.

Older parturients frequently choose epidural analgesia (when available).[17] Commonly, they wish to remain alert and "involved" in their labor and delivery. If she receives a segmental epidural for pain relief, the patient will still be able to feel the sacral pressure at the end of the first stage and therefore maintain the urge to push, a component that is pyschologically important to many educated parturients. After delivery with epidural analgesia, these new mothers appear more alert and rested, in comparison to when intravenous medication or no analgesia is employed, allowing them to interact (bond) more effectively with a much awaited neonate. In the absence of pregnancy complications, the older mother can choose from the anesthetic methods presented earlier in this chapter or in Chapter 6 for vaginal delivery or cesarean section.

Anesthesia for Pregnancy Termination

Unfortunately, not all of these pregnancies have a happy ending. Following substantiation of abnormal cytogenetic studies, the parturient may choose to terminate the pregnancy. The participation of anesthesia personnel should be optional, based on the anesthesiologist's and anesthetist's moral and ethical views.

By the time termination is performed, many of these pregnancies have progressed to the second trimester. Prostaglandins E_2 or $F_{2\alpha}$ are widely used to initiate labor and delivery by means of insertion (suppository or gel) into the vagina next to the cervix. Subsequently, the prostaglandin produces cervical softening, uterine contractions, cervical dilatation, and expulsion of the products of conception. Retained products of conception frequently require postpartum curettage.

The need for anesthesia during this time period varies among patients. Contractions and/or curettage can be quite painful. Patients commonly receive intravenous analgesics (i.e., narcotics) and sedatives (barbiturates, phenothiazines, or benzodiazepines) during this time. The obstetrician frequently prescribes antiemetic and antidiarrheal agents prophylactically due to the very high incidence of nausea, vomiting, and diarrhea induced by the prostaglandins. If the induction becomes prolonged, a lumbar epidural anesthetic will assist in making the parturient more comfortable during this psychologically difficult time.

During the anesthetic evaluation, the side effects of prostaglandins should be recognized. Increases in body temperature and white blood cell count often occur and must be clinically differentiated from infection (which may be a contraindication to epidural placement). Rarely, a consumptive coagulopathy develops following the use of prostaglandins to terminate pregnancy;[36] therefore, the patient care team should obtain a coagulation screen (platelet count and fibrinogen level) prior to regional anesthesia.

If an epidural is in place, it can then be used to provide anesthesia for the curettage if needed. When profound analgesia is not required until the time of curettage, a subarachnoid block suffices nicely if no coagulation abnormalities are present. A paracervical block, which patients readily accept when combined with intravenous sedation, also provides good anesthesia for this procedure.

Summary

The young pregnant adolescent (less than 16 years old) challenges the obstetric and anesthesia teams. Prenatal counseling should be available concerning nutrition and the signs and symptoms of premature labor. Childbirth preparation classes and a visit to the labor and delivery area allay the parturient's fear and anxiety. During the labor and delivery period, the continual presence of a support person to reassure the patient decreases anxiety and may lessen analgesic requirements. Intravenous narcotics are commonly administered for pain relief; however, as labor progresses, a lumbar epidural anesthetic provides more intense analgesia during this psychologically difficult time. These parturients do not experience an increased cesarean section rate despite a higher incidence of pelvic inlet contraction; thus, a vaginal delivery usually ensues.

The elderly gravida (over 35 years old) may present with maternal disease resulting from the aging process itself (hypertension, cardiac disease, etc.). Age also increases the risk of fetal anomalies, especially Down's syndrome, and these parturients are more prone to experience complications during labor as well as delivery, the latter leading to a higher rate of forceps and cesarean deliveries. This chapter presents obstetric and anesthetic considerations for delivery of the elderly gravida as well as for prostaglandin termination of pregnancy.

The anticipation of potential maternal complications during these pregnancies as well as the labor and delivery period should aid the health care team in optimizing the final outcome of the pregnancy—a healthy baby and a happy mother.

References

1. Safro, IL: Adolescent sexuality, pregnancy, and childbearing. In Smith, PB and Mumford, DM (eds): Adolescent Pregnancy: Perspectives for the Health Professional. GK Hall & Co, Boston, 1980, p 32.
2. Baldwin, W: Adolescent pregnancy and childbearing: An overview. Semin Perinatol 5:1, 1981.
3. Carey, WB, McCann-Sanford, T and Davidson EC, Jr: Adolescent age and obstetric risk. Sem Perinatol 5:9, 1981.
4. Lawrence, RA and Merritt, TA: Infants of adolescent mothers: Perinatal, neonatal, and infancy outcome. Sem Perinatol 5:19, 1981.
5. Coates, JB, III: Obstetrics in the very young adolescent. Am J Obstet Gynecol 108:68, 1970.
6. Lewis, BV and Nash, PJ: Pregnancy in patients under 16 years. Br Med J 2:733, 1967.
7. Duenhoelter, JH, Jimenez, JM and Baumann, G: Pregnancy performance of patients under fifteen years of age. Obstet Gynecol 46:49, 1975.
8. Utian, WH: Obstetrical implications of pregnancy in primigravidae aged 16 years or less. Br Med J 2:734, 1967.
9. Zackler, J, Andelman, SL and Bauer, F: The young adolescent as an obstetric risk. Am J Obstet Gynecol 103:305, 1969.
10. Fielding, JE: Adolescent pregnancy revisited. N Engl J Med 299:893, 1978.
11. Battaglia, FC, Frazier, TM and Hellegers, AE: Obstetric and pediatric complications of juvenile pregnancy. Pediatrics 32:902, 1963.
12. Leppert, PC, Namerow, PB and Horowitz, E: Cesarean section deliveries among adolescent mothers enrolled in a comprehensive prenatal care program. Am J Obstet Gynecol 152:623, 1985.
13. Gibbs, RF: Informed consent: The changing concepts. Legal Perspect Anesth 2:1, 1982.
14. Gibbs, RF: The evolving concept of informed consent. Legal Perspect Anesth 5:1, 1985.
15. Bromage, PR: Aging and epidural dose requirements: Segmental spread and predictability of epidural analgesia in youth and extreme age. Br J Anaesth 41:1016, 1969.
16. Urdang, L and Flexner, SB: The Random House Dictionary of the English Language. Random House, New York, 1968.
17. Kirz, DS, Dorchester, W and Freeman, RK: Advanced maternal age: The mature gravida. Am J Obstet Gynecol 152:7, 1985.
18. Adams, MM, Oakley, GP, Jr and Marks, JS: Maternal age and births in the 1980s. JAMA 247:493, 1982.
19. Verp, MS and Simpson, JL: Amniocentesis for cytogenetic studies. In Filkins, K and Russo, JF (eds): Human Prenatal Diagnosis. Marcel Dekker Inc, New York, 1985, p 13.
20. Booth, RT and Williams, GL: Elderly primigravidae. J Obstet Gynaecol Br Commonw 71:249, 1964.
21. Horger, EO, III and Smythe, AR, II: Pregnancy in women over forty. Obstet Gynecol 49:257, 1977.
22. Kessler, I, et al: The problem of the older primipara. Obstet Gynecol 56:165, 1980.
23. Posner, LB, Chidiac, JE and Posner, AC: Pregnancy at age 40 and over. Obstet Gynecol 17:194, 1961.
24. Koren, Z, Zuckerman, H and Brzezinski, A: Pregnancy and delivery after forty. Obstet Gynecol 21:165, 1963.
25. Blum, M: Is the elderly primipara really at high risk? J Perinat Med 7:108, 1979.
26. Waters, EG and Wagner, HP: Pregnancy and labor experiences of elderly primigravidas. Am J Obstet Gynecol 59:296, 1950.
27. Randall, LM and Taylor, JC: Elderly primigravid women. Am J Obstet Gynecol 57:1210, 1949.
28. Kajanoja, P and Widholm, O: Pregnancy and delivery in women aged 40 and over. Obstet Gynecol 51:47, 1978.
29. Jacobson, L: The elderly primigravida: A study of 543 cases. Acta Obstet Gynecol Scand 42:244, 1963.
30. Higdon, AL: Pregnancy in the woman over forty. Am J Obstet Gynecol 80:38, 1960.
31. Hankins, GDV, et al: Myocardial infarction during pregnancy: A review. Obstet Gynecol 65:139, 1985.
32. Friedman, EA and Sachtleben, MR: Relation of maternal age to the course of labor. Am J Obstet Gynecol 91:915, 1965.
33. Morrison, I: The elderly gravida. Am J Obstet Gynecol 121:465, 1975.
34. Grimes, DA and Gross, GK: Pregnancy outcomes in black women aged 35 and older. Obstet Gynecol 58:614, 1981.
35. Davidson, EC, Jr and Fukushima, T: The age extremes for reproduction: Current implications for policy change. Am J Obstet Gynecol 152:467, 1985.
36. Pritchard, JA, MacDonald, PC and Gant, NF: Williams' Obstetrics. Appleton-Century-Crofts, Norwalk, CO, 1985, pp 482–483.

CHAPTER 25

THE TRAUMATIZED OBSTETRIC PATIENT

JOHN W. BRYANT, M.D.
A. SCOTT WHEELER, M.D.

Trauma is a growing problem as the 20th century closes. Enclosed within thin sheetmetal or fiberglass, individuals hurtle down highways and along crowded streets at increasing speeds, severely injuring themselves or others. The pregnant woman and her fetus are not immune to accidental injuries, which, according to Patterson,[1] occur in 6 to 7 percent of all pregnancies as the modern woman takes on more hazardous jobs, travels extensively, and participates in competitive sports and conditioning programs.[2] The protuberant abdomen, loosened pelvic joints, easy fatigability, and fainting spells also increase her risk of injury.[3] Many injuries are catastrophic.

The National Safety Council in 1982 listed trauma as the most frequent cause of death in women under 35 years of age (or during childbearing years), citing 36 deaths per 100,000 women.[4] In comparison, maternal mortality from other causes approximates 15 deaths per 100,000 pregnancies,[4] suggesting that trauma poses a greater threat to young women than various other complications of pregnancy (e.g., toxemia, hemorrhage, infection). Motor vehicle deaths are 10 times more frequent than any other type.[5] Violent assault, suicide, falls, and burns are the next most likely causes of catastrophic injury.[4]

Therefore, trauma is a major health hazard for pregnant women and their fetuses. This chapter discusses (1) the pathophysiology of trauma as related to pregnancy, (2) initial assessment and resuscitation of mother and fetus in the field and emergency room, and (3) anesthetic management in the operating room. Hopefully, the reader will gain valuable information about effective management of life-threatening trauma. Those interested in anesthesia for less catastrophic injuries are referred to Chapter 27.

Pathophysiology of Trauma and Pregnancy

Depending on extent and duration of injury, a severely traumatized individual may sustain reversible or irreversible damage of one or more organ systems. Compromised organ function may be a direct result of tissue damage or an indirect result of cellular malfunction caused by hypoxemia, anemia, and hypoperfusion. Severe, long-standing intracellular hypoxia depletes energy stores and may lead to generalized loss of cell membrane integrity, producing a state of irreversible shock. Therefore, respiratory insufficiency and cardiovascular failure can cause severe morbidity and death, even when other major organs are not irreversibly traumatized. Hypothermia, which frequently develops when traumatized individuals go unnoticed for significant periods out of doors, also reduces tissue perfusion and cellular activity. Treatment in cold emergency areas and resuscitation with large volumes of fluid (at room temperature) further decrease core temperature, promote the development of cardiac arrhythmias, and alter distribution and elimination of drugs. Uncorrected hypovolemia stimulates peripheral vascular reflex activity and catecholamine release, both of which decrease perfusion of splanchnic tissues, kidneys, muscles, and so forth, while attempting to preserve coronary and cerebral blood flow. Reflex tachycardia increases myocardial oxygen consumption, which may be poorly tolerated in individuals with cardiac disease. Of significant concern is the appearance of disseminated intravascular coagulation (DIC) occurring when tissue trauma or a transfusion reaction releases thromboplastin and activates procoagulant factors. Fibrin deposition in the microcirculation impairs organ perfusion, and consumption of clotting factors attenuates hemostasis and facilitates hemorrhage (Chap. 15). Circulating levels of platelets and clotting factors (especially V and VIII) may also become inadequate and promote additional bleeding when blood products and crystalloids are used to replace massive blood loss (in excess of 1.5 times the blood volume).

Due to the physiologic alterations of pregnancy (Chap. 1) the gravid patient may respond differently to catastrophic injury. Yet few studies prospectively assess maternal outcome following severe trauma. Crosby and Costiloe[6] compiled data on 441 pregnant victims of both severe and minor automobile collisions, noting maternal death in 15 cases (3.4 percent) and nonfatal, major injuries in 26 patients (6.1 percent). Major causes of death included (1) head trauma, seven cases, three of which were combined with orthopedic injuries, and (2) exsanguinating hemorrhage, six cases, resulting from ruptured major arteries, disrupted intraperitoneal organs, or extraperitoneal bleeding from pelvic fractures. Of the 26 nonfatal, severe traumas, five were life-threatening pelvic fractures and two were life-threatening liver lacerations. Therefore, head trauma and hemorrhage from ruptured arteries, pelvic fractures, and damaged thoracoabdominal viscera constitute the greatest risks to women severely injured in auto accidents. Blunt abdominal trauma sufficient to cause pelvic fracture may portend an especially poor prognosis during pregnancy,[1] presumably due to the increased pelvic vascularity developing during gestation.

In regard to fetal outcome (gestational age over 12 weeks), Crosby and Costiloe[6] noted comparable death rates in mother and fetus following severe automobile accidents, concluding that the leading cause of fetal death was maternal death. Abruptio placentae accounted for most fetal wastage when the mother survived. Maternal and fetal mortality rates were highest when the mother failed to wear a seat belt and was ejected during the collision.[6] Shoulder harnesses obviate previous concerns about possible uterine, placental, and fetal trauma produced by lap belts.[7] While prone to trauma during automobile collisions, the pregnant uterus may protect the other abdominal organs, especially midline viscera such as the stomach, pancreas, diaphragm, and mesentery, by providing a cushion between these structures and the abdominal wall (point of impact).[3,8] However, hemorrhage from a ruptured uterus or separated placenta often jeopardizes maternal and fetal survival, especially when coupled with significant bleeding from other tissues.

In addition to the expanding uterus, other anatomic and physiologic changes of pregnancy (Chap. 1) can modify the mother's response to injury. Therefore, physicians attending a pregnant trauma victim must be cognizant of several complicating factors, including the following:[9]

1. Pregnancy may change the pattern or severity of trauma.
2. Pregnancy may alter the signs and symptoms of a particular injury as well as results of laboratory tests used in diagnosis and therapy.
3. Management of a traumatized parturient should be modified to accommodate and pre-

serve physiologic changes induced by pregnancy.

4. Trauma may initiate pathologic conditions peculiar to pregnancy (e.g., abruptio placentae, amniotic fluid embolism, ruptured uterus).

5. A pregnancy-related disease may occur coincidentally with trauma and complicate the diagnosis and therapy of some injuries (e.g., eclampsia complicating possible head trauma).[9]

CARDIOVASCULAR SYSTEM

During pregnancy, cardiac output increases to 6 to 7 liters per min as heart rate increases concomitantly by 15 to 20 beats per min and reaches 80 to 90 beats per min at term. Mean arterial pressure decreases by 10 to 15 mmHg, and systemic vascular resistance decreases substantially. Therefore, the trauma team should anticipate somewhat lower blood pressure values in pregnant than in nonpregnant individuals. Conversely, elevated blood pressure in the pregnant patient is never normal. Hypertension usually reflects catecholamine release secondary to pain, anxiety, hypoxemia, and/or hypercarbia but may be the result of simultaneous pregnancy-induced hypertension. Catecholamine release, especially when associated with hypovolemia and hypoxia, constricts the uterine arteries, decreases placental perfusion, and produces fetal hypoxia.[10] Greiss and Coworkers[11] demonstrated a 10- to 20-percent decrease in uterine blood flow in gravid ewes following a 30- to 35-percent decrease in maternal blood volume. During this period, maternal blood pressures did not change. These data demonstrate that, in trauma victims, normal or elevated maternal blood pressures may not guarantee normal placental perfusion. The fetus can be severely jeopardized while the mother appears stable.[4] Since the fetus may deteriorate before the mother in response to maternal hypoxia and hypovolemia, continuous electronic fetal heart rate monitoring is necessary.

While often using blood pressure measurements to determine cardiovascular status and to assess the effects of fluid resuscitation, the trauma team must also remember that the 40-percent increase in maternal blood volume markedly improves the mother's tolerance to hemorrhage.[2] The pregnant woman may maintain normal blood pressure and a relatively low heart rate during substantial hemorrhage,[12] sometimes causing underestimation of blood loss. Thus, the pregnant trauma victim may require substantially more fluid and blood replacement than the nonpregnant individual for restoration of normal blood volume and tissue perfusion during periods of hypovolemic shock.[4] In such cases, serial measurements of central venous pressure and/or pulmonary capillary wedge pressure are most helpful in determining appropriate volumes of fluid replacement. Alpha-agonistic vasopressors decrease uterine perfusion. If required, centrally acting vasopressors such as ephedrine, mephentermine, and low-dose dobutamine are preferable since they restore blood pressure while preserving uterine perfusion.[1]

In the late second and third trimesters, the gravid uterus impairs cardiovascular function when the mother is supine (Chap. 1). Occlusion of the inferior vena cava by the gravid uterus decreases right ventricular filling pressures and cardiac output, resulting in hypotension and decreased uterine blood flow. Aortic compression further decreases uterine perfusion. Hypovolemia accentuates these effects; so that, in the pregnant trauma victim, the supine position must be avoided.[9] Therefore the uterus should always be displaced to the left during resuscitative or diagnostic maneuvers by tilting the bed 15 to 20 degrees or by placing a wedge under the right hip.

COMPOSITION OF BLOOD

The hypervolemia of pregnancy increases the mother's tolerance to hemorrhage but also demands a greater volume of fluid replacement for restoration of a stable cardiovascular system. Patient care team members must remember that the dilutional anemia of pregnancy often complicates initial assessment of degree of hemorrhage, if based upon hematocrit or hemoglobin values. This is especially so in women with poor prenatal nutrition, who may have hematocrit and hemoglobin values below 30 percent and 10 g per dl, respectively, prior to a traumatic event.

Gestationally related increases in circulating levels of fibrinogen and Factors VII, VIII, and IX and decreases in plasminogen activator substances are of benefit during hemorrhage but increase the risk of thromboembolic disease when pelvic or lower extremity fractures necessitate immobilization.[2] In such cases, the prophylactic use of low-dose heparin warrants consideration after hemorrhage ceases.

Disseminated intravascular coagulation (DIC) may develop rapidly when trauma is associated with abruptio placentae, severe pregnancy-induced hypertension (pre-eclampsia), or amniotic fluid embolism (Chap. 15). Efforts to control bleeding from traumatized tissues are difficult and can be facilitated temporarily only by administration of clotting factors (fresh frozen plasma, cryoprecipitate, platelets, etc.). Termination of pregnancy and removal of the placenta promptly resolves DIC and may be necessary to save the mother's life.

Posttraumatic infection is a serious threat to patients who survive their injuries. The physiologic leukocytosis of pregnancy — that is, white blood counts of 10,000 to 25,000 in response to minimal stress — may cloud the interpretation of elevated white counts for infection screening postoperatively.[2]

PULMONARY SYSTEM

During gestation, several important respiratory changes can diminish maternal survival during trauma. For example, increased vascularity and congestion of the respiratory tract accentuate upper airway bleeding in response to head, neck, or thoracic injury while markedly narrowing the false vocal cords. These changes increase the likelihood of airway obstruction and difficult tracheal intubation in traumatized parturients. Epistaxis occurs more frequently following placement of nasal airways or nasotracheal tubes. Furthermore, the decreased functional residual capacity (FRC) enhances the development of hypoxemia and oxyhemoglobin desaturation during periods of apnea or complete airway obstruction. Rapid establishment of a good airway and reinstitution of adequate ventilation with supplemental oxygen therefore assume primary importance in unconscious gravidas. For example, maternal hemoglobin saturation decreases to less than 77 percent even when tracheal intubation requires as little as 30 sec (of apnea).[13] In mothers requiring surgery, a decreased FRC increases the rate of induction and emergence from inhalation anesthesia.[13] Also of concern is the decreased buffering capacity of blood, resulting from renal excretion of bicarbonate ions (to compensate for respiratory alkalosis) and the physiologic decrease in hemoglobin levels.[13] Metabolic acidosis thus develops more rapidly during periods of hypoxia and hypoperfusion. The patient care team must assess the effects of controlled ventilation, either manual or mechanical, with frequent arterial blood gas measurements and avoid the detrimental effects of excessive hyperventilation and hypocarbia on uterine blood flow and fetal oxygenation. Arterial carbon dioxide tensions are best maintained at 30 to 35 mmHg.

GASTROINTESTINAL SYSTEM

Pregnancy distorts the lower esophageal sphincter and delays gastric emptying (Chap. 1). Placental gastrin increases gastric hydrochloric acid secretion. These changes place traumatized pregnant women at high risk for regurgitation and aspiration of gastric contents when head injuries or cerebral ischemia reduce the level of consciousness. Cricoid pressure and rapid tracheal intubation with a cuffed tube usually protect the lungs against aspiration of acid and/or food particles.

Of importance to the trauma surgeon is the enlarged uterus, which pushes small bowel in a cephalad direction resulting in variable anatomic findings. Compartmentalization of small intestine into the upper abdomen increases risk of intestinal injury in gravidas who sustain penetrating wounds to the upper abdomen or lower thorax.[1] The lax abdominal musculature of pregnancy often diminishes the signs of peritoneal irritation (guarding and rigidity). Paracentesis procedures require extreme caution due to the gravid uterus and resulting displacement of bowel.[9]

GENITOURINARY SYSTEM

The gravid uterus may cause bilateral ureteral dilation and incomplete bladder emptying.[1] Urinary tract infections occur more frequently, a possible source of post-traumatic fever. The full bladder compressed between the uterus and pelvis is more vulnerable to rupture during pelvic trauma. At the same time, urinary system assessment with ureteropyelography (IVP) is more difficult in pregnancy.[4] Blood urea nitrogen and serum creatinine values decrease during gestation; values in excess of 10 mg per dl and 0.8 mg per dl, respectively, indicate compromised renal function.

The information above demonstrates how physiologic changes of pregnancy generate patient care problems in maternal assessment, interpretation of laboratory studies, and appropriate management of trauma. The reader is referred to Chapter 1 for background information on normal physiologic changes in other systems.

Assessment and Resuscitation

At the scene of the accident, properly trained health care professionals must initiate the ABCs of trauma at the earliest possible moment, while continuing to assess the patient. Airway evaluation is particularly vital since obstruction by blood, vomitus, swollen tissues, and so forth rapidly produce maternal and fetal hypoxia. A member of the resuscitation team should carefully examine the mouth and neck of lethargic and obtunded individuals, clear the pharynx as necessary, and control the airway, when indicated, with an oral airway, endotracheal tube, or cricoid thyroidotomy. In unconscious patients, the trachea must be protected from aspiration of foreign bodies, food particles, or gastric acid, which is best accomplished by use of cricoid pressure and rapid nasal or oral intubation with a cuffed, 6.0- to 7.0-mm tube. Such maneuvers require experienced personnel since additional airway stimulation or trauma may aggravate swelling and bleeding or produce laryngospasm. Possible cervical spine injury in patients with obvious head and neck trauma mandates careful manipulation of the head during airway management procedures. Certainly, a second pair of skilled hands as well as the availability of suction and a variety of laryngoscope blades and endotracheal tubes facilitate difficult intubation.

When the patient arrives in the emergency room, the capability to perform fiberoptic intubation or jet ventilation through a transtracheal cannula is advised. Not infrequently a cervical collar and backboard remain in place until neck roentgenograms rule out cervical and upper thoracic spine fractures. Cervical collars complicate orotracheal intubation. Awake, nasal intubation then becomes ideal, despite the risk of epistaxis, but can be difficult in combative, disoriented patients. Fiberoptic intubation sometimes provides an alternative but may be an exercise in futility when blood or traumatized tissues occupy the hypopharynx. In some cases pharmacologic intervention can be considered for tracheal intubation, *if anatomy of mouth and neck is normal.* A standard, rapid-sequence approach with low-dose ketamine (0.25 to 0.5 mg per kg), etomidate (0.1 to 0.2 mg per kg), or thiopental (2 to 3 mg per kg), succinylcholine, and cricoid pressure follows preoxygenation by mask in the responsive individual. One best avoids ketamine in those with increased intracranial pressure. Unconsciousness eliminates the need for amnestic agents (ketamine, etomidate, etc.), especially when hemodynamics are unstable. To facilitate this approach, we position sand bags near both sides of the head and place axial traction to the sides of the head manually, following which an assistant removes the top of the cervical collar, if present, and applies cricoid pressure. Induction drugs are then given, with suction, laryngoscope, and endotracheal tubes in readiness. The trachea is rapidly intubated, and the cuff is inflated immediately.

In severely injured patients, establishment and maintenance of a good airway is the most important initial intervention. Yet, certain airway management techniques are fraught with danger, especially when attempted by inexperienced personnel. Those unskilled in tracheal intubation should remember the value of evacuation of upper airway matter, use of an oral airway to avoid soft-tissue obstruction, and administration of supplemental oxygen by mask until more experienced personnel arrive.

Following establishment of a good airway, arterial oxygenation is enhanced by use of nasal cannulae or face mask in spontaneously breathing subjects. When apparent hypoventilation exists, assisted or controlled ventilation with a snugly-fitted face mask or an endotracheal tube begins, using a ventilation system (e.g., Ambu bag, Mapelson D). Arterial blood gas determinations guide the resuscitation team regarding supplemental oxygen and ventilation requirements. Arterial oxygen levels are best maintained above 80 mmHg, while a $PaCO_2$ of 30 to 35 mmHg helps preserve uterine blood flow. Severe metabolic acidosis (pH <7.20) necessitates sodium bicarbonate administration, especially when hemodynamics are poor. Hypernatremia, hypokalemia, and increased affinity of hemoglobin for oxygen, possibly occurring secondary to sodium bicarbonate, mandate judicious administration.

Once the airway is secured and good ventilation and oxygenation are provided, a trauma team member should place a nasogastric tube and evacuate the stomach.[14] Oral gastric tubes are best in patients with nasal or maxillofacial trauma. More importantly, sufficient intravenous access must be provided, preferably by means of two, large-bore (14- to 16-gauge) cannulae placed percutaneously in the upper extremities. If this is not possible, direct venisection via cut-down and insertion of 12-gauge or 8-French feeding cannulae is an alternative. Other possible access sites include subclavian, internal or external jugular, and femoral veins, which are percutaneously cannulated. Catheters are sutured with 2.0 silk if time allows. Approximately 50 ml of blood is then drawn for important laboratory values (Table 25–1).[15]

In the young, healthy pregnant patient restoration of blood volume is the key to cardiovascular resuscitation. In hypotensive patients, approximately 2000 ml of balanced salt solution are infused over 3 to 5 min *with the mother maintained in left lateral tilt position*.[15] If blood pressure and pulse fail to return to acceptable levels, we rapidly administer colloid (e.g., 1000 ml Plasmanate or hetastarch) and consider additional intravenous lines.[15] The existence of a jugular, subclavian, or femoral catheter allows determination of central venous pressure. When type-specific blood is available and hematocrit/hemoglobin levels indicate severe anemia (HGB <8 g per dl), four units of packed cells are infused every 10 to 15 min until hemodynamic parameters stabilize and/or central venous pressure reaches 8 to 12 cm H_2O.[15] When possible, blood is *both* typed and crossmatched to avoid maternal exposure to foreign, red-cell antigens (e.g., ABO, Rh), which may produce erythroblastosis fetalis at a later time. However, profound hypovolemic shock dictates use of type-specific, uncrossmatched blood, when necessary for maternal and fetal survival. Following successful resuscitation, amniocentesis later in pregnancy determines the extent of fetal red cell hemolysis. Warming of fluids and blood products, a trauma room temperature of 22 to 25°C, and use of overhead heating lamps help prevent maternal hypothermia.

During cardiovascular resuscitation, continual assessment with automated blood pressure readings (i.e., Dinamap), and continuous maternal electrocardiographic monitoring constitute the standard of care. Absence of pulse and/or blood pressure indicates the initiation of measures as defined by the Advanced Cardiac Life Support (ACLS) protocol.[14] External cardiac compression combined with intravenous cardiotonic agents may become necessary until circulating blood volume is sufficiently restored. Additionally, MAST trousers are acceptable for use in the first trimester of pregnancy, and leg trousers can be used throughout gestation.[12]

When time allows, rectal examination is performed to exclude obvious urethral injury, a Foley catheter is placed, and urine is sent for urinalysis.[15] The presence or absence of fetal heart tones should be determined by fetoscope or by Doppler. The obstetrician or obstetrics nurse then places external devices necessary for continuous, electronic fetal heart rate monitoring. In our center, the initial assessment-resuscitation process includes the following radio-

Table 25–1. INITIAL BATTERY OF LABORATORY TESTS FOR VICTIMS OF SEVERE TRAUMA

Complete blood count, including platelet count
Prothrombin time, partial thromboplastin time, fibrinogen level, fibrin degradation product levels
Serum sodium, potassium, chloride, blood urea nitrogen, creatinine, glucose, amylase levels
Blood alcohol level
Type and crossmatch for minimum of six units packed red blood cells
Arterial blood gas values
Urinalysis

graphs: anterior chest, cervical spine, KUB, and, in all blunt abdominal traumas, a single-shot pyelogram with 50 to 100 ml of intravenous contrast material. Fetal radiation exposures must be considered and are best avoided, if possible, by placing a lead apron over the mother's abdomen.[15]

Having completed the procedures described above, members of the trauma team—specifically the surgeon and obstetrician—proceed with definitive diagnosis and triage. Following initial resuscitation, the stabilized patient should be rapidly transferred (most expeditiously by helicopter) to a center containing facilities and personnel required for complete surgical, obstetric, and anesthetic management, including intensive maternal and fetal surveillance/care postoperatively.

Surgical Assessment

In many trauma centers today, definitive assessment includes assignment of a trauma score to each patient. Table 25–2 outlines the scoring method used in our hospital. Such methods often include the Glasgow Coma Scale and Total Trauma Score.[16] Results of these scoring methods generally correlate well with patient outcome[17] and, thus, can be used by the surgical team to determine operability. In comatose patients with significant head trauma, neurologic evaluation includes computed tomography (CT scan) of the head unless precluded by life-threatening injuries or ongoing hemorrhage. Intracranial hemorrhage must be considered and treated surgically before proceeding with surgical correction of less life-threatening abdominal or orthopedic injuries.[4] On the other hand, the surgeon will defer CT scan of the head until later in subjects requiring immediate surgery for treatment of massive hemorrhage. All trauma team members must consider the possibility of increased intracranial pressure (ICP) in any patient with head trauma and make necessary therapeutic adjustments (mannitol in normovolemic subjects, steroids, hyperventilation, etc.). When feasible, direct monitoring of ICP, fetal heart rate, and arterial blood gas values assist the determination of an optimal degree of hyperventilation.

Blunt or penetrating chest injuries may produce rib fractures, hemothorax, pneumothorax, pulmonary contusions, cardiac injuries, hemomediastinum, and/or pericardial temponade. Disruption of great vessels often leads to hemorrhagic shock and requires immediate correction.[4] Trauma victims with flail chest receive endotracheal intubation and positive pressure ventilation for internal splinting.[15] The coexistence of pulmonary contusion often necessitates a high fraction of inspired oxygen (FIO_2) and positive end expiratory pressure (PEEP). Additionally, these modalities are required in the comatose patient with aspiration pneumonitis. Suspected tension pneumothorax requires immediate needle thoracocentesis at the second intercostal space, just lateral to the mid-clavicular line.[15] Chest tubes are placed when roentgenograms confirm the presence of hemothorax or pneumothorax. Some surgeons place prophylatic chest tubes when trauma patients with multiple rib fractures are to receive positive-pressure ventilation for prolonged periods.[15] In all patients with significant chest trauma, possible cardiac damage necessitates a 12-lead electrocardiogram (ECG). Evidence of myocardial damage or ischemia warrants serial determination of ECG and cardiac enzyme levels, and, when time allows, placement of a Swan-Ganz catheter provides assessment of cardiac function. The surgeon must expeditiously perform exploratory thoracotomy for treatment of cardiac lacerations with tamponade, ruptured major vessels, large open chest wounds, or damage to the trachea or thoracic esophagus. In pregnant women, penetrating injuries to the lower chest may be associated with injury to small intestines.[1] Diaphragmatic trauma bears consideration as well.

Obvious abdominal trauma associated with hypotension usually indicates peritoneal lavage, which is the principal determinant of whether a pregnant trauma victim requires laparotomy. The enlarged uterus and lax abdominal muscles often complicate clinical abdominal examination. Return of blood, fecal material, small-bowel contents, or bloody amniotic fluid during lavage mandates immediate laparotomy.[18] Cowley and Dunham[19] recommend the following as minimal criteria for laparotomy: (1) erythrocyte count >100 cells per mm^3 of lavage fluid; (2) leukocyte count >5 cells per mm^3; (3) presence of gastrointestinal contents such as

Table 25–2. TRAUMA SCORING SYSTEM AT CARRAWAY METHODIST MEDICAL CENTER

Trauma score		
A. Glascow Coma Scale	14–15	5
	11–13	4
	8–10	3
	5–7	2
	3–4	1
B. Respiratory rate	10–24/min	4
	25–35/min	3
	36/min or more	2
	1–9/min	1
	None	0
C. Respiratory expansion	Normal	1
	Retractive, shallow	0
D. Systolic BP	90 mmHg or more	4
	70–89 mmHg	3
	50–69 mmHg	2
	0–49 mmHg	1
	No pulse	0
E. Capillary refill	Normal	2
	Delayed	1
	None	0
Total trauma score	(A+B+C+D+E)	1–16
Glascow Coma Scale		
Eye-opening response	Spontaneous	4
	To voice	3
	To pain	2
	None	1
Best motor response	Obeys command	6
	Localizes pain	5
	Withdraws from pain	4
	Flexion response	3
	Extension response	2
	None	1
Best verbal response	Oriented	5
	Confused	4
	Inappropriate words	3
	Incomprehensible sounds	2
	None	1
Total		3–15

vegetable fibers, bile, and bacteria; or (4) elevated amylase levels in lavage fluid, which indicates small-bowel injury. Free air under the diaphragm (on an upright chest roentgenogram), progressive abdominal distension associated with a decreasing hematocrit, or perforation of the abdominal wall also necessitates laparotomy.[18]

Blunt abdominal trauma may rupture intraperitoneal viscera (including the uterus), lacerate intra-abdominal blood vessels, and cause retroperitoneal hemorrhage. Blunt injuries to the left upper quadrant frequently injure the spleen. Buchsbaum[20] reported a 15-percent maternal mortality rate in a series of splenic ruptures. In patients with pelvic trauma, retroperitoneal hemorrhage occurs frequently and becomes life-threatening when hematoma formation progresses. External compression can be attempted with MAST trousers,[15] but laparotomy and aortic compression are necessary for control of a rapidly expanding hematoma.[4] These maneuvers have obvious implications regarding uteroplacental perfusion. If the hematoma does not expand and vital signs and hematocrit levels stabilize after transfusion, retroperitoneal hemorrhage requires observation only.

In pregnant women with gunshot wounds to the abdomen, Buchsbaum[20] notes a relatively low maternal mortality when compared with an expected death rate of 10 percent. The enlarged uterus serves as a protective mechanism by absorbing and dissipating missile energy. However, maternal bowel and bladder injury occurs frequently. Fetal injury and perinatal mortality rates approximate 60 to 70 percent when the bullet enters the uterus, often causing direct fetal trauma and premature delivery.[20] As a result, gunshot wounds to the lower abdomen require aggressive surgical management. Hysterotomy and/or hysterectomy are not always necessary and depend on findings at laparotomy,[2] during which a properly retracted uterus should not obscure the operative field. Stab wounds to the abdomen also carry a relatively low maternal mortality (1 to 2 percent).[1] Although the gravid uterus may protect against knife injuries, upper abdominal injuries are associated with an increased incidence of viscus trauma.

Severe back trauma and less severe blunt or penetrating abdominal injuries can damage the urinary tract. Bladder rupture frequently accompanies pelvic fracture, while urethral obstruction can result from retroperitoneal hemorrhage. Findings suggestive of urinary damage or bruising over the flank region indicates evaluation with IVP, which is usually safe when systolic blood pressure exceeds 70 mmHg.[4] Integrity of the bladder is evaluated by injecting 300 ml cystografin via Foley catheter for pelvic roentgenograms. Renal pedicle damage necessitates open debridement, hemostasis, ureteral takedown, and drainage.[4]

Burns secondary to fires, explosions, scalding water, or electrical accidents are associated with a maternal mortality rate of 37 percent when the burn involves more than 60 percent of the mother's surface area. On the other hand, maternal deaths do not occur when a burn involves less than 60 percent of body surface area.[2] The treatment method at Brooke Army Burn Center[2] includes immediate removal of clothing and enclosure of the patient in sterile sheets. Chemical burns are treated with copious saline irrigation. Fluid requirements generally consist of lactated Ringer's solution, 40 ml for each 1 percent of area burned per 24 hours. One half of this daily amount is given in the first 8-hour period. Patients with second- or third-degree burns of face or neck receive an endotracheal tube for provision of a good airway.[15] This is especially important in those sustaining inhalation injuries to airway mucosa. Fiberoptic bronchoscopy assesses the extent of damage. High-voltage electrical burns can produce many problems, but muscle damage leading to release of myoglobin and myoglobinuria is often overlooked.[15] When urine assays reveal myoglobin, diuresis induced by mannitol and furosemide is advised. Renal function and intravascular fluid losses (from diurectic agents) require close observation and aggressive management.[12]

Victims of motor vehicle accidents frequently sustain multiple injuries, including long-bone fractures. Femoral fractures, which usually require abdominal casting or a hip spica cast for fixation in nonpregnant patients, are better managed by open fixation to avoid compromised uterine growth, difficulties in fetal assessment, or management problems during labor and delivery.[4] The patient care team must remain cognizant of possible fat embolization syndrome resulting from long-bone fractures and necessitating supportive modalities regarding pulmonary, cardiac, and neurologic function.[21]

The gravid patient with a fractured mandible, which requires a wiring procedure, must receive expert airway management. Preoperative ranitidine, 50 mg intravenously, and sodium citrate, 30 ml orally, decrease the likelihood of acid aspiration. The use of intramuscular or intravenous glycopyrrolate, phenyleprine spray to the nasal mucosa, and a thoroughly lubricated 6.0- to 7.0-mm nasotracheal tube help prevent epistaxis. In patients with reasonable range of mandibular motion, an intravenous induction prior to nasotracheal intubation, rather than an awake intubation, minimizes maternal stress, catecholamine release, and decreased uterine perfusion. Application of cricoid pressure throughout induction prevents passive regurgitation of gastric contents.

Urologic, orthopedic, pulmonary, abdominal, and head-neck injuries frequently require multiple roentgenograms. Although possible fetal effects generate concern, x-ray procedures are performed as indicated for maternal diagnosis and treatment. The surgeon best avoids the use of fluoroscopy, which produces substantial radiation exposures.

Obstetric Assessment

While the trauma surgeon stabilizes the severely injured patient, the obstetrician must remember that, even though efforts may not succeed in maternal resuscitation, it may be possible to save the fetus. This demands effective communication between the surgeon, obstetrician, and anesthesiologist.

The obstetrician's concerns include possible premature placental separation, a ruptured uterus, ruptured amniotic membranes, and direct fetal injury.[4] Real-time ultrasonography is portable and provides assessment of fetal movement, cardiac motion, and gestational age in the trauma room (Chap. 3). The experienced ultrasonographer can also detect fetal injuries. However, a B-mode unit more accurately determines fetal size and gestational age, intrauterine death, and placental location as well as the presence of soft-tissue masses and retroplacental or pelvic hematomas. Evaluation of the fetus, placenta, and uterus should be performed with either method when time allows. As important, constant fetal heart rate monitoring—initially with fetoscope and subsequently with an electronic monitor—must begin at admission and continue throughout the emergency-room period, intraoperatively, and postoperatively.

Following traumatic placental separation, the obstetrician weighs the risk of maternal bleeding and fetal hypoxia against the risk of prematurity when determining the need for delivery (see Chaps. 15 and 17). Partial placental separations often subside during conservative management, which includes close maternal and fetal monitoring and usually results in a healthy infant. Furthermore, small abruptions rarely produce disseminated intravascular coagulopathy (DIC). In contrast, large or complete placental separation produce an unacceptable risk of maternal and fetal mortality. For example, clinical symptoms such as mild to moderate external bleeding and premature labor may occur following placental separation of less than 25 percent, while maternal shock, uterine tetany, severe fetal distress, and DIC accompany abruptions exceeding 50 percent of placental surface area.[3] Maternal and fetal status combined with other ongoing events guide the obstetrician's recommendations about the propriety of immediate versus delayed delivery. The presence of DIC almost certainly warrants immediate delivery.

Traumatic rupture of amniotic membranes initially creates little maternal risk but requires documentation with speculum examination and use of nitrazine paper and a fern test. Rupture calls for close observation for infection (amnionitis); however, the coexistence of multiple trauma negates the usefulness of body temperature measurements and white blood cell counts. Amnionitis can produce devastating maternal and fetal effects (see Chap. 22) and dictates vaginal or abdominal delivery. Ruptured membranes in the presence of a dilated cervix predispose to umbilical cord prolapse. Diagnosis rests on the presence of fetal distress (bradycardia) and an umbilical cord noted within the vagina on speculum or digital examination. Generally, immediate abdominal delivery provides the best chance for survival of the viable fetus following prolapse of the umbilical cord.

Abdominal exploration does not always mandate hysterotomy and evacuation of the fetus. To the contrary, cesarean delivery becomes necessary only when (1) the uterus is ruptured; (2) fetal distress supersedes the risk of premature delivery; (3) the gravid uterus significantly impairs surgical exposure and the concomitant surgical pathology threatens maternal survival; or (4) maternal death is imminent. Minor perforations or superficial lacerations of the gravid uterus may bleed significantly but usually allow for easy repair during laparotomy. Hysterectomy becomes indicated when a severely damaged uterus cannot be repaired or substantial hemorrhage from a ruptured uterus cannot be controlled.[2] As an alternative, hypogastric artery ligation often decreases uterine arterial perfusion pressure sufficiently to allow surgical hemostasis and, thus, preserves the woman's ability to bear children.[2]

During blunt, low abdominopelvic trauma, skull fracture is the most common fetal injury and usually takes place during maternal pelvic fracture.[2,12] Fetal clavicular and lower-extremity fractures are also frequent.[3] Roentgenograms of abdomen and pelvis generally reveal fetal orthopedic and cranial injuries. However, nonlethal soft-tissue damage may go unnoticed. Soft-tissue wounds heal more slowly in utero than postpartum.[3] If noted, life-threatening fetal injuries justify cesarean delivery of the relatively mature infant (>1500 g). A pediatric surgeon or orthopedist, pediatrician, and another anesthesia team should be summoned to attend the injured fetus soon after delivery.

When maternal death appears imminent, members of the trauma team should proceed expeditiously with cesarean section to salvage the fetus. Ritter and coworkers[22] reported reasonable fetal outcome following 120 postmortem cesarean sections. In contrast, Behney and associates[23] evaluated results of 72 such procedures, noting that 27 infants survived delivery. Of these babies, 16 subsequently expired, and 11 survived. In another study, Weber and coworkers[18] closely followed seven infants delivered postmortem, finding that three babies died immediately, two premature infants born within 5 min of the mother's death survived with acceptable neurologic function, and two term infants born 15 min after the mother's death survived but had severe mental retardation. These data corroborate Patterson,[1] who proposes advanced gestational age and a short maternal death–to–fetal delivery interval as the critical factors determining outcome. Little chance of good survival exists when this interval exceeds 15 min. Until delivery, maternal fluid resuscitation, inotropic support with intravenous ephedrine, alkali therapy with sodium bicarbonate, positive-pressure ventilation with pure oxygen, and other resuscitative measures should continue unabated to preserve placental perfusion and fetal oxygenation. Immediately following delivery, successful neonatal resuscitation requires the expertise of at least two individuals.

When severe maternal trauma leads to intrauterine fetal demise, the obstetrician induces labor with oxytocin or prostaglandin, preferably within 7 to 10 days, but at a time when the mother's condition is stable.[12]

Anesthetic Management

Following initial resuscitation and evaluation, the trauma team transports the mother to the operating room. Gravidas must remain in left lateral tilt position during transport, and life support measures must continue. Additionally, a battery-powered electrocardiograph and blood pressure monitor should continuously assess hemodynamics during transport of unstable patients.

When the trauma victim enters the operating room, many necessary tasks require effective communication, cooperation, and efficiency among nursing and physician personnel. Members of the trauma team and emergency room staff can assist the anesthesia team by continuing to infuse blood products, giving interim reports on patient status, helping with additional intravenous access, and, when necessary, placing monitors. In most cases, at least two experienced anesthesia personnel are required for resuscitation and administration of anesthesia in the catastrophically injured patient. In some circumstances, three to four individuals seem insufficient, which emphasizes that drugs and equipment must be thoroughly prepared ahead of time and all members must work together efficiently.

On the operating table, left uterine displacement continues. One anesthesia team member separates and identifies intravenous lines and fluid bags, while another connects the intubated patient to pure oxygen delivered by a semiclosed circle absorber system and a ventilator initially set at 100 ml per kg per min. Unintubated patients breathe 100 percent oxygen by clear anesthesia mask. The nauseated patient should receive metaclopramide, 10 mg, intravenously. Another individual simultaneously places necessary anesthesia monitors (Table 25–3). Central venous pressure, Swan-Ganz, and radial artery monitors are often feasible only after initiation of anesthesia and correction of severe hypovolemia. However, an available anesthesia member or surgeon can place a ra-

Table 25–3. INITIAL ANESTHESIA MONITORING IN SEVERE TRAUMA

Stethoscope, precordial or esophageal
Electrocardiograph
Automated blood pressure
Temperature, nasal or esophageal
Oxygen, end-tidal or inspired
Carbon dioxide, end-tidal
Pulse oximetry
Peripheral nerve stimulator
Urine output
Fetal heart rate (electronically when possible)

dial artery line, percutaneously or by cut-down, provided surgical preparations continue. Prior to induction, suction the nasogastric tube in unintubated patients to remove additional gastric fluids then inject 30 ml sodium citrate, 0.3 M, or Bicitra intragastrically to increase pH.

In the unconscious, hypotensive, and previously intubated gravida neuromuscular blockade with intravenous pancuronium or vecuronium prevents movement and provides surgical relaxation until the anesthesia team restores intravascular volume and can maintain relatively normal blood pressure values. Until then, additional anesthetic agents may potentiate hypotension.

A more complex situation occurs, however, in unintubated conscious or responsive patients with moderate hypovolemia and hypotension, and especially those with cervical spine fracture or facial trauma. Anesthetic induction then requires judicious consideration of the preferred method of airway management (awake intubation versus intubation under intravenous analgesia/anesthesia). Head and neck trauma usually indicates awake nasal or oral intubation or at least requires direct laryngoscopic evaluation of the hypopharynx and supraglottic area prior to intravenous induction. Nasopharyngeal application of local anesthetic plus a vasoconstrictor agent (phenylephrine) decreases the chance for epistaxis and facilitates nasal intubation (6.5- to 7.0-mm tube) performed either blindly or with a fiberoptic laryngoscope. Immediately following awake intubation hypnotic agents such as midazolam, diazepam, scopolamine, ketamine (0.25 to 0.5 mg per kg), or etomidate (0.2 to 0.15 mg per kg) are given to minimize awareness.[18] Intravenous muscle relaxants are then administered to facilitate surgery. Of the nondepolarizing agents, vecuronium (0.8 to 1.0 mg per kg) provides the most stable hemodynamic parameters.[24]

In conscious, hypovolemic individuals without head trauma and deemed suitable for intravenous induction, we use the following approach: (1) defasciculation and preoxygenation until the end-tidal oxygen monitor or mass spectrometer reveals thorough denitrogenation; (2) induction with etomidate (0.1 to 0.15 mg per kg), ketamine (0.25 to 0.5 mg per kg), or midazolam (0.05 to 0.1 mg per kg) followed by cricoid pressure and intravenous succinylcholine (1.5 to 2.0 mg per kg); (3) rapid orotracheal intubation with a 7.0- to 7.5-mm endotracheal tube; (4) immediate insufflation of the cuff with 8 to 10 ml of air; (5) controlled ventilation, 100 ml per kg per min, with pure oxygen; (6) reassessment of blood pressure and pulse; and (7) additional administration of hypnotic agent or light isoflurane (0.5 to 1.0 percent) in oxygen to prevent recall. However, halogenated agents are best avoided until hemodynamic parameters are stable. Furthermore, prudence dictates against the use of halothane in subjects prone to develop hepatic ischemia or enflurane in those with urinary tract damage.

Following induction, resuscitation continues with rapid infusion of intravenous fluids and blood, while one anesthesia team member places a 14- or 16-gauge CVP catheter via the external or internal jugular approach and cannulates a radial artery for continuous blood pressure measurements and blood sampling. The CVP line provides a site for subsequent placement of a 7F Swan-Ganz catheter. Arterial blood gas values are then obtained and ventilator adjustments made as necessary to keep maternal $PaCO_2$ levels between 30 and 35 mmHg. A dilemma arises in patients with head trauma, who may have increased intracranial pressure. Hyperventilation is preferred to decrease cerebral blood flow and prevent intracranial hypertension, yet also decreases uterine blood flow and fetal oxygenation. If fetal survival is anticipated, moderate hyperventilation to a $PaCO_2$ of 26 to 30 mmHg seems justified.

To prevent hypothermia, the anesthesia team administers intravenous fluids through warmers, maintains the mother on a blanket warmer set at 37°C, employs lower fresh gas inflow rates (<3 liters per min), and places a heat-moisture exchanger (HME) between endotracheal tube and Y-piece. Most important, room temperature remains at or is increased to approximately 22°C. Otherwise, hypothermia develops and shifts the maternal oxyhemoglobin saturation curve leftward, increases systemic vascular resistence, decreases cardiac output, and decreases uterine blood flow. Severe hypothermia (<32°C) sometimes induces ventricular fibrillation.

During the initial anesthetic and resuscitation period, documentation of patient parameters is important but should not delay more necessary interventions. We routinely record data from most monitoring methods (see Table 25–3) either every 5 min (blood pressure and pulse) or every 15 min (temperature, oxygen concentration, end-tidal carbon dioxide tension, oximetry results, CVP and pulmonary artery pressure values, fetal heart rate, and ventilation settings) on the anesthesia graphics sheet. Blood loss and urine output are recorded every 30 min. Arterial blood gas measurements, hematocrit levels, clotting studies, and electrolytes are sampled when indicated, with blood gas and hematocrit values usually documented hourly. Using these measurements the anesthesia team makes necessary adjustments in both resuscitation maneuvers and maintenance of anesthesia. For example, fluid infusion rates decrease when blood pressure exceeds 100/60 mmHg, CVP increases to 8 to 10 mmHg, and urine output exceeds 1 ml per kg per hour. A comparison of end-tidal oxygen levels and arterial oxygen concentrations allows computation of venous admixture and shunt fraction ($\dot{Q}s/\dot{Q}t$), which determine FIO_2 requirements. A progressive or acute decrease in both pulse oximetry (percent saturation of tissue hemoglobin) and end-tidal PCO_2 levels indicates decreased biventricular cardiac output especially when arterial PO_2 concurrently exceeds 80 mmHg. Acutely decreasing oximetry values suggest decreased delivery of oxygen to tissues due to impaired left ventricular output. Concomitant reductions in end-tidal CO_2 imply decreased right ventricular output, pulmonary hypoperfusion, and, thus, decreased delivery of CO_2 to the lungs. In that case, the anesthesia team reassesses CVP and hematocrit levels to determine volume status and/or administers inotropes to improve cardiac function. Intravenous ephedrine is preferred because of its minimal effect on uterine vascular resistance. However, compounds with α-agonist properties (epinephrine and high doses of dopamine or dobutamine)[25] are given as necessary for maternal survival. ECG and blood pressure findings of cardiac arrest dictate external or internal cardiac compression; defibrillation may be necessary. Chest tubes are placed following the symptoms of tension pneumothorax (i.e., hypotension, venous distension and increased CVP, decreased pulmonary compliance and unilaterally decreased breath sounds, cyanosis, and decreased pulse oximetry). Deleterious changes in fetal heart rate, such as acute bradycardia, indicate placental hypoperfusion and severe fetal hypoxia.

When resuscitation efforts stabilize the mother, the anesthetist should deepen anesthesia with halogenated agents, nitrous oxide, and/or narcotics to prevent maternal awareness and minimize catecholamine release. Halogenated agents are maintained at relatively low levels (e.g., halothane 0.5 percent, enflurane 1.0 percent, isoflurane 0.75 percent) to avoid significant maternal and fetal cardiovascular depression.[26] Bowel trauma, pneumothorax, high shunt fraction, or intracranial air countraindicates nitrous oxide, but nitrous oxide is preferable to halogenated drugs, especially halothane and enflurane, for patients with increased intracranial pressure. Intravenous narcotics such as fentanyl and sufentanil produce little effect on maternal cardiovascular function, decrease requirements for halogenated agents, and warrant consideration in the resuscitated, hypertensive gravida. However, the anesthesia team defers the use of opiates when the surgeon or obstetrician plans delivery during laparotomy. Fluid overload, leading to pulmonary edema and hypoxia, may necessitate intravenous furosemide. Hypokalemia requires intravenous potassium.

In the severely injured mother, the anesthesia team initially strives to optimize maternal cardiopulmonary physiology to restore and preserve organ perfusion and oxygenation, and necessarily places less emphasis on anesthetic effects in the fetus. This should not be the case, however, in less severely traumatized women who enter the operating room with a minimal degree of cardiopulmonary compromise. Anesthesia team members must then recognize possible anesthetic effects on the developing embryo or fetus and on uterine blood flow (see Chap. 27). When appropriate, members of the patient care team should consider regional anesthesia which produces little fetal drug exposure and obviates the possibility of aspiration pneumonitis. Supplementation of regional blocks with suitable intravenous sedatives and narcotics deserves consideration in the anxious, alert gravida in the second or third trimester of pregnancy. For example, we recently employed continuous lumbar epidural blockade using lidocaine and bupivacaine, combined with intravenous midazolam, fentanyl, and nasal oxygen, to provide anesthesia for repair of hip fracture at 34 weeks' gestation. Epidural morphine produced excellent postoperative analgesia for 72 hours. Such management resulted in a grateful mother and a healthy fetus.

When the anesthesia team or the alert mother with good cardiopulmonary function prefers general anesthesia, we commonly employ the method used for cesarean section (Chap. 6): (1) oral administration of clear antacid; (2) precurarization and thorough preoxygenation; (3) a rapid-sequence induction with thiopental (3 to 4 mg per kg) or ketamine (0.8 to 1.0 mg per kg), succinylcholine (1.5 to 2.0 mg per kg), and cricoid pressure; (4) placement of a cuffed, 7.0- to 7.5-mm orotracheal tube; and (5) maintenance with isoflurane (0.75 percent), halothane (0.5 percent), or enflurane (1.0 percent) and nitrous oxide (40 to 50 percent), oxygen, and muscle relaxant. Controlled ventilation begins at 100 ml per kg per min but changes as necessary to produce an end-tidal carbon dioxide level of 28 to 32 mmHg. When the surgical team plans to avoid intraoperative delivery, fentanyl or sufentanil can be given intravenously during preoxygenation and after intubation to blunt the pressor response to tracheal intubation and surgical stimulation, respectively. One should anticipate a transient diminution in beat-to-beat variability of fetal heart rate following intravenous narcotics or sedatives. The anesthesia team defers use of intravenous opiates and tranquilizers until after delivery and stands by to assist the newborn if delivery is planned.

Recovery Room Management

At completion of surgery, the anesthesiologist and nurse anesthetist discontinue anesthetic drugs while making plans for patient transport and recovery room care. Recovery room nurses receive instruction regarding patient status, necessary ventilator settings, and required laboratory studies. The obstetrician and/or obstetrics nurse provides an electronic monitor to continuously assess fetal heart rate and to note onset of uterine contractions (premature labor). All gravidas in the second or third trimester are transported and maintained in lateral tilt position while controlled ventilation continues with supplemental oxygen. Hypothermia and shivering, hemodynamic instability, a high shunt fraction, and continuing hemorrhage rule against extubation. Muscle relaxants are not reversed when the patient-care team plans prolonged ventilation. However, extubation can be considered in the stable mother following reversal of muscle relaxants, the presence of relatively normal end-tidal CO_2 tensions and adequate oxygen levels, and the return of responsiveness or consciousness.

The compromised mother with continuing hemorrhage requires the assistance of at least two experienced recovery room personnel. If necessary, resuscitation efforts continue unabated throughout the recovery room period and in the intensive care unit. Standard laboratory assessment initially includes complete blood count, electrolytes, blood urea nitrogen and creatinine, clotting parameters, and arterial blood gas values. A chest roentgenogram determines position of the endotracheal tube and central lines (CVP and Swan-Ganz). Pharmaceuticals are given as needed for maternal cardiopulmonary stability. Clotting factors and platelets may be required following massive transfusion and dilution of clotting factors. Continuing hemorrhage necessitates additional blood transfusions given through blood warmers. All efforts are made to reverse hypothermia (application of warm blankets, room temperature at 22 to 25°C, etc.). Narcotics and sedatives are judiciously administered when required for postoperative pain or for maternal tolerance to mechanical ventilation.

Table 25–4. IMPORTANT MANAGEMENT REQUIREMENTS DURING SEVERE TRAUMA

Initial resuscitation
- Provide a good airway.
- Assure adequate ventilation.
- Initiate cardiac resuscitation (ACLS) (Use left lateral tilt position).
- Gain intravenous access with peripheral or central venous lines.
- Restore intravascular volume with crystalloid, colloid, and blood.

Surgical assessment
- CNS: Glasgow Coma Scale, CT scan; assess ICP.
- Chest: chest x-ray, chest tubes, blood gases, ECG.
- Abdominal: gastric tube, peritoneal lavage, foley catheter, IVP.
- Burns: assess degree, surface area, possible pulmonary effects.
- Skeletal: x-rays of neck, long bones; shield fetus.
- Fetus: presence of fetal heart tones, ultrasonography.
- Obtain appropriate laboratory tests (see Table 25–1).

Anesthesia management
- Continue resuscitation using left lateral tilt position.
- Control airway, continue ventilation; give muscle relaxants if endotracheal tube exists.
- Obtain further IV access if indicated; monitor central venous pressure for fluid requirements.
- Anesthesia as indicated by cerebral, pulmonary, and hemodynamic status; thorough monitoring (see Table 25–3); place radial artery cannula.
- Optimize maternal cardiopulmonary physiology; place Swan-Ganz catheter.

Summary

In the double tragedy of the catastrophically traumatized pregnant patient, the anesthesia team is uniquely qualified to assure the best possible outcome. We have the knowledge of the physiologic changes of pregnancy, the pathophysiology of trauma, and the requirement for surgical exposure. Daily we manipulate the dynamics of the clotting system, control massive fluid shifts, and anticipate the physiologic reaction to anesthetic agents. Our ability to control and manage the airway, gain access to the intravascular compartment, and provide pharmacologic cardiac support is unsurpassed. Thus, the caring, well trained anesthesiologist and nurse-anesthetist are indispensable to the trauma team as well as the mother and fetus. Table 25–4 summarizes important requirements in the management of severely traumatized pregnant women.

References

1. Patterson, RM: Trauma in pregnancy. Clin Obstet Gynecol 27:32, 1984.
2. Baker DP: Trauma in the pregnant patient. Surg Clin North Am 1:235, 1982.
3. Crosby, WM: Trauma during pregnancy: Maternal and fetal injury. Obstet Gynecol Surv 29:683, 1974.
4. Crosby, WM: Traumatic injuries during pregnancy. Clin Obstet Gynecol 26:902, 1983.
5. Jackson, FC: Accidental injury: The problem and the initiatives. In Buchsbaum, HJ: Trauma in Pregnancy. WB Saunders, Philadelphia, 1979, p 121.
6. Crosby, WM and Costiloe, JP: Safety of lap belt restraint for pregnant victims of automobile collisions. New Engl J Med 29:683, 1974.
7. Crosby, WM, King, AL and Stout, LC: Fetal survival following impact: Improvement with shoulder harness restraint. Am J Obstet Gynecol 112:1101, 1972.
8. Griswold, RA and Collier, HS: Blunt abdominal trauma. Internat Abstr Surg 112:309, 1961.
9. Cruikshank, DP: Anatomic and physiologic alterations of pregnancy that modified the response to trauma. In Buchsbaum, HJ (ed): Trauma in Pregnancy. Philadelphia, WB Saunders, 1979, p 21.
10. Cosmi, EV and Shnider, SM: Obstetric anesthesia and uterine blood flow. In Shnider, SM and Levinson, G (eds): Anesthesia for Obstetrics. Williams & Wilkins, Baltimore, 1979, p 23.
11. Greiss, FC, et al: Uterine vascular responses to hemorrhage during pregnancy. Obstet Gynecol 77:569, 1966.
12. Haycock, CE: Emergency care of the pregnant traumatized patient. Emerg Med Clin North Am 2:849, 1984.
13. Sexton, J: Surgery in a gravid patient. J Oral Surg 36:878, 1970.
14. Par, MS, III: Adult advanced cardiac life support. JAMA 255:2933, 1986.
15. Resuscitation/Receiving Unit Protocol. Carraway Methodist Medical Center, Birmingham, Alabama, 1986.
16. Hawkins, MO, et al: The trauma score: A self-assessment guide. Alabama Med 55:44, 1986.

17. Neel, K: The trauma rush. Emergency 31:35, 1985.
18. Weber, CE, et al: Postmortem cesarean section. Am J Obstet Gynecol 110:158, 1971.
19. Cowley, RA and Dunham, CM: Shock, trauma, critical care manual. University Park Press, Baltimore, 1982.
20. Buchsbaum, HJ: Accidental injury complicating pregnancy. Am J Obstet Gynecol 102:752, 1968.
21. Wilson, RF: Trauma. In Shoemaker, WE, Thompson, WK and Halbrook, PR (eds): Textbook of Critical Care. WB Saunders, Philadelphia, 1984, p 907.
22. Ritter, J, et al: Postmortem cesarean section. JAMA 175:715, 1961.
23. Behney, CA, et al: Cesarean section delivery after death of the mother. JAMA 176:617, 1961.
24. Savarese, JT: Do the newer muscle relaxants offer any advantage over the old? Refresher Course Lectures, Annual Meeting, ASA, San Francisco. 221:2, 1984.
25. Fishburne, JI, et al: Vascular and uterine responses to dobutamine and dopamine in the gravid ewe. Am J Obstet Gynecol 137:944, 1980.
26. Pulahniuk, RJ and Shnider, SM: Maternal and fetal cardiovascular and acid-base changes during halothane and isoflurane anesthesia in the pregnant ewe. Anesthesiology 41:462, 1974.

CHAPTER 26

SUBSTANCE ABUSE

NANCY KENEPP, M.D.

Since a large portion of the drug abusing population is of child-bearing age, substance abuse occurs frequently during pregnancy, especially in urban areas. It affects the well being of the entire pregnancy, from prenatal care and fetal development to intrapartum management and postnatal neurobehavioral development. Each drug influences anesthetic management in the peripartum period differently. Parenteral self-administration implies a different constellation of complications. The etiology of substance abuse, related problems in pregnancy, specific drug effects, and their implications for anesthetic care are presented in this chapter.

Etiology of Substance Abuse

INCIDENCE

Drug abuse encompasses occasional recreational use, addiction, and inadvertent or suicidal overdose. Table 26–1 lists commonly abused substances grouped by their major cerebral and sympathomimetic effects. More mothers abuse nonnarcotic drugs than narcotics.[1] According to the University of Michigan's Institute for Social Research Survey[2] of 15,200 high school students in 1986, hallucinogens and ethanol are the most frequently abused substances. Alcohol utilization remains unchanged from the previous year (with 65 percent of respondents employing it in the month previous to the survey) as does smoking (with 30 percent). Marijuana use decreased compared with previous years, but 50 percent still employ it and 25 percent do so regularly. Other illicit stimulants and inhalants are equally utilized: in the last month, 20 percent had tried each. Use of opiates (9 percent), sedatives (10 percent), and Quaalude (5 percent) all declined. Twelve percent of high school students report using cocaine in the previous year; 6 percent in the previous month; whereas daily cocaine use is 0.4 percent. Four percent reported employing "crack."

INITIATING FACTORS

Drug experimentation reflects social acceptability, peer attitude, availability, risk, curiosity, and individual tendency to accept social norms.[3]

Table 26–1. COMMONLY ABUSED SUBSTANCES: APPROXIMATE CNS AND CENTRAL SYMPATHETIC EFFECTS

Class	CNS Depressants	CNS Stimulants	Opiate Receptor Agents	Antidepressants
1. (Central sympathetic stimulation)	Antihistamines, sedatives	Amphetamines, cocaine	Phencyclidine, nitrous oxide	Tricyclics, MAO inhibitors
2. (Little or no central sympathetic effect)	Marijuana	Nicotine, LSD	Phenothiazines, butero-phenones	Lithium
3. (Central sympathetic depression)	Ethanol, sedatives, barbiturates		Narcotics, benzodiazepines	

For example, in some American Indian villages, 25 percent of children between 5 and 15 years inhale gasoline fumes.[4] Abusers often progress from cigarettes and alcohol to marijuana, then to cocaine, hallucinogens, and other drugs.[5] Interestingly, progression is unlikely without early use of marijuana. Maternal psychoactive or illicit drug use favors progression in their offspring. Abuse also correlates with adolescent depressive symptomatology and dropping out of school.[6] Pre-existing psychopathology is not a requisite for drug abuse. Neither reported consumption nor laboratory tests reliably assess the degree of abuse with recreational use.[7]

Addictive Drugs

Addiction increases the frequency of toxic reactions, medical-psychological complications, overdose, and death. A biopsychosocial phenomenon justified by physiologic and behavioral theory, addiction maintenance depends on conditioning to environmental stimuli and reinforcing the consequences of drug use (pleasurable effects, termination of initial aversive effect of the drug, social reinforcement, relief of acute or protracted withdrawal symptoms).[8] In youths, social status reinforcement is instrumental in maintaining drug use until tolerance to initial aversive effects develops. Environmental conditioning ranks importantly in the development of relapse after discontinuing drug use. Although personality characteristics vary, abusers are more impulsive and rebellious with respect to social norms and have less tolerance for frustration.

PHARMACOLOGY OF ADDICTIVE DRUGS

Addictive drugs share the capacity to produce tolerance and dependence. Drug disposition tolerance varies according to species and genetic make-up, while pharmacodynamic tolerance relates to drug dependence. Tolerance can develop with a single dose of drug, and all sites of action may not be equally tolerant.[9] Thus, the chance for drug-induced organ damage increases as the minimum "high" dose increases. Dependence, characterized by rebound hyperexcitability or depression, may also develop with a single dose. With short-acting compounds rebound symptoms occur while the initial drug effect wanes, reinforcing drug-seeking behavior. Minimal symptoms accompany discontinuation of long-acting drugs. Protracted abstinence syndrome, a general sense of distress following pharmacologic withdrawal, relates to environmental conditioning. Cross-dependence, which consists of withdrawal symptom suppression while maintaining dependence, is the basis of methadone substitution therapy, multiple drug abuse, and inadvertent drug overdose. Cross-dependence with alcohol accounts for 50 percent of narcotic overdoses.[10]

PATHOPHYSIOLOGY OF ADDICTIVE DRUGS

Major hazards of addictive drugs usually follow parenteral administration and include transmission of communicable diseases, infection from shared equipment, and toxic or allergic reactions to the drug or contaminants. Table 26–2

Table 26–2. COMPLICATIONS OF PARENTERAL DRUG ABUSE

Hepatitis	Bacterial endocarditis
Tricuspid insufficiency	Cellulitis
Septic phlebitis	Septic pulmonary infarct
Pulmonary hypertension	AIDS
Pulmonary edema	Superficial or deep abscess
Foreign body emboli	Cerebral abscess
Lymphedema	Vertebral osteomyelitis
Bullous pulmonary damage	Pneumonia
Pulmonary abscess	Tetanus

lists reported complications.[11,12] In New York City, 70 percent of AIDS patients abuse drugs, and the incidence of AIDS equals that of endocarditis among addicts admitted to hospitals.[13]

ADDICTIVE DRUGS IN PREGNANCY

Psychosocial Effects

The drug abuser's unstable environment hinders adequate nutrition and prenatal care. A part of the fetal abuse spectrum—failure to protect the child from chemical assault—may be an antecedent to child abuse.[14] Intervention proves most successful in programs designed to handle all women's needs rather than merely those of the mother and fetus.[15]

Pharmacologic Effects

Maternal. Physiologic changes in body water, plasma volume, and drug metabolism and sensitivity alter drug biodisposition and pharmacodynamics in pregnancy, with consequences relevant for drug effect, half-life, peak concentration after a single dose, and fetal exposure.[16] Specific effects on maternal (or paternal) physiology alter fertility, placental implantation, uterine blood flow, and placental function.

Placental. Placental metabolism resembles hepatic biodegradation of drugs, but substrate specificity and enzyme quantity remain restricted. The environmentally determined quantity and quality of enzymes changes in smokers.[17,18]

Fetal. Exogenous drugs induce fetal liver enzymes, which may transform naturally occurring substances such as steroids and alter embryogenesis. Fetal effects occur primarily from the drug or its metabolic products or, secondarily, from drug-induced functional changes, as with behavioral teratogens.[19]

Neonatal. Decreased neonatal metabolic capabilities prolong drug effects and thereby increase the likelihood of infant intoxication and/or withdrawal. Necessary treatment of withdrawal syndrome with a specific drug agonist, based on a symptom scoring system, may additionally prolong neonatal drug exposure.[20]

Pathophysiologic Effects

Maternal. Drug-obtaining behavior stresses mothers physically and mentally. Maternal nutrition is suboptimal. Increased sensitivity to depressants in pregnancy invites overdose and/or impaired placental exchange. The physiologic changes of pregnancy amplify the cardiovascular and respiratory depressant effects of drugs.

Placental. Drug-induced changes in placental blood flow threaten fetal well being. Abnormal fetal and neonatal behavioral development may occur from altered brain neurochemistry mediated by drug interactions with placental and brain neurotransmitter receptors. In humans, placental neuroreceptors vary widely in drug abusers, whereas they remain fairly constant in the pregnant nonuser. Substance abuse may disrupt the normal receptor-mediated messages for brain development.[21]

Fetal. Substance abuse adversely affects the unborn child through specific toxic effects and nonspecific effects from unstable environment and poor prenatal care.[22] Specific toxic effects may include functional changes, which are nonspecific to the class of drug, or drug-specific behavioral changes.[23] Functional changes include alteration of the normal patterns of enzyme development with subsequent functional abnormalities, or imprinting of hepatic metabolism of a compound, resulting in a functional change. For example, imprinting of hepatic metabolism of steroids produces feminization.[19]

Nonspecific environmental effects on oxygen content in infants born to smoking, alcoholic, and drug-dependent mothers might cause growth retardation.

Neonatal. Infants of drug abusers are smaller and have more apnea, aspiration, weight loss, and hyperbilirubinemia.[2] Newborn withdrawal symptoms associate with excessive neonatal weight loss.[24] Alterations in infant neurobehavior and neurochemistry result in long-term changes in behavior. Hepatitis and AIDS may be transmitted transplacentally.[25]

ANESTHETIC IMPLICATIONS IN DRUG ADDICTION

The peripartum period calls for supporting addiction since withdrawal is stressful, reducing uterine blood flow and increasing fetal risk and the likelihood of cesarean delivery. Anesthetic risk is greater during withdrawal than during supported addiction; also one can expect more cesarean sections for fetal distress among withdrawing patients.

Metabolic Interactions

The abused agent may alter anesthetic metabolism. For example, ethanol increases enflurane defluorination.[26] In turn, anesthetic agents may induce increased hepatic metabolism of the abused agent, producing withdrawal or drug-seeking behavior.[27] Both halothane and spinal anesthesia induce hepatic microsomal enzyme activity.[28] Alternatively, anesthetics may block drug metabolism by reducing available receptors or enzymes, just as halothane decreases benzodiazepine metabolism.[29]

Physiologic Interactions

Clinicians reserve administration of anesthesia for situations providing a benefit appropriate to the risk. Pharmacologic drug interactions adversely affect cardiovascular, respiratory, uteroplacental, and fetal function. Fortunately, endogenous feedback systems usually balance and correct drug-induced abnormalities over time, so that careful titration of anesthetic agents to avoid gross abnormalities evades morbidity. However, the possible complications of parenteral drug abuse (see Table 26–2) may complicate the administration of and response to anesthesia.

Addicts may tolerate stress poorly, because tolerance depresses the response to endogenous opioids. Addicts receive more analgesia and anesthesia for labor than control patients; yet those receiving anesthesia deliver infants with better Apgar scores than those not receiving anesthesia.[30] Transcutaneous oxygen and ECG monitoring of laboring parturients helps identify patients requiring anesthetic intervention. Although epidural and spinal narcotics have not been studied in this population, patients taking sympathomimetic drugs interacting with adrenergic agonist agents would benefit from these procedures. One should avoid extensive sympathetic blockade during regional analgesia in such patients. Parenteral narcotic administration increases respiratory depression, a likely occurrence in those abusing drugs cross-dependent with narcotics. Table 26–3 outlines basic anesthetic guidelines.

Depressant Agents

ETHANOL

Pharmacology

The tocolytic and teratogenic effects of ethanol stimulated intense research on its use in pregnancy. Ethanol depresses the central nervous system (CNS). Metabolic and pharmacodynamic tolerance have genetic origins, and tolerance does not elevate the lethal blood level.[31] Ethanol has cross-tolerance with most CNS depressants, including general anesthetics, but not with narcotics. Acute intoxication increases sensitivity to cross-tolerant drugs, and chronic use decreases sensitivity.

Metabolic drug interactions with acute alcohol intoxication include inhibition of hepatic cytochrome p450–dependent drug oxidation, which increases the levels of drugs predominantly excreted by hepatic metabolism (e.g., propranolol, lidocaine). Drugs inhibiting acetaldehyde metabolism increase ethanol-induced CNS depression and flushing. In contrast, chronic abuse stimulates hepatic oxidation and decreases availability of drugs metabolized by the liver.

Ethanol enhances conversion of dihomogam-

Table 26–3. ANESTHETIC MANAGEMENT OF DRUG ABUSERS

Abnormality	Management
Coma	Intubate to protect airway, assess respiratory, cardiovascular status, Glasgow coma scale, administer specific antagonist.
Respiratory depression	Monitor blood gases invasively or noninvasively, administer specific antagonist, intubate, assisted ventilation, avoid additional respiratory depressants.
Hypotension	Monitor blood pressure invasively, O_2 saturation, consider cardiac output, venous O_2 saturation invasively, assess cause: bradycardia, vasodilation, myocardial depression, myocardial ischemia, hypovolemia.
Bradycardia	Atropine, isuprel, pacemaker.
Vasodilation	α-Adrenergic agonist, hydration.
Myocardial depression	Ephedrine, dopamine, epinephrine, digitalis, amrinone, calcium, delivery of infant, intra-aortic balloon pump.
Myocardial ischemia	Monitor ECG and ST segment, consider blood pressure and cardiac output invasively, control tachycardia: β-adrenergic or calcium channel blocker, vasodilator: nitroglycerin, provide analgesia.
Hypertension	Monitor ECG and ST segment, treat: hydralazine, nitroglycerin, nitroprusside, trimethaphan.
Hypovolemia	Monitor CVP, administer crystalloid, albumin, blood.
Seizures	Ventilate, administer thiopental, or diazepam, intubate to protect airway.
Combative	Monitor cardiovascular and respiratory function, correct as necessary, then sedate.
Fetal Distress	Assess respiratory and cardiovascular function, correct if possible, consider uterine relaxation: amyl nitrate, or magnesium, deliver fetus with another anesthesiologist to assist neonatal care.

malinolenic acid (DGLA) to prostaglandin E_1 (PGE_1) and acutely increases PGE_1. Ethanol also blocks δ-6-desaturase, a necessary component for replenishment of DGLA. Addicts may drink to replenish low PGE_1 levels. Absent PGE_1 causes fibrosis, cardiomyopathy, reproductive failure, gastritis, and pancreatitis. Lithium, diphenylhydantoin, and zinc deficiency, which also produce decreased PGE_1, all produce fetal alcohol syndrome (FAS).[32]

Withdrawal Stages. Tremor, hypertension, anxiety, and tachycardia appear within 6 to 24 hours; prominent autonomic hyperactivity and hallucinations, indicating stage two, follow. Seizures, stage three, are more common in binge drinkers, apparently due to "kindling" caused by repeated withdrawal.[33] Delirium tremens proves life-threatening and necessitates pharmacologic treatment, regardless of the dangers of fetal drug exposure. Phenobarbitol and clonidine are the preferred treatment drugs since benzodiazepines are possible teratogens, paraldehyde causes acidosis, and phenothiazides do not prevent delirium tremens. In humans, the serotonin agonist drugs zymeledine and citalopram act effectively and, in animals, 5-hydroxytryptamine precursors, intracerebral and postsynaptic agonist agents, and uptake inhibitors are effective.[34]

Metabolic Causes of Alcoholic Morbidity. Ethanol dehydrogenase conversion to acetaldehyde represents the rate-limiting step of ethanol metabolism, occurring only if aldehyde dehydrogenase removes acetaldehyde, since the equilibrium reaction leans toward the formation of ethanol. Five genes determine multiple isoenzymes of alcohol dehydrogenase. Racial variations in acetaldehyde dehydrogenase activity are responsible for flushing reactions.[35,36] Excessive liver or muscle acetaldehyde oxidation causes oxygen radical peroxidation of lipid, producing hepatitis, myopathy, cardiomyopathy, and damage to other tissues and membranes.[37]

Pathophysiology

The obstetric anesthesiologist must consider the damaging effects of alcohol abuse on body organs. Table 26–4 outlines the pathophysiology of alcoholism. Myopathy may exacerbate residual neuromuscular blockade or the motor block of regional anesthesia. Muscle cell mem-

Table 26–4. PATHOPHYSIOLOGY OF ALCOHOL

Site	Pathophysiology
CNS	Acute: depression, "partially anesthetized"; chronic: myelopathy, polyneuropathy, Wernike-Korsakoff, cerebellar degeneration, cortical damage, withdrawal seizures
Lungs	Acute: respiratory failure, intrapulmonary shunting, surfactant and macrophage inhibition, aspiration pneumonia; chronic: ventilation-perfusion mismatch, intrapulmonary shunting, chronic infection
Cardiovascular	Acute: myocardial depression, abnormal electrophysiology, arrhythmia, cellular damage; chronic: alcoholic and nutritional myopathy, increased catecholamines, hypertension
Hepatic	Acute: cellular damage, hypoglycemia from inhibition gluconeogenesis, decreased drug metabolism; chronic: fatty infiltration, hepatitis, enzyme induction, cirrhosis, portal hypertension, decreased hepatic blood flow, decreased drug metabolism, protein and coagulation factor synthesis
Gastrointestinal	Gastritis, esophagitis, malabsorption, pancreatitis, bleeding esophageal varices
Nutritional	Dietary deficiencies, malabsorption, vitamin deficiencies
Hematologic	Coagulopathy—multifactorial, platelet, leukocyte, and erythrocyte dysfunction.
Electrolytes	Acute: diuresis with sodium and potassium loss; chronic: antidiuresis with sodium retention, hypokalemia, hypomagnesemia, intracellular calcium derangement
Muscular	Myopathy
Endocrine	Alterations of insulin, cortisone, aldosterone, catecholamines, growth hormone, prolactin, and luteinizing hormone
Ophthalmic	Abnormal zinc and vitamin A reduce dark adaptation.

brane damage or intracellular phosphate deficiency produce acute myopathy accompanied by myoglobinuria. Chronic alcoholic myopathy is associated with selective atrophy of type II muscle fibers.[38] Patients with cardiomyopathy may not tolerate depressant anesthetics. Acutely, ethanol alters cardiac mechanical function and electrophysiologic properties. Chronic consumption produces progressive dysfunction and congestive cardiomyopathy.[39] Pulmonary involvement increases the likelihood of hypoxemia. Alcohol use affects pulmonary vasculature, causing shunting and ventilation-perfusion mismatch. Myelopathy, characterized by progressive spastic paraparesis, may occur with signs of both lateral and dorsal column involvement.[40] Nutritional polyneuropathy occurs commonly. Both myelopathy and polyneuropathy may compound recovery from regional analgesia. Rapid correction of hyponatremia may cause iatrogenic central pontine myelinolysis.[41] Coagulopathy may limit application of regional anesthetics. Ineffective thrombopoiesis and increased platelet destruction produce thrombocytopenia. Qualitative platelet abnormalities include decreased procoagulant-, cyclic AMP-, and MAO activity, a smaller nucleotide storage pool, and decreased release and aggregation. Endocrine abnormalities alter the response to stress and anesthetic agents. Cortisol, aldosterone, prolactin, epinephrine, and norepinephrine secretion increase while growth hormone decreases.[42] Reproductive capacity diminishes in both males and females.

Pregnancy and Ethanol Abuse

Maternal Effects. In pregnant rats, ethanol consumption decreases maternal production of growth hormone.[43] In humans, serum γ-glutamyl transpeptidase correlates with degree of ethanol consumption, and decreases in serum levels of α-fetoprotein and pregnancy-specific β-1-glycoprotein have predictive value for development of FAS.[44,45]

Uteroplacental Effect. Alcohol has no effect on umbilical artery impedance.[46] Ethanol ingestion inhibits placental transport of α-aminobutyric acid.[47] The former fact confirms the absence of a direct effect of ethanol on placental blood flow, whereas the latter implies that alcohol ingestion impairs transfer of nutrients across the placenta. Placental alcohol metabolism resembles hepatic metabolism of alcohol.[48]

Fetal Effect. Maternal consumption of more than 90 ml of absolute alcohol per day produces intrauterine growth retardation and developmental deficits in a dose-dependent fashion. First trimester exposure relates to developmental defects, and third trimester abuse is associated with growth retardation.[49] Although PGE_1 deficiency accounts for fetal morbidity,[32] it fails to explain how paternal exposure also causes growth retardation, decreased cerebral weight, and decreased cerebral incorporation of DNA, RNA, and leucine.[50] In rats, ethanol decreases fetal brain levels of tyrosine, increases levels of serotonin, histamine, 5-hydroxyindoleacetic acid and norepinephrine,[51] and reduces the size of the vermal cerebellum.[52] Ethanol ingestion in the third trimester delays the expected rises in the lecithin/sphingomyelin (L/S) ratio and amniotic levels of PG (phosphatidylglycerol) in humans, probably by damaging fetal alveolar cell membranes or altering phospholipid metabolism.[53]

Neonatal Effect. Acute or chronic fetal ethanol intoxication can depress the newborn. Ethanol withdrawal causes agitation, excess crying, irritability, excess sweating, and seizures beginning within 24 hours. Treatment consists of supportive care supplemented as necessary with phenobarbitol, diazepam, or chlorpromazine.

Fetal Alcohol Syndrome. Antenatal alcohol exposure produces a syndrome consisting of growth deficiency, major and minor anomalies, mental and motor performance derangements, and fetal and perinatal wasteage. The prominent facial anomalies are a drawn appearance, midface hypoplasia, diminished philtrum, and small mandible. At age 1, linear growth and weight gain are 65 and 35 percent of expected values, respectively, despite normal growth hormone levels.[49,54] Variability of occurrence represents an important aspect, with full expression in one or two live births per thousand and partial involvement in three to five per thousand. Since intestinal transport of L-valine is normal in the rat, nutrient absorption deficiency likely does not cause growth deficiency.[55] FAS may be representative of a large group of defects produced by agents capable of inducing placental enzymes or altering neurotransmitter receptors.

Obstetric and Anesthetic Considerations

Obstetrics. Mothers require assistance in curtailing alcohol use. Discontinuing ethanol during the third trimester lessens the effect on Brazelton neonatal assessment scores, but acute withdrawal increases catecholamine levels and probably reduces placental blood flow.[49] Fluctuating ethanol levels seem especially detrimental to the fetus.

Anesthesia for Chronic Ethanol Abusers. The sober alcoholic needs anesthesia tailored to suit her pathophysiology. Narcotic analgesia might exacerbate hypoxia, resulting from ethanol-related increased pulmonary shunting. Liver impairment may alter the rate of narcotic metabolism. Myelopathy and neuropathy may confuse evaluation of neurologic deficit following regional anesthesia, and myopathy increases the incidence of backache. Coagulopathy increases the risk of epidural hematoma. Liver disease can affect local anesthetic metabolism. Metabolism of amide local anesthetics is normal, providing the prothrombin time remains within normal limits. Decreased liver production of cholinesterase prolongs 2-chloroprocaine metabolism.

These considerations also apply to spinal or epidural anesthesia for cesarean section. Here, the mother will generally benefit by remaining conscious during the procedure. Tolerance to CNS depressants increases the likelihood of patient awareness during general anesthesia. However, increasing the dose of barbiturate to assure unconsciousness may cause hypotension and neonatal depression.[56] Ventilation-perfusion mismatch increases the risk of hypoxia during induction or positive-pressure ventilation. Decreased pseudocholinesterase prolongs succinylcholine-induced paralysis. An increased volume of distribution decreases the potency of nondepolarizing muscle relaxants but prolongs the duration of action in the presence of impaired hepatic metabolism. The MAC for inhalational anesthetics increases in chronic alcoholics, but effects on uterine muscle (relaxation) may not change. Enflurane defluorination rises with chronic ethanol ingestion, increasing concern about fluoride toxicity.[26] Peripheral neuropathy may cause hypotension, while hypomagnesemia may produce arrhythmias. Withdrawal induces sympathetic hyperactivity. A recent report indicates that alcoholic hepatitis does not increase anesthetic morbidity for superficial operations.[57]

Anesthesia for Acute Intoxication. Acute intoxication impairs patient co-operation, alters fluid and electrolyte balance, increases gastric acid, and increases general anesthetic potency. Epidural block is safer for the alert and cooperative patient, but ethanol will impair local anesthetic metabolism.[27] Since any degree of sedation increases the risk of hypoventilation and pulmonary aspiration, uncooperative or depressed patients undergoing cesarean section should receive general endotracheal anesthesia with a rapid-sequence approach using cricoid pressure. Even ethanol levels below 100 mg per dl can depress myocardial contractility; reduced doses of etomidate are preferable to sodium pentothal for induction. Glucose administration will prevent maternal reactive hypoglycemia, which often follows acute intoxication. After delivery of the child, anesthetic agents can be titrated as needed. Enflurane defluorination decreases during acute intoxication but increases as serum ethanol levels decrease.[26] Isofluorane interferes least with alcohol metabolism. A member of the anesthesia team should be available to assist in the care of the neonate, since depression appears likely.

BARBITURATES

Pharmacology

Barbiturates depress short synaptic pathways in the central reticular core of the brain stem and block EEG arousal from brain stem stimulation. Most commonly, their abuse relates to potentiation of other drugs or relief of withdrawal symptoms. Metabolic and pharmacodynamic tolerance develop, but the lethal dose remains unaltered, increasing the threat of overdose. Cross-tolerance to ethanol develops. Intoxication resembles ethanol intoxication and irritability, moroseness, and quarrelsomeness commonly occur.

Treatment of Overdose and Withdrawal. Management of overdose entails cardiopulmonary support. Alkalinization of urine or hemodialysis speeds elimination of the agents and, hence, recovery. Hypotension and hypovolemia may require several liters of intravenous fluid and vasopressors for correction.

Withdrawal symptoms for barbiturates resemble those for glutethimide, meprobamate, and methaqualone. Weakness, anxiety, insomnia, tremors, hyperreflexia, muscle twitching, and paroxysmal EEG abnormalities occur initially and progress to seizures, delirium, visual hallucinations, hyperpyrexia, and orthostatic hypotension. Eighty percent of patients convulse. Administration of barbiturates does not immediately reverse withdrawal symptomatology, so substitution therapy, most frequently with pentobarbital or phenobarbital, is necessary throughout pregnancy.

Pregnancy

Uteroplacental and Fetal Effects. Maternal cardiovascular changes may compromise placental perfusion during intoxication or withdrawal. No clear-cut evidence exists of fetal developmental damage in humans, although barbiturates are behavioral teratogens in animals. Barbiturate exposure in early gestation reduces brain weight and changes brain biochemistry and neuromorphology in animals, a situation resembling FAS. Levels of hormones, vitamins, and other biologically active macromolecules diminish due to induction of hepatic metabolizing enzymes.[58]

Neonatal Effects. Fetal hepatic enzyme induction decreases neonatal bilirubin levels. Infants of addicts or epileptics using phenobarbital are passively addicted but not tolerant.[58] Withdrawal symptoms may not surface until as long as a week after birth. Treatment consists of conservative measures and administration of paregoric or phenobarbital. In animals, maternal barbiturate consumption causes long-lasting disturbances in activity, learning performance, sexual behavior, and reproductive function in offspring.[58]

Obstetric and Anesthesia Considerations

Obstetric. Although abstinence remains less critical than with ethanol, health professionals should encourage patients to reduce ingestion, especially in the first trimester. Patients taking barbiturates chronically should continue to do so during pregnancy. Close fetal surveillance becomes necessary.

Anesthesia for Chronic Abuse. Residual levels of drug may increase sensitivity to narcotics. Conduction anesthesia is preferable for labor and cesarean section. Awareness may occur during induction of general anesthesia because of tolerance. However, increasing the dose of thiopental may depress the fetus and endangers the mother, who lacks tolerance to cardiac depressant effects of barbiturates. Chronic barbiturate use does not increase the MAC for inhalation anesthetics.

Anesthesia for Acute Intoxication. Intubation of unconscious patients provides adequate maternal and fetal oxygenation and prevents aspiration of gastric contents. Invasive cardiovascular monitoring with radial and pulmonary arterial catheters guides the physician in assessing fluid requirements and use of vasopressors. Acutely intoxicated patients may be hypotensive and severely hypovolemic. Central venous pressure monitoring will assist administration of adequate intravenous fluids. No sedation should occur initially, but small increments of antihistamine sedatives or phenothiazines may control combative behavior in mild or moderately intoxicated patients. The anesthetist should not attempt conduction anesthesia until the patient becomes stable and reasonably sober. Patients requiring cesarean section should receive general anesthesia. Intubation is accomplished without further maternal cardiovascular or fetal central nervous system depression. The patient's condition may require induction with only 0.1 mg per kg ketamine, or even succinylcholine alone, depending on the suspected degree of myocardial depression. Patients receiving vasopressors should not receive sedation under any circumstances. After delivery, inhalation agents or short-acting narcotic titration follows, as indicated by the reaction to surgical stimuli. Although MAC for inhalation anesthetics does not increase, their cardiovascular depressant effects are potentiated. As with chronic barbiturate abuse, narcotic sensitivity increases in acute intoxication. Once the patient regains full consciousness, extubation may proceed.

SEDATIVES

Sedative use, dependence, and withdrawal resemble barbiturate or alcohol abuse. However, sedatives have fewer cardiovascular depressant effects.

Propanediol Carbamates

Because meprobamate and tybamate are less potent than barbiturates, physicians use them less frequently for sedative purposes. As with barbiturates, meprobamate induces hepatic enzymes, and withdrawal symptoms are similar. Tolerance does not affect the lethal dose. Meprobamate potentiates narcotics and relieves ethanol withdrawal symptoms, but does not represent a good barbiturate substitute. Several studies associate increased risk of fetal malformation with maternal use of meprobamate in the first trimester.[59]

Methaqualone

The most abused agent in the sedative group, methaqualone has antitussive, antihistaminic, and antispasmodic qualities as well as hypnotic, sedative, and anticonvulsant effects. Addicts experience promotion of unreserved interpersonal relationships and aphrodisiac qualities. Like barbiturates, methaqualone induces enzymes, produces tolerance, and potentiates other depressant drugs. Overdosage causes cardiac and respiratory depression, extrapyramidal signs, and convulsions. Barbiturates should not be used to control convulsions. Dialysis remains ineffective.

Antihistamine Sedatives

Methapyriline, pyrilamine, diphenhydramine, and tripelennamine are central depressants, producing central adrenergic stimulation as well as anticholinergic and local anesthetic effects. They have a relatively short duration of action, and tolerance and dependence do not occur. Individuals abuse these drugs to potentiate narcotics and alleviate alcohol withdrawal symptoms.[60] Excessive doses produce central stimulation with excitement, ataxia, hallucinations, convulsions, fixed dilated pupils, and flushed facies. Cardiac depression and respiratory impairment are minimal. Treatment is supportive; thiopental or diazepam provides effective therapy for convulsions. With the exception of the piperazine derivatives, these drugs reportedly have no teratogenicity.

Miscellaneous Sedatives

These drugs also exhibit a high frequency of dependence and include chloral hydrate, paraldehyde, ethchlorvinyl, ethinamate, and piperidinediones (glutethimide, methypyrlon). Glutethimide has prominent anticholinergic effects. Addiction to paraldehyde associates with metabolic acidosis, a reason to avoid its use as an alcohol or narcotic substitute in either mother or neonate.

Obstetric and Anesthetic Considerations

Treatment resembles that for barbiturate addiction and acute intoxication. Management goals are similar regarding anesthetic care. Patients using meprobamate in the first trimester need encouragement to stop use altogether or switch to a less teratogenic drug. Patients abusing antihistamine sedatives do not require anticholinergic drugs.

Agents Acting at Opiate Receptors

NARCOTICS

Pharmacology

Agonist narcotics bind primarily to mu opioid receptor sites and alter CNS sodium channel configuration.[61] Narcotic binding of opiate receptors in the hypothalamus inhibits secretion of luteinizing hormone–releasing hormone and decreases plasma levels of luteinizing hormone (LH) and testosterone.[62] In the same manner, ACTH suppression occurs. Tolerance to opiate receptor agonist agents decreases the duration and intensity of analgesic, euphorigenic, and other CNS depressant effects and increases the lethal dose. Heroin, pentazocine, and methadone constitute the most frequently abused drugs. The known efficacy of buccal administration may increase morphine abuse.[63]

Treatment of Intoxication. Naloxone reverses coma, hypoventilation, and hypotension from narcotic overdose but must be given as a continuous intravenous infusion because of its short duration of action.[64] Nalbuphine seems preferred because of its long half-life, but requires additional investigation.[65] The benzodiazepine antagonist 3-hydroxymethyl-b-carboline (3HMC) reverses narcotic respiratory depression without reversing analgesia; it may become highly utilized in the future.[66]

Treatment of Withdrawal. Table 26–5 lists symptoms of narcotic withdrawal. Addicts may abuse clonidine to alleviate symptoms during self-withdrawal; however, unsupervised use of clonidine may harm the fetus. At present, methadone substitution is the treatment of choice. Narcotics can be withdrawn immediately after substitution begins or after a 6- to 18-month period of stabilization. Investigators[67] are examining the hyperprolactinemic effect of sulpiride as a substituting agent. During the protracted abstinence syndrome, patients become insensitive to respiratory stimulation produced by carbon dioxide, overconcerned about discomfort, unable to tolerate stress, and have a poor self-image.

Pregnancy

Maternal and Uteroplacental Effects. Maternal narcotic usage elevates carbon dioxide and decreases the oxygen content of blood. Passively addicted infants develop respiratory dis-

Table 26–5. NARCOTIC WITHDRAWAL SYMPTOMS OF MOTHER AND NEONATE

Maternal	Neonate
Anxiety	Occasional seizure
Nervousness	Excessive crying
Jittery behavior	Jittery behavior
Tremor	Tremor
Gooseflesh	Irritability
Lacrimation	Hyperactive reflexes
Yawning	Yawning
Rhinorrhea	Sneezing
Sweating	Sweating
Increased respirations	Increased respirations
Hypotension	Alkalosis
Hypertension	Hypocapnia
Tachycardia	Fever
Weakness	Increased stools
Vomiting	Vomiting
Dehydration	Dehydration
Anorexia	Uncoordinated sucking
Weight loss	Increased flexor tone
Depression	Disorganized responses

tress syndrome less frequently. Accelerated differentiation of alveolar epithelium, induced by elevated levels of prolactin in cord serum of addicts, may explain the decreased incidence of respiratory distress syndrome.[68] In heroin addiction, where sympathetic tone may become excessive between doses, the incidence of abruptio placentae approaches 25 percent.[69]

Fetal Effect. Enzyme induction and cardiovascular instability induced by withdrawal may account for some of the adverse effects of opiates on human development. For example, morphine administered during pregnancy causes early maturation of female fetuses and interferes with postnatal physical growth and neurobehavioral development in rats.[70] When given to rats beginning at the time of conception, α-acetyl methadol (LAAM; an agonist similar to methadone) shortens gestation, whereas when given 3 weeks prior to conception, it has no deleterious effect.[71] Doses of LAAM sufficient to increase ethylmorphine N-demethylase levels decrease maternal weight gain and increase fetal mortality.[72] Naloxone administration during gestation increases stillbirth rates and decreases pup size, weight, and postnatal weight gain.[71]

Neonatal Effects. Antenatal exposure to narcotics increases infant morbidity, mainly from prematurity and meconium aspiration. Eighty percent of infants exhibit some of the withdrawal symptoms listed in Table 26–5. These symptoms coincide with a dramatic increase in plasma β-endorphin, β-lipoprotein, and metenkephalin concentrations.[73] The Brazleton Neonatal Behavioral Assessment Scale, Moro score, and/or Neonatal Narcotic Withdrawal Index gauge severity of withdrawal and help to determine the advisability of treatment.[74–76] Although withdrawal symptoms are generally best treated with a specific agonist, in neonates, phenobarbital and paregoric are the pharmacologic agents most commonly employed. In one survey,[76] seven of 62 infants treated with phenobarbital demonstrated seizure activity before 1 month of age, whereas none developed seizures with use of paregoric. Another survey[77] demonstrated a shorter treatment period with phenobarbital, while a third[78] found no difference between the former drugs and proved diazepam alone inadequate. Thus, paregoric most effectively prevents seizures, and phenobarbital best suppresses symptoms. Successful management with clonidine has been reported, but remains investigational.[79]

Neonatal Outcome. Morbidity and mortality during pregnancy are minimal when mothers receive treatment in methadone clinics.[69] Passive neonatal addiction induces tolerance to the influence of endogenous opioids on breathing. Thus, ventilatory response to carbon dioxide diminishes and sudden infant death syndrome appears five to ten times more frequently.[80] Infants of narcotics abusers have low weight at birth but catch up in all parameters but head circumference by 9 months and have normal Bayley scores at age 2.[1] However, an increased incidence of central motor dysfunction persists at 2 to 5 years.[81]

Obstetric and Anesthetic Considerations

Obstetric. Patients should receive substitution therapy at a methadone clinic during pregnancy.[82] Minimizing the methadone dose in the third trimester limits the toxicologic risk to the fetus.[83] Careful surveillance of fetal growth and viability using ultrasonography is advisable.

Anesthesia for Methadone Maintenance. Controlled methadone usage interferes minimally with anesthesia but residual disease from parenteral abuse may persist and influence anesthesia outcome (see Tables 26–2, 26–3). Anesthesia plans should reflect those for other patients with similar medical problems. Narcotics are not contraindicated; conversely, hypotension during general anesthesia may relate to acute withdrawal associated with inadequate narcotic. Intravenous short-acting narcotics such as fentanyl supplement methadone maintenance. Respiratory morbidity from use of epidural or intrathecal narcotics might increase because of concurrent use of parenteral narcotic maintenance therapy. Interestingly, epidural administration of butorphenol produced withdrawal symptoms in one patient.[84]

Anesthesia for Heroin Abuse. Parenteral abusers require isolation precautions for AIDS and hepatitis. Some arrive in labor intoxicated and hypotensive. Others arrive with uterine hyperactivity, which frequently occurs during abstinence. Since hypoxia and hypercarbia generate concern, maternal oxygen saturation monitoring with a pulse oximeter or transcutaneous monitoring of partial pressures of oxygen and carbon dioxide during labor aids evaluation. Naloxone infusions reduce narcosis, and methadone administration controls withdrawal.

The choice of analgesia for labor depends on the patient's pathophysiology. Co-operative patients with normal coagulation and stable neurologic, cardiovascular, and pulmonary function will benefit from epidural blocks. AIDS may contraindicate an indwelling epidural catheter because impaired immunity increases the likelihood of infection resulting from attraction of blood-borne pathogens to the catheter. A single epidural dose of local anesthetic and narcotic combined might more appropriately suit patients with AIDS. Narcotics and sedatives are not contraindicated as long as their titration proceeds carefully, in conjunction with monitoring of oxygen saturation.

The patient's medical problems dictate anesthetic plans for cesarean section (see Tables 26–2 and 26–3). Conduction anesthesia (with epidural or spinal blockade) avoids interaction of opiates with general anesthetics. If using general anesthesia, nalbuphine or naloxone can reverse excess narcotic during recovery. However, administration of antagonists requires careful titration to avoid inducing acute withdrawal.

Anesthesia for Acute Intoxication. The patient may require no further analgesia for labor. Supplemental epidural block avoids further maternal respiratory compromise and fetal depression. Patients with significant depression need stabilization during labor with carefully titrated doses of naloxone or nalbuphine. Narcotic reversal is counterproductive if general anesthesia proves necessary. Induction of general anesthesia in narcotized patients requires less barbiturate.

AGONIST ANTAGONIST ANALGESICS

Pharmacology

Opioid agonist antagonist drugs act primarily as antagonists at mu receptors and as agonist agents at kappa receptors (see Table 26–6). Usually mixed agonist binding at mu receptors reverses endogenous and exogenous agonist agents, while kappa receptor binding produces analgesia without respiratory depression. Drugs acting primarily as kappa receptor agonist agents produce sedation rather than the euphoria characteristic of mu receptor agonist drugs and cause less physical dependency than mu agonists. Naloxone administration reverses mixed agonist drugs (pentazocine, butorphanol, buprenorphine, and nalbuphine). Pentazocine abuse occurs extensively. Withdrawal symptoms are mild and generally do not require substitution of methadone.[60]

Pregnancy

Fetal effects of agonist-antagonist drugs parallel those of opioids (mu agonists). Buprenorphine causes postconception implantation loss and early fetal death in rats as well as extra rib formation in rabbits. Maternal pentacozine and pyribenzamine abuse produce growth retardation and abstinence symptoms in 35 percent of human infants.[60]

Table 26–6. PHYSIOLOGIC EFFECTS AND AGONISTS OF DIFFERENT OPIATE RECEPTORS

Receptor	Physiology	Agonist
Mu	Euphoria, analgesia, respiratory depression, miosis, bradycardia	β-Endorphin, morphine
Kappa	Sedation, analgesia, no respiratory depression, miosis	Dynorphin, bremazocine, ketocyclazocine, ethyl ketazocine
Sigma	Tachycardia, tachypnea, vasomotor stimulation, dysphoria, hallucinations	Phencyclidine, SKF 10047 (N-allylnormetazocine)
Delta	Analgesia, modulates mu receptor	Leu-enkephalin, β-endorphin, dadle (Tyr-DAla-Gly-Phe-DLeu), pentazocine (?), ketamine (?)
Epsilon	?	β-Endorphin

Obstetric and Anesthetic Considerations

Management is comparable to mu agonist management. Pentazocine abusers often use other drugs to potentiate its effects; the anesthesia team should consider the importance of multiple drug use relative to anesthetic drug interactions. Decreased responsiveness to mu agonist drugs induced by mixed agonists decreases the effectiveness of short-acting agents like fentanyl in the peripartum period.

NITROUS OXIDE

Nitrous oxide is a partial mu, kappa, and sigma agonist.[85] Inhibiting enkephalinase can prevent tolerance.[86] In comparison to opiate agonist agents, addiction to nitrous oxide occurs infrequently. Myelopathy is the most prominent complication of chronic nitrous oxide exposure. Nitrous oxide inhibits fetal DNA replication by oxidation of vitamin B_{12}, thereby preventing methionine synthesis. Although administration of large amounts of folinic acid should bypass the block of thiamine synthesis, its efficacy remains uncertain. Some[87] have recommended avoiding nitrous oxide administration during pregnancy; administration prior to term, especially early in gestation, seems inadvisable.

BENZODIAZEPINES

Pharmacology

Benzodiazepines stimulate opiate receptors and depress central parasympathetic and sympathetic outflow by potentiating "GABA-ergic" activity.[61] Substance abusers use these to enhance narcotics or relieve ethanol withdrawal. Pharmacodynamic tolerance develops within 24 hours, but negligible hepatic enzyme induction occurs. These agents produce no severe cardiovascular or respiratory depression. Benzodiazepines depress nocturnal gastric acid excretion. Intoxication produces drowsiness, ataxia, and hostility. Owing to their long half-lives, withdrawal symptoms and seizures occur only with high doses. Additional benzodiazepines, rather than barbiturates, are the best treatment for withdrawal symptoms.[88] Treatment of overdose is mainly supportive. The patient may need tracheal intubation and assisted ventilation to ensure an adequate airway and good maternal oxygenation. Physostigmine partially antagonizes the CNS effects, and some behavioral effects reverse after administration of opiate antagonists such as naloxone.

Pregnancy

Fetal Effects. Benzodiazepines cause teratogenic and embryotoxic effects in animals. Amoxepine in rats and rabbits possesses embryotoxic and fetotoxic activity and decreases postnatal survival. Diazepam reduces the number of pregnancies and surviving offspring, and produces skeletal deformities in rodents. Several human studies[59] indicate an increased risk of congenital malformations, such as cleft palate, with first trimester exposure to chlordiazepoxide or diazepam.

Neonatal Effects. Benzodiazepines increase fetal heart rate, decrease fetal heart rate variability, and induce neonatal hypotonia and hypothermia with maternal administration of as little as 2.5 mg of diazepam. The neonatal half-life of diazepam and its active metabolite, desmethyldiazepam, approaches 4 days (100 hours). Benzodiazepines are established neurobehavioral teratogens in animals.[23] Transient neonatal neurobehavioral changes occur in human infants exposed to diazepam. Neonatal withdrawal occurs. Although bilirubin-albumin uncoupling by the carrier sodium benzoate is negligible with small maternal doses, maternal parenteral abuse might produce kernicterus in the neonate.

Obstetric and Anesthetic Considerations

Benzodiazepine abusers require the same care as barbiturate addicts, with special emphasis on abstinence in the first trimester. Anesthetic plans resemble those of barbiturate abuse, with less concern for cardiovascular depression. Halothane inhibits benzodiazepine metabolism.[29]

PHENOTHIAZINES AND BUTEROPHENONES

Pharmacology

Buterophenones (e.g., droperidol, haldol) have much in common with phenothiazines but produce fewer adrenergic effects. Both inhibit reuptake of norepinephrine and 5-hydroxytryptamine in the cerebral cortex, and both attenuate dopamine activation of adenylate cyclase in the limbic system and caudate nucleus. Mickelson and others[89] attribute antihallucinatory effects to binding on sigma opiate receptors. The agents produce peripheral adrenergic agonist effects and cholinergic and α-adrenergic blocking effects. Minimal hepatic microsomal enzyme induction and physical dependency develop. Noted for antipsychotic and neuroleptic effects, buterophenones also enhance the effects of narcotic and hypnotic agents.

Treatment of Overdose. Coma, seizures, extra pyramidal effects, respiratory depression, hypotension, arrhythmias, and fever occur during overdosage. Treatment consists of management of these symptoms and cardiopulmonary support. Amphetamine, aminophylline, and caffeine reverse CNS depression. Direct-acting α-adrenergic agonists reverse hypotension; beta agonists such as epinephrine may produce paradoxical hypotension by dilating central vessels.

Pregnancy

Phenothiazines appear to have embryocidal, but not teratogenic, activity. Neonatal chlorpromazine kinetic studies describe a two-compartment model with a 35-hour rapid half-life and a 77-hour elimination half-life. In one case report,[90] the infant of a mother treated with chlorpromazine and lithium exhibited severe neurologic depression for 8 days. Phenothiazines increase the development of neonatal jaundice, cause hyporeflexia, or hyperreflexia, and produce extrapyramidal signs in newborns. Long-term neurobehavioral effects have not been documented.

Obstetric and Anesthetic Considerations

Obstetrics. Phenothiazines probably cause less harm than the agents they potentiate. Mothers abusing drugs during pregnancy need no warning about the use of phenothiazines.

Anesthesia. Phenothiazines potentiate CNS depressants, including narcotics, and decrease narcotic requirements during labor. To avoid conditions requiring maternal administration of adrenergic-agonist drugs, the obstetric anesthesiologist must gradually establish the level of anesthesia, or refractory hypotension may accompany conduction block. Mephentermine offers more effective treatment than ephedrine because it possesses more α-agonist activity. Epidural analgesia appears preferable to spinal anesthesia for cesarean section, since hypotension occurs less frequently with the latter. Phenothiazines have local anesthesia-like antiarrhythmic effects, which might interact with bupivacaine to increase the likelihood of myocardial toxicity. Because etomidate causes less cardiovascular depression than sodium pentothal physicians prefer it for induction during periods of hypotension. The patient needs no additional anticholinergic agents since phenothiazines have anticholinergic properties.

Antidepressants

This chapter includes a discussion of antidepressant agents because of their toxicity, anesthetic interactions, and overdose frequency in substance abusers.

TRICYCLIC ANTIDEPRESSANTS

Pharmacology

Tricyclic antidepressants produce anticholinergic effects and decrease blood pressure. They block uptake of norepinephrine and 5-HT by adrenergic nerve terminals in the CNS, but dopamine receptors remain unaffected. Acute overdose causes hyperpyrexia, hypertension, seizures, and coma, all of which are treated with α-adrenergic blocking agents, diazepam, and physostigmine. Tricyclic-induced arrhythmias, except those produced by amitryptyline, respond to propranolol and lidocaine. Those caused by the direct local anesthetic effect of amitriptyline reverse with alkalinization by administration of sodium bicarbonate,[91] or perhaps bretylium.

Pregnancy

Decreased blood pressure, orthostatic hypotension, and arrhythmias can interfere with uteroplacental blood flow. Trimiprimine and imiprimine also have embryotoxic effects producing major congenital anomalies in rats and rabbits. These are best discontinued as soon as possible following conception.

Obstetric and Anesthetic Considerations

Tricyclic antidepressants augment pressor effects of sympathetic amines, decreasing dose requirements of ephedrine. Tricyclics prolong hexobarbitol-induced sleep time, increase sensitivity to anesthetic agents, and sensitize the myocardium to epinephrine. However the mother generally tolerates the usual induction dose of sodium pentothal well. Anticholinergic effects, especially tachycardia, are prominent.

MONOAMINE OXIDASE (MAO) INHIBITORS

Pharmacology

MAO inhibitors elevate mood, inhibit hepatic microsomal enzymes, and increase biogenic amines, especially 5-HT. Overdose produces hyperpyrexia, agitation, hallucination, hyperreflexia, convulsions, hypertension, and hypotension. Conservative management usually shows success.

Pregnancy

Like tricyclic antidepressants, MAO inhibitors lower blood pressure and potentially reduce placental blood flow. Phenylzine reduces mouse litter size and produces growth retardation in dogs and rats. MAO imhibitors are not teratogenic.

Obstetric and Anesthetic Considerations

MAO inhibitors contraindicate meperidine administration due to the possibility of severe malignant hypertension with simultaneous use of the drugs. Mandatory discontinuation for 2 weeks avoids other anesthetic interactions, but anesthetic morbidity does not increase in patients taking MAO inhibitors undergoing emergency procedures.[92] Most recommend only direct alpha agonists for treatment of severe hypotension, as MAO inhibitors markedly potentiate indirect-acting catecholamines. One must give alpha agonists judiciously in pregnant women, due to possible disruptions in uterine blood flow. MAO inhibitors interfere with drug detoxification, thereby potentiating the effect of central depressants and local anesthetics. They also prolong the anticholinergic effect.

LITHIUM

Pharmacology

Lithium, a sodium substitute, slows the sodium pump in excitable membranes 10- to 25-fold. It inhibits activation of adenylate cyclase in the CNS, alters GABA and glutamate concentrations, and modifies hormonal responses. Adenylate cyclase inhibition increases renal excretion of sodium, potassium, water, and 17-hydroxycorticosteroids, leading to inhibition of antidiuretic hormone. Lithium inhibits thyroid iodine release by suppressing thyrotropin activation of adenylate cyclase. It causes sodium retention, increases intravascular volume, and depresses the T wave on ECG. Overdose produces circulatory collapse, bradycardia, coma, and seizures. Treatment includes cardiovascular support, correction of electrolyte imbalance, and acceleration of renal excretion by sodium bicarbonate, aminophylline, or osmotic diuretic administration.

Pregnancy

In pregnancy, a low-salt diet or natriuretics can initiate toxicity by decreasing serum sodium, thereby limiting renal excretion. Lithium alters maternal cellular lithium transport and increases fetal red blood cell choline.[93] An insulin-like effect, probably also related to adenylate cyclase inhibition, depletes fetal liver glycogen. Maternal lithium use causes neonatal goiter, FAS, Ebstein's anomaly, and CNS depression at birth.[32] Lithium has a bimodal excretion curve with a slow phase lasting 10 to 14 days in adults; neonatal elimination should take place over a prolonged period. Workers report severe neurologic depression in a neonate exposed to lithium and chlorpromazine.[90]

Obstetric and Anesthetic Considerations

Obstetric. If possible, discontinue lithium or substitute it with tricyclic antidepressants during pregnancy. If continued lithium administration proves necessary, monitor serum levels frequently and adjust dosage to accommodate changes in total body water and renal excretion. Hypothyroidism may require thyroid replacement. Patients with hyperemesis or transient gastrointestinal disease with vomiting or diarrhea require treatment with intravenous hydration to avoid lithium toxicity caused by decreased renal excretion associated with dehydration and hyponatremia. Mild toxicity responds to hydration and sodium bicarbonate administration. Treatment of hypotension may call for large doses of ephedrine, as lithium depresses the response to norepinephrine. Comatose patients require intubation for airway protection and to insure adequate maternal ventilation. Since lithium is excreted in breast milk, mothers taking lithium should avoid breast feeding.

Anesthetic. Since lithium produces CNS depression, administration of narcotics and sedatives for labor increases maternal and fetal sedation. Hypothyroidism may potentiate sensitivity to CNS depressants. Dehydration associated with diaphoresis or sweating may elevate lithium levels by decreasing excretion. Nausea and vomiting associated with toxicity may mimic labor. Epidural block benefits labor and cesarean section; however, intravenous isotonic fluid administration for prevention of hypotension can increase lithium excretion. Because treatment of hypotension may require large doses of ephedrine, epidural block is preferable to spinal anesthesia for cesarean section. Sensitivity to general anesthetics increases, and one should consider making necessary adjustments in anesthetic doses, as response to vasopressors is sluggish, especially in the hypothyroid patient. Etomidate will produce less hypotension on induction of general anesthesia than thiopental. Potential interaction with neuromuscular blockers, specifically succinylcholine and pancuronium, appears not to be a clinical problem, although neuromuscular blockade requires careful monitoring.

Hallucinogens

MARIJUANA

Pharmacology

Marijuana affects acetylcholine turnover in the CNS by a GABA-ergic mechanism,[94] producing sleepiness, ataxia, and decreased motor and cognitive ability. Marijuana interferes with secretion of luteinizing hormone, follicle-stimulating hormone, and prolactin, and produces oligospermia. A β-adrenergic agonist, marijuana increases heart rate, myocardial work load, plasma volume, and postural hypotension. Propranolol blocks its peripheral effects. The serum half-life of marijuana extends for days. Tolerance develops to some behavioral effects and, as with opiates, the lethal dose increases. No cross-tolerance develops with hallucinogens, but some exists to ethanol.

Marijuana abuse improves self-perception and produces euphoria, relaxation, and temporal disintegration. Higher doses may trigger paranoid feelings, delusions, and hallucinations.[94] Mild sympathomimetic effects accompanying intoxication call for conservative treatment. Diazepam is preferable for sedation, since chlorpromazine potentiates postural hypotension and barbiturates potentiate hallucinations. No recognized withdrawal syndrome occurs, but irritability, restlessness, insomnia, and nervousness accompany discontinuation.

Pregnancy

Marijuana reduces maternal weight gain and food and water consumption in rats. Neonatal birth weight and weight at 21 days decreases, while postnatal mortality increases.[95] Maternal and paternal exposure in animals affect developmental and reproductive functions of offspring.[94] In humans, marijuana dose-dependently reduces gestation time,[96] and is linked with a higher incidence of meconium staining and shorter height at age 8 months.[97,98] Marijuana and/or tobacco affects visual processing in the human infant.[99]

Obstetric and Anesthetic Considerations

Anesthesia for Chronic Abuse. Because unintoxicated marijuana users have chronic bronchitis and bronchoconstriction, they require the same anesthetic care as cigarette smokers. Regional rather than general anesthesia is best for cesarean section. As with asthmatics, avoid anesthetics that cause bronchoconstriction, if possible.

Anesthesia for Acute Intoxication. Tachycardias up to 140 beats per minute, resulting from sympathomimetic effects, occur commonly. Patients may already have sufficient analgesia for vaginal delivery when severely intoxicated. With epidural block, use of mephentermine rather than ephedrine to reduce hypotension may avoid further tachycardia. If the patient needs general anesthesia, keep in mind her greater sensitivity to sodium pentothal and halothane; marijuana reduces MAC for all general anesthetics. For asthmatics, etomidate is the preferred induction agent, since it does not produce bronchoconstriction and does not increase fetal depression. Pre-existing dry mouth and tachycardia negate the need for anticholinergics. Marijuana-induced microsomal dechlorinase increases halothane metabolism.[100]

INHALANTS

Chemical fumes cause excitation, euphoria, and hallucinations[4] (Table 26–7). Usually children having no other available substances abuse them, but their use is increasing.[2] Tolerance can develop. Complications of inhalants include stupor, coma, convulsions, and hepatic and renal failure. Death from pulmonary edema or cardiac arrythmia can occur acutely during inhalation. Choice of anesthesia primarily depends upon renal and hepatic function. Although epidural analgesia promotes hepatic and renal blood flow better than general anesthesia, patients with severe hepatic or renal failure require general anesthesia for cesarean section. Coagulopathy accompanies severe hepatic and renal failure, and intravenous administration of large amounts of crystalloid may provoke pulmonary edema in patients with renal failure. General anesthesia, necessary in the stuporous patient, protects the airway and facilitates oxygenation and ventilation.

Table 26–7. COMMONLY USED INHALANTS

Acetone	Toluene
Aliphatic acetates	Alcohols
Benzene	Carbon tetrachloride
Trichloroethane	Trichloroethylene
Ethyl ether	Vinyl ether
Xylene	Freon-12

CYCLOHEXYLAMINES (PHENCYCLIDINE)

Pharmacology

Phencyclidine (PCP) is a potent psychomimetic agent capable of producing a state indistinguishable from schizophrenia. The compound binds to a low-affinity sigma opiate receptor site,[89,101–103] and chlorthiazine and haloperidol may directly antagonize it. Like ketamine, its autonomic side effects include hypertension, tachycardia, diaphoresis, nausea, and hyperthermia; but unlike ketamine, PCP also causes seizures.[104] PCP users usually smoke it together with tobacco or marijuana. Slurred speech, ataxia, clonus, and tremors accompany intoxication. Severe psychotic reactions appear more often in naive users.

Pregnancy

Investigators[105] report PCP detection in breast milk, amniotic fluid, and neonatal urine in the first few days of life. Neonatal symptoms include jitteriness, hypotonicity, vomiting, and diarrhea unrelieved by phenobarbital. In a clinical report,[106] microcephaly occurred in one of two exposed infants. Abnormal ventilation during sleep and neurobehavior occur at birth, but Bayley scores at age two appear normal.[1,78,107]

Obstetric and Anesthetic Effects

Obstetric. Pregnant women should be encouraged to abstain from use of PCP to avoid behavioral teratogenicity.

Anesthesia for Chronic Abuse. These users receive the same anesthesia as normal patients, except that sedation with chlorthiazine may produce hypotension and bradycardia. Psychosis can recur during emergence from anesthesia.

Anesthesia for Acute Intoxication. Hyperthermia-induced PCP intoxication increases both maternal and fetal oxygen consumption, and may compromise fetal well being. Customary antipyretic medications control this condition during labor, and a cooling blanket is useful during general anesthesia. Acute intoxication with PCP potentiates narcotics and sympathomimetic agents. Narcotic analgesic administration during labor necessitates pulse oximetry, as for narcotic addiction. Reduced doses of ephedrine treat hypotension during spinal or epidural anesthesia. Hallucinating patients require general anesthesia. Induction of general anesthesia with sodium pentothal best depresses a more severe hypertensive response to intubation during PCP intoxication. Phencyclidine inhibits pseudocholinesterase; cautious administration of succinylcholine using a neuromuscular block monitor will avoid prolonged neuromuscular blockade produced by depressed succinylcholine metabolism.

OTHER HALLUCINOGENS

The drugs discussed here are of two sorts: (1) indolalkylamines (lysergic acid diethylamide, LSD; psilocybin; and psilocin) and (2) phenylethylamines (mescaline; nutmeg; and 2,5-dimethoxy-4-methylamphetamine, STP).

Pharmacology

The most potent of these agents, LSD, reduces central 5-hydroxytryptamine turnover and induces or compels states of altered perception, thought, or feeling. Metabolized by hepatic microsomes, it has a half-life of 175 minutes, but effects last for 12 hours. Agents are cross-tolerant among themselves. LSD produces sympathomimetic and analgesic effects as well as muscle weakness, decreased creatinine clearance, and possible chromosomal damage. Lethal overdoses in humans rarely occur; animals die of respiratory failure and hyperthermia. Barbiturates or diazepam counteracts psychosis. STP produces euphoria and enhanced self-awareness without perceptual distortion or hallucinations. One should avoid sedation with chlorpromazine, as it may potentiate hallucinations and can be lethal. Repeated doses of STP cause CNS toxicity.[100]

Pregnancy

In animals, LSD causes abortions, deformities, and stillbirths, while in humans it increases the rate of abortions and congenital anomalies. American Indians with long histories of mescaline abuse experience no adverse fetal effects.

Obstetric and Anesthetic Considerations

Anesthesia for Chronic Abuse. Anesthesia generally resembles that for normal patients. The ability of these hallucinogens (in residual amounts) to potentiate narcotics and sympathomimetic agents necessitates administering anesthetics in small, titrated doses. Chronic use of phenylethylamine hallucinogens, like amphetamine, decreases MAC for general inhalational anesthetics. Psychosis can recur postoperatively.

Anesthesia for Acute Intoxication. LSD decreases plasma cholinesterase and may increase the duration of action of 2-chloroprocaine and succinylcholine. The prominence of hyperthermic and anticholinergic effects contraindicates administration of anticholinergic agents. Careful monitoring of body temperature with use of a cooling blanket may control hyperthermia. Although the transient curare-like effects of mescaline in dogs has not been reported in humans, smaller doses of nondepolarizing agents and use of a peripheral nerve stimulator to monitor neuromuscular blockade are advisable.

Stimulants

COCAINE

Pharmacology

Cocaine inhibits reuptake of norepinephrine at nerve endings. In addition to producing analgesia and local anesthesia, cocaine accelerates and desynchronizes the EEG and increases blood pressure, respiration, and uterine tone. Chronic intranasal or parenteral use produces serious consequences including seizures, depression, and paranoia.[109] Cocaine-induced coronary artery spasm causes focal endothelial injury and platelet aggregation, resulting in acute vascular platelet thrombosis and chronic intimal proliferation with myocardial infarction.[110–112] Pseudomembraneous colitis and cerebrovascular accidents can occur at a young age.[113]

Treatment of Intoxication, Overdose, and Addiction. Victims die from seizures and respiratory failure but may appear to have sustained a myocardial infarction. Table 26–8 lists symptoms of cocaine toxicity. Beta-adrenergic blocking agents control tachycardia. Unopposed α-adrenergic stimulation can develop, produce hypertension, and require treatment with nitroprusside.[114] Psychosis responds to neuroleptics or lithium, although the former does not reduce euphoria.[115] Cocaine's rewarding effects hypothetically result from acute activation of dopamine pathways and its addicting effects, from dopamine depletion. Thus administration of dopamine agonist drugs prevents cocaine craving.[116,117]

Pregnancy

Uteroplacental Effect. Cocaine increases norepinephrine levels, decreases uterine blood flow, and increases uterine contractility. Abruptio placentae and labor can occur immediately following self-administration of intravenous cocaine.[118] In pregnant sheep, doses of intravenous cocaine producing serum levels comparable to those in humans increased maternal blood pressure 32 to 37 percent and fetal blood pressure 12 percent. Uterine blood flow decreases 36 to 42 percent for 15 minutes, and maternal norepinephrine levels increase 210 percent.[119]

Fetal and Neonatal Effects. Increased pregnancy resorption, reduced maternal and fetal weight, eye defects, skeletal defects, cryptorchidism, and hydronephrosis emerge with intraperitoneal injection of cocaine into pregnant animals.[120,121] In humans, cocaine abuse increases the frequency of spontaneous abortions; patient-reported abortion rates approximate 36 to 46 percent.[118] Intravenous cocaine also induces perinatal cerebral infarction.[122] In a study of pregnancy outcome, Chasnoff and coworkers[118] note sudden infant death syndrome (SIDS) in one infant and prune belly syndrome (a defect related to genitourinary development at 5 weeks') in another whose mother abused cocaine at 5 weeks' gestation. Additionally, Brazelton assessments reveal significant depression of interactive behavior and poor organizational response to environmental stimuli.[118]

Obstetric and Anesthetic Considerations

Obstetrics. Health workers should advise cocaine abusers that cocaine endangers the life and development of the fetus, and that its use should be curtailed.

Anesthesia for Chronic Abuse. Patients require thorough evaluation for evidence of coronary artery disease, including ECG and possibly cardiac enzyme evaluation as well as echocardiography. In addition to the usual monitoring, ECG leads II and V, ST segment trends, and possibly transesophageal echocardiography can detect ischemia. The abuser's catecholamine depletion and sluggish response to ephedrine dictate performing an epidural block using gradual extension to avoid hypotension, rather than

Table 26–8. SIGNS OF COCAINE TOXICITY

CNS	Psychological	Cardiovascular	Miscellaneous
Delirium	Irritability	Arrhythmia	Fever
Convulsions	Restlessness	Pallor	Diaphoresis
Hyperreflexia	Tenseness	Tachycardia	
Tremor	Anxiety	Hypertension	Dry mouth
Dizziness	Garrulousness	Angina	
Hallucinations	Euphoria	Headache	Dilated pupils
Coma	Insomnia	Flushing	
	Panic		
Cerebral hemorrhage	Suicidal or homicidal ideation	Circulatory collapse	

instituting spinal anesthesia for cesarean section. Cocaine abusers display increased sensitivity to CNS depressants and decreased MAC. Etomidate produces less hypotension than thiopental during induction of general anesthesia. Measures appropriate for patients with identified coronary artery disease include use of nitroglycerine and β-adrenergic or calcium channel blockers, to control heart rate and prevent vasospasm, and avoidance of ketamine and nitrous oxide.

Anesthesia for Acute Toxicity. Since cocaine increases uterine contractility, labor occurs frequently in intoxicated addicts. The patient may require little anesthesia, since cocaine produces systemic analgesia. Even though neuroleptic agents such as droperidol or haldol depress the fetus, the patient may need them to control psychotic behavior. Epidural analgesia during labor will reverse vasoconstriction-associated reductions of uterine blood flow and will prevent further decreases associated with pain. Local anesthetics may potentiate the toxicity of cocaine, which itself is a local anesthetic ester primarily metabolized by the liver. Since plasma cholinesterase does not significantly metabolize cocaine, 2-chloroprocaine is a good choice for cesarean section. Spinal anesthesia minimizes the risk of local anesthetic toxicity. However, depletion of intravascular volume and uncertain response to sympathomimetic agents because of catecholamine depletion increase the risk of hypotension with spinal anesthesia. In addition to the monitoring recommended for chronic cocaine abuse, central venous pressure monitoring facilitates correction of intravascular volume deficits.

Most cases of abruptio placentae call for general anesthesia. The presence of cocaine during general anesthesia can precipitate myocardial infarction (according to isolated case reports) or can be relatively benign (in reports of mean blood pressure response).[123–125] With severe cocaine toxicity, maternal blood volume and pressure control — via fluid, propranalol, and/or sodium nitroprusside — must precede anesthesia. Thiopental induction limits catecholamine release in response to tracheal intubation, but etomidate is safer with hypovolemia. In the presence of acute cocaine toxicity, patients should not receive agents that either potentiate catecholamines (ketamine) or sensitize the myocardium (halothane); such substances will exacerbate cocaine toxicity.

Narcotics and nitrous oxide complicate anesthesia maintenance in amphetamine abusers, due to the sympathomimetic effects of nitrous oxide, which potentiate the ability of amphetamines to increase MAC.[126] Since amphetamine increases catecholamine response in a manner similar to that of cocaine one can expect nitrous oxide to complicate maintenance of anesthesia during cocaine toxicity. Additionally, patients with impaired coronary arterial flow should not receive nitrous oxide. If ECG signs of myocardial ischemia appear, the measures indicated in the discussion of chronic cocaine abuse may be necessary. Neuroleptic agents such as droperidol or thorazine facilitate maintenance of post-delivery anesthesia, since they possess both sedative and α-adrenergic blocking effects and do not influence uterine contractility.

AMPHETAMINES

Pharmacology

Amphetamines stimulate release and inhibit reuptake of catecholamines peripherally and centrally, resulting in increased blood pressure, respirations, and uterine tone, and decreased appetite. Methamphetamine produces more CNS and fewer cardiovascular effects than amphetamine. Tolerance to amphetamine develops only to central and not to cardiovascular effects. Abuse results from mood elevation and fatigue reduction. Weight loss, bruxism, face picking, suspiciousness, stereotyped repetitious or disorganized behavior, and paranoid schizophrenia characterize chronic abuse. Psychotic symptoms appear slower than with cocaine, possibly because amphetamine metabolites contribute to psychosis development. Users take increasing doses until aberrant behavior prevents them from obtaining additional drug. Within a few hours of cessation, they sleep for 12 to 18 hours, awakening hungry and depressed. Depression causes a new "run." Narcotics delay the "crash."

Treatment of Overdose. Overdose produces severe chest pain, toxic paranoid syndrome, seizures, unconsciousness, and death from respiratory failure. Toxic symptoms resemble those for cocaine and call for similar treatment.

Ammonium chloride urine acidification accelerates excretion.

Pregnancy

Acute amphetamine administration in rats and monkeys disrupts normal parental care behavior patterns.[127] Congenital anomalies accompany amphetamine abuse in animals. The human infant is small for gestational age. Amphetamine abusers deliver prematurely in 25 percent of cases, and their neonates have a perinatal mortality rate of 7.5 percent.[128] Neonatal withdrawal produces excessive drowsiness and occasional seizures.

Obstetric and Anesthetic Considerations

Obstetric. As with cocaine, mothers should abstain from amphetamines during pregnancy. Known users require close surveillance of fetal growth and placental function with ultrasonography and nonstress or biophysical profile monitoring during gestation.

Anesthesia for Chronic Abuse. Amphetamine abusers respond poorly to indirect-acting sympathomimetic agents, increasing the hazards of hypotension during conduction anesthesia. The dose requirements (ED50) for intravenous and inhalation agents decreases. With general anesthesia, etomidate causes less cardiovascular depression than sodium pentothal.

Anesthesia for Acute Intoxication. The comatose patient requires intubation for airway protection and assisted ventilation for respiratory failure. Preoperatively, neuroleptics or barbiturates stabilize paranoid patients. As with cocaine, patients benefit from careful monitoring for evidence of myocardial ischemia, although coronary artery disease appears less often with amphetamine abuse. The hypovolemic patient should undergo CVP monitoring. Whereas cocaine levels invariably decrease, continued absorption of oral amphetamine may increase its toxicity during labor. Epidural analgesia maintains or improves uterine blood flow. Anesthetists prefer epidural to spinal block since vasoconstriction and volume depletion occur in these patients. As with cocaine, the ED50 for general anesthetics increases, and amphetamine sensitizes the myocardium to catecholamines. Thiopental induction attenuates the hypertensive response to intubation, but etomidate is safer during hypovolemia. Some workers[126] report difficulty maintaining anesthesia with nitrous oxide and fentanyl.

TOBACCO

Pharmacology

Nicotine, the active agent in tobacco, stimulates the CNS and autonomic ganglia, triggering release of epinephrine from the adrenal medulla. In large doses, it produces ganglionic blockade. Tolerance develops to some of its effects. Withdrawal symptoms, including irritability, aggressiveness, hostility, depression, and concentration difficulties result from environmental conditioning rather than from pharmacologic dependence.

Pregnancy

Maternal and Uteroplacental Effects. Smoking alters the hypothalamic-pituitary axis, inhibiting release of LH and prolactin and decreasing fertility and gestational length. Growth retardation and neonatal mortality increase.[129] Nicotine and cotinine appear in amniotic fluid, fetal serum, and placental tissues throughout pregnancy, with fetal nicotine levels exceeding maternal.[130] Nicotine increases umbilical and fetal aortic flow.[131] Microscopically, placentas of heavy smokers exhibit atrophic hypovascular villi. Dehydroepiandrosterone sulfate (DHA-S) loading tests reveal reduced conversion to estradiol, indicating that placental impairment from nicotine-induced vasoconstriction produces growth retardation.[132] Nicotine also decreases placental uptake of α-aminobutyric acid.[47]

Fetal and Neonatal Effects. In rats, nicotine retards embryo cell cleavage, reducing cell numbers.[133] Maternal smoking suppresses postnatal DNA synthesis, especially in the cerebellum, provoking developmental abnormalities in rats.[134] A study[135] of audiogenic seizures in newborn mice indicates that CNS development lags with nicotine exposure. In humans at term, fetal heart rate increases and variability decreases.[136] Nicotine affects visual processing in human infants antenatally exposed to marijuana and tobacco.[99]

Obstetric and Anesthetic Considerations

Obstetric. Patients should stop smoking during pregnancy. Even in late gestation some benefits occur from discontinuation since nicotine and carbon monoxide elimination span only a 12- to 24-hour period.[137] Thus, oxygen transport to the placenta should improve.

Anesthesia. Smoking on the day of surgery increases gastric volume and increases risk for aspiration.[138] Smoking produces chronic bronchitis, elevates carbon monoxide levels, and increases the likelihood of hypoxia during intubation and bronchospasm thereafter. Regional anesthesia avoids airway difficulties.

Polydrug Abuse

PHARMACOLOGY

Few substance abusers use a single agent. The baseline pattern of tobacco, ethanol, and marijuana persists as the abuser advances to more potent drugs. Ten percent of ethanol abusing clinic patients screen positive for other drugs.[139] Easily obtained CNS depressants reduce the need for expensive narcotics; thus, screening patients at a methadone clinic uncovered heroin, cocaine, benzodiazepine, tricyclic antidepressant, and PCP use.[140] Combinations of agents may potentiate effects of individual substances. For example, barbiturates and amphetamine together produce more euphoria than either drug alone. Amphetamine prolongs and potentiates LSD. Also, combinations may avoid undesirable side effects: narcotics or depressants moderate cocaine's sympathetic effect. Depressants hide withdrawal symptoms when abuse becomes socially unacceptable; thus, weekend binge drinkers get through the week on benzodiazepines. In many cases, polydrug abuse continues throughout pregnancy.[1,78,80]

PREGNANCY

Both nicotine and alcohol inhibit placental α-aminobutyric acid transport, and their effects are additive, indicating that fetal growth retardation caused by these substances may be additive.[47] Passively addicted infants with abstinence symptoms have increased weight loss and regain their birth weight later than expected.[24] Overnight pneumograms show abnormalities in neonates with polydrug exposure.[80] Infants exposed to mixed nonnarcotic drugs demonstrate irritability and deficits in state control at birth but possess no difference in Bayley scores at 2 years.[1,141] Motor dysfunction persists at 2- to 5-year follow-up examinations.[81]

Obstetric and Anesthesia Considerations

The "safety" of single versus polydrug abuse is not established. Total fetal drug exposure should be minimized.

The predominant drug determines anesthesia, but plans may need modification to accommodate the potential interactions with a second substance. Unless withdrawal begins, longer intervals between ingestion and anesthesia result in less complications. Pulse oximetry or transcutaneous blood gas monitoring detects unexpected respiratory depression during labor. Monitoring CVP assists in differentiating drug-induced and hypovolemic tachycardia. Spinal anesthesia for cesarean section avoids potential drug interactions, but has value only in the absence of dehydration and in the presence of unaffected responses to sympathetic agonist agents. Anesthetics administered in small doses and titrated to effect avoid severe reactions.

Summary

Multiple drug abuse during pregnancy, not uncommon, emanates from progressive behavioral reinforcement and pharmacologic tolerance and dependence. Maternal health, fertility, prenatal care, placental function, fetal development, neonatal morbidity, and child behavior all undergo adverse affects from drug abuse. Metabolic and pharmacologic drug interactions and altered maternal physiology affect anesthesia. Ethanol produces multisystem maternal pathophysiology, cross-tolerance with general anesthetics, and FAS. Barbiturates are behavioral teratogens in animals. Tolerance to CNS, but not circulatory, depressant effects complicates anesthesia in barbiturate abusers. Narcotics produce abortion and premature birth unless the patient receives stable concentrations of methadone.

Narcotic reversal agents facilitate anesthesia. Benzodiazepines, established behavioral teratogens in animals, are also associated with congenital anomalies in humans. They help control hallucinogenic psychosis and withdrawal symptoms, but prolonged fetal depression limits their use for anesthesia. The interaction of phenothiazines, tricyclic antidepressants, and MAO inhibitors with sympathetic amines increases the risk of conduction blocks. Lithium use should discontinue during pregnancy. Marijuana, PCP, and LSD, behavioral teratogens in animals, alter neonatal neurobehavior in humans. Collectively, they possess sympathomimetic properties and potentiate general anesthetic CNS depression. Cocaine and amphetamine cause abortion, abruptio placentae, and acute neurobehavioral abnormalities. Anesthesia is complicated acutely by severe central sympathetic stimulation and chronically by depletion of catecholamines. In addicts, collectively, the choice and technique of anesthesia for vaginal delivery and cesarean section depends upon the degree of intoxication and the possible anesthetic interaction involved with each agent.

References

1. Chasnoff, IJ, et al: Prenatal drug exposure: Effects on neonatal and infant growth and development. Neurobehav Toxicol Teratol 8:357, 1986.
2. University of Michigan Institute for Social Research 1986 Survey. *The Philadelphia Inquirer*. Feb 24, 1987, p B1.
3. Kulberg, A: Substance abuse: Clinical identification and management. Pediatr Clin North Am 33:325, 1986.
4. Remington, G and Hoffman, BF: Gas sniffing as a form of substance abuse. Can J Psychiatry 29:31, 1984.
5. Semlitz, L and Gold, MS: Adolescent drug abuse. Diagnosis, treatment, and prevention. Psychiatr Clin North Am 9:455, 1986.
6. Yamaguchi, K and Kandel, DB: Patterns of drug use from adolescence to young adulthood. III: Predictors of progression. Am J Public Health 74:673, 1984.
7. Little, RE, et al: Agreement between laboratory tests and self-reports of alcohol, tobacco, caffeine, marijuana and other drug use in post-partum women. Soc Sci Med 22:91, 1986.
8. Keeley, KA and Solomon, J: New perspectives on the similarities and differences of alcoholism and drug abuse. Curr Alcohol 8:99, 1981.
9. Adler, MW and Geller, EB: Contributions of neuropharmacology to understanding mechanisms of tolerance and dependence. Natl Inst Drug Abuse Res Monogr Ser 54:27, 1984.
10. Kreek, MJ: Opioid interactions with alcohol. Adv Alcohol Subst Abuse 3:35, 1984.
11. Goldstein, DS, et al: Bullous pulmonary damage in users of intravenous drugs. Chest 89:266, 1986.
12. Sapico, FL and Montgomerie, JZ: Vertebral osteomyelitis in intravenous drug abusers: Report of three cases and review of the literature. Rev Infect Dis 2:196, 1980.
13. Maayan, S, et al: Acquired immunodeficiency syndrome (AIDS) in an economically disadvantaged population. Arch Intern Med 145:1607, 1985.
14. Condon, JT: The spectrum of fetal abuse in pregnant women. J Nerv Ment Dis 174:509, 1986.
15. Marsh, JC and Miller, NA: Female clients in substance abuse treatment. Int J Addict 20:995, 1985.
16. Mucklow, JC: The fate of drugs in pregnancy. Clin Obstet Gynaecol 13:161, 1986.
17. Pelkonen, O and Moilanen, ML: The specificity and multiplicity of human placental xenobiotic-metabolizing monooxygenase system studied by potential substrates, inhibitors and gel electrophoresis. Med Biol 57:306, 1979.
18. Gottlieb, K and Manchester, DK: Twin study methodology and variability in xenobiotic placental metabolism. Teratogenesis Carcinog Mutagen 6:253, 1986.
19. Lucier, GW, Lui, EM and Lamartiniere, CA: Metabolic activation/deactivation reactions during perinatal development. Environ Health Perspect 29:7, 1979.
20. Committee on Drugs of the American Academy of Pediatrics: Neonatal drug withdrawal. Pediatrics 72:895, 1983.
21. Perry, BD, et al: Prenatal exposure to drugs of abuse in humans: Effects on placental neurotransmitter receptors. Neurobehav Toxicol Teratol 6:295, 1984.
22. Ericksson, M, Larsson, G and Zetterstrom, R: Abuse of alcohol, drugs and tobacco during pregnancy: Consequences for the child. Paediatrician 8:228, 1979.
23. Martin, JC: Irreversible changes in mature and aging animals following intrauterine drug exposure. Neurobehav Toxicol Teratol 8:335, 1986.
24. Weinberger, SM, et al: Early weight-change patterns in neonatal abstinence. Am J Dis Child 140:829, 1986.
25. Rubinstein, A, et al: Acquired immunodeficiency with reversed T4/T8 ratios in infants born to promiscuous and drug-addicted mothers. JAMA 249:2350, 1983.
26. Pantuck, EJ, et al: Inhibition and stimulation of enflurane metabolism in the rat following a single dose or chronic administration of ethanol. Anesthesiology 62:255, 1985.
27. Reilly, CS, et al: The effect of halothane on drug disposition: Contribution of changes in intrinsic drug metabolizing capacity and hepatic blood flow. Anesthesiology 63:70, 1985.
28. Loft, S: Increased hepatic microsomal enzyme activity after surgery under halothane or spinal anesthesia. Anesthesiology 62:11, 1985.
29. Bell, LE, Slattery, JT and Calkins, DF: Effect of halothane-oxygen anesthesia on the pharmacoki-

netics of diazepam and its metabolites in mice. J Pharmacol Exp Ther 233:94, 1985.

30. Silver, H, et al: Addiction in pregnancy: High risk intrapartum management and outcome. Society for Obstetric Anesthesia and Perinatology, Abstracts of Scientific Papers. Salt Lake City, 1986, p 57.
31. Erwin, VG and McClearn, GE: Genetic influences on alcohol consumption and actions of alcohol. Curr Alcohol 8:405, 1981.
32. Horrobin, DF: A biochemical basis for alcoholism and alcohol-induced damage including the fetal alcohol syndrome and cirrhosis: Interference with essential fatty acid and prostaglandin metabolism. Med Hypotheses 6:929, 1980.
33. Pinel, JP: Alcohol withdrawal seizures: Implications of kindling. Pharmacol Biochem Behav 13(Suppl)1:225, 1980.
34. Naranjo, CA, Sellers, EM and Lawrin, MO: Modulation of ethanol intake by serotonin uptake inhibitors. J Clin Psychiatry 47(Suppl)1:16, 1986.
35. Li, TK and Bosron, WF: Genetic variability of enzymes of alcohol metabolism in human beings. Ann Emerg Med 15:997, 1986.
36. Chan, AW: Racial differences in alcohol sensitivity. Alcohol Alcohol 21:93, 1986.
37. Garcia-Bunuel, L: Lipid peroxidation in alcoholic myopathy and cardiomyopathy. Med Hypotheses 13:217, 1984.
38. Martin, F and Peters, TJ: Alcoholic muscle disease. Alcohol Alcohol 20:125, 1985.
39. Segel, LD, et al: Alcohol and the heart. Med Clin North Am 68:147, 1984.
40. Sage, JI, Van Uitert, RL and Lepore, FE: Alcoholic myelopathy without substantial liver disease: A syndrome of progressive dorsal and lateral column dysfunction. Arch Neurol 41:999, 1984.
41. Nakada, T and Knight, RT: Alcohol and the central nervous system. Med Clin North Am 68:121,1984.
42. Ylikahri, RH, Huttunen, MO and Harkonen, M: Hormonal changes during alcohol intoxication and withdrawal. Pharmacol Biochem Behav 13(Suppl)1:131, 1980.
43. Lee, M and Wakabayashi, K: Pituitary and thyroid hormones in pregnant alcohol-fed rats and their fetuses. Alcoholism (NY) 10:428, 1986.
44. Reyes, E: The role of gamma-glutamyl transpeptidase in alcoholism. Neurobehav Toxicol Teratol 7:171, 1985.
45. Halmesmaki, E, et al: Alpha-fetoprotein, human placental lactogen, and pregnancy-specific beta 1-glycoprotein in pregnant women who drink: Relation to fetal alcohol syndrome. Am J Obstet Gynecol 155:598, 1986.
46. Erskine, RL and Ritchie, JW: The effect of maternal consumption of alcohol on human umbilical artery blood flow. Am J Obstet Gynecol 154:318, 1986.
47. Fisher, SE, Atkinson, M and Van Thiel, DH: Selective fetal malnutrition: The effect of nicotine, ethanol, and acetaldehyde upon in vitro uptake of alpha-aminoisobutyric acid by human term placental villous slices. Dev Pharmacol Ther 7:229, 1984.
48. Rice, PA, et al: The effect of ethanol on the production of lactate, triglycerides, phospholipids, and free fatty acids in the perfused human placenta. Am J Obstet Gynecol 155:207, 1986.
49. Smith, IE, et al: The effect of volume and duration of prenatal ethanol exposure on neonatal physical and behavioral development. Neurobehav Toxicol Teratol 8:375, 1986.
50. Tanaka, H, Suzuki, N and Arima, M: Experimental studies on the influence of male alcoholism on fetal development. Brain Dev 4:1, 1982.
51. Mena, MA, Martin del Rio, R and Herrera, E: The effect of long-term ethanol maternal ingestion and withdrawal on brain regional monoamine and amino acid precursors in 15-day-old rats. Gen Pharmacol 15:151, 1984.
52. Nathaniel, EJ, et al: Prenatal ethanol exposure and cerebellar development in rats. Exp Neurol 93:601, 1986.
53. Halvorsen, PR, Gross, TL and Sokol, RJ: The effect of heavy maternal alcohol intake on amniotic fluid phospholipids in late pregnancy. Am J Perinatol 2:173, 1985.
54. Sokol, RJ: Alcohol and abnormal outcomes of pregnancy. Can Med Assoc J 125:143, 1981.
55. Ghishan, FK, Henderson, G and Meneely, R: Intestinal function in infant rats: Effect of maternal chronic ethanol ingestion. J Nutr 111:1124, 1981.
56. Dundee, JW, et al: The "induction" dose of thiopentone: A method of study and preliminary illustrative results. Anaesthesia 37:1176, 1982.
57. Zinn, SE, Fairly, HB and Glenn, JD: Liver function in patients with mild alcoholic hepatitis, after enflurane, nitrous oxide-narcotic, and spinal anesthesia. Anesth Analg 64:487, 1985.
58. Fishman, RH and Yanai, J: Long-lasting effects of early barbiturates on central nervous system and behavior. Neurosci Biobehav Rev 7:19, 1983.
59. Milkovich, L and van den Berg, BJ: Effects of prenatal meprobamate and chlordiazepoxide hydrochloride on human embryonic and fetal development. N Engl J Med 291:1268, 1974.
60. von Almen, WF II and Miller, JM, Jr: "Ts and Blues" in pregnancy. J Reprod Med (US) 31:236, 1986.
61. Martin, WR: Pharmacology of opioids. Pharmacol Rev 35:283, 1983.
62. Cicero, TJ: Effects of exogenous and endogenous opiates on the hypothalamic-pituitary-gonadal axis in the male. Fed Proc 39:2551, 1980.
63. Bell, MD, et al: Buccal morphine: A new route for analgesia? Lancet 1:71, 1985.
64. Bradberry, JC and Raebel, MA: Continuous infusion of naloxone in the treatment of narcotic overdose. Drug Intell Clin Pharm 15:945, 1981.
65. Magruder, MR, Delaney, RD and DiFazio, CA: Reversal of narcotic induced respiratory depression with nalbuphine hydrochloride. Anesthesiol Rev 9:34, 1982.
66. Naughton, N, et al: A benzodiazepine antagonist inhibits the cerebral metabolic and respiratory depressant effects of fentanyl. Life Sci 36:2239, 1985.
67. Patti, F, et al: Effect of sulpiride on chronic abstinence syndrome in addicted patients. Clin Neuropharmacol (United States) 9:469, 1986.
68. Parekh, A, et al: Intrauterine exposure to narcotics

and cord blood prolactin concentrations. Obstet Gynecol 57:447, 1981.
69. Finnegan, LP: Effects of maternal opiate abuse on the newborn. Fed Proc 44:2314, 1985.
70. Lapointe, G and Nosal, G: Morphine treatment during rat pregnancy: Neonatal and preweaning consequences. Biol Neonate 42:22, 1982.
71. Lichtblau, L and Sparber, SB: Opiate withdrawal in utero increases neonatal morbidity in the rat. Science 212:943, 1981.
72. Mercurio, SD, Lichtblau, L and Sparber, SB: Separation of hepatic N-demethylase-inducing and opioid dependence-producing doses of levo-alpha-acetylmethadol in the pregnant rat. Life Sci 33:1127, 1984.
73. Panerai, AE, et al: Plasma beta-endorphin, beta-lipotropin, and met-enkephalin concentrations during pregnancy in normal and drug-addicted women and their newborn. J Clin Endocrinol Metab 57:537, 1983.
74. Green, M and Suffet, F: The Neonatal Narcotic Withdrawal Index: A device for the improvement of care in the abstinence syndrome. Am J Drug Alcohol Abuse 8:203, 1981.
75. Chasnoff, IJ and Burns, WJ: The Moro reaction: A scoring system for neonatal narcotic withdrawal. Dev Med Child Neurol 26:484, 1984.
76. Kandall, SR, et al: Opiate vs CNS depressant therapy in neonatal drug abstinence syndrome. Am J Dis Child 137:378, 1983.
77. Carin, I, et al: Neonatal methadone withdrawal: Effect of two treatment regimens. Am J Dis Child 137:1166, 1983.
78. Kaltenbach, K and Finnegan, LP: Neonatal abstinence syndrome, pharmacotherapy and developmental outcome. Neurobehav Toxicol Teratol (US) 8:353, 1986.
79. Hoder, EL, et al: Clonidine treatment of neonatal narcotic abstinence syndrome. Psychiatry Res 13:243, 1984.
80. Ward, SL, et al: Abnormal sleeping ventilatory pattern in infants of substance-abusing mothers. Am J Dis Child 140:1015, 1986.
81. Doberczak, TM, et al: Peripheral nerve conduction studies in passively addicted neonates. Arch Phys Med Rehabil 67:4, 1986.
82. Senay, EC: Methadone maintenance treatment. Int J Addict 20:803, 1986.
83. Offidani, C, et al: Methadone in pregnancy: Clinical-toxicological aspects. J Toxicol Clin Toxicol 24:295, 1986.
84. Weintraub, SJ and Naulty, JS: Acute abstinence syndrome after epidural injection of butorphanol. Anesth Analg 64:452, 1985.
85. Gillman, MA: Nitrous oxide — an opioid addictive agent: Review of the evidence. Am J Med 81:97, 1986.
86. Rupreht, J, et al: Enkephalinase inhibition prevented tolerance to nitrous oxide analgesia in rats. Acta Anesth Scand 28:617, 1984.
87. Mazze, RI, et al: Reproduction and fetal development in mice chronically exposed to nitrous oxide. Teratology 26:11, 1982.
88. Rosenberg, HC and Chiu, TH: Time course for development of benzodiazepine tolerance and physical dependence. Neurosci Biobehav Rev 9:123, 1985.
89. Mickelson, MM and Lahti, RA: Demonstration of non-opioid sigma binding with (d)3H-SKF 10047 in guinea pig brain. Res Commun Chem Pathol Pharmacol 47:255, 1985.
90. Nielsen, HC, et al: Chlorpromazine excretion by the neonate following chronic in utero exposure. Pediatr Pharmacol (NY) 3:1, 1983.
91. Sasyniuk, BI, Jhamandas, V and Valois, M: Experimental amitriptyline intoxication: Treatment of cardiac toxicity with sodium bicarbonate. Ann Emerg Med 15:1052, 1986.
92. el-Ganzouri, AR, et al: Monoamine oxidase inhibitors: Should they be discontinued preoperatively? Anesth Analg 64:592, 1985.
93. Mallinger, AG, et al: Lithium treatment during pregnancy: A case study of erythrocyte choline content and lithium transport. J Clin Psychiatry 44:381, 1983.
94. Husain, S and Khan, I: An update on cannabis research. Bull Narc 1985 37:3, 1985.
95. Abel, EL, Dintcheff, BA and Day, N: Effects of marijuana on pregnant rats and their offspring. Psychopharmacology (Berlin) 71:71, 1980.
96. Fried, PA, Watkinson, B and Willan, A: Marijuana use during pregnancy and decreased length of gestation. Am J Obstet Gynecol 150:23, 1984.
97. Greenland, S, et al: Effects of marijuana on human pregnancy, labor, and delivery. Neurobehav Toxicol Teratol 4:447, 1982.
98. Barr, HM, et al: Infant size at 8 months of age: Relationship to maternal use of alcohol, nicotine, and caffeine during pregnancy. Pediatrics 74:336, 1984.
99. Tansley, BW, Fried, PA and Mount, HT: Visual processing in children exposed prenatally to marijuana and nicotine: a preliminary report. Can J Public Health 77(Suppl)1:72, 1986.
100. Berman, ML and Bochantin, JF: Effect of delta-9 tetrahydrocannabinol (marihuana) on liver microsomal dechlorinase activity: A preliminary report. Anesth Analg 51:929, 1972.
101. Sircar, R, et al: Characterization and autoradiographic visualization of (+)-[3H]SKF10,047 binding in rat and mouse brain: Further evidence for phencyclidine/"sigma opiate" receptor commonality. J Pharmacol Exp Ther 237:681, 1986.
102. Mendelsohn, LG, et al: Sigma opioid receptor: Characterization and co-identity with the phencyclidine receptor. J Pharmacol Exp Ther 233:597, 1985.
103. Murray, TF and Leid, ME: Interaction of dextrorotatory opioids with phencyclidine recognition sites in rat brain membranes. Life Sci 34:1899, 1984.
104. Leccese, AP, et al: The convulsant and anticonvulsant effects of phencyclidine (PCP) and PCP analogues in the rat. Behav Brain Res 19:163, 1986.
105. Kaufman, KR, et al: PCP in amniotic fluid and breast milk: Case report. J Clin Psychiatry 44:269, 1983.
106. Strauss, AA, Modaniou, HD and Bosu, SK: Neonatal manifestations of maternal phencyclidine (PCP) abuse. Pediatrics 68:550, 1981.
107. Howard, J, Kropenske, V and Tyler, R: The long-

term effects on neurodevelopment in infants exposed prenatally to PCP. Natl Inst Drug Abuse Res Monogr Ser 64:237, 1986.
108. Woolverton, WL: A review of the effects of repeated administration of selected phenylethylamines. Drug Alcohol Depend 17:143, 1986.
109. Washton, AM and Tatarsky, A: Adverse effects of cocaine abuse. Natl Inst Drug Abuse Res Monogr Ser 49:247, 1984.
110. Simpson, RW and Edwards, WD: Pathogenesis of cocaine-induced ischemic heart disease: Autopsy findings in a 21-year-old man. Arch Pathol Lab Med 110:479, 1986.
111. Howard, RE, Hueter, DC and Davis, GJ: Acute myocardial infarction following cocaine abuse in a young woman with normal coronary arteries. JAMA 254:95, 1985.
112. Pasternack, PF, Colvin, SB and Baumann, FG: Cocaine-induced angina pectoris and acute myocardial infarction in patients younger than 40 years. Am J Cardiol 55:847, 1985.
113. Fishel, R, et al: Cocaine colitis: Is this a new syndrome? Dis Colon Rectum 28:264, 1985.
114. Ramoska, E and Sacchetti, AD: Propranolol-induced hypertension in treatment of cocaine intoxication. Ann Emerg Med 14:1112, 1985.
115. Scott, ME and Mullaly, RW: Lithium therapy for cocaine-induced psychosis: A clinical perspective. South Med J 74:1475, 1981.
116. Dackis, CA, et al: Bromocriptine treatment for cocaine abuse: The dopamine depletion hypothesis. Int J Psychiatry Med 15:125, 1985.
117. Dackis, CA and Gold, MS: Pharmacological approaches to cocaine addiction. J Subst Abuse Treat 2:139, 1985.
118. Chasnoff, IJ, et al: Cocaine use in pregnancy. N Engl J Med 313:666, 1985.
119. Moore, TR, et al: Hemodynamic effects of intravenous cocaine on the pregnant ewe and fetus. Am J Obstet Gynecol 155:883, 1986.
120. Fantel, AG and Macphail, BJ: The teratogenicity of cocaine. Teratology 26:17, 1982.
121. Mahalik, MP, Gautieri, RF and Mann, DE, Jr: Teratogenic potential of cocaine hydrochloride in CF-1 mice. J Pharm Sci 69:703, 1980.
122. Chasnoff, IJ, et al: Perinatal cerebral infarction and maternal cocaine use. J Pediatr 108:456, 1986.
123. Barash, PG, et al: Is cocaine a sympathetic stimulant during general anesthesia? JAMA 243:1437, 1980.
124. Chiu, YC, et al: Myocardial infarction with topical cocaine anesthesia for nasal surgery. Arch Otolaryngol Head Neck Surg 112:988, 1986.
125. el-Din, AS and Mostafa, SM: Severe hypertension during anaesthesia for dacryocystorhinostomy. Anaesthesia 40:787, 1985.
126. Michel, R and Adams, AP: Acute amphetamine abuse: Problems during general anaesthesia for neurosurgery. Anaesthesia 34:1016, 1979.
127. Piccirillo, M, et al: Amphetamine and maternal behavior: Dose-response relationships. Psychopharmacology (Berlin) 70:195, 1980.
128. Eriksson, M, Larsson, G and Zetterstrom, R: Amphetamine addiction and pregnancy. II: Pregnancy, delivery and the neonatal period. Socio-medical aspects. Acta Obstet Gynecol Scand 60:253, 1981.
129. Weisberg, E: Smoking and reproductive health. Clin Reprod Fertil 3:175, 1985.
130. Luck, W, et al: Extent of nicotine and cotinine transfer to the human fetus, placenta, and amniotic fluid of smoking mothers. Dev Pharmacol Ther 8:384, 1985.
131. Sindberg, EP and Marsal, K: Acute effects of maternal smoking on fetal blood flow. Acta Obstet Gynecol Scand 63:391, 1984.
132. Mochizuki, M, et al: Effects of smoking on fetoplacental-maternal system during pregnancy. Am J Obstet Gynecol 149:413, 1984.
133. Mitchell, JA and Hammer, RE: Effects of nicotine on oviductal blood flow and embryo development in the rat. J Reprod Fertil 74:71, 1985.
134. Slotkin, TA, et al: Effects of maternal nicotine injections on brain development in the rat: Ornithine decarboxylase activity, nucleic acids and proteins in discrete brain regions. Brain Res Bull 17:41, 1986.
135. Al-Hachim, GM and Mahmoud, FA: Prenatal nicotine and CNS development. Epilepsia 26:661, 1985.
136. Sindberg, EP, et al: Acute effects of maternal smoking on fetal heart beat intervals. Acta Obstet Gynecol Scand 63:385, 1984.
137. Pearce, AC and Jones, RM: Smoking and anesthesia: Preoperative abstinence and perioperative morbidity. Anesthesiology 61:576, 1984.
138. Wright, DJ and Pandya, A: Smoking and gastric juice volume in outpatients. Can Anaesth Soc J 26:328, 1979.
139. Kania, J and Kofoed, L: Drug use by alcoholics in outpatient treatment. Am J Drug Alcohol Abuse 10:529, 1984.
140. Kaul, B and Davidow, B: Drug abuse patterns of patients on methadone treatment in New York City. Am J Drug Alcohol Abuse 8:17, 1981.
141. Chasnoff, IJ, et al: Maternal nonnarcotic substance abuse during pregnancy: Effects on infant development. Neurobehav Toxicol Teratol 6:277, 1984.

CHAPTER 27

NONOBSTETRIC SURGERY IN THE PREGNANT PATIENT

HILDA PEDERSEN, M.B., Ch.B., F.F.A.R.C.S.

The frequency of surgery in pregnant women, undertaken for reasons unrelated to parturition itself, is variously estimated to be 1.6 to 2.2 percent of all pregnancies[1,2] or up to 50,000 procedures per year in this country.[3] During the first two trimesters, the most common surgical conditions, apart from trauma, are lesions involving torsion, rupture, or hemorrhage of ovarian cysts (1 in 2500)[4] and acute appendicitis (0.07 percent of pregnancies).[5] Perforation, peritonitis, and thrombophlebitis, complications that can result from delayed diagnosis in the pregnant woman presenting with an acute abdomen, may increase anesthetic hazard. Breast tumors probably constitute the next most common reason for surgery during pregnancy.[4] Anesthesia to facilitate correction of an incompetent cervix (Shirodkar suture, McDonald procedure) during the first or second trimester has become fairly routine. Increasingly frequent reports of successful surgery in pregnant women with intracranial tumors and aneurysms, cardiac valvular disease, pheochromocytoma, hyperthyroidism, etc., make timely the consideration of the basic objectives in anesthetic management, the aim being to provide the most favorable outcome for mother and baby.

Risks of anesthesia and surgery for both mother and fetus may be related to alterations in maternal physiology, possible teratogenicity of anesthetic agents, the influence of anesthetic agents and/or techniques on uteroplacental perfusion, the surgical condition itself and its therapy, and potential abortion or premature delivery.

Four major studies attempted to relate surgery and anesthesia during human pregnancy to fetal outcome, as determined by anomalies, premature labor, or intrauterine demise.[1,2,6,7] Although they failed to correlate surgery and anesthetic exposure with congenital anomalies, all demonstrated increased fetal mortality, particularly following operations during the first trimester. No particular anesthetic agent or technique was implicated, and it seemed that the condition that necessitated surgery was the most relevant factor: mortality was highest after pelvic surgery.

A report in 1963 on a population of 18,493 pregnant women, 67 of whom had operations during pregnancy, showed a fetal mortality rate of 11.2 percent, survival being poorest when the procedure was performed for cervical incompetence.[6] Surgical manipulations of the uterus and procedures performed for management of cervical incompetence represent major factors initiating premature labor.[8] In 1965, a study among 9073 parturients, of whom 1.6 percent had surgery, found an 8.8 percent incidence of premature labor (and perinatal mortality of 7.5 percent), in the surgical group compared with only 2 percent in the control group.[1] More recently, pregnancy outcome following surgery in 287 dental assistants or dentist's wives out of a population of 12,929, showed that surgery during pregnancy was associated with a significant increase in spontaneous abortion rates compared to those not undergoing surgery (8 percent versus 5.1 percent).[2] In an attempt to answer the questions raised by these findings, a review was taken of the entire population of the Canadian province of Manitoba between the years 1971 and 1978.[7] State health insurance records identified 2565 pregnant women who had surgery during this period. Each patient was matched with a woman of similar age, living in the same area, with a pregnancy-related condition without surgical intervention, and documented the outcome of pregnancy (i.e., normal delivery, abnormal delivery, or abortion), surgical procedure, type of anesthesia used (none, local, general, or nerve block), and incidence of congenital anomalies. As in earlier studies, surgery during pregnancy did not increase the incidence of congenital anomalies. However, the risk of spontaneous abortion rose in women who received general anesthesia for surgery during the first or second trimester. This was most evident following gynecologic surgery, but it also occurred after other procedures. In contrast to earlier studies, few underwent cervical cerclage, suggesting that factors other than the obstetric condition might be important. Results also might have been influenced by the small number of obstetric and gynecologic procedures performed under anesthesia other than general, so that the effect of the site of surgery alone could not be evaluated. The authors emphasize the multiplicity of factors other than choice of anesthetic agent (e.g., diagnostic x-rays, antibiotics, analgesics, infection, decreased uterine perfusion, stress) that might account for the increased risk of abortion.

The study of the effects of chronic exposure to subanesthetic concentrations of inhalation agents on pregnancy offers a different approach to the question of outcome. Evidence originates from animal studies and from epidemiologic surveys carried out on operating room personnel and their children. The first report, coming from Russia in 1967, noted that an unusually large number of spontaneous abortions occurred among anesthesiologists.[9] Studies followed in Denmark, Finland, the United Kingdom, and this country. A nationwide survey conducted by the American Society of Anesthesiologists found a higher incidence of cancer and spontaneous abortion among female anesthesia personnel as well as more congenital abnormalities in their infants.[10] Furthermore, the last of these misfortunes also applied, though to a lesser degree, to unexposed wives of male operating room personnel. Another study, involving nurse-anesthetists, suggested a higher-than-expected incidence of cancer.[11] All of these studies have been disputed[12,13] because of possible statistical inaccuracies and inappropriate control groups. Another survey conducted among dentists and their female assistants compared the incidence of spontaneous abortions and congenital abnormalities among those exposed to inhalation anesthetics and those using only local anesthetics in their daily practice.[14] More complications occurred among assistants and wives of dentists exposed to inhalation agents. Because of the controversy surrounding this issue, the American Society of Anesthesiologists recently commissioned an independent review by a group of epidemiologists.[15] This group challenged the data from most of the selected surveys for a variety of reasons, including responder bias, inappropriate control groups, failure to document exposure levels or to verify medical data, and inability to ascertain which of the many operating room environmental factors might be to blame. The group concluded that although exposed women appeared to have an increased risk of abortion (and, to a much lesser extent, congenital anomalies), the increase could be accounted for by bias and uncontrolled variables. Two subsequent studies avoided some of these problems by matching information from a questionnaire with that obtained from medical records or registries of abortions, births, and congenital malformations.[16,17] Neither study found significant deviations from expected rates of threatened abortion in exposed women. In addition, no differences in birth weight distribution, perinatal mortality, or congenital malformations between exposed and unexposed women were detected.[17] The authors point out that their results do not eliminate the possibility of reproductive hazard relating to working in operating rooms, since very early abortions not requiring hospitalization, congenital abnormalities not apparent at birth, and infertility might have been missed.

Physiologic Changes in Pregnancy

During pregnancy changes occur in practically every organ system, being largely induced by hormonal secretions from the corpus luteum and placenta. Later adaptations relate to the mechanical effects of the steadily enlarging uterus in the second and third trimesters. Since Chapter 1 describes these changes, only a few points will be emphasized here.

BLOOD VOLUME AND CONSTITUENTS

Both plasma volume and red cell volume begin to increase between the 6th and 13th week of pregnancy. Plasma volume increases 40 to 50 percent, and total blood volume increases 25 to 50 percent above normal.[18] The lesser rise in red cell volume (20 percent) leads to a decline in red cell count, hemoglobin, and hematocrit.

Other significant changes include a rise in plasma fibrinogen[19] and platelets,[20] which, in association with marked increases in activity of several clotting factors, predispose the pregnant woman to thromboembolic phenomena.[21]

In both pregnancy and the puerperium serum cholinesterase activity declines,[22,23] but this reduced activity of normal enzyme probably does not cause prolonged apnea following moderate doses of succinylcholine (50 to 400 mg).[24]

HEMODYNAMIC CHANGES

Cardiac output and heart rate gradually increase until, at 30 to 34 weeks, the cardiac output reaches its peak of 30 to 50 percent above normal. From this time onward, inferior vena caval compression becomes increasingly important and accounts for the "supine hypotensive syndrome" characterized by arterial hypotension, tachycardia, pallor, and faintness seen in approximately 10 percent of supine pregnant women at term.[25] Pregnancy-related engorgement of the intervertebral plexus reduces the volume of epidural and subarachnoid spaces and may contribute to the 20- to 30-percent reduction in drug requirement observed during regional anesthesia.

RESPIRATORY SYSTEM

Capillary engorgement occurs throughout the respiratory tract of most pregnant women.[26] Nasal breathing may become more difficult, and the risk of bleeding following nasotracheal intubation or placement of nasopharyngeal airways increases.

After the fifth month of pregnancy expiratory reserve volume, residual volume, and functional residual capacity (FRC) decrease.[27] Net minute ventilation increases soon after conception, reaching a maximum of 50 percent above normal nonpregnant levels during the second or third month.[28] Dead space does not change significantly; therefore, at term alveolar ventilation exceeds that of the nonpregnant state by about 70 percent. Increased alveolar ventilation, along with decreased FRC, enhances maternal uptake and elimination of inhalation anesthetics.[29] Decreased FRC and increased metabolic rate predispose the mother to hypoxemia, even during a brief period of airway obstruction, or apnea.[30]

GASTROINTESTINAL TRACT

During pregnancy the enlarging uterus gradually pushes the stomach and intestines upward. Evacuation of a watery meal may be delayed by 60 percent from the 34th week onward.[31] Pain, anxiety, narcotics, and belladonna alkaloids potentiate this delay. The administration of general anesthesia enhances the risk of regurgitation and aspiration during pregnancy, rendering rapid induction, cricoid pressure, and endotracheal intubation necessary in all patients undergoing general anesthesia during the last two trimesters of pregnancy.

Effects of Anesthetic Agents and Techniques on the Embryo and Fetus

DIRECT EFFECTS

Following recognition that anesthetics may depress cell growth and division, evidence has been accumulating regarding the cellular effects of these agents and their metabolic products. Halothane, in concentrations of 0.7 percent or higher, interferes with the synthesis of DNA.[32,33] Studies indicate that abnormal products of cell division may follow exposure to a variety of anesthetics.[10] The mechanisms by which cytotoxicity — whether the effects be mutagenic, teratogenic, or carcinogenic — may occur have been of growing interest.

Work in small animals exposed to toxic substances and anesthetics shows a dose-related response, the first change being decreased fertility and increased fetal death. With increasing dose, the number of surviving fetuses with anomalies increases, the peak incidence occurring at a dose that causes 50 percent fetal death.[34] The teratogenic effects vary markedly between species, and also within the same species. The stage of development at the time of exposure proves crucial, with dramatic sensitivity at certain times, and little or no effect at later times.[34,35] The period of organogenesis is most critical (15 to 56 days in humans), but a particular sensitivity of the central nervous system to external factors may exist later, during the period of myelination. C^{14}-labeled cholesterol administered in the newborn period persists in the white matter of rabbits for 1 year. This high metabolic stability of constituents of myelin sheaths and other brain substances suggests that exposure to agents that detrimentally affect myelin formation could produce prolonged sequelae. Several experiments have demonstrated that brief intrauterine exposure of rats to halothane adversely affects postnatal learning behavior and causes CNS cellular degeneration and decreased brain weight. Findings with enflurane are inconsistent.[36–38]

In man, many congenital malfunctions show a pattern of multifactorial inheritance. Maldevelopment results from a combination of factors within one individual, such as hereditary predisposition, sensitivity to a given drug, and exposure at a vulnerable time in development.

INDIRECT EFFECTS

The adequacy of the uteroplacental circulation is easily affected by drugs and anesthetic procedures. Decreased placental perfusion pressure or increased vascular resistance may result in placental hypoperfusion and fetal asphyxia.

Maternal systemic hypotension secondary to epidural or spinal anesthesia, aortocaval compression in the supine position, or hemorrhage may reduce perfusion pressure across the intervillous space. Usually the placental vasculature is widely dilated, consequently perfusion pressure constitutes the major determinant of uterine blood flow.[39] However, with low concentrations of general anesthetics, such as halothane and isoflurane, a small drop in maternal blood pressure may be associated with increased uterine blood flow because of uterine muscle relaxation and decreased uterine vascular resistance.[40]

Increased uterine activity may result in reduced placental perfusion. Alpha-adrenergic drugs such as methoxamine[41] or ketamine[42] (in doses above 1.1 mg per kg) may increase uterine tone.

The mechanical effects of severe maternal hyperventilation may reduce uterine blood flow,[43] and hypocapnia may compromise fetal oxygenation by causing direct constriction of the umbilical vessels and a leftward shift of the maternal oxyhemoglobin dissociation curve.

Epinephrine and norepinephrine infusion results in decreased uterine blood flow and deterioration of fetal condition in experimental animals.[44,45] Local anesthetic solutions containing epinephrine or maternal pain and apprehension may have a similar effect on the fetus.

The increased risk due to rapid depletion of oxygen in the pregnant woman has already been mentioned. High inspired oxygen concentrations should be administered to the mother before induction of general anesthesia and during regional anesthesia. No evidence exists that maternal hyperoxia at normal atmospheric pressures can produce retrolental fibroplasia or premature closure of the ductus arteriosus in utero.

Specific Drugs and Agents

Exposure to specific drugs commonly used by anesthesiologists is examined, bearing in mind the difficulty of extrapolating laboratory data to the clinical situation as seen in man. The concentrations and duration of exposure usually greatly exceeded those used clinically and most studies were performed in lower animals, such as the chick embryo or rat, in which gestation or organogenesis are very brief.

Very large numbers of patients must be exposed to a suspected teratogen before its safety can be ascertained. A large prospective study that attempted to determine association between maternal drug exposure and neonatal abnormalities highlights the difficulties in proving causal relationships.[46] Complicating factors include the frequency of maternal exposure to a multiplicity of drugs; the difficulty in separating the effects of the underlying pathology and surgical treatment from those of the drug administered; differing degrees of risk with stage of gestation; and the variety, rather than the consistency, of anomalies which appear in association with one agent.

PREMEDICATION AND SEDATION

Anticholinergics

Atropine, scopolamine, and glycopyrrolate are not teratogenic.[47]

Tranquilizers and Sedatives

Several of the phenothiazines and other tranquilizers are teratogenic in rats and rabbits.[48–50] A wide spectrum of malformations follows the use of pentobarbital and phenobarbital in mice but not in rats or rabbits.[35,51] Species differences and variations in experimental method may explain the disparate results.

Several retrospective studies indicate an association between minor tranquilizers taken during pregnancy and increased risk of congenital anomalies. Meprobamate (Equanil) or chlordiazepoxide (Librium) exposure during the first 6 weeks of gestation causes significantly more anomalies than when other or "no drugs" are used.[52] In contrast, Hartz and associates[53] could not detect a difference in fetal outcome between exposed and unexposed groups after ingestion of meprobamate or chlordiazepoxide in early pregnancy. Several reports describe a relationship between diazepam (Valium) and oral clefts,[54,55] but the most recently published studies do not confirm this.[56] A prospective study of more than 50,000 human pregnancies in which approximately 1300 patients had taken various doses of phenothiazines during the first 4 months of pregnancy, showed no evidence of adverse effects on perinatal mortality, birth weight, congenital abnormalities, or intelligence at 4 years of age.[57]

The "control group" does not have the anxiety or stress causing the need for medication. Stress in the study groups may be the causative factor for anomalies, not the tranquilizer itself. Obviously final conclusions cannot yet be made regarding the use of minor tranquilizers in early pregnancy.

Narcotics

Central nervous system malformations have followed maternal administration of several narcotics in hamsters.[58] The investigators employed different doses given by single injection 4 days before killing the animals and chronic exposure for a few days before death. Increased maternal doses of heroin and methadone increased the number of abnormal fetuses, but multiple doses of morphine and meperidine failed to produce more anomalies above a certain dose level. In other animal studies methadone given to pregnant mice on day 9 produced central nervous system malformations in embryos;[59] negative results were obtained in rats and rabbits.[60] In contrast, rats exposed to morphine produced growth-retarded offspring with increased fetal mortality.[61,62] Interestingly, these studies revealed that narcotic antagonists (nalorphine and naloxone) could block the teratogenic effects in hamsters.[58]

It remains doubtful whether these data are relevant with respect to anesthetic exposure of pregnant patients, with the possible exception of high-dose narcotic anesthesia, as used in cardiac surgery. Although the offspring of narcotic-addicted mothers show growth retardation and behavioral problems, they do not display an increased incidence of congenital abnormalities.

H_2 Blockers

As already stated, alterations in gastric anatomy and function increase the pregnant patient's risk for aspiration should she lose protective airway reflexes. Although women of less than 20 weeks' gestation stand no more risk from low pH or high gastric volume than comparable nonpregnant surgical patients,[63] it remains unknown at which week of gestation the risk of aspiration becomes significant. However, in the second half of pregnancy, it seems judicious to use histamine$_2$ blockers (such as cimetidine; or ranitidine, which appears to be associated with fewer drug interactions and side effects.)[64] Cimetidine, through binding of its imidazole group to cytochrome P-450, inhibits the metabolism of a number of drugs, such as propranolol, diazepam, librium, and amide local anesthetics.

Metoclopramide

Intravenous metoclopramide, a dopamine antagonist, accelerates gastric emptying, decreases mean gastric volume, and increases lower esophageal sphincter tone.[63,66] Ranitidine and metoclopramide may prove to be a useful combination for premedication, but the effectiveness of the latter drug as a prophylactic antiemetic varies extremely.[67]

INTRAVENOUS ANESTHETICS

Thiopental and Methohexital

Both agents are frequently used for induction of anesthesia. The elimination half-life of sodium thiopental increases in pregnant women at term due to a larger-than-normal volume of distribution.[68] As they are normally used in the operating room, barbiturates are unlikely to compromise the fetus.

Ketamine

This is useful for inducing anesthesia when substantial maternal hypotension and/or hypovolemia develop. Low doses do not significantly affect uterine activity, whereas larger doses during the first two trimesters, but not at term, raise uterine tone and can endanger the fetus.[69,70]

Etomidate

This induction agent has a rapid onset and short duration of action and produces less myocardial depression than thiopental.[71] However, etomidate may blunt the patient's adrenal stress response to surgery and, since placental transfer has been substantiated, may be of limited usefulness in pregnancy.[72,73]

MUSCLE RELAXANTS

Although all commonly used muscle relaxants cross the placenta to some degree, the only evidence of adverse fetal effects consists of a study showing musculoskeletal deformities involving the joints after infusion of d-tubocurarine into chick embryos between the 7th and 15th days of incubation.[74]

The commonest complications of the use of muscle relaxants relate to cardiac arrhythmias and hypotension secondary to histamine release. Pregnant patients have decreased levels of plasma pseudocholinesterase but ample reserve persists to eliminate succinylcholine rapidly.[75]

INHALATION AGENTS

Nitrous Oxide

Nitrous oxide has been extensively studied following the 1955 observation that patients with tetanus developed leukopenia after being exposed to nitrous oxide for several days. Subsequent investigations showed a concentration-dependent inhibition of hematopoiesis in rats.[76,77] Numerous studies have demonstrated significant effects on fetal growth, skeletal development, and death rate in both pregnant rats and incubating chicks exposed to concentrations of from 50 to 80 percent nitrous oxide for periods ranging from hours to days.[78,79] Whether adverse effects at such high doses were caused by the anesthetic itself or the accompanying physiologic derangements is unknown. In a study of prolonged exposure of rats to subanesthetic concentrations of nitrous oxide or room air, Vieira and associates[80] found that 1000 ppm of nitrous oxide resulted in a higher incidence of fetal resorptions, skeletal malformations, and smaller fetuses than air. Since these concentrations do not produce anesthesia, this study supports the conclusion that nitrous oxide may be teratogenic. In contrast to the above findings with high dosage or prolonged exposure, concentrations of 50 percent or less for periods of less than 24 hrs produced no adverse fetal effects.[81,82]

Although the mechanism of the teratogenic effect of nitrous oxide remains uncertain, it may be due to the inhibitory effect of the agent on methionine synthetase activity.[83] Nitrous oxide irreversibly oxidizes vitamin B_{12}, a cofactor of this enzyme, to an inactive form. Inhibition of methionine synthetase has been detected in liver biopsy specimens obtained from surgical patients after exposure to 50 to 70 percent nitrous oxide for 1.25 to 2.75 hours.[84] A dose-dependent decrease in both maternal and fetal methionine synthetase activity occurs following exposure of pregnant rats to 10 to 50 percent nitrous oxide for periods ranging from 60 to 240 min.[85] Perhaps failure of this enzyme to convert homocysteine to the essential amino acid methionine may lead to abnormalities of myelination of nerve fibers. Furthermore, inhibition of methionine synthesis decreases thymidine production, which in turn can lead to decreased DNA synthesis and inhibition of cell division. This explains the megaloblastic anemia that results from chronic, but not acute, exposure to nitrous oxide.

Because of the evidence that nitrous oxide adversely affects methionine synthetase activity, some authorities have recommended that pregnant women should not receive it in the first two trimesters.[86,87] However, a recent study demonstrated no significant changes in plasma methionine concentrations following exposure to 60–70 percent nitrous oxide for up to 4 hours.[88] Similarly, in another study, bone marrow function remained normal in patients administered 50 percent nitrous oxide for up to 6 hours for routine surgery.[89]

A review of approximately 400 in vitro fertilization procedures, in which ova were retrieved under general (nitrous oxide) or local anesthesia showed no differences in pregnancy rates.[90] Two other reviews of exposure to nitrous oxide, this time for cervical cerclage, also showed no effects of the agent on fetal outcome.[91,92]

A recent editorial points out that definitive clinical studies which might help to elucidate the dilemma surrounding the use of nitrous oxide during pregnancy remain to be done, but that the anesthesiologist should not be deterred from administering the agent to pregnant women.[93] We concur with this conclusion.

Halogenated Agents

Exposing pregnant rats to halothane 0.8 percent for 12 hours at various times during gestation increases the incidence of anomalous skeletal development and fetal death.[94] Briefer administration of halothane 0.6 percent for 3 hours in pregnant hamsters on day 11 of gestation reduces fetal weight and age, and increases the number of abortions.[95] Other investigations failed to show these teratogenic effects in rats, rabbits, and mice exposed for brief periods to subanesthetic concentrations of this drug, but anesthetic concentrations (1 percent) proved lethal to fetuses, while prolonged exposure (5 days per week for 9 weeks, up to 4 MAC hours daily) led to no teratogenic effects at lower doses, decreased ossification at higher doses, and skeletal variants at the highest dose.[96,97] The animals in the last study exhibited extreme hypothermia, and the authors concluded that hypothermia, rather than the anesthetic itself, caused the teratogenic effects.

Subanesthetic concentrations of enflurane are not teratogenic. Mice exposed to 1 percent enflurane for 4 hours per day on days 6 to 15 of gestation had more cleft palates and minor skeletal and visceral abnormalities.[98] In a subsequent study by the same authors, teratogenic changes following exposure to 0.6-percent isoflurane in mice resembled those found with enflurane, but cleft palate occurred six times more frequently (12 percent and 1.9 percent).[99] Because mice readily develop cleft palate, its occurrence as an isolated finding suggests that this might be a species-specific response. In an attempt to clarify the results from earlier studies, rats were exposed to 0.75 MAC halothane, isoflurane, or enflurane, 0.55 MAC nitrous oxide, or a known teratogen, retinoic acid, for two 6-hour periods at three different stages of pregnancy.[100] No major morphologic abnormalities occurred in any of the anesthetic groups. An increased number of resorptions (equivalent to spontaneous abortion in humans) in animals exposed to nitrous oxide were the only positive finding.

Since a single exposure to an anesthetic agent seems unlikely to result in fetal abnormality, the selection of agent should be based on surgical requirements. Halothane, enflurane, and isoflurane can decrease uterine activity, and these agents may be recommended for use during abdominal surgery, particularly in late pregnancy, during expected uterine manipulation. Pregnant ewes administered 1.0 to 1.5 MAC halothane or isoflurane demonstrated an increase in uterine blood flow despite mild hypotension because of decreased uterine vascular resistance.[40] However, 2 MAC significantly decreases maternal blood pressure, cardiac output, and uterine blood flow, along with fetal blood pressure, heart rate, pH, base excess, and oxygen saturation. Isoflurane may affect the fetus more adversely than halothane in spite of similar decreases in maternal blood pressure. In sheep, halothane 1.5 percent did not compromise fetal cardiac output or regional blood flow to vital organs, and fetal oxygenation and acid-base status remained stable.[101] In contrast, 2 percent isoflurane significantly reduced fetal placental blood flow, which resulted in progressive fetal acidosis.[102]

LOCAL ANESTHETICS

These drugs stabilize cell membranes and may affect cell mitosis at certain stages of development. Sturrock and Nunn compared the cytotoxic effects of procaine, lidocaine, and bupivacaine on cultures of hamster lung fibroblasts and found decreased cell survival with ED 50 values at concentrations as low as one tenth those used clinically.[103] No evidence exists that local anesthetics cause teratogenesis in animals or man.

The local anesthetic prilocaine may produce maternal or fetal methemoglobinemia, and fetal red blood cells display an increased susceptibility to a number of oxidants.[104]

VASOACTIVE DRUGS

In a retrospective study of 3082 pregnancies, exposure to sympathomimetic agents significantly increased the incidence of minor malformations in the offspring.[105] In chick embryos there was a direct relationship between drug concentration and anomaly formation, especially of the cardiovascular system, and this increased with greater β-receptor activity (isoproterenol > epinephrine > norepinephrine).[106] Propranolol at adequate β-blocking doses completely inhibited the formation of those anomalies.

Alpha-adrenergic agonists can constrict uterine and placental vasculature, causing fetal asphyxia.[107,108] Indirectly acting adrenergic agonists such as ephedrine improve uterine blood flow when given during maternal hypotension[75] and may be the best vasopressors for use during general or regional anesthesia.

HYPOXIA, HYPERCARBIA, AND OTHER FACTORS

The cytotoxicity of anesthetic agents and adjuvants associates closely with biodegradation, which, in turn, is influenced by oxygenation and hepatic blood flow. Thus the complications that may occur during anesthesia, such as maternal hypoxia, hypotension, hypocarbia or hypercarbia and electrolyte disturbances, may be more critical to teratogenesis than the anesthetic agents per se. Certainly hypoxia has been well documented as a teratogen in the chick embryo,[109] mouse,[110] and rat,[111] and hypercarbia results in congenital anomalies in rats.[112] The role of carbohydrate metabolism on embryonic development is also important. Forty-eight hours of fasting and the administration of insulin to pregnant rats on day 7, 9, or 11 of gestation have produced a large number of skeletal deformities.[113]

Hyperbaric oxygen (100 percent at 2 atmospheres for 3 hours, or 3 atmospheres for 2 hours) in the hamster caused a significant number of congenital anomalies.[114] In rabbits, hyperbaric oxygen administered in late pregnancy produced retrolental fibroplasia, retinal detachment, and stillbirth.[115] High concentrations of oxygen at normal pressure have not been shown to be teratogenic in experimental animals.

Recommendations for Anesthetic Care

In general, physicians agree that only emergency surgery should be performed during pregnancy. The possibility of pregnancy should be considered in all female surgical patients of reproductive age, so that the urgency of the proposed operation can be rationally evaluated. Based on the already described maternal and fetal hazards, the following approach to anesthesia seems indicated:

1. Personal reassurance during the preanesthetic visit and adequate sedation and premedication should allay apprehension. A thorough but reassuring discussion of the hazards of anesthesia is important for the patient and her family, for they probably have many fears for the unborn baby. They should be informed of the low incidence of fetal loss, and the relevance of animal studies should be put into proper perspective. As far as is known, the mother's disease and the nature of surgery affect the outcome more than any particular anesthetic technique, and the patient should know that her baby will be monitored, if possible, during the procedure and that tocolytic agents such as ritodrine or terbutaline will be used, if necessary, to suppress uterine contractility.

2. Pain should be relieved whenever present. Avoid acetylsalicylic acid (and other nonsteroidal anti-inflammatory agents) since they inhibit prostaglandin synthesis and may stimulate in utero closure of the ductus arteriosus.

3. Administration of 15 to 30 ml of antacid within an hour prior to induction of anesthesia raises the gastric pH above the critical level. Clear antacids seem to be better tolerated when aspirated. Ranitidine and metoclopramide may be useful.

4. Beginning in the second trimester, mothers should not be transported or placed on the operating table in the supine position. The lateral decubitus position or left uterine displacement minimizes the risk of aortocaval compression.

5. Rapid intravenous infusion of at least 1 liter of crystalloid solution prior to induction helps to prevent hypotension related to spinal or epidural anesthesia. If maternal blood pressure falls more than 15 to 20 percent despite pretreatment, a predominantly β-adrenergic vasopressor, such as ephedrine, should be promptly administered intravenously.

6. Careful denitrogenation should precede general anesthesia to avoid maternal and fetal hypoxemia during induction and intubation.

7. The application of cricoid pressure and rapid endotracheal intubation with a cuffed tube will minimize the risk of aspiration.

8. To reduce fetal hazard, particularly during the first trimester, choose drugs with a long history of safety. These include thiopental, morphine, meperidine, muscle relaxants, and low concentrations of nitrous oxide. However, ketamine, 0.5 to 0.75 mg per kg, might be preferable to thiopental as an induction agent in the face of severe hypovolemia. In low doses, ketamine should have minimal effect on uterine tone, particularly in late pregnancy.[70] Halothane or other volatile agents may offer the specific advantage of relaxing the uterus during procedures involving the pelvic organs, particularly the uterus itself (e.g., cervical cerclage—Shirodkar or McDonald procedure).

9. In order to avoid maternal hyperventilation, monitor arterial blood gases or end-expiratory PCO_2.

10. Prevent hypovolemia by adequate intravenous replacement of fluid in order to preserve uteroplacental blood flow.

11. It is advisable to monitor the fetal heart rate continuously throughout surgery and anesthesia, providing that the placement of the transducer does not encroach upon the surgical field.[116,117] Using the directional Doppler apparatus, monitoring becomes technically feasible from the 16th week of pregnancy. Uterine tone may also be monitored with an external tocodynamometer if the uterus has grown enough to reach the umbilicus or above.

12. Special procedures, such as hypothermia and induced hypotension, might be needed to facilitate surgery, despite potential fetal hazard. Successful fetal outcome following both procedures for intracranial operations has been reported.[118,119] Numerous reports exist of cardiopulmonary bypass being performed during pregnancy, with generally good outcome.[120–123] Persistent fetal bradycardia and loss of beat-to-beat variability occurred frequently throughout the period of bypass, despite acceptable maternal oxygenation and acid-base balance. One survey reported only one maternal death in 86 procedures using extracorporeal circulation and more than 80-percent survival of fetuses.[123] The author suggested that the procedures

might be safer when fetal heart and uterine monitoring were used, and perfusion hypothermia was avoided. At this time little work has been done to determine the fetal effects of cardiopulmonary bypass.

References

1. Shnider, SM and Webster, GM: Maternal and fetal hazards of surgery during pregnancy. Am J Obstet Gynecol 92:891, 1965.
2. Brodsky, JB, et al: Surgery during pregnancy and fetal outcome. Am J Obstet Gynecol 138:1165, 1980.
3. Cohen, EN, Bellville, JW and Brown, BS: Anesthesia, pregnancy and miscarriage: A study of operating room nurses and anesthetists. Anesthesiology 35: 343, 1971.
4. Levine, W and Diamond, B: Surgical procedures during pregnancy. Am J Obstet Gynecol 81:1046, 1962.
5. Babaknia, A, Parsa, H and Woodruff, JD: Appendicitis during pregnancy. Obstet Gynecol 50:40, 1977.
6. Smith, BE: Fetal prognosis after anesthesia during gestation. Anesth Analg 42:521, 1963.
7. Duncan, PG, et al: Fetal risk of anesthesia and surgery during pregnancy. Anesthesiology 64:790, 1986.
8. Delaney AG: Anesthesia in the pregnant woman. Clin Obstet Gynecol 26:795, 1983.
9. Vaisman, AL: Working conditions in surgery and their effect on the health of anesthesiologists. Eksp Khir Anest 3:44, 1967.
10. Ad Hoc Committee on the Effect of Trace Anesthetics on the Health of Operating Room Personnel, American Society of Anesthesiologists: Occupational disease among operating room personnel: A national study. Anesthesiology 41:321, 1974.
11. Corbett, TH, et al: Incidence of cancer among Michigan nurse-anesthetists. Anesthesiology 38:260, 1973.
12. Walts, LF, Forsythe, AB and Moore JG: Critique: Occupational disease among operating room personnel. Anesthesiology 42:608, 1975.
13. Fink, BR and Cullen, BF: Anesthetic pollution: What is happening to us? Anesthesiology 45:79, 1976.
14. Cohen, EN, Brown, BW and Wu, M: Anesthetic health hazards in the dental operatory. Anesthesiology 51:S256, 1976.
15. Buring, JE, Hennekens, CH and Mayrent, SL: Health experiences of operating room personnel. Anesthesiology 62:325, 1985.
16. Axelsson, G and Rylander, R: Exposure to anesthetic gases and spontaneous abortion: Response bias in postal questionnaire study. Int J Epidemiol 11:250, 1982.
17. Ericson, HA and Källén, AJB: Hospitalization for miscarriage and delivery outcome among Swedish nurses working in operating rooms, 1973–1978. Anesth Analg 64:981, 1985.
18. Lund, CJ and Donovan, JC: Blood volume during pregnancy. Am J Obstet Gynecol 98:393, 1967.
19. Longo, LD, Caillouette, JC and Russell, KP: Fibrinogen deficiencies in pregnancy. Obstet Gynecol 14:97, 1959.
20. Mor, A, et al: Platelet counts in pregnancy and labor: A comparative study. Obstet Gynecol 16:338, 1960.
21. Marx, GF and Orkin, LR: Physiology of Obstetric Anesthesia. Charles C Thomas, Springfield, IL, 1969.
22. Shnider, SM: Serum cholinesterase activity during pregnancy, labor and the puerperium. Anesthesiology 26:335, 1965.
23. Hazel, B and Monier, D: Human serum cholinesterase: Variations during pregnancy and post-partum. Canad Anaesth Soc J 18:272, 1971.
24. Wildsmith, JAW: Serum pseudocholinesterase, pregnancy and suxamethonium. Anaesthesia 27:90, 1972.
25. Howard, BK, Goodson, JH and Mengert, WF: Supine hypotensive syndrome of late pregnancy. Obstet Gynecol 1:371, 1953.
26. Bonica, JJ: Principles and Practices of Obstetric Analgesia and Anesthesia. F.A. Davis, Philadelphia, 1967.
27. Cugell, DW, et al: Pulmonary function in pregnancy. I: Serial observations in normal women. Am Rev Tuberc 67:568, 1953.
28. Anderson, GJ, et al: The maternal oxygen tension and acid-base status during pregnancy. J Obstet Gynaecol Br Commonw 76:16, 1969.
29. Moya, F and Smith, BE: Uptake, distribution and placental transport of drugs and anesthetics. Anesthesiology 26:465, 1965.
30. Archer, GW and Marx, GF: Arterial oxygenation during apnoea in parturient women. Br J Anaesth 46:358, 1974.
31. Davison, JS, Davison, MC and Hay, DM: Gastric emptying time in late pregnancy and labour. J Obstet Gynaecol Br Commonw 77:37, 1970.
32. Jackson, SJ: The metabolic effect of halothane on mammalian hepatoma cells in vitro. II: Inhibition of DNA synthesis. Anesthesiology 39:405, 1973.
33. Sturrock, J and Nunn, JF: Effects of halothane on DNA synthesis and the presynthetic phase (GI) in dividing fibroblasts. Anesthesiology 45:413, 1976.
34. Smith, BE: Teratogenicity of inhalation anesthetics. In: Progress in Anesthesiology. London, Excerpta Medica, 1970, p 589.
35. Smith, BE: Teratogenic capabilities of surgical anesthesia. Adv Teratol 3:127, 1968.
36. Chalon, J, et al: Intrauterine exposure to halothane increases murine postnatal autotolerance to halothane and reduces brain weight. Anesth Analg 62:565, 1983.
37. Chalon, J, et al: Exposure to halothane and enflurane affects learning function of murine progeny. Anesth Analg 60:794, 1981.
38. Peters, MA and Hudson, PM: Postnatal development and behavior in offspring of enflurane exposed pregnant rats. Arch Int Pharmacody Ther 256:134, 1982.
39. Greiss, FC, Jr: Pressure-flow relationship in the gra-

vid uterine vascular bed. Am J Obstet Gynecol 96:41, 1966.
40. Palahniuk, RJ and Shnider, SM: Maternal and fetal cardiovascular and acid-base changes during halothane and isoflurane anesthesia in the pregnant ewe. Anesthesiology 41:462, 1974.
41. Vasicka, A, et al: Spinal and epidural anesthesia: fetal and uterine response to acute hypo- and hypertension. Am J Obstet Gynecol 90:800, 1964.
42. Galloon, S: Ketamine for obstetric delivery. Anesthesiology 44:522, 1976.
43. Levinson, G, et al: Effects of maternal hyperventilation on uterine blood flow and fetal oxygenation and acid-base status. Anesthesiology 40:340, 1974.
44. Adamsons, K, Mueller-Heubach, E and Myers, RE: Production of fetal asphyxia in the rhesus monkey by administration of catecholamines to the mother. Am J Obstet Gynecol 109:148, 1971.
45. Rosenfeld, CR, Barton, MD and Meschia, G: Effects of epinephrine on distribution of blood flow in the pregnant ewe. Am J Obstet Gynecol 124:156, 1976.
46. Slone, D, et al: Maternal drug exposure and fetal abnormalities. Clin Pharmacol Therap 14:648, 1973.
47. Shepard, TH: Catalog of Teratogenic Agents, ed 3. Johns Hopkins University Press, Baltimore, 1980.
48. Roux, C: Action tératogène de la prochlorpérazine. Arch Franc Pédiatr 16:968, 1959.
49. Robson, JM and Sullivan, FM: The production of foetal abnormalities in rabbits by imipramine. Lancet 1:638, 1963.
50. Tonge, SR: Permanent alterations in catecholamine concentrations in discrete areas of brain in the offspring of rats treated with methylamphetamine and chlorpromazine. Br J Pharmacol 47:425, 1973.
51. Goldman, AS and Yakovac, WC: Prevention of salicylate teratogenicity in immobilized rats by certain central nervous system depressants. Proc Soc Exp Biol Med 115:693, 1964.
52. Milkovich, L and van den Berg, BJ: Effects of prenatal meprobamate and chlordiazepoxide hydrochloride on human embryonic and fetal development. N Engl J Med 291:1268, 1974.
53. Hartz, SC, et al: Antenatal exposure to meprobamate and chlordiazepoxide in relation to malformations, mental development and childhood mortality. N Engl J Med 292:726, 1975.
54. Saxén, I and Saxén, L: Association between maternal intake of diazepam and oral clefts. Lancet 2:498, 1975.
55. Safra, MJ and Oakley, GP: Association between cleft lip with or without cleft palate and prenatal exposure to diazepam. Lancet 2:478, 1975.
56. Rice, SA and Pellegrini, M: Teratology of fixed agents. In Baden, JM and Brodsky, JB (eds): The Pregnant Surgical Patient. Futura Publishing Co., Mt Kisco, NY, 1985, pp 53–82.
57. Slone, D, et al: Antenatal exposure to the phenothiazines in relation to congenital malformations, perinatal mortality rate, birth weight, and intelligence quotient score. Am J Obstet Gynecol 128:486, 1977.
58. Geber, WF and Schramm, LC: Congenital malformations of the central nervous system produced by narcotic analgesics in the hamster. Am J Obstet Gynecol 123:705, 1975.
59. Jurand, A: Teratogenic activity of methadone hydrochloride in mouse and chick embryos. J Embryol Exp Morphol 30:449, 1973.
60. Markham, JK, Emerson, JL and Owen, NV: Teratogenicity studies of methadone HCl in rats and rabbits. Nature 233:342. 1971.
61. Steele, WJ and Johannesson, T: Effects of prenatally-administered morphine on brain development and resultant tolerance to the analgesic effect of morphine in offspring of morphine-treated rats. Acta Pharmacol Toxicol 36:243, 1975.
62. Davis, WM and Lin, CH: Prenatal morphine effects on survival and behaviour of rat offspring. Res Commun Chem Pathol Pharmacol 3:205, 1972.
63. Wyner, J and Cohen, SE: Gastric volume in early pregnancy: Effect of metoclopramide. Anesthesiology 57:209, 1982.
64. Breen, KJ, et al: Effects of cimetidine and ranitidine on hepatic drug metabolism. Clin Pharmacol Ther 31:297, 1982.
65. Wood, M, et al: The effect of cimetidine on anesthetic metabolism and toxicity. Anesth Analg 65:481, 1986.
66. Cohen, SE, Woods, WA and Wyner, J: Antiemetic efficacy of droperidol and metoclopramide. Anesthesiology 60:67, 1984.
67. Rao, TLK, Suseela, M and El-Etr, AA: Metoclopramide and cimetidine to reduce gastric pH and volume. Anesth Analg 63:264, 1984.
68. Morgan, DJ, et al: Pharmacokinetics and plasma binding of thiopental. II: Anesthesiology 54:474, 1981.
69. Marx, GF, Hwang, HS and Chandra, P: Postpartum uterine pressures with different doses of ketamine. Anesthesiology 50:163, 1979.
70. Oats, JN, Vasey, DP and Waldron, BA: Effects of ketamine on the pregnant uterus. Br J Anaesth 51:1163, 1979.
71. Kissin, I, et al: Inotropic and anesthetic potencies of etomidate and thiopental in dogs. Anesth Analg 62:961, 1983.
72. Wagner, RL and White, PF: Etomidate vs thiopental: Comparative effects on adrenocortical function (abstr). Anesthesiology 61:353, 1984.
73. Suresh, MS, et al: Etomidate pharmacokinetics during cesarean section (abstr). Anesthesiology 65:388, 1986.
74. Drachman, DB and Coulombre, AJ: Experimental clubfoot and arthrogryposis multiplex congenita. Lancet 2:523, 1962.
75. Conklin, KA and Murad, SHN: Pharmacology of drugs in obstetric anesthesia. Semin Anesth 1:83, 1982.
76. Green, CD and Eastwood, DW: Effects of nitrous oxide inhalation on hemopoiesis in rats. Anesthesiology 24:341, 1963.
77. Anderson, NB: The effect of CNS depressants on mitosis. Acta Anaesth Scand Supplement XXII 10:1, 1966.
78. Fink, BR, Shepard, TH and Blandau, RJ: Terato-

genic activity of nitrous oxide. Nature 214:146, 1967.
79. Smith, BE, Gaub, MI and Moya, F: Teratogenic effects of anesthetic agents: Nitrous oxide. Anesth Analg 44:726, 1965.
80. Vieira, E, et al: Effects of low concentrations of nitrous oxide on rat fetuses. Anesth Analg 59:175, 1980.
81. Pope, WDB, et al: Fetotoxicity in rats following chronic exposure to halothane, nitrous oxide or methoxyflurane. Anesthesiology 48:11, 1978.
82. Mazze, RI, et al: Reproduction and fetal development in mice chronically exposed to nitrous oxide. Teratology 26:11, 1982.
83. Chanarin, I: Cobalamins and nitrous oxide: A review. J Clin Pathol 33:909, 1980.
84. Koblin, DD, et al: Nitrous oxide inactivates methionine synthetase in human liver. Anesth Analg 61:75, 1982.
85. Baden, JM, Serra, M and Mazze, RI: Inhibition of fetal methionine synthase by nitrous oxide. Br J Anaesth 56:523, 1984.
86. Nunn, JF and Chanarin, I: Nitrous oxide inactivates methionine synthetase. In Eger, EI, II (ed): Nitrous Oxide/N_2O. Elsevier, New York, 1985, p 221.
87. Eger, EI, II: Should we not use nitrous oxide? In: Eger, EI, II (ed): Nitrous Oxide/N_2O. Elsevier, New York, 1985, p 339.
88. Nunn, JF, et al: Effect of short-term administration of nitrous oxide on plasma concentration of methionine, tryptophan, phenylalanine, and S-adenosyl methionine in man. Br J Anaesth 58:1, 1986.
89. O'Sullivan, H, et al: Human bone marrow biochemical function and megaloblastic hematopoiesis after nitrous oxide anesthesia. Anesthesiology 55:645, 1981.
90. Belaisch-Allart, JC, et al: Various techniques for oocyte recovery in an in vitro fertilization and embryo transfer program. J Vitro Fert Embryo Transfer 2:99, 1985.
91. Crawford, JS and Lewis, M: Nitrous oxide in early human pregnancy. Anaesthesia 41:900, 1986.
92. Aldridge, LM and Tunstall, ME: Nitrous oxide and the fetus: a review and the results of a retrospective study of 175 cases of anaesthesia for insertion of Shirodkhar suture. Br J Anaesth 58:1348, 1986.
93. Mazze, RI: Nitrous oxide during pregnancy (editorial). Anaesthesia 41:897, 1986.
94. Basford, AB and Fink, BR: The teratogenicity of halothane in the rat. Anesthesiology 29:1167, 1968.
95. Bussard, DA, et al: Fetal changes in hamsters anesthetized with nitrous oxide and halothane. Anesthesiology 41:275, 1974.
96. Kennedy, GL, et al: Reproductive and teratologic studies with halothane. Toxicol Appl Pharmacol 35:467, 1976.
97. Wharton, RS, et al: Fetal morphology in mice exposed to halothane. Anesthesiology 51:532, 1979.
98. Wharton, RS, Mazze, RI and Wilson, AI: Reproduction and fetal development in mice chronically exposed to enflurane. Anesthesiology 54:505, 1981.
99. Mazze, RI, et al: Effects of isoflurane on reproduction and fetal development in mice. Anesth Analg 63:249, 1984.
100. Mazze, RI, et al: Reproductive and teratogenic effects of nitrous oxide, halothane, isoflurane and enflurane in Sprague-Dawley rats. Anesthesiology: 63:A439, 1985.
101. Biehl, DR, et al: Effect of halothane on cardiac output and regional flow in the fetal lamb in utero. Anesth Analg 62:489, 1983.
102. Biehl, DR, et al: The uptake of isoflurane by the foetal lamb in utero: Effect on regional blood flow. Can Anaesth Soc J 30:581, 1983.
103. Sturrock, JE and Nunn, JF: Cytotoxic effects of procaine, lignocaine and bupivacaine. Br J Anaesth 51:273, 1979.
104. Adamsons, K and Joelsson, I: The effects of pharmacologic agents upon the fetus and newborn. Am J Obstet Gynecol 96:437, 1966.
105. Heinonen, OP, Slone, O and Shapiro, S: Birth defects and drugs in pregnancy. Publishing Sciences Group, Littleton, MA, 1977, p 516.
106. Hodach, RJ, et al: Aortic arch anomalies associated with administration of epinephrine in chick embryos. Teratology 9:203, 1974.
107. Callendar, K, et al: Dopamine administration in the normotensive pregnant ewe. Obstet Gynecol 51: 586, 1978.
108. Rosenfeld, CR, Barton, MD and Meschia, G: Effects of epinephrine on distribution of blood flow in the pregnant ewe. Am J Obstet Gynecol 124:156, 1976.
109. Grabowski, CT and Paar, JA: The teratogenic effects of graded doses of hypoxia on the chick embryo. Am J Anat 103:313, 1958.
110. Ingalls, TH, Curley, FJ and Prindle, RA: Anoxia as a cause of fetal death and congenital defect in the mouse. Am J Dis Child 80:34, 1960.
111. Haring, OM: The effects of prenatal hypoxia on the cardiovascular system in the rat. Arch Pathol 80: 351, 1965.
112. Haring, OM: Cardiac malformations in rats induced by exposure of the mother to carbon dioxide during pregnancy. Circ Res 8:1218, 1960.
113. Hannah, RS and Moore, KL: Effects of fasting and insulin on skeletal development in rats. Teratology 4:135, 1971.
114. Ferm, BH: Teratogenic effects of hyperbaric oxygen. Proc Soc Exp Biol Med 116:975, 1964.
115. Fujikura, T: Retrolental fibroplasia and prematurity in newborn rabbits induced by maternal hyperoxia. Am J Obstet Gynecol 90:854, 1964.
116. Katz, JD, Hook, R and Barash, PG: Fetal heart rate monitoring in the pregnant patient under surgery. Am J Obstet Gynecol 125:267, 1976.
117. Liu, PL, et al: Foetal monitoring in parturients undergoing surgery unrelated to pregnancy. Can Anaesth Soc J 32:525, 1985.
118. Hehre, FW: Hypothermia for operations during pregnancy. Anesth Analg 44:424, 1965.
119. Kofke, WA, Wuest, HP and McGinnis, LA: Cesarean section following ruptured cerebral aneurysm and neuroresuscitation. Anesthesiology 60:242, 1984.
120. Estafanous, FG and Buckley, S: Management of anes-

thesia for open heart surgery during pregnancy. Cleve Clin Q 43:121, 1976.

121. Trimakas, AP, et al: Fetal monitoring during cardiac pulmonary bypass for removal of a left atrial myxoma during pregnancy. Johns Hopkins Med J 144:156, 1979.

122. Bahary, CM, et al: Tococardiography in pregnancy during extracorporeal bypass for mitral valve replacement. Israel J Med Sci 16:395, 1980.

123. Becker, RM: Intracardiac surgery in pregnant women. Ann Thorac Surg 36:453, 1983.

CHAPTER 28

IN VITRO FERTILIZATION

FRED J. SPIELMAN, M.D.

The concept of in vitro fertilization (IVF) and embryo transfer has interested reproductive physiologists for several decades. In 1959 Chang[1] achieved success with extracorporeal fertilization in rabbits. During the following years veterinarians utilized this technique with cattle, sheep, pigs, and horses.[2] Edwards and Steptoe originally devised the technique for human IVF for relief of otherwise incorrectable tubal infertility.[3] In England, after 109 embryo transfers, the first two live births occurred in 1978 and 1979. The Department of Obstetrics and Gynecology at Eastern Virginia Medical School achieved success by 1981 and became the first IVF center in the United States. By 1981, an increasing number of centers reported births following IVF, and by 1982 IVF had produced over 100 children. Presently this technique has resulted in over 2000 babies worldwide. Although only 10 years have passed since the birth of the first human conceived through IVF, the method has emerged as an effective option for many infertile couples.[4]

Currently more than 50 American medical centers offer IVF and many more plan to do so in the future.[5] More than 25 programs exist in Great Britain.[6] In 1982, the Board of Directors of the American Fertility Society recognized IVF as an acceptable treatment for infertility in couples in which the wife has absent or irreparable damage of the fallopian tubes.[7]

IVF circumvents the blocked fallopian tubes by harvesting the mature egg, most commonly via laparoscopy, just prior to its discharge from the follicle. Following transfer to an external medium, exposure to sperm takes place, fertilization occurs, and development ensues in a controlled environment. Finally, the fertilized egg is returned to the uterine cavity for continued maturation.[8]

IVF and embryo transfer are labor-intensive undertakings which require as many as 20 staff members. Successful IVF programs necessitate integration of physicians and technologists with diverse skills, including a reproductive endocrinologist to supervise and monitor follicular development, a surgeon skilled in laparoscopy, oocyte retrieval and embryo transfer, and technicians to prepare the required special growth media. Hospital laboratories must be able to perform daily assays for hormones.[9] During the course of a treatment cycle, the IVF team must function 7 days a week. All of this points to the advantage of associating IVF with a large hospital, especially one connected with academic medicine.[8]

The surgeon and the patient often incorrectly classify the surgery and anesthesia required with IVF as minor events since oocyte retrieval requires a small skin incision, can be accomplished quickly, and takes place in an ambulatory surgery environment. However, the ability to perform a safe and successful anesthetic for IVF calls for attention to many important aspects of the procedure. Recovery from anesthesia must occur rapidly, with a minimum of side effects. The anesthesiologist must understand and cope with the physiologic implications of pneumoperitoneum, Trendelenburg position, and the use of intraperitoneal carbon dioxide, while minimizing the risks of aspiration of gastric contents, gas embolism, hypoxia, hypercarbia, and nerve damage that may accompany these major physiologic alterations.

Obstetric Considerations for in Vitro Fertilization

PATIENT SELECTION AND EVALUATION

Initially, only women with damaged or absent fallopian tubes qualified for IVF. Recently the indications for IVF have broadened to include male factors, endometriosis, cervical mucus abnormalities, and unexplained long-term infertility. Although artificial insemination with donor sperm is effective in patients with oligospermia, a rather common cause of infertility, many couples reject this alternative since IVF gives them a chance to have their own child.[4] Patients with endometriosis who have failed to conceive following surgery and hormone therapy are excellent candidates for IVF. Unexplained infertility may be due to defects in the sperms' fertilizing ability, the oocytes' ability to be fertilized, or the ability of the embryo to implant in the uterus.[10]

Usually, laparoscopy is a relatively safe, low-risk procedure; however, it should not be performed on patients for whom anesthesia would be contraindicated or on patients with chronic medical problems that render pregnancy unsafe.

Pretreatment screening of all couples insures that no alternative therapy exists and that a reasonable chance of success with IVF can be anticipated.[10] Initially the IVF team carefully reviews the infertility history, including past evaluations and medical and surgical treatment. For patients with a history of extensive pelvic surgery and abdominal adhesions, a screening laparoscopy and/or an hysterosalpingogram may be necessary to establish the feasibility and safety of ovum aspiration.[4]

Diabetes mellitus, thyroid disease, and hypertension should be properly controlled during the pre-conception period. Patient counseling with regard to dietary habits, smoking, and alcohol consumption increases the chances of a successful outcome of pregnancy.[5] Finally, an andrology survey of the partner is an important area of investigation, to determine the adequacy of motile sperm and to rule out infection.[11]

IN VITRO FERTILIZATION PROTOCOL

The process of IVF involves obtaining mature oocytes and incubating them with sperm. Transfer of the embryos into the uterine cavity follows, where they implant and pregnancy progresses naturally.[4]

Follicular Stimulation and Aspiration

An attempt to stimulate multiple ovarian follicles represents the initial procedure in IVF. Most programs employ combinations of clomiphene citrate, human chorionic gonadotropin (hCG), follicle-stimulating hormone (FSH; Metrodin), or gonadotropin-releasing hormone (GRH) to induce oocyte recruitment with the goal of aspirating preovulatory oocytes just before their release from the follicle. Oocyte collection takes place as close as possible to the time of expected ovulation to avoid immature oocytes (if done too early) or spontaneous ovulation (if done too late).[12] Daily cervical mucus analysis and serum estrogen levels help determine the best time for oocyte aspiration. Ideally, ultrasound examination will reveal a minimum of two follicles more than 15 mm in diameter just prior to aspiration.

Oocyte Aspiration

The surgeon usually aspirates the follicles early in the morning to prevent emergencies from delaying the procedure and he must obtain a large number of oocytes since the pregnancy rate improves as the number of embryos transferred to the uterus increases. The surgeon aspirates only follicles measuring more than 10 mm; smaller follicles tend to contain immature oocytes, which have a lower fertilization rate.[12]

Follicle aspiration may be achieved by laparoscopy or by ultrasonographically guided aspiration via the abdomen or vagina. The abdominal approach takes place through a full bladder; the transvaginal technique passes through the fornix by culdocentesis. Direct visualization of the ovaries is the major advantage of the laparoscopic technique. Unfortunately, laparoscopy usually requires general anesthesia with its associated morbidity, and the presence of adhesions occasionally renders the ovaries inaccessible, decreasing the success of the procedure. Although laparoscopy has served as the traditional and most widely employed method, over the past few years, the ultrasonographically guided technique has emerged as a viable alternative.[12] The transvaginal approach causes fewer complications than the transabdominal method. Aspiration can be performed from either freely mobile ovaries or those bound by adhesions. Ultrasound recovers fewer oocytes than laparoscopy; however both methods produce a similar number of successful pregnancies.[13]

Semen Preparation

The partner donates semen 2 to 4 hours before insemination after abstaining from sex for 3 to 5 days. Technicians liquefy the semen, mix it with insemination medium, and incubate it for about 30 min in an atmosphere of 5-percent carbon dioxide prior to inseminating oocytes with over one million sperm in 3 cc of insemination medium.[14]

Fertilization, Cleavage, and Embryo Transfer

Examination of the follicular contents occurs in a laboratory adjacent to the operating room. Following identification and isolation from the follicular fluid the oocyte is placed in an organ culture dish containing the sperm, insemination medium, and fetal serum. Transfer occurs most commonly when the embryo reaches the four- to eight-cell stage. An earlier transfer offers the theoretical advantages of shortening the time the embryo remains in an artificial medium and hastening the time of return to a more natural environment. Later transfer, however, allows more precise control and monitoring of the embryo's development. Transfer usually takes place 40 to 50 hours after insemination.[14]

Once normal embryo development has been confirmed the patient moves to a room next to the surgical suite and is positioned appropriately for embryo transfer. An anterior uterus calls for a knee-chest position while a posterior uterus indicates the dorsal lithotomy position in order to keep the fundus lower than the cervix. The embryos are placed in a transfer catheter and introduced into the uterine cavity. After transfer, the patient remains prone or supine for 4 hours and then remains relatively inactive for the next 48 hours.[4] Embryo transfer requires minimal medication; a small dose of diazepam or midazolam suffices for particularly anxious patients. Commencing on the day of embryo transfer, many IVF centers administer progesterone suppositories or injections to ensure adequate endometrial development.

OUTCOME OF IN VITRO FERTILIZATION PREGNANCIES

In the early years of IVF (1978 to 1981) the pregnancy rate ranged from 1 to 8 percent, but a steady rise in successful outcome has followed, with the rate currently standing at 15 to 20 percent. Several factors account for the improved outcome. More precise monitoring of the ovulatory process has permitted the harvesting of a large number of mature oocytes. Hormonal stimulation of follicles has improved oocyte recovery, and multiple embryo transfers have also added to the better pregnancy statistics.[15] If the uterus receives one embryo, the chance of a pregnancy is about 10 percent; two embryos increase this to 15 percent; three, to 20 percent; and four to more than 25 percent.[6] Women 40 years or older experience pregnancy rates of less than 10 percent. Success increases to 12 percent in women between 30 to 39 years of age and is highest in those under 30 years. Difficulty in stimulating ovulation may partially account for the lower success rates in older women; however, the reduced quality of the ova and endometrium may also play a significant role.[16]

The extraordinary nature of conception in pregnancies achieved with IVF raises the possibility of the increased risk of producing fetal abnormalities, such as multiple gestation, abortions, ectopic pregnancy, and chromosomal abnormalities. Several factors probably contribute to a greater obstetric risk in IVF than in natural pregnancy. The women tend to be older, often have a history of previous reproductive losses or endocrine problems, and frequently have undergone tubal surgery.[17]

After pregnancy is well established, obstetric care requires no specific precautions. The decision to routinely perform amniocentesis remains controversial. Two cases of spontaneous abortion have already been reported following complications of amniocentesis in IVF patients. Most centers perform this test only for usual indications, such as advanced maternal age, history of neural tube defects, or to detect certain sex-linked carrier states.[18] Ultrasonographic studies are less controversial. Although no evidence suggests that a viable pregnancy calls for an ultrasound examination, given the benign nature of the test and the newness of the IVF process, most centers use this screening technique.[5]

Multiple Gestation

Multiple gestation occurs 10 times more often following IVF than in natural cycles because of the practice of transferring many embryos.[18] Multiple gestation predisposes to an increased rate of prematurity, pregnancy-induced hypertension, and fetal loss. Multiple pregnancy presents a real concern and may have a rate as high as 25 to 35 percent. Overall, multiple gestation rates stand at 10 percent for twins, 1.4 percent for triplets, and 0.3 percent for quadruplets. The risk of multiple conceptions limits the number of embryos transferred. Most IVF programs transfer a maximum of three to four embryos, which gives an excellent chance of success and limits the multiple pregnancy rate to 15 to 25 percent.[16]

Ectopic Pregnancy

Ectopic pregnancy following IVF occurs three times more often than in the normal population. Retrograde transport of the embryo, excessive volume of transfer medium, a forceful injection close to or into the tubal ostium, pre-existing tubal disease, and previous tubal surgery account for the increased rate.[16]

Congenital Malformations

A possible increased risk for congenital malformations represents a major concern with IVF. Factors influencing the chance of chromosomal abnormalities and congenital malformations in IVF pregnancies include advanced age, drugs used to stimulate ovulation, and the procedures to prepare the sperm and oocyte, including mechanical manipulation, artificial growth media, exposure to light, and fluctuating temperatures. Based on the limited data available, no evidence of an increase in the incidence of congenital malformations after IVF exists; final conclusions await larger numbers of conceptions.[16,18]

Spontaneous Abortion

Inclusion of those cases in which maternal blood levels of B-hCG increase initially and then decline pushes the incidence of spontaneous abortion after IVF to 50 to 80 percent. Most of these "abortions," actually represent "failed chemical pregnancies," indicating early problems with implantation rather than early abortion after successful implantation.[17] In contrast, spontaneous abortion after the absence of one menstrual period occurs in 12 to 30 percent of IVF pregnancies. The likely causes of abortion include chromosomal abnormalities of the embryo, inadequate function of the corpus luteum, and insufficient development of the endometrium. Remember, however, that approximately 15 percent of normal conceptions result in spontaneous abortions.

Cesarean Section

No evidence suggests that a favorable outcome requires a cesarean section, providing that the pregnancy has been uncomplicated.[5] IVF pregnancies do, however, result in a high cesarean section rate (33 to 56 percent)[18,19] because of increased numbers of multiple gestations, older maternal age, and increased incidence of pregnancy-induced hypertension. The pregnancy-induced hypertension most likely reflects the older age, multiple gestation, and primigravidity of the typical IVF patient. The obstetrician's concern for the "premium nature" of these pregnancies also contributes to the unusually high incidence of cesarean section.[20]

It is vital to follow up the progress of children conceived by IVF in order to detect any adverse outcomes in their physical and psychological development. There should also be some assessment of the parent-child relationship. Only careful study of thousands of IVF pregnancies and the children will provide definite conclusions about the fetal and maternal risks of the procedure.

Anesthetic Considerations

OOCYTE RETRIEVAL

Despite the low mortality and morbidity associated with laparoscopy, the occasional occurrence of a catastrophic complication indicates that follicular aspiration carries some risk. Aspiration of follicles via laparoscopy requires the creation of the pneumoperitoneum; if done incorrectly this may result in a significant number of complications. The lower margin of the umbilicus is the ideal site for the insertion of the veress needle, followed by the trocar, sleeve, and laparoscope. This relatively avascular area is the thinnest portion of the abdominal wall, and adhesions rarely occur in this location.[21] An incorrectly placed needle may insufflate the abdominal wall, the retroperitoneum, the mesentery, the omentum, or the bowel.

Pneumoperitoneum

Carbon dioxide and nitrous oxide are used for producing the pneumoperitoneum. High solubility, which permits rapid absorption of any gas remaining postoperatively and gives a margin of safety if accidentally injected intravascularly, makes carbon dioxide the gas of choice. The theoretical possibility of altering the pH of the follicular fluid is the main concern with the use of carbon dioxide. The transperitoneal pressure gradient into the blood may produce hypercarbia. Nitrous oxide is not absorbed during pneumoperitoneum in quantities sufficient to cause hypoxia, nor does it sustain combustion.[22] Nitrous oxide proves especially helpful when performing the operation with local analgesia since it causes less diaphragmatic and peritoneal irritation than carbon dioxide.[23]

Trendelenburg Position

Laparoscopy requires that the patient assume the Trendelenburg position. This head-down position allows the abdominal organs to gravitate toward the diaphragm and out of the pelvis, making the ovaries easily visualized and accessible. Meticulous care and proper positioning reduce the severity of soft-tissue and neurologic complications associated with this operative requirement. One of the patient's arms should be at her side so that the surgeon can be in the optimal position to operate. The superficial course of the ulnar nerve dictates that the elbow be adequately padded. Shoulder rests prevent the patient from sliding off when the operating table is tilted more than 45 degrees. Brachial plexus injury is the most common neural complication of Trendelenburg position. Shoulder braces can depress the clavicle into the retroclavicular space, causing direct compression and stretching of the nerve roots. Prevention depends on careful positioning of the arms at the patient's side, or, if extended, the arm must not be hyperextended. Caution the surgeon about leaning on the patient's extended arm, and place the shoulder rest at the acromioclavicular junction and not over the clavicle.[24]

Cardiac Physiology and Complications

Laparoscopy alters cardiac physiology. Severe hypotension and cardiac arrest rarely occur, but less significant changes such as mild reduction of arterial pressure and cardiac output happen commonly. These cardiovascular changes result from the head-down position and pneumoperitoneum.[25] Increased intra-abdominal pressure reduces venous return; when this pressure exceeds 30 mmHg, significant decreases in central venous, arterial, and pulse pressures occur, as well as a small decrease in cardiac output.[26] The pneumoperitoneum sequesters blood in the legs and reduces the circulating blood volume. Routine intraoperative blood pressure and heart rate monitoring may not indicate a drop in cardiac output because compensatory mechanisms usually operate effectively in healthy women.[25] At the conclusion of the operation the patient should be returned slowly to the horizontal position, to allow gradual shunting of blood from the thorax and upper extremities into the lower extremities. This will decrease the incidence and severity of hypotension.[24]

Pulmonary Physiology and Complications

The Trendelenburg position and pneumoperitoneum produce cephalad pressure on the diaphragm and significantly reduce vital capacity. Restriction of lung capacity and increased pulmonary blood volume result from the head-down tilt. These factors decrease pulmonary compliance, diminish functional residual capacity, and compromise aeration of the lower lobes, all of which may cause postoperative atelectasis.[27]

Alexander, Noe, and Brown[28] reported a significant rise in $PaCO_2$ and a fall in pH in patients who underwent laparoscopy with general anesthesia when carbon dioxide produced the pneumoperitoneum. Increased absorption of carbon dioxide from the peritoneal cavity caused the hypercarbia. The blood rapidly absorbs carbon dioxide because of the high difference in partial pressures between the pneumoperitoneum and the blood perfusing the abdomen. Spontaneous ventilation can lead to significant hypercarbia because of diminished alveolar ventilation and exogenous carbon dioxide. Controlled ventilation and the use of a respirometer and end-tidal gas analyzer obviate this problem.

Steep Trendelenburg position requires endotracheal intubation. The position of the endotracheal tube should be confirmed after the Trendelenburg position is assumed since the mediastinum may shift cephalad, causing the endotracheal tube to pass into a bronchus.[23]

Gas embolism rarely occurs but represents a potentially fatal complication of laparoscopy. Intravascular injection of gas may follow direct needle or trocar placement into a vessel or may develop indirectly from insufflation of gas into an abdominal organ. A high index of suspicion when cardiac arrhythmias and hypotension occur aids early diagnosis. The characteristic auscultatory changes in heart sounds occur later (mill-wheel murmur). Precordial Doppler ultrasound provides the most sensitive method for detecting a gas embolism. End-tidal gas analysis also is helpful.[29]

Pneumothorax is another potentially serious complication. The gas may dissect retroperitoneally through congenital foramina and produce a pneumomediastinum, or it may enter the chest cavity through defects in the diaphragm or weak points of the aortic and esophageal hiatus. Cyanosis, hypotension, subcutaneous emphysema, or an increase in the peak inspiratory pressure are signs of pneumothorax. Awake patients may complain of dyspnea and chest pain. Hyperresonance on chest percussion and absent or diminished breath sounds constitute further evidence of pneumothorax.[30]

Hemorrhage

Hemorrhage from laparoscopy accounts for almost half of all complications. Blood vessel injuries range from minor bleeding from superficial vessels to massive hemorrhage due to lacerations of major retroperitoneal vessels. Either the verres needle or the trocar may be responsible for trauma.[31] The blind insertion of the needle and trocar demands strict attention to anatomic landmarks and safe insertion techniques including the use of sharp instruments, adequately established pneumoperitoneum, elevation of the abdominal wall, avoidance of lateral insertion of the needle and trocar, and Trendelenburg position.

ANESTHETIC TECHNIQUE FOR FOLLICULAR ASPIRATION

Premedication

Oocyte retrievals are usually outpatient procedures; therefore, the anesthetic administered must ensure that the patient will recover quickly and be well enough to leave the medical center within a few hours after the procedure. With these goals in mind, many anesthesiologists avoid premedication with sedatives or long-acting narcotics. The preanesthetic visit may alleviate anxiety more effectively than any drugs. Providing the patient with a pleasant waiting area and permitting continued support from a relative or friend until the time of surgery will help the patient remain calm.[32]

Ong[33] demonstrated that nonobese adult outpatients undergoing elective surgery face a greater risk of aspiration than inpatients because of larger volumes of highly acidic gastric contents. Manchikanti and colleagues[34] have shown that 88 percent of unpremedicated patients have a gastric pH less than 2.5 and 56 percent have gastric volumes greater than 25 cc with a pH less than 2.5. They also observed that premedication with diazepam, hydroxyzine, or prochlorperazine does not alter the pH or gastric volumes as compared to no premedication. These results have prompted anesthesiologists to consider the administration of antacids, histamine-receptor antagonists, and gastroprokinetic drugs such as metoclopramide to all patients undergoing IVF. Nevertheless, no convincing evidence exists that prophylactic therapy eliminates pulmonary damage or reduces anesthesia-related mortality if aspiration occurs.

In recent years gynecologists have successfully employed local, regional, and general anesthesia for laparoscopy. The ideal anesthetic for follicular aspiration does not cause oocyte toxicity, minimizes the stress of the laparoscopy, permits rapid recovery, has no effects following repeated administration, and causes minimal side effects.[14]

Local Anesthesia

Local anesthesia offers the advantages of reduced anesthesia time, faster postoperative recovery, less nausea and vomiting, fewer postoperative complications, and lower costs when compared with other anesthetic techniques.[35,36] The awake patient facilitates early awareness of complications such as carbon dioxide embolus, pneumothorax, and hemorrhage. Finally, the surgeon can demonstrate anatomy and pathology directly to the patient by means of a fiberoptic teaching extension. Local anesthesia for follicular aspiration, although technically easy, is unsuitable for most patients. Unlike laparoscopy for tubal ligation, follicular aspiration requires multiple puncture sites and considerable abdominal and pelvic organ manipulation. The steep Trendelenburg position and necessarily large pneumoperitoneum make breathing difficult. The severe head-down tilt causes intracranial blood stasis resulting in significant discomfort. The patient undergoing laparoscopic oocyte retrieval with local anesthesia must be cooperative, calm, and able to withstand mild to moderate pain during the procedure.

For the transabdominal approach for follicular aspiration, local anesthetics are infiltrated in the suprapubic area. For the transvaginal approach, the vaginal wall is anesthetized. The anesthesiologist administers small incremental doses of short-acting narcotics and sedatives as required for patient comfort. Numerous drugs and drug combinations have served to supplement local anesthesia. Unanimity of opinion regarding superiority of one type of drug therapy has not evolved. The administration of the drugs in appropriate doses with proper patient monitoring is most important.

Intravenous sedation requires trained personnel to monitor the patient's airway, ventilation, and other vital functions; all narcotics and most sedatives can depress respiration. Therefore, anesthesia personnel should attend the surgical procedure.

Regional Anesthesia

Regional anesthesia, frequently used for laparoscopic tubal ligation and diagnostic laparoscopy, is rarely employed for oocyte retrieval. Spinal and epidural analgesia have the advantages of reducing the need for sedatives and narcotics and produce excellent muscle relaxation. Regional anesthesia avoids the postoperative discomforts of general anesthesia such as sore throat, muscle pains, and airway trauma. Recovery time from general anesthesia is longer than from regional. However, surgical manipulation, steep Trendelenburg position, and pneumoperitoneum often make spontaneous ventilation difficult. Many outpatient centers avoid spinal anesthesia in young women for fear of post–lumbar puncture headaches, while other centers do not administer epidural anesthesia since the block takes a relatively long time to administer and "set-up."

General Anesthesia

In spite of the recent popularity of local and regional anesthesia, the vast majority of laparoscopic follicular aspirations are performed using general anesthesia. It provides excellent muscle relaxation, the ability to control ventilation, elimination of patient anxiety, complete analgesia and amnesia, and a still operative field. No ideal technique exists for general anesthesia for follicular aspiration. Regardless of the method chosen, patient safety and comfort plus quick discharge from the outpatient center should be the goals. The general anesthesia technique should minimize nausea, headache, sore throat, and muscle pains.[32]

Although pregnancies have followed the use of oocytes obtained after prolonged general anesthesia, the harvesting team should prepare the abdomen and all necessary equipment prior to the induction of anesthesia to minimize exposure time.[12]

Following an intravenous induction, oxygen, nitrous oxide, and small amounts of potent inhalation agents, short-acting narcotics and muscle relaxants commonly provide anesthesia. The use of steep Trendelenburg position, high intra-abdominal filling pressure, low pH, and large volumes of gastric contents mandate tracheal intubation.

Induction of anesthesia with short-acting barbiturates represents the most common and suitable technique. Endler and associates[37] have demonstrated thiamylol in the follicular fluid as early as 13 minutes after injection. Nitrous oxide proves particularly useful in the outpatient setting by decreasing the requirement for the longer-acting agents.[32] Prolonged nitrous oxide exposure can interfere with DNA synthesis and therefore detrimentally affect early embryonic development. Since nitrous oxide inhibits methionine synthesis activity, Roizen and coworkers[38] investigated whether it affects oocyte function. They concluded that nitrous oxide does not decrease success rates or increase chromosomal abnormalities.

Intubation and surgery require muscle relaxation. The use of an intermediate-duration, nondepolarizing relaxant such as vecuronium or atracurium for both intubation and surgery will avoid the use of succinylcholine, thereby eliminating myalgias. Outpatients experience a significantly greater incidence and severity of muscle pains than inpatients.

The use of a small amount of potent inhalation agent ensures patient amnesia. Isoflurane has the lowest blood-gas coefficient (1.3) and the shortest elimination time. It also undergoes the least metabolism, reducing patient exposure to metabolites that might have the potential for delayed toxicity.[32,39] In comparing halothane, enflurane, and isoflurane for a short anesthetic, no single agent appears to be superior in facilitating quick discharge from the recovery room.[40]

Intraoperative narcotics reduce the necessary concentration of potent inhalation agent while minimizing pain at the end of surgery. The narcotic employed must have a rapid onset, short duration, and produce minimal cardiovascular depression. Fentanyl has these favorable characteristics. The onset of analgesia follows intravenous administration within 2 min, and pain relief lasts about 45 min. Doses of 1 to 2 μg per kg usually suffice.[32]

Postoperative Pain

Following laparoscopy, all patients experience some discomfort. Incisional pain, diffuse abdominal discomfort, and referred shoulder pain are the most common symptoms reported by patients. With succinylcholine use, generalized myalgia commonly develops. Since incisional and abdominal discomfort are usually mild, the appearance of moderate to severe pain raises the possibility of a subcutaneous or subfascial hematoma.[6] Irritation of the peritoneum underlying the diaphragm causes pain referred to the shoulder because diaphragmatic sensory innervation travels by way of the phrenic nerve. Regional anesthesia reduces the incidence of postoperative pain and facilitates its control. When required, small doses of analgesics given intravenously provide the safest and most efficacious method of pain control in the recovery room. Fentanyl, 12.5 to 50 μg, usually brings rapid relief of discomfort without delaying discharge.

Postoperative Nausea and Vomiting

Nausea and vomiting commonly follow general anesthesia and can be severe enough to require hospitalization, particularly after laparoscopy, which causes diaphragmatic irritation. A number of antiemetics have been used in an attempt to control the nausea and vomiting. The intraoperative administration of droperidol, 0.625 to

1.25 mg intravenously, has achieved considerable success.[41] Nitrous oxide increases middle ear pressure and distends the gastrointestinal tract and thereby may increase vomiting. Lonie and Harper[42] studied the effects of nitrous oxide on postoperative vomiting in women undergoing laparoscopy. They observed that patients receiving nitrous oxide had a significantly higher incidence of vomiting than women who did not receive the anesthetic.

Future of in Vitro Fertilization

Since the first IVF baby was delivered, many changes and improvements have taken place. Although the pregnancy rate for IVF now approaches 25 percent, many technical and theoretical problems remain to be solved. Among these are determining the best method for stimulating multiple follicles and improving the monitoring to insure retrieval of the most mature oocytes. Better media and culture environment could improve in vitro embryo growth. It is also important to reduce embryo trauma during transfer to the uterus.[15,43]

Excess embryos may be frozen and subsequently thawed and transferred. Presently only about half of the embryos survive freezing and thawing.[43] Cryopreservation of human embryos, therefore, requires further study. Screening embryos for genetic disease will be an area of intense investigation. Workers are developing DNA probes to detect genetic abnormalities. IVF could be offered to couples at risk of genetic disease. Two or more cells could be removed from the embryo and tested for an abnormal or absent gene.[43]

Despite the necessary time commitment, the operative risks involved, and the costs of up to $5000 per cycle (plus $2500 for screening), IVF offers a reasonable chance of pregnancy for couples who were previously believed to be infertile.

Summary

This chapter summarizes important aspects of IVF, including its history, indications, technical aspects, and outcome. Oocyte retrieval requires the presence of an anesthesiologist. Laparoscopic aspiration performed under general anesthesia reduces patient anxiety and provides excellent muscle relaxation, operating conditions, and ability to control ventilation. Endotracheal intubation is mandatory. Although no specific anesthetic regimen is required, oxygen, nitrous oxide, and small doses of potent inhalation agents and short-acting narcotics provide intraoperative analgesia and amnesia, and minimize postoperative discomfort. Knowledge of the physiologic changes that occur with the Trendelenburg position and pneumoperitoneum, and vigilance for signs of hemorrhage and gas embolism are essential to avoiding serious complications.

References

1. Chang, MC: Fertilization of rabbit ova in vitro. Nature 184:877, 1959.
2. Garcia, JE: In vitro fertilization. Obstet Gynecol Annu 14:45, 1985.
3. Steptoe, PC and Edwards, RG: Reimplantation of a human embryo with subsequent tubal pregnancy. Lancet 1:880, 1976.
4. Halme, J: In vitro fertilization: A new treatment for infertility. In Hammond, MG and Talbert, LM (eds): Infertility: A Practical Guide for the Physician. Medical Economics, Oradell, NJ, 1985.
5. Gonik, G: Pregnancy management following in vitro fertilization and embryo transfer. In Wolf, DP and Quigley, MM (eds): Human In Vitro Fertilization and Embryo Transfer. Plenum Press, New York, 1984, p 365.
6. Richards, T: IVF update. Br Med J 292:1156, 1986.
7. The American Fertility Society Annual Meeting, Las Vegas, March 20, 1982.
8. Grobstein, C, Flower, M and Mendeloff, J: External human fertilization: An evaluation of policy. Science 222:127, 1983.
9. Wolf, DP and Quigley, MM: Historical background and essentials for a program in in vitro fertilization and embryo transfer. In Wolf, DP and Quigley, MM (eds): Human In Vitro Fertilization and Embryo Transfer. Plenum Press, New York, 1984, p 1.
10. Quigley, MM: Patient screening and selection. In Wolf, DP and Quigley, MM (eds): Human In Vitro Fertilization and Embryo Transfer. Plenum Press, New York, 1984, p 37.
11. Jones, JW, Jr: In vitro fertilization. In Buttram, VC, Jr and Reiter, RC (eds): Surgical Treatment of the Infertile Female. Williams & Wilkins, Baltimore, 1985, p 355.
12. DeCherney, AH and Lavy, G: Oocyte recovery methods in in-vitro fertilization. Clin Obstet Gynecol 29:171, 1986.
13. Allart, JB, et al: Oocyte recovery under local anaesthesia. In Testart, J and Frydman, R (eds): Human In

Vitro Fertilization: Actual Problems and Prospects. Elsevier Science Publishers, Amsterdam, 1985, p 53.
14. Acosta, AA and Garcia, JE: Extracorporeal fertilization and embryo transfer. In Aiman, J (ed): Infertility: Diagnosis and Management. Springer-Verlag, New York, 1984, p 215.
15. Marrs, RP: In vitro fertilization's future looks bright. Cont Obstet Gynecol 20:135, 1982.
16. Laufer, N and Navot, D: Human in vitro fertilization. In DeCherney, AH (ed): Reproduction Failure. Churchill Livingstone, Edinburgh, 1986, p 219.
17. Walters, WAW: Pregnancy and its management. In Trounson, A and Wood, C (eds): In Vitro Fertilization and Embryo Transfer. Churchill Livingstone, Edinburgh, 1984, p 205.
18. Lancaster, PAL: Obstetric outcome. Clin Obstet Gynecol 12:847, 1985.
19. Andrews, MC, et al: An analysis of the obstetric outcome of 125 consecutive pregnancies conceived in vitro and resulting in 100 deliveries. Am J Obstet Gynecol 154:848, 1986.
20. Wood, C, et al: Clinical features of eight pregnancies resulting from in vitro fertilization and embryo transfer. Fertil Steril 38:22, 1982.
21. Cali, RW: Laparoscopy. Surg Clin North Am 60:407, 1980.
22. Corbett, TH, et al: End-expired nitrous oxide levels after pneumoperitoneum. Anesth Analg 53:527, 1974.
23. Rolbin, SH: Anesthesia for postpartum sterilization surgery. In Shnider, SM and Levinson, G (eds): Anesthesia for Obstetrics. Williams & Wilkins, Baltimore, 1986, p 182.
24. Schiller, WR: The Trendelenburg position. In Martin, JT (ed): Positioning in Anesthesia and Surgery. WB Saunders, Philadelphia, 1978, p 89.
25. Borten, M: Laparoscopic Complications: Prevention and Management. BC Decker, Inc., Toronto, 1986, p 186.
26. Motew, M, et al: Cardiovascular effects and acid-base and blood gas changes during laparoscopy. Am J Obstet Gynecol 115:1002, 1973.
27. Borten, M: Laparoscopic Complications: Prevention and Management. BC Decker, Inc., Toronto, 1986, p 198.
28. Alexander, GP, Noe, FE and Brown, EM: Anesthesia for pelvic laparoscopy. Anesth Analg 48:14, 1969.
29. Borten, M: Laparoscopic Complications: Prevention and Management. BC Decker, Inc., Toronto, 1986, p 266.
30. Doctor, NH and Hussain, Z: Bilateral pneumothorax associated with laparoscopy: A case report of a rare hazard and review of literature. Anaesthesia 28:75, 1973.
31. Borten, M: Laparoscopic Complications: Prevention and Management. BC Decker, Inc., Toronto, 1986, p 298.
32. Lichtiger, M, Wetchler, BV and Philip, BK: The adult and geriatric patient. In Wetchler, BV (ed): Anesthesia for Ambulatory Surgery. JB Lippincott Co., London, 1985, p 175.
33. Ong, BY, Palahniuk, RJ and Cumming, M: Gastric volume and pH in outpatients. Can Anaesth Soc J 25:36, 1978.
34. Manchikanti, L, et al: Assessment of effect of various modes of premedication on acid aspiration risk factors in outpatient surgery. Anesth Analg 66:81, 1987.
35. Spielman, FJ, et al: Pharmacokinetic and pharmacodynamics of local analgesia for laparoscopic tubal ligations. Am J Obstet Gynecol 146:821, 1983.
36. Spielman, FJ, et al: Local versus general anesthesia for laparoscopic tubal sterilization. Anesthesiology 63:A253, 1985.
37. Endler, GC, et al: Follicular fluid levels of sodium thiamylal during laparoscopy for oocyte retrieval. Abstracts of Society for Anesthesia and Perinatology, 1986, p 135.
38. Roizen, MF, et al: Effect of nitrous oxide on in vitro fertilization success rate. Anesth Analg 64:274, 1985.
39. Wade, JG and Stevens, WC: Isoflurane: An anesthetic for the eighties? Anesth Analg 60:666, 1981.
40. Wetchler, BV: Problem solving in the postanesthesia care unit. In Wetchler, BV (ed): Anesthesia for Ambulatory Surgery. JB Lippincott Co., London, 1985, p 275.
41. Wetchler, BV, Collins, IS and Jacob, L: Antiemetic effects of droperidol on the ambulatory surgery patient. Anesthesiol Rev 9:23, 1982.
42. Lonie, DS and Harper, NJN: Nitrous oxide anaesthesia and vomiting: The effect of nitrous oxide anaesthesia on the incidence of vomiting following gynaecological laparoscopy. Anaesthesia 41:703, 1986.
43. Jones, GS: Update on in vitro fertilization. Endocrinol Rev 5:62, 1984.
44. Wood, C and Trounson, A: Current state and future of IVF. Clin Obstet Gynecol 12:753, 1985.

INDEX

An "*f*" in italics indicates a figure. A "*t*" in italics indicates a table.